Anaesthesia and Intensive Care A–Z

An Encyclopaedia of Principles and Practice

To
Gill, Emma and Abigail

to
Alison, Jonathan and Sophie

and to

Geraldine

Commissioning Editor: Alison Taylor
Development Editor: Clive Hewat
Project Manager: Elouise Ball
Design Direction: George Ajayi
Illustration Manager: Bruce Hogarth

Anaesthesia and Intensive Care A–Z

An Encyclopaedia of Principles and Practice

Steven M Yentis BSc, MBBS, FRCA, MD, MA
Consultant Anaesthetist, Chelsea and Westminster Hospital;
Honorary Senior Lecturer, Imperial College London, UK

Nicholas P Hirsch MBBS, FRCA, FRCP
Consultant Anaesthetist, The National Hospital for Neurology and Neurosurgery;
Honorary Senior Lecturer, The Institute of Neurology, Queen Square, London, UK

Gary B Smith BM, FRCA, FRCP
Consultant in Critical Care, Portsmouth Hospitals NHS Trust;
Professor, University of Bournemouth, UK

FOURTH EDITION

CHURCHILL LIVINGSTONE

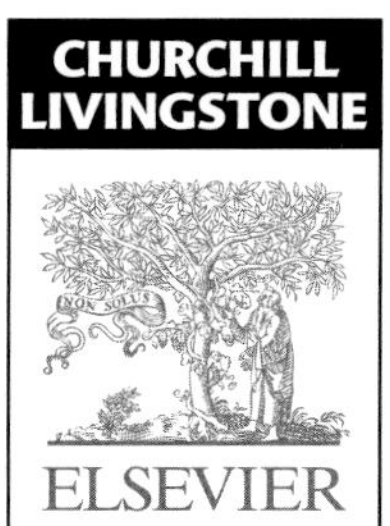

EDINBURGH LONDON NEW YORK OXFORD PHILADELPHIA ST LOUIS SYDNEY TORONTO 2009

CHURCHILL
LIVINGSTONE
ELSEVIER

ISBN: 9780443067853
Reprinted 2009

British Library Cataloguing in Publication Data
A catalogue record for this book is available from the British Library

Library of Congress Cataloging in Publication Data
A catalog record for this book is available from the Library of Congress

Notice
Knowledge and best practice in this field are constantly changing. As new research and experience broaden our knowledge, changes in practice, treatment and drug therapy may become necessary or appropriate. Readers are advised to check the most current information provided (i) on procedures featured or (ii) by the manufacturer of each product to be administered, to verify the recommended dose or formula, the method and duration of administration, and contraindications. It is the responsibility of the practitioner, relying on their own experience and knowledge of the patient, to make diagnoses, to determine dosages and the best treatment for each individual patient, and to take all appropriate safety precautions. To the fullest extent of the law, neither the Publisher nor the Authors assume any liability for any injury and/or damage to persons or property arising out or related to any use of the material contained in this book.

The Publisher

The Publisher's policy is to use **paper manufactured from sustainable forests**

Printed in China

Preface

In the 15 years since the publication of the first edition of our textbook, we have been delighted to find that it has been adopted by both trainees and established practitioners alike. Whilst our original idea was to produce a readily accessible source of information for those sitting the Royal College of Anaesthetists' Fellowship examinations, it is now obvious that the book appeals to a far wider readership. We hope that the *A–Z* will continue to be useful to all staff who help us care for patients on a daily basis, as well as to anaesthetists and intensivists of all grades.

The difference between the list of entries in the first edition and those in the current one continues to increase, with a huge expansion of new entries and revision of existing ones. This change acknowledges the enormous breadth of information needed to satisfy the vast range of activities performed by our anaesthetic, intensive care, nursing and other colleagues, and also reflects the ever-changing field in which we work.

The publication of a textbook requires the support of a multitude of people. We are indebted to our colleagues, both junior and senior, who have gently criticised previous editions; their suggestions have been invaluable and have directly resulted in changes found in each new edition over the years. We also thank the staff of Elsevier and their predecessors for their support during the life of this project. Finally, our enthusiasm for the *A–Z* would have been impossible to sustain without the unending support of our families and, as before, this edition is dedicated to them.

SMY
NPH
GBS

Acknowledgements

We are grateful to the publishers, editors and authors concerned for permission to reproduce or modify the following Figures and Tables:

Figure 2b: from Bowman WC (1990) *Pharmacology of Neuromuscular Function*, 2nd edn, Wright, Bristol

Figures 80, 81 and 96: from Soni N (1989) *Anaesthesia and Intensive Care*, Heinemann, Oxford

Figure 84: from Samsoon GLT and Young JRB (1987) Difficult tracheal intubation: a retrospective study. *Anaesthesia*, **42**, 482–6

Figure 87: from Parbrook GD, Davis PD and Parbrook EO (1990) *Basic Physics and Measurement in Anaesthesia*, 3rd edn, Butterworth-Heinemann, Oxford

Figure 120: from the British Medical Association and the Royal Pharmaceutical Association (1998) *British National Formulary*, London

Figure 133: from Ross Russell RW and Wiles CM (1985) *Neurology*, Heinemann, Oxford

Figure 148: from Lentner C (ed.) (1981) *Geigy Scientific Tables*, 8th edn, vol. 1, Ciba-Geigy, Basle

Figure 156: from Howell RS (1980) Piped medical gas and vacuum systems. *Anaesthesia*, **35**, 676–98

Table 5: from Knaus WA, Draper EA, Wagner DP and Zimmerman JE (1985) APACHE II: a severity of disease classification system for acutely ill patients. *Crit Care Med*, **13**, 818–29

Explanatory notes

Arrangement of text

Entries are arranged alphabetically, with some related subjects grouped together to make coverage of one subject easier. For example, entries relating to tracheal intubation may be found under **I** as in **Intubation, awake, Intubation, blind nasal**, etc.

Cross-referencing

Bold type indicates a cross reference. An abbreviation highlighted in bold type refers to an entry in its fully spelled form. For example, '... **ARDS** may occur ...' refers to the entry **Acute respiratory distress syndrome**. Further instructions appear in italics.

References

Reference to a suitable article is provided at the foot of the entry where appropriate.

Proper names

Where possible, a short biographical note is provided at the foot of the entry when a person is mentioned. Dates of birth and death are given, or the date of description if these dates are unknown. No dates are given for contemporary names. Where more than one eponymous entry occurs, e.g. **Haldane apparatus** and **Haldane effect**, details are given under the first entry. The term 'anaesthetist' is used in the English sense, i.e. a medical practitioner who practises anaesthesia; the terms 'anesthesiologist' and 'anaesthesiologist' are not used.

Drugs

Individual drugs have entries where they have especial relevance to, or may by given by, the anaesthetist or intensivist. Where many different drugs exist within the same group, for example β-adrenergic receptor antagonists, those which may be given intravenously have their own entry, whilst the others are described under the group description. The reader is referred back to entries describing drug groups and classes where appropriate.

Recommended International Non-proprietary Names (rINNs)

Following work undertaken by the World Health Organization, recent European law requires the replacement of existing national drug nomenclature with rINNs. For most drugs, rINNS are identical to the British Approved Name (BAN). The Medicines Control Agency (UK) has proposed a two-stage process for the introduction of rINNs. For substances where the change is substantial, both names will appear on manufacturers' labels and leaflets for a number of years, with the rINN preceding the BAN on the drug label. For drugs where the change presents little hazard, the change will be immediate. For some drugs which do not appear in either of the above two categories, the British (or USP) name may still be used.

There are over 200 affected drugs, many of them no longer available. Affected drugs that are mentioned in this book (though not all of them have their own entries) are listed below – though please note that in common with the British Pharmacopoeia, the terms 'adrenaline' and 'noradrenaline' will be used throughout the text in preference to epinephrine and norepinephrine respectively, because of their status as natural hormones. Thus (with the exception of adrenaline and noradrenaline) the format for affected drugs is rINN (BAN), e.g. **Tetracaine hydrochloride** (Amethocaine). Non-BAN, non-rINN names are also provided for certain other drugs (for example **Isopreterenol**, *see Isoprenaline*) to help direct non-UK readers or those unfamiliar with UK terminology.

continued over page

continued

BAN	*rINN*
Adrenaline	Epinephrine
Amethocaine	Tetracaine
Amoxycillin	Amoxicillin
Amphetamine	Amfetamine
Amylobarbitone	Amobarbital
Beclomethasone	Beclometasone
Benzhexol	Trihexyphenidyl
Benztropine	Benzatropine
Busulphan	Busulfan
Cephramandole	Ceframandole
Cephazolin	Cefazolin
Cephradine	Cefradine
Chlormethiazole	Clomethiazole
Chlorpheniramine	Chlorphenamine
Corticotrophin	Corticotropin
Cyclosporin	Ciclosporin
Dicyclomine	Dicycloverine
Dothiepin	Dosulepin
Ethamsylate	Etamsylate
Ethacrynic acid	Etacrynic acid
Frusemide	Furosemide
Indomethacin	Indometacin
Lignocaine	Lidocaine
Methohexitone	Methohexital
Methylene blue	Methylthioninium chloride
Noradrenaline	Norepinephrine
Oxpentifylline	Pentoxifylline
Phenobarbitone	Phenobarbital
Sodium cromoglycate	Sodium cromoglicate
Sulphadiazine	Sulfadiazine
Sulphasalazine	Sulfasalazine
Tetracosactrin	Tetracosactide
Thiopentone	Thiopental
Tribravarin	Ribavarin
Trimeprazine	Alimemazine

Abbreviations

ACE inhibitors angiotensin converting enzyme inhibitors
ACTH adrenocorticotrophic hormone
ADP adenosine diphosphate
AIDS acquired immune deficiency syndrome
cAMP cyclic adenosine monophosphate
APACHE acute physiology and chronic health evaluation
ARDS acute respiratory distress syndrome
ASA American Society of Anesthesiologists
ASD atrial septal defect
ATP adenosine triphosphate
BP blood pressure
$CMRO_2$ cerebral metabolic rate for oxygen
CNS central nervous system
CO_2 carbon dioxide
COPD chronic obstructive pulmonary disease
CPAP continuous positive airway pressure
CPR cardiopulmonary resuscitation
CSE combined spinal-extradural
CSF cerebrospinal fluid
CT computed tomography
CVA cerebrovascular accident
CVP central venous pressure
CVS cardiovascular system
CXR chest X-ray
DIC disseminated intravascular coagulation
DNA deoxyribonucleic acid
2,3-DPG 2,3-diphosphoglycerate
DVT deep vein thrombosis
ECF extracellular fluid
ECG electrocardiography
EEG electroencephalography
EMG electromyography
ENT ear, nose and throat
FEV_1 forced expiratory volume in 1 second
$F_{I}O_2$ fractional inspired concentration of oxygen
FRC functional residual capacity
FVC forced vital capacity
G gauge
GABA γ-aminobutyric acid
GFR glomerular filtration rate
GIT gastrointestinal tract
GTN glyceryl trinitrate
HCO_3^- bicarbonate
HDU high dependency unit
HIV human immunodeficiency virus
5-HT 5-hydroxytryptamine
ICP intracranial pressure
ICU intensive care unit
IgA, IgG, etc. immunoglobulin A, G, etc.
im intramuscular
IMV intermittent mandatory ventilation
IPPV intermittent positive pressure ventilation
iv intravenous
IVRA intravenous regional anaesthesia
JVP jugular venous pressure
MAC minimal alveolar concentration
MAP mean arterial pressure
MH malignant hyperthermia
MI myocardial infarction
MODS multiple organ dysfunction syndrome
MRI magnetic resonance imaging
mw molecular weight
NHS National Health Service
NICE National Institute for Health and Clinical Excellence
NMDA N-methyl-D-aspartate
N_2O nitrous oxide
NSAID non-steroidal anti-inflammatory drug
O_2 oxygen
ODA/P operating department assistant/practitioner
P_{CO_2} partial pressure of carbon dioxide
PE pulmonary embolus

PEEP positive end-expiratory pressure

***P*o$_2$** partial pressure of oxygen

PONV postoperative nausea and vomiting

pr per rectum

RNA ribonucleic acid

RS respiratory system

sc subcutaneous

SIRS systemic inflammatory response syndrome

SLE systemic lupus erythematosus

SVP saturated vapour pressure

SVR systemic vascular resistance

SVT supraventricular tachycardia

TB tuberculosis

TENS transcutaneous electrical nerve stimulation

TIVA total intravenous anaesthesia

TPN total parenteral nutrition

TURP transurethral resection of prostate

UK United Kingdom

US(A) United States (of America)

VF ventricular fibrillation

$\dot{V}/\dot{Q}$ ventilation/perfusion

VSD ventricular septal defect

VT ventricular tachycardia

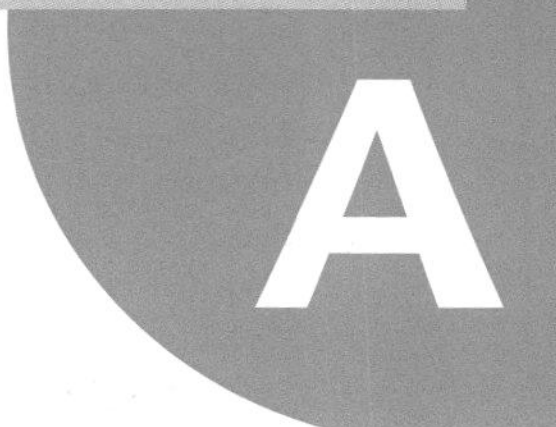

A severity characterisation of trauma (ASCOT). Trauma scale derived from the Glasgow coma scale, systolic BP, revised trauma score, abbreviated injury scale and age. A logistic regression equation is used to provide a probability of mortality. Excludes patients with a very poor or very good prognosis. Has been claimed to be superior to the trauma revised injury severity score system although more complex.
Champion HR, Copes WS, Sacco WJ, et al (1996). J Trauma; 40: 42–8

A–adO_2, *see Alveolar–arterial oxygen difference*

ABA, *see American Board of Anesthesiology*

Abbott, Edward Gilbert, *see Morton, William*

Abbreviated injury scale (AIS). Trauma scale first described in 1971 and updated many times since. Comprises a classification of injuries with each given a 6-digit code (the last indicating severity, with 1 = minor and 6 = fatal). The codes are linked to International Classification of Diseases codes, thus aiding standardisation of records. The anatomical profile is a refinement in which the locations of injuries are divided into four categories; the AIS scores are added and the square root taken to minimise the contribution of less severe injuries.
Copes WS, Lawnick M, Champion HR, Sacco WJ (1988). J Trauma; 28: 78–86

Abciximab. Monoclonal antibody preparation used as an antiplatelet drug and adjunct to aspirin and heparin in high risk patients undergoing percutaneous transluminal coronary angioplasty. Consists of Fab fragments of immunoglobulin directed against the glycoprotein IIb/IIIa receptor on the platelet surface. Inhibits platelet aggregation and thrombus formation; effects last 24–48 h after infusion. Careful consideration of risks and benefits should precede use since risk of bleeding is increased. Licensed for single use only.
- Dosage: 250 μg/min iv 10–60 min (up to 24 h in unstable angina) before angioplasty with 125 μg/kg/min (up to 10 μg/min for 12 h afterwards).
- Side effects: bleeding, hypotension, nausea, bradycardia. Thrombocytopenia occurs rarely.

Abdominal compartment syndrome. Combination of increased intra-abdominal pressure and organ dysfunction, e.g. following abdominal trauma or extensive surgery, resulting from haemorrhage, leakage of oedema fluid and/or massive intestinal oedema. May also follow liver transplantation and acute pancreatitis. Intra-abdominal pressures above 20–25 cmH_2O may be associated with reduced venous return and cardiac output, impaired ventilation, reduced renal blood flow and oliguria. Increased CVP may lead to raised ICP. Diagnosed clinically and by measuring intra-abdominal pressure via a bladder catheter or nasogastric tube, using a water column manometer.

Management includes laparotomy and leaving the abdomen open and/or using silastic material to cover the abdominal contents. Paracentesis may be effective if raised intra-abdominal pressure is due to accumulation of fluid, e.g. ascites. Full resuscitation must be performed before decompression as rapid release of pressure may result in sudden washout of inflammatory mediators from ischaemic tissues, causing acidosis and hypotension.
Malbrain ML, Cheatham ML, Kirkpatrick A, et al (2006). Intensive Care Med; 32: 1722–1732, and Cheatham ML, Malbrain ML, Kirkpatrick A (2007). Intensive Care Med; 33: 951–62
See also, Compartment syndromes

Abdominal decompression. Technique in obstetric analgesia whereby negative pressure is applied to the abdomen in order to reduce labour pain and possibly shorten labour. Thought to act by making the uterus more spherical during contractions, thus contracting with less force. Now rarely used.
See also, Obstetric analgesia and anaesthesia

Abdominal field block. Technique using 100–200 ml local anaesthetic agent, involving infiltration of the skin, subcutaneous tissues, abdominal muscles and fascia. Provides analgesia of the abdominal wall and anterior peritoneum, but not of the viscera. Now rarely used. Rectus sheath block, transversus abdominis plane block, iliac crest block and inguinal hernia field block are more specific blocks.

Abdominal sepsis, *see Intra-abdominal sepsis*

Abdominal trauma. May be blunt (e.g. road traffic accidents) or penetrating (e.g. stabbing, bullet wounds). Often carries a high morbidity and mortality because injuries may go undetected. May lead to massive intra-abdominal blood loss or abdominal compartment syndrome. The abdomen can be divided into three areas:
  - intrathoracic: protected by the bony thoracic cage. Contains the spleen, liver, stomach and diaphragm. Injury may be associated with rib fractures. The diaphragm may also be injured by blows to the lower abdomen (which impart pressure waves to the diaphragm) or by penetrating injuries of the chest.
  - true abdomen: contains the small and large bowel, bladder and, in the female, uterus, fallopian tubes and ovaries.
  - retroperitoneal: contains the kidneys, ureters, pancreas and duodenum. May result in massive blood loss from retroperitoneal venous injury.
- Management:
  - basic resuscitation as for trauma generally.
  - initial assessment: examination of the anterior abdominal wall, both flanks, back, buttocks, perineum (and in

men, the urethral meatus) for bruises, lacerations, entry and exit wounds. Signs may be masked by unconsciousness, spinal cord injury or the effects of alcohol or drugs. Abdominal swelling usually indicates intra-abdominal haemorrhage; abdominal guarding or rigidity usually indicates visceral injury. Absence of bowel sounds may indicate intra-peritoneal haemorrhage or peritoneal soiling with bowel contents. Colonic or rectal injuries may cause blood pr. A high index of suspicion is required for retroperitoneal injuries since examination is difficult.
- imaging: abdominal X-ray may reveal free gas under the diaphragm (erect or semi-erect; may also be visible on chest X-ray) or laterally (lateral decubitus X-ray); other investigations include pelvic X-ray and urological radiology if indicated (e.g. iv urogram, etc.), CT and MRI scanning and ultrasound.
- peritoneal lavage is indicated in blunt abdominal trauma associated with:
  - altered pain response (head injury, spinal cord injury, drugs, etc.).
  - unexplained hypovolaemia following multiple trauma.
  - equivocal diagnostic findings.
- insertion of a nasogastric tube and urinary catheter (provided no urethral injury; a suprapubic catheter may be necessary).
- indications for laparotomy include penetrating injuries, obvious intra-abdominal haemorrhage, signs of bowel perforation or a positive peritoneal lavage.

See also, Pelvic trauma

ABO blood groups. Discovered in 1900 by Landsteiner in Vienna. Antigens may be present on red blood cells, with antibodies in the plasma (Table 1). The antibodies, mostly type-M immunoglobulins, develop within the first few months of life, presumably in response to naturally occurring antigens of similar structure to the blood antigens. Infusion of blood containing an ABO antigen into a patient who already has the corresponding antibody may lead to an adverse reaction; hence the description of group O individuals as universal donors, and of group AB individuals as universal recipients.
[Karl Landsteiner (1868–1943), Austrian-born US pathologist]
See also, Blood cross-matching; Blood groups; Blood transfusion

ABPI, *see Ankle Brachial Pressure Index*

Abruption, *see Antepartum haemorrhage*

Absolute risk reduction. Indicator of treatment effect in clinical trials. For a reduction in incidence of events from a% to b%, it equals (a–b)%. Does not give an indication of the magnitude of a or b.
See also, Meta-analysis; Number needed to treat; Odds ratio; Relative risk reduction

Table 1 Antigens and antibodies in ABO blood groups

Group	*Incidence in UK (%)*	*Red cell antigen*	*Plasma antibody*
A	42	A	Anti-B
B	8	B	Anti-A
AB	3	A and B	None
O	47	None	Anti-A and anti-B

Abuse of anaesthetic agents. May occur because of easy access to potent drugs by operating theatre or ICU staff. Opioid analgesic drugs are the most commonly abused agents, but others include benzodiazepines and inhalational anaesthetic agents. Abuse may be suggested by behavioural or mood changes, or excessive and inappropriate requests for opioids. Main considerations include the safety of patients, counselling and psychiatric therapy for the abuser, and legal aspects of drug abuse. May be associated with alcoholism.
Berry CB, Crome IB, Plant M, Plant M (2000). Anaesthesia; 55: 946–52
See also, Misuse of Drugs Act; Sick doctor scheme; Substance abuse

Acarbose. Inhibitor of intestinal alpha glucosidases and pancreatic amylase; used in the treatment of diabetes mellitus, usually in combination with a biguanide or sulfonylurea. Delays digestion and absorption of starch and sucrose. Has a small blood glucose lowering effect.
- Dosage: 50 mg orally once daily, increasing up to 200 mg 8 hourly.
- Side effects include flatulence and diarrhoea, and rarely hepatic dysfunction. Contraindicated in pregnancy and inflammatory bowel disease.

See also, Meglitinides; Thiazolidinediones

Accessory nerve block. Performed for spasm of trapezius and sternomastoid muscles (there is no sensory component to the nerve). 5–10 ml local anaesthetic agent is injected 2 cm below the mastoid process into the sternomastoid muscle, through which the nerve runs.

Accident, major, *see Incident, major*

ACD, Acid–citrate–dextrose solution, *see Blood storage*

ACD-CPR, Active compression decompression CPR, *see Cardiac massage; Cardiopulmonary resuscitation*

ACE, Angiotensin converting enzyme, *see Renin/angiotensin system*

ACE anaesthetic mixture. Mixture of alcohol, chloroform and diethyl ether, in a ratio of 1:2:3 parts, suggested in 1860 as an alternative to chloroform alone. Popular into the 1900s as a means of reducing total dose and side effects of any one of the three drugs.

ACE inhibitors, *see Angiotensin converting enzyme inhibitors*

Acetaminophen, *see Paracetamol*

Acetazolamide. Carbonic anhydrase inhibitor, which reduces bicarbonate formation and hydrogen ion excretion, thereby creating a metabolic acidosis. Also a weak diuretic, but rarely used as such. Used to treat glaucoma, metabolic alkalosis, altitude sickness and childhood epilepsy. Useful in the treatment of severe hyperphosphataemia because it leads to urinary excretion of phosphate. May be used to lower ICP by reducing CSF production. Has been used to alkalinise the urine in tumour lysis syndrome or to enhance excretion in drug intoxications, e.g. with salicylates.
- Dosage: 0.25–0.5 g orally/iv, once/twice daily.

Acetylcholine (ACh). Neurotransmitter, the acetyl ester of the base choline (Fig. 1). Synthesised from acetylcoenzyme

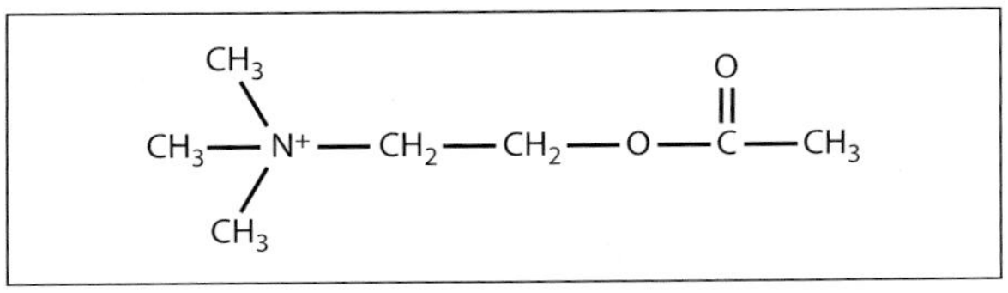

$$(CH_3)_3N^+—CH_2—CH_2—O—\overset{O}{\overset{\|}{C}}—CH_3$$

Fig. 1 Structure of acetylcholine

A and choline in nerve ending cytoplasm; the reaction is catalysed by choline acetyltransferase. Choline is actively transported into the nerve and acetylcoenzyme A is formed in mitochondria. ACh is stored in vesicles.

- ACh is the transmitter at:
  - autonomic ganglia.
  - parasympathetic postganglionic nerve endings.
  - sympathetic postganglionic nerve endings at sweat glands and some muscle blood vessels.
  - the neuromuscular junction.
  - many parts of the CNS where it has a prominent role in learning.

Has either muscarinic or nicotinic actions, depending on the acetylcholine receptors involved. ACh is hydrolysed to choline and acetate by acetylcholinesterase on the postsynaptic membrane. Other esterases also exist, e.g. plasma cholinesterase.

See also, Muscarine and muscarinic receptors; Neuromuscular transmission; Nicotine and nicotinic receptors; Parasympathetic nervous system; Sympathetic nervous system; Synaptic transmission

Acetylcholine receptors. Transmembrane proteins activated by acetylcholine (ACh). ACh receptors may be muscarinic or nicotinic (Fig. 2a). Injected ACh first stimulates muscarinic receptors. As the dose is increased, nicotinic receptors are stimulated; i.e. parasympathetic stimulation and sweating precedes effects at ganglia and the neuromuscular junction (NMJ).

The structure of the postsynaptic (nicotinic) receptors at the NMJ has been identified largely through work on the electric eel. Each receptor consists of five glycosylated protein subunits which project into the synaptic cleft. The subunits have been designated α (mw 40 000), β (mw 49 000), γ (mw 60 000) and δ (mw 67 000). The γ subunit is thought to be replaced by an ε subunit in mammals. The subunits span the postsynaptic membrane and form a cylinder around a central ion channel (Fig. 2b). The two α subunits of each receptor carry the binding sites for ACh. Occupation of these sites causes a configurational change of the subunits, thus opening the ion channel; cations (mainly sodium, potassium and calcium) flow through the channel according to their concentration gradients and thus generate an action potential. Non-depolarising neuromuscular blocking drugs at normal doses reduce the number of receptors available to ACh. At higher doses they may also block the ion channel. Muscarinic receptors are G protein-coupled receptors.

Neuronal forms of ACh receptors are more heterogenous with a large number of subunit configurations.

See also, Muscarine and muscarinic receptors; Neuromuscular transmission; Nicotine and nicotinic receptors; Parasympathetic nervous system; Sympathetic nervous system; Synaptic transmission

Acetylcholinesterase. Enzyme present in the basement postsynaptic membranes of cholinergic synapses and neuromuscular junctions. Also found in red blood cells and the placenta. Converts acetylcholine (ACh) into acetate

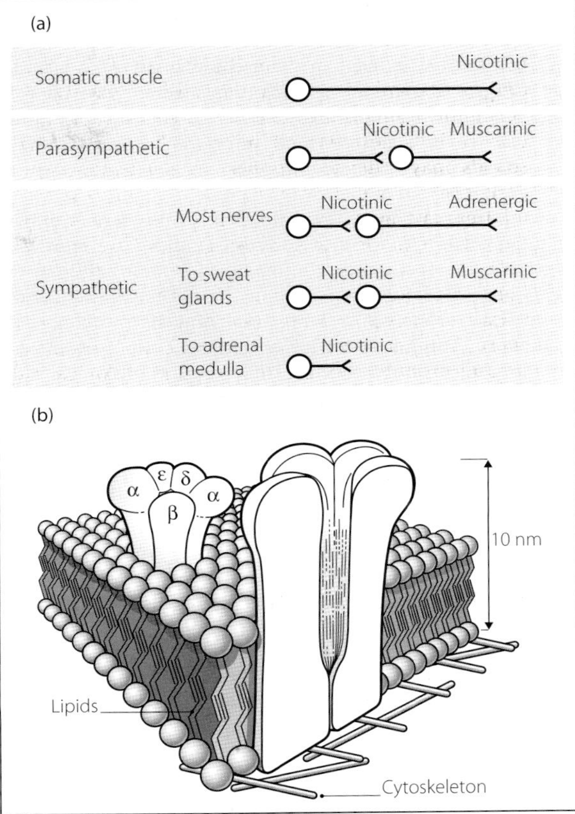

Fig. 2 (a) Types of acetylcholine receptors. (b) Structure of nicotinic acetylcholine receptor

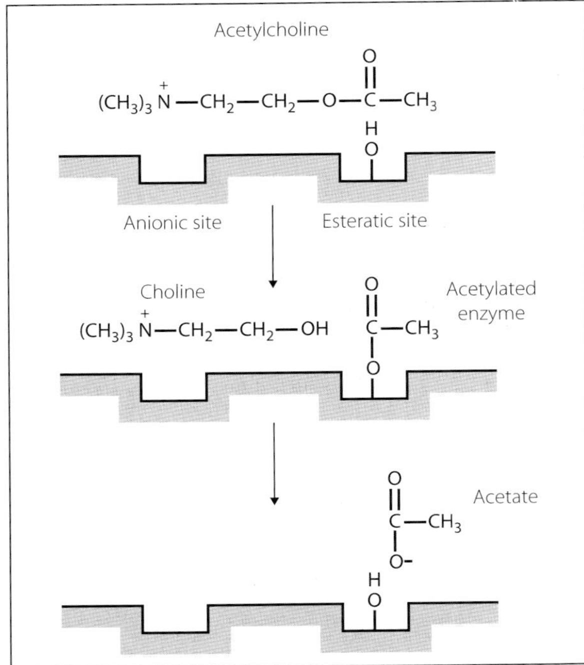

Fig. 3 Action of acetylcholinesterase

and choline, thus terminating its action. The $N(CH_3)_3^+$ part of ACh binds to the anionic site of the enzyme, and the acetate end of ACh forms an intermediate bond at the esteratic site. Choline is liberated, and the intermediate substrate/enzyme complex is then hydrolysed to release acetate (Fig. 3).
See also, Acetylcholinesterase inhibitors; Neuromuscular transmission; Synaptic transmission

Acetylcholinesterase inhibitors. Substances which increase acetylcholine (ACh) concentrations by inhibiting acetylcholinesterase. Used clinically for their action at the neuromuscular junction in myasthenia gravis and in the reversal of non-depolarising neuromuscular blockade. Concurrent administration of an antimuscarinic agent, e.g. atropine or glycopyrronium, reduces unwanted effects of increased ACh concentrations at muscarinic receptors. Effects at ganglia are minimal at normal doses. Central effects may occur if the drug readily crosses the blood–brain barrier, e.g. physostigmine (used to treat the central anticholinergic syndrome).
Have also been used to treat tachyarrhythmias.
- Classification:
  - prosthetic: competitive inhibition at the anionic site of the enzyme prevents binding of ACh, e.g. edrophonium, tetrahydroaminocrine.
  - oxydiaphoretic: acts as a substrate for the enzyme; the reaction proceeds as far as the intermediate substrate/enzyme complex. Hydrolysis of the complex and thus reactivation of the enzyme is slow.
    Examples:
    - neostigmine, physostigmine (few hours).
    - pyridostigmine (several hours).
    - distigmine (up to a day).

    Organophosphorus compounds act as oxydiaphoretic inhibitors, but the substrate/enzyme complex is minimally hydrolysed; inhibition lasts for weeks until new enzyme is synthesised.

Acetylcholinesterase inhibitors augment depolarising neuromuscular blockade and may cause depolarising blockade in overdose. They may also cause bradycardia, hypotension, agitation, miosis, increased GIT activity, sweating and salivation.

Centrally acting acetylcholinesterase inhibitors (e.g. donepezil, rivastigmine, galantamine) are used for symptomatic treatment of Alzheimer's dementia. Of potential anaesthetic relevance because of their side effects (including nausea, vomiting, fatigue, muscle cramps, increased creatine kinase, convulsions, bradycardia, confusion) and enhancement of the actions of suxamethonium.
[Alois Alzheimer (1864–1915), German neurologist and pathologist]
See also, Neuromuscular transmission; Organophosphorus poisoning

N-Acetylcysteine. Derivative of the naturally occurring amino acid, L-cysteine. A free radical scavenger, it acts as an antidote in paracetamol poisoning, probably by restoring depleted hepatic stores of glutathione or by acting as an alternative substrate for a toxic metabolite of paracetamol. Also used as an ocular lubricant.

Has been investigated for a possible role in protection against myocardial reperfusion injury, treatment of fulminant hepatic failure, and treatment of MODS, acute lung injury and neuropsychiatric complications of carbon monoxide poisoning. Has also been used as a mucolytic because of its ability to split disulphide bonds in mucus glycoprotein.
- Dosage:
  - paracetamol poisoning: 150 mg/kg (to a maximum of 12 g) in 200 ml 5% dextrose iv over 15 min, followed by 50 mg/kg in 500 ml dextrose over 4 h, then 100 mg/kg in 1 litre dextrose over 16 h.
  - to reduce viscosity of airway secretions: 200 mg 8 hourly, orally. Has been delivered by nebuliser.
- Side effects: rashes, anaphylaxis. Has been associated with bronchospasm in asthmatics.

Achalasia. Disorder of oesophageal motility caused by idiopathic degeneration of nerve cells in the myenteric plexus or vagal nuclei. Results in dysphagia and oesophageal dilatation. A similar condition may result from American trypanosomal infection (Chagas' disease). Aspiration pneumonitis or repeated chest infections may occur. Achalasia is treated by mechanical distension of the lower oesophagus or by surgery. Heller's cardiomyotomy (longitudinal myotomy leaving the mucosa intact) may be undertaken via abdominal or thoracic approaches. Preoperative respiratory assessment is essential. Patients are at high risk of aspirating oesophageal contents, and rapid sequence induction must be performed.
[Carlos Chagas (1879–1934), Brazilian physician; Ernst Heller (1877–1964), German surgeon]
See also, Aspiration of gastric contents; Induction, rapid sequence

Achondroplasia. Skeletal disorder, inherited as an autosomal dominant gene, although most cases arise by spontaneous mutation. Results in dwarfism, with normally sized trunk and shortened limbs. Flat face, bulging skull vault and spinal deformity may make tracheal intubation difficult, and the larynx may be smaller than normal. Obstructive sleep apnoea may occur. Foramen magnum and spinal canal stenoses may be present. The former may result in cord compression on neck extension; the latter may make central regional blockade difficult and reduce volume requirements for epidural anaesthesia.

Aciclovir. Antiviral drug; an analogue of nucleoside 2′-deoxyguanosine. Inhibits viral DNA polymerase; active against herpes viruses and used in the treatment of encephalitis, varicella zoster (chickenpox/shingles) and postherpetic neuralgia, and for prophylaxis and treatment of herpes infections in immunocompromised patients. Treatment should start at onset of infection; the drug does not eradicate the virus but may markedly attenuate the clinical infection.
- Dosage:
  - as topical cream, 5 times daily.
  - 200–800 mg orally, 2–5 times daily in adults.
  - 5–10 mg/kg 8 hourly iv, infused over 1 h.
- Side effects: rashes, GIT disturbances, hepatic and renal impairment, blood dyscrasias, headache, dizziness, severe local inflammation after iv use, confusion, convulsions, coma.

Acid. Substance which yields hydrogen ions in solution.

Acidaemia. Arterial pH < 7.35 or hydrogen ion concentration > 45 nmol/l.
See also, Acid–base balance; Acidosis

Acid–base balance. Maintenance of stable pH in body fluids is necessary for normal enzyme activity, ion distribution and protein structure. Normally, blood pH is maintained at 7.35–7.45 (hydrogen ion (H^+) concentration 35–45 nmol/l); intracellular pH changes with extracellular pH. During normal metabolism of neutral substances, organic acids are produced which generate hydrogen ions.

- Maintenance of pH depends on:
  - buffers in tissues and blood, which minimise the increase of H^+ concentration.
  - regulation by kidneys and lungs; the kidneys excrete about 60–80 mmol and the lungs about 15–20000 mmol H^+ per day.

Because of the relationship between CO_2, carbonic acid, bicarbonate (HCO_3^-) and H^+, and the ability to excrete CO_2 rapidly from the lungs, respiratory function is important in acid–base balance:

$$H_2O + CO_2 \rightleftharpoons H_2CO_3 \rightleftharpoons HCO_3^- + H^+$$

Thus hyper- and hypoventilation cause alkalosis and acidosis respectively. Similarly, hyper- or hypoventilation may compensate for non-respiratory acidosis or alkalosis respectively, by returning pH towards normal.

Sources of H^+ excreted via the kidneys include lactic acid from blood cells, muscle and brain, sulphuric acid from metabolism of sulphur-containing proteins, and acetoacetic acid from fatty acid metabolism.

- The kidney can compensate for acid–base disturbances in three ways:
  - by regulating the amount of HCO_3^- reabsorbed. 80–90% of filtered HCO_3^- is reabsorbed in the proximal tubule:
    - filtered sodium ion is exchanged for H^+ across the tubule cell membrane.
    - filtered HCO_3^- and excreted H^+ form carbonic acid.
    - carbonic acid is converted to CO_2 and water by carbonic anhydrase on the cell membrane.
    - CO_2 and water reform carbonic acid (catalysed again by carbonic anhydrase) within the cell.
    - carbonic acid releases HCO_3^- and H^+.
    - HCO_3^- passes into the blood; H^+ is exchanged for sodium ion, etc.
  - by forming dihydrogen phosphate from monohydrogen phosphate in the distal tubule ($HPO_4^{2-} + H^+ \rightarrow H_2PO_4^-$). The H^+ is supplied from carbonic acid, leaving HCO_3^- which passes into the blood.
  - by combination of ammonia, passing out of the cells, with H^+, supplied as above. The resultant ammonium ions cannot pass back into the cells.

In acid–base disorders, the primary change determines whether a disturbance is respiratory or metabolic. The direction of change in H^+ concentration determines acidosis or alkalosis. Renal or respiratory compensation attempts to restore normal pH, not reverse the primary change. For example, in the Henderson–Hasselbalch equation:

$$\text{pH} = \text{p}K_a + \log\frac{[HCO_3^-]}{[CO_2]}$$

adjustment of the HCO_3^-/CO_2 concentration ratio restores pH towards its normal value, e.g.:

- primary change: increased CO_2; leads to decreased pH (respiratory acidosis).
- compensation: HCO_3^- retention by kidneys; increased ammonium secretion, etc.

An 'alternative approach' suggested by Stewart in 1983 focuses on the strong ion difference to explain the underlying processes rather than the above 'traditional approach' which concentrates more on interpretation of measurements. It is based on the degree of dissociation of ions in solution, in particular the effects of strong ions and weak acids, and the role of bicarbonate as a marker of acid–base imbalance rather than a cause.

[Peter Stewart (1921–1993), Canadian physiologist]

See also, Acid; Base; Blood gas tensions; Breathing, control of; Davenport diagram; Siggaard-Andersen nomogram

Acid–citrate–dextrose solution, *see Blood storage*

Acidosis. A process in which arterial pH < 7.35 (or hydrogen ion > 45 mmol/l), or would be < 7.35 if there were no compensatory mechanisms of acid–base balance.
See also, Acidosis, metabolic; Acidosis, respiratory

Acidosis, metabolic. Acidosis due to metabolic causes, resulting in an inappropriately low pH for the measured arterial $P\text{CO}_2$.

- Caused by:
  - increased acid production:
    - ketone bodies, e.g. in diabetes mellitus.
    - lactate, e.g. in shock, exercise.
  - acid ingestion: e.g. salicylate poisoning.
  - failure to excrete hydrogen ion (H^+):
    - renal failure.
    - distal renal tubular acidosis.
    - carbonic anhydrase inhibitors.
  - loss of bicarbonate:
    - diarrhoea.
    - gastrointestinal fistulae.
    - proximal renal tubular acidosis.
    - ureteroenterostomy.
- May be differentiated by the presence or absence of an anion gap:
  - anion gap metabolic acidosis occurs in renal failure, lactic acidosis, ketoacidosis, rhabdomyolysis and following ingestion of certain toxins (e.g. salicylates, methanol, ethylene glycol).
  - non-anion gap (hyperchloraemic) metabolic acidosis is caused by the administration of chloride-containing solutions (e.g. saline) in large volumes, amino acid solutions, diarrhoea, pancreatic fistulae, ileal loop procedures, after rapid correction of a chronically compensated respiratory alkalosis or renal tubular acidosis.
- Primary change: increased H^+/decreased bicarbonate.
- Compensation:
  - hyperventilation: plasma bicarbonate falls by about 1.3 mmol/l for every 1 kPa acute decrease in arterial $P\text{CO}_2$, which usually does not fall below 1.3–1.9 kPa (10–15 mmHg).
  - increased renal H^+ secretion.
- Effects:
  - hyperventilation (Kussmaul breathing).
  - confusion, weakness, coma.
  - cardiac depression.
  - hyperkalaemia.
- Treatment:
  - of underlying cause.
  - bicarbonate therapy is reserved for treatment of severe acidaemia (e.g. pH under 7.1) because of problems associated with its use.

    If bicarbonate is required, a formula for iv infusion is:

    $$\frac{\text{base excess} \times \text{body weight (kg)}}{3}\ \text{mmol}$$

    Half this amount is given initially.
  - other agents under investigation include sodium dichloroacetate, Carbicarb (sodium bicarbonate and carbonate in equimolar concentrations) and THAM (2-amino-2-hydroxymethyl-1,3-propanediol).

Morris CG, Low J (2008). Anaesthesia; 63: 294–301 and 396–411

See also, Acidaemia; Acid–base balance

Acidosis, respiratory. Acidosis due to increased arterial $P\text{CO}_2$. Caused by alveolar hypoventilation.

- Primary change: increased arterial $P\text{CO}_2$.
- Compensation:
  - initial rise in plasma bicarbonate due to increased carbonic acid formation and dissociation.
  - increased acid secretion/bicarbonate retention by the kidneys. In acute hypercapnia, bicarbonate concentration increases by about 0.7 mmol/l per 1 kPa rise in arterial $P\text{CO}_2$. In chronic hypercapnia it increases by 2.6 mmol/l per 1 kPa.
- Effects: those of hypercapnia.
- Treatment: of underlying cause.

See also, Acidaemia; Acid–base balance

ACLS, *see Advanced Cardiac Life Support*

Acquired immune deficiency syndrome (AIDS), *see Human immunodeficiency viral infection*

Acromegaly. Disease caused by excessive growth hormone secretion after puberty; usually caused by a pituitary adenoma but ectopic secretion may also occur. Incidence is 6–8 per million population.

- Features:
  - enlarged jaw, tongue and larynx; widespread increase in soft tissue mass; enlarged feet and hands. Nerve entrapment may occur, e.g. carpal tunnel syndrome.
  - respiratory obstruction, including sleep apnoea.
  - tendency towards diabetes mellitus, hypertension and cardiac failure (may be due to cardiomyopathy). Thyroid and adrenal impairment may occur.

  Apart from the above diseases, acromegaly may present difficulties with tracheal intubation and maintenance of the airway.

Treatment is primarily pituitary surgery with or without subsequent radiotherapy. Some patients respond to bromocriptine or somatostatin analogues.

Smith M, Hirsch NP (2000). Br J Anaesth; 85: 3–14

ACT, Activated clotting time, *see Coagulation studies*

Acta Anaesthesiologica Scandinavica. Official journal of the Scandinavian Society of Anaesthesiology and Intensive Care Medicine, first published in 1957.

ACTH, *see Adrenocorticotrophic hormone*

Actin. One of the protein components of muscle (mw 43 000). In muscle, arranged into a double strand of thin filaments (F-actin) with globular 'beads' (G-actin), to which myosin binds, along their length. Present in all cells as microfilaments.

See also, Muscle contraction

Action potential. Sequential changes in transmembrane potential that result in the propagation of electrical impulses in excitable cells (Fig. 4a).

- Stages involved are summarised as follows:
  - A: depolarisation of the membrane by 15 mV (threshold level).
  - B: rapid depolarisation to +40 mV.
  - C: repolarisation, rapid at first then slow.
  - D: hyperpolarisation.
  - E: return to the resting membrane potential.

Depolarisation causes opening of sodium channels and entry of sodium ions into the cell, which causes further depolarisation. Sodium permeability then falls. Potassium permeability increases slowly and helps bring about repolarisation. Normal ion distribution is restored due to action of the sodium/potassium pump. The action potential is followed by a refractory period.

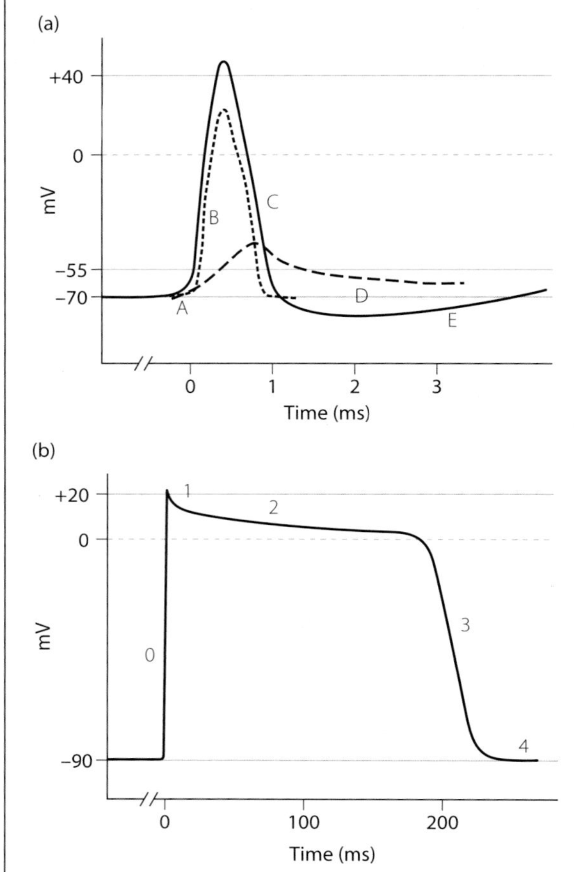

Fig. 4 (a) Nerve action potential (solid) showing changes in sodium (dotted) and potassium (dashed) conductance. (b) Cardiac action potential (see text)

Action potentials in nerve and other cells involve similar changes; in cardiac muscle, however, a plateau follows depolarisation, brought about by calcium entry. The refractory period is thus lengthened (Fig. 4b).

- There are five phases of the cardiac action potential:
  - phase 0: fast depolarisation and sodium entry.
  - phase 1: onset of repolarisation due to sodium channel closure.
  - phase 2: plateau due to calcium entry.
  - phase 3: repolarisation.
  - phase 4: resting membrane potential. In pacemaker cells, there is slow spontaneous depolarisation, due to decreased potassium permeability, leading to initiation of impulses.

See also, Nerve conduction

Activated charcoal, *see Charcoal, activated*

Activated clotting time, *see Coagulation studies*

Activated protein C, *see Drotrecogin alfa; Protein C*

Activation energy. Energy required to initiate a chemical reaction. For ignition of explosive mixtures of anaesthetic

agents the energy may be provided by sparks, e.g. from build-up of static electricity or electrical equipment. Combustion of cyclopropane requires less activation energy than that of diethyl ether. Activation energy is less for mixtures with O_2 than with air, and least for stoichiometric mixtures of reactants.
See also, Explosions and fires

Active compression/decompression cardiopulmonary resuscitation, *see Cardiac massage; Cardiopulmonary resuscitation*

Active transport. Energy-requiring transport of particles across cell membranes. Protein 'pumps' within the membranes utilise energy which is usually supplied by ATP metabolism, in order to move ions and molecules, often against concentration gradients. A typical example is the sodium/potassium pump.

Acupuncture. Use of fine needles (usually 30–33 G) to produce healing and pain relief. Originated in China thousands of years ago, and closely linked with the philosophy and practice of traditional Chinese medicine. Thus abnormalities in the flow of Qi (Chi: the life energy that circulates around the body along meridians, nourishing the internal organs) result in imbalance between Yin and Yang, the two polar opposites present in all aspects of the universe. Internal abnormalities may be diagnosed by pulse diagnosis (palpation of the radial arteries at different positions and depths). The appropriate organ is then treated by acupuncture at specific points on the skin, often along the meridian named after, and related to, that organ. Yin and Yang, and flow of Qi, are thus restored.

Modern Western acupuncture involves needle insertion at sites chosen for more 'scientific' reasons; e.g. around an affected area, at trigger points found nearby, or more proximally but within the appropriate dermatome. These may be combined with distant or local traditional points, although conclusive evidence for the existence of acupuncture points and meridians has never been shown. The needles may be left inserted and stimulated manually, electrically or thermally to increase intensity of stimulation. Pressure at acupuncture points (acupressure) may produce similar but less intense stimulation.

- Possible mechanisms:
  - local reflex pathways at spinal level.
  - closure of the 'gate' in the gate control theory of pain.
  - central release of endorphins/enkephalins, and possibly involvement of other neurotransmitters.
  - modulation of the 'memory' of pain.

Still used widely in China. Increasingly used in the West for chronic pain, musculoskeletal disorders, headache and migraine, and other disorders in which modern Western medicine has had little success. Claims that acupuncture may be employed alone to provide analgesia for surgery are now viewed with scepticism, although it has been used to provide analgesia and reduce PONV (e.g. 5 minutes' stimulation at the point P6 (Pericardium 6: 1–2 inches (2.5–5 cm) proximal to the distal wrist crease, between flexor carpi radialis and palmaris longus tendons).
Wang SM, Kain ZN, White P (2008). Anesth Analg; 106: 602–10 and 611–21

Acute cortical necrosis, *see Renal failure*

Acute crisis resource management, *see Crisis resource management*

Acute demyelinating encephalomyelopathy, *see Demyelinating diseases*

Acute life-threatening events – recognition and treatment (ALERT). Multiprofessional course developed in an effort to reduce the incidence of potentially avoidable cardiac arrests, admissions to ICU and in-hospital deaths. Aimed especially at pre-registration house officers, ward nurses and physiotherapists, but suitable for other clinical groups. Based on principles of many life-support training programmes (e.g. ALS, ATLS, APLS, CCrISP), its development embraces both clinical governance and multiprofessional education. Uses a structured and prioritised system of patient assessment and management to assist ward staff to recognise patients at risk of deterioration and those who are already seriously ill. Using a system of assessment similar to that of CCrISP, participants are taught to manage life-threatening events and to organise subsequent care.
Smith GB, Osgood VM, Crane S (2002). Resuscitation; 52: 281–6
See also, Early warning scores; Medical emergency team; Outreach team

Acute lung injury (ALI). Syndrome of inflammation and increased permeability of lung tissue associated with a variety of clinical, radiological and physiological abnormalities that cannot be explained by, but may coexist with, left atrial or pulmonary capillary hypertension. Associated with sepsis, multiple trauma, aspiration pneumonitis, multiple blood transfusion, pancreatitis, cardiopulmonary bypass and fat embolism. Onset is usually within 2–3 days of the precipitating illness or injury, although direct lung insults usually have a shorter insult-to-onset time. Acute respiratory distress syndrome (ARDS) is now regarded to be the most severe form of ALI. Both ARDS and ALI have similar diagnostic features which include:
  - acute onset.
  - bilateral diffuse infiltrates seen on the chest X-ray.
  - pulmonary wedge pressure ≤ 18 mmHg or absence of clinical evidence of left atrial hypertension.
  - arterial hypoxaemia resistant to oxygen therapy alone ($P_aO_2/F_IO_2 < 39.9$ kPa [300 mmHg] for definition of ALI; < 26.6 kPa [200 mmHg] for definition of ARDS), regardless of the level of PEEP.

The definitions of ALI and ARDS are increasingly being challenged.
Other features:
  - reduced respiratory compliance, lung volumes and increased work of breathing.
  - $\dot{V}/\dot{Q}$ mismatch and increased shunt.
  - pulmonary vascular resistance may be raised.
  - an air bronchogram may be seen on the chest X-ray.
  - in uncomplicated ALI, plasma oncotic pressure is normal.
  - MODS may occur and is a common cause of death.
- Pathophysiology: ALI results from damage to either the lung epithelium or endothelium. Two pathways of injury exist:
  - direct effects of an insult on lung cells, e.g. aspiration, smoke inhalation.
  - indirect result of an acute systemic inflammatory response involving both humoral (activation of complement, coagulation and kinin systems; release of mediators including cytokines, oxidants, nitric oxide, etc.) and cellular (neutrophils, macrophages and lymphocytes) components. Pulmonary infiltration by neutrophils leads to interstitial fibrosis, possibly as a

result of damage caused by free radicals. Examples include sepsis, pancreatitis, fat embolism, etc.
Histopathological findings can be divided into three phases: exudative (oedema and haemorrhage), proliferative (organisation and repair) and fibrotic.

- Treatment is largely supportive:
  - general support: nutrition, DVT prophylaxis, prevention of infection, etc.
  - O_2 therapy (trying where possible to keep F_IO_2 below 0.6). CPAP is often helpful as it improves FRC.
  - ventilatory support: IPPV may be necessary if CPAP is ineffective. PEEP is often required, but airway pressure is often already high because of reduced compliance, increasing the risk of barotrauma and impaired cardiac output. CO_2 elimination may demand increasing minute volumes but this too risks ventilator-associated lung injury. This has led to the development of lung protection strategies including low-frequency minute volume ventilation with extracorporeal CO_2 removal, permissive hypercapnia and the use of smaller than normal tidal volumes. Other ventilatory strategies used to minimise ventilator-associated lung injury in ALI include inverse ratio ventilation (at I:E ratios of up to 4:1), airway pressure release ventilation and high frequency ventilation. Extracorporeal membrane oxygenation has been used with varying success.
  - posture of the patient: prone ventilation may improve oxygenation in some patients.
  - fluid restriction is usually instituted to reduce lung water, although avoidance of initial fluid overload is thought to be more important. Diuretics have been used, with careful monitoring of renal function.
  - vasodilator drugs have been used to decrease pulmonary vascular resistance, e.g. prostacyclin. Nitric oxide has also been used to produce pulmonary vasodilatation, but there is, as yet, little evidence of long-term benefit.
  - fears over leakage of colloids into pulmonary interstitial spaces, with subsequent exacerbation of oedema, are balanced by possible advantages of colloids in maintaining oncotic pressure.
  - corticosteroid therapy is controversial. There appears to be no benefit to their prophylactic administration, nor in high-dose, short-term therapy at the onset of ALI/ARDS. However, corticosteroids may have a role in non-resolving ARDS.
  - free radical scavengers, antiprostaglandins and antiproteases have been investigated.

Wheeler AP, Bernard GR (2007). Lancet; 369: 1553–64

Acute phase response. A reaction of the haemopoietic and hepatic systems to inflammation or tissue injury, assumed to be of benefit to the host. There is a rise in the number/activity of certain cells (neutrophils, platelets) and plasma proteins (e.g. fibrinogen, complement, C-reactive protein, plasminogen, haptoglobin) involved in host defence, whilst there is a reduction in proteins which have transport and binding functions (e.g. albumin, haemoglobin, transferrin). Initiated by actions of cytokine mediators such as interleukins (IL-1α, IL-1β, IL-6 and IL-11), tumour necrosis factors (α and β) and leukaemia inhibitory factor.

Serum levels of acute phase proteins (e.g. C-reactive protein) can be helpful in diagnosis, monitoring and prognosis of certain diseases. The rise in fibrinogen levels causes an elevation in ESR. The fall in albumin is due to redistribution and decreased hepatic synthesis.

Acute physiology, age, chronic health evaluation, *see APACHE III scoring system*

Acute physiology and chronic health evaluation, *see APACHE/APACHE II scoring systems*

Acute physiology score (APS). Physiological component of severity of illness scoring systems, such as APACHE II/III and Simplified APS. Weighted values (e.g. 0 to 4 in APACHE II) are assigned to each of a range of physiological variables (e.g. temperature, mean arterial blood pressure, serum creatinine) on the basis of its derangement from an established 'normal' range, as measured either upon ICU admission or within 24 h of entry. The sum of all assigned weighted values for the physiological variables that comprise a given scoring system constitutes the acute physiological score. The higher the acute physiology score, the sicker the patient.
See also, Mortality/survival prediction on intensive care unit; Simplified acute physiology score

Acute respiratory distress syndrome (ARDS). Previously termed adult respiratory distress syndrome, despite the process also occurring in children. First described in 1967 as non-cardiogenic pulmonary oedema secondary to conditions not primarily affecting the lungs (e.g. shock, sepsis, pancreatitis, massive blood transfusion, fat embolism). Now regarded as the most severe form of acute lung injury (ALI). Distinguished from ALI purely on the P_aO_2/F_IO_2 ratio which is < 26.6 kPa (200 mmHg) for ARDS.

Pathophysiology, treatment, etc. is as for ALI. Histological appearances are similar to respiratory distress syndrome of the newborn, hence its name. Overall mortality of ARDS is approximately 50–60% but depends on the underlying cause; it is highest following aspiration pneumonitis or sepsis. Early deaths are rare, and patients dying late in the course of the illness usually die with hypoxaemia not because of it. For survivors, residual pulmonary impairment is possible but rarely severe.

Wheeler AP, Bernard GR (2007). Lancet; 369: 1553–64

Acute tubular necrosis, *see Renal failure*

Acyclovir, *see Aciclovir*

Addiction, *see Alcoholism; Substance abuse*

Addison's disease, *see Adrenocortical insufficiency*

ADEM, Acute demyelinating encephalomyelopathy, *see Demyelinating diseases*

Adenosine. Nucleoside, of importance in energy homeostasis at the cellular level. Reduces O_2 consumption, increases coronary blood flow, causes vasodilatation and slows atrioventricular conduction (possibly via increased potassium conductance and reduced calcium conductance). Also an inhibitory CNS neurotransmitter.

Has become the drug of choice for treatment of SVT (including that associated with Wolff–Parkinson–White syndrome) and diagnosis of other tachyarrhythmias by slowing atrioventricular conduction. Its short half-life (8–10 s) and lack of negative inotropism make it an attractive alternative to verapamil. Unclassified as an antiarrhythmic drug.

Has also been used as a directly acting vasodilator drug in hypotensive anaesthesia. Increases cardiac output, with stable heart rate. Its effects are rapidly reversible on stopping the infusion.

- Dosage:
  - SVT: 3 mg by rapid iv injection; if unsuccessful after 1–2 min this is followed by 6 mg and then 12 mg.
  - hypotensive anaesthesia: 50–300 μg/kg/min. ATP has also been used.
- Side effects are usually mild and include flushing, dyspnoea and nausea. Bronchoconstriction may occur in asthmatics. Bradycardia is resistant to atropine. Adenosine's action is prolonged in dipyridamole therapy (because uptake of adenosine is inhibited) and reduced by theophylline and other xanthines (because of competitive antagonism). Transplanted hearts are particularly sensitive to adenosine's effects.

Adenosine monophosphate, cyclic (cAMP). Cyclic adenosine 3′,5′-monophosphate, formed from ATP by the enzyme adenylate cyclase. Activation of surface receptors may cause a guanine nucleotide regulatory protein (G protein) to interact with adenylate cyclase with resultant increases in intracellular cAMP levels (Fig. 5). Many substances act on surface receptors in this way, including catecholamines (β effects), vasopressin, ACTH, histamine, glucagon, parathyroid hormone and calcitonin.

Some substances inhibit adenylate cyclase via an inhibitory regulatory protein, e.g. noradrenaline at α_2-adrenergic receptors.

cAMP causes phosphorylation of proteins, particularly enzymes, by activating protein kinases. Phosphorylation changes enzyme activity and therefore cell metabolism; thus the intracellular concentration of cAMP determines cell activity, and cAMP acts as a 'second messenger'.

cAMP is inactivated by phosphodiesterase to 5′-AMP. Phosphodiesterase inhibitors, e.g. aminophylline and enoximone, increase cAMP levels.

Adenosine triphosphate and diphosphate (ATP and ADP). ATP is the most important high-energy phosphate compound. When hydrolysed to form ADP, it releases large amounts of energy which may be utilised in many cellular processes, e.g. active transport, muscle contraction, etc. Its phosphate bonds are formed using energy from catabolism; aerobic glycolysis generates 38 moles of ATP per mole of glucose, and anaerobic glycolysis yields 2 moles of ATP.

Other high-energy phosphate compounds include phosphorylcreatine (in muscle), ADP itself, and other nucleotides.
See also, Cytochrome oxidase system; Metabolism; Tricarboxylic acid cycle

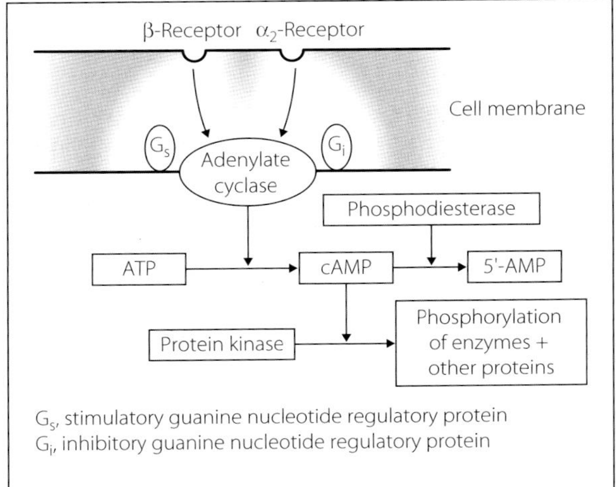

Fig. 5 cAMP involvement in transmembrane signalling

Adenylate cyclase, *see Adenosine monophosphate, cyclic*

ADH, Antidiuretic hormone, *see Vasopressin*

Adhesion molecules. Molecules normally sited on cell surfaces, involved in embryogenesis, cell growth and differentiation, and wound repair. Also mediate endothelial cell/leucocyte adhesion, transendothelial migration and cytotoxic T cell-induced lysis. Four major families exist: integrins, cadherins, selectins (named after the tissues in which they were discovered: L-selectin (leucocytes), E-selectin (endothelial cells), P-selectin (platelets)) and members of the immunoglobulin superfamily.

In general, contact between an adhesion receptor and the extracellular milieu results in the transmission of information allowing the cell to interact with its environment. Defective interactions involving adhesion molecules are implicated in disease (e.g. certain skin diseases, metastasis of cancer cells). Many pathogens use adhesion receptors to penetrate tissue cells. Overexpression of intravascular adhesion molecules or receptors has been implicated in rheumatoid arthritis and rejection of transplanted organs. Control of vascular integrity and defence against invasive pathogens requires regulation of adhesive interactions among blood cells and between blood cells and the vessel walls. Circulating leucocytes bind to the selectins of activated endothelial cells, become activated by chemoattractants and migrate through intracellular gaps to the site of inflammation. Thus adhesion molecules play a part in the inflammatory response in sepsis.

Adiabatic change. Volume change of a gas in which there is no transfer of heat to or from the system. Sudden compression of a gas without removal of resultant heat causes a rise in temperature. This may occur in the gas already present in the valves and pipes of an anaesthetic machine when a cylinder is turned on (hence the danger of explosion if oil or grease is present). Sudden adiabatic expansion of a gas results in cooling, as in the cryoprobe.
See also, Isothermal change

Adjustable pressure-limiting valves. Valves which open to allow passage of expired and surplus fresh gas from a breathing system, but close to prevent indrawing of air. Ideally the opening pressure should be as low as possible to reduce resistance to expiration, but not so low as to allow the reservoir bag to empty through it. Most contain a thin disc held against its seating by a spring, as in the original Heidbrink valve. Adjusting the tension in the spring, usually by screwing the valve top, alters the pressure at which the valve opens. The valve must be vertical in order to function correctly.

Modern valves, even when screwed fully down, will open at high pressures (60 cmH_2O). Most are now encased in a hood for scavenging of waste gases.
[Jay A Heidbrink (1875–1957), US anaesthetist]
See also, Anaesthetic breathing systems; Non-rebreathing valves

ADP, *see Adenosine triphosphate and diphosphate*

Adrenal gland. Situated on the upper pole of the kidney, each gland is composed of an outer cortex and an inner medulla. The cortex consists of the outer zona glomerulosa (secreting aldosterone), the middle zona fasciculata (secreting glucocorticoids) and inner zona reticularis (secreting sex hormones). Hypersecretion may result in hyperaldosteronism, Cushing's syndrome and virilisation/feminisation respectively. Hyposecretion causes adrenocortical insufficiency.

The adrenal medulla is thought to be derived from a sympathetic ganglion in which the postganglionic neurones have lost their axons, and secrete catecholamines into the bloodstream. Hypersecretion results in phaeochromocytoma.
See also, Sympathetic nervous system

Adrenaline (Epinephrine). Catecholamine, acting as a hormone and neurotransmitter in the sympathetic nervous system and brainstem pathways. Synthesised and released from the adrenal gland medulla and central adrenergic neurones (*for structure, synthesis and metabolism, see Catecholamines*). Called epinephrine in the USA because the name adrenaline, used in other countries, was too similar to the US-registered trade name Adrenalin that referred to a specific product (both adrenaline (Latin) and epinephrine (Greek) referring to the location of the adrenal gland 'on the kidney').

Stimulates both α- and β-adrenergic receptors; displays predominantly β-effects at low doses, α- at higher doses. Low dose infusion may lower BP by causing vasodilatation in muscle via β_2-receptors, despite increased cardiac output via β_1-receptors. Higher doses cause α-mediated vasoconstriction and increased systolic BP, although diastolic pressure may still decrease.

- Clinical uses:
  - with local anaesthetic agents, as a vasoconstrictor.
  - in anaphylactic reaction, cardiac arrest, bronchospasm.
  - as an inotropic drug.
  - in glaucoma (reduces aqueous humour production).
  - in croup.

Adrenaline may cause cardiac arrhythmias, especially in the presence of hypercapnia, hypoxia and certain drugs, e.g. halothane, cyclopropane and cocaine. During halothane anaesthesia, suggested maximal dosage of adrenaline is 10 ml 1:100 000 solution (100 μg) in 10 min, or 30 ml (300 μg) in 1 h. More dilute solutions should be used if possible. Adrenaline should not be used for ring blocks of digits or for penile nerve blocks, because of possible ischaemia to distal tissues.

- Dosage:
  - anaphylaxis: 0.1 mg iv (1 ml 1:10 000 solution), repeated as required. The recommended initial route in general medical guidelines is usually im (0.5–1.0 ml 1:1000 solution), reflecting the risks of iv administration without appropriate monitoring.
  - cardiac arrest: 1 mg (10 ml 1:10 000) iv.
  - by infusion: 0.01–0.15 μg/kg/min initially, increasing as required.
  - croup: 0.4 ml/kg nebulised up to 5 ml maximum, repeated after 30 min if required.

  Subcutaneous injection in shocked patients results in unreliable absorption. Adrenaline may be administered via a tracheal tube in 2–3 times the iv dose.

See also, Tracheal administration of drugs

α-Adrenergic receptor agonists. Naturally occurring agonists include adrenaline and noradrenaline which stimulate both α_1- and α_2-adrenergic receptors.

Methoxamine and phenylephrine are synthetic α_1-receptor agonists, used to cause vasoconstriction, e.g. to correct hypotension in spinal anaesthesia.

Clonidine acts on central α_2-receptors. Clonidine and other α_2-receptor agonists (e.g. dexmedetomidine) have been shown to reduce pain sensation and reduce requirements for general anaesthetics and have also been used for sedation in ICU. Other α_2-receptor agonists (e.g. xylazine, detomidine and medetomidine) have been used in veterinary practice as anaesthetic agents for many years.

β-Adrenergic receptor agonists. Agonists include adrenaline and isoprenaline which stimulate both β_1- and β_2-adrenergic receptors. Dopamine and dobutamine act mainly at β_1-receptors.

Salbutamol and terbutaline predominantly affect β_2-receptors, and are used clinically to cause bronchodilatation in asthma, and as tocolytic drugs in premature labour. Foroterol and salmeterol are longer acting agents given by inhalation for chronic asthma. Ritodrine is also used as a tocolytic drug. Some β_1-receptor effects are seen at high doses, e.g. tachycardia. They have been used in the treatment of cardiac failure and cardiogenic shock; stimulation of vascular β_2-receptors causes vasodilatation and reduces afterload.

α-Adrenergic receptor antagonists (α-Blockers). Usually refer to antagonists which act exclusively at α-adrenergic receptors.

- Drugs may be:
  - selective:
    - α_1-receptors, e.g. prazosin, doxazosin, terazosin, indoramin, phenoxybenzamine. Tamsulosin acts specifically at α_{1A}-receptors and is used in benign prostatic hypertrophy.
    - α_2-receptors: yohimbine.
  - non-selective, e.g. phentolamine.

Labetalol and carvedilol (a drug with similar effects) are antagonists at both α- and β-receptors. Other drugs may also act at α-receptors as part of a range of effects, e.g. chlorpromazine, droperidol.

Antagonism may be competitive, e.g. phentolamine, or non-competitive and therefore longer-lasting, e.g. phenoxybenzamine.

Used to lower BP and reduce afterload by causing vasodilatation. Compensatory tachycardia may occur.

- Side effects: postural hypotension, dizziness, tachycardia (less so with the selective α_1-antagonists, possibly because the negative feedback of noradrenaline at α_2-receptors is unaffected). Tachyphylaxis may occur.

β-Adrenergic receptor antagonists (β-Blockers). Competitive antagonists at β-adrenergic receptors.

- Actions:
  - reduce heart rate, force of contraction and myocardial O_2 consumption.
  - increase coronary blood flow by increasing diastolic filling time.
  - antiarrhythmic action results from β-receptor antagonism and possibly a membrane-stabilising effect at high doses.
  - antihypertensive action (not fully understood but may involve reductions in cardiac output, central sympathetic activity, and renin levels).
  - some have partial agonist activity (intrinsic sympathomimetic activity), e.g. pindolol, acebutolol, celiprolol and oxprenolol.
  - practolol, atenolol, metoprolol, betaxolol, bisoprolol, nebivolol and acebutolol are relatively cardioselective, but all will block β_2-receptors at high doses. Celiprolol has β_1-receptor antagonist and β_2-receptor agonist properties, thus causing peripheral vasodilatation in addition to cardiac effects.
  - labetalol and carvedilol have α- and β-receptor blocking properties. The former is available for iv administration and is widely used for acute reduction in BP.

- Half-lives:
  - esmolol: a few minutes. Hydrolysed by esterases, e.g. in red blood cells.
  - metoprolol, oxprenolol, pindolol, propranolol, timolol: 2–4 h.
  - atenolol, practolol, sotalol: 6–12 h.
  - nadolol: 24 h.

Most are readily absorbed by mouth, and undergo extensive first-pass metabolism. Practolol, atenolol, celiprolol, nadolol and sotalol are water soluble and largely excreted unchanged in the urine; propranolol and metoprolol are lipid soluble and almost completely metabolised in the liver.

- Uses:
  - hypertension, ischaemic heart disease, MI, arrhythmias, hyperthyroidism, anxiety, migraine prophylaxis. Have been shown to improve outcome in cardiac failure when added to ACE inhibitor therapy.
  - perioperatively: to reduce the hypertensive response to laryngoscopy; to treat perioperative hypertension, tachycardias and myocardial ischaemia; in hypotensive anaesthesia. Following a number of clinical studies, the use of pre- and postoperative β-agonists has been advocated as a means of reducing perioperative cardiovascular morbidity and mortality in high risk patients. However, this has been questioned because of fears over adverse effects, uncertainties over methodological aspects of the studies, and incompatibility of this approach with goal-directed inotrope therapy.
- Side effects:
  - cardiac failure, especially in combination with other negative inotropes.
  - bronchospasm and peripheral arterial insufficiency, via blockade of β_2-receptors.
  - increased risk of diabetes when used to treat hypertension and reduced cardiovascular (β_1) and metabolic (β_2) response to hypoglycaemia in diabetics.
  - sleep disturbances: less likely with water-soluble drugs.
  - oral practolol was withdrawn because of the oculomucocutaneous syndrome following its use. The iv preparation has been withdrawn for commercial reasons.

β-Adrenergic receptor antagonist poisoning. Uncommon, but overdosage is hazardous because of these drugs' narrow therapeutic ratio. General features include decreased myocardial contractility and failure, bradycardia, cardiac conduction defects, hypotension, bronchospasm, coma and convulsions, the latter two especially with propranolol. Sotalol may cause ventricular tachyarrhythmias. Hypoglycaemia is rare.

- Treatment:
  - as for poisoning and overdoses generally.
  - CVS effects may require CPR, glucagon (2–20 mg (50–150 μg/kg in children) iv followed by 50 μg/kg/h) or iv infusion of isoprenaline. Atropine is often ineffective but should be tried in vagal-blocking doses (3 mg iv (40 μg/kg in children)). Cardiac pacing may be required.

Adrenergic receptors. Group of G protein-coupled receptors, activated by adrenaline and other catecholamines, and divided into α- and β-receptors. Further subdivided into $\beta_1/\beta_2/\beta_3$ and α_1/α_2 receptors (Table 2).

Their effects are mediated by 'second messengers': α_1-receptor effects by increases in intracellular calcium ion concentration, α_2-receptor effects by reducing intracellular cAMP, and β_1- and β_2-receptor effects by increasing cAMP. There is evidence for mixed receptor populations at both pre- and postsynaptic membranes. α_2-Receptors have been further subdivided into α_{2A} (responsible for central regulation of BP, sympathetic activity, pain processing and alertness), α_{2B} (causes vasoconstriction) and α_{2C} (thought to be involved in behavioural responses).

Insel P (1996). N Engl J Med; 334: 580–5

See also, α-Adrenergic receptor agonists; β-Adrenergic receptor agonists; α-Adrenergic receptor antagonists; β-Adrenergic receptor antagonists; Sympathetic nervous system

Table 2 Classification and actions of adrenergic receptors

Receptor type	*Site*	*Effect of stimulation*
α_1	Vascular smooth muscle	Contraction
	Bladder smooth muscle (sphincter)	Contraction
	Radial muscle of iris	Contraction
	Intestinal smooth muscle	Relaxation, but contraction of sphincters
	Uterus	Variable
	Salivary glands	Viscous secretion
	Liver	Glycogenolysis
	Pancreas	Decreased secretion of enzymes, insulin and glucagon
α_2	Presynaptic membranes of adrenergic synapses	Reduced release of noradrenaline
	Postsynaptic membranes	Smooth muscle contraction
	Platelets	Aggregation
β_1	Heart	Increased rate and force of contraction
	Adipose tissue	Breakdown of stored triglycerides to fatty acids
	Juxtaglomerular apparatus	Increased renin secretion
β_2	Vascular smooth muscle (muscle beds)	Relaxation
	Bronchial smooth muscle	Relaxation
	Intestinal smooth muscle	Relaxation
	Bladder sphincter	Relaxation
	Uterus	Variable; relaxes the pregnant uterus
	Salivary glands	Watery secretion
	Liver	Glycogenolysis
	Pancreas	Increased insulin and glucagon secretion
β_3	Adipose tissue	Lipolysis

Adrenocortical insufficiency. May be due to:

- primary adrenal failure (Addison's disease) due to:
  - autoimmune disease (most common cause). May be associated with other autoimmune disease, e.g. diabetes, thyroid disease, pernicious anaemia, vitiligo.
  - TB, amyloidosis, metastatic infiltration, haemorrhage, drugs or infarction, e.g. in shock. Waterhouse–Friderichsen syndrome comprises bilateral adrenal cortical haemorrhage associated with severe meningococcal disease.
- secondary adrenal failure due to:
  - corticosteroid therapy withdrawal.
  - ACTH deficiency, e.g. due to surgery, head injury, tumours, infarction of the pituitary or the hypothalamus.

- Features:
  - acute: hypotension and electrolyte abnormalities (hyponatraemia, hyperkalaemia, hypochloraemia, hypercalcaemia and hypoglycaemia), muscle weakness. In critically ill patients, treatment of occult adrenocortical

insufficiency may be necessary for reversal of hypotension that is resistant to vasopressor drugs.
- chronic: weight loss, vomiting, diarrhoea, malaise, postural hypotension, increased risk of infection, muscle weakness. Dark pigmentation in scars and skin creases occur in primary disease. Acute insufficiency (crises) may develop following stress, e.g. infection, surgery, or any critical illness.

Diagnosed by measurement of plasma cortisol and ACTH levels, including demonstration of an impaired cortisol response following tetracosactide (tetracosactin) (synthetic ACTH terminal portion).

- Treatment:
  - acute: CPR, iv saline, hydrocortisone 100 mg 6 hourly iv (preferably as the sodium succinate).
  - chronic: hydrocortisone 20–30 mg/day, fludrocortisone 50–300 µg/day, both orally. Typically, both are required in primary insufficiency but only hydrocortisone in secondary insufficiency, although this may not always hold true.

[Thomas Addison (1793–1860) and Rupert Waterhouse (1873–1958), English physicians; Carl Friderichsen (1886–1979), Danish paediatrician]

Adrenocorticotrophic hormone (ACTH). Polypeptide hormone (39 amino acids; mw 4500) secreted by corticotropic cells of the anterior pituitary gland in response to corticotropin releasing factor secreted by the hypothalamus. Release of ACTH is highest in the early morning and is increased by emotional and physical stress, including surgery. It increases corticosteroid synthesis in the adrenal glands, particularly glucocorticoids but also aldosterone. ACTH production is inhibited by glucocorticoids (i.e. negative feedback). ACTH or its synthetic analogue tetracosactide (tetracosactin) has been used in place of corticosteroid therapy in an attempt to reduce adrenocortical suppression, and is used for diagnostic tests in endocrinology. It has also been used to treat post-dural puncture headache although this is not supported by evidence.
See also, Stress response to surgery

Adult respiratory distress syndrome, *see Acute respiratory distress syndrome*

Advance decision (Advance directive; 'Living will'). Statement, usually written, which provides for a mentally competent person to refuse certain future medical treatments, usually involving life saving therapies, if he/she were subsequently to become mentally or physically incompetent. The directive may be triggered by certain background conditions such as dementia, persistent vegetative state and terminal disease, or acute events including cardiorespiratory arrest, pneumonia, acute renal failure, major CVA or spinal cord injury. Legal and ethical issues relate to competence (capacity) of the individual, the possibility of changing one's mind, advances in medicine or techniques since the directive was written, the refusal of what might be considered basic care (e.g. feeding), difficulties anticipating the specific circumstances that may arise and therefore be covered, and the objections of doctors and other healthcare staff. Previously commonly referred to as advance directives, they were renamed 'advance decisions' in the Mental Capacity Act 2005, which enshrined them into statute for the first time. From April 2007, in order to be legally valid, an advance decision must:
- be made by a person ≥ 18 years old, with the capacity to make it.
- specify the treatment to be refused (can be in lay terms) and the circumstances in which this refusal would apply.
- be made freely without the influence of anyone else.
- be unaltered from when it was made.

White SM, Baldwin TJ (2006). Anaesthesia; 61: 381–9

Advanced (Cardiac) Life Support (ACLS/ALS). System of advanced management of cardiac arrest and its training to paramedics, doctors, nurses and other healthcare professionals. Also encompasses the recognition and management of peri-arrest arrhythmias and post-resuscitation care. In the UK, ALS courses are run by the Resuscitation Council (UK). In the USA, the American Heart Association runs ACLS courses.
See also, Advanced life support, adult; Basic life support, adult; Cardiopulmonary resuscitation

Advanced life support, adult. Component of CPR involving specialised equipment, techniques (e.g. tracheal intubation), drugs, monitoring, 100% oxygen, etc. Airway management may include use of tracheal intubation, laryngeal mask airway, Combitube or, rarely, tracheostomy. Recommendations of the European Resuscitation Council (2005):
- attention to 'ABC' of basic life support ± advanced airway management, if there is a delay in getting a defibrillator. Defibrillation should take place without delay for a witnessed or in-hospital cardiac arrest; for out-of-hospital unwitnessed arrest, 2 min of CPR should precede defibrillation. A precordial thump should be considered for witnessed, monitored collapse when a defibrillator is not immediately available.
- actions then depend on the initial rhythm:
  - 'shockable' i.e. VF/pulseless VT:
    - defibrillation: a single shock of 150–200 J (biphasic) or 360 J (monophasic) followed by immediate resumption of CPR without reassessing the rhythm or feeling for a pulse. After 2 min of CPR, reassess and if indicated, subsequent shocks of 150–360 J (biphasic) or 360 J (monophasic). If it is unclear whether the rhythm is asystole or fine VF, continue basic life support and do not attempt defibrillation.
    - adrenaline 1 mg iv if VF/VT persists after a second shock, then 1 mg every 3–5 min if it still persists.
    - consider and correct potentially reversible causes (see below); if not already done, secure the airway, administer oxygen, get iv access. Cardiac massage and ventilation at 30:2; compressions should be uninterrupted once the airway has been secured.
    - in refractory VF despite three shocks, consider amiodarone 300 mg as an iv bolus; 150 mg as a second bolus followed by 900 mg/24 h. Lidocaine 1 mg/kg is an alternative if amiodarone is unavailable, but should not be used in addition (maximum 3 mg/kg in the first hour). Consider use of different paddle positions/contacts, different defibrillator, buffers, etc. if refractory. Magnesium sulphate 8 mmol may be indicated in hypomagnesaemia, torsade de pointes or digoxin toxicity.
  - 'non-shockable' i.e. asystole or pulseless electrical activity (PEA):
    - adrenaline 1 mg as soon as venous access obtained, repeated every 3–5 min. CPR for 2 min. Consider and correct potentially reversible causes; cardiac massage and ventilation as for VF (see above).
    - reassess after 2 min and repeat the above if necessary. Consider use of atropine 3 mg if pulse rate is less than 60/min, cardiac pacing, buffers, etc. if refractory.

- potentially reversible causes (4 'H's and 4 'T's): hypoxaemia, hypovolaemia, electrolyte and metabolic disorders (especially hyper-/hypokalaemia), hypothermia, tension pneumothorax, cardiac tamponade, toxic/therapeutic disturbances (poisoning and overdoses), thromboembolic/mechanical obstruction (PE). A fifth 'H' (hydrogen ions, i.e. acidosis) and a fifth 'T' (coronary thrombosis) have also been suggested.
- drugs are usually given iv, preferably via a central vein. Peripheral lines should be flushed with 20 ml saline after each drug. Tracheal administration of drugs is possible, using 2–3 times the iv doses of atropine, lidocaine and adrenaline (each diluted in 10 ml saline).
- consider buffers, e.g. bicarbonate 50 ml 8.4% solution in severe acidosis (pH < 7.1 or base excess exceeding -10), or specific conditions, e.g. tricyclic antidepressant drug poisoning, hyperkalaemia.
- if unsuccessful, CPR is generally discontinued after 30–60 min depending on the circumstances (longer in treatable conditions and in children).
- post-arrest care:
  - checking of arterial blood gases, electrolytes and chest X-ray.
  - transfer to ICU and cardiorespiratory support as required. MODS may occur.
  - therapeutic hypothermia to 32–34°C for 12–24 h improves outcome in unconscious adult patients with spontaneous circulation after out-of-hospital cardiac arrest due to VF, and possibly for other out-of-hospital arrest rhythms or in-hospital arrest.
- special situations:
  - trauma, choking, near-drowning, electrocution, anaphylactic reaction.
  - paediatric and neonatal CPR (*see Cardiopulmonary resuscitation, paediatric; Cardiopulmonary resuscitation, neonatal*).

- Recent changes/controversies:
  - calcium not recommended routinely because it reduces coronary and cerebral blood flow.
  - intracardiac injection not recommended because of the risk of trauma.
  - hyperglycaemia is thought to worsen the effects of cerebral hypoxia. Avoidance of glucose solutions during CPR has been suggested.
  - high dose adrenaline and bretylium no longer recommended.
  - the decision to stop CPR may be difficult in certain circumstances, as may the decision not to start, e.g. terminally ill, elderly patients, etc. Regular consideration of do not resuscitate orders has been suggested as routine. Advance decisions may specify conditions under which patients do or do not wish to be resuscitated.
  - there has been recent controversy over whether relatives of cardiac arrest victims should witness resuscitation attempts; discomfort of staff and possible hindrance of CPR may be offset by the beneficial effects of relatives' seeing that adequate efforts have been expended and their being able to be present if the patient dies.
  - manipulation of intrathoracic pressure has been suggested in order to improve cardiac output (*see Cardiac massage*).
  - vasopressin has been suggested as an alternative to adrenaline but there is no firm evidence to support it.

Complications include trauma to abdominal organs, ribs, etc. and those associated with tracheal intubation/attempted intubation, vascular access, etc.

European Resuscitation Council (2005). Resuscitation; 67 Suppl 1: S39–86

See also, Acute Cardiac Life Support; Brainstem death; Cough-CPR; Resuscitation Council (UK)

Advanced Life Support in Obstetrics (ALSO). Training system developed in the USA and administered by the American Association of Family Physicians; introduced in the UK as part of the Maternal and Neonatal Emergency Training (MANET) project. Aimed at training medical and midwifery staff in the practical management of maternal and neonatal emergencies and provision of life support for the mother and child. Similar to other CPR training systems (e.g. ACLS, ATLS) in its approach and structure.

See also, Cardiopulmonary resuscitation, neonatal

Advanced Paediatric Life Support (APLS). System of management of the sick or injured child, devised by specialists in paediatrics, accident and emergency medicine, anaesthesia and paediatric surgery in the UK and administered by the Advanced Life Support Group. The system integrates basic and advanced resuscitation techniques, similar to those employed in ALS/ACLS and ATLS, to permit the assessment and treatment of paediatric emergencies (e.g. airway obstruction, cardiac arrest, hypothermia, convulsions, poisoning and trauma). Incorporates assessment of the airway, breathing and circulation with special emphasis on determining if the child has failure of respiration or circulation. Stresses the anatomical and physiological differences between adults and children whilst emphasising paediatric normal ranges (e.g. for weight, cardiorespiratory parameters). Underlines the usefulness of specific interventions (e.g. insertion of an intraosseous needle).

See also, Cardiopulmonary resuscitation, paediatric

Advanced Trauma Life Support (ATLS). System of trauma management devised by physicians in Nebraska, USA in 1978 and adopted by the American College of Surgeons in 1979. Based on the concept of reducing morbidity and mortality in the first ('Golden') hour following trauma during which patients may die from potentially survivable injuries (airway obstruction, hypovolaemia, pneumothorax, cardiac tamponade, etc.), by teaching all members of the trauma team the same algorithms and procedures which are then carried out by rote on every patient. Has been criticised (mainly by senior doctors) because of its very didactic nature, although this is one of its strengths since those most likely to be in the 'front line' of trauma care are traditionally junior doctors who lack the expertise and judgement of their seniors.

Consists of the following phases:

- preparation.
- triage.
- primary survey: incorporates assessment of the integrity and function of the airway, cervical spine, breathing, circulation and neurological status. The patient is fully exposed to detect all life-threatening injuries, with resuscitation taking place in tandem with the primary survey. The need for radiographs of the chest, lateral cervical spine and pelvis should be considered during the primary survey but should not delay resuscitation (the cervical spine is assumed to require immobilisation for any injury above the clavicles until proven otherwise). This takes place simultaneously with the primary survey.
- resuscitation of life-threatening conditions.
- secondary survey: the patient is fully examined from 'head to toe' to exclude injuries to scalp, cranium, face, neck, shoulders, chest, abdomen, perineum, long

bones, spine and spinal cord. Special procedures (e.g. abdominal ultrasound, diagnostic peritoneal lavage, iv pyelogram, CT of brain) may be undertaken during this phase, prior to planning of definitive care.
- continued post-resuscitation monitoring and re-evaluation.
- definitive care: e.g. surgery, ICU admission or transfer to a specialist centre.

ATLS courses are administered in the USA by the American College of Surgeons and by the Royal College of Surgeons of England in the UK.

Carmont MR (2005). Postgrad Med J; 81: 87–91

Adverse drug reactions. Undesired drug effects, usually divided into:
- predictable (type A) dose-related side effects, e.g. hypotension following thiopental.
- unpredictable (type B; idiosyncratic) usually less common reactions. These are unrelated to known pharmacological properties of a drug (i.e. not due to common side effects or overdose), usually involving the immune system in some way (but not always, e.g. MH).

Suspected adverse reactions are voluntarily reported to the Medicines and Healthcare products Regulatory Agency on yellow cards, introduced in 1964 and updated in 2000. The yellow card system was extended to nurse reporters in 2002. Specific yellow cards for reporting anaesthetic drug reactions were introduced in 1988, to encourage reporting of serious reactions to established drugs and any reaction to new drugs. Anaesthetists give many different drugs iv to large numbers of patients, and therefore reactions are often seen. Reactions may be more likely if drugs are given quickly and in combination.

- Mechanisms:
  - on first exposure:
    - direct histamine release, e.g. tubocurarine, atracurium, thiopental, Althesin.
    - alternative pathway complement activation, e.g. Althesin.
  - apparently on first exposure: prior sensitisation by other (e.g. environmental) antigens may cause crossover sensitivity to subsequently administered drugs; e.g. reactions to dextrans may involve prior exposure to bacterial antigens.
  - requiring prior exposure:
    - anaphylactic reaction, e.g. to thiopental.
    - classical pathway complement activation, e.g. Althesin. Other drugs dissolved in Cremophor EL may crossreact.

Features range from mild skin rash to anaphylaxis. First exposure reactions tend to be milder and more frequent than those requiring prior exposure.

Reported incidence varies between countries and according to definitions but severe allergic reactions are thought to occur in about 1:10 000 to 1:20 000 cases.

- Management:
  - immediate medical management as for anaphylaxis.
  - testing:
    - a plain blood sample should be taken as soon as possible and at 1 h and 6 h after the reaction for mast cell tryptase levels if an anaphylactic/anaphylactoid reaction is suspected (99% of plasma tryptase arises from mast cells; plasma levels are therefore normally under 1 ng/ml; $\leq$ 15 ng/ml suggests an anaphylactoid reaction and > 20 ng/ml suggests an anaphylactic reaction). Tryptase is stable in solution and its half-life is 2.5 h, so if samples at exactly 1 h and 6 h are not taken, back-calculation to the time of the reaction should still be possible if the samples' actual times are accurately recorded. Histamine, complement and immunoglobulin levels may also be useful.
    - prick testing (placement of a drop of solution on to the skin of the forearm and gently lifting the underlying skin with a needle) has been suggested as the most useful investigation for specific agents. Since 'neat' solutions may cause flares in normal subjects, 1:10 dilutions or lower should also be used. A wide range of drugs should be tested. Waiting for ~6 months after the reaction has been suggested in order to allow recovery of the immune system.
    - radioallergosorbent testing (RAST; utilises radioactive-linked anti-immunoglobulin antibodies directed against specific antigen binding sites) may demonstrate specific antibodies against suxamethonium and penicillins; testing for other anaesthetic drugs is no longer considered specific enough. RAST may also be useful in latex allergy.
    - the role of other tests, e.g. *in vitro* basophil studies, is controversial.

Mertes PM, Laxenaire MC (2002). Eur J Anaesth; 19: 240–62

AF, *see Atrial fibrillation*

Affinity. Extent to which a drug binds to a receptor. A drug with high affinity binds more strongly than one with lower affinity, whatever its intrinsic activity.

Afterload. Ventricular wall tension required to eject stroke volume during systole.
- For the left ventricle, afterload is increased by:
  - an anatomical obstruction, e.g. aortic stenosis.
  - raised SVR.
  - decreased elasticity of the aorta and large blood vessels.
  - increased ventricular volume (greater tension is needed to produce the necessary pressure (Laplace's law)).

Increased afterload results in increased myocardial work and O_2 consumption, and decreased stroke volume. Reduction of afterload may be achieved with vasodilator drugs.

See also, Preload

Agonist. Substance which binds to a receptor to cause a response within the cell. It has high affinity for the receptor and high intrinsic activity.

A partial agonist binds to the receptor, but causes less response; it may have high affinity, but it has less intrinsic activity. It may therefore act as a competitive antagonist in the presence of a pure agonist.

An agonist–antagonist causes agonism at certain receptors and antagonism at others.

See also, Dose–response curves; Receptor theory

Agranulocytosis, *see Leucocytes*

AGSS, Anaesthetic gas scavenging system, *see Scavenging*

AIDS, Acquired immunodeficiency syndrome, *see Human immunodeficiency viral infection*

Air. Dry natural air contains by volume:

Nitrogen	78.03%	Hydrogen	0.001%
O_2	20.99%	Helium	0.0005%
Argon	0.93%	Krypton	0.0001%
CO_2	0.03%	Xenon	0.000008%
Neon	0.0015%		

'Medical' air may be supplied by a compressor or in cylinders. The latter (containing air at 137 bar) are grey with black and white shoulders. Piped air is normally at 4 bar.

Air embolism. Introduction of air bubbles into the circulation, usually into veins (although arterial air embolism has been caused by prolonged flushing of arterial lines in neonates). A potential risk when venous pressure is lower than atmospheric pressure. It may occur during any surgery when an open vein is raised above the heart; it is particularly likely in neurosurgery with the patient in the sitting position since the dural sinuses do not collapse. May also occur during central venous cannulation (minimised by tilting the patient head-down) or removal of a CVP line. Procedures involving insufflation or injection of gas, e.g. laparoscopy, epidural anaesthesia using loss of resistance to air, laser surgery with gas-cooled probes, may also lead to embolism. N_2O diffuses into bubbles, increasing their volume and exacerbating their effects. Morbidity and mortality are dependent on the volume of the air entrained and the rate of accumulation.

Air in the heart is compressed with each beat and not expelled, causing foaming and interruption of blood flow. Pulmonary vessels may become obstructed. Small bubbles may have little effect. Paradoxical air emboli pass to the systemic circulation via the pulmonary vascular bed or cardiac septal defects (a probe-patent foramen ovale exists in 20–30% of patients at autopsy). The bubbles may obstruct the coronary or cerebral vessels.

- Clinical features:
  - reduced cardiac output.
  - tachycardia.
  - cyanosis.
  - bronchospasm and pulmonary oedema may occur. Dyspnoea, coughing and chest pain are common in the awake patient.
  - tinkling sounds on auscultation, e.g. with an oesophageal/precordial stethoscope; large amounts of air may cause a 'mill-wheel' murmur. Embolism may be detected by a precordial Doppler probe, transcranial Doppler ultrasound or by transoesophageal echocardiography, although the extreme sensitivity of these techniques may reveal many tiny bubbles which are of disputed clinical significance.
  - sudden reduction of end-tidal CO_2 due to increased dead space and decreased cardiac output. End-tidal nitrogen monitoring has also been used to monitor air embolism.
  - raised pulmonary artery resistance and pressure.
  - signs of right-sided strain on the ECG; ventricular ectopics or fibrillation may occur.
- Treatment:
  - to prevent further embolism:
    - seal veins.
    - flood the wound with fluid.
    - increase venous pressure using head-down tilt, iv fluids, jugular venous compression, PEEP. The latter and the antigravity suit have been advocated for prevention of air embolism in neurosurgery in the sitting position. The use of the modified sitting position with the legs placed horizontally may decrease the incidence.
  - once air has entered the circulation:
    - CPR if required.
    - stop N_2O.
    - the head-down, left lateral position is said to increase the likelihood of air remaining in the right atrium.
    - remove air from the right atrium or ventricle via a central line. Special wide-bore, multi-holed catheters are available for this purpose, although whether these are necessary is controversial.
    - hyperbaric O_2 has been used to reduce the size of the embolism and improve oxygenation.

Similar concerns exist during CVP line placement and removal. For the latter, use of plastic occlusive dressings has been suggested as preferable to use of gauze, since the latter may not prevent indrawing of air.

Mirski MA, Lele AJ, Fitzsimmons L Toung TJK (2007). Anesthesiology; 106: 164–77

Airway. The upper airway includes the mouth, nose, pharynx and larynx. Maintenance of the airway in the unconscious or anaesthetised patient is achieved by combined flexion of the neck and extension at the atlantooccipital joint (the 'sniffing position'), and lifting the angles of the mandible forward. The tongue is lifted forward by the genioglossus muscle which is attached to the back of the point of the jaw; the hyoid bone and larynx are pulled forward by the hyoglossus, mylohyoid, geniohyoid and digastric muscles. Upward pressure on the soft tissues of the floor of the mouth may cause obstruction, particularly in children, and should be avoided. In the lateral (recovery) position, the tongue and jaw fall forward under gravity, improving the airway. Airway obstruction during anaesthesia has traditionally been attributed to the tongue falling back against the posterior pharyngeal wall. Radiological and electromyographic studies suggest that obstruction by the soft palate or epiglottis secondary to reduced local muscle activity may also be responsible.

Hillman DR, Platt PR, Eastwood PR (2003). Br J Anaesth; 91: 31–9

See also, Airways; Tracheobronchial tree

Airway exchange catheter. Device placed into the trachea both to maintain oxygenation after tracheal extubation (i.e. inserted through the tracheal tube before the latter is removed), and to facilitate reintubation should it be required. Available devices share similar features: they are long, hollow catheters, able to be attached to an O_2 supply at their proximal end (e.g. using a detachable 15 mm connector) and stiff enough to act as a guide for a tracheal tube passed over them. The distal end may be angulated, allowing the catheter also to be used as a bougie, e.g. during direct laryngoscopy. A specific type of exchange catheter (the Aintree catheter) has been designed for exchanging a laryngeal mask airway with a tracheal tube via a flexible fibrescope.

Airway obstruction. Obstruction may occur at the mouth, pharynx, larynx, trachea and large bronchi. It may be caused by the tongue falling backwards, laryngospasm, strictures, tumours and soft tissue swellings, oedema, infection (e.g. diphtheria, epiglottitis) and foreign objects, including teeth and anaesthetic equipment. Hypotonia of the muscles involved in upper airway maintenance is common during anaesthesia. During IPPV, mechanical obstruction may occur at any point along the breathing system.

Airway obstruction results in hypoventilation and increased work of breathing. It may present as an acute medical emergency requiring immediate management.

- Features:
  - spontaneous ventilation:
    - dyspnoea, noisy respiration, stridor.
    - use of accessory muscles of respiration, with tracheal tug, supraclavicular and intercostal indrawing, and paradoxical 'see-saw' movement of abdomen and chest.

- tachypnoea, tachycardia and other features of hypoxaemia, hypercapnia and respiratory failure.
- pulmonary oedema may occur if negative intrathoracic pressures are excessive.
- during anaesthesia, poor movement of the reservoir bag may occur.

- IPPV:
  - increased airway pressures with reduced chest movement; noisy respiration or wheeze.
  - features of hypoxaemia and hypercapnia may be present.

- Management:
  - O_2 therapy (increased F_IO_2 during anaesthesia).
  - spontaneous ventilation:
    - general measures in unconscious/anaesthetised patients:
      - turn to the lateral position if practical.
      - correct positioning of the head, elevation of the jaw, and use of oropharyngeal or nasopharyngeal airways. Tracheal intubation may be required as below.
    - specific treatment, e.g.:
      - antibacterial drugs for infection.
      - fresh frozen plasma or C1 esterase inhibitor for hereditary angioedema.
      - nebulised adrenaline for croup.
      - Heimlich manoeuvre for choking.
    - increasing gas flow: helium–O_2 mixtures.
    - bypassing the obstruction: tracheal intubation, tracheostomy or cricothyrotomy. The last two may be difficult if the anatomy is distorted.
  - IPPV:
    - causes of increased airway pressure and hypoventilation other than obstruction due to equipment (e.g. bronchospasm, pneumothorax, inadequate neuromuscular blockade and coughing) should be considered.
    - while ventilating by hand, all tubing should be checked for kinks. A suction catheter will not pass down the tracheal tube if the latter is obstructed, e.g. by kinks, mucus, herniated cuff, etc. If auscultation of the chest does not suggest bronchospasm or pneumothorax, the cuff should be deflated and the tracheal tube pulled back slightly. If ventilation does not improve, the tube should be removed and ventilation attempted by facepiece.
- Anaesthesia for patients with airway obstruction:
  - preoperatively:
    - preoperative assessment for the above features and management as above.
    - useful pre-induction investigations include:
      - radiography, including tomograms, thoracic inlet views and CT scanning.
      - arterial blood gas analysis.
      - flow–volume loops.
    - premedication may aid smooth induction of anaesthesia but excessive sedation should be avoided.
  - perioperatively:
    - anaesthesia should be induced with facilities for resuscitation and tracheostomy/cricothyrotomy available.
    - patients with upper airway obstruction usually adopt the optimal head and neck position for maximal air movement; muscle relaxation caused by iv induction may therefore lead to sudden complete obstruction. It may be impossible to ventilate the patient by facepiece, and tracheal intubation may be difficult or impossible. IV anaesthetic agents should therefore be avoided. Similarly, neuromuscular blocking drugs should not be used until the airway has been secured. Inhalational induction, classically with halothane (nowadays, sevoflurane) and N_2O/O_2 (or O_2 alone if obstruction is severe) should be employed. Deep anaesthesia is achieved slowly; if obstruction worsens, anaesthesia is allowed to lighten. Full monitoring is mandatory.
    - tracheal intubation is performed without paralysis; lidocaine spray may be useful.
    - awake intubation with a flexible endoscope is an alternative, although complete obstruction may occur if airflow is already critically impaired. Tracheostomy using local anaesthesia is another option.
  - postoperatively: as for difficult intubation (*see Intubation, difficult*).

Classical management of patients with large airway compression, e.g. by mediastinal tumours, also employs inhalational induction and anaesthesia. This avoids acute exacerbation of airway obstruction caused by sudden muscle relaxation.

In the recovery room or casualty department, all unconscious patients should be positioned in the recovery position, to protect them from aspiration and airway obstruction.

See also, Intubation, awake

Airway pressure. Pressure within the breathing system and tracheobronchial tree. Useful as an indicator of mechanical obstruction to expiration during spontaneous ventilation. During IPPV, airway pressures may indicate disconnection, level of PEEP, mechanical obstruction, decreased lung compliance or increased airway resistance, and the risk of barotrauma. The pressure measured at the mouth may considerably exceed alveolar pressure during positive pressure breaths, especially if airway resistance and gas flow rates are high. During expiration, mouth pressure falls to zero, but alveolar pressure may lag behind. In some ventilators airway pressure is measured in the expiratory limb of the breathing system.

Airway pressure release ventilation (APRV). CPAP with intermittent release to ambient pressure (or a lower level of CPAP) causing expiration. Spontaneous ventilation may continue between APRV breaths. Allows reduction of mean airway pressure, and has been used to support respiration in ARDS. Weaning is achieved by reducing the frequency of CPAP release until the patient is breathing spontaneously with CPAP maintained.

Bray JG, Cane RD (1992). Curr Opin Anaesth; 5: 855–8

Airway resistance.

$$\text{Resistance} = \frac{\text{driving pressure}}{\text{gas flow}}$$

Driving pressure is the difference between alveolar and mouth pressures, and may be measured using the body plethysmograph. Alternatively, gas flow may be halted repeatedly for a tenth of a second at a time with a shutter; during the brief period of no flow, alveolar pressure may be measured at the mouth. Gas flow can be measured with a pneumotachograph.

Most of the resistance resides in the large and medium-sized bronchi; severe damage to the small airways may occur before a measurable increase in resistance.

At low lung volumes, the radial traction produced by lung parenchyma surrounding the airways, and which holds them open, is reduced; thus airway calibre is reduced, and resistance increased. During forced expiration, some airways may close, causing air trapping. Bronchoconstriction, and increased density or viscosity of the inspired gas, increase resistance (density because flow is not purely laminar in the airways). Resistance is increased in chronic bronchitis due to airway narrowing and bronchoconstriction. In emphysema the airways close because of lung parenchymal destruction.

Airway resistance increases during anaesthesia; this may be caused by bronchospasm, reduction in FRC and lung volume, or by the tubes and connections of the breathing system.

See also, Closing capacity; Compliance

Airways. Devices placed in the upper airway (but not into the larynx); used to:
- relieve airway obstruction.
- prevent biting and occlusion of the tracheal tube.
- support the tracheal tube.
- allow suction.
- act as a conduit for fibreoptic intubation.
- facilitate CPR.

Thus usually employed during anaesthesia and in unconscious patients.
- Types:
  - oropharyngeal: Guedel's airway is most commonly used. Modifications include a side port for attachment to a fresh gas source (Waters' airway), 15 mm connectors for attachment to a breathing system, caps with side ports, and airways used for fibreoptic intubation (Fig. 6). A cuffed oropharyngeal airway (COPA) with a 15 mm connector was described in 1991 but is not widely used. Oropharyngeal airways are the commonest cause of damage to teeth in anaesthetised patients. They must be placed with care, particularly in children where soft tissue damage can easily occur.
  - oral supraglottic: designed to be placed close to, but above, the larynx, resulting in a better seal and therefore the ability to control ventilation. Include (Fig. 7):
    - laryngeal mask airway: the most widely used.
    - laryngeal tube: requires less mouth opening. Has two cuffs, inflated by a single inflation tube. Available in seven sizes, suitable for babies up to adults. Performs better for IPPV in studies than for spontaneous ventilation. A new double-lumen version (laryngeal tube Sonda) is similar in function to the Combitube (*see Oesophageal obturators and airways*).
  - i-gel: similar in function to the laryngeal mask airway but the 'cuff' is made of soft gel and non-inflatable; incorporates a gastric channel and bite block. Available in sizes 3–5.
  - others have been described but are not widely used:
    - Airway Management Device (AMD): has a single lumen and two cuffs, inflated independently. The lower cuff compresses the device's lumen when inflated; when the cuff is deflated, a suction catheter may be passed into the oesophagus. Available in three adult sizes.

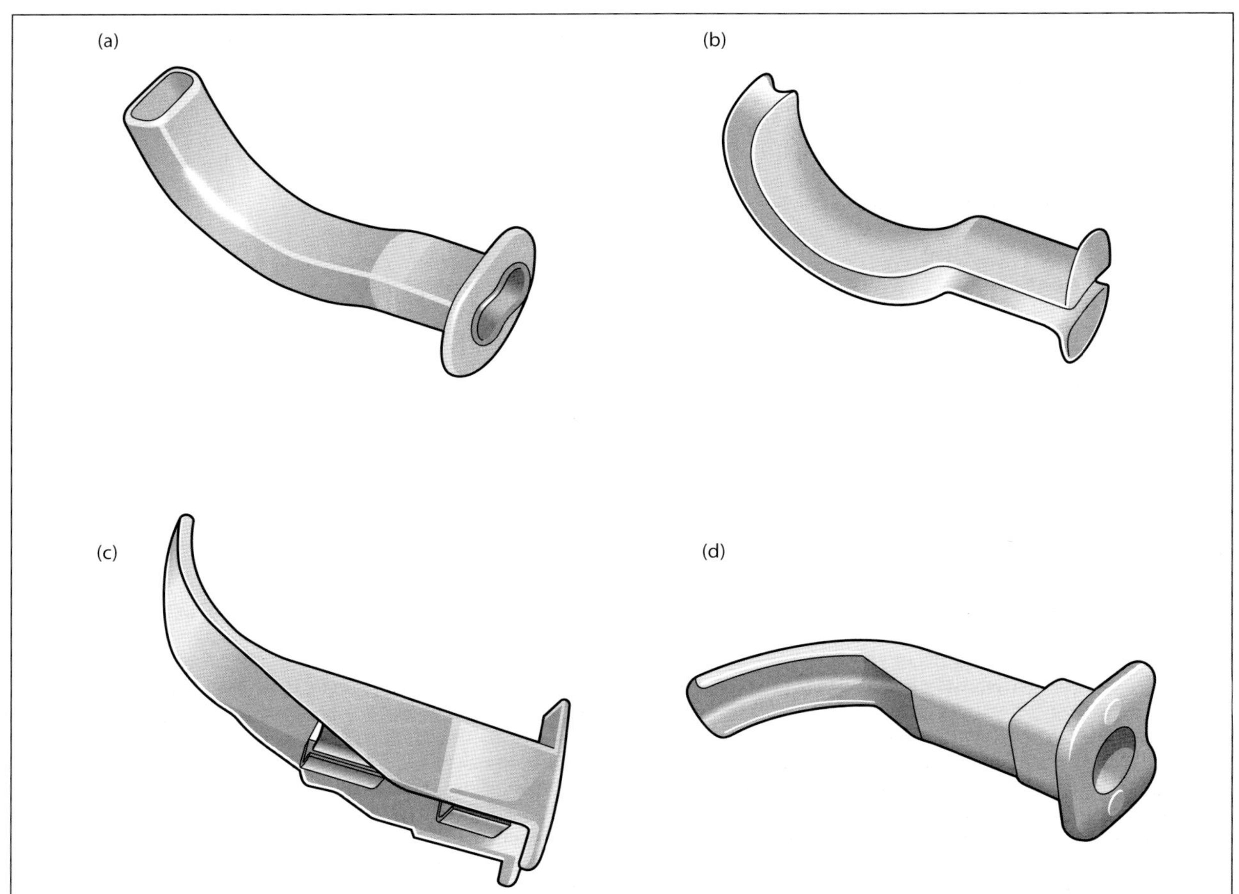

Fig. 6 Examples of oropharyngeal airways: (a) Guedel; (b) Berman; (c) Ovassapian; (d) Williams. The latter three are used for fibreoptic intubation; the Berman and Ovassapian allow the airway to be removed without dislodging the tracheal tube once placed

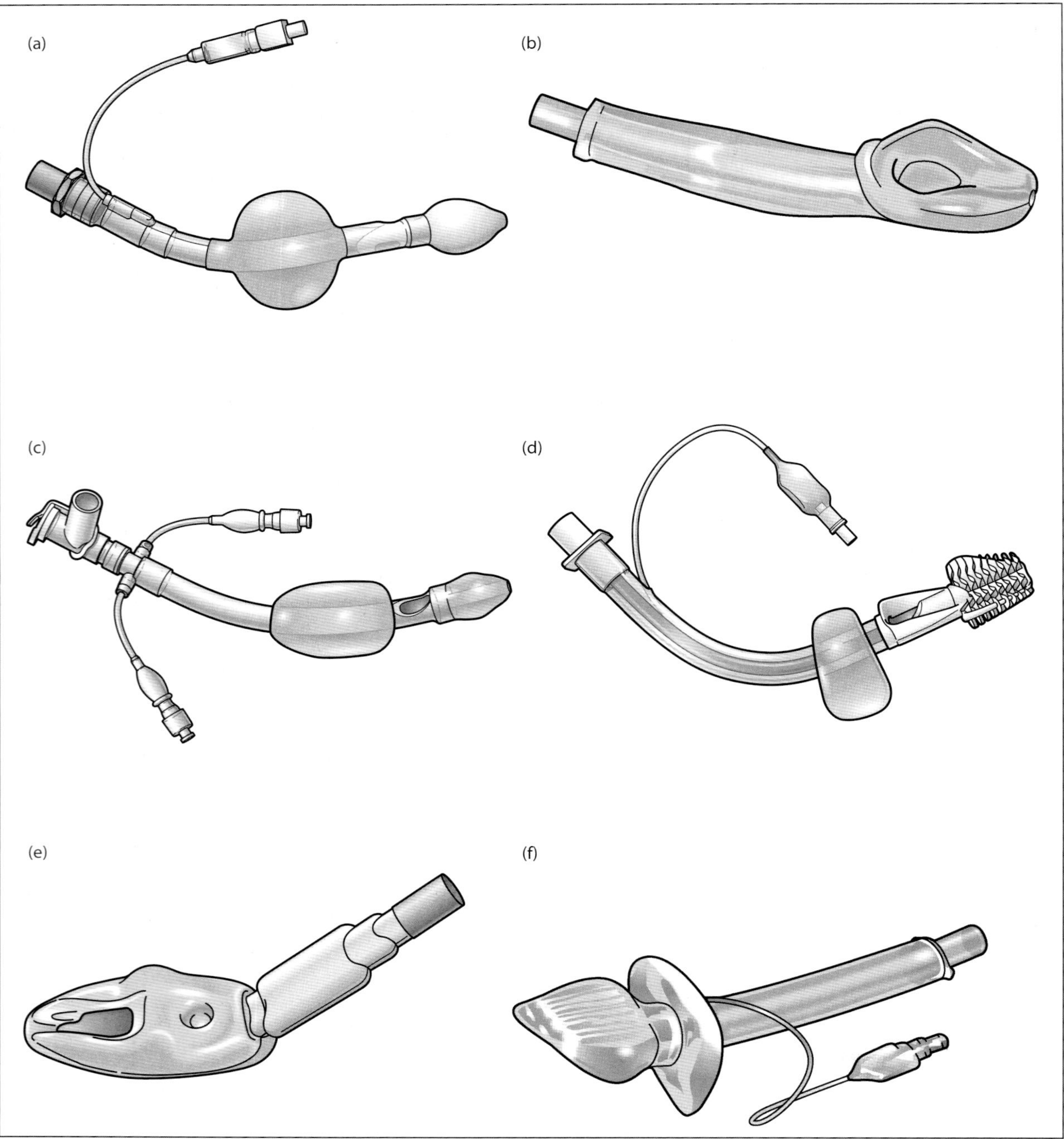

Fig. 7 Examples of supraglottic airways: (a) laryngeal tube; (b) i-gel; (c) AMD; (d) PAXpress; (e) SLIPA; (f) Cobra. (See Fig. 95 for laryngeal mask airway)

- PAXpress: similar to the laryngeal mask airway but with a gilled pharyngeal portion instead of a cuff. More traumatic on insertion. Available in one size, for all adults.
- Streamlined Liner of the Pharyngeal Airway (SLIPA): similar to the laryngeal mask airway but with a soft hollow pharyngeal portion instead of a cuff, which acts both as a seal and as a sump for collecting liquid should regurgitation occur. Available in six adult sizes (47–57), corresponding to the width of the thyroid cartilage.
- Cobra: single-use device similar in function to the laryngeal mask airway; available in eight sizes.

▸ nasopharyngeal: usually smooth non-cuffed tubes with a flange to prevent pushing them completely into the nose. Avoids risk to capped teeth, but may cause epistaxis. Cuffed nasal airways may be held in place by the inflated cuff, and allow attachment to a breathing system.

Insertion of an airway may cause gagging, coughing and laryngospasm unless the patient is comatose or adequately anaesthetised; these may also occur on waking.

[Robert Alvin Berman (1914–1999), US anaesthetist; Andranik Ovassapian, Iranian-born US anaesthetist; R Tudor Williams, Canadian anaesthetist]

McIntyre JWR (1996). Can J Anaesth; 43: 629–35

AIS, *see Abbreviated injury scale*

Albendazole. Agent used in conjunction with surgery to treat hydatid disease. May be used alone if surgical treatment is deemed impossible.

- Dose 800 mg orally/day in divided doses for 28 days, followed by a 14-day treatment-free period. Up to 3 cycles may be given.
- Side effects: GIT upset, headache, dizziness, hepatic impairment, pancytopenia.

Albumin. Protein (mw 69 000), the major constituent of plasma protein (normal plasma levels: 35–50 /l). Important in the maintenance of plasma oncotic pressure, as a buffer, and in the transport of various molecules such as bilirubin, hormones, fatty acids, etc. and drugs. It is synthesised by the liver and removed from the plasma into the interstitial fluid. It may then pass via lymphatics back to the plasma, or into cells to be metabolised. May have a role as a free radical scavenger. Albumin depletion occurs in severe illness, infection, trauma, etc. Available for transfusion as 4.5% and 20% solutions. Has been used as a colloid when providing iv fluid therapy for critically ill patients but hypoalbuminaemia in these patients usually results from increased metabolism of circulating albumin; administration does not generally result in maintained plasma albumin levels and no improvement in outcome has been found when compared with cheaper alternatives. In 1998 a meta-analysis suggested that critically ill patients treated with albumin might have a greater mortality than those given alternatives, although whether this was caused by the albumin (or whether this was in fact true) caused considerable controversy. Since then, at least one large randomised study of albumin versus saline for fluid resuscitation has shown that, in a heterogeneous adult ICU population, iv albumin administration is safe, but confers no clear advantage over saline.

Nicholson JP, Wolmarans MR, Park GR (2000). Br J Anaesth; 85: 599–610

See also, Blood products; Protein-binding

Albuterol, *see Salbutamol*

Alcohol, *see Alcohols*

Alcohol poisoning. Problems, features and management depend on the alcohols ingested:

- ethanol: commonly complicates or precipitates acute illness or injury, especially trauma. Results in depressed consciousness (hindering assessment of head injury, etc.), potentiation of depressant drugs, and a lack of inhibition. Patients are often uncooperative. Other effects of acute intoxication include vasodilatation, tachycardia, arrhythmias, vomiting, reduced lower oesophageal sphincter pressure, gastric irritation, delayed gastric emptying, hypoglycaemia (typically 6–36 h after ingestion, especially in a starved or malnourished individual), metabolic acidosis, dehydration (has a diuretic effect), coma and convulsions. Intoxication occurs at blood levels ~100–150 mg/dl (22–33 mmol/l), loss of muscle coordination at ~150–200 mg/dl (33–43 mmol/l), decreased level of consciousness at ~200–300 mg/dl (43–65 mmol/l), and death at ~300–500 mg/dl (65–109 mmol/l). The fatal adult dose is about 300–500 ml absolute alcohol (500–1200 ml strong spirits) within 1 h.

  Management is mainly supportive as for poisoning and overdoses. A traditional emergency department remedy consists of naloxone and glucose but is not generally recommended. Haemodialysis has been used in severe poisoning. Features of alcoholism require attention if present.
- methanol: toxic effects result from formaldehyde (converted to carbon monoxide) and formic acid, produced by hepatic metabolism of methanol. Features occur after 8–36 h and include intoxication, vomiting, abdominal pain, coma, visual disturbances, severe metabolic acidosis with a large anion gap and osmolar gap, and hyperglycaemia. About 10 ml pure methanol may result in permanent blindness, with the fatal adult dose around 30 ml (methylated spirits contains 5% methanol and 95% ethanol, the latter causing the most toxicity). Blood levels greater than 500 mg/ml (15 mmol/l) indicate severe poisoning.

  Management includes gastric lavage if within 2 h of ingestion, administration of bicarbonate, inhibition of further methanol metabolism with ethanol (50 g orally/iv followed by 10–20 g/h iv to produce blood levels of 100–200 g/dl (20–30 mmol/l)). More recently, fomepizole has gained acceptance as an alternative to alcohol and may reduce the need for haemodialysis, which may still be required in severe cases. Folic acid or its metabolites have also been used (utilised in formate metabolism). Haemodialysis has been used in severe poisoning.
- isopropanol: effects are caused by the alcohol itself, not its metabolites. Effects are similar to those of ethanol but longer lasting. Gastritis, renal tubular acidosis, myopathy and haemolysis may occur.

  Management is with gastric lavage if within 2 h of ingestion and supportive thereafter.
- ethylene glycol: toxic effects result from glycoaldehyde, glycolate and oxalate, produced by metabolism of the parent compound. Glycoaldehyde causes cerebral impairment, glycolate and oxalate produce severe metabolic acidosis (oxalate may also cause renal damage). The fatal adult dose is ~100 g although patients have survived much larger doses. Features include intoxication, vomiting, haematemesis, coma, convulsions, depressed reflexes, myoclonus, nystagmus, papilloedema and ophthalmoplegia within the first 12 h; tachycardia, hypertension, pulmonary oedema and cardiac failure within the next 12 h; and renal failure over the subsequent 2–3 days. Investigations may reveal severe lactic acidosis, a large anion gap and osmolar gap, hypocalcaemia and hyperkalaemia. Blood levels exceeding ~200 mg/l (~35 mmol/l) indicate severe poisoning.

  Management includes haemodialysis, ethanol and fomepizole as for methanol; thiamine and pyridoxine have also been used.

Alcohol withdrawal. May be precipitated by acute illness or surgery, even if regular intake of alcohol (ethanol) is apparently not excessive and without the other features of alcoholism. Includes:

- tremulousness, agitation, nausea, vomiting: usually within 6–8 h of abstinence. The most common features seen.
- hallucinations: usually visual; occur 10–30 h after abstinence and in under 10% of cases.
- convulsions: occur up to 48 h after abstinence and in about 5% of cases.
- delirium tremens: includes the above symptoms plus confusion, disorientation, sweating, tachycardia and hypertension. Occurs up to 2–3 days after abstinence and in about 5% of cases.

Management includes reassurance although sedative drugs, e.g. benzodiazepines, carbamazepine, clomethiaziole, may be required. More recently, clonidine has been used successfully to smooth withdrawal. Vitamin B_6 supplements are usually administered, but if there is a risk of encephalopathy a mixture of vitamins is best prescribed.

Kosten TR, O'Connor PG (2003). N Engl J Med; 348: 1786–95

Alcoholism. Form of substance abuse in which there is narrowing of the drinking repertoire (loss of day-to-day variation in drinking habits), increased tolerance to alcohol (ethanol), symptoms of alcohol withdrawal when intake is stopped, a craving for alcohol and drinking in the early part of the day/middle of the night. May precipitate admission to hospital as a consequence of acute alcohol poisoning or intoxication, or impaired organ function resulting from chronic abuse; may also complicate the management of incidental disease or surgery.

- Effects of chronic alcohol intake:
  - cerebral/cerebellar degeneration, peripheral neuropathy, psychiatric disturbances (Wernicke's encephalopathy, Korsakoff's psychosis).
  - withdrawal may lead to tremor, anxiety, hallucinations, convulsions, delirium tremens.
  - gastritis, peptic ulcer disease, oesophageal varices; may lead to gastrointestinal haemorrhage.
  - pancreatitis.
  - fatty liver, hepatic enzyme induction, cirrhosis causing hepatic failure, coagulopathy.
  - malnutrition, immunodeficiency.
  - myopathy, cardiomyopathy.

[Karl Wernicke (1848–1904), German neurologist; Sergei Korsakoff (1853–1900), Russian neurologist and psychologist]

Alcohols. Group of aliphatic (i.e. non-cyclic) organic chemicals containing one or more hydroxyl (–OH) groups and which form esters (containing the –O–O– linkage) with acids. Used as solvents and cleaning agents. Those of particular medical/anaesthetic relevance include:

- ethanol (ethyl alcohol; C_2H_5OH): commonly referred to as 'alcohol'; widely drunk throughout the world and often abused resulting in acute toxicity or alcoholism. Used in the past as an anaesthetic agent and as a tocolytic drug. May be added to irrigant solution to monitor the latter's uptake during TURP. Also used for destructive injection, e.g. into neural tissue in chronic pain management. In the ICU, iv alcohol may be used to treat methanol poisoning; it may also be useful for sedating alcoholics (1–10 g/h of a 5–10% solution).

  Metabolised mostly to acetaldehyde, then acetate, acetylcoenzyme A and finally CO_2 and water via the tricarboxylic acid cycle. 5% is excreted unchanged, mostly in the urine but also in the breath. The rate of metabolism is 10 ml/h at concentrations above 100 mg/dl (22 mmol/l); below this level it is subject to first order kinetics with a half-life of about 1 h (*see Michaelis–Menten kinetics*). Produces 30 kJ/g (7 Cal/g); it has been used as an iv energy source.
- methanol (methyl alcohol; CH_3OH): derived from distillation of wood or from coal or natural gas. Used in the petroleum and paint industries. Contained with ethanol in methylated spirits. Extremely toxic if ingested.
- isopropanol (isopropyl alcohol; $(CH_3)_2CHOH$): used as a solvent and to clean the skin before invasive procedures. Oxidised in the liver to acetone.
- ethylene glycol (glycol; $(CH_2OH)_2$): used as an antifreeze.
- propylene glycol ($CH_3.CHOH.CH_2OH$): used as a solvent in drugs, e.g. etomidate, GTN.

All are CNS depressants, rapidly absorbed from the upper GIT (also by inhalation and, to varying degrees, percutaneously) and metabolised by hepatic alcohol dehydrogenase to the aldehyde; all except isopropanol are metabolised further to the corresponding acid by aldehyde dehydrogenase.

See also, Alcohol poisoning; Alcohol withdrawal

Alcuronium chloride. Non-depolarising neuromuscular blocking drug, introduced in 1961 and withdrawn in the UK in 1994. Caused mild histamine release and hypotension, but anaphylaxis, when it occurred, was often severe.

Aldosterone. Mineralocorticoid hormone secreted by the cortex of the adrenal gland in response to reduced renal blood flow (via renin/angiotensin system), trauma and anxiety (via ACTH release), and hyperkalaemia and hyponatraemia (direct effect on the adrenal cortex). Increases sodium reabsorption from urine, sweat and saliva. Acts on the sodium/potassium pump via intracellular messenger RNA production. Renal effects are in the distal tubule and collecting ducts: sodium and water are retained, with potassium and hydrogen ions lost in exchange for sodium ions.

Hyperaldosteronism results in hypertension and hypokalaemia. In cardiac failure and cirrhosis, aldosterone levels may be raised, although the mechanism is unclear.

Aldosterone antagonists, e.g. spironolactone, potassium canrenoate and eplerenone, cause sodium loss and potassium retention.

ALERT, *see Acute life-threatening events – recognition and treatment*

Alfentanil hydrochloride. Opioid analgesic drug derived from fentanyl, with 10–20% of the latter's potency. Developed in 1976. Has faster onset of action than fentanyl (within 1 minute) because it is mostly (90%) unionized at body pH. Although its clearance is only 50% that of fentanyl, it has a shorter duration of action because of its lower volume of distribution. Has minimal cardiovascular effects, although bradycardia and hypotension may occur. Other effects are similar to those of fentanyl. Metabolised in the liver to noralfentanil.

- Dosage:
  - for spontaneously breathing patients, up to 500 µg initially, followed by increments of 250 µg. Slow injection reduces the incidence of apnoea.
  - 30–50 µg/kg to obtund the hypertensive response to tracheal intubation. Up to 125 µg/kg is used in cardiac surgery.
  - for infusion, a loading dose of 50–100 µg/kg, followed by 0.5–1 µg/kg/min. Higher rates have been used in TIVA. The infusion is discontinued 10–30 min before surgery ends. Also used for sedation in ICU at 30–60 µg/kg/h initially.

Alimemazine tartrate (Trimeprazine). Phenothiazine-derived antihistamine drug, used for premedication in children. More sedative than other antihistamines. Has antiemetic properties.

- Dosage: up to 2 mg/kg orally 1–2 h preoperatively.
- Side effects include dry mouth, circumoral pallor and dizziness. May cause postoperative restlessness due to antanalgesia. Has been implicated in causing prolonged respiratory depression on rare occasions.

Aliskiren, *see Renin/angiotensin system*

Alkalaemia. Arterial pH > 7.45 or H^+ concentration < 35 nmol/l.
See also, Acid–base balance; Alkalosis

Alkalosis. A process in which arterial pH > 7.45 (or H^+ concentration < 35 nmol/l), or would be > 7.45 if there were no compensatory mechanisms of acid–base balance.
See also, Alkalosis, metabolic; Alkalosis, respiratory

Alkalosis, metabolic. Inappropriately high pH for the measured arterial $P\text{CO}_2$.

- Caused by:
  - acid loss, e.g. vomiting, nasogastric aspiration.
  - base ingestion:
    - bicarbonate (usually iatrogenic).
    - citrate from blood transfusion.
    - milk-alkali syndrome.
    - forced alkaline diuresis.
  - potassium/chloride depletion leading to acid urine production.
- Primary change: increased bicarbonate/decreased hydrogen ion.
- Compensation:
  - hypoventilation: reaches its maximum within 24 h, usually with an upper limit for arterial $P\text{CO}_2$ of 7–8 kPa (50–60 mmHg). Initial increase in HCO_3^- is about 0.76 mmol/l per kPa change in arterial $P\text{CO}_2$ above 5.3 kPa (1 mmol/l per 10 mmHg above 40) although the level of compensatory change is less predictable than in metabolic acidosis.
  - decreased renal acid secretion.
- Effects:
  - confusion.
  - paraesthesia/tetany (reduced free ionised calcium concentration due to altered protein-binding).
- Treatment:
  - correction of ECF and potassium depletion.
  - rarely, acid therapy, e.g. ammonium chloride or hydrochloric acid: deficit = base excess × body weight (kg) mmol.

See also, Acid–base balance

Alkalosis, respiratory. Alkalosis due to decreased arterial $P\text{CO}_2$. Caused by alveolar hyperventilation, e.g. fear, pain, hypoxia, or during IPPV.

- Primary change: decreased arterial $P\text{CO}_2$.
- Compensation:
  - initial fall in plasma bicarbonate due to decreased carbonic acid formation and dissociation.
  - decreased acid secretion/increased bicarbonate excretion by the kidneys.

    In acute hypocapnia, bicarbonate concentration falls by about 1.3 mmol/l per 1 kPa fall in arterial $P\text{CO}_2$. In chronic hypocapnia the fall per 1 kPa is 4.0 mmol/l.
- Effects: those of hypocapnia.
- Treatment: of underlying cause.

See also, Acid–base balance

Alkylating drugs, *see Cytotoxic drugs*

Allen's test. Originally described for assessing arterial flow to the hand in thromboangiitis obliterans. Modified for assessment of ulnar artery flow prior to radial arterial cannulation. The ulnar and radial arteries are compressed at the wrist, and the patient asked to clench tightly and open the hand, causing blanching. Pressure over the ulnar artery is released; the colour of the palm normally takes less than 5–10 s to return to normal, with over 15 s considered abnormal. A similar manoeuvre may be performed with the radial artery before ulnar artery cannulation. Although widely performed, it is inaccurate in predicting risk from ischaemic damage.
[Edgar Van Nuys Allen (1900–1961), US physician]

Allergic reactions, *see Adverse drug reactions*

Allodynia. Pain from a stimulus that is not normally painful.

Alpha-adrenergic . . ., *see α-Adrenergic . . .*

Alprostadil. Prostaglandin E_1, used to maintain patency of a patent ductus arteriosus in neonates with congenital heart disease in whom the ductus is vital for survival, e.g. pulmonary atresia/stenosis, Fallot's tetralogy, coarctation, transposition of the great arteries.

- Dosage: 50–100 ng/kg/min initially via the umbilical artery or iv, reduced to the lowest effective dose.
- Side effects include apnoea, brady- or tachycardia, hypotension, pyrexia, diarrhoea, convulsions, DIC, hypokalaemia. Undiluted preparation reacts with plastic containers so care in preparation is required.

ALS, *see Advanced Cardiac Life Support; Advanced life support, adult; Advanced Life Support in Obstetrics; Advanced Paediatric Life Support; Advanced Trauma Life Support; Neonatal Resuscitation Programme*

ALSO, *see Advanced Life Support in Obstetrics*

Alteplase (rt-PA, tissue-type plasminogen activator). Fibrinolytic drug, used in acute management of MI and PE and being investigated for use in acute ischaemic stroke. Becomes active when it binds to fibrin, converting plasminogen to plasmin which dissolves the fibrin. Thought to be non-immunogenic.

- Dosage:
  - within 6 h of MI: 15 mg iv followed by 50 mg/30 min, then 35 mg/60 min.
  - within 6–12 h of MI: 10 mg then 50 mg/60 min, then 40 mg/2 h.
  - PE: 10 mg followed by 90 mg/2 h.
  - acute stroke (within 3 h): 0.9 mg/kg (up to 90 mg); 10% by iv injection, the remainder by infusion.

Maximum dose: 1.5 mg/kg if under 65 kg body weight.

- Side effects: as for fibrinolytic drugs.

Althesin. IV anaesthetic agent introduced in 1971, composed of two corticosteroids, alphaxalone 9 mg/ml and alphadolone 3 mg/ml. Withdrawn in 1984 because of a high incidence of adverse drug reactions, mostly minor but occasionally severe. These were thought to be due to Cremophor EL, the solubilising agent. Previously widely used because of its rapid onset and short duration of action; still used in veterinary practice.

Altitude, high. Problems include:

- lack of O_2: e.g. atmospheric pressure at 18 000 ft (5486 m) is half that at sea level. $F_{I}O_2$ is constant, but $P\text{O}_2$ is lowered. This effect is offset initially by the shape of the oxyhaemoglobin dissociation curve, which maintains haemoglobin saturation above 90% up to 10 000 ft. Compensatory changes due to hypoxia include hyperventilation, increased erythropoietin secretion resulting in polycythaemia, increased 2, 3-DPG, proliferation of peripheral capillaries, and alterations in intracellular

oxidative enzymes. Alkalaemia is reduced after a few days, via increased renal bicarbonate loss. CSF pH is returned towards normal. Pulmonary vasoconstriction may result in right heart strain. High altitude illness is thought to be related to acute hypoxia and alkalosis; it consists of headache, malaise, nausea, diarrhoea, and may lead to pulmonary or cerebral oedema.
- low temperatures, e.g. ambient temperature is −20°C at 18 000 ft.
- expansion of gas-containing cavities, e.g. inner ear.
- decompression sickness.
- anaesthetic apparatus at high altitude:
  - vaporisers: SVP is unaffected by atmospheric pressure, thus the partial pressure of volatile agent in the vaporiser is the same as at sea level. Because atmospheric pressure is reduced, the delivered concentration is increased from that marked on the dial, but since anaesthetic action depends on alveolar partial pressure, not concentration, the same settings may be used as at sea level. However, reduced temperature may alter vaporisation.
  - flowmeters: since atmospheric pressure is reduced, a given amount of gas occupies a greater volume than at sea level; i.e. has reduced density. Thus a greater volume is required to pass through a Rotameter flowmeter to maintain the bobbin at a certain height, because it is the number of gas molecules hitting the bobbin that support it. The flowmeters therefore under-read at high altitudes. However, since the clinical effects depend on the number of molecules, not volume of gas, the flowmeters may be used as normal.

Basnyat B, Murdoch DR (2003). Lancet; 361: 1967–74

Altitude, low. Problems are related to high pressure:
- those of hyperbaric O_2 (*see Oxygen, hyperbaric*).
- inert gas narcosis.
- neurological impairment, e.g. tremor, disorientation.
- pressure reversal of anaesthesia.
- effects on equipment:
  - implosion of glass ampoules, etc.
  - deflation of air-filled tracheal tube cuffs, etc.
  - functioning of vaporisers and flowmeters is normal as above.

Alveolar air equation. In its simplified form:

$$\text{alveolar } P\text{O}_2 = F_I\text{O}_2(P_\text{B} - P_\text{A}\text{H}_2\text{O}) - \frac{P_\text{A}\text{CO}_2}{R}$$

$$\text{or } P_I\text{O}_2 - \frac{P_\text{A}\text{CO}_2}{R}$$

where P_B = ambient barometric pressure.
P_AH_2O = alveolar partial pressure of water (normally 6.3 kPa (47 mmHg)).
P_ACO_2 = alveolar PCO_2; approximately equals arterial PCO_2.
R = respiratory exchange ratio, normally 0.8.
P_IO_2 = inspired PO_2.

Useful for estimating alveolar PO_2, e.g. when determining alveolar–arterial O_2 difference, shunt fractions, etc. The equation also illustrates how hypercapnia may lower P_AO_2. Another form of the equation allows for differences between inspired and expired gas volumes, and is unaffected by inert gas exchange:

$$\text{alveolar } P\text{O}_2 = P_I\text{O}_2 - P_\text{A}\text{CO}_2 - \left(\frac{P_I\text{O}_2 - P_\text{E}\text{O}_2}{P_\text{E}\text{CO}_2}\right)$$

where P_EO_2 = mixed expired PO_2
P_ECO_2 = mixed expired PCO_2

Alveolar–arterial oxygen difference (A–ado_2). Alveolar PO_2 minus arterial PO_2. Useful as a measure of $\dot{V}/\dot{Q}$ mismatch and shunt. Alveolar PO_2 is estimated using the alveolar air equation; arterial PO_2 is measured directly. The small shunt and $\dot{V}/\dot{Q}$ mismatch in normal subjects results in a normal A–ado_2 of less than 2.0 kPa (15 mmHg) breathing air; this may reach 4.0 kPa (30 mmHg) in the elderly. It increases when breathing high O_2 concentrations because the shunt component is not corrected; i.e. normally up to 15 kPa (115 mmHg) breathing 100% O_2.

Alveolar gases. Normal alveolar gas partial pressures and intravascular gas tensions are shown in Table 3. End-tidal gas approximates to alveolar gas in normal subjects and may be monitored, e.g. during anaesthesia.
See also, End-tidal gas sampling

Alveolar gas transfer. Depends on:
- alveolar ventilation.
- diffusion across alveolar membrane, fluid interface and capillary endothelium (normally less than 0.5 μm).
- solubility of gases in blood.
- cardiac output.

For gases transferred from the bloodstream to the alveolus, e.g. CO_2, and anaesthetic vapours during recovery, the same factors apply, but in reverse order.

With normal cardiac output, blood cells take about 0.75 s to pass through pulmonary capillaries. O_2 transfer is usually complete within 0.25 s; part of the time is taken for the reaction with haemoglobin. CO_2 diffuses 20 times more quickly through tissue layers; transfer is also complete within 0.25 s. Transfer of highly soluble gases, e.g. carbon monoxide, is limited by diffusion between alveolus and capillary, since large volumes can be taken up by the blood once they reach it. Transfer of insoluble gases, e.g. N_2O, is limited by blood flow from alveoli, since capillary blood is rapidly saturated.
See also, Carbon dioxide transport; Diffusing capacity; Oxygen transport

Alveolar hypoventilation syndrome, *see Obesity hypoventilation syndrome*

Alveolar ventilation. Volume of gas entering the alveoli per minute; normally about 4–4.5 l/min. Equals (tidal volume minus dead space) × respiratory rate; thus rapid small breaths result in a much smaller alveolar ventilation than slow deep breaths, even though minute ventilation remains constant. In the upright position, apical alveoli receive less ventilation than basal ones, because the former are already expanded by gravity and are thus less able to expand further on inspiration. Since all the exhaled CO_2 comes from the alveoli, the amount exhaled in a minute equals alveolar ventilation × alveolar concentration of CO_2. Thus alveolar (and hence arterial) CO_2 concentration is inversely proportional to alveolar ventilation, at any fixed rate of CO_2 production.
See also, Ventilation/perfusion mismatch

Table 3 Normal respiratory gas partial pressures and tensions in kPa (mmHg)

	Inspired	Alveolar	Arterial	Venous	Expired
O_2	21 (160)	14 (106)	13.3 (100)	5.3 (40)	15 (105)
CO_2	0.03 (0.2)	5.3 (40)	5.3 (40)	6.1 (46)	4 (30)
Nitrogen	80 (600)	74 (560)	74 (560)	74 (560)	75 (570)
H_2O	Variable	6.3 (47)	6.3 (47)	6.3 (47)	6.3 (47)

Alveolitis. Generalised inflammation of lung parenchyma. Classified into:

- cryptogenic fibrosing alveolitis: cause is unknown, therefore a disease of exclusion. Characterised by differing amounts of inflammation and fibrosis of the pulmonary air spaces and interstitium. Most common at 50–60 years and in smokers. Possible, but unproven, triggers include viral infection and exposure to metal dusts or wood fires. Has an aggressive course with 50% mortality at 5 years, despite therapy.

  Symptoms include progressive dyspnoea without wheeze, dry cough, weight loss and lethargy. Clubbing occurs in 70–80%. Most striking signs are the very distinctive, fine, end-expiratory crepitations heard at the lung bases and mid-axillary lines. Progresses to central cyanosis, pulmonary hypertension, cor pulmonale and a restrictive pattern of pulmonary impairment as for pulmonary fibrosis. Chest X-ray may reveal small lung fields with reticulonodular shadowing at lung peripheries and bases. CT scanning, radioisotope scanning and lung biopsy may help with the diagnosis.

  There is no specific treatment, although corticosteroids and cyclophosphamide or azathioprine may be used. Ciclosporin has theoretical benefits. Lung transplantation may be possible.
- extrinsic allergic alveolitis (hypersensitivity pneumonitis): causative agents include aspergillus (farmer's lung, malt-worker's lung), pituitary extracts (pituitary snuff taker's lung), avian proteins (bird-fancier's lung), etc. May be:
  - acute: requires initial sensitisation to an antigen. Subsequent exposure results in repeated episodes of dyspnoea, cough, malaise, fever, chills, aches and lethargy. Wheezing is uncommon. Severity depends on the dose of antigen; in very severe cases, life-threatening respiratory failure occurs. Recovery is accelerated by corticosteroids.
  - chronic: less dramatic onset, with a slow increase in dyspnoea with minimal other systemic upset and no acute episodes. May cause cor pulmonale.

  Chest X-ray may be normal, but widespread ground-glass appearance in mid- and lower zones is common. Lung function is as above although it may be normal between acute attacks. Other investigations and treatment as above.
- drug-induced alveolitis: patients may present with acute cough, fever and dyspnoea or with slowly progressive dyspnoea. Causal agents include: O_2, nitrofurantoin, paraquat, amiodarone and cytotoxic drugs.
- others: include physical agents (e.g. radiation), connective tissue diseases.

All forms may lead to pulmonary fibrosis, which may also occur without generalised alveolitis, e.g. following local disease or aspiration of irritant substances.

Alveolus. Terminal part of the respiratory tree; the site of gas exchange. About 3×10^8 exist in both lungs, with estimated total surface area 70–80 m^2. Their walls are comprised of a capillary meshwork covered in cytoplasmic extensions of type I pneumocytes. Traditionally thought to conform to the bubble model; i.e. spherical in structure with a thin water lining, with surfactant molecules preventing collapse. Electron microscopy, and experimental and mathematical models, have led to alternative theories, e.g. pooling of water at septal corners with dry areas of surfactant in between, and surface tension helping return water to interstitial fluid.

Amantadine hydrochloride. Drug with both antiparkinsonian and antiviral effects. In Parkinson's disease, it improves tremor, rigidity and mild dyskinesia, but only in a small percentage of sufferers. Has been used for the treatment of herpes zoster infections, both during the acute phase and in the treatment of postherpetic pain. May also be used for prophylaxis of influenza A in very selective groups (e.g. unimmunised patients, healthcare workers during an epidemic).

- Dosage:
  - parkinsonism: 100 mg orally, once daily (doubled after 1 week).
  - herpes zoster: 100 mg twice daily for 14 days.
  - influenza A: 100 mg/day for 4–5 days as treatment, 100 mg/day for 6 weeks as prophylaxis.
- Side effects: nausea, dizziness, convulsions, hallucinations, GIT disturbance.

Ambu-bag, *see Self-inflating bags*

Ambu-E valve, *see Non-rebreathing valves*

American Board of Anesthesiology (ABA). Recognised as an independent Board by the American Board of Medical Specialties in 1941, having been an affiliate of the American Board of Surgery since 1938. Issues the Diploma of the ABA.

American Society of Anesthesiologists (ASA). Formed from the American Society of Anesthetists in 1945, to distinguish 'anesthesiologists' from 'anesthetists'. The American Society of Anesthetists had been formed in 1936 from the New York Society of Anesthetists, which until 1911 had been the Long Island Society of Anesthetists, founded in 1905. The ASA is concerned with improving the standards, education and audit of anaesthesia, and publishes the journal *Anesthesiology*.

Amethocaine, *see Tetracaine*

Amfetamine poisoning. Overdosage of amfetamines may cause nervousness, hyperactivity, tachycardia, hypertension, hallucinations and hyperthermia. Intracranial haemorrhage may accompany acute severe hypertension. The toxic dose is not well defined as there is a wide variation in response related to tolerance in chronic abusers. Diagnosis is made on the history and clinical grounds, supported by qualitative laboratory analysis (plasma levels are unhelpful in guiding management). Patients should have continuous ECG and core temperature monitoring, and urine analysed for myoglobin. Treatment includes general supportive care as for poisoning and overdoses, and the use of chlorpromazine and β-adrenergic receptor antagonists (although β_2-receptor mediated vasoconstriction in skeletal muscle vessels may increase BP). Forced acid diuresis increases excretion but this should not be undertaken if there is associated rhabdomyolysis.

Amfetamines (Amphetamines). Group of drugs related to adrenaline, causing stimulation of the central and sympathetic nervous systems. Commonly abused, they cause addiction and are controlled drugs. Used in narcolepsy. May increase MAC of inhalational anaesthetic agents.
See also, Amfetamine poisoning

Amikacin. Antibacterial drug; an aminoglycoside with bactericidal activity against some Gram-positive and many Gram-negative organisms including pseudomonas. Indicated for the treatment of serious infections caused by Gram-negative bacilli resistant to gentamicin. Not absorbed from the GIT, it must be given parenterally. Excreted via the kidney.

- Dosage: 7.5 mg/kg im or slowly iv, 12 hourly (8 hourly in severe infection) up to 15 g over 10 days. One hour (peak) concentration should not exceed 30 mg/l and pre-dose (trough) level should be less than 10 mg/l.
- Side effects: as for gentamicin.

Amino acids. Organic acid components of proteins; they produce polypeptide chains by forming peptide bonds between the amino group of one and the carboxyl group of another, with the elimination of water.

Amino acids from the breakdown of ingested and endogenous proteins form an amino acid pool from which new proteins are synthesised. Amino acids are involved in carbohydrate and fat metabolism; amino groups may be removed or transferred to other molecules (deamination and transamination respectively). Deamination results in the liberation of ammonia, which may be excreted as urea, or taken up by other amino acids to form amides.

Eight dietary amino acids are essential for life in humans: valine, leucine, isoleucine, threonine, methionine, phenylalanine, tryptophan and lysine. Arginine and histidine are required for normal growth. Other amino acids may be synthesised from carbohydrate and fat breakdown products.

Glutamine, the most abundant amino acid in the body, appears to have a key role in muscle synthesis and immune function, as a neurotransmitter and as a major metabolic fuel for the enterocytes. Inclusion of glutamate in enteral feeds appears to reduce gut permeability and prevents the mucosal atrophy that occurs when food is not given by the enteral route.

Synthetic crystalline amino acid solutions (containing the *l*-isomers) are used as a nitrogen source during TPN. The composition of solutions varies considerably by manufacturer, although all provide the essential, and most of the non-essential, amino acids. Enteral feed solutions also include a mixture of amino acids.

See also, Nitrogen balance

γ-Aminobutyric acid (GABA). Inhibitory neurotransmitter found in many parts of the CNS. Binds to specific GABA receptors, causing opening of chloride channels and chloride entry into cells. The GABA receptor complex is closely associated with receptor sites for picrotoxin, which closes the chloride channels, and benzodiazepines, which augment the opening induced by GABA. Many anticonvulsant drugs facilitate the action of GABA, suggesting its role in the regulation of central activity and epilepsy. GABA may also be involved in presynaptic inhibition at many central synapses. The significance of a second GABA receptor, activation of which increases potassium conductance, is uncertain.

GABA receptors have received recent attention as a possible site of action of anaesthetic agents. The type A ($GABA_A$) receptor, a pentameric collection of glycoprotein subunits, responds to low concentrations of anaesthetics by potentiating the effect of GABA at the receptor whereas high concentrations directly activate the receptor. It appears that different anaesthetic agents interact with different subunits of the receptor (e.g. etomidate binds with the β subunit).

Aminoglycosides. Group of bactericidal antibacterial drugs. Includes amikacin, gentamicin, kanamycin, neomycin, netilmicin, streptomycin and tobramycin.

Active against some Gram-positive and many Gram-negative organisms. Amikacin, gentamicin and tobramycin are also active against pseudomonas.

Not absorbed from the GIT; must be given parenterally. Excretion is via the kidney and delayed in renal impairment. Side effects include ototoxicity (especially with concurrent furosemide therapy) and nephrotoxicity. In pregnancy, they may cross the placenta and cause fetal ototoxicity. They may also impair neuromuscular function and therefore avoidance has been suggested in myasthenia gravis. Monitoring of plasma levels should ideally be performed in all cases but is especially important in the elderly, children, those with renal impairment, the obese, and if high dosage or prolonged treatment is used. Monitored using 1 h (peak) and pre-dose (trough) samples.

2-Amino-2-hydroxymethyl-1,3-propanediol (THAM). Buffer solution which acts both intra- and extracellularly. Acts by consuming (rather than producing) CO_2 via the following reaction:

$$(CH_2OH)_3C{-}H_2 + HA \rightleftharpoons (CH_2OH)_3C{-}NH^{3+} + A^-$$

Has been used in the control of metabolic acidosis (e.g. post cardiac arrest) or increased ICP, but is not currently recommended for clinical practice.

Holmdahl M, Wicklund L, Wetterburg T, et al (2000). Acta Anaesthesiol Scand; 44: 524–7

Aminophylline. Phosphodiesterase inhibitor, a mixture of theophylline and ethylenediamine. Much more soluble than theophylline alone, hence its use iv. Used as a bronchodilator drug (but not as first line therapy), and as an inotropic drug especially in paediatrics.

Causes bronchodilatation, increased diaphragmatic contractility, vasodilatation, increased cardiac output (direct effect on the heart), diuresis (direct effect on the kidney), and CNS stimulation.

- Dosage:
  - 100–500 mg 6–12 hourly, orally (depending on the preparation), usually as slow-release preparations. Rectal preparations are no longer used, as they were associated with proctitis and unpredictable response.
  - for emergency iv use, injection of 5–7 mg/kg over 30 min may be followed by an infusion of 0.5 mg/kg/h (up to 1 mg/kg/h in smokers), with ECG monitoring. Dosage should be reduced in cardiac and hepatic failure, and during therapy with cimetidine, erythromycin and ciprofloxacin. Phenytoin, carbamazepine and other enzyme inducers may decrease its half-life.
- Side effects: arrhythmias, agitation and convulsions, GIT disturbances.

Care should be taken when patients already on oral treatment are given iv aminophylline, since the drug has a low therapeutic ratio. Plasma levels should be measured; therapeutic range is 10–20 mg/l.

Aminopyridine. Originally 4-aminopyridine, a drug previously used to reverse non-depolarising neuromuscular blockade, and to treat myasthenic syndrome. Does not inhibit acetylcholinesterase, but acts presynaptically to increase acetylcholine release, thereby increasing the force of muscle contraction. It also enters the brain and may cause convulsions. Replaced by 3,4-diaminopyridine, which does not cross the blood–brain barrier.

Amiodarone hydrochloride. Class III antiarrhythmic drug, used for treating supraventricular and ventricular arrhythmias. Acts by prolonging the cardiac action potential and refractory period. Causes minimal myocardial depression. Half-life is over 4 weeks. Acts rapidly following iv administration.

- Dosage:
  - 200 mg orally, thrice daily for 1 week, reducing to twice daily then once daily for maintenance.
  - as an iv infusion: 5 mg/kg over 20–120 min followed by up to 1.2 g/24 h, with ECG monitoring. Bradycardia may occur. May cause inflammation of peripheral veins. The dose should be reduced after 1–2 days.
- Side effects: prolonged administration commonly results in corneal microdeposits (reversible, and rarely affecting vision), and may cause photosensitivity, peripheral neuropathy, hyper- or hypothyroidism, hepatitis and pulmonary fibrosis.

Amitriptyline hydrochloride. Tricyclic antidepressant drug, used in endogenous depression. Has marked sedative effects and thus well suited for patients with agitated depression. Also used in chronic neuropathic pain management, especially when pain prevents sleeping at night. Antidepressant and analgesic effects become apparent after 2–4 weeks' treatment.

- Dosage:
  - depression: 75 mg orally/day (less in the elderly), in divided doses or as a single dose at night, increased up to 150–200 mg/day.
  - pain: 25–75 mg at night.
- Side effects: muscarinic effects include arrhythmias, heart block, dry mouth, urinary retention, blurred vision, constipation; hypersensitivity, blood dyscrasias, hepatic impairment, confusion and convulsions may also occur. Should be avoided in cardiovascular disease.

See also, Tricyclic antidepressant drug poisoning

Ammonia (NH_3). Colourless pungent-smelling gas, highly soluble in water. Toxic to all human cells. Produced in the GIT by the action of enteric organisms on dietary proteins and amino acids, and detoxified by transformation in the liver into urea. Normal blood level is 100–200 mg/l; levels rise in the presence of severe liver disease or a portal–systemic blood shunt. Ammonia intoxication causes tremor, slurred speech, blurred vision and coma. There is a loose association between blood ammonia level and the degree of hepatic encephalopathy in hepatic failure. Rare genetic disorders of the urea cycle (e.g. ornithine carbamoyltransferase deficiency) lead to hyperammonaemia; similarly, treatment with sodium valproate may result in raised ammonia levels due to interference with the urea cycle.

Ammonia is also produced in the proximal tubule of the kidney from the breakdown of glutamine. It combines intracellularly with H^+ to form the ammonium ion (NH^{4+}) which is secreted by the proximal tubule cells into the tubular filtrate, thereby facilitating regulation of acid–base balance and cation conservation. Ammonia formed from the dissociation of NH^{4+} is reabsorbed, recycled and resecreted, primarily by the collecting tubule.

See also, Nitrogen balance

Amnesia. Impairment of memory. May occur with intracranial pathology, dementia, metabolic disturbances, alcoholism and psychological disturbances. May be caused by head injury and drugs. Patients who recover from critical illness may have poor recall of events afterwards.

Retrograde amnesia (between the causative agent/event and the last memory beforehand) is common after head injury. Anterograde amnesia (loss of memory for the period following the causative agent/event) may occur after head injury, and is common after administration of certain drugs, typically benzodiazepines and hyoscine. Awareness during anaesthesia, with amnesia preventing subsequent recall, may be more common than previously thought.

Amniotic fluid embolism. Condition traditionally said to be caused by entry of amniotic fluid and fetal cells into the maternal circulation, triggering an inflammatory response similar to an anaphylactoid reaction. Usually occurs during labour or delivery although it can present up to 48 h post-partum and also during Caesarean section. Said to be more common in multiparous, older women, and with forceful labour, although this has been questioned. Typical features include cyanosis, vomiting, drowsiness, convulsions and shock, with DIC and acute lung injury. The aetiology is unclear since fetal elements may be found in the circulation of apparently unaffected women and not all 'typical' clinical cases are confirmed pathologically or immunologically. Treatment is supportive. Although rare (~1–2:100 000 births), it carries a high mortality (traditionally quoted at 40–80%, although more recent series suggest a mortality of 15–20%), and thus remains a significant cause of maternal death.

Moore J, Baldisseri MR (2005). Crit Care Med; 33 (Suppl 10): S279–85

Amoebiasis, *see Tropical diseases*

Amoxicillin (Amoxycillin). Derivative of ampicillin, differing only by one hydroxyl group; has similar antibacterial activity but oral absorption is better and unaffected by food in the stomach. Enteral administration produces higher plasma and tissue levels than ampicillin. Combined with β-lactamase inhibitor clavulanic acid in co-amoxiclav.

- Dosage: 250–500 mg orally, 500 mg im or 500 mg–1 g iv, 8 hourly.
- Side effects: as for ampicillin.

Ampere. SI unit of current. Defined as the current flowing in two straight parallel wires of infinite length, 1 metre apart in a vacuum, which will produce a force of 2×10^{-7} newtons/metre length on each of the wires.

[Andre Ampère (1775–1836), French physicist]

Amphetamine poisoning, *see Amfetamine poisoning*

Amphetamines, *see Amfetamines*

Amphotericin (Amphotericin B). Polyene antifungal drug, active against most fungi and yeasts. Not absorbed enterally. Highly protein-bound, it penetrates tissues poorly. Administered orally as a treatment for intestinal candidiasis, or iv for systemic fungal infections. Amphotericin is available encapsulated in liposomes or as a complex with sodium cholesteryl sulphate, both of which reduce its toxicity.

- Dosage: 100–200 mg orally, 6 hourly. The iv dose (1–5 mg/kg/day) depends upon the formulation.
- Side effects: renal and hepatic impairment, nausea and vomiting, electrolyte disturbance especially hypokalaemia, arrhythmias, blood dyscrasias, convulsions, peripheral neuropathy, visual and hearing disturbances. A test dose is recommended before iv administration because of the risk of anaphylactic reaction.

Ampicillin. Broad-spectrum semisynthetic bactericidal penicillin. Active against many Gram-positive and negative organisms but ineffective against β-lactamase producing bacteria. Only moderately well absorbed orally (~50% of dose) and this is further diminished by food in the gut. Excreted into bile and urine.

- Dosage: 250 mg–1 g orally, 6 hourly; 500 mg iv or im, 4–6 hourly.
- Side effects: nausea, rash, diarrhoea.

Amrinone lactate. Phosphodiesterase inhibitor, used as an inotropic drug. Active iv and orally. Increases cardiac output and reduces SVR via inhibition of cardiac and vascular muscle phosphodiesterase. MAP and heart rate are unaltered. Half-life is 3–6 h. Not available in the UK. Milrinone, a more potent derivative, is less likely to cause side effects (e.g. GIT upset, thrombocytopenia).

Amylase. Group of enzymes secreted by salivary glands and the pancreas. Salivary amylase (an α-amylase – ptyalin) breaks down starch at an optimal pH of 6.7; consequently it is inactivated by gastric acid. In the small intestine, both salivary and pancreatic α-amylase act on ingested polysaccharides.

Plasma amylase measurements may be useful for the diagnosis of numerous conditions, particularly acute pancreatitis. About 35–40% of total plasma amylase activity is contributed by the pancreatic isoenzyme. Amylase levels > 5000 U/l are suggestive of acute pancreatitis (peak reached within 24–48 h); intra-abdominal emergencies (e.g. perforated peptic ulcer, mesenteric infarction) are usually associated with lower plasma levels.

See also, Carbohydrates

Anaemia. Reduced haemoglobin concentration; usually defined as less than 13 g/dl for males, 12 g/dl for females. In children, the figure varies; 18 g/dl (1–2 weeks of age); 11 g/dl (6 months–6 years); 12 g/dl (6–12 years).

- Caused by:
  - reduced production:
    - deficiency of iron, vitamin B_{12}, folate.
    - chronic disease, e.g. malignancy, infection.
    - endocrine disease, e.g. hypothyroidism, adrenocortical insufficiency.
    - bone marrow infiltration, e.g. leukaemia, myelofibrosis.
    - aplastic anaemia, including drug-induced, e.g. chloramphenicol.
    - reduced erythropoietin secretion, e.g. renal failure.
    - abnormal red cells/haemoglobin, e.g. sideroblastic anaemia, thalassaemia.
  - increased haemolysis.
  - haemorrhage:
    - acute.
    - chronic.
- Investigated by measuring the size and haemoglobin content of erythrocytes:
  - hypochromic, microcytic: e.g. thalassaemia, iron deficiency including chronic haemorrhage, chronic disease.
  - normochromic, macrocytic: vitamin B_{12} or folate deficiency, alcoholism.
  - normochromic, normocytic: chronic disease, e.g. infection, malignancy, renal failure, endocrine disease; aplastic anaemia, bone marrow disease or infiltration.

Other investigations include examination of blood film (e.g. for sickle cells, parasites, reticulocytes suggesting increased breakdown or haemorrhage, etc.), measurement of platelets and white cells, bone marrow aspiration and further blood tests, e.g. iron, vitamin B_{12}, etc.

- Effects:
  - reduced O_2 carrying capacity of blood: fatigue, dyspnoea on exertion, angina.
  - increased cardiac output, to maintain O_2 flux: palpitations, tachycardia, systolic murmurs, cardiac failure. Reduced viscosity increases flow but turbulence is more likely.
  - increased 2,3-DPG.
  - maintenance of blood volume by haemodilution.

Unexpected anaemia should be investigated before routine surgery. The traditional minimal 'safe' haemoglobin concentration for anaesthesia has been 10 g/dl, unless surgery is urgent; below this level, reduced O_2 carriage was felt to outweigh the advantage of reduced blood viscosity and increased flow. More recently, 7–10 g/dl has been suggested, reflecting the concerns over the complications of transfusion (except in ischaemic heart disease, in which postoperative mortality increases as preoperative haemoglobin concentration falls below around 10 g/dl). Reduction of cardiac output during anaesthesia is particularly hazardous. F_IO_2 of 0.5 is often advocated to reduce risk of perioperative hypoxia by increasing the O_2 reserve within the lungs.

In the ICU, recent evidence suggests that lowering the threshold for transfusion from 10 g/dl to 7 g/dl may decrease mortality, organ dysfunction and cardiac complications.

Transfused stored blood takes up to 24 h to reach its full O_2 carrying capacity; ideally transfusion should occur at least 1 day preoperatively. Slow transfusion also minimises the risk of fluid overload in chronic anaemia.

Anaerobic infection. Caused by:

- obligate anaerobes: only grow in the absence of O_2.
- microaerophilic organisms: only grow under conditions of reduced O_2 tension.
- facultative anaerobes: capable of growing aerobically or anaerobically.

The most important anaerobic bacteria include species of clostridium, bacteroides and actinomycoses. Predisposing factors for anaerobic infection include disruption of mucosal barriers, impaired blood supply, tissue injury and necrosis. Most infecting organisms are endogenous. Infections are accompanied by foul-smelling, putrid pus. Specimens for analysis of possible anaerobic infections may require special anaerobic transport systems as some anaerobic species die if exposed to O_2. Metronidazole is especially active against anaerobes.

Anaerobic threshold. Measure of overall cardiopulmonary capacity, obtained from cardiopulmonary exercise testing. Derived from the inflection point of the oxygen consumption/carbon dioxide production curve obtained during maximal exercise (Fig. 8), taking into account the respiratory exchange ratio. Represents the point at which respiration

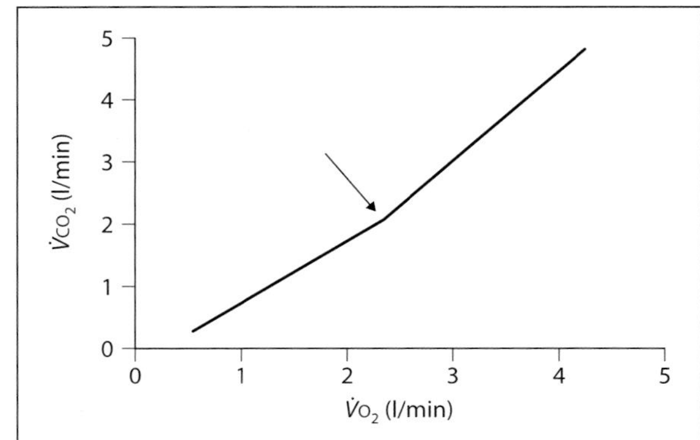

Fig. 8 Anaerobic threshold (arrowed)

switches from aerobic to anaerobic; i.e. more carbon dioxide is produced per oxygen molecule consumed. Has been used to predict outcome from major surgery, an anaerobic threshold of < 10–11 ml/kg/min indicating a greater risk of death, especially if associated with high risk surgery and/or ischaemic heart disease.

Wheeler AP, Bernard GR (2007). Lancet; 369: 1553–64

Anaesthesia. Official journal of the Association of Anaesthetists of Great Britain and Ireland, first published in 1946.

Anaesthesia (from Greek: an + aisthesis; without feeling). Term suggested by Oliver Wendell Holmes in 1846 to describe the state of sleep produced by ether; the word had been used previously to describe lack of feeling, e.g. due to peripheral neuropathy. He introduced derived words, e.g. 'anaesthetic agent'.

Anaesthesia and Intensive Care. Official journal of the Australian Society of Anaesthetists (formed in 1935) since its launch in 1972. Also the official journal of the Australian and New Zealand Intensive Care Society and the New Zealand Society of Anaesthetists.

Anaesthesia, balanced, *see Balanced anaesthesia*

Anaesthesia crisis resource management, *see Crisis resource management*

Anaesthesia, depth of. Anaesthesia is generally accepted as being a continuum in which increasing depth of anaesthesia results in loss of consciousness, recall, and somatic and autonomic reflexes. Some would argue that, whilst these are the effects of anaesthetic drugs in increasing dosage, 'anaesthesia' itself occurs at a particular undefined point, and is therefore either present or absent.

Assessment is important in order to avoid inadequate anaesthesia with awareness and troublesome reflexes, or overdose.

- Methods of assessment:
  - clinical:
    - stages of anaesthesia (*see Anaesthesia, stages of*).
    - signs of light anaesthesia:
      - lacrimation.
      - tachycardia.
      - hypertension.
      - sweating.
      - reactive dilated pupils.
      - movement, laryngospasm, etc.

      These signs may be altered by anaesthetic drugs themselves, and by others, e.g. opioids, atropine, neuromuscular blocking drugs.
    - isolated forearm technique.
  - EEG:
    - conventional EEG: bulky and difficult to interpret. Poor correlation between different anaesthetic agents.
    - cerebral function monitor and analysing monitor: easier to use and read, but less informative than conventional EEG.
    - power spectral analysis: graphic display of complicated data; easier to interpret than conventional EEG. Recently, monitors displaying derivations such as bispectral index or entropy (describing non-linear dynamics) have been introduced. These monitors display single numbers that are claimed to represent global activity and allow titration of anaesthesia in order to keep the value within defined limits and thus reduce both awareness and overdosage, although their place is controversial.
  - evoked potentials: similar effects are produced by different anaesthetic agents.
  - oesophageal contractility: affected by smooth muscle relaxants and ganglion blocking drugs, also by disease, e.g. achalasia.
  - EMG: particularly of the frontalis muscle. Requires separate monitoring of peripheral neuromuscular blockade in addition.

Bruhn J, Myles PS, Sneyd R, Struys MMRF (2006). Br J Anaesth; 97: 85–94

Anaesthesia dolorosa. Pain in an anaesthetic area, typically following destructive treatment of trigeminal neuralgia. Unpleasant symptoms, ranging from paraesthesia to severe pain, develop in the area of the face rendered anaesthetic, and may be more distressing than the original symptoms. Anaesthesia dolorosa may develop many months after the lesion, and is often refractory to further treatment, including surgery. Limited success has been reported with gabapentin.

Anaesthesia, history of.
- Early attempts at pain relief:
  - opium used for many centuries, especially in the Far East. First injected iv by Wren in 1665.
  - use of other plants and derivatives for many centuries, e.g. cocaine (cocada), mandragora, alcohol.
  - acupuncture.
  - unconsciousness produced by carotid compression.
  - analgesia produced by cold (refrigeration anaesthesia), compression and ischaemia: 1500–1600s.
  - mesmerism: 1700–1800s.
- General anaesthesia:
  - effects of diethyl ether on animals described by Paracelsus: 1540.
  - understanding of basic physiology, especially respiratory and cardiovascular, and isolation of many gases, e.g. O_2, CO_2, N_2O: 1600–1700s.
  - N_2O suggested for analgesia by Davy in 1799.
  - CO_2 inhalation to produce insensibility described by Hickman in 1824.
  - use of diethyl ether for anaesthesia by Long, Clarke: 1842.
  - use of N_2O for anaesthesia by Wells, Colton: 1844.
  - first public demonstration of ether anaesthesia in Boston by Morton: October 16th 1846 (*see Bigelow; Holmes; Warren*).
  - first UK use in Dumfries and London: December 19th 1846 (*see Boott*). Used in London by Squire two days later (*see Liston*).
  - chloroform introduced by Simpson: 1847.
  - first deaths, e.g. Greener: 1848.
  - development in UK led by Snow, then Clover.
  - rectal administration of anaesthetic agents described.
  - iv anaesthesia produced with chloral hydrate by Oré: 1872.
  - ether versus chloroform: the former was favoured in England and northern USA, the latter in Scotland and southern USA. Other agents introduced (*see Inhalational anaesthetic agents*). Boyle machine described 1917.
  - iv anaesthesia popularised by Weese, Lundy and Waters: 1930s (*see Intravenous anaesthetic agents*). Neuromuscular blockade introduced by Griffith: 1942. Halothane introduced 1956.
  - UK pioneers: Hewitt, Macewen, Magill, Rowbotham, Macintosh (first UK professor), Hewer, Organe.

- USA pioneers: Waters (first university professor), Guedel, Mckesson, Crile, McMechan, Lundy.
- UK: Association of Anaesthetists founded 1932; DA examination 1935; Faculty of Anaesthetists 1948; FFARCS examination 1953; College of Anaesthetists 1988; Royal College of Anaesthetists 1992.
- USA: American Society of Anesthesiologists founded 1945.
- World Federation of Societies of Anaesthesiologists founded 1955.

- Local anaesthesia:
  - cocaine isolated 1860.
  - topical anaesthesia produced by Koller: 1884.
  - spinal anaesthesia by Corning: 1885; Bier: 1898.
  - epidural anaesthesia 1901.
  - pioneers: Braun, Lawen, Labat.

[Sir Christopher Wren (1632–1723), English scientist and architect; Helmut Weese (1897–1954), German pharmacologist]

See also, Cardiopulmonary resuscitation; Intermittent positive pressure ventilation; Intensive care, history of; Intubation, tracheal; Local anaesthetic agents

Anaesthesia, mechanism of. The precise mechanism is unknown, but theories are as follows:

- anatomical level:
  - ascending reticular activating system is thought to be the most likely site, but cerebral cortex, olfactory cortex, hippocampus and limbic system are probably involved.
  - spinal cord is also affected by anaesthetics.
  - synaptic sites are thought to be more important than axonal sites, since the former are blocked more easily than the latter at clinically effective concentrations of anaesthetic agent. Agents are thought to modify presynaptic release of neurotransmitter, and/or postsynaptic binding. They may modulate overall synaptic function by delaying certain impulses only, or by a global effect. Reduced excitation is thought to be mainly responsible, but increased inhibitory activity has also been shown.
- cellular level: membranes are thought to be the likeliest site of action, although anaesthetics have been shown to interact with microtubules and other cytoplasmic structures. Summary of evidence;
  - potency of volatile agents is related to their lipid solubility (Meyer–Overton rule), hence the suggestion of membrane lipids as the target site. However, this does not explain the cut-off effect or the lack of potentiation of anaesthetics by heat.
  - membrane or other proteins may be affected by anaesthetics. Interaction with certain proteins has also been shown to be related to potency. Specific molecule systems may be involved. Recently, attention has focused on type A GABA receptors ($GABA_A$ receptors) as a specific site of action of anaesthetic agents. The ion channels consist of five subunits with the putative site for anaesthetic action near the middle of the transmembrane protein complex; different receptor subunits may confer different sensitivities to anaesthetics. Binding is thought to cause a conformational change in the receptor and open the channel, enhancing inhibitory chloride activity. Other receptor systems may also be affected, e.g. the opioid system.
  - membrane expansion by anaesthetics to beyond a critical volume has been postulated, supported by pressure reversal of anaesthesia in tadpoles and some other animal experiments. The multisite expansion hypothesis has been suggested to account for differences between different agents and experimental conditions; it proposes that different agents act at various sites within the membrane to cause membrane expansion and alter fluidity. The function of membrane pumps and configuration of ionic channels are thus altered.
- other theories, now thought to be less important:
  - clathrate theory (water hydrates of anaesthetic agents).
  - Ferguson's thermodynamic activity theory: related activity to the chemical composition of the agent concerned, by determining the energy contained within the chemical bonds of its molecules. Related to lipid solubility and other physical properties.
  - Bernard suggested that anaesthetics caused intracellular protein coagulation.

[J Ferguson (described 1939), English scientist]

Postgraduate Educational Issue (2002). Br J Anaesth; 89: 1–183

Anaesthesia, one lung, *see One-lung anaesthesia*

Anaesthesia Practitioners, *see Physician's Assistants (Anaesthesia)*

Anaesthesia, stages of. In 1847, Snow described five stages of narcotism, although a less detailed classification had already been described. The classic description of anaesthetic stages was by Guedel in 1937 in unpremedicated patients, breathing diethyl ether in air:

- stage 1 (analgesia):
  - normal reflexes.
  - ends with loss of the eyelash reflex and unconsciousness.
- stage 2 (excitement):
  - irregular breathing, struggling.
  - dilated pupils.
  - vomiting, coughing and laryngospasm may occur.
  - ends with the onset of automatic breathing and loss of the eyelid reflex.
- stage 3 (surgical anaesthesia):
  - plane I:
    - until eyes centrally placed with loss of conjunctival reflex.
    - swallowing and vomiting depressed.
    - pupils normal/small.
    - lacrimation increased.
  - plane II:
    - until onset of intercostal paralysis.
    - regular deep breathing.
    - loss of corneal reflex.
    - pupils becoming larger.
    - lacrimation increased.
  - plane III:
    - until complete intercostal paralysis.
    - shallow breathing.
    - light reflex depressed.
    - laryngeal reflexes depressed.
    - lacrimation depressed.
  - plane IV:
    - until diaphragmatic paralysis.
    - carinal reflexes depressed.
- stage 4 (overdose):
  - apnoea.
  - dilated pupils.

With modern agents and techniques, the stages often occur too rapidly to be easily distinguished.

The stages may be seen in reverse order on emergence from anaesthesia.
See also, Anaesthesia, depth of

Anaesthesia, total intravenous, *see Total intravenous anaesthesia*

Anaesthetic accidents, *see Anaesthetic morbidity and mortality*

Anaesthetic agents, *see Inhalational anaesthetic agents; Intravenous anaesthetic agents; Local anaesthetic agents*

Anaesthetic breathing systems.
- Definitions:
  - open: unrestricted ambient air as the fresh gas supply.
  - semi-open: as above, but some restriction to air supply, e.g. enclosed mask.
  - closed: totally closed circle system.
  - semi-closed: air intake prevented but venting of excess gases allowed. Classified by Mapleson into five groups, A to E, in 1954; a sixth (F) was added later (Fig. 9).
- Mapleson's classification (excludes open drop techniques, circle systems, and use of non-rebreathing valves):
  - Mapleson A (Magill attachment):
    - efficient for spontaneous ventilation, because exhaled dead space gas is reused at the next inspiration, and exhaled alveolar gas passes out through the valve. Thus fresh gas flow (FGF) theoretically may equal alveolar minute volume (70 ml/kg/min).
    - inefficient for IPPV, because some fresh gas is lost through the valve when the bag is squeezed, and exhaled alveolar gas may be retained in the system and rebreathed. High gas flows are therefore needed (2–3 × minute volume).
  - Mapleson B and C: rarely used, other than for resuscitation. Inefficient; thus 2–3 × minute volume is required.
  - Mapleson D:
    - inefficient for spontaneous ventilation, because exhaled gas passes into the reservoir bag with fresh gas, and may be rebreathed unless FGF is high. Suggested values for FGF range from 150 to 250 ml/kg/min; resistance to breathing may be a problem at high FGF.
    - efficient for IPPV; exhaled dead space gas passes into the bag and is reused but when alveolar gas reaches the bag, the bag is full of fresh gas and dead space gas; alveolar gas is thus voided through the valve. Theoretically, 70 ml/kg/min will maintain normocapnia.
  - Mapleson E (Ayre's T-piece): used for children, because of its low resistance to breathing. To prevent breathing of atmospheric air, the reservoir limb should exceed tidal volume. A FGF of 2–3 × minute volume is required to prevent rebreathing. May be used for IPPV by intermittent occlusion of the reservoir limb outlet.
  - Mapleson F (Jackson Rees Modification): adapted from Ayre's T-piece. The bag allows easier control of ventilation, and its movement demonstrates breathing during spontaneous ventilation. Suggested FGF: 2–3 × minute volume for spontaneous ventilation. For IPPV, 200 ml/kg has been suggested, although more complicated formulae exist.
- Modifications include:
  - coaxial versions of the A and D systems (Lack and Bain respectively): the valve is accessible to the anaesthetist for adjustment and scavenging, and the tubing is longer and lighter.

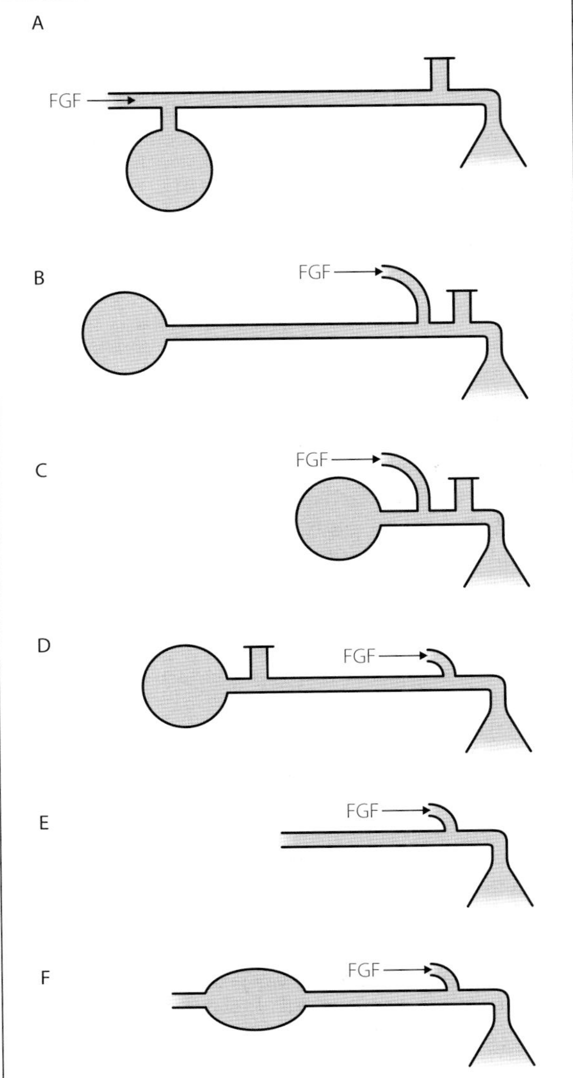

Fig. 9 Classification of anaesthetic breathing systems (see text)

  - Humphrey ADE system: valve and bag are at the machine end, with a lever incorporated within the valve block; may be converted into type A, D or E systems depending on requirements.
  - enclosed afferent reservoir system: resembles the Mapleson D with an additional reservoir placed on the FGF limb. This reservoir is enclosed within a chamber which connects to the main limb such that compressing the original reservoir bag (e.g. manually) causes the additional reservoir to be compressed too, increasing the tidal volume delivered. The system (in a more sophisticated form, including a bellows as the additional reservoir) has been incorporated within a ventilator system; although it has been shown to be efficient during both spontaneous and controlled ventilation it is not widely used.

British and International Standard taper sizes of breathing system connections are 15 mm for tracheal tube connectors and paediatric components, and 22 mm for adult components. Some components have both external tapers of 22 mm, and internal tapers of 15 mm. Some paediatric equipment has

8.5 mm diameter fittings, although not standard. Upstream parts of connections are traditionally 'male', and fit into the 'female' downstream parts.

[William W Mapleson, Cardiff physicist; Philip Ayre (1902–1980), Newcastle anaesthetist; Gordon Jackson Rees (1918–2000), Liverpool anaesthetist; David Humphrey, South African physiologist and anaesthetist]

Conway CM (1985). Br J Anaesth; 57: 649–57

See also, Adjustable pressure-limiting valve; Catheter mounts; Coaxial anaesthetic breathing systems; Facepieces; Tracheal tubes; Valveless anaesthetic breathing systems

Anaesthetic drug labels, *see Syringe labels*

Anaesthetic machines. Term commonly refers to machines providing continuous flow of anaesthetic gases (c.f. **intermittent flow anaesthetic machines**). The original **Boyle** machine was developed in 1917 at St Bartholomew's Hospital, although similar apparatus was already being used in America and France.

- Usual system:
  - **piped gas supply** or **cylinders**.
  - pressure gauges may indicate pipeline, cylinder or regulated (reduced) pressure (*see Pressure measurement*).
  - **pressure regulators** provide constant gas pressure, usually about 400 kPa (4 bar) in the UK. Pipelines are already at this pressure.
  - **flowmeters**, usually **Rotameters**.
  - **vaporisers**.
  - pressure relief valve downstream from the vaporisers protects the flowmeters from excessive pressure; it opens at about 38–40 kPa. May be combined with a non-return valve.
  - O_2 flush; bypasses flowmeters and vaporisers, delivering at least 35 l/min.
  - **O_2 failure warning device**.
  - **ventilators**, **monitoring** equipment, **suction equipment**, and various **anaesthetic breathing systems** may be incorporated. Some machines contain microprocessors for digitalised control of functions, e.g. gas flow.
- Modern safety features reduce the risk of:
  - delivering hypoxic gas mixtures:
    - to avoid incorrect gas delivery:
      - **pin index system** for cylinders and non-interchangeable connectors for piped gas outlet.
      - colour coding of pipelines and cylinders.
      - O_2 analyser.
      - O_2 flowmeter control is bigger and has a different profile from others; it is positioned in the same place on all machines (i.e. on the left in the UK; on the right in the USA).
      - linkage between N_2O and O_2 Rotameters, so that less than 25% O_2 cannot be 'dialed up', e.g. **Quantiflex apparatus** and newer machines.
    - to avoid O_2 leak: O_2 flowmeter feeds downstream from the others; thus a cracked CO_2 Rotameter leaks N_2O in preference to O_2.
    - to avoid risk of O_2 delivery failure:
      - O_2 pressure gauge.
      - O_2 failure warning device; preferably switching off other gas flows and allowing air to be breathed.
      - O_2 analyser.
  - delivering excessive CO_2 (e.g. caused by the CO_2 flowmeter opened fully, with the bobbin hidden at the top of the flowmeter tube):
    - maximal possible CO_2 flow is limited, e.g. to 500 ml/min.
    - bobbin is clearly visible throughout the length of the Rotameter tube.
    - CO_2 cylinder is connected to the machine only when specifically required.
  - delivering excessive pressures:
    - **adjustable pressure limiting valve** on breathing systems: modern ones produce maximal pressures of 70 cmH_2O when fully closed. Many ventilators also have cut-off maximal pressures.
    - distensible **reservoir bag**; maximal pressure attainable is about 60 cmH_2O. Pressure reaches a plateau as the bag distends, falling slightly (**Laplace's law**) before bursting.
- Other safety features:
  - switches to prevent **soda lime** being used with **trichloroethylene** (older machines).
  - **key filling system** for vaporisers.
  - negative and positive pressure relief valves within **scavenging** systems.
  - **antistatic precautions**.

Thompson PW, Wilkinson DJ (1985). Br J Anaesth; 57: 640–8

See also, Checking of anaesthetic equipment

Anaesthetic morbidity and mortality. Complications during and following anaesthesia are difficult to quantify, since many may be related to surgery or other factors. Many are avoidable, and may be more disturbing to the patient than the surgery itself.

- Examples:
  - **PONV**.
  - **sore throat**.
  - headache: often related to perioperative dehydration and starvation. **Post-dural puncture headache**.
  - damage to **teeth**, mouth, **eyes**, etc.
  - backache: especially after lithotomy position. Reduced by lumbar pillows.
  - muscle pains following **suxamethonium**.
  - thrombophlebitis/pain at injection or infusion sites.
  - extravasation of injectate/intra-arterial injection.
  - drowsiness, disorientation.
  - **blood transfusion** hazards.
  - **nerve injury** and damage related to **positioning of the patient**.
  - burns, e.g. from **diathermy**.
  - falls during transfer from/to trolleys, etc.
  - **awareness**.
  - tracheal intubation difficulties (*see Intubation, complications of*).
  - **adverse drug reactions**, e.g. **halothane hepatitis**, **MH**.
  - drug overdose.
  - renal impairment, e.g. following uncorrected hypotension.
  - cardiovascular complications: **MI**, **hypertension/hypotension**, **air embolism**, **arrhythmias**.
  - respiratory complications: **hypoventilation**, **atelectasis**, **chest infection**, **PE**, **pneumothorax**, **aspiration pneumonitis**, **airway obstruction**, **bronchospasm**.
  - psychological changes.
  - severe neurological complications: **CVA**, brain damage, spinal cord infarction; they often follow severe hypotension/cardiac arrest/hypoxia.
  - **death**.
- Mortality may be related to anaesthesia, surgery, or the medical condition of the patient. Mortality studies in the UK, USA, Canada, Scandinavia, Europe and Australia have all implicated similar factors:

- preoperatively:
  - inadequate assessment.
  - hypovolaemia and inadequate resuscitation.
- perioperatively:
  - aspiration.
  - inadequate monitoring.
  - intubation difficulties.
  - delivery of hypoxic gas mixtures and equipment failure.
  - inexperience/inadequate supervision.
- postoperatively:
  - inadequate observation.
  - hypoventilation due to respiratory depression, residual neuromuscular blockade, and respiratory obstruction.
- Morbidity and mortality are thus reduced by:
  - thorough preoperative assessment and adequate resuscitation.
  - checking of anaesthetic equipment and drugs.
  - adequate monitoring.
  - anticipation of likely problems.
  - attention to detail.
  - adequate recovery facilities.
  - adequate supervision/assistance.

Clear contemporaneous record-keeping promotes careful perioperative monitoring and assists retrospective analysis of complications and future anaesthetic management.
See also, Audit; Confidential Enquiries into Maternal Deaths, Report on; Confidential Enquiry into Perioperative Deaths

Anaesthetic rooms (Induction rooms). Usual in the UK but not used in many other countries.

- Advantages:
  - quiet area for induction of anaesthesia, teaching, etc.
  - less frightening for the patient than lying on the operating table. Allows parents to be present during induction of anaesthesia in children.
  - anaesthetists' domain; i.e. without pressure from surgeons, etc.
  - store for anaesthetic drugs, equipment, etc.
  - increased throughput of the operating suite, if another anaesthetist is available to start whilst previous cases are being completed in theatre.
- Disadvantages:
  - expensive duplication of equipment is required, e.g. anaesthetic machine, monitoring, scavenging, etc.
  - monitoring is disconnected during transfer of the patient.
  - transfer and positioning for surgery is more hazardous with the patient anaesthetised than when awake.
  - equipment, iv fluids, drugs, etc. may not be immediately available in the operating theatre.

The above disadvantages lead many anaesthetists to induce anaesthesia in the operating theatre for high risk patients. Continued existence of anaesthetic rooms is controversial. Holding areas capable of processing many patients at once (allowing premedication and performance of regional blocks) have been suggested as an alternative.
Meyer-Witting M, Wilkinson DJ (1992). Anaesthesia; 47: 1021–2

Anaesthetic simulators. Training devices that duplicate artificially the conditions likely to be encountered during operations. Useful in the development of diagnostic and therapeutic skills, decision making, team training, analysing tasks and errors, and assessing risks. Allow prospective and repeated observation and analysis of actions rather than retrospective assessment. Individual components, e.g. mannikins, may be used to teach specific skills (part-task trainers), or combined within the setting of an entire operating suite with monitoring equipment and controlled with computers (high-fidelity simulation), often interacting through a mathematical model.

Are now widely used in areas other than anaesthesia, e.g. obstetrics, emergency medicine and surgery.

Despite the best efforts, simulators may not always reflect real conditions accurately. For instance, some activities may be easier to perform on simulators than in the operating room; conversely, some may be more difficult. Reality is further impeded by the need to model average 'patients' who may not respond in the 'extreme' ways of some real patients; equally, subjects' responses may be different when they are aware that they are working with a simulator. The cost of sophisticated simulators and the labour-intensive staffing requirements are further disincentives. Nevertheless, simulation has become an established part of training programmes in many countries, and has also been studied as a means of assessing practitioners.
Wong AK (2004). Can J Anaesth; 51: 455–64
See also, Crisis resource management

Analeptic drugs. Drugs causing stimulation of the CNS as their most prominent action (many other drugs also have stimulant properties, e.g. aminophylline).

- Mechanism of action:
  - block inhibition, e.g. strychnine (via glycine antagonism), picrotoxin (via GABA antagonism).
  - increase excitation, e.g. doxapram, nikethamide.

Doxapram and nikethamide increase respiration via stimulation of peripheral chemoreceptors. All the analeptics may cause cardiovascular stimulation, and convulsions at sufficient doses.

Analgesia. Lack of sensation of pain from a normally painful stimulus.
See also, Analgesic drugs

Analgesic drugs. May be divided into:

- opioid analgesic drugs.
- inhibitors of prostaglandin synthesis:
  - NSAIDs.
  - paracetamol.
- others:
  - inhalational anaesthetic agents, e.g. N_2O, trichloroethylene.
  - ketamine.
  - nefopam, ethoheptazine.
  - local anaesthetic agents.
- adjuncts: i.e. reduce pain or pain sensation by alternative means: e.g. antidepressant drugs, corticosteroids, carbamazepine, gabapentin, muscle relaxants, e.g. diazepam, etc. Used widely in chronic pain management. Caffeine is often included in oral analgesic preparations.

Analgesic drugs are distinguished from anaesthetic agents by their ability to reduce pain sensation without inducing sleep; thus N_2O is a good analgesic but a poor anaesthetic, and halothane has poor analgesic properties but is a potent anaesthetic. In practice the distinction is not precise, as analgesic drugs, e.g. opiates, will cause unconsciousness at high doses, and anaesthetic drugs, e.g. halothane, will abolish pain sensation at deep planes of anaesthesia.

Anaphylactic reaction. Type I immune reaction, resulting from an antigen–antibody reaction on the surface of mast

cells. Cross-linking of two immunoglobulin type-E (reagin) molecules by the antigen results in the release of histamine and other vasoactive substances, e.g. kinins, 5-HT and leukotrienes. Type-G immunoglobulin may also be involved. True anaphylaxis requires previous exposure to the antigen responsible, sometimes many exposures; e.g. anaphylaxis to thiopental classically occurs after more than 10 exposures. However, in 80% of cases no prior exposure is evident. More common in women, which has led to the suggestion that exposure to cosmetics may 'prime' the reaction. Incidence is estimated at 1 in 10–20 000 anaesthetics. Agents most commonly implicated are the neuromuscular blocking drugs (70%) especially suxamethonium and vecuronium, latex (10%), colloids (5%) and antibacterial drugs (3%). Mortality is approximately 5%. Has been classified clinically into five grades:
- I: cutaneous: erythema, urticaria, angio-oedema.
- II: as above plus hypotension, tachycardia, bronchospasm.
- III: as above but severe; collapse, arrhythmias.
- IV: cardiac and/or respiratory arrest.
- V: death.

- Treatment:
    - CPR, especially iv fluids and O_2 administration.
    - adrenaline im (0.5–1.0 ml of 1:1000 every 10 min as required) or iv (0.5–1.0 ml of 1:10 000 slowly, repeated as required). IV infusion of adrenaline or noradrenaline may be required after initial treatment. Alternative vasoconstrictors, e.g. metaraminol, have been successfully used in resistant cases.
    - secondary treatment includes antihistamine drugs, e.g. chlorphenamine 10–20 mg slowly iv (H_2-receptor antagonists, e.g. ranitidine 50 mg slowly iv should be considered), and hydrocortisone 100–500 mg iv. Bicarbonate therapy may be required according to blood gas analysis.

Subsequent testing is as for adverse drug reactions in general.

Kroigaard M, Garvey LH, Gillberg L (2007). Acta Anaesthesiol Scand; 51: 655–70

Anaphylactoid reaction. Although clinically similar to an anaphylactic reaction, anaphylactoid reactions do not involve immunoglobulin cross-linkage. Underlying mechanisms include the release of vasoactive substances, e.g. histamine, by:
- direct histamine release from mast cells. Radiological contrast media are one of the most common causes. Neuromuscular blocking drugs may also cause it, especially atracurium, tubocurarine.
- complement activation, via either classical or alternative pathways. Althesin may cause either.

Direct histamine release and alternative pathway complement activation do not require prior exposure to the causative agent, whereas true anaphylaxis does.

Management is as for anaphylaxis.

Hepner DL, Castells MC (2003). Anesth Analg; 97: 1381–95

See also, Adverse drug reactions

Aneroid gauge, *see Pressure measurement*

Anesthesia and Analgesia. Oldest current journal of anaesthesia, first published in 1922 as *Current Researches in Anesthesia and Analgesia* (the journal of the National Anesthesia Research Society, which became the International Anesthesia Research Society in 1925). Also the official journal of the Society of Cardiovascular Anesthetists, the Society of Pediatric Anesthesia, the Society of Ambulatory Anesthesia, the International Society for Anaesthetic Pharmacology, the Society for Technology in Anesthesia and the Anesthesia Patient Safety Foundation.

Craig DB, Martin JT (1997). Anesth Analg; 85: 237–47

Anesthesiology. Journal of the American Society of Anesthesiologists, first published in 1940. Also the official journal of the Society of Obstetric Anesthesia and Perinatology, and the American Society of Critical Care Anesthetists.

Anesthesiology. American term describing the practice of anaesthesia by trained physicians (anesthesiologists) as opposed to others who might administer anaesthetics (e.g. nurse anesthetists). Formally accepted as a specialty by the American Medical Association in 1940. In the UK, the term 'anaesthetist' implies medical qualification.

Angina, *see Ischaemic heart disease; Myocardial ischaemia*

Angio-oedema. Tissue swelling resulting from allergic reactions. Spread of oedema through subcutaneous tissue often involves the periorbital region, lips, tongue and oropharynx. Life-threatening airway obstruction may occur. Common precipitants include plants, foodstuffs (e.g. shellfish, nuts) and drugs (especially angiotensin converting enzyme inhibitors). Acute swelling often settles after about 6 h, although treatment of a severe life-threatening attack should follow the management of an anaphylactic reaction.

Certain forms of angio-oedema result from a deficiency of C1-esterase inhibitor, either acquired or hereditary. Colicky abdominal pain or severe respiratory obstruction are frequent clinical pictures. Treatment of attacks resulting from these forms includes androgens, e.g. danazol, plasminogen inhibitors or replacement of C1-esterase inhibitor (as fresh frozen plasma or in a synthetic form).

See also, Complement, Hereditary angio-oedema

Angioplasty, *see Percutaneous transluminal coronary angioplasty*

Angiotensin II receptor antagonists. Antihypertensive drugs, also being investigated for treatment of heart failure; competitively inhibit angiotensin II at its AT_1 receptor subtype on arteriolar smooth muscle, thus less likely than angiotensin converting enzyme inhibitors to cause systemic side effects including those related to interaction with other hormone systems (e.g. involving kinins), or renin/angiotensin system imbalance. However, may cause hypotension or hyperkalaemia, and should be used with caution in renal artery stenosis. Other side effects include rash, urticaria, angio-oedema, myalgia, GIT disturbance and dizziness. Losartan was the first to be developed, valsartan, candesartan, eprosartan, irbesartan and telmisartan subsequently.

Angiotensin converting enzyme inhibitors (ACE inhibitors). Originally isolated from snake venom. Used in the treatment of hypertension and cardiac failure, they have been shown to reduce mortality in cardiac failure associated with MI. They block the action of angiotensin converting enzyme; apart from converting angiotensin I to angiotensin II, this enzyme breaks down kinins, naturally occurring vasodilators. The ACE inhibitors cause vasodilatation and a drop in BP, which may be profound after the first dose. Side effects include hypotension, rashes, leucopenia, renal and hepatic damage, loss of taste, angio-oedema, pancreatitis, GIT disturbance, myalgia, dizziness, headache and cough. Severe hypotension may follow induction of anaesthesia or perioperative haemorrhage, especially if the patient is fluid and/or sodium depleted (e.g. taking diuretics). Should be used with caution in patients with renovascular disease.

Captopril and enalapril were the first and second ACE inhibitor introduced respectively; newer ones include cilazapril, fosinopril, lisinopril, moexipril, perindopril, quinapril, ramipril and trandolapril.
See also, Renin/angiotensin system

Angiotensins, *see Renin/angiotensin system*

Animal bites, *see Bites and stings*

Anion gap. Difference between measured cation and anion concentrations in the plasma. Sodium concentrations exceed chloride plus bicarbonate concentrations by 4–11 mmol/l (the range has changed in recent years as modern methods of measuring electrolytes give rise to higher normal values for chloride concentrations). Anionic proteins, phosphate and sulphate make up the difference. Of use in the differential diagnosis of metabolic acidosis; anionic gap increases when organic anions accumulate, e.g. in lactic acidosis, ketoacidosis, uraemia. It does not increase in acidosis due to loss of bicarbonate or intake of hydrochloric acid. Not an infallible tool since other cations such as potassium, calcium and magnesium may influence the calculation. Anion gap has also been compared to alterations in plasma bicarbonate levels ($\delta AG/\delta HCO_3^-$ ratio). It has also been calculated for urine electrolytes.

Ankle Brachial Pressure Index (ABPI). Measure of peripheral vascular disease, calculated by dividing the systolic pressure in the leg (best results are obtained if the dorsalis pedis and posterior tibial artery pressures are averaged) by the systolic pressure in the arms (average of left and right brachial artery pressures). Normally 0.91–1.3, with values > 1.3 suggesting poor arterial compressibility due to medial arterial calcification while values of < 0.9, < 0.7 and < 0.4 indicate mild, moderate and severe disease respectively. Has been used to predict cardiovascular morbidity and mortality and distinguish atherosclerosis from other causes of leg pain.

Ankle, nerve blocks. Useful for surgery distal to the ankle.
- Nerves to be blocked are as follows (Fig. 10):
  - tibial nerve (L5–S3): lies posterior to the posterior tibial artery, between flexor digitorum longus and flexor hallucis longus tendons. Divides into lateral and medial plantar nerves behind the medial malleolus. Supplies the anterior and medial parts of the sole of the foot. A needle is inserted lateral to the posterior tibial artery at the level of the medial malleolus, or medial to the Achilles tendon if the artery cannot be felt. It is passed anteriorly and 5–10 ml local anaesthetic agent injected as it is withdrawn.
  - sural nerve (L5–S2): formed from branches of the tibial and common peroneal nerves. Accompanies the short saphenous vein behind the lateral malleolus and supplies the posterior part of the sole, the back of the lower leg, the heel and lateral side of the foot. Subcutaneous infiltration is performed from the Achilles tendon to the lateral malleolus, using 5–10 ml solution.
  - deep and superficial peroneal nerves (both L4–S2): the deep peroneal nerve supplies the area between the first and second toes. It lies between anterior tibial (medially) and extensor hallucis longus (laterally) tendons, lateral to the anterior tibial artery. A needle is inserted between these tendons; a click may be felt as it penetrates the extensor retinaculum. 5 ml solution is injected. The superficial peroneal nerve is blocked by subcutaneous infiltration from the lateral malleolus to the front of the tibia. It supplies the dorsum of the foot.
  - saphenous nerve (L3–4): the terminal branch of the femoral nerve; blocked by subcutaneous infiltration above and anterior to the medial malleolus. It supplies the medial side of the ankle joint.

Ankylosing spondylitis. Disease characterised by inflammation and fusion of the sacroiliac joints and lumbar vertebrae; may also involve the thoracic and cervical spine. Commonest in males, with a high proportion carrying tissue type antigen HLA B27.
- Features:
  - backache and stiffness. Spinal cord compression may occur; atlantoaxial subluxation or cervical fracture may also occur. Spinal/epidural anaesthesia may be difficult.
  - restricted ventilation if thoracic spine or costovertebral joints are severely affected; increased diaphragmatic movement usually preserves good lung function. Pulmonary fibrosis is rare.
  - tracheal intubation may be difficult due to a stiff or rigid neck, or temporomandibular joint involvement.
  - aortitis may occur (in less than 5% of chronic sufferers), causing aortic regurgitation. Cardiomyopathy and conduction defects are rare.
  - amyloidosis may occur.

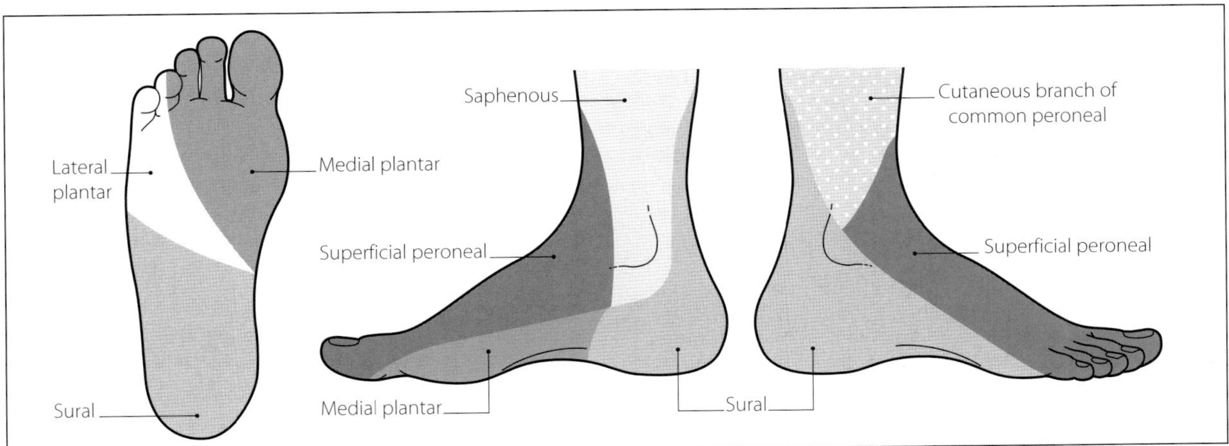

Fig. 10 Cutaneous innervation of the ankle and foot

Anorexia nervosa. Psychiatric condition, most common in young women. Characterised by loss of weight, distortion of body image and amenorrhoea; the last results from weight loss, and psychological and endocrine factors.
- Anaesthetic considerations:
  - electrolyte disturbances, especially hypokalaemia, are associated with laxative abuse or self-induced vomiting.
  - tendency towards hypothermia, hypotension and bradycardia.
  - reduced lean body mass.
  - anaemia.
  - rare complications: myopathy, cardiomyopathy, peripheral neuritis, hepatic impairment, gastric dilatation.

Treatment includes behavioural and psychotherapy; chlorpromazine has also been used.
Seller CA, Ravalia A (2003). Anaesthesia; 58: 437–43

Anrep effect. Intrinsic regulatory mechanism of the heart in response to acute increases in afterload. Initial reduction in stroke volume and increase in left ventricular diastolic pressure are followed by restoration to near original values.
[Gleb V Anrep (1890–1955), Russian-born Egyptian physiologist]
Yentis SM (1998). J Roy Soc Med; 91: 209–12

Anrep, Vassily (1852–1927). Russian scientist and medico-politician. Described the pharmacology of cocaine in 1880 and was the first person to describe the numbing effect of sc injection; he went on to perform the first nerve blocks (intercostal), publishing his results in Russian in 1884 but failing to publicise his work more widely. His son Gleb described the Anrep effect.
Yentis SM (1999). Anesthesiology; 90: 890–5

Antacids. Used to relieve pain in peptic ulcer disease, hiatus hernia and gastro-oesophageal reflux by increasing gastric pH. Used preoperatively in patients at high risk from aspiration of gastric contents, e.g. in obstetrics, and have been used on ICU as prophylaxis against stress ulcers. Many preparations are available; sodium citrate is most commonly used in anaesthetic practice. Chronic overuse of antacids may result in alkalosis, hypercalcaemia (calcium salts), constipation (aluminium salts) and diarrhoea (magnesium salts).

Antagonist. Substance that opposes the action of an agonist.
- Antagonism may be:
  - competitive: the substance reversibly binds to a receptor, and causes no direct response within the cell (i.e. has no intrinsic activity), but may cause a response by displacing an agonist, e.g. naloxone.
  - non-competitive: as above but with irreversible binding, e.g. phenoxybenzamine.
  - physiological: opposing actions are produced by binding at different receptors, e.g. histamine and adrenaline causing bronchoconstriction and bronchodilatation respectively.

See also, Dose–response curves; Receptor theory

Antanalgesia. Increased sensitivity to painful stimuli caused by small doses of depressant drugs, e.g. thiopental. Thought to result from suppression of the inhibitory action of the ascending reticular activating system, allowing increased cortical responsiveness (decreased pain threshold). Larger doses depress the activating system and induce sleep. Antanalgesia may also occur as blood drug levels fall, e.g. causing postoperative restlessness when barbiturates or alimemazine are used as premedication, especially in children.

Antecubital fossa (Cubital fossa). Triangular fossa, anterior to the elbow joint (Fig. 11).
- Borders:
  - proximal: a line between the humeral epicondyles.
  - lateral: brachioradialis muscle.
  - medial: pronator teres.
  - floor: supinator and brachialis muscles, with the joint capsule behind.
  - roof: deep fascia with the median cubital vein and medial cutaneous nerve on top.
- Contents from medial to lateral (embedded in fat):
  - median nerve.
  - brachial artery, dividing into radial and ulnar arteries.
  - biceps tendon.
  - posterior interosseus and radial nerves.

The bicipital aponeurosis lies between the superficial veins and deeper structures, protecting the latter during venepuncture. Damage may still be caused to nerves and arteries during this procedure; anomalous branches are relatively common. Accidental intra-arterial injection of drugs is a particular hazard.
See also, Venous drainage of arm

Antepartum haemorrhage (APH). Defined as vaginal bleeding after 22 weeks' gestation. Occurs in up to 5% of all pregnancies. Most cases are not severe and are associated with various conditions including infection. Two conditions affecting the placenta are of particular importance to the anaesthetist since they may cause sudden and severe collapse and rapid exsanguination, although this extreme is fortunately rare:
  - placenta praevia: the placenta encroaches upon or covers the cervical os. Presents with vaginal bleeding, usually in the third trimester; there may be fetal distress.

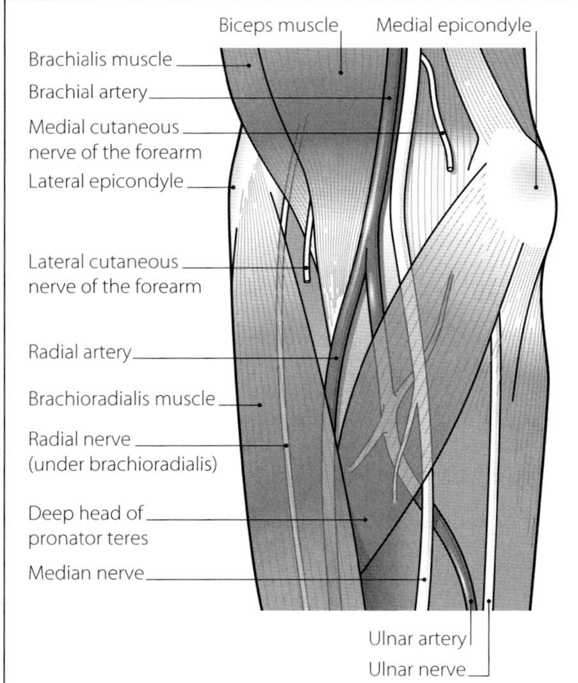

Fig. 11 Anatomy of the antecubital fossa

Unless the mother is at risk of exsanguination, delivery of the fetus by Caesarean section should wait until adequate blood has been obtained and appropriate staff are present, since the mother is not at risk of developing coagulopathy unless massive transfusion is required. In its most severe form, the placenta invades (placenta accreta) or even penetrates (placenta percreta) the uterine wall; haemorrhage may be torrential and require hysterectomy. Placenta accreta/percreta is more common if there has been prior uterine surgery, e.g. myomectomy or Caesarean section, the risk increasing with each previous procedure.

- placental abruption: haemorrhage behind the placenta. May present with abdominal pain and fetal distress, usually in the third trimester; vaginal bleeding is not always present. Caesarean section should not be delayed since there is a risk of developing DIC if the fetus is not delivered, this risk increasing the longer the wait. Has been associated with renal cortical necrosis.

Anaesthetic management includes standard resuscitation and techniques of obstetric analgesia and anaesthesia; the choice of regional versus general anaesthesia depends on the cardiovascular stability, estimated blood loss, presence of fetal distress, whether there is a coagulopathy and the preferences of the anaesthetist, obstetrician and patient. Postpartum observation is important since adequate fluid balance and renal output must be maintained; in addition placenta praevia in particular predisposes to postpartum haemorrhage since the uterine lower segment is not able to contract as effectively as the more muscular upper segment.

Anterior spinal artery syndrome. Infarction of the spinal cord due to anterior spinal artery insufficiency. May follow profound hypotension, e.g. in spinal or epidural anaesthesia. May also occur after aortic surgery. Results in lower motor neurone paralysis at the level of the lesion, and spastic paraplegia with reduced pain and temperature sensation below the level. Because the posterior spinal arteries supply the dorsal columns and posterior horns, joint position sense and vibration sensation are preserved.

Anthrax, *see Biological weapons*

Antiarrhythmic drugs. Classified by Vaughan Williams into four classes, depending on their effects on the action potential *in vitro* (Table 4). A fifth class has been suggested which includes a number of miscellaneous drugs (e.g. digoxin, and other cardiac glycosides, adenosine, magnesium) which do not fit into the standard four classes. More usefully classified for clinical purposes according to their site of action:

- atrioventricular node: calcium channel blocking drugs, digoxin, β-adrenergic receptor antagonists, adenosine (used for supraventricular arrhythmias).
- atria, ventricles and accessory pathways: quinidine, procainamide, disopyramide, amiodarone (used for supraventricular and ventricular arrhythmias).
- ventricles only: lidocaine (lignocaine), mexiletine, phenytoin (used for ventricular arrhythmias).

[EM Vaughan Williams, English pharmacologist]

See also, individual arrhythmias

Antibacterial drugs. Drugs used to kill bacteria (bactericidal) or inhibit bacterial replication (bacteriostatic).

Antibiotics are synthesised by micro-organisms and kill or inhibit other micro-organisms. Drugs synthesised *in vitro*, e.g. sulphonamides, are not antibiotics.

Table 4 Classification of antiarrhythmic drugs

Class	*Action*	*Examples*
I	Slow depolarisation rate by inhibiting sodium influx	
a	Prolong action potential	Quinidine Procainamide Disopyramide
b	Shorten action potential	Lidocaine Mexiletine Phenytoin
c	No effect on action potential	Flecainide Propafenone Encainide
II	Diminish effect of catecholamines	β-adrenergic receptor antagonists Bretylium
III	Prolong action potential, without affecting depolarisation rate	Amiodarone Sotalol Bretylium
IV	Inhibit calcium influx	Calcium channel blocking drugs
V	Miscellaneous	Digoxin Adenosine Magnesium

- Main groups:
  - β-lactams: bactericidal; act by inhibiting cell wall synthesis. Include penicillins, cephalosporins, aztreonam, carbapenems.
  - macrolides: bacteriostatic; act by inhibiting protein synthesis. Include erythromycin and related drugs.
  - aminoglycosides: bactericidal; inhibit protein synthesis. Include gentamicin, netilmicin.
  - tetracyclines: bacteriostatic; inhibit protein synthesis.
  - sulphonamides and trimethoprim: each alone is bacteriostatic; the combination (co-trimazole) is bactericidal.
  - 4-quinolones: bactericidal; impair nucleic acid replication. Include nalidixic acid and ciprofloxacin.
  - glycopeptides, e.g. teicoplanin and vancomycin: bactericidal.
  - others, e.g. clindamycin, chloramphenicol, metronidazole, polimixins, fusidic acid, linezolid, quinupristin/dalfopristin.
  - antituberculous drugs.

Choice of antibacterial drug depends on the organism involved (or suspected), the severity of the condition and the site of the infection. In many conditions, initial therapy is based on a 'best guess' principle with broad-spectrum drugs, narrower therapy being continued when the results of culture and sensitivity studies are known. The requirement for prompt treatment in severe illness may conflict with the need to obtain adequate samples for culture before therapy is started. Much concern exists about the increasing problem of bacterial resistance.

See also, Antifungal drugs; Antiviral drugs

Antibiotics, *see Antibacterial drugs*

Antibodies, *see Immunoglobulins*

Anticholinergic drugs. Strictly, should include all drugs impairing cholinergic transmission, although the term usually refers to antagonists of acetylcholine at muscarinic receptors. Antagonists at nicotinic receptors are classified as either ganglion blocking drugs or neuromuscular blocking drugs. Effects include tachycardia, bronchodilatation, mydriasis, reduced gland secretion, smooth muscle relaxation, and sedation or restlessness. Anaesthetic uses include the treatment of bradycardia, as a component of premedication and antagonism of the cardiac effects of acetylcholinesterase inhibitors.

- In anaesthesia, the most commonly used agents are atropine, hyoscine and glycopyrronium. Comparison of actions:
  - atropine:
    - central excitation.
    - greater action than hyoscine on the heart, bronchial smooth muscle and GIT.
  - hyoscine:
    - central depression; amnesia (may cause excitement in the elderly).
    - greater action than atropine on the pupil and sweat, salivary and bronchial glands.
  - glycopyrronium:
    - minimal central effects (quaternary ammonium ion; crosses the blood–brain barrier less readily than atropine and hyoscine, both tertiary ions).
    - similar peripheral actions to atropine, but with greater antisialagogue effect and less effect on the heart. Less antiemetic action than hyoscine and atropine.
    - longer duration of action.
- Other uses of anticholinergic drugs include:
  - antispasmodic effect (on bowel and bladder), e.g. propantheline.
  - ulcer healing, e.g. pirenzepine.
  - bronchodilatation, e.g. ipratropium.
  - mydriasis and cycloplegia (dilatation of pupil and paralysis of accommodation), e.g. atropine.

Anticholinergic antiparkinsonian drugs, e.g. benzatropine, procyclidine, orphenadrine, are used for their central effects.
See also, Acetylcholine receptors; Central anticholinergic syndrome; Muscarine and muscarinic receptors; Nicotine and nicotinic receptors

Anticholinesterases, *see Acetylcholinesterase inhibitors*

Anticoagulant drugs. Mechanisms of action:

- prevent synthesis of coagulation factors, e.g. warfarin.
- inhibit existing factors, e.g. heparin.
- inhibit platelet aggregation, i.e. antiplatelet drugs.
- break down circulating fibrinogen, e.g. ancrod (snake venom derivative; not commonly used).

Fibrinolytic drugs break down thrombus once formed. Warfarin and heparin are more effective at preventing venous thrombus than arterial thrombus, as the former contains relatively more fibrin. Antiplatelet drugs are more effective in arterial blood, where thrombus contains many platelets and little fibrin.

Anticonvulsant drugs. Postulated mechanism is via:

- neuronal sodium channel blockade, e.g. phenytoin, lamotrigine, sodium valproate, carbamazepine.
- enhancement of GABA receptor activation or increase in synaptic GABA levels, e.g. barbiturates, benzodiazepines, gabapentin, vigabatrin.
- calcium channel blockade, e.g. carbamazepine, ethosuximide.
- unknown action: levetiracetam.

First line management of status epilepticus involves use of iv lorazepam. Diazepam, phenytoin, fosphenytoin and thiopental are also used.

- For treatment of epilepsy, certain drugs are more likely to succeed:
  - generalized (grand mal) or partial seizures: phenytoin, phenobarbital, primidone, carbamazepine, benzodiazepines.
  - petit mal: ethosuximide, clonazepam, sodium valproate.

Vigabatrin, gabapentin, lamotrigine and levetiracetam are used as add-on drugs in resistant cases.

For patients undergoing surgery, anticonvulsant therapy should continue up to operation, and recommence as soon as possible postoperatively. If oral therapy is delayed postoperatively, parenteral administration may be substituted. Phenobarbital and phenytoin cause hepatic enzyme induction and increase certain drug metabolism.

Antidepressant drugs. Most increase central amine concentrations (e.g. dopamine, noradrenaline, 5-HT), supporting the theory that depression results from amine deficiency. Further evidence is that central depletion (e.g. by reserpine) may cause depression.

- May be classified thus:
  - tricyclic antidepressant drugs: block noradrenaline uptake from synapses.
  - selective serotonin reuptake inhibitors (SSRIs): specifically block reuptake of 5-HT, e.g. fluoxetine. Nefazodone blocks serotonin uptake and its receptors, whilst venlafaxine is a serotonin and noradrenaline reuptake inhibitor.
  - monoamine oxidase inhibitors (MAOIs): prevent catecholamine breakdown.
  - others, e.g. lithium (mechanism of action is unknown), reboxetine (selective noradrenaline reuptake inhibitor), mirtazapine (presynaptic α_2-antagonist).

Perioperative problems arising from concurrent antidepressant therapy may occur, particularly with MAOIs.

Antidiuretic hormone, *see Vasopressin*

Antiemetic drugs. Most act on the vomiting centre directly, e.g. antihistamine and anticholinergic drugs, or on the chemoreceptor trigger zone (CTZ), e.g. phenothiazines, butyrophenones and metoclopramide (Fig. 12). The latter group are dopamine receptor antagonists. In addition, metoclopramide increases lower oesophageal sphincter tone and gastric emptying by a peripheral action. Metoclopramide in very high dosage is thought to act via central 5-HT receptors; this has led to the development of 5-HT_3 receptor antagonists.

Dopamine antagonists are suitable for treatment of vomiting associated with morphine, which stimulates the CTZ. Increased vestibular stimulation of the vomiting centre, e.g. in motion sickness, is best treated with drugs acting on the vomiting centre, e.g. hyoscine. Sedation is a common side effect, particularly of antihistamines, anticholinergic drugs and phenothiazines. In addition, phenothiazines may cause hypotension, and all dopamine antagonists may cause dystonic reactions.

Dexamethasone 4–8 mg has been shown in many studies to have an antiemetic effect although its mechanism of action is uncertain. Cannabis derivatives have been used in the treatment of chemotherapy-induced emesis. More recently, the neurokinin-1 receptor antagonists have been developed

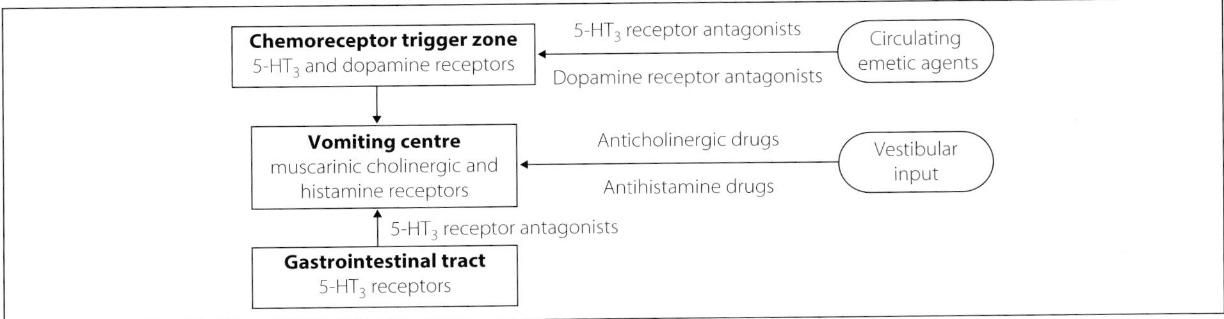

Fig. 12 Site of action of different antiemetic drugs

as antiemetic drugs, initially licensed for use in cancer chemotherapy.
See also, Postoperative nausea and vomiting

Anti-endotoxin antibodies. Antibodies directed against various parts of Gram-negative endotoxins; they have been investigated as possible treatments of severe sepsis. Theoretically, antibodies against the inner core of endotoxin (which is conserved among many different bacteria) should be useful in protecting against many organisms. They have conferred protection against Gram-negative infection in animal models, but their place in clinical practice is controversial. One (HA-1A; Centoxin) was introduced in 1991 for use in humans, but was withdrawn in 1993 following evidence that it might increase mortality in patients without Gram-negative bacteraemia. Another, E5, produced conflicting results in human trials and was never released.

Antifibrinolytic drugs. Drugs which prevent dissolution of fibrin. Include ε-aminocaproic acid (no longer available in the UK) and tranexamic acid, which inhibit plasminogen activation and thus reduce fibrinolysis. Sometimes used to reduce bleeding after prostatectomy and dental extraction and in uncontrollable postoperative haemorrhage in ICU.
See also, Coagulation

Antifungal drugs. Heterogeneous group of drugs active against fungi; includes:
- polyenes (amphotericin, nystatin).
- imidazoles (e.g. clotrimazole, ketoconazole, miconazole).
- triazoles (fluconazole, itraconazole, voriconazole).
- others (caspofungin, flucytosine, griseofulvin).

Antigen. Substance which may provoke an immune response, then react with the cells or antibodies produced. Usually a protein or carbohydrate molecule. Some substances (called haptens), too small to provoke immune reactions alone, may combine with host molecules, e.g. proteins, to form a larger antigenic combination.

Antigravity suit. Garment used to apply pressure to the lower half of the body, in order to increase blood volume in the upper half and prevent hypotension, e.g. in the sitting position in neurosurgery. Systolic BP and CVP are increased; the latter may aid prevention of air embolism. Modern suits are inflated pneumatically around the legs and abdomen, to a pressure of 2–8 kPa.

Military antishock trousers (MAST) have been used in trauma to produce similar effects. They also splint broken bones and apply pressure to bleeding points.

Antihistamine drugs. Refers to H_1 histamine receptor antagonists.
- Uses:
  - prevention or treatment of allergic disorders, e.g. hay fever, urticaria, drug reactions, e.g. chlorphenamine.
  - for sedation or in premedication, e.g. promethazine and alimemazine.
  - prevention/treatment of nausea and vomiting, e.g. cinnarizine, cyclizine (act on vomiting centre).

They have anticholinergic effects (e.g. dry mouth, blurring of vision, urinary retention). Newer drugs, e.g. terfenadine, cross the blood–brain barrier to a lesser extent, causing less sedation.
See also, H_2 receptor antagonists

Antihypertensive drugs. Drugs used to reduce BP may act at different sites (Fig. 13):
- diuretics: reduce ECF volume initially and also cause vasodilatation (1).
- vasodilator drugs: act on the vascular smooth muscle (2), either directly, e.g. hydralazine, sodium nitroprusside,

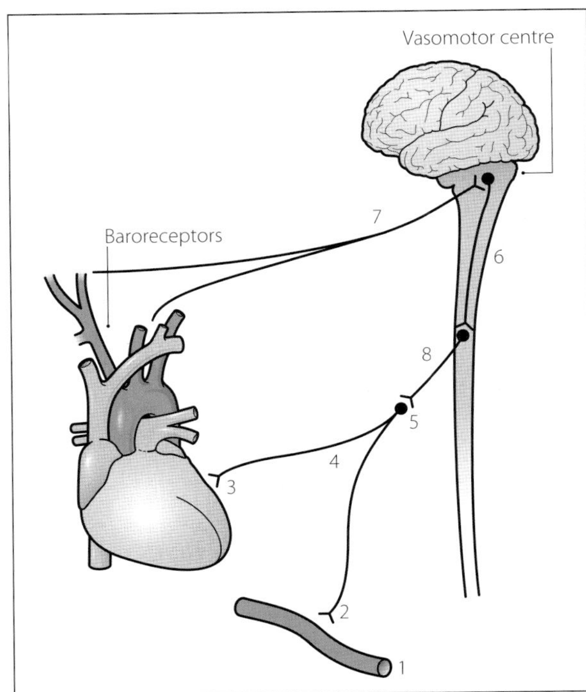

Fig. 13 Sites of action of antihypertensive drugs (see text)

or indirectly, e.g. α-adrenergic receptor antagonists, calcium channel blocking drugs, angiotensin II receptor antagonists. Angiotensin converting enzyme inhibitors also decrease water and sodium retention.

- β-adrenergic receptor antagonists: lower cardiac output (3).
- adrenergic neurone blocking drugs (4): e.g. guanethidine depletes nerve endings of noradrenaline, preventing its release. Reserpine prevents storage and release of noradrenaline. α-Methyl-p-tyrosine inhibits dopa formation from tyrosine.
- ganglion blocking drugs (5).
- centrally acting drugs (6): reduce sympathetic activity, e.g. reserpine, α-methyldopa, clonidine, moxonidine.

In addition, anaesthetic agents and techniques may reduce BP; e.g. halothane depresses baroreceptor activity (7) and also reduces sympathetic activity and cardiac output; spinal and epidural anaesthesia block sympathetic outflow (8).

In the treatment of hypertension, thiazide diuretics, β-adrenergic receptor antagonists and oral vasodilators (except for α-adrenergic receptor antagonists) are used most commonly. More recently, the AB/CD algorithm has been suggested: ACE inhibitors or β-antagonists for 'high renin' hypertension, typically younger and non-black patients, and calcium channel blocking drugs and/or diuretics for 'low renin' hypertension, typically older and black patients. NICE guidelines (2006) suggest an ACE inhibitor initially for young patients, and a thiazide or calcium blocker in older or black patients, with combination therapy if required (β- and α-antagonists as fourth line drugs).

Ganglion blockers, adrenergic neurone blocking drugs and the centrally acting drugs are seldom used, because of their side effects.

In the treatment of a hypertensive crisis, vasodilator drugs are often given iv. For patients undergoing surgery, antihypertensive drugs should be continued up to operation, and recommenced as soon as possible postoperatively.

See also, Hypotensive anaesthesia

Anti-inflammatory drugs, *see Non-steroidal anti-inflammatory drugs; Corticosteroids*

Antimalarial drugs. Used for:

- prophylaxis: no drugs give absolute protection against malaria. Treatment should begin at least 1 week prior to travel to an endemic area and continued for at least 4 weeks after leaving. Drugs used depend upon the area to be visited and include chloroquine, proguanil, mefloquine and doxycycline.
- treatment:
  - falciparum malaria: chloroquine is not used because of worldwide resistance. Quinine, mefloquine and halofantrine are the main treatments. Halofantrine is rarely used today; it can cause prolonged Q–T syndrome. Mefloquine is contraindicated in epilepsy. Artemether with lumefantrine has recently been introduced.
  - benign malaria: chloroquine is the drug of choice ± primaquine.

Baird JK (2005). N Engl J Med; 352: 1565–77

Antimitotic drugs, *see Cytotoxic drugs*

Antiparkinsonian drugs. Treatment of Parkinson's disease is directed towards increasing central dopaminergic activity, or decreasing cholinergic activity:

- increasing dopamine:
  - levodopa: crosses the blood–brain barrier and is converted to dopamine by dopa decarboxylase. Decarboxylase inhibitors (carbidopa, benserazide), which do not cross the blood–brain barrier, prevent peripheral dopamine formation, thus reducing the dose of levodopa required and the incidence of side effects. Entacapone prevents peripheral breakdown of levodopa by inhibiting catechol-O-methyl transferase and is used in combination with decarboxylase inhibitors in severe cases.

    Levodopa is most effective for bradykinesia. Its use may be limited by nausea and vomiting, dystonic movements, postural hypotension and psychiatric disturbances. Improvement is usually only temporary and may exhibit 'on–off' effectiveness.
  - bromocriptine, lisuride, pergolide and apomorphine: dopamine agonists. Ropinirole is a selective D_2 receptor agonist. Pramipexole is a D_2 and D_3 agonist.
  - amantadine: increases release of endogenous dopamine.
  - selegiline: monoamine oxidase inhibitor type B.
  - amfetamines have been used.
- anticholinergic drugs, e.g. atropine, benzatropine, trihexyphenidyl, procyclidine: most effective for rigidity, tremor, and treatment of drug-induced parkinsonism. For acute drug-induced dystonic reactions, benzatropine 1–2 mg or procyclidine 5–10 mg may be given iv.

There is a higher risk of intraoperative arrhythmias and labile BP in patients taking these drugs.

Antiphospholipid syndrome, *see Coagulation disorders*

Antiplatelet drugs. Reduce platelet adhesion and aggregation, thereby inhibiting intraluminal thrombus formation. May act via different mechanisms:

- inhibition of platelet cyclo-oxygenase and thromboxane α_2 production; may be reversible, e.g. prostacyclin, or irreversible, e.g. low dose aspirin, and other NSAIDs.
- increased intraplatelet cAMP levels, e.g. dipyridamole.
- inhibition of glycoprotein IIb/IIIa complex activation (the site at which fibrinogen, von Willebrand factor and adhesive proteins bind to platelets); may be reversible, e.g. abciximab, eptifibatide, tirofiban (all given iv), or irreversible, e.g. clopidogrel, ticlopidine (both taken orally).

Used to improve cerebral, peripheral and coronary blood supply in vascular disease, and to prevent thromboembolism. Glycoprotein IIb/IIIa inhibitors are recommended for high risk patients with unstable angina or non-Q wave MI and for those undergoing percutaneous transluminal coronary angioplasty. Dextran also has an antiplatelet action and has been used to prevent postoperative DVT and PE.

Patients receiving these drugs who present for surgery may be at increased risk of bleeding. The place of regional anaesthesia in such patients is controversial because of the possibly increased risk of spinal haematoma.

See also, Anticoagulant drugs; Coagulation

Antispasmodic drugs. Used as adjunctive therapy in the management of non-ulcer dyspepsia, irritable bowel syndrome and diverticular disease. Also administered during GIT endoscopy and radiology, and when constructing bowel anastomoses.

Include:

- antimuscarinic agents (e.g. atropine, dicycloverine, hyoscine, propantheline). Produce dry mouth, blurred

vision, urinary retention and constipation. Also relax the oesophageal sphincter, causing gastrooesophageal reflux.
- others: e.g. alverine, mebeverine, peppermint oil: direct intestinal smooth muscle relaxants.

Antispasmodics should not be used in patients with ileus.

Antistatic precautions. Employed in operating suites, to prevent build-up of static electricity with possible sparks, explosions and fires. Surfaces and materials should have relatively low electrical resistance, to allow leakage of charge to earth, but not so low as to allow electrocution and electrical burns.

- Precautions include:
  - avoidance of wool, nylon, silk, etc., which may generate static charge. Cotton blankets and clothing are suitable (resistance is very low in moist atmospheres).
  - antistatic rubber (containing carbon) for tubing, etc. Coloured black with yellow labels for identification. Resistance is 100 000–10 000 000 ohms/cm.
  - terrazzo floor (stone pieces embedded in cement and polished): resistance should be 20 000–5 000 000 ohms between two points 60 cm apart.
  - trolleys and other equipment have conducting wheels; staff wear antistatic footwear.

Sparks are more likely in cold dry atmospheres, therefore relative humidity should exceed 50% and temperature exceed 20°C.

The requirement for expensive antistatic flooring and other precautions has been questioned, since the use of flammable anaesthetic agents such as cyclopropane and diethyl ether has ceased in the UK, and although fires may still occur with other substances (e.g. alcohol skin cleansers), ignition is usually caused by a high energy source such as diathermy or laser rather than static electricity.

Antithrombin III. Cofactor of heparin and natural inhibitor of coagulation. Often deficient in critical illness such as sepsis hence its investigation as a possible treatment, though evidence suggests that therapy causes no improvement in outcome whilst increasing bleeding complications.

Torossian A, Graf J, Bauhofer (2007). Br Med J; 335: 1219–20

Antituberculous drugs. Used for:

- prophylaxis: advised for susceptible close contacts or following treatment of TB in immunocompromised patients. Comprises isoniazid daily for 6 months alone, or combined with rifampicin daily for 3 months.
- treatment: carried out in two phases:
  - initial phase (2 months) using at least three drugs: intended to reduce the number of viable organisms as quickly as possible to avoid resistance. Usually includes isoniazid, rifampicin, pyrazinamide and ethambutol (the last added if resistance is thought likely). Streptomycin is rarely used today but sometimes added if resistance to isoniazid is present.
  - continuation phase (further 4 months) using two drugs: intended to eradicate the bacteria from the body (longer treatment may be required in bone, joint, CNS and resistant infections). Usually comprises continuation of isoniazid and rifampicin therapy.

Other drugs used in resistant cases or when side effects are limiting include capreomycin, cycloserine, azithromycin, clarithromycin, 4-quinolones and rifabutin.

Treatment must be supervised if non-compliance is suspected since partial completion of treatment courses is a major factor in producing resistance. During use of antituberculous drugs (especially pyrazinamide, isoniazid and rifampicin), monitoring of liver function is mandatory. Streptomycin and ethambutol should be avoided in patients with renal impairment.

Chan ED, Iseman MD (2002). Br Med J; 325: 1282–6

Antiviral drugs. Heterogeneous group of drugs with generally non-specific actions. Parenteral use is usually reserved for severe life-threatening systemic infections, especially in immunocompromised patients. Available drugs can best be classified according to the infections in which they are used:

- herpes simplex/varicella zoster:
  - aciclovir: purine nucleoside analogue; after phosphorylation, it inhibits viral DNA polymerase. Phosphorylated by, and therefore active against, herpes simplex and varicella zoster viruses. Early initiation of treatment is important. May be useful in HIV infection. May be given topically, orally or iv; side effects include GIT upset, rashes, and deteriorating renal and liver function.
  - famciclovir, valaciclovir, idoxuridine, inosine, amantadine: used for herpes and zoster infection of the skin and mucous membranes.
- HIV:
  - nucleoside reverse transcriptase inhibitors: e.g. zidovudine, abacavir, zalcitabine, didanosine, stavudine, lamivudine, tenofovir.
  - protease inhibitors: e.g. indinavir, ritonavir, lopinavir, nelfinavir, amprenavir, saquinavir. May cause metabolic derangement including hyperlipidaemia and redistribution of body fat, insulin resistance and hyperglycaemia.
  - non-nucleoside reverse transcriptase inhibitors: e.g. efavirenz, nevirapine. May cause severe skin reactions and hepatic impairment.
- cytomegalovirus: ganciclovir, valganciclovir, foscarnet.
- respiratory syncitial virus: tribavirin.

In addition, interferons are used in hepatitis infections.

Antoine equation. Describes the theoretical variation of SVP with temperature. Empirically relates SVP to three constants, derived from experimental data for each substance.
[C Antoine (described 1888), French scientist]

Aortic aneurysm, abdominal. Manifestation of peripheral vascular disease, most often due to atherosclerosis. Usually occurs in males over 60 years old. Often presents with abdominal or back pain, or as an asymptomatic, pulsatile abdominal swelling, increasingly detected by ultrasound screening. May rupture or dissect acutely leading to death; leakage is amenable to urgent surgical intervention. Elective surgery is indicated when the diameter of the aneurysm exceeds 5 cm. The traditional open procedure is usually performed via an abdominal incision from xiphisternum to pubis. Alternatives include endoluminal repair, in which a graft is placed via percutaneous arterial puncture, or a semi-laparoscopic method, in which much of the mobilisation is achieved via small incisions before grafting. Preparation should be as for the open technique since the risk of proceeding or of severe, sudden haemorrhage is always present. Endoluminal repair in particular has been shown to reduce blood loss, organ dysfunction, hospital stay and early mortality, although mortality at 1 year is thought to be the same as after open repair.

- Anaesthetic considerations for elective repair:
  - preoperative assessment is particularly directed to the effects of widespread atherosclerosis, i.e. affecting

coronary, renal, cerebral and peripheral arteries. Hypertension is also common.
- perioperatively:
  - monitoring: ECG; direct arterial, central venous and possibly pulmonary artery pressure measurement; temperature; urine output.
  - at least two large bore iv cannulae.
  - warming blanket and warming of iv fluids. Humidification of inspired gases.
  - cardiovascular responses:
    - hypertension during tracheal intubation.
    - increased afterload caused by aortic cross-clamping. Hypertension and left ventricular failure may occur. Anticipatory use of vasodilator drugs may help to reduce hypertension and left ventricular strain.
    - reduction of afterload, return of vasodilator metabolites from lower part of the body, and possible haemorrhage following aortic unclamping (declamping syndrome). Myocardial contractility is reduced by the acidotic venous return. Anticipatory volume loading prior to unclamping, with termination of vasodilator therapy before slow controlled release of the clamp, may reduce hypotension. Bicarbonate therapy is guided by arterial acid–base analysis; it is often not required if clamping time is less than 1–1.5 h.
  - blood loss and effects of massive blood transfusion.
  - postoperative visceral dysfunction:
    - renal failure may follow aortic surgery; it is more likely to occur after suprarenal cross-clamping. Mannitol, furosemide or dopamine is often given before aortic clamping, to encourage diuresis.
    - GIT ischaemia and infarction may occur if the mesenteric arterial supply is interrupted. The anterior spinal artery syndrome may also occur.

    Attempts to reduce the effects of renal and GIT ischaemia have also included hypothermia and use of metabolic precursors, e.g. inosine.
- postoperatively: ICU or HDU. Elective IPPV may be required. Epidural analgesia is often used.

- For emergency surgery, the following are important:
  - preinduction monitoring and insertion of lines.
  - preparation and towelling of the patient before induction.
  - availability of blood, O negative if necessary.
  - rapid sequence induction. Etomidate or ketamine is often used.

Abdominal muscular relaxation following induction of anaesthesia may result in decreased abdominal 'tamponade' of the leaking aneurysm, resulting in further haemorrhage and hypotension. Prognosis is generally poor.

See also, Aortic aneurysm, thoracic; Blood transfusion, massive; Induction, rapid sequence

Aortic aneurysm, thoracic. Usually results from aortic dissection. Surgical approach is via left thoracotomy; one-lung anaesthesia facilitates surgery. Concurrent aortic valve replacement may be required. General anaesthetic management is as for abdominal aneurysm repair. Cardiovascular instability may be more dramatic because of the proximity of the aortic clamp to the heart, and the reduction of venous return and cardiac output during surgical manoeuvres. Complications include haemorrhage and infarction of spinal cord, liver, gut, kidneys and heart. Perioperative drainage of CSF is commonly performed to reduce spinal cord ischaemia. Operative techniques may include atriofemoral cardiopulmonary bypass, or use of a shunt across the clamped aortic section.

See also, Aortic aneurysm, abdominal

Aortic bodies. Peripheral chemoreceptors near the aortic arch. Similar in structure and function to the carotid bodies. Afferents pass to the medulla via the vagus.

Aortic coarctation, *see Coarctation of aorta*

Aortic counter-pulsation balloon pump, *see Intra-aortic counter-pulsation balloon pump*

Aortic dissection. Passage of blood into the aortic wall, usually involving the media of the vessel. Degeneration of this layer is usually caused by atherosclerosis but is also seen in Marfan's syndrome and Ehlers–Danlos syndrome. Often associated with hypertension. Dissection may involve branches of the aorta, including the coronary arteries. Additionally, rupture into pericardium, pleural cavity, mediastinum or abdomen may occur. May also follow chest trauma. Classified according to site:
- type I: starts in the ascending aorta, extending proximally to the aortic valve and distally around the aortic arch (least common).
- type II: limited to the ascending aorta.
- type III: starts near the left subclavian artery, extending along the descending aorta.

- Features:
  - severe tearing central chest pain; may mimic MI. May radiate to the back or abdomen.
  - signs of aortic regurgitation.
  - signs of haemorrhage or cardiac tamponade.
  - progressive loss of radial pulses and CVA may indicate extension along the aortic arch. Coronary artery involvement may cause MI. Renal vessels may be involved.
  - chest X-ray may reveal a widened mediastinum or pleural effusion. Echocardiography, CT/MRI scanning and aortography may be used in diagnosis.
- Management:
  - analgesia.
  - control of BP, e.g. using vasodilator drugs.
  - surgery is increasingly employed, especially if the aortic valve is involved, dissection progresses or rupture occurs. Management: as for thoracic aortic aneurysm.

[Edward Ehlers (1863–1937), Danish dermatologist; Henri Alexandre Danlos (1844–1912), French dermatologist]

See also, Aortic aneurysm, thoracic

Aortic regurgitation. Retrograde flow of blood through the aortic valve during diastole. Causes left ventricular hypertrophy and dilatation, with greatly increased stroke volume. Later, compliance decreases and end-diastolic pressure increases, with ventricular failure.
- Caused by:
  - rheumatic fever; usually affects the mitral value too.
  - aortic dissection.
  - endocarditis (especially acute regurgitation).
  - Marfan's syndrome.
  - congenital defect (associated with aortic stenosis).
  - chest trauma, ankylosing spondylitis, rheumatoid disease, syphilis.
- Features:
  - collapsing pulse with widened pulse pressure (water hammer). Bobbing of the head in synchrony with the pulse (Musset's sign) may occur.
  - early diastolic murmur, high pitched and blowing. Loudest in expiration and with the patient leaning forward, and heard at the left sternal edge, sometimes at the apex. The 3rd heart sound may be present. A thrill is absent. An aortic ejection murmur is usually present, radiating

to the neck; a mid-diastolic mitral murmur may be present due to obstruction by aortic backflow (Austin Flint murmur).
- left ventricular failure.
- angina is usually late.
- investigations: ECG may show left ventricular hypertrophy; chest X-ray may show ventricular enlargement/failure. Echocardiography and cardiac catheterisation are also useful.

- Anaesthetic management:
  - antibiotic prophylaxis as for congenital heart disease.
  - general principles: as for cardiac surgery/ischaemic heart disease. Myocardial ischaemia and left ventricular failure may occur.
  - the following should be avoided:
    - bradycardia: increases time for regurgitation.
    - peripheral vasoconstriction and increased diastolic pressure: increases afterload and therefore regurgitation. Peripheral vasodilatation reduces regurgitation and increases forward flow.
  - cardioplegia solution is infused directly into the coronary arteries during cardiac surgery, since if injected into the aortic root it will enter the ventricle.
  - left ventricular end-diastolic pressure may be much greater than measured pulmonary capillary wedge pressure, if the mitral valve is closed early by the regurgitant backflow.
  - postoperative hypertension may occur.

[Austin Flint (1812–1886), US physician; Alfred de Musset (1810–1857), French poet]

See also, Heart murmurs; Preoperative assessment; Valvular heart disease

Aortic stenosis. Narrowed aortic valve with obstruction to the left ventricular outflow, resulting in a pressure gradient between the left ventricle and aortic root. Initially, left ventricular hypertrophy and increased force of contraction maintain stroke volume. Compliance is decreased. Coronary blood flow is decreased due to increased left ventricular end-diastolic pressure and involvement of the coronary sinuses, whilst left ventricular work increases. Ultimately, contractility falls, with left ventricular dilatation and reduced cardiac output.

- Caused by:
  - rheumatic fever: may present at any age (usually also involves the mitral valve).
  - congenital bicuspid valve: usually presents in middle age.
  - degenerative calcification: usually in the elderly.
- Features:
  - angina (30–40%), syncope, left ventricular failure.
  - sudden death.
  - low volume slow-rising pulse with reduced pulse pressure (plateau pulse). AF usually signifies coexistent mitral disease.
  - ejection systolic murmur, radiating to the neck. Loudest in the aortic area, with the patient sitting forward in expiration. The second heart sound is quiet, with reversed splitting if stenosis is severe (due to delayed left ventricular emptying). A thrill, 4th sound and ejection click may be present.
  - investigations: ECG may show left ventricular hypertrophy; chest X-ray may show ventricular enlargement/failure, possibly with calcification and poststenotic dilatation. Echocardiography and cardiac catheterisation are especially useful. The gradient across the valve exceeds 50 mmHg in severe stenosis, falling as left ventricular failure supervenes. Normal valve area is 2.6–3.5 cm^2; in moderate and severe stenosis the area is reduced to $<$ 1.0 and $<$ 0.7 cm^2 respectively.
- Anaesthetic management:
  - antibiotic prophylaxis as for congenital heart disease.
  - general principles: as for cardiac surgery/ischaemic heart disease. Myocardial ischaemia, ventricular arrhythmias and left ventricular failure may occur.
  - the following should be avoided:
    - loss of sinus rhythm: atrial contraction is vital to maintain adequate ventricular filling.
    - peripheral vasodilatation: cardiac output is fixed, therefore BP may fall dramatically causing myocardial ischaemia.
    - excessive peripheral vasoconstriction: further reduces left ventricular outflow.
    - tachycardia: ventricular filling is impaired and coronary blood flow reduced.
    - myocardial depression.
  - postoperative hypertension may occur.

See also, Heart murmurs; Preoperative assessment; Valvular heart disease

Aortocaval compression (Supine hypotension syndrome). Compression of the great vessels against the vertebral bodies by the gravid uterus in the supine position in late pregnancy. Vena caval compression reduces venous return and cardiac output with a compensatory increase in SVR; this may be symptomless ('concealed'), or associated with hypotension, bradycardia or syncope ('revealed'). Reduced placental blood flow may result from the reduced cardiac output, vasoconstriction and compression of the aorta. During uterine contractions, the compression may worsen (Poseiro effect). Reduced cardiac output is more likely to occur if vasoconstrictor reflexes are impaired, e.g. during regional or general anaesthesia. May be reduced by tilting the mother to one side, e.g. with a wedge. Up to 45° tilt may be required. Left lateral tilt is usually preferable.

See also, Obstetric analgesia and anaesthesia

Aortovelography. Use of a Doppler ultrasound probe in the suprasternal notch to measure blood velocity and acceleration in the ascending aorta. Used for cardiac output measurement, but inaccurate.

APACHE scoring system (Acute physiology and chronic health evaluation). Tool described in 1981 for assessing the severity of illness of individual patients and predicting the risk of hospital mortality for groups of patients treated in ICUs. Consists of two parts: an acute physiology score (APS) and an assessment of the patient's pre-illness health status. The APS is combined with the pre-admission health status (assigned A–D by reviewing his/her medical history for details from the previous 6 months) to give the final APACHE score, e.g. 36-B. Rarely used now because of acknowledged superiority of other systems, e.g. APACHE II, APACHE III, SAPS, MPM.

Wong DT, Knaus WA (1991). Can J Anaesth; 38: 374–83

See also, Mortality/survival prediction on intensive care unit

APACHE II scoring system (Acute physiology and chronic health evaluation; version II). Revised version of the prototype APACHE scoring system, described in 1985. Internationally, the most frequently used intensive care severity of illness scoring system. The number of physiological measurements used in the acute physiology score has been reduced to 12, chosen using a combination of subjective clinical opinion and objective statistical analysis. Weightings are allocated for the degree of derangement of each physiological parameter in the first 24 h after ICU admission (range 0–4), age and chronic health (Table 6). Definitions of chronic health are more specific than in the original APACHE system. The assigned weights for all physiological measurements, age and chronic health are summated to give an APACHE II score (maximum 71), which is further integrated with the patient's diagnosis to calculate the estimate of hospital mortality.

APACHE II has been validated in many large centres and is thought to be a reliable method for estimating group outcome amongst ICU patients. Survival rates of 50% have been reported for an admission score of about 25 points, with 80% mortality for scores above 35 points. More recently, repeated assessments (i.e. change in APACHE II score over time) have been used to chart patients' progress.

Wong DT, Knaus WA (1991). Can J Anaesth; 38: 374–83

See also, APACHE III scoring system, Mortality/survival prediction on intensive care unit

APACHE III scoring system (Acute physiology, age and chronic health evaluation). Latest version of the APACHE scoring system introduced in 1991 in an attempt to improve upon the risk prediction available with APACHE II. Consists of a numerical score (range 0–299) reflecting the weights assigned to the variables of three principal data categories: physiological measurements, chronological age (the emphasis on age reflected in the reassignment of the second 'A' in 'APACHE') and chronic health status. APACHE III uses data from 16 physiological measurements. Weighting of physiological abnormalities is considerably more complex than in earlier versions of the APACHE system and physiological abnormalities have a greater relative importance in the APACHE III score and predictive equations. The chronic health component has been modified and is based on 7 variables referring to the presence or absence of haematological malignancies, lymphoma, AIDS, metastatic cancer, immunosuppression, hepatic failure and liver cirrhosis.

APACHE III uses 78 mutually exclusive disease definitions to group patients according to the principal reason for ICU admission. Patients admitted directly from the operating or recovery room are classified as operative (surgical), and are further subdivided according to the urgency of the operation (elective versus emergency). All other patients are classified as non-operative (medical). In order to assess the impact of therapeutic interventions before ICU admission, additional information about the patient's treatment location immediately prior to admission was integrated into the APACHE III model. The APACHE III score is integrated with the patient's diagnosis and source prior to ICU to calculate the estimate of hospital mortality. Although its performance is slightly better than that of APACHE II, APACHE III is less widely used because the predictive equations it employs are commercially protected.

Wong DT, Knaus WA (1991). Can J Anaesth; 38: 374–83

See also, Mortality/survival prediction on intensive care unit

Apgar scoring system. Widely used method of evaluating the condition of the neonate, described in 1953. Points are awarded up to a maximum total of 10 according to clinical findings (Table 5). Assessments are commonly performed at 1 and 5 min after birth, but may be repeated as necessary. Colour may be omitted from the observed signs to give a maximum score of 8 (Apgar minus colour score).

[Virginia Apgar (1909–1975), US anaesthetist]

Table 5 Apgar scoring system

Sign	*Score 0*	*Score 1*	*Score 2*
Heart rate	Absent	<100	>100
Respiratory effort	Absent	Weak cry	Strong cry
Muscle tone	Limp	Poor tone	Good tone
Reflex irritability	No response	Some movement	Strong withdrawal
Colour	Blue, pale	Pink body, blue extremities	Pink

APLS, *see Advanced Paediatric Life Support*

Apneustic centre, *see Breathing, control of*

Apnoea. Absence of breathing. Causes are as for hypoventilation. Results in hypercapnia and hypoxaemia. The rate of onset and severity of hypoxaemia are related to the F_IO_2, FRC and O_2 consumption. Thus preoxygenation delays the onset of hypoxaemia following apnoea. In pregnancy, hypoxaemia develops more quickly, due to reduced FRC and increased O_2 consumption.

Alveolar $P\text{CO}_2$ rises at about 0.5 kPa/min (3.8 mmHg/min) when CO_2 production is normal.

In paediatrics, prematurity is a major cause of recurrent apnoea. In newborn animals, induced hypoxaemia results in vigorous efforts to breathe, followed by primary apnoea and bradycardia, then secondary (terminal) apnoea after a few gasps. During primary apnoea, gasping and possibly spontaneous respiration may be induced by stimulation; the gasp reflex is also active. During secondary apnoea, active resuscitation and oxygenation are required to restore breathing.

See also, Cardiopulmonary resuscitation, neonatal; Sleep apnoea

Apnoeic oxygenation. Method of delivering O_2 to the lungs by insufflation during apnoea. A catheter is passed into the trachea, its tip lying at the carina. O_2 passed through it at 4–6 l/min reaches the alveoli mainly by mass diffusion, with O_2 utilised faster than CO_2 is produced. The technique does not remove CO_2, which rises at a rate of approximately 0.5 kPa/min (3.8 mmHg/min) at normal rates of CO_2 production. Hypercapnia may therefore occur during prolonged procedures.

May be used to maintain oxygenation, e.g. during bronchoscopy, or during the diagnosis of brainstem death.

See also, Insufflation techniques

Apomorphine hydrochloride. Alkaloid derived from morphine, with a powerful agonist action at both D_1 and D_2 dopamine receptors. Used to treat refractory motor fluctuations in Parkinson's disease which are inadequately controlled by levodopa or other dopaminergic drugs. Overdosage causes respiratory depression which is reversed by naloxone. Causes intense stimulation of the chemoreceptor trigger zone resulting in vomiting. Needs to be prescribed with an antiemetic drug. Has previously been used as an emetic drug to empty the stomach, but rarely used now because of the superior safety profile of ipecachuana.

- Dosage: 3–30 mg/day as sc boluses (max 10 mg per bolus) or 1–4 mg/h sc by infusion, up to 100 mg/day (changing the injection site every 12 h).
- Side effects: vomiting, salivation, worsening dyskinesia, sedation, local ulceration.

Table 6 APACHE II scoring system

Physiological variable	High abnormal range +4	+3	+2	+1	0	Low normal range +1	+2	+3	+4
Temperature – rectal (°C)	≥41°	39°–40.9°		38.5°–38.9°	36°–38.4°	34°–35.9°	32°–33.9°	30°–31.9°	≤29.9°
Mean arterial pressure (mmHg)	>160	130–159	110–129		70–109		50–69		≤49
Heart rate (ventricular response)	≥180	140–179	110–139		70–109		55–69	40–54	≤39
Respiratory rate (non-ventilated or ventilated)	≥50	35–49		25–34	12–24	10–11	6–9		≤5
Oxygenation: A–aO_2 or P_aO_2 (kPa (mmHg))									
(a) F_IO_2 ≥0.5 record A–aO_2	>67 (>500)	47–66.9 (350–499)	27–46.9 (300–349)		<27 (<200)				
(b) F_IO_2 <0.5 record only P_aO_2					>9.3 (>70)	8.1–9.3 (61–70)		7.3–8.0 (55–60)	<7.3 (<55)
Arterial pH	≥7.7	7.6–7.69		7.5–7.59	7.33–7.49		7.25–7.32	7.15–7.24	<7.15
Serum sodium (mmol/l)	≥180	160–179	155–159	150–154	130–149		120–129	111–119	≤110
Serum potassium (mmol/l)	≥7	6–6.9		5.5–5.9	3.5–5.4	3–3.4	2.5–2.9		<2.5
Serum creatinine (μmmol/l (mg/100 ml)) (Double point score for *acute* renal failure)	>301 (≥3.5)	170–300 (2–3.4)	130–169 (1.5–1.9)		50–129 (0.6–1.4)		<50 (<0.6)		
Haematocrit (%)	≥60		50–59.9	46–49.9	30–45.9		20–29.9		<20
White blood count (total/mm^3) (in 1000s)	≥40		20–39.9	15–19.9	3–14.9		1–2.9		<1
Glasgow coma scale (GCS) Score = 15 minus actual GCS									
A Total Acute Physiology Score (APS) Sum of the 12 individual variable points									
Serum HCO_3^-, (venous mmol/l) (Not preferred, use if no ABGs)	≥52	41–51.9		32–40.9	22–31.9		18–21.9	15–17.9	<15

B AGE POINTS

Assign points to age as follows:

AGE (years)	Points
≤44	0
45–54	2
55–64	5
65–74	5
≥75	6

C CHRONIC HEALTH POINTS

If the patient has a history of severe organ system insufficiency or is immunocompromised assign points as follows:

(a) for non-operative or emergency postoperative patients +5 points or

(b) for elective postoperative patients +2 points

DEFINITIONS

Organ insufficiency or immunocompromised state must have been evident *prior* to this hospital admission and conform to the following criteria:

LIVER: Biopsy-proven cirrhosis and documented portal hypertension; episodes of past upper GI bleeding attributed to portal hypertension, or prior episodes of hepatic failure/encephalopathy/coma

CARDIOVASCULAR: New York Heart Association Class IV (inability to perform physical activity)

RESPIRATORY: Chronic restrictive, obstructive, or vascular disease resulting in severe exercise restriction, i.e. unable to climb stairs or perform household duties, or documented chronic hypoxia, hypercapnia, secondary polycythaemia, severe pulmonary hypertension (>40 mmHg), or respiratory dependency

RENAL: Receiving chronic dialysis

IMMUNOCOMPROMISED: The patient has received therapy that suppresses resistance to infection, e.g. immunosuppression, chemotherapy, radiation, long-term or recent high dose corticosteroids, or has a disease that is sufficiently advanced to suppress resistance to infection, e.g. leukaemia, lymphoma, AIDS

APACHE II SCORE

Sum of **A** + **B** + **C**

A APS points

B Age points

C Chronic health points

Total APACHE II

Aprepitant. Neurokinin-1 receptor antagonist, licensed as an antiemetic drug as part of combination therapy (with a corticosteroid and a 5-HT_3 receptor antagonist) in cancer chemotherapy. Has been studied in PONV.
- Dosage: 125 mg, 80 mg and 80 mg orally on 3 successive days.
- Side effect: hiccups, fatigue.

Aprotinin. Proteolytic enzyme inhibitor. Inhibits:
  - plasmin (at low dose, causing reduced fibrinolysis).
  - kallikrein (at higher dose, causing reduced coagulation).
  - trypsin.

Intermediate doses cause reduced platelet aggregation. Has been used to reduce perioperative blood loss, e.g. in cardiac surgery. May also be useful in the treatment of haemorrhage due to hyperplasminaemia (e.g. during dissection of malignant tumours, in acute promyelocytic leukaemia and following thrombolytic therapy). Its usefulness in acute pancreatitis is unproven. The manufacturers ceased marketing it in 2007 pending investigation of claims that its use increases mortality following cardiac surgery.
- Dosage:
  - cardiac surgery: 2 000 000 units iv before sternotomy (50 000 units slowly to test for allergy, followed by 1 950 000 units over 20 min) then 500 000/h by infusion until surgery ends.
  - hyperplasminaemia: 500 000–1 000 000 units over 5–10 min, followed by 200 000 units hourly as required.

Hypersensitivity reactions may occur.

APRV, *see Airway pressure release ventilation*

APS, *see Acute physiology score*

Apudomas. Tumours of amine precursor uptake and decarboxylation (APUD) cells. APUD cells are present in the anterior pituitary gland, thyroid gland, adrenal gland medulla, GIT, pancreatic islets, carotid body and lung. Originally thought to arise from neural crest tissue; now thought to be derived from endoderm. They have similar structural and biochemical properties, secreting polypeptides and amines. They may secrete hormones which cause systemic disturbances, e.g. insulin, glucagon, catecholamines, 5-HT, somatostatin, gastrin and vasoactive intestinal peptide.
See also, Carcinoid syndrome; Multiple endocrine adenomatosis; Phaeochromocytoma

Arachidonic acid. Essential fatty acid synthesised from phospholipids and metabolised by lipoxygenase and cyclo-oxygenase to leukotrienes and endoperoxides respectively (Fig. 14). Endoperoxides form prostaglandins, prostacyclin and thromboxanes via separate pathways. The pathways are inhibited by corticosteroids and NSAIDs as shown.

Arachidonic acid may also undergo peroxidation during oxidative stress, under the action of free radicals, with the production of isoprostanes.

Arachnoiditis. Inflammation of the arachnoid and pial meninges. Has occurred after spinal and epidural anaesthesia; antiseptic solutions and preservatives in drug solutions (e.g. sodium bisulphite) have been implicated. Also occurs after radiotherapy, trauma and myelography with oil-based contrast media. May occur months or years after the insult. Progressive fibrosis may cause spinal canal narrowing, ischaemia and permanent nerve damage. The cauda equina is usually affected, with pain, muscle weakness, and loss of sphincter control. May rarely spread cranially. Response to treatment is generally poor.
See also, Cauda equina syndrome

ARAS, *see Ascending reticular activating system*

ARDS, *see Acute respiratory distress syndrome*

Argatroban. Hirudin, studied as an alternative to heparin. Similar to lepirudin but excreted via the liver as opposed to the kidneys. Half-life is 30–60 min, thus requiring administration by continuous infusion.

Arginine vasopressin/argipressin, *see Vasopressin*

Arm–brain circulation time. Time taken for a substance injected into an arm vein (traditionally antecubital) to reach the brain. If a bile salt is injected, the time until arrival of the bitter taste at the tongue may be measured (normally 10–20 s; this may be greatly prolonged when cardiac output is reduced). Useful conceptually when comparing different iv induction agents; thus thiopental acts 'within one arm–brain circulation time', whereas midazolam takes longer.

Arrhythmias. Disturbances in normal sinus rhythm.
- Classification:
  - disorders of impulse formation:
    - supraventricular:
      - sinus arrhythmia, bradycardia and tachycardia.
      - SVT.
      - sick sinus syndrome.
      - AF, atrial flutter, atrial ectopic beats.
    - junctional arrhythmias.
    - VF, ventricular tachycardia, ventricular ectopic beats.
  - disorders of impulse conduction:
    - slowed/blocked conduction (e.g. heart block).
    - abnormal pathway of conduction (e.g. Wolff–Parkinson–White syndrome).

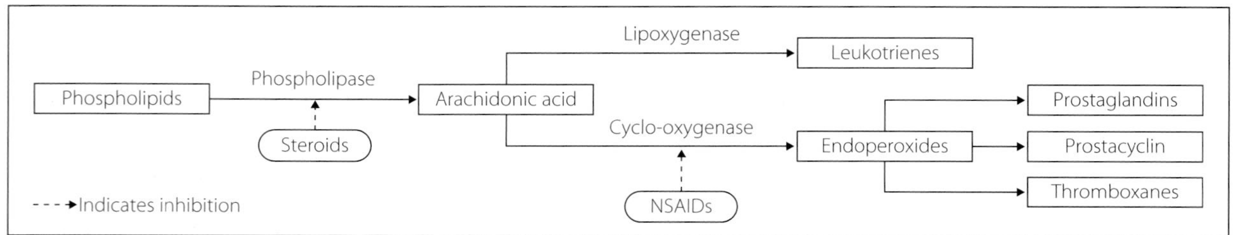

Fig. 14 Arachidonic acid pathways

Arrhythmias, especially tachycardias, are common in acute illness. During anaesthesia, ECG monitoring is mandatory. Bradycardia, junctional rhythm and ventricular ectopic beats (including bigemini) are common, but usually not serious.

- Arrhythmias are more likely with:
  - pre-existing cardiac disease.
  - hypoxaemia and hypercapnia.
  - acid–base disturbances.
  - electrolyte abnormalities, especially of potassium, calcium, magnesium.
  - drugs, e.g. inotropic drugs, antiarrhythmic drugs, theophylline, cocaine. During anaesthesia, halothane sensitises the myocardium to catecholamines.
  - mechanical stimulation of heart chambers (e.g. central venous/pulmonary artery catheterisation).
  - pacemaker malfunction.
  - certain diseases, e.g. thyrotoxicosis, subarachnoid haemorrhage.
  - manoeuvres which activate powerful reflex pathways, e.g. during dental surgery, oculocardiac reflex, visceral manipulation, tracheobronchial suctioning.

Special Supplement (2000). Crit Care Med; 28: N115–80

Arterial blood pressure. The pulsatile ejection of the stroke volume gives rise to the arterial waveform, from which systolic, diastolic and mean arterial pressures may be determined.

MAP = cardiac output × SVR

Thus arterial pressure may vary with changes in cardiac output (stroke volume × heart rate) and vascular resistance.

- Control of BP:
  - short term:
    - intrinsic regulatory properties of the heart: Anrep effect, Bowditch effect, Starling's law.
    - autonomic pathways involving baroreceptors, vasomotor centre and cardioinhibitory centre.
    - hormonal mechanisms:
      - renin/angiotensin system.
      - vasopressin.
      - adrenaline and noradrenaline as part of the sympathetic response.
  - intermediate/long term: renin/angiotensin system, aldosterone, vasopressin, atrial natriuretic peptide, endocannibinoids.

See also, Arterial blood pressure measurement; Diastolic blood pressure; Hypertension

Arterial blood pressure measurement. First attempted by Hales in 1733, who inserted pipes several feet long into the arteries of animals. The BP cuff was introduced by Riva-Rocci in 1896. Measurement and recording of BP was introduced into anaesthetic practice by Cushing in 1901.

- May be direct or indirect:
  - direct:
    - gives a continuous reading; i.e. changes may be noticed rapidly.
    - provides additional information from the shape of the arterial waveform.
    - requires arterial cannulation.
    - requires calibration and zeroing of the monitoring system.
    - resonance and damping may cause inaccuracy.
  - indirect:
    - palpation (unreliable).
    - mercury or aneroid manometer attached to a cuff: the brachial artery is palpated and the cuff inflated to 30–60 mmHg above the pressure at which the pulsation disappears, i.e. well above systolic pressure. Cuff pressure is released at 2–3 mmHg/s, and pressure measured by detecting pulsation by using the Korotkoff sounds, a pulse detector or Doppler probe. The cuff width must be 20% greater than the arm's diameter or half its circumference; narrower cuffs will over-read. Error may arise between different observers. BP should be recorded to the nearest 2 mmHg.
    - oscillotonometer.
    - automatic measuring devices which use the same cuff for inflation and detection of movement of the arterial walls. Consecutive pulsations are compared, and complex circuitry prevents error from patient movement, etc. Systolic and MAP are usually measured and diastolic pressure calculated. Tend to over-read when pressures are high, and under-read when low. Inconsistencies occur if the cardiac cycle is irregular, e.g. in atrial fibrillation.
    - Finapres device: a cuff is inflated around a finger, and its pressure varied continuously to keep its volume constant, using infra-red photometry to measure volume. Cuff pressure is proportional to finger arterial pressure; a continuous display of the arterial pressure waveform is obtained. May be unreliable if peripheral vascular disease is present.
    - continuous arterial tonometry: a pressure transducer is positioned over the radial artery, compressing it against the radius. The transducer output voltage is proportional to the arterial BP, which is displayed as a continuous trace. Periodic calibration is performed using an automatic oscillometric cuff on the arm.

[Stephen Hales (1677–1761), English curate and naturalist; Scipione Riva-Rocci (1863–1937), Italian physician]

See also, Pressure measurement

Arterial cannulation. Used for direct arterial BP measurement, and to allow repeated arterial blood gas analysis. Peripheral cannulation, e.g. of radial and dorsalis pedis arteries, produces higher peak systolic pressure than more central cannulation, but is usually preferred because of reduced complication rates. Other sites available include brachial, ulnar, posterior tibial and femoral arteries. Allen's test is often performed before radial artery catheterisation, but is of doubtful value. Continuous slow flushing with heparinised saline (3–4 ml/h) reduces blockage and is preferable to intermittent injection. The need for addition of heparin has been questioned. Flushing with excessive volumes of solution may introduce air into the carotid circulation, especially in children.

- System consists of:
  - cannula: ischaemia, emboli and tissue necrosis are uncommon if a 20–22 G parallel-sided Teflon cannula is used, and removed within 24–48 h.
  - connecting catheter: short and stiff to reduce resonance.
  - transducer placed level with the heart. Requires calibration and zeroing.
  - electrical monitor and connections. An adequate frequency response of less than 40 Hz is required.

Bubbles, clots and kinks may cause damping.

Intravascular transducers may be placed within large arteries, but are expensive and not routinely used.

Arterial gas tensions, *see Blood gas tensions*

Arterial waveform. The shape of the pressure wave recorded directly from the aorta differs from that recorded from smaller arteries; the peak systolic pressure and pulse pressure increase, and the dicrotic notch becomes more apparent, peripherally (Fig. 15a). The aorta and large arteries are distended by the stroke volume during its ejection; during diastole, elastic recoil maintains diastolic blood flow (Windkessel effect). Smaller vessels are less compliant and therefore less distensible; thus the pressure peaks are higher and travel faster peripherally. In the elderly, decreased aortic compliance results in higher peak pressures.

- Abnormal waveforms (Fig. 15b):
  - anacrotic: aortic stenosis.
  - collapsing:
    - hyperdynamic circulation, e.g. pregnancy, fever, anaemia, hyperthyroidism, arteriovenous fistula.
    - aortic regurgitation.
  - bisferiens: aortic stenosis + aortic regurgitation.
  - alternans: left ventricular failure.
  - excessive damping: e.g. air bubble.
  - excessive resonance: e.g. catheter too long or flexible.
- Information that may be derived from the normal waveform:
  - arterial BP.
  - stroke volume and cardiac output, from the area under the systolic part of the waveform.
  - myocardial contractility, as indicated by rate of pressure change per unit time (dP/dt).
  - outflow resistance; estimated by the slope of the diastolic decay. A slow fall may occur in vasoconstriction, a rapid fall in vasodilatation.
  - hypovolaemia is suggested by a low dicrotic notch, narrow width of the waveform and large falls in peak pressure with IPPV breaths.

[Windkessel, German, 'wind-chamber']

See also, Arterial blood pressure; Cardiac cycle; Mean arterial pressure

Arteriovenous oxygen difference. Difference between arterial and mixed venous O_2 content, normally 5 ml O_2/100 ml blood. Increased with low cardiac ouput or exercise (high O_2 extraction). Decreased with peripheral arteriovenous shunting, or when tissue O_2 extraction is impaired, e.g. sepsis or cyanide poisoning.

See also, Oxygen transport

Arthritis, *see Connective tissue diseases; Rheumatoid arthritis*

Articaine hydrochloride (Carticaine). Local anaesthetic agent containing both ester and amide groups, first used clinically in 1974. Although used in Canada and continental Europe for several years, was only introduced in the UK (only in combination with adrenaline) in 2001. Chemically similar to prilocaine and of similar potency. Suggested as being particularly suitable for dental anaesthesia because of its low toxicity (maximal safe dose 7 mg/kg), an ability to diffuse readily through tissues and its metabolism by blood and tissue esterases. Elimination half-life is about 1.6 h, with 50% excreted in the urine. Duration of action is about 2–4 h.

Artificial heart, *see Heart, artificial*

Artificial hibernation, *see Lytic cocktail*

Artificial ventilation, *see Expired air ventilation; Intermittent positive pressure ventilation*

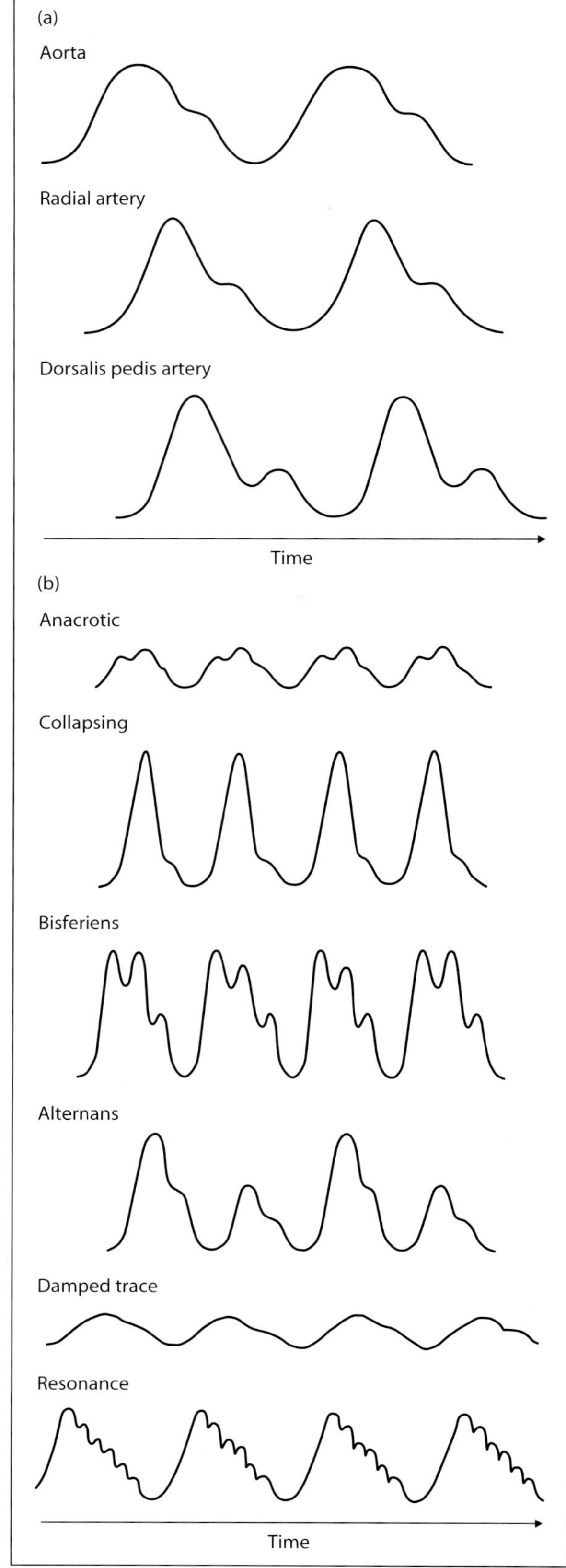

Fig. 15 (a) Arterial tracing from different sites. (b) Abnormal arterial waveforms

ASA physical status. Classification system adopted by the American Society of Anesthesiologists in 1941 for categorising preoperative physical status. Originally with six categories (the last two referring to emergency cases), a seventh (moribund patient) was later added and in 1962 the ASA adopted a modified five-category system with the postscript 'E' indicating emergency surgery. A sixth category was added in 1984/5 in the ASA's relative value guide for billing purposes:

- 1: normal healthy patient.
- 2: mild systemic disease.
- 3: severe systemic disease.
- 4: severe systemic disease that is a constant threat to life.
- 5: moribund patient; not expected to survive without the operation.
- 6: declared brain-dead organ donor.

Extremes of age, smoking and late pregnancy are sometimes taken as criteria for category 2.

Although not an indicator of anaesthetic or operative risk, there is reasonable correlation with overall outcome. Widely used in clinical trials to standardise fitness of patients. However, use of the scoring system may be inconsistent between anaesthetists; thus the same patient may be assigned to different categories depending on who performs the assessment.
See also, Preoperative assessment

Ascending cholangitis, *see Cholangitis, acute*

Ascending reticular activating system (ARAS). Ascending neural system which affects cerebral cortical activity; it extends from the medulla to the midbrain. Its main pathway is the central tegmental tract, conveying impulses to the hypothalamus and thalamus and then to the cortex. Any lesion interrupting the ARAS tends to cause coma. Because of close proximity to other brainstem nuclei, lesions often cause cardiovascular or respiratory disturbances. Anaesthetic agents are thought to produce their effect by blocking impulses from the ARAS.

Ascites. Excessive free fluid within the abdominal cavity; may exceed 20–30 l in extreme cases. Initially asymptomatic but features include weight gain, abdominal discomfort, fullness in the patient's flanks, shifting dullness to percussion and a fluid thrill. May be sufficient to restrict ventilation if gross, via increased intra-abdominal pressure or pleural effusions. There may be dependent oedema despite evidence of hypovolaemia.

Causes include hepatic failure, cardiac failure, abdominal malignancy, hepatic vein or portal vein occlusion, constrictive pericarditis, nephrotic syndrome, malnutrition, pancreatitis, trauma (haemoperitoneum), ovarian hyperstimulation syndrome and bacterial peritonitis. Analysis of the ascitic fluid may help in the differential diagnosis, as for pleural effusion.

Management includes treatment of the underlying cause, reducing sodium intake, diuretics (traditionally spironolactone and furosemide) and paracentesis. Fluid often reaccumulates; if losses are severe and continuous the fluid may be recirculated into the venous system via a simple shunt or following filtration in an extracorporeal circuit.

ASCOT, *see A severity characterisation of trauma*

Aspiration of gastric contents. Potentially a risk in all unconscious, sedated or anaesthetised patients, as lower oesophageal sphincter tone decreases and laryngeal reflexes are depressed. Aspiration may follow passive regurgitation of gastric contents or vomiting, and is not necessarily prevented by the presence of a cuffed tracheal or tracheostomy tube.

- Factors predisposing to aspiration:
  - full stomach:
    - recent oral intake. In all but extreme emergencies, patients are starved of food for 4–6 h before anaesthesia, although recent evidence suggests that total fluid restriction may be unnecessary.
    - gastrointestinal obstruction.
    - gastrointestinal bleeding.
    - ileus.
    - trauma/shock/anxiety/pain. After trauma, gastric emptying may be delayed for several h, especially in children.
    - hiatus hernia.
    - drugs, e.g. opioid analgesic drugs.
    - pregnancy.
  - inefficient lower oesophageal sphincter:
    - hiatus hernia.
    - drugs, e.g. opioids, atropine.
    - pregnancy with heartburn.
    - presence of a nasogastric tube.
  - raised intra-abdominal pressure:
    - pregnancy.
    - lithotomy position.
    - obesity.
  - oesophagus not empty:
    - achalasia.
    - strictures.
    - pharyngeal pouch.
  - ineffective laryngeal reflexes:
    - general anaesthesia/sedation.
    - topical anaesthesia.
    - neurological disease.
- May result in:
  - stimulation of the airway(s) causing breath-holding, cough, bronchospasm.
  - impaired laryngoscopy if it occurs during induction of anaesthesia.
  - obstruction of the upper airway by solid or semi-solid matter causing complete or partial airway obstruction.
  - obstruction of smaller airways causing distal atelectasis.
  - aspiration pneumonitis.

Silent and continuous aspiration of small amounts of material may cause repeated episodes of moderate respiratory impairment, especially in patients with chronically impaired protective reflexes. The diagnosis may be easy to confuse with other conditions, e.g. repeated small PEs or chest infections.

- Measures to reduce risk:
  - starvation.
  - empty stomach:
    - via nasogastric tube.
    - metoclopramide.
    - apomorphine-induced vomiting.
  - increase lower oesophageal sphincter tone, e.g. with metoclopramide, prochlorperazine.
  - rapid sequence induction of anaesthesia.
  - induction in the lateral or sitting position.
  - reduction of the severity of aspiration pneumonitis: e.g. H_2 receptor antagonists, antacids, proton pump inhibitors.
- If aspiration occurs:
  - the patient should be placed in the head-down lateral position.
  - material is aspirated from the pharynx and larynx, and O_2 administered.

- tracheal intubation may be necessary to protect the airway, and to allow tracheobronchial suction.
- further management is as for aspiration pneumonitis.

Ng A, Smith G (2001). Anesth Analg; 93: 494–513
See also, Induction, rapid sequence

Aspiration pneumonitis (Mendelson's syndrome). Inflammatory reaction of lung parenchyma following aspiration of gastric contents, originally described in obstetric patients. A 'critical' volume of 25 ml of aspirate, of pH 2.5, has been suggested to be required to produce the syndrome, although these figures have been disputed since they are based on animal studies. The more acidic the inhaled material, the less volume is required to produce pneumonitis.

Particulate antacids, e.g. magnesium trisilicate, may themselves be associated with pneumonitis if aspirated.

The acid gastric contents cause chemical injury and loss of surfactant. Pneumonitis occurs within hours of aspiration, with decreased FRC and pulmonary compliance, pulmonary hypertension, shunt and increased extravascular lung water. Features include dyspnoea, tachypnoea, tachycardia, hypoxia and bronchospasm, with or without pyrexia. Crepitations and wheezes may be heard on chest auscultation. Irregular fluffy densities may appear on the chest X-ray from 8 to 24 h. Movement of fluid into the lungs results in hypovolaemia and hypotension. The syndrome is often considered part of the ARDS spectrum. Differential diagnosis includes cardiac failure, sepsis, PE, amniotic fluid embolism and fat embolism.

Treatment is mainly supportive with O_2 therapy, bronchodilator drugs, and removal of aspirate and secretions by physiotherapy and suction. Bronchoscopy may be required to remove large particulate matter. Secondary infection may occur, and prophylactic antibacterial drugs are sometimes given although this is controversial. Use of high dose corticosteroids is declining but inhaled corticosteroids may be beneficial for treatment of bronchospasm. CPAP or IPPV with PEEP may be required in severe cases. Mortality is high.

[Curtis L Mendelson (1913–2002), US obstetrician]
Marik PE (2001). N Engl J Med; 344: 665–71

Aspirin. Acetylsalicylic acid, synthesised in the early 1900s in Germany. Commonest salicylate in use. Uses, effects, pharmacokinetics, etc. as for salicylates. Used widely as an antiplatelet drug. Should not be given to children under 16 years of age, and inadvisable in adolescents, because of the risk of Reye's syndrome.

- Dosage:
  - analgesia: 300–900 mg orally 4–6 hourly, up to a total of 4 g daily.
  - secondary prevention of thrombotic cerebrovascular or CVS disease: 75–100 mg once daily, orally.
  - acute MI: 150–300 mg once daily, orally.
  - following cardiac surgery: 75–100 mg once daily, orally.

Over-the-counter sale of 300 mg tablets/capsules in the UK is limited to packs of 32 (packs of 100 tablets/capsules may be purchased from pharmacists in special circumstances).
See also, Salicylate poisoning

Assisted ventilation. Positive pressure ventilation supplementing each spontaneous breath made by the patient. May be useful during transient hypoventilation caused by respiratory depressant drugs in spontaneously breathing anaesthetised patients. Also used in ICU, e.g. in weaning from ventilators.

- Different modes:
  - assist mode ventilation: delivery of positive pressure breaths triggered by inspiratory effort.
  - assist-control mode ventilation: assist mode ventilation against a background of regular IPPV.
  - inspiratory pressure support.
  - inspiratory volume support.
  - proportional assist ventilation.

Association of Anaesthetists of Great Britain and Ireland. Founded in 1932 to represent anaesthetists' interests and to establish a diploma in anaesthetics (DA examination). Prior to this, the London Society of Anaesthetists (founded 1893) had formed the Anaesthetic Section of the Royal Society of Medicine in 1908, its purpose to advance the science and art of anaesthesia. Also publishes the journal *Anaesthesia* and regular guidelines on various aspects of anaesthetic practice. Has over 10 000 members. The Group of Anaesthetists in Training (GAT; formerly the Junior Anaesthetists Group; JAG) has over 3500 members.
Helliwell PJ (1982). Anaesthesia; 37: 913–23

Asthma. Reversible airways obstruction, resulting from bronchoconstriction, bronchial mucosal oedema and mucus plugging. Causes high airways resistance, hypoxaemia, air trapping, and increased work of breathing. Two main forms exist:

- extrinsic allergic: begins in childhood; may have an associated family history of atopy (e.g. hayfever, eczema), is episodic and tends to respond to therapy.
- intrinsic: adult onset; no allergic family history. Nasal polyps are common and exacerbations occur with infection and aspirin. Less responsive to treatment.

Patients' bronchi show increased sensitivity to triggering agents, constricting when normal bronchi may not. During anaesthesia, surgical stimulation or stimulation of the pharynx or larynx may cause bronchospasm.

- Chronic drug treatment:
  - β_2-adrenergic receptor agonists, e.g. salbutamol.
  - aminophylline and related drugs.
  - corticosteroids.
  - sodium cromoglicate.
  - anticholinergic drugs, e.g. ipratropium.
  - leukotriene receptor antagonists: their role is uncertain.
- Acute severe asthma:
  - signs of a severe attack:
    - inability to talk.
    - tachycardia > 110/min.
    - tachypnoea > 25/min.
    - pulsus paradoxus > 10 mmHg.
    - peak expiratory flow rate (PEFR) < 50% of predicted normal.
  - signs of life-threatening attack:
    - silent chest on auscultation.
    - cyanosis.
    - bradycardia.
    - exhausted, confused or unconscious patient.
  - arterial blood gas measurement: hypoxaemia, largely from $\dot{V}/\dot{Q}$ mismatch, may be severe. It may worsen following bronchodilator treatment due to increased dead space and $\dot{V}/\dot{Q}$ mismatch. Arterial $P\text{CO}_2$ is usually reduced because of hyperventilation, but may rise in severe cases, indicating requirement for IPPV. There is poor correlation between FEV_1 and arterial $P\text{CO}_2$.
  - other problems: pneumothorax, infection, dehydration. Hypokalaemia is common due to corticosteroids, catecholamine administration, and respiratory alkalosis.

- general medical and ICU management:
  - first-line therapies:
    - humidified O_2 with high F_IO_2 is required.
    - nebulised salbutamol 2.5–5 mg or terbutaline 5–10 mg 4 hourly; iv salbutamol 250 μg may be given, followed by 5–20 μg/min, although in general, iv administration of $β_2$-agonists is thought to have no advantage over the inhaled route.
    - nebulised ipratropium 0.1–0.5 mg is traditionally alternated with $β_2$-agonists, although in modern practice they are often combined in the same nebuliser.
    - corticosteroids; e.g. hydrocortisone 100–200 mg 4 hourly iv, or by infusion.
  - second-line therapies:
    - magnesium sulphate 1.2–2.0 g iv over 20 min has recently been introduced to UK guidelines as a one-off treatment.
    - aminophylline 3–6 mg/kg iv, followed by 0.5 mg/kg/h (with caution if the patient is already taking theophyllines).
    - diethyl ether, halothane, ketamine and adrenaline have been used in resistant cases.
- supportive therapies:
  - antibacterial drugs, physiotherapy, iv rehydration.
  - IPPV:
    - intubation may provoke cardiac arrhythmias in severe hypoxia/hypercapnia.
    - sedation and muscle relaxation are required to aid IPPV.
    - high inflation pressures risk barotrauma and decreased cardiac output.
    - a flow generator ventilator is required, to ensure adequate tidal volumes.
    - because expiration may not be complete before the next breath, FRC increases with 'gas trapping', usually reaching equilibrium after 5–10 breaths. Despite the resultant auto-PEEP (intrinsic PEEP) and traditional teaching that PEEP should not be used in asthma because of the increased risk of barotrauma, PEEP has been applied to good effect and may actually reduce FRC by an unknown mechanism.
    - adequate ventilation may be difficult; permissive hypercapnia is often practised. Gas exchange may be improved by a slow inspiratory flow rate, low minute volume (6–8 l/min) and low ventilatory rate (12–14/min). Expiration should occupy at least 50% of the ventilatory cycle duration.
- bronchopulmonary lavage has been used.

- Anaesthetic management of patients with asthma:
  - preoperatively:
    - preoperative assessment is directed towards respiratory function, frequency and severity of attacks, and drug therapy (including corticosteroids).
    - investigations: chest X-ray; PEFR/spirometry (especially pre- and postbronchodilator); arterial blood gas analysis.
    - premedication: although many opioid analgesic drugs may release histamine, they are commonly prescribed, particularly pethidine. Antihistamines are often used. Anticholinergic drugs may reduce parasympathetically induced bronchospasm, but excessive drying of secretions may be disadvantageous.
    - nebulised bronchodilators may be given with premedication. Preoperative physiotherapy may also be useful. Steroid cover may be required.
  - perioperatively:
    - regional anaesthesia is often suitable.
    - thiopental has been implicated as causing bronchospasm, although this is controversial. Propofol, etomidate and ketamine are suitable alternatives. Halothane and other volatile agents cause bronchodilatation. Tubocurarine and atracurium may cause histamine release, whilst vecuronium, pancuronium and fentanyl do not.
    - tracheal intubation and the presence of a tracheal tube may cause bronchospasm. This may be reduced by spraying the larynx and trachea with lidocaine; iv lidocaine, 1–2 mg/kg, has been used to reduce the incidence of bronchospasm on intubation and extubation. Alternatively, techniques avoiding tracheal intubation may be employed.
    - β-adrenergic receptor antagonists should be avoided.
    - dehydration should be avoided.

See also, Bronchodilator drugs

Astrup method. Used for the analysis of blood acid–base status. The pH of a blood sample is measured, and the sample equilibrated with two gases of different CO_2 concentration, usually 4% and 8%. pH is measured after each equilibration, and the standard bicarbonate and base excess calculated. The original CO_2 tension is calculated from the pH of the original sample, using the Siggaard-Andersen nomogram. [Poul Astrup (1915–2000), Danish chemist]

Asystole. Absent cardiac electrical activity. Common in cardiac arrest due to hypoxia or exsanguination, especially in children. Must be distinguished from accidental ECG disconnection. Management: as in CPR.

Atelectasis. Absence of gas from part of, or all of, the lung. Caused by inadequate aeration of alveoli, with subsequent absorption of gas. The latter occurs because the total partial pressure of dissolved gases in venous blood is less than atmospheric pressure; gas trapped behind obstructed airways, e.g. by secretions, is therefore slowly absorbed. Nitrogen, being relatively insoluble in blood, tends to splint alveoli open when breathing air. Absorption atelectasis may follow high F_IO_2, since O_2 is readily absorbed into the blood and the nitrogen has been washed out of the alveoli.

Has been shown by CT scanning to occur in dependent parts of the lung during anaesthesia in normal patients, contributing to impaired gas exchange. May also follow accidental endobronchial placement of a tracheal tube. It may persist postoperatively, particularly in patients with poor lung function and sputum retention, and when chest movement is reduced, e.g. by pain after upper abdominal surgery or fractured ribs. Hypoxaemia, tachypnoea and tachycardia result, with reduced air entry to the affected area of lung, which may then become infected. Treatment of atelectasis includes physiotherapy, incentive spirometry, humidification, intermittent lung inflations using a ventilator, CPAP and, occasionally, bronchoscopy.

Duggan M, Kavanagh BP (2005). Anesthesiology; 102: 838–54

Atenolol. Water-soluble β-adrenergic receptor antagonist, available for oral and iv administration. Relatively selective for $β_1$-receptors. Uses and side effects are as for β-adrenergic receptor antagonists in general.

- Dosage:
  - hypertension: 50 mg/day orally; angina and arrhythmias: 50–100 mg/day.
  - acute arrhythmias: 150 μg/kg iv over 20 min, repeated 12 hourly as required.

- after acute MI: 5–10 mg slowly iv, then 50 mg iv after 15 min and 12 h, then 100 mg/day orally.
- perioperatively in patients at risk from ischaemic heart disease: 5–10 mg iv before surgery, then 50–100 mg orally during the hospital stay (up to a week).

- Side effects: as for β-adrenergic receptor antagonists.

Atherosclerosis. Disease involving the intima of medium and large arteries, resulting in fat accumulation and fibrous plaques which narrow the vessel lumen. Further stenosis may follow thrombosis and haemorrhage. Thought to be at least partly inflammatory in aetiology, although the precise roles of proinflammatory and prothrombotic mediators are uncertain. Causes ischaemic heart disease, cerebrovascular disease, and peripheral arterial insufficiency, especially in the legs. Thus patients with peripheral vascular disease frequently have occult atherosclerotic disease involving other organs.

A rigid arterial tree results in a high systolic arterial BP with normal diastolic pressure, a common finding in the elderly, since virtually all elderly patients have some atherosclerosis. Antihypertensive treatment is not usually required in these patients.

Hansson GK (2005). N Engl J Med; 352: 1685–95

ATLS, *see Advanced Trauma Life Support*

Atmosphere. Unit of pressure. One atmosphere equals 760 mmHg (101.33 kPa), the average barometric pressure at sea level.
See also, Bar

ATN, Acute tubular necrosis, *see Renal failure*

Atopy. Tendency to asthma, hay fever, eczema and other allergic conditions, including adverse drug reactions. Sufferers are sensitive to antigens which usually cause no reaction in normal subjects. May be familial. IgE levels may be raised. Drugs associated with histamine release should be avoided.

ATP, *see Adenosine triphosphate and diphosphate*

ATPD and ATPS. Ambient temperature and pressure, dry; and ambient temperature and pressure, saturated with water vapour. Used for standardising gas volume measurements.

Atracurium besylate. Non-depolarising neuromuscular blocking drug, first used in 1980. A bisquaternary nitrogenous plant derivative. Initial dose: 0.3–0.6 mg/kg. Intubation is possible approximately 90 s after a dose of 0.5 mg/kg. Effects last 20–30 min. Supplementary dose: 0.1–0.2 mg/kg. Has been given by iv infusion at 0.3–0.6 mg/kg/h. May cause histamine release, usually mild but severe reactions have been reported (an isomer of atracurium, cisatracurium, has similar neuromuscular properties but causes less histamine release). At body temperature and pH, undergoes spontaneous Hofmann elimination to laudanosine. Up to 50% ester hydrolysis also occurs. Often considered the drug of choice in renal or hepatic impairment. Its cardiostability, low risk of accumulation and spontaneous reversal are also advantages. Stored at 2–8°C; at room temperature, activity decreases by only a few per cent per month.

Atrial ectopic beats. Impulses arising from abnormal pacemaker sites within the atria. The P waves are usually abnormal, and arise early in the cardiac cycle. They are usually conducted to the ventricles in the normal way, producing normal QRS complexes (Fig. 16). Very early ectopics may produce abnormal QRS complexes, because the ventricular conducting system may still be refractory when the ectopic impulse reaches it. The resultant QRS may then be mistaken for a ventricular ectopic beat. Several ectopic sites may give rise to the 'wandering pacemaker', producing differently shaped P waves with differing PR intervals. Rarely require treatment.
See also, Arrhythmias; Electrocardiography

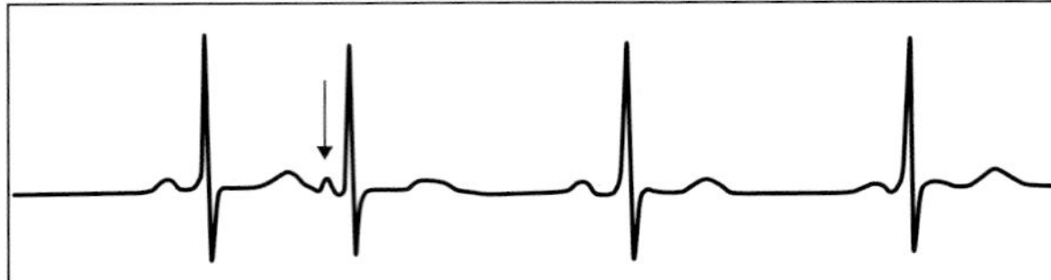

Fig. 16 Example of an atrial ectopic beat (arrowed)

Atrial fibrillation (AF). Lack of coordinated atrial contraction, resulting in impulses from many different parts of the atria reaching the atrioventricular (AV) node in quick succession, only some of which are transmitted. Ventricular response may be fast, resulting in inadequate ventricular filling, and reduced stroke volume and cardiac output. Cardiac failure, hypotension and systemic emboli from intra-atrial thrombus may occur.

- Features:
  - irregularly irregular pulse. Ventricular rate depends upon the conducting ability of the atrioventricular node; usually rapid, the ventricular activity is slow and regular if complete heart block exists.
  - no P waves on the ECG (Fig. 17).
- May be idiopathic or caused by:
  - ischaemic heart disease (most common cause), including acute MI.
  - mitral valve disease.
  - hyperthyroidism.
  - PE.
  - cardiomyopathy.
  - thoracic surgery/central venous cannulation.
  - acute hypovolaemia.
- Treatment:
  - drug therapy is aimed at reducing AV node conduction and ventricular rate. Sinus rhythm may be restored. Examples include digoxin (usually drug of choice), β-adrenergic receptor antagonists, verapamil, diltiazem, amiodarone and disopyramide.
  - cardioversion especially if recent onset (< 3 days).
  - anticoagulation should be considered if AF has persisted for more than 2–3 days, especially before cardioversion. In chronic AF, aspirin or warfarin is used depending on the absence or presence of other risk factors, e.g. diabetes.

See also, Arrhythmias

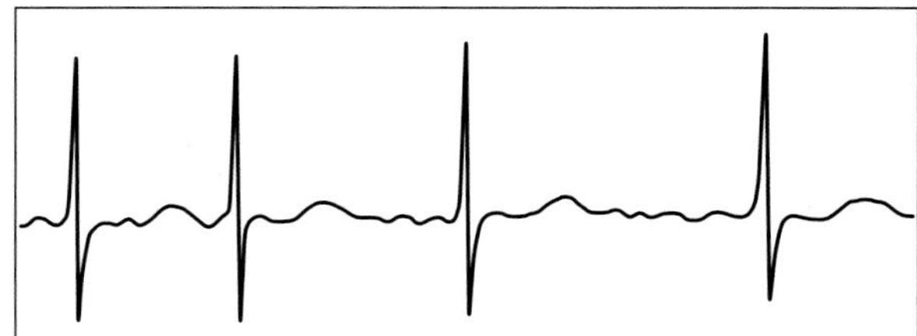

Fig. 17 Atrial fibrillation

Atrial flutter. Arrhythmia resulting from rapid atrial discharge (usually 300/min), caused by a re-entrant circuit within the atria and usually initiated by an atrial ectopic beat. May be paroxysmal or sustained. Commonly occurs with 4:1 or 2:1 atrioventricular block; i.e. with ventricular rates 75/min or 150/min respectively.

- Features:
  - usually regular pulse.
  - saw-tooth flutter (F) waves on the ECG (Fig. 18); with 2:1 block the second flutter wave of each pair may be hidden in the QRS or T waves, leading to the incorrect diagnosis of sinus tachycardia. Carotid sinus massage may slow the ventricular rate enough to reveal rapid flutter waves.
- Causes: as for AF.
- Treatment:
  - aimed at restoring sinus rhythm: cardioversion using low energy (25–50 J), rapid atrial pacing, and drug therapy as for AF.
  - digoxin may convert flutter to AF.

See also, Cardiac pacing

Atrial natriuretic peptide (ANP). Hormone isolated from the right atrium; similar peptides are present in the cardiac ventricles and vascular endothelium. Released in response to atrial stretching, e.g. in fluid overload (i.e. not to increased atrial pressure *per se*), sympathetic stimulation and presence of angiotensin II.

- Actions:
  - increases GFR, and urinary sodium and water excretion. Decreases reabsorption of sodium ions in the proximal convoluted tubule of the nephron.
  - relaxes vascular smooth muscle; renal vessels are more sensitive than others.
  - inhibits plasma renin activity and aldosterone release.
  - releases free fatty acids from adipose tissue.

Thought to act via specific receptors. ANP and related peptides have been investigated as markers of cardiac failure and myocardial ischaemia. Inhibition of their breakdown has been investigated as possible therapy in hypertension, cardiac failure and myocardial ischaemia, whilst infusion of ANP has been investigated for its renal protective effect in oliguric acute tubular necrosis. A synthetic ANP is available.

de Lemos JA, McGuire DK, Drazner MH (2003). Lancet; 362: 316–22

See also, B-type natriuretic hormone

Atrial septal defect (ASD). Accounts for up to 15% of congenital heart disease.

- Normal septal development is as follows:
  - the septum primum grows down from the top of the heart, separating the right and left halves of the common atrium.
  - the foramen secundum appears in its upper part.
  - the septum secundum grows down to the right of the septum primum, usually just covering the foramen secundum.
  - the foramen ovale is formed from the foramen secundum and overlapping septum secundum.
- Features of ASD:
  - pulmonary flow murmur with or without a tricuspid murmur, increasing on inspiration. Fixed splitting of the second heart sound.
  - right ventricular hypertrophy, right bundle branch block and right axis deviation may be present.
  - pulmonary hypertension.

Over 90% of defects are secundum ASDs; they may present in later life with pulmonary hypertension, right-sided cardiac failure, Eisenmenger's syndrome and AF. Suturing of the defect is usually quick if a patch is not required.

Ostium primum defects may involve the atrioventricular valves; they often present early. Repair is more complicated. Valve regurgitation and conduction defects may follow surgery.

- Anaesthetic management: as for congenital heart disease and cardiac surgery.

See also, Heart murmurs; Preoperative assessment

Atrial stretch receptors, *see Baroreceptors*

Atrioventricular block, *see Heart block*

Atrioventricular dissociation. Unrelated ventricular and atrial activity. The term is usually reserved for when the ventricular rate exceeds the atrial rate, to distinguish it from complete heart block (in which the reverse occurs). Ventricular activity may arise from the atrioventricular node or an ectopic pacemaker. It may occur during bradycardia as an escape mechanism, and during anaesthesia. On the ECG, P waves and QRS complexes are unrelated, the former more widely spaced than the latter (Fig. 19). Rarely clinically significant.

See also, Arrhythmias

Atrioventricular node, *see Heart, conducting system*

Atropine sulphate. Anticholinergic drug, an ester of tropic acid and tropine. Found in the deadly nightshade. Used to reduce muscarinic effects of acetylcholinesterase inhibitors, for premedication, and in the treatment of bradycardia and asystole. Has also been used as an antispasmodic drug and as a mydriatic.

- Effects:
  - CVS:
    - tachycardia (may cause bradycardia initially; thought to be due to central vagal stimulation). BP rises only if initially low due to bradycardia.
    - cutaneous vasodilatation (cause unknown).

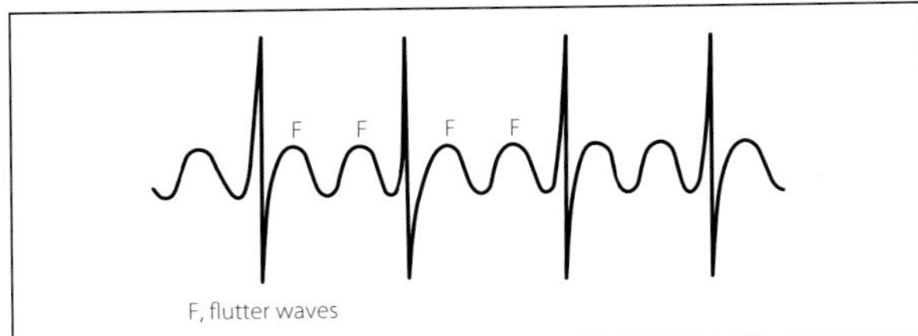

Fig. 18 Atrial flutter

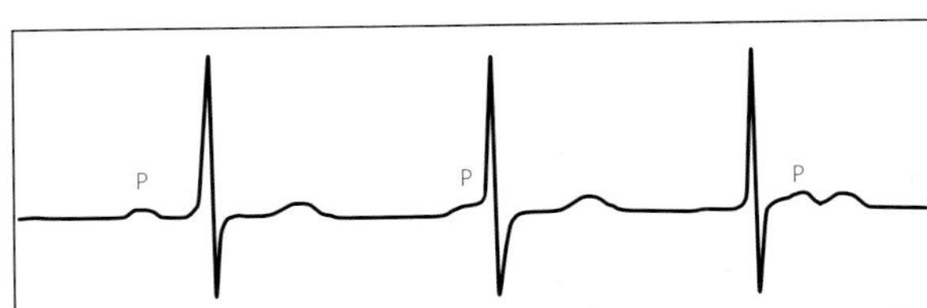

Fig. 19 Atrioventricular dissociation

- CNS:
  - excitement, hallucinations and hyperthermia, especially in children.
  - antiparkinsonian effect.
- RS:
  - bronchodilatation and increased dead space.
  - reduced secretions.
- GIT:
  - reduced salivation.
  - reduced motility.
  - reduced secretion.
  - reduced lower oesophageal sphincter tone.
- others:
  - reduced sweating.
  - mydriasis and cycloplegia.
  - reduced bladder and ureteric tone.
- Standard doses:
  - 0.1–0.6 mg increments iv for bradycardia. A larger maximum dose (3 mg) has been recommended for the management of peri-arrest arrhythmias, in order to block the vagus completely.
  - 0.3–0.6 mg im as premedication; 0.01–0.02 mg/kg for children.
  - 0.01–0.02 mg/kg when given with acetylcholinesterase inhibitors.
  - 3 mg during asystole.
  - 0.6–1.2 mg orally at night in irritable bowel disease, diverticulitis.

May be administered via the tracheal tube in twice the iv dose.

Atropine should be avoided in pyrexial patients, particularly children.

Applied directly to the eye, it may provoke closed-angle glaucoma in susceptible patients, the iris obstructing drainage of aqueous humour when the pupil is dilated.

See also, Anticholinergic drugs, for comparison with hyoscine and glycopyrronium; Tracheal administration of drugs

Audioanaesthesia (White noise/sound). Multifrequency sound, played to patients through headphones in order to reduce pain, e.g. in obstetrics. The volume is increased during contractions, with or without soft music in between. Has been employed to reduce awareness during Caesarean section. Now rarely used.

See also, Obstetric analgesia and anaesthesia

Audit. Systematic process by which medical practice is assessed and improved. Involves the following steps:
- of a particular aspect of practice (e.g. reducing PONV).
- assessment of how that practice is carried out (e.g. measuring nausea scores, recording usage of antiemetics).
- judgement by peer review whether certain standards are being met (e.g. deciding in advance that more than 10% of patients suffering severe nausea is unacceptable. National standards exist for many areas of practice, e.g. issued by professional bodies).
- identification of areas for improvement where practice is substandard (e.g. prophylactic antiemetics not being given for high risk surgery).
- addressing the deficiency (e.g. education, institution of protocols).
- reassessment after a period to check that practice has improved and standards are being met; i.e. 'closing the audit loop'. In order to be effective, specific audits require repeating regularly.

Audit (is the correct management being used?) should be distinguished from research (what is the correct management?) although both may involve similar methods of data collection and analysis.
- Anaesthetic/ICU applications include monitoring:
  - organisation of services, e.g. appropriate allocation of trainees, cancellation of surgery because of insufficient staff, leave allocations, costs, etc.
  - management of patients' drug usage, clinical policies, etc.
  - complications, e.g. unplanned admission to ICU, specific events.

Methods include analysis of currently held data (e.g. anaesthetic record-keeping) or specific studies into particular aspects of care (e.g. National Confidential Enquiry into Patient Outcome and Death and Confidential Enquiries into Maternal Deaths). Audit is now a mandatory part of medical practice in the UK, despite controversy over its value in relation to costs.

See also, Quality assurance; Risk management

Auriculotemporal nerve block, *see Mandibular nerve blocks*

Auscultatory gap. During auscultatory arterial BP measurement, the Korotkoff sounds may disappear at a point below systolic pressure, to reappear at a lower pressure before disappearing again at diastolic pressure. The significance is unknown, but it emphasises the importance of palpating the artery before auscultation, in order to ensure that the absence of sounds is because the pressure is above systolic, and not within the 'silent' gap.

Australia antigen, *see Hepatitis*

Autoimmune disease. Characterised by activation of the immune system, directed against host tissue. May involve antibody production, attacking intracellular, extracellular or cell membrane antigens. Pathogenesis is not fully understood, but involves imbalance of suppressor and helper T lymphocyte cell function. May affect specific organs, e.g. adrenocortical insufficiency, or many tissues, e.g. connective tissue diseases.
- May follow triggering agents, e.g.:
  - drugs: SLE-like syndrome after procainamide or hydralazine therapy, haemolytic anaemia after α-methyldopa therapy.
  - infection: haemolysis following mycoplasma pneumonia, rheumatic fever following streptococcal infection. Viral infections are often implicated.

Genetic factors are also important, hence the association between certain diseases and HLA types, e.g. myasthenia gravis, thyroid disease, pernicious anaemia and vitiligo. More than one of these diseases may occur in the same patient, suggesting common mechanisms. Testing for autoantibodies may be useful in the diagnosis and treatment of these conditions.

Autologous blood transfusion, *see Blood transfusion, autologous*

Autonomic hyperreflexia. Increased sensitivity of sympathetic reflexes in patients with spinal cord injury above T5/6. Cutaneous or visceral stimuli below the level of the lesion may result in mass discharge of sympathetic nerves, causing sweating, vasoconstriction and hypertension, with high levels of circulating catecholamines. Baroreceptor stimulation results in compensatory bradycardia. Distension of hollow viscera, especially of the bladder, is a potent stimulus.

It may also occur during abdominal surgery and labour. Onset of susceptibility is usually within a few weeks of injury.

In anaesthesia, both general and regional techniques have been used; spinal anaesthesia has been suggested as the technique of choice, if appropriate. Control of hypertension has been successfully achieved with vasodilator drugs. Hypotension may also occur.

Autonomic nervous system. System which regulates non-voluntary bodily functions, by means of reflex pathways. Efferent nerves contain medullated fibres which leave the brain and spinal cord to synapse with non-medullated fibres in peripheral ganglia. Closely related to the CNS, both anatomically and functionally; thus sensory input may affect autonomic activity and also consciousness and voluntary behaviour, e.g. pain, temperature, sensation, etc.

- Divided into the parasympathetic and sympathetic nervous systems, on the basis of anatomical, pharmacological and functional differences (Fig. 20):
  - parasympathetic:
    - output in cranial and sacral nerves; ganglia near to target organs.
    - acetylcholine released as a transmitter at pre- and postganglionic nerve endings.

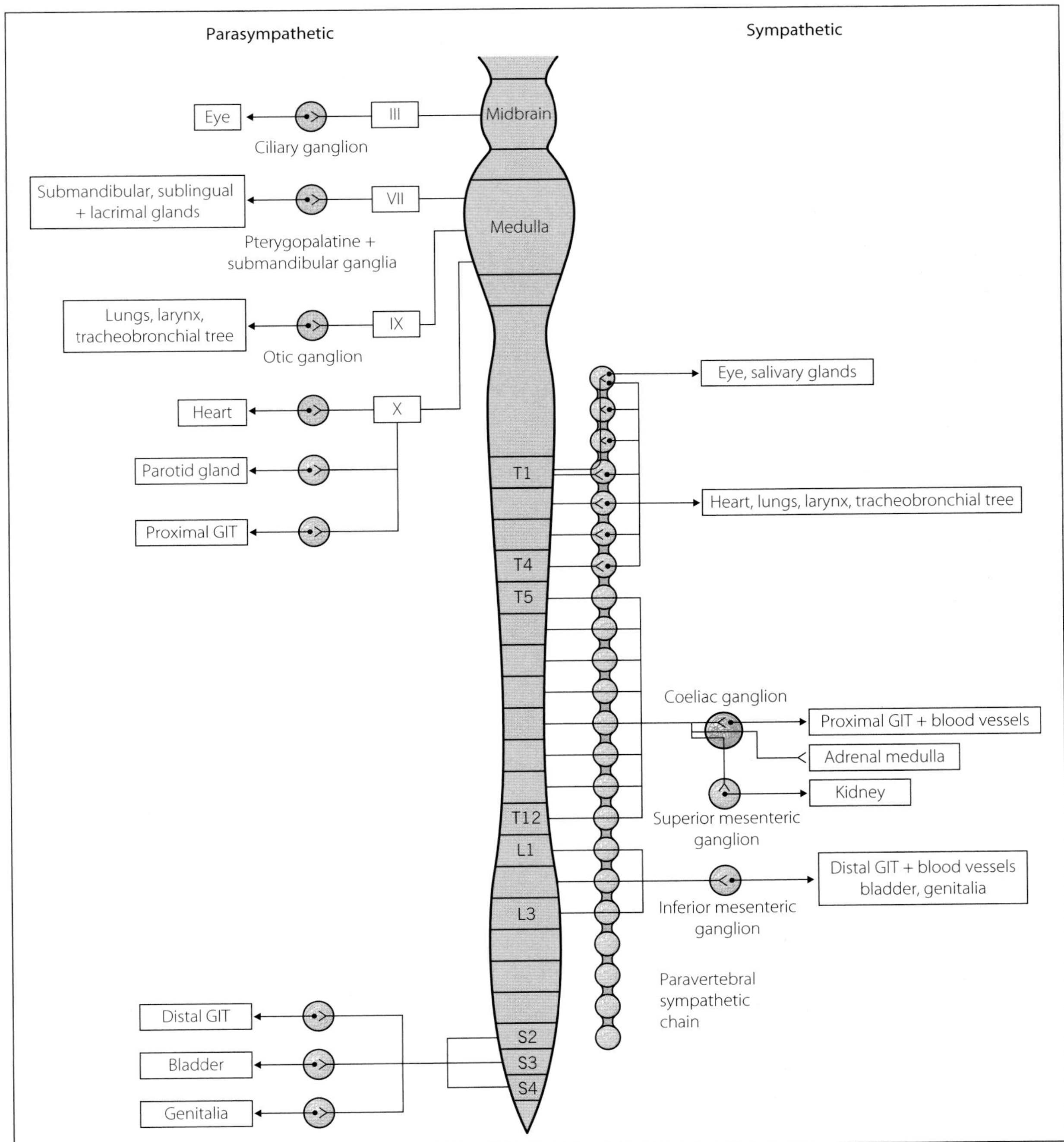

Fig. 20 Autonomic nervous system

- increases GIT activity, and reduces arousal and cardiovascular activity.
- sympathetic:
  - output in thoracic and lumbar segments of the spinal cord; ganglia form the sympathetic trunk.
  - acetylcholine released at preganglionic nerve endings, **adrenaline** and **noradrenaline** (in general) at postganglionic nerve endings.
  - increases arousal and cardiovascular activity ('fight or flight' reaction), reduces visceral activity.

Some organs receive only sympathetic innervation (e.g. piloerector muscles, adipose tissue, **juxtaglomerular apparatus**), others only parasympathetic innervation (e.g. lacrimal glands); most are under dual control.

Autonomic neuropathy. May be:
- central:
  - primary, e.g. progressive autonomic failure (Shy–Drager syndrome).
  - secondary to **CVA**, infection, drugs, etc.
- peripheral, e.g. due to **diabetes mellitus**, amyloidosis, **autoimmune diseases**, **porphyria**, **Guillain–Barré syndrome**, **myasthenic syndrome**.

Results in postural hypotension, cardiac conduction defects, bladder dysfunction and GIT disturbances including delayed gastric emptying. Diabetics with autonomic neuropathy have increased risk of perioperative cardiac or respiratory arrest.

- Useful bedside tests of autonomic function include:
  - pulse and BP measurement lying and standing; a postural drop of over 30 mmHg indicates autonomic dysfunction.
  - **Valsalva manoeuvre**.
  - effect of breathing on pulse rate (normally slows on expiration).
  - sustained hand grip (normal response: tachycardia and over 15 mmHg increase in diastolic BP).

ECG is useful for the latter two tests. Other tests include observation of sweating and pupillary responses, and catecholamine studies.

Patients with autonomic neuropathy are at risk of developing severe hypotension during anaesthesia, particularly with **spinal** or **epidural anaesthesia**, and **IPPV**. They may also show reduced response to **hypoglycaemia**. There may be increased risk of **aspiration of gastric contents**.

[George Shy (1919–1967) and Glenn Drager (1917–1967), US neurologists]

See also, Peripheral neuropathy

Autoregulation. The regulation of tissue **blood flow** by the tissues themselves, e.g. kidney, brain and heart.
- Several theories exist:
  - myogenic theory: postulates that muscle in the vessel wall contracts as intraluminal pressure increases, thus maintaining wall tension by reducing radius, in accordance with **Laplace's law**.
  - metabolic theory: argues that vasodilator substances (**nitric oxide**, **hydrogen ions**, CO_2, **adenosine**, etc.) accumulate in the tissues at low blood flow; the resultant vasodilatation results in increased flow and the vasodilator metabolites are washed away.
  - tissue theory: states that as blood flow increases, the vessels are compressed by the increased amount of interstitial fluid that has accumulated.

Usually occurs at MAP of 60–160 mmHg in normotensive subjects; it may be impaired by volatile anaesthetic agents, **vasodilator drugs** or disease states (e.g. **cerebral blood flow** in **head injury**).

See also, Systemic vascular resistance

Autotransfusion, *see Blood transfusion, autologous*

Average, *see Mean*

Avogadro's hypothesis. At constant temperature and pressure, equal volumes of all ideal gases contain the same number of molecules. One **mole** of a substance at standard temperature and pressure contains 6.023×10^{23} particles (Avogadro's number), and one mole of a gas occupies 22.4 litres.

[Count Amedeo Avogadro (1776–1856), Italian scientist]

AVP, Arginine vasopressin, *see Vasopressin*

AVPU scale. Simple scale of responsiveness, commonly used to assess the neurological status of patients, e.g. following **trauma**, **cardiac arrest**, etc. Records whether the patient is alert (A), responsive only to vocal (V) or painful (P) stimuli, or unresponsive (U). Easier and faster to perform than other more complicated **trauma scales** and systems such as the **Glasgow coma scale**.

Awareness. Ability to recall events occurring during general anaesthesia. Twice as common when **neuromuscular blocking drugs** are used with 'light anaesthesia'. Ranges from being wide awake but paralysed, to showing evidence of being awake perioperatively but without conscious recall (wakefulness; amnesic wakefulness). Signs of light anaesthesia (tachycardia, sweating, hypertension, large pupils, lacrimation) may not be present. The incidence is uncertain because of the range of possible aware states and the different methods of detection; figures of 0.01–0.03% conscious awareness with pain and 0.1–0.2% reporting on postoperative interview have been estimated. **Post-traumatic stress disorder** may rarely result postoperatively; it has been suggested that psychiatric referral should be arranged routinely in cases of awareness but this has been disputed.

Dreams, often vivid and unpleasant, may represent a subconscious form of awareness. Postoperative interview or hypnosis may reveal recall of pain, events, comments or specific messages played to patients. The significance of non-conscious recall is unknown; beneficial effects of encouraging messages during surgery have been reported. It may be **memory** of awareness, rather than the awareness itself, which is affected by anaesthesia. Similarly, it has been suggested that intense surgical stimulation may be able to 'rouse' patients from levels of anaesthesia (resulting in awareness) which might be adequate for less intense stimulation.

- Associated with:
  - administration of low doses (< 0.8 **MAC**) of volatile anaesthetic agents, e.g. in **Caesarean section** or anaesthesia for moribund patients, especially when **premedication** is omitted.
  - delay in reaching adequate blood levels of inhalational agents, e.g. during nitrogen washout in low flow breathing systems.
  - reliance on iv agents given by bolus without inhalational agents, leading to awareness between doses; e.g. during **bronchoscopy**, or repeated attempts at difficult intubation.
  - equipment failure.

Use of high dose opioid drugs may not prevent awareness, although the patient may not feel pain.

May be reduced by adequate **checking of equipment**, the use of amnesic drugs, e.g. **hyoscine** or **benzodiazepines**, and the addition of a small amount of volatile agent to inspired gases.

See also, Anaesthesia, depth of; Isolated forearm technique; Traumatic neurotic syndrome

Axillary venous cannulation. Route of central venous cannulation, usually used when alternative sites are unsuitable. Advantages include venous puncture outside the ribcage, thus reducing the risk of pneumothorax, and the ability to compress directly the axillary artery if accidentally punctured. A number of techniques have been described, classified into:

- proximal: with the arm abducted to 45°, a needle is introduced 3 fingers' breadth (5 cm) below the coracoid process and directed at the junction of the medial ¼ and lateral 3/4 of the clavicle.
- distal: with the arm abducted to 90°, a needle is introduced 1 cm medial to the axillary arterial pulsation in the axilla. The medial cutaneous nerve may be at risk with this approach.

Ayre's T-piece, *see Anaesthetic breathing systems*

Azathioprine. Non-specific cytotoxic drug, used as an immunosuppressive drug in organ transplantation, myasthenia gravis and inflammatory disease. Metabolised to mercaptopurine.

- Dose: 3–5 mg/kg orally/iv initially; maintenance 1–4 mg/kg per day.
- Side effects: myelosuppression, fever, rigors, arthralgia, myalgia, interstitial nephritis, liver toxicity. Monitoring of therapy requires regular full blood counts. The iv preparation is alkaline and very irritant.

Azeotrope. Mixture of two or more liquids whose components cannot be separated by distillation. The boiling point of each is altered by the presence of the other substance, thus the components share the same boiling point, and the vapour contains the components in the same proportions as in the liquid mixture. Halothane and ether form an azeotrope, when mixed in the ratio of 2:1 by volume.

Azidothymidine, *see Zidovudine*

Azithromycin. Macrolide, similar to erythromycin but less active against Gram-positive bacteria and more active against certain Gram-negative ones. Used in respiratory and other infections and as an antituberculous drug in resistant TB. Extensively tissue bound.

- Dosage: 500 mg orally once daily, for 3 days.
- Side effects: as for clarithromycin.

AZT, Azidothymidine, *see Zidovudine*

Aztreonam. Monocyclic β-lactam (monobactam) active against Gram-negative aerobes (including pseudomonas) but not Gram-positive organisms; thus reserved for specific (as opposed to 'blind') therapy. Causes less induction of, and resistant to, β-lactamases. Synergistic with aminoglycosides against many bacteria.

- Dosage: 0.5–1.0 g iv over 3–5 min or by deep im injection, 6–8 hourly (or 2 g iv 12 hourly); in severe infections 2 g iv 6–8 hourly.
- Side effects: as for penicillin. May cause phlebitis and pain on injection.

Azumolene sodium. Analogue of dantrolene; has been investigated as an alternative because of its greater water solubility and a smaller volume of administration.

B

BACCN, *see British Association of Critical Care Nurses*

Backward failure, *see Cardiac failure*

Baclofen. Skeletal muscle relaxant, used to treat muscle spasticity, e.g. following spinal injury and in multiple sclerosis. Acts at the spinal cord and centrally.

- Dosage: 5 mg orally, 8 hourly, increased slowly up to 100 mg/day. Has also been given intrathecally: 25–50 μg over 1 minute, increased by 25 μg/24 h up to 100 μg to establish an effective dose, then 12–2000 μg/day by infusion for maintenance.
- Side effects: sedation, nausea, confusion, convulsions, hypotension, GIT upset, visual disturbances, rarely hepatic impairment.

Bacteraemia. Presence of bacteria in the blood. May be present in SIRS and sepsis, but is not necessary for either diagnosis to be made.
See also, blood cultures; endotoxins

Bacteria. Ubiquitous micro-organisms with a bilayered cytoplasmic membrane, a double-stranded loop of DNA and, in most cases, an outer cell wall containing muramic acid. Responsible for many diseases; mechanisms include the initiation of inflammatory pathways by endotoxins or exotoxins; direct toxic effects on/destruction of tissues or organ systems; impairment of host defensive mechanisms; invasion of host cells; and provocation of autoimmune processes. Early claims that bacterial infections had been conquered by the development of antibacterial drugs are now seen as premature in light of the increasing problem of bacterial resistance. Divided and classified according to their ability to be stained by crystal violet after iodine fixation and alcohol decolorisation (Gram staining), various aspects of their metabolism and their morphology:

- Gram-positive: cell wall consists of peptidoglycan (made up of glucosamine, muramic acid and amino acids), lipoteichoic acid and polysaccharides; include:
  - aerobes:
    - cocci, e.g. staphylococci, enterococci, streptococci species.
    - bacilli, e.g. bacillus, corynebacterium, mycobacterium species.
  - anaerobes:
    - cocci, e.g. peptococcus species.
    - bacilli, e.g. actinomyces, propionibacterium, clostridium species.
- Gram-negative: have an additional outer cell wall layer containing lipopolysaccharide (endotoxin); include:
  - aerobes:
    - cocci, e.g. neisseria species.
    - bacilli, e.g. enterobacteria (enterobacter, escherichia, klebsiella, proteus, salmonella, serratia, shigella, yersinia), vibrio, acinetobacter, pseudomonas, brucella, bordetella, campylobacter, haemophilus, helicobacter, legionella, chlamydia, rickettsia, mycoplasma, leptospira, treponema species.
  - anaerobes:
    - cocci, e.g. veillonella species.
    - bacilli, e.g. bacteroides species.

Bacteria may also be classified according to antigenic properties of the cell surface, and by their susceptibility to various viral phages and antibiotics.
[Hans Gram (1853–1938), Danish physician]
See also, individual infections

Bacterial contamination of breathing equipment, *see Contamination of breathing equipment*

Bacterial resistance. Ability of bacteria to survive in the presence of antibacterial drugs. An increasing problem of huge significance in terms of cost, pressure on development of new antibiotics and the (lack of) ability to treat infections both in critically ill patients and the community as a whole.

- Mechanisms:
  - impermeability of the cell wall to the drug, e.g. pseudomonas and many antibiotics.
  - lack of intracellular binding site for the antibiotic, e.g. *Streptococcus pneumoniae* and penicillin resistance.
  - lack of target metabolic pathways, e.g. vancomycin is only effective against Gram-positive organisms because it affects synthesis of the peptidoglycan cell wall components that Gram-negative bacteria do not possess.
  - production of specific enzymes against the drug, e.g. penicillinase.

Resistance may be a natural or acquired property. Bacteria may acquire resistance via activation of a dormant gene or transfer of the responsible gene from other bacteria (horizontal evolution).

Factors which increase the likelihood of resistance occurring include indiscriminate use of antibacterial drugs, inappropriate choice of drug and use of suboptimal dosage regimens (including poor compliance by users, e.g. long-term anti-TB drug therapy). Regular consultation with microbiologists, use of antibiotic guidelines and infection control procedures, and microbiological surveillance may limit the problem. In the UK, the Department of Health has run several campaigns to increase awareness of the problem and encourage sensible prescribing of antibiotics.

Resistance may also occur in other organisms although the problem is greatest in bacteria.
Shorr AF, Lipman J (2007). Crit Care Med; 35: 299–301

Bacterial translocation. Passage of bacteria across the bowel wall via lymphatics into the hepatic portal circulation, and thence possibly into the systemic circulation. Has been implicated in the pathophysiology of intra-abdominal or generalised sepsis and MODS, with increased bowel wall permeability resulting from reduced blood flow or increased oxygen demand allowing bacteria or their components (e.g. endotoxins) to enter the circulation and stimulate various inflammatory mediator pathways including cytokines. The inflammatory response may thus be initiated or maintained. Resting the bowel is thought to increase the chances of bacterial translocation; therefore early enteral feeding of critically ill patients (especially with a glutamine-enriched feed) is believed to be beneficial.

Although much evidence supports the occurrence of bacterial translocation, its actual significance in SIRS and MODS is disputed.

De-Souza DA, Greene LJ (2005). Crit Care Med; 33: 1125–35

Bactericidal/permeability-increasing protein. Protein normally released by activated polymorphonuclear leucocytes. Binds to and neutralises endotoxin and is bactericidal against Gram-negative organisms (by increasing permeability of bacterial cell walls). May have a role in the future treatment of severe Gram-negative infections, e.g. meningococcal disease. Lipopolysaccharide-binding protein is closely related.

See also, Sepsis; Sepsis syndrome; Septic shock; Systemic inflammatory response syndrome

Bain breathing system, *see Coaxial anaesthetic breathing systems*

Bainbridge reflex. Reflex tachycardia following an increase in venous pressure, e.g. following rapid infusion of fluid. Does not occur in transplanted hearts, suggesting true reflex pathways. Of unknown significance.

[Francis Bainbridge (1874–1921), English physiologist]

Balanced anaesthesia. Concept of using combinations of drugs and techniques (e.g. general and regional anaesthesia) to provide adequate analgesia, anaesthesia and muscle relaxation (triad of anaesthesia). Each drug reduces the requirement for the others, thereby reducing side effects due to any single agent, and also allowing faster recovery. Arose from Crile's description of anociassociation in 1911, and Lundy's refinement in 1926.

Ballistocardiography. Detection of body motion resulting from movement of blood within the body with each heartbeat. Used to measure cardiac output and stroke volume, and in the investigation of cardiac disease, but technically difficult to perform accurately.

Balloon pump, *see Intra-aortic counter-pulsation balloon pump*

Bar. Unit of pressure. Although not an SI unit, commonly used when referring to the pressures at which anaesthetic gases are delivered from cylinders and piped gas supplies.

$$1 \text{ bar} = 10^5 \text{ N/m}^2\text{(Pa)} = 10^6 \text{dyne/cm}^2$$
$$= 14.5 \text{ lb/in}^2 \approx 1 \text{ atm}$$

Baralyme. Calcium hydroxide 80% and barium octahydrate 20%. Used to absorb CO_2. Although less efficient than soda lime, it produces less heat and is more stable in dry atmospheres. Used in spacecraft. Carbon monoxide production has occurred when volatile agents containing the CHF_2 moiety (desflurane, enflurane or isoflurane) are passed over dry warm baralyme, e.g. at the start of a Monday morning operating session following prolonged passage of dry gas through the absorber.

Barbiturate poisoning. Causes CNS depression with hypoventilation, hypotension, hypothermia and coma. Skin blisters and muscle necrosis may also occur.

- Treatment:
  - general measures as for poisoning and overdoses.
  - of the above complications.
  - forced alkaline diuresis, dialysis or haemoperfusion may be indicated.

Now rare, with the declining use of barbiturates.

See also, Forced diuresis

Barbiturates. Drugs derived from barbituric acid, itself derived from urea and malonic acid and first synthesised in 1864. The first sedative barbiturate, diethyl barbituric acid, was synthesised in 1903. Many others have been developed since, including phenobarbital in 1912, hexobarbital in 1932 (the first widely used iv barbiturate), thiopental in 1934, and methohexital (methohexitone) in 1957.

- Substitutions at certain positions of the molecule confer hypnotic or other properties to the compound (Fig. 21). Chemical classification:
  - oxybarbiturates: as shown. Slow onset and prolonged action, e.g. phenobarbital.
  - thiobarbiturates: sulphur atom at position 2. Rapid onset, smooth action, and rapid recovery, e.g. thiopental.
  - methylbarbiturates: methyl group at position 1. Rapid onset and recovery, with excitatory phenomena, e.g. methohexital.
  - methylthiobarbiturates: both substitutions. Very rapid, but too high an incidence of excitatory phenomena to be useful clinically.

  Long side groups are associated with greater potency and convulsant properties. Phenyl groups confer anticonvulsant action.
- Divided clinically into:
  - long acting, e.g. phenobarbital.
  - medium acting, e.g. amobarbital.
  - very short acting, e.g. thiopental.

  Speed of onset of action reflects lipid solubility, and thus brain penetration. The actions of long- and medium-acting drugs are terminated by metabolism; the shorter duration of action of thiopental and methohexital is due to redistribution within the body.
- Actions:
  - general CNS depression, especially cerebral cortex and ascending reticular activating system.
  - central respiratory depression (dose related).
  - antanalgesia.
  - reduction of rapid eye movement sleep (with rebound increase after cessation of chronic use).
  - anticonvulsant or convulsant properties according to structure.
  - cardiovascular depression. Central depression is usually mild; the hypotension seen after thiopental is largely due to direct myocardial depression and venodilatation.
  - hypothermia.

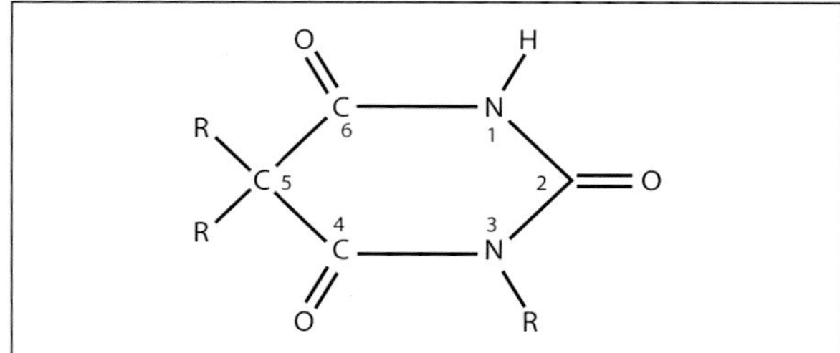

Fig. 21 Structure of the barbiturate ring

Hepatic metabolism is followed by renal excretion. Cause hepatic enzyme induction.

Contraindicated in porphyria.

Used mainly for induction of anaesthesia, and as anticonvulsant drugs. Have been largely replaced by benzodiazepines for use as sedatives and hypnotics, as the latter drugs are safer.

See also, Barbiturate poisoning

Barker, Arthur E (1850–1916). English Professor of Surgery at University of London. Helped popularise spinal anaesthesia in the UK. In 1907, became the first to use hyperbaric solutions of local anaesthetic agents, combined with alterations in the patient's posture, to vary the height of block achieved. Used specially prepared solutions of stovaine (combined with 5% glucose) from Paris.

Lee JA (1979). Anaesthesia; 34: 885–91

Baroreceptor reflex (Pressoreceptor, Carotid sinus or Depressor reflex). Reflex involved in the short-term control of arterial BP. Increased BP stimulates baroreceptors in the carotid sinus and aortic arch, increasing afferent discharge which is inhibitory to the vasomotor centre and excitatory to the cardioinhibitory centre in the medulla. Vasomotor inhibition (reduced sympathetic activity) and increased cardioinhibitory activity (vagal stimulation) results in a lowering of BP and heart rate. The opposite changes occur following a fall in BP, with sympathetic stimulation and parasympathetic inhibition. Resultant peripheral vasoconstriction occurs mainly in non-vital vascular beds, e.g. skin, muscle, GIT.

The reflex is reset within 30 min if the change in BP is sustained. It may be depressed by certain drugs, e.g. halothane and possibly propofol.

See also, Valsalva manoeuvre

Baroreceptors. Stretch receptors in the walls of blood vessels and heart chambers. Respond to distension caused by increased pressure, and are involved in control of arterial BP.

- Exist in many sites:
  - carotid sinus and aortic arch:
    - at normal BP, discharge slowly. Rate of discharge is increased by a rise in BP, and by increased rate of rise.
    - send afferent impulses via the carotid sinus nerve (branch of glossopharyngeal nerve) and vagus (afferents from aortic arch) to the vasomotor centre and cardioinhibitory centre in the medulla. Raised BP invokes the baroreceptor reflex.
  - atrial stretch receptors:
    - found in both atria.
    - some discharge during atrial systole, causing tachycardia; these may be involved in the Bainbridge reflex. Others discharge during diastolic distension (more so when venous return is increased or during IPPV). Discharge results in reduced sympathetic activity, and increased urine flow via inhibition of vasopressin release.
  - ventricular stretch receptors: stimulation causes reduced sympathetic activity in animals, but the clinical significance is doubtful. May also respond to chemical stimulation (Bezold–Jarisch reflex).
  - pulmonary stretch receptors:
    - stimulation results in bradycardia and hypotension, but to a lesser extent than systemic baroreceptor stimulation. Respiratory rate is reduced.
    - exact site is unknown.
  - coronary baroreceptors: importance is uncertain.

Other baroreceptors may be present in the mesentery, affecting local blood flow.

Barotrauma. Physical injury caused by excessive pressure; the term usually refers to pneumothorax, pneumomediastinum, pneumoperitoneum or subcutaneous emphysema resulting from passage of air from the tracheobronchial tree and alveoli into adjacent tissues. Risk of barotrauma is increased by raised airway pressures, e.g. with IPPV and PEEP (especially if excessive tidal volume or air flow is delivered, or if the patient 'fights the ventilator'). High frequency ventilation may reduce the risk. Diseased lungs with reduced compliance are more at risk of developing barotrauma, e.g. in asthma, ARDS; limiting inspiratory pressures at the expense of reduced minute volume and increased arterial CO_2 is increasingly used to reduce the risk of barotrauma in these patients (permissive hypercapnia). Evidence of pulmonary interstitial emphysema may be seen on the chest X-ray (perivascular air, hilar air streaks and subpleural air cysts) before development of severe pneumothorax. In all cases, N_2O will aggravate the problem.

Risk of barotrauma during anaesthesia is reduced by various pressure-limiting features of anaesthetic machines and breathing systems.

Anzueto A, Frutos-Vivar F, Esteban A, et al (2004). Intensive Care Med; 30: 612–9

See also, Emphysema, subcutaneous; Ventilator-associated lung injury

Basal metabolic rate (BMR). Amount of energy liberated by catabolism of food per unit time, under standardised conditions (i.e. a relaxed subject at comfortable temperature, 12–14 h after a meal, corrected for age, sex and surface area).

- Determined by measuring:
  - heat produced by the subject enclosed in an insulated room, the outside walls of which are maintained at constant temperature. The heat produced raises the temperature of water passing through coils in the ceiling, allowing calculation of BMR.
  - O_2 consumption: the subject breathes via a sealed circuit (containing a CO_2 absorber) from an O_2 filled spirometer. As O_2 is consumed, the volume inside the spirometer falls, and a graph of volume against time is obtained. O_2 consumption per unit time is corrected to standard temperature and pressure. Average energy liberated per litre of O_2 consumed = 20.1 kJ (4.82 Cal; some variation occurs with different food sources); thus BMR may be calculated. A similar derivation can be obtained electronically by the bedside 'metabolic cart', e.g. when calculating energy balance in critically ill patients.

Normal BMR (adult male) is 197 kJ/m^2/h (40 Cal/m^2/h). BMR values are often expressed as percentages above or below normal values obtained from charts or tables.

- Metabolic rate is increased by:
  - circulating catecholamines, e.g. due to stress.
  - muscle activity.
  - raised temperature.
  - hyperthyroidism.
  - pregnancy.
  - recent feeding (specific dynamic action of foods).
  - age and sex (higher in males and children).

Measurement of metabolic rate under basal conditions eliminates many of these variables.

See also, Metabolism

Basal narcosis, *see Rectal administration of anaesthetic agents*

Base. Substance which can accept hydrogen ions, thereby reducing hydrogen ion concentration.

Base excess/deficit. Amount of acid or base (in mmol) required to restore 1 litre of blood to normal pH at $P\text{CO}_2$ of 5.3 kPa (40 mmHg) and at body temperature. By convention, its value is negative in acidosis and positive in alkalosis. May be read from the Siggaard-Andersen nomogram. Useful as an indication of severity of the metabolic component of acid–base disturbance, and in the calculation of the appropriate dose of acid or base in its treatment. For example, in acidosis:

total bicarbonate deficit (mmol) = base deficit (mmol/l) × 'treatable' fluid compartment (l); estimated to be 30% of body weight, comprised of ECF and exchangeable intracellular fluid

$$= \text{base deficit} \times \frac{\text{body weight}}{3}$$

Because of problems associated with bicarbonate administration, half the calculated deficit is given initially.
See also, Acid–base balance; Blood gas tensions

Basic life support, adult (BLS). Component of CPR without any equipment or drugs (i.e. suitable for anyone to administer). Known as the 'ABC' of resuscitation. Use with simple equipment, e.g. airways, facepieces, self-inflating bags, oesophageal obturators, laryngeal mask airway, etc. has been defined as 'basic life support with airway adjuncts'. Latest international recommendations (2005):

- ensure own safety and that of the victim.
- assess: e.g. shake the victim, ask if he/she is alright, etc. If responsive, leave the patient in the same position (provided safe) and get help. If unresponsive, shout for help, turn the patient onto his/her back, open the airway and remove any obstruction.
- Airway: tilt the head back and lift the chin. Remove food, dentures, etc. from the airway. Use airway adjuncts if available.
- Breathing: check first – look, listen and feel for up to 10 s. If breathing, turn into the recovery position unless spinal cord injury is suspected. Summon help; a solo rescuer should 'phone first' since the chance of successful defibrillation falls with increasing delay (although children, trauma or drowning victims, and poisoned or choking patients may benefit from 1 minute of CPR before calling for help). If not breathing, summon help and on returning, start cardiac massage; after 30 compressions give two slow effective breaths (700–1000 ml, each over 1 s) followed by another 30 compressions. Rapid breaths are more likely to inflate the stomach. Cricoid pressure should be applied if additional help is available. Risk of HIV infection, hepatitis, etc. is considered negligible. Inflating equipment and 100% O_2 should be used if available.
- Circulation: apply external cardiac massage (4–5 cm chest depressions) at 100/min, with the hands in the centre of the chest, stopping only if the patient starts breathing. External bleeding should be stopped and the feet raised.
- if there is a second rescuer, they should swap every 1–2 min to minimise fatigue. The recommended ratio of compressions:breaths is now 30:2 for both single- and two-operator CPR. Chest-compression-only CPR is acceptable if the rescuer is unable or unwilling to give rescue breaths.
- in cases of choking, encourage coughing in conscious patients; clear the airway manually and use ≤ 5 back slaps then ≤ 5 abdominal thrusts (Heimlich manoeuvre) if not breathing or unable to speak, repeated as necessary; use basic life support (as above) if the patient becomes unconscious.

All medical and paramedical personnel should be able to administer basic life support (ideally every member of the public). Ability of hospital staff has been consistently shown to be poor. Regular training sessions are thought to be necessary, using training mannikins.
European Resuscitation Council (2005). Resuscitation; 67 (Suppl 1): S1–190
See also Advanced life support, adult; Cardiac arrest; Cardiopulmonary resuscitation, neonatal; Cardiopulmonary resuscitation, paediatric; International Liaison Committee on Resuscitation; Resuscitation Council (UK)

BASICS, *see British Association for Immediate Care*

Batson's plexus. Valveless epidural venous plexus composed of anterior and posterior longitudinal veins, communicating at each vertebral level with venous rings which pass transversely around the dural sac. Also communicates with basivertebral veins passing from the middle of the posterior surface of each vertebral body, and with sacral, lumbar, thoracic and cervical veins. It thus connects pelvic veins with intracranial veins. Provides an alternative route for venous blood to reach the heart from the legs. Originally described to explain a route for metastatic spread of tumours. Distends when vena caval venous return is obstructed, e.g. in pregnancy, thus reducing the space available for local anaesthetic solution in epidural anaesthesia.
[Oscar V Batson (1894–1979), US otolaryngologist]
See also, Epidural space

Beclometasone dipropionate (Beclomethasone). Inhaled corticosteroid, used to prevent bronchospasm in asthma by reducing airway inflammation.

- Dosage: 100–800 μg 6–12 hourly, depending on severity, and preparation of drug. A nebuliser preparation is available but is relatively inefficient since the drug is poorly soluble.
- Side effects: as for corticosteroids, although systemic uptake is low. Hoarse voice and oral candidiasis may occur with high dosage.

Becquerel. SI unit of radioactivity. One becquerel = amount of radioactivity produced when one nucleus disintegrates per second.
[Antoine Becquerel (1852–1908), French physicist]

Bed sores, *see Decubitus ulcers*

Bee stings, *see Bites and stings*

Beer–Lambert law. Combination of two separate laws describing absorption of monochromatic light by a transparent substance through which it passes:

- Beer's law: intensity of transmitted light decreases exponentially as concentration of substance increases.
- Lambert's law: intensity of transmitted light decreases exponentially as distance travelled through the substance increases.

Forms the basis for spectrophotometric techniques, e.g. enzyme assays, oximetry, near infra-red spectroscopy.
[August Beer (1825–1863) and Johann Lambert (1728–1777), German physicists]

Bell–Magendie law. The dorsal roots of the spinal cord are sensory, the ventral roots motor.

[Sir Charles Bell (1774–1842), Scottish surgeon; François Magendie (1783–1855), French physiologist]

Bellows. The term may apply to bellows incorporated into ventilators or to hand-operated devices. The latter have been used in CPR and animal experiments for several centuries. More modern devices allow manual controlled ventilation, and are either applied directly to the patient's face or used in draw-over techniques.

- Examples:
  - Cardiff bellows: mainly used for resuscitation (rarely used now, self-inflating bags being preferred).
    Design:
    - concertina bellows with a facepiece at one end.
    - non-rebreathing valve between the bellows and face-piece.
    - one-way valve at the other end of the bellows which prevents air or O_2 leaks during compression, whilst allowing fresh gas entry during expansion.
  - Oxford bellows (Fig. 22): used for resuscitation or draw-over anaesthesia.
    Design:
    - concertina bellows mounted on a block containing one-way valves.
    - held open by an internal spring, but may be manually compressed. Expansion draws in air or O_2 through a side port.
    - unidirectional gas flow is ensured by the one-way valves, one on either side of the bellows. A non-rebreathing valve is required between the bellows and patient.

    In earlier models, an O_2 inlet opened directly into the closed bellows system. This could allow build-up of excessive pressure, with risk of barotrauma.

Bends, *see Decompression sickness*

Benzatropine mesylate (Benztropine). Anticholinergic drug, used to treat acute dystonic reactions and Parkinson's disease, especially drug-induced.

- Dosage:
  - 1–4 mg orally, daily.
  - 1–2 mg iv/im, repeated as required.

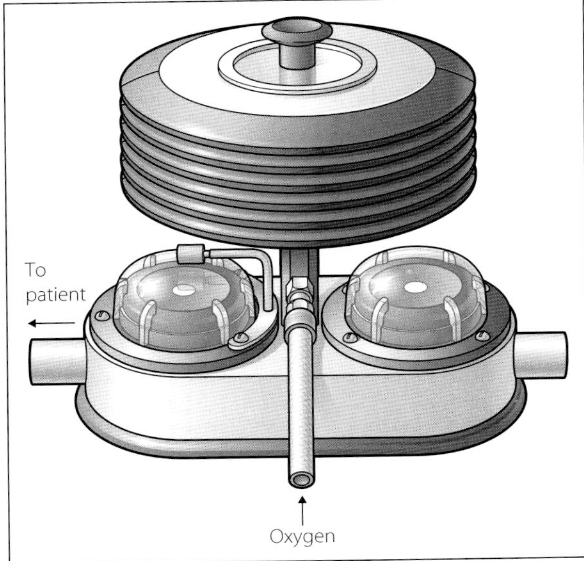

Fig. 22 Oxford bellows

- Side effects: sedation, dry mouth, blurred vision, GIT upset, urinary retention, tachycardia. May make tardive dyskinesia worse.

Benzodiazepine poisoning. Commonest overdose involving prescription drugs. Generally considered to be less serious than overdose with other sedatives, although death may occur, usually due to respiratory depression and aspiration of gastric contents. Of the benzodiazepines, temazepam is most sedating, and oxazepam least sedating, when taken in overdose. Often accompanied by alcohol poisoning.

Features are mainly those of CNS depression; hypoventilation and hypotension may also be present. Treatment is largely supportive. Flumazenil may be used but large doses may be required and the effects may be temporary; acute withdrawal and convulsions may be provoked in patients on chronic benzodiazepine therapy.

Benzodiazepines. Group of drugs with sedative, anxiolytic and anticonvulsant properties. Also cause amnesia and muscle relaxation. Act by enhancing GABA-mediated inhibition in the brain and spinal cord, especially the limbic system and ascending reticular activating system. Thought to activate specific receptors forming part of the $GABA_A$ receptor complex, enhancing the increase in chloride ion conductance caused by GABA itself.

- Anaesthetic uses:
  - premedication, e.g. diazepam, temazepam, lorazepam.
  - sedation, e.g. diazepam, midazolam.
  - as anticonvulsant drugs, e.g. diazepam, lorazepam, clonazepam.
  - induction of anaesthesia, e.g. midazolam.
- Half-life:
  - midazolam: 1–3 h.
  - oxazepam: 3–8 h.
  - temazepam: 6–8 h.
  - lorazepam: 12 h.
  - diazepam, clonazepam: 24–48 h.

Metabolism often produces active products with long half-lives, e.g. diazepam to temazepam and nordiazepam (the latter has a half-life of up to 900 h and is itself metabolised to oxazepam). In chronic use, benzodiazepines have largely replaced barbiturates as hypnotics and anxiolytics, since they cause fewer and less serious side effects. Overdosage is also less dangerous, usually requiring supportive treatment only. Hepatic enzyme induction is rare. A chronic dependence state may occur, with withdrawal featuring tremor, anxiety and confusion. Flumazenil is a specific benzodiazepine antagonist.
See also, Benzodiazepine poisoning

Benztropine, *see Benzatropine*

Benzylpenicillin (Penicillin G). Antibacterial drug, the first penicillin. Used mainly in infections caused by Gram-positive and negative cocci although its use is hampered by increasing bacterial resistance. The drug of choice in meningococcal disease, gas gangrene, tetanus, anthrax and diphtheria. Inactivated by gastric acid, thus poorly absorbed orally.

- Dosage: 0.6–1.2 g im/slowly iv, 6 hourly; up to 2.4 g 4–6 hourly in meningococcal meningitis or anthrax.
- Side effects: allergic reactions, convulsions following high doses or in renal failure.

Bernard, Claude (1813–1878). French physiologist, whose many contributions to modern physiology include

demonstrating that the liver could synthesise glucose, proving that pancreatic secretions could digest food, discovering vasomotor nerves, and investigating the effects of curare at the neuromuscular junction. Also suggested the concept of 'internal environment' (*milieu interieur*) and homeostasis.
Lee JA (1978). Anaesthesia; 33: 741–7

Bernoulli effect. Reduction of pressure when a fluid accelerates through a constriction. As velocity increases during passage through the constriction, kinetic energy increases. Total energy remains the same, therefore potential energy (hence pressure) falls. Beyond the constriction, the pressure rises again. A second fluid may be entrained through a side arm into the area of lower pressure, causing mixing of the two fluids (Venturi principle).
[Daniel Bernoulli (1700–1782), Swiss mathematician]

Bert effect. Convulsions caused by acute O_2 toxicity, seen with hyperbaric O_2 therapy (3 atm).
[Paul Bert (1833–1896), French physiologist]
See also, Oxygen therapy, hyperbaric

Beta-adrenergic . . . , *see β-Adrenergic . . .*

Beta-lactams, *see β-Lactams*

Bethanidine sulphate. Antihypertensive drug no longer available, with similar actions to guanethidine, but shorter acting.

Bezold–Jarisch reflex. Bradycardia, vasodilatation and hypotension following stimulation of ventricular receptors by ischaemia or drugs, e.g. nicotine and veratridine. Thought to involve inhibition of the baroreceptor reflex. Although of disputed clinical significance, a role in regulation of BP and the response to hypovolaemia has been suggested. The reflex may be activated during myocardial ischaemia or MI, and in rare cases of unexplained cardiovascular collapse following spinal/epidural anaesthesia.
[Albert von Bezold (1836–1868), German physiologist; Adolf Jarisch (1850–1902), Austrian dermatologist]
Campagna JA, Carter C (2003). Anesthesiology; 98: 1250–60

Bicarbonate. Anion present in plasma at a concentration of 24–33 mmol/l, formed from dissociation of carbonic acid. Intimately involved with acid–base balance, as part of the major plasma buffer system. Filtered in the kidneys and reabsorbed to a variable extent, according to acid–base status. 80% of filtered bicarbonate is reabsorbed in the proximal tubule via formation of carbonic acid, which in turn forms CO_2 and water aided by carbonic anhydrase. The bicarbonate ion itself does not pass easily across cell membranes.

- Sodium bicarbonate may be administered iv to raise blood pH in severe acidosis, but with potentially undesirable effects:
  - increases formation of CO_2, which passes readily into cells (unlike bicarbonate), worsening intracellular acidosis.
  - increased blood pH shifts the oxyhaemoglobin dissociation curve to the left, with increased affinity of haemoglobin for O_2 and impaired O_2 delivery to the tissues.
  - solutions contain 1 mmol sodium ions per mmol bicarbonate ions, representing a significant sodium load.
  - 8.4% solution is hypertonic: increased plasma osmolality may cause arterial vasodilatation and hypotension.
  - severe tissue necrosis may follow extravasation.

For these reasons, treatment is usually reserved for pH below 7.1–7.2.

- Dose: $\frac{\text{base deficit} \times \text{body weight (kg)}}{3}$ mmol

  Half of this dose is given initially.

Presented as 8.4%, 4.2% and 1.26% solutions (1000 mmol/l, 500 mmol/l and 150 mmol/l respectively).
See also, Base excess/deficit

Bier, Karl August Gustav (1861–1949). Renowned German surgeon, Professor in Bonn and then Berlin. Introduced spinal anaesthesia using cocaine, describing its use on himself, his assistant and a series of patients, in 1899. Gave a classic description of the post-dural puncture headache he later suffered, and suggested CSF leakage during the injection as a possible cause. Also introduced IVRA, using procaine, in 1908. As consulting surgeon during World War I, he introduced the German steel helmet.
van Zundert A, Goerig M (2000). Reg Anesth Pain Med; 25: 26–33

Bier's block, *see Intravenous regional anaesthesia*

Bigelow, Henry Jacob (1818–1890). US surgeon at the Massachusetts General Hospital, Boston, he sponsored Wells' abortive attempt at anaesthesia in 1845 and promoted and published the first account of Morton's use of diethyl ether anaesthesia for surgery in 1846. Described several operations and the intraoperative events that occurred during them. Later, as a Professor, he became renowned for many contributions to surgery, including inventing a urological evacuator.

Biguanides. Hypoglycaemic drugs, used to treat non-insulin dependent diabetes mellitus. Act by decreasing gluconeogenesis and by increasing glucose utilisation peripherally. Require some pancreatic islet cell function to be effective. May cause lactic acidosis, especially in renal or hepatic impairment. Lactic acidosis is particularly likely with phenformin, which is now unavailable in the UK. Metformin, the remaining biguanide, is used as first-line treatment in obese patients in whom diet alone is unsuccessful, or when a sulphonylurea alone is inadequate.

Biliary tract. Bile produced by the liver passes to the right and left hepatic ducts which unite to form the common hepatic duct. This is joined by the cystic duct which drains the gallbladder, to form the common bile duct; the latter drains into the duodenum (with the pancreatic duct) through the ampulla of Vater, the lumen of which is controlled by the sphincter of Oddi. Both infection of the biliary tree (cholangitis) and inflammation of the gallbladder (cholecystitis) may occur during critical illness.
[Ruggero Oddi (1845–1906), Italian physiologist and anatomist; Abraham Vater (1684–1751), German anatomist and botanist]
See also, Jaundice

Binding of drugs, *see Pharmacokinetics; Protein-binding*

Bioavailability. Extent and rate of uptake of active drug by the body. Expressed as a percentage, assuming iv injection provides 100% bioavailability. For an orally administered dose, it equals the area under the resultant concentration-against-time curve divided by that for an iv dose. Low values of bioavailability occur with poorly absorbed drugs, or those that undergo extensive first-pass metabolism. Various formulations of the same

drug may have different bioavailability. 'Bioinequivalence' is a statistically significant difference in bioavailability, whereas 'therapeutic inequivalence' is a clinically important difference, e.g. as may occur with different preparations of **digoxin**.
See also, Pharmacokinetics

Biofeedback. Technique whereby bodily processes normally under involuntary control, e.g. heart rate, are displayed to the subject, enabling voluntary control to be learnt. Has been used to aid relaxation, and in chronic **pain management** when increased muscle tension is present, using the **EMG** as the displayed signal.

Bioimpedance cardiac output measurement, *see Impedance plethysmography*

Biological weapons. Living organisms or infected material derived from them, used for hostile purposes, either by certain nations in 'legitimate' biological warfare or by (bio)terrorists. The agents depend for their effects on their ability to multiply in the person, animal or plant attacked. Although not pathognomonic of a bioterrorist attack, the following should raise suspicion:

- an unusual clustering of illness in time or space.
- an unusual age distribution of a common illness (e.g. apparent chickenpox in adults).
- a large epidemic.
- disease that is more severe than expected.
- an unusual route of exposure.
- disease outside its normal transmission season.
- multiple simultaneous epidemics of different diseases.
- unusual strains or variants of organisms or antimicrobial resistance patterns.

Potential diseases include:

- anthrax: Gram-negative bacillus causing fever, skin eschars and associated lymphadenopathy, chest pain, dry cough, nausea and abdominal pain, followed by sepsis, shock, widened mediastinum, hemorrhagic pleural effusions, and respiratory failure. Mortality rates vary depending on exposure: approximately 20% for cutaneous anthrax without antibiotics, 25–75% for gastrointestinal anthrax and over 80% for inhalation anthrax.
- pneumonic plague: Gram-negative bacillus causing mucopurulent sputum, chest pain and hemoptysis. Mortality if untreated approaches 100%.
- tularaemia: Gram-negative coccobacillus causing bronchopneumonia, pleuritis and hilar lymphadenopathy. Overall mortality for virulent strains is 5–15%, but up to 30–60% in pulmonic or septicaemic tularaemia without antibiotics.
- viral haemorrhagic fevers: influenza-like illness with haemorrhage, petechiae, and ecchymoses or multiple organ failure. Mortality approaches 100% for the most virulent forms.
- **botulism**: a paralytic illness characterised by symmetric, descending flaccid paralysis of motor and autonomic nerves, usually beginning with the cranial nerves. Mortality is approximately 6% if appropriately treated.
- smallpox: febrile illness followed by a generalised macular or papular-vesicular-pustular eruption. Mortality is approximately 30%.

Management includes specific and general supportive measures; consideration should also be directed towards protection of staff, decontamination of clinical areas and equipment, disposal of bodies and other aspects of major incidents.
White SM (2002). Br J Anaesth; 89: 306–24
See also, Incident, major; Chemical weapons

Biotransformation, *see Pharmacokinetics*

BIPAP. Bi-level positive airway pressure, *see Non-invasive positive pressure ventilation*

Bispectral index, *see Power spectral analysis*

Bisphosphonates. Group of drugs used in Paget's disease, osteoporosis, metastatic bone disease and **hypercalcaemia**; they are adsorbed on to hydroxyapatite crystals, interfering with bone turnover and thus slowing the rate of **calcium** mobilisation. The following may be given iv by slow infusion, e.g. in severe hypercalcaemia of malignancy:

- disodium pamidronate: 15–60 mg, given once or divided over 2–4 days, up to a maximum of 90 mg in total.
- ibandronic acid: 2–4 mg by a single infusion.
- sodium clodronate: 300 mg/day for 7–10 days or 1.5 g by a single infusion.
- zoledronic acid: 4–5 mg (depending on the preparation) over 15 min by a single infusion.

Side effects include **hypocalcaemia**, **hypophosphataemia**, pyrexia, flu-like illness, vomiting and headache. Blood dyscrasias, hyper- or hypotension, renal and hepatic dysfunction may rarely occur, especially with disodium pamidronate.
[Sir James Paget (1814–1899), English surgeon]

Bites and stings. May include animal bites, and animal or plant stings. Problems are related to:

- local tissue **trauma** itself: damage to vital organs, haemorrhage, oedema, etc. Importance varies with the size, location and number of the wound(s).
- effect of venom or toxin delivered: may cause an intense immune and inflammatory reaction, usually with severe pain and swelling. Systemic features usually present within 1–4 h; they may vary but typically include:
  - cardiovascular: hypertension (from **neurotransmitter** release), hypotension (from cardiac depression, **hypovolaemia**, vasodilatation), **arrhythmias**.
  - respiratory: **bronchospasm**, **pulmonary oedema**, **respiratory failure** (type I or II), **airway obstruction** (from oedema).
  - gastrointestinal: nausea, vomiting.
  - neurological: confusion, **coma**, **convulsions**.
  - neuromuscular: **cranial nerve** palsies and peripheral **paralysis** (from pre- or postsynaptic neuromuscular junction blockade), muscle spasms (from neurotransmitter release), **rhabdomyolysis**.
  - haematological: **coagulation disorders**, **haemolysis**.
  - renal: impairment from **myoglobinuria**, hypotension and direct nephrotoxicity.
- wound infection, either introduced at the time of injury or acquired secondarily.
- systemic transmitted disease, e.g. **tetanus**, **rabies**, plague.

Venoms are typically mixtures of several compounds, including enzymes and other proteins, amino acids, peptides, carbohydrates and lipids. The age and health of the victim, and the site and route of envenomation, may affect the severity of the injury. Identification of the offending animal or plant is particularly important, since prognosis and management may vary considerably between species. Certain species' venoms may be identified by blood testing.

- Management:
  - initial resuscitation as for trauma, **anaphylaxis**. Rapid transfer of victims of envenomation to hospital is the most important prehospital measure. Jewellery, etc.

should be removed from the affected limb as swelling may be marked.

- specific management according to the animal/plant involved. Measures include:
  - removing venom from the wound, e.g. suction to snake bites. Mechanical devices exist to prevent wound contamination with mouth organisms or poisoning the rescuer through oral lesions, etc. Some authorities suggest avoidance of suction altogether in case it increases systemic absorption of venom.
  - reducing further absorption, e.g. venous tourniquets (arterial if the venom is especially poisonous); compression and immobilisation of snake bites. Use of ice treatment is controversial in snake bites, but is thought to be beneficial in scorpion stings.
  - neutralisation of venom already absorbed. Many antivenoms are derived from horses, and severe allergic reactions may occur.
- general supportive management according to the system affected. IV fluids are usually required. Blood should be taken early as certain venoms and antivenoms may interfere with grouping. Frequent assessment of all systems and degree of swelling are important. Antitetanus immunisation should be given. Broad-spectrum anti-bacterial drugs are often given.

Bivalirudin. Recombinant hirudin used as anticoagulant in patients undergoing percutaneous transluminal coronary angioplasty.

- Dosage: 750 μg/kg iv initially followed by 1.75 mg/kg/h for up to 4 h after procedure.
- Side effects: bleeding, hypotension, angina, headache.

Bladder washouts. Main types used in ICU:

- to remove debris and exclude catheter blockage as a cause of oliguria: sterile saline. Various solutions are available to remove phosphate deposits.
- to dissolve blood clots: sterile saline or sodium citrate 3% irrigation. Streptokinase-streptodornase enzyme preparation may also be used (allergic reactions and burning may occur).
- for urinary tract infection: chlorhexidine 1:5000 (may cause burning and haemorrhage); ineffective in pseudomonal infections. Saline may also be used. Amphotericin may be used in fungal infection.

Also used to treat local malignancy.

Blast injury, *see Chest trauma*

Bleeding time, *see Coagulation studies*

Bleomycin. Antibiotic cytotoxic drug, given iv or im to treat lymphomas and certain other solid tumours. Causes little myelosuppression but skin and allergic reactions are common. May cause dose-dependent progressive pulmonary fibrosis, thought to be exacerbated if high concentrations of O_2 are administered, e.g. for anaesthesia. Suspicion of fibrosis (chest X-ray changes or basal crepitations) is an indication to stop therapy.

Blood. Cell formation occurs in the liver, spleen and bone marrow prior to birth, after which it occurs in bone marrow only. In adults, active bone marrow is confined to vertebrae, ribs, sternum, ilia and humeral and femoral heads. Stem cells differentiate into mature cellular components over many cell divisions. Primary stem cells may give rise to the lymphocyte series of stem cells or to secondary stem cells. The secondary stem cells may give rise to the erythrocyte, granulocyte, monocyte or megakaryocyte series of stem cells (the latter forming platelets).

See also, Blood volume; Leucocytes; Plasma

Blood, artificial. Man-made solutions capable of gas transport and O_2 delivery to the tissues. Attractive because the complications of blood transfusion and the need for blood cross-matching may be avoided. Two types have been investigated:

- haemoglobin solutions:
  - must be free of red cell debris (stroma free) to avoid renal damage, which has also occurred with certain stroma-free solutions. Other effects may include impairment of macrophage activity, vasoconstriction and activation of various inflammatory pathways. Free haemoglobin solutions are also hyperosmotic and are quickly broken down in the blood.
  - the oxyhaemoglobin dissociation curve of free haemoglobin is markedly shifted to the left of that for intra-erythrocyte haemoglobin, reducing its usefulness.
  - must be stored in O_2-free atmosphere to avoid oxidisation to methaemoglobin.

  Various modifications of the haemoglobin molecule have been made in order to prolong its half-life from under 1 h to over 24 h, including polymerisation with glutaraldehyde, linking haemoglobin with hydroxyethyl starch or dextran, cross-linking the α or β chains, and fusing the chains end-to-end (the latter has been done with recombinant human haemoglobin). Bovine haemoglobin, and encapsulation of haemoglobin within liposomes, has also been used. Many of these preparations are currently undergoing clinical trials.
- perfluorocarbon solutions (e.g. Fluosol DA20) carry dissolved O_2 in an amount directly proportionate to its partial pressure, and have been used to supplement O_2 delivery in organ ischaemia due to shock, arterial (including coronary) insufficiency and haemorrhage. Have been used for liquid ventilation. Even with high F_IO_2, O_2 content is less than that of haemoglobin (newer compounds may be more efficient at O_2 carriage). Accumulation in the reticuloendothelial system is of unknown significance. Clinical trials are currently in progress.

Squires JE (2002). Science; 295: 1002–5

Blood–brain barrier. Physiological boundary between the bloodstream and CNS, preventing transfer of substances from plasma to brain. The original concept was suggested by the lack of staining of brain tissue by aniline dyes given systemically. Arises because of tight junctions between capillary endothelial cells in the brain and epithelial cells in the choroid plexus; glial cells also impede passage of hydrophilic molecules. Active transport may still occur. Certain areas of the brain lie outside the barrier, e.g. the hypothalamus and areas lining the third and fourth ventricles (including the chemoreceptor trigger zone).

The ability of chemicals to cross the barrier is proportional to their lipid solubility, and inversely proportional to molecular size and charge. Water, O_2 and CO_2 cross freely; charged ions and larger molecules take longer to cross unless lipid soluble. All substances eventually penetrate the brain; the rate of penetration is important clinically. Some drugs only cross the barrier in their unionised, non-protein-bound form, i.e. a small proportion of the injected dose, e.g. thiopental. Neuromuscular blocking drugs are charged, and cross to a very limited extent. Glycopyrronium, being charged, crosses to a lesser extent than atropine.

The effectiveness of the barrier in neonates is less than in adults, hence the increased passage of drugs, e.g. opioid analgesic drugs, and other substances, e.g. bile salts causing kernicterus. Meningitis may reduce the integrity of the barrier.

Blood cross-matching. Necessary to avoid reactions caused by transfusion of blood into a recipient whose plasma contains antibodies against the transfused blood. ABO and Rhesus are the most relevant blood group systems clinically, although others may be important.

Antibodies may be naturally occurring, e.g. ABO system, or only acquired after exposure, e.g. Rhesus.

- General method:
  - if red cells have serum added which contains antibody against them, agglutination of the cells occurs.
  - serum of known identity is used to identify the recipient's blood group (ABO and Rhesus).
  - recipient's serum is screened for atypical antibodies against other groups.
  - recipient's serum is added to red cells from each donor unit (i.e. cross-match).

Full cross-matching takes up to an hour. Emergency ABO and Rhesus typing takes just a few minutes but may not prevent minor incompatibilities. Uncross-matched O Rhesus negative blood is reserved for life-threatening emergencies. Antibody screening with selection of appropriate donor blood without formal cross-matching has been suggested, being cheaper and time-saving. FFP is not cross-matched, but chosen as type-specific (ABO) so that antibodies are not infused into a recipient who might have the corresponding antigens on their cells. Platelets are suspended in plasma so are also selected as type specific, but in this case according to Rhesus typing too.

UK colour coding for labelling of blood for transfusion was replaced by a black and white lettering system in 1992.

See also, Blood transfusion

Blood cultures. Performed to detect circulating micro-organisms. Blood is taken under aseptic conditions and injected into (usually two) bottles containing culture medium, for aerobic and anaerobic incubation. Diluting the sample at least 4–5 times in the culture broth reduces the antimicrobial activity of serum and of any circulating drugs. Changing the hypodermic needle between taking blood and injection into the bottles is not now thought to be necessary, although contamination of the needle and bottles must be avoided. Sensitivity depends on the type of infection, the number of cultures and volume of blood taken. At least 2–3 cultures, each using at least 10–30 ml blood, are usually recommended. More samples may be required when there is concurrent antibacterial drug therapy (the sample may be diluted several times or the drug removed in the laboratory to increase the yield) or when endocarditis is suspected. False-positive results may be suggested by the organism recovered (e.g. *Bacillus* species, coagulase-negative staphylococci, diphtheroids), their presence in only a single culture out of many and after prolonged incubation, and a high level of suspicion.

Many different culture systems exist, some directed at particular organisms. Different systems may be used together to increase their yield. Modern microbiological techniques may involve automatic alerting of staff when significant microbial growth interrupts passage of light through the bottles. The organisms may then be identified and sensitivity to antimicrobials determined.

See also, Sepsis

Blood filters. Devices for removing microaggregates during blood transfusion. Platelet microaggregates form early in stored blood, with leucocytes and fibrin aggregates occurring after 7 days' storage. Pulmonary microembolism has been suggested as a cause of pulmonary dysfunction following transfusion.

- Types of filters:
  - screen filters: sieves with pores of a certain size.
  - depth filters: remove particles mainly by adsorption. Pore size varies, and effective filtration may be reduced by channel formation within the filter.
  - combination filters.

Most contain woven fibre meshes, e.g. of polyester or nylon.

Standard iv giving sets suitable for blood transfusion contain screen filters of 170 μm pore size. Filtration of microaggregates requires microfilters of 20–40 μm pore size. The general use of microfilters is controversial; by activating complement in transfused blood they may increase formation of microaggregates within the recipient's bloodstream. They add to expense, increase resistance to flow and may cause haemolysis. They have, however, been shown to be of use in extracorporeal circulation.

Blood flow. For any organ:

$$\text{Flow} = \frac{\text{perfusion pressure}}{\text{resistance}}$$

Perfusion pressure depends not only on arterial and venous pressures, but also on local pressures within the capillary circulation.

- Resistance depends on:
  - vessel radius, controlled by humoral, neural and local mechanisms (autoregulation).
  - vessel length.
  - blood viscosity. Reduced peripherally due to plasma skimming, which results in blood with reduced haematocrit leaving vessels via side branches. Reduced in anaemia.

Flow is normally laminar; i.e. it roughly obeys the Hagen–Poiseuille equation, although blood vessels are not rigid, arterial flow is pulsatile and blood is not an ideal fluid. Turbulent flow may occur in constricted arteries and in hyperdynamic circulation, particularly in anaemia, when viscosity is reduced (*see Reynolds' number*).

- Measurement:
  - direct measurement of blood from the arterial supply.
  - electromagnetic flow measurement.
  - Doppler measurement.
  - indirect methods:
    - Fick principle.
    - dilution techniques.
    - plethysmography.

Approximate blood flow to, and O_2 consumption of, various organs are shown in Table 7.

Blood/gas partition coefficients, *see Partition coefficients*

Table 7 Blood flow to and O_2 consumption of heart, brain and kidneys

	Blood flow		O_2 consumption	
Organ	(ml/min)	(ml/100 g tissue/min)	(ml/min)	(ml/100 g tissue/min)
Heart	250	80	30	10
Brain	700	50	50	3
Kidneys	1200	400	20	6

Blood gas tensions. Normal values:

- arterial blood:
  - O_2 13.3 kPa (100 mmHg)
  - CO_2 5.3 kPa (40 mmHg)
- mixed venous blood:
  - O_2 5.3 kPa (40 mmHg)
  - CO_2 6.1 kPa (46 mmHg)

Inaccuracy may result from excess heparin (acidic), bubbles within the sample, inadvertent venous sampling (when arterial sampling is intended), and metabolism by blood cells. The latter is reduced by rapid analysis after taking the sample, or storage of the sample in ice.

O_2, CO_2 and pH electrodes require maintenance at 37°C.

Arterial blood gas analysis usually provides values for O_2 and CO_2 tensions, bicarbonate and standard bicarbonate concentrations, pH and base excess.

- Suggested plan for interpretation:
  - oxygenation:
    - knowledge of the F_IO_2 is required before interpretation is possible.
    - calculation of the alveolar PO_2 (from alveolar gas equation).
    - calculation of the alveolar–arterial O_2 difference.
  - acid–base balance:
    - identification of acidaemia or alkalaemia, representing acidosis or alkalosis respectively.
    - identification of a respiratory component by looking at the CO_2 tension.
    - identification of a metabolic component by looking at the base excess/deficit or standard bicarbonate (both are corrected to a normal CO_2 tension, thus eliminating respiratory factors).
    - knowledge of the clinical situation helps to decide whether the respiratory or metabolic component represents the primary change.

See also, Carbon dioxide measurement; Carbon dioxide transport; Oxygen measurement; Oxygen transport

Blood groups. Each individual's red cells bear certain antigens capable of producing an antibody response in another person. Some are only present on red cells, e.g. Rhesus antigens; others are also present on other tissue cells, e.g. ABO antigens. Immunoglobulins may occur naturally, e.g. ABO and Lewis, or following exposure to the antigen, e.g. Rhesus; they are usually IgG or IgM. Administration of blood cells to a recipient who has the corresponding antibody causes haemolysis and a severe reaction.

Minor blood groups may be important clinically following ABO typed uncross-matched blood transfusion, or multiple transfusions; an atypical antibody in a recipient makes the finding of suitable donor blood difficult. Minor groups include the Kell, Duffy, Lewis and Kidd systems. Many more have been described; the significance of such diversity is unclear.

See also, Blood cross-matching

Blood loss, perioperative. Important as a guide to perioperative and potential postoperative fluid requirements, and also as indicator of potential development of a coagulation disorder related to massive blood transfusion.

- Methods of estimation:
  - clinical judgement of the patient's volume status.
  - observation of wound and swabs.
  - weighing swabs and subtracting their dry weight. Weighing swabs may underestimate blood loss if fluid is lost by evaporation or soaked into drapes. Overestimation may occur if saline, etc. is weighed without correction.
  - measuring sucker loss.
  - washing of all swabs, drapes, etc. in a known volume of water and measuring haemoglobin concentration. Volume of blood lost may then be calculated. Measurement of potassium released from lysed cells has also been used.
  - measurement of blood volume.

Replacement with blood has been suggested if losses exceed 15–20% of blood volume in adults, or 10% in children, although greater losses may be allowed if the preoperative haemoglobin concentration is high. Recent guidelines suggest that under stable conditions, a haemoglobin concentration of 7–10 g/dl should be a general indication for blood transfusion, depending on the circumstances. Until blood transfusion becomes necessary, losses may be replaced with colloid or crystalloid solutions (the latter in about 2–3 times the volume of the former).

- Blood loss may be reduced by:
  - hypotensive anaesthesia.
  - tourniquets.
  - local infiltration with vasopressor drugs.
  - appropriate positioning, e.g. head-up for ENT surgery.
  - spinal and epidural anaesthesia.
- Bleeding may be increased by:
  - raised venous pressure:
  - raised intrathoracic pressure, e.g. due to respiratory obstruction, coughing, straining.
  - fluid overload and cardiac failure.
  - inappropriate positioning.
  - venous obstruction.
  - hypercapnia.
  - coagulation disorders:
    - pre-existing.
    - dilutional coagulopathy.
    - incompatible blood transfusion.
    - anticoagulant drugs.
    - DIC.
  - hypertension.
  - poor surgical technique.

See also, Blood transfusion, massive; Haemorrhage

Blood patch, epidural. Injection of 10–20 ml autologous venous blood, immediately after removal from a peripheral vein under sterile conditions, into the epidural space for the relief of post-dural puncture headache. Blood is thought to seal the dura, preventing further CSF leak although cranial displacement of CSF resulting from epidural injection is thought to be important, at least initially. Maintaining the supine position for at least 2 h after patching is thought to increase the chance of success, by reducing 'dislodgement' of the clot from the dural puncture site. Should be avoided if the patient is febrile, in case of bacteraemia and subsequent epidural abscess. The sending of blood for culture at the time of patching has also been suggested, in case infection does occur. Flushing the epidural needle with saline as the needle is withdrawn may prevent a continuous clot from lying between the epidural space and skin, thus reducing risk of epidural contamination.

Spectacular results have been claimed for blood patching, even when performed up to several months after dural puncture. Relief of headache may occur immediately or within 24 h. Prophylactic use has been less consistently successful. Complications are rare, and include bradycardia, back and neck ache, root pain, pyrexia, tinnitus and vertigo. Subsequent epidural anaesthesia is thought to be unaffected.

Blood pressure, *see Arterial blood pressure; Diastolic blood pressure; Mean blood pressure; Systolic blood pressure*

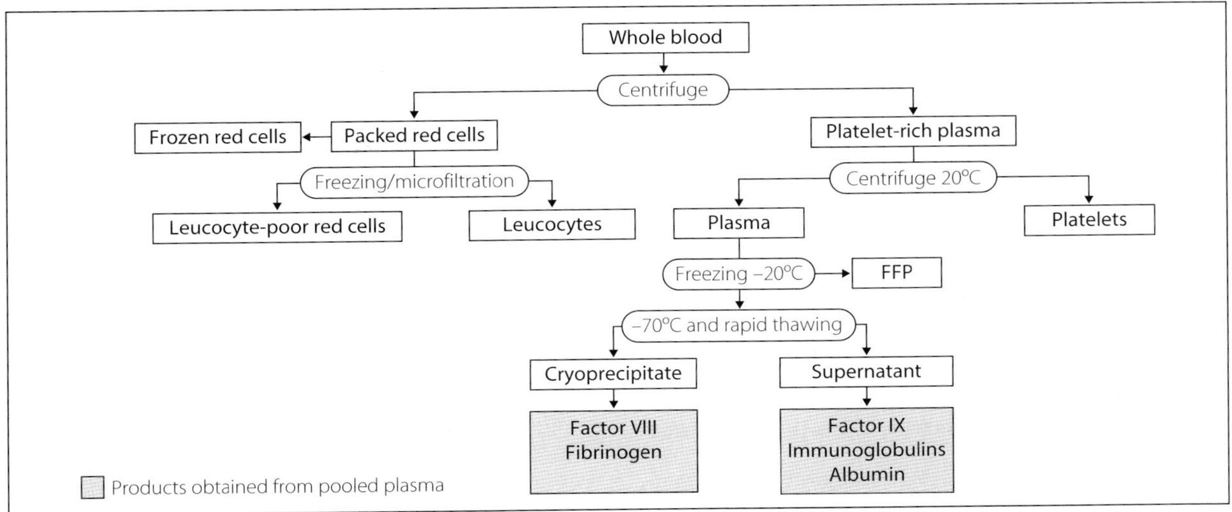

Fig. 23 Blood products available from whole blood

Blood products. Many products may be obtained from donated blood (Fig. 23), including:

- whole blood: shelf-life of 35 days. 70 ml citrate preservative solution is added to 420 ml blood. It is the source from which all other blood products are derived and is therefore a precious commodity. Consequently the use of whole blood for blood transfusion is restricted in the UK. Heparinised whole blood (lasts for 2 days) has been used for paediatric cardiac surgery.
- packed red cells (plasma reduced): haematocrit is approximately 0.6–0.7. Produced by removing 150–200 ml citrated plasma from a unit of whole blood. Whole blood is now routinely depleted by ~250 ml plasma per unit, and the red cells resuspended in 100 ml SAG-M (saline–adenine–glucose–mannitol) solution, to give a final haematocrit of ~0.6–0.7. Shelf life is 35 days. Since 1998, routinely depleted of leucocytes to decrease the risk of transmitting variant Creutzfeldt-Jakob disease.
- microaggregate-free blood: leucocytes, platelets and debris removed (i.e. the 'buffy coat'). Used to prevent reactions to leucocyte and platelet antigens.
- leucocytes: separated from blood donated by patients whose leucocyte count has been increased by pretreatment with corticosteroids, or those with chronic granulocytic leukaemia.
- frozen blood: used by the armed forces but too expensive and time-consuming for routine use. Glycerol is added to prevent haemolysis. Requires thawing and washing. May be stored for many years.
- platelets: either obtained from single donors by plateletpheresis (one donation yielding 1–3 therapeutic doses) or from multiple units of donated whole blood (one unit of platelets derived from four donors). Last for 3–5 days. Transfusion is usually restricted to patients with a platelet count of 50×10^9/l or less, unless platelet function is abnormal. 6 units usually increase the platelet count by $20–30 \times 10^9$/l. Filtered by microfilters; ordinary iv giving sets are suitable. Require ABO cross-matching. Contains citrate.
- fresh frozen plasma (FFP): lasts for a year. Requires thawing and must be ABO compatible. Contains all the clotting factors. Also a source of plasma cholinesterase. Viral infection risk is as for whole blood. In the UK, one unit of FFP is derived from plasma from a single donor, and FFP for children born after 1995 is derived from unpaid US donors. Contains citrate. Once thawed, can be stored at 4°C and given within 24 h, or kept at room temperature and given within 4 h.
- cryoprecipitate: obtained by slowly thawing FFP. Frozen and stored at –20°C; thawed immediately before use. Rich in factor VIII, fibrinogen and von Willebrand's factor. 10 bags increase fibrinogen levels by ~1 g/l. Viral infection risk is as for whole blood. Cross-matched as for FFP.
- human albumin solution (HAS; previously called plasma protein fraction, PPF): shelf-life of about 2 years. Heat-treated to kill viruses. Contains virtually no clotting factors. Available as 4.5% and 20% (salt-poor albumin) solutions; both contain 140–150 mmol/l sodium but the latter contains less sodium per gram of albumin. UK supplies are now sourced from the USA.
- fibrinogen. Rarely used. Concentrated from donor pools, therefore with higher risk of viral infections.
- factor concentrates, e.g. VIII and IX. Now obtained by recombinant gene engineering, so the risk of viral infection is removed. Previously, the risk was as for fibrinogen. Recombinant activated factor VII (rFVIIa) is available for the treatment of patients with acquired or congenital haemophilia, and inhibitors to factors VIII or IX of the clotting cascade. Factor VIIa enhances thrombin generation on the surfaces of activated, but apparently not inactivated, platelets, and appears to have only a local effect with no action on systemic coagulation. Its use is now being suggested for reversing haemorrhage after trauma, over-anticoagulation and haemorrhagic CVA.

See also, Blood, artificial; Blood storage

Blood storage. Viability of red cells is defined as at least 70% survival 24 h post-transfusion.

- The following occur in stored blood:
  - reduced pH, as low as 6.7–7.0, mainly due to high $P\text{CO}_2$.
  - increased lactic acid.
  - increased potassium ion concentration, up to 30 mmol/l.
  - reduced ATP and glucose consumption.
  - shift to the left of oxyhaemoglobin dissociation curve (Valtis–Kennedy effect).

- reduced 2,3-DPG levels.
- reduced viability of other blood constituents, e.g. platelets and leucocytes, and formation of microaggregates. Coagulation factors V and VIII are almost completely destroyed, XI is reduced, and IX and X are reduced after 7 days.

- Storage solutions:
  - ACD (acid–citrate–dextrose): trisodium citrate, citric acid and dextrose. Introduced in the 1940s. Red cell survival is 21 days. 2,3-DPG is greatly reduced after 7 days.
  - CPD (citrate–phosphate–dextrose): citrate, sodium dihydrogen phosphate and dextrose. Described in the late 1950s. Red cell survival: 28 days. 2,3-DPG is greatly reduced after 14 days.
  - CPD-A. Addition of adenine increases red cell ATP levels. Red cell survival: 35 days. 2,3-DPG is low after 14 days.
  - SAG-M (saline 140 mmol/l, adenine 1.5 mmol/l, glucose 50 mmol/l and mannitol 30 mmol/l). Used to resuspend concentrated red cells after removal of plasma from CPD anticoagulated blood, allowing a greater amount of plasma to be removed for other blood products. Has similar preserving properties to CPD-A. Mannitol prevents haemolysis. BAGPM (bicarbonate-added glucose–phosphate–mannitol) is similar.

Storage at 2–6°C is best for red cells but platelets and clotting factors are reduced. 22°C is best for platelets (survival time 3–5 days). Freezing of blood is expensive and time-consuming, but allows storage for many years. It requires 2 hours' thawing, and removal of glycerol (used to prevent haemolysis).

After rewarming and transfusion, potassium is taken up by red cells. 2,3-DPG levels are restored within 24 h.

Plastic collection bags, permeable to CO_2 without altering the blood itself, were introduced in the 1960s. In the closed triple bag system, blood passes from the donor to the first collection bag, from which plasma and red cells are passed into separate bags if required. The closed system prevents exposure to air and infection.

Before transfusion, the correct identity of the unit of blood (including expiry date) and of the patient must be confirmed (including the wearing of an identification band). The integrity of the bag should be checked. Blood left out of the fridge for more than 30 min should be transfused within 4 h or discarded. Details of each unit given and the total volume transfused should be recorded in the patient's notes and/or anaesthetic record.

See also, Blood products; Blood transfusion

Blood substitutes, *see Blood, artificial*

Blood tests, preoperative, *see Investigations, preoperative*

Blood transfusion. Reports of transfusion between animals, and between animals and man, date from the seventeenth century. Transfusions between men were performed in the early nineteenth century. Adverse reactions in recipients, and clotting of blood, were major problems. ABO blood groups were discovered in 1900; improvements in blood cross-matching and anticoagulation followed.

In the UK, the National Blood Transfusion Service relies on voluntary donors, and is increasingly hard-pressed to meet demand for blood and blood products. Perioperative use accounts for about 50% of total blood usage. Recent guidelines suggest that under stable conditions, a perioperative haemoglobin concentration of 7–10 g/dl should be a general indication for blood transfusion, depending on the circumstances.

- Complications of transfusion:
  - immunological (reactions are associated with 2% of all transfusions):
    - immediate haemolysis (e.g. ABO incompatibility). Incidence is 1 in 250 000–1 000 000. Features include rapid onset of fever, back pain, skin rash, hypotension and dyspnoea. DIC and renal failure may occur. Hypotension and increased oozing of blood from wounds may be the only indication of incompatible transfusion in an anaesthetised patient. Immediate treatment is as for anaphylactic reaction, although the underlying mechanisms are different. Samples of recipient and donor blood should be taken for analysis. Mortality is up to 50%. Most cases arise from clerical errors (e.g. incorrect labelling or administration to the wrong patient).
    - delayed haemolysis (e.g. minor groups). Usually occurs 7–10 days after transfusion, with fever, anaemia and jaundice. Renal failure may occur.
    - reactions to platelets and leucocytes (HLA antigens). Slow onset of fever, dyspnoea and tachycardia; shock is rare.
    - reactions to donor plasma proteins (often immunoglobulin A). May cause anaphylactic reactions. Transfusion-related acute lung injury (TRALI), a form of ALI caused by donor antibodies reacting with recipient leucocyte antigens, occurs in 1:5000–10 000 transfusions.
    - graft-versus-host disease in immunosuppressed patients.
    - febrile reactions of unknown aetiology, with or without urticaria.
    - infusion of Rhesus positive blood into Rhesus negative women of child-bearing age may cause haemolytic disease of the newborn in future pregnancies.
    - increased mortality has been reported in patients undergoing surgery for colonic cancer, who receive perioperative transfusion. The mechanism is unknown but may be associated with a substance contained in plasma. Plasma reduced blood has been suggested as a better alternative to whole blood, if transfusion is absolutely necessary in this group.
  - infective:
    - hepatitis. Donors are excluded for 1 year after hepatitis or jaundice. Donor blood is routinely screened for hepatitis B surface antigen. Routine serological testing for hepatitis C was introduced in 1991. Hepatitis A is not tested for, as no carrier state exists. If post-transfusion hepatitis occurs, the donor may be traced and further investigated. Risk of transmission is approximately 1 in 500 000 for hepatitis B and 1 in 32 million for hepatitis C, per unit transfused.
    - HIV infection. At-risk groups are excluded from donating blood. Antibody testing of donor blood has been routine in the UK since 1985. Both cellular components and plasma may transmit HIV. HIV-2 screening began in 1990. Risk of contracting HIV is thought to be 1 in 4–7 million units.
    - human T cell leukaemia and lymphoma virus type I (HTLV-I) transmission may follow blood transfusion; screening is performed in the USA, Canada, Japan, Brazil and several European countries but not in the UK. Malignancy uncommonly follows infection.
    - malaria. Donors are excluded within 6 months of visiting endemic areas. For the following 5 years, plasma only is collected, unless cleared by antibody testing.

- syphilis. Donors with past history are excluded. Blood is routinely screened.
- cytomegalovirus. Antibody testing is available for immunocompromised patients but not routine. About 55% of the population are CMV positive.
- glandular fever: donors are excluded for 2 years.
- brucellosis: donors with past history are excluded.
- bacterial contamination of donor units may result in fever and cardiovascular collapse. Gram-negative organisms are often responsible, e.g. pseudomonas or coliforms. Platelet concentrates harbouring staphylococcus, yersinia and salmonella have been reported. Incidence is about 1 in 500 000.
- transmission of the new variant Creutzfeldt–Jakob disease (vCJD) by contaminated blood has been reported although the importance of this route is unknown, especially since vCJD is still very rare. Routine removal of 95% of white blood cells from blood for transfusion (leucodepletion) was instituted in the UK in 1998 in an attempt to reduce the risk. In 2002 it was announced in the UK that FFP for neonates and children born after 1995 (who should not have been exposed to BSE via the food chain) would be obtained from unpaid US blood donors. In 2004, after the death of a patient who possibly contracted vCJD via transfused blood, UK donors were banned from giving blood if they had received a transfusion after 1980.

- metabolic:
  - hyperkalaemia: rarely a problem, unless with rapid transfusion in hyperkalaemic patients, as potassium is rapidly taken up by red cells after infusion and warming.
  - citrate toxicity: citrate is normally metabolised to bicarbonate within a few minutes. Rapid transfusion of citrated blood may cause hypocalcaemia, and calcium administration may be required. Alkalosis may follow citrate metabolism to bicarbonate. With the modern practice of using SAG-M (saline–adenine–glucose–mannitol) solution, citrate toxicity is rare unless large volumes of plasma or platelet preparations are given, since these do contain citrate.
  - acidosis due to transfused blood is rarely a problem (see above).
- circulatory overload and cardiac failure. More likely in the elderly, and in the correction of chronic anaemia. Diuretics, e.g. furosemide 40 mg, may be given with transfusion.
- hypothermia. Rapid infusion of cold blood may cause cardiac arrest. All transfused blood should be warmed, especially when infused rapidly. Excessive heat may cause haemolysis.
- in the ICU, recent evidence suggests that lowering the threshold for transfusion from 10 g/dl to 7 g/dl may decrease mortality, organ dysfunction and cardiac complications.
- impaired O_2 delivery to tissues, due to the leftward shift of oxyhaemoglobin dissociation curve in stored blood which lasts up to 24 h – possibly even 'pulling' O_2 from the tissues. In addition, red cells in stored blood are thought to be more likely to cause blockage of capillaries owing to their reduced physical flexibility, further impairing O_2 delivery.
- impaired coagulation caused by dilution and/or consumption of circulating clotting factors and platelets. DIC is rare.
- microaggregates (*see Blood filters*).
- thrombophlebitis and extravasation.
- air embolism.
- iron overload (chronic transfusions).
- interaction when stored blood is administered following iv fluids, e.g. clotting (gelatin solutions, Hartmann's solution), haemolysis (dextrose solutions).

Klein HG, Spahn DR, Carson JL (2007). Lancet; 370: 415–26

See also, Blood groups; Blood storage; Blood transfusion, massive; Intravenous fluid administration; Rhesus blood groups

Blood transfusion, autologous. Transfusion of a patient's own, pre-donated, blood. Interest in it has increased over the last decade because of fears over transfusion reactions and transmission of infection, and an increasing shortfall between demand and the supply of blood donors.

- Different methods used:
  - 2–6 units are taken over a period of days or weeks before surgery. Concurrent oral iron therapy ensures an adequate bone-marrow response. Erythropoietin has been used. Pre-transfusion testing varies between centres, from ABO grouping to full cross-matching. Labelling of blood must be meticulous and this requirement, together with wastage of unused blood (which may be up to 20%), results in the administration costs being higher than for allogeneic transfusion. Only suitable for elective surgery.
  - perioperative haemodilution: simultaneous collection of blood and replacement of removed volume with colloid or crystalloid. The collected blood is available for transfusion when required, usually during or shortly after blood loss has stopped.
  - peri- or postoperative retransfusion of blood salvaged from the operation site during surgery. Washing and filtering removes debris and contaminants. Methods range from simple collecting systems to expensive centrifuging machines. Can potentially salvage large volumes of blood but fears have been expressed over activation of coagulation and inflammatory factors in the transfused blood.

Vanderlinde ES, Heal JM, Blumberg N (2002). BMJ; 324: 772–5

See also, Blood transfusion

Blood transfusion, massive. Definitions vary but include:
- transfusion of 10 units of blood within 6 h.
- transfusion of 5 units of blood within 1 h.
- replacement of blood volume with transfused blood within 24 h.

- Adverse effects are those of blood transfusion generally; in particular:
  - impaired O_2 delivery to tissues.
  - impaired coagulation. Fresh frozen plasma and platelets should be given only when there is clinical and laboratory evidence of abnormal coagulation.
  - hypothermia.
  - hypocalcaemia (if rapid transfusion).
  - hyperkalaemia may occur although this is rarely a problem; hypokalaemia may follow potassium uptake by red cells.
  - metabolic acidosis may occur initially; alkalosis may follow as citrate is metabolised to bicarbonate (rare with modern blood products).
  - hypovolaemia or fluid overload.
  - ARDS may follow many situations where large blood transfusions are required.

See also, Blood products; Blood storage

Blood urea nitrogen (BUN). Nitrogen component of blood urea. Gives an indication of renal function in a similar way to urea measurement. Normally 1.5–3.3 mmol/l (10–20 mg/dl).

Blood volume. Measured by dilution techniques; plasma volume is found by injecting a known dose of marker (e.g. albumin labelled with dyes or radioactive iodine) into the blood and measuring plasma concentrations. Rapid exchange of albumin between plasma and interstitial fluid leads to slight overestimation using this method; larger molecules, e.g. immunoglobulin, may be used.

$$\text{Total blood volume} = \text{plasma volume} \times \frac{100}{100 - \%\text{haematocrit}}$$

Red cell volume may be found by labelling erythrocytes with radioactive markers, e.g. ^{51}Cr.

Total blood volume is approximately 70 ml/kg in adults, 80 ml/kg in children and 90 ml/kg in neonates (although the latter may vary widely, depending on how much blood is returned from the placenta at birth. The formula: [% haematocrit + 50] ml/kg has been suggested for neonates).

- Distribution (approximate):
  - 60–70% venous
  - 15% arterial
  - 10% within the heart
  - 5% capillary.

Jones JG, Wardrop CAJ (2000). Br J Anaesth; 84: 226–35

Bloody tap, *see Epidural anaesthesia*

Blow-off valve, *see Adjustable pressure-limiting valve*

BMI, Body mass index, *see Obesity*

BMR, *see Basal metabolic rate*

Bodok seal. Metal-edged rubber bonded disk, used to prevent gas leaks from the cylinder/yoke interface on anaesthetic machines.

Body mass index, *see Obesity*

Body plethysmograph. Airtight box, large enough to enclose a human, used to study lung volumes and pressures. Once a subject is inside, air pressure and volume may be measured before and during respiration.

- May be used to measure:
  - FRC: the subject makes inspiratory effort against a shutter. Box volume is decreased due to lung expansion, and box pressure increased because of the decrease in volume. Applying Boyle's law:

    original pressure × volume = new pressure × new volume

    where new volume = original volume – change in lung volume.

    Thus change in lung volume may be calculated. If airway pressures are also measured:

    original airway pressure × resting lung volume = new airway pressure × new lung volume

    where resting lung volume = FRC
    new volume = FRC + change in lung volume.

    Thus FRC may be calculated.
  - airway resistance:

    $$= \frac{\text{alveolar pressure} - \text{mouth pressure}}{\text{airflow}}$$

    The subject breathes the air in the box. Box volume is reduced by the change in alveolar volume during inspiration, measured as above. Lung volume may be measured at the same time, as above:

    lung volume × starting alveolar pressure = new lung volume × new alveolar pressure;

    where starting alveolar pressure = box pressure, and new lung volume = lung volume + alveolar volume.

    Alveolar pressure may thus be calculated. Also, mouth pressure = box pressure, and flow may be measured using a pneumotachograph.
  - pulmonary blood flow: the subject breathes from a bag containing N_2O and O_2 within the box. As the N_2O is taken up by the blood, the volume of the bag decreases. Since N_2O uptake is flow limited (*see Alveolar gas transfer*), uptake occurs in steps with each heartbeat. The decrease in bag size therefore occurs in steps, and is calculated by measuring bag pressure, and box volume and pressure. If the N_2O carrying capacity of blood is known, pulmonary blood flow may be calculated and displayed as a continuous trace showing pulsatile flow.

Body surface area, *see Surface area, body*

Bohr effect. Shift to the right of the oxyhaemoglobin dissociation curve associated with a rise in blood $P\text{CO}_2$ and/or fall in pH. Results in lower affinity of haemoglobin for O_2, favouring O_2 delivery to the tissues, where CO_2 levels are high.

The double Bohr effect refers to pregnancy, when CO_2 passes from fetal to maternal blood at the placenta, causing the following changes:

- maternal blood: CO_2 rises, i.e. shift of curve to right and reduced O_2 affinity.
- fetal blood: CO_2 falls, i.e. shift of curve to left and increased O_2 affinity.

The net effect is to favour O_2 transfer from maternal to fetal blood.

[Christian Bohr (1855–1911), Danish physiologist]

See also, Oxygen transport

Bohr equation. Equation used to derive physiological dead space.

Expired CO_2 = inspired CO_2 + CO_2 given out by lungs,
or: $F_E \times V_T = (F_I \times V_T) + (F_A \times V_A)$,

where F_E = fractional concentration of CO_2 in expired gas
F_I = fractional concentration of CO_2 in inspired gas
F_A = fractional concentration of CO_2 in alveolar gas
V_T = tidal volume
V_A = alveolar component of tidal volume.

Since inspired CO_2 is negligible, it may be ignored:

i.e. $F_E \times V_T = F_A \times V_A$

But $V_A = V_T - V_D$, where V_D = dead space

Therefore: $F_E \times V_T = F_A \times (V_T - V_D)$
$= (F_A \times V_T) - (F_A \times V_D)$
or: $F_A \times V_D = (F_A \times V_T) - (F_E \times V_T)$
$= V_T\,(F_A - F_E)$

$$\text{Therefore } \frac{V_D}{V_T} = \frac{F_A - F_E}{F_A}$$

Since partial pressure is proportional to concentration:

$$\frac{V_D}{V_T} = \frac{P_A\text{CO}_2 - P_E\text{CO}_2}{P_A\text{CO}_2}$$

where $P_A\text{CO}_2$ = alveolar partial pressure of CO_2
$P_E\text{CO}_2$ = mixed expired partial pressure of CO_2

Since alveolar $P\text{CO}_2$ approximately equals arterial $P\text{CO}_2$,

$$\frac{V_D}{V_T} = \frac{P_a\text{CO}_2 - P_E\text{CO}_2}{P_a\text{CO}_2}$$

where P_aCO_2 = arterial partial pressure of CO_2.
See also, Bohr effect

Boiling point (bp). Temperature of a substance at which its SVP equals external atmospheric pressure. Additional heat does not raise the temperature further, but provides the latent heat of vaporisation necessary for the liquid to evaporate. If external pressure is raised, e.g. within a pressure cooker, bp is also raised; thus the maximal temperature attainable is raised, and food cooks more quickly.

Bone marrow harvest. Taking of bone marrow for bone marrow transplantation, from either a healthy donor (allograft) or the patient-recipient prior to radio- or chemotherapy (autograft). Usually performed under general anaesthesia, especially in children, although local anaesthetic techniques may be used.

- Anaesthetic considerations:
  - preoperatively:
    - allografts: donors are usually fit.
    - autografts: usually performed for blood malignancy; i.e. patients may be anaemic, thrombocytopenic, etc. and prone to infections. Cardiovascular, respiratory and renal function may be impaired. Drug treatment may include cytotoxic drugs and corticosteroids.
  - perioperatively:
    - marrow is usually taken from the posterior and anterior iliac crests and sternum, requiring positioning first supine, then prone, although the lateral position may suffice. Tracheal intubation and IPPV is usually employed. Avoidance of N_2O has been suggested but this is controversial.
    - an iv cannula is mandatory, since large volume losses, initially from marrow cavity but eventually from the vascular compartment, must be replaced. Autologous blood transfusion is usually performed, especially for allografts. Non-autologous blood is irradiated prior to transfusion to kill any leucocytes present. The volume of marrow harvested is up to 20–30% of estimated blood volume, to provide the required leucocyte count.
    - heparin may be given to stop the marrow clotting; it may also protect against fat embolism which may occur during harvesting.
  - postoperatively: large volumes of iv fluids are often required.

Bone marrow transplantation. Performed for leukaemias, lymphomas, certain solid tumours, and various non-malignant disorders including aplastic anaemia, haemoglobinopathies and rare genetic diseases. Involves donation of bone marrow (usually under general anaesthesia), and its subsequent infusion via a central vein into the recipient, whose own bone marrow has been ablated with chemotherapy ± radiotherapy.

- May be one of three types:
  - autologous: the recipient's own bone marrow is taken and treated to remove neoplastic cells before being frozen and stored while ablation is performed. Mortality is up to 10%.
  - syngeneic: the donor and recipient are identical twins. Treatment of the collected cells is not required.
  - allogeneic: the donor is HLA-matched as closely as possible to the recipient; they usually come from the same family or racial group. Mortality is up to 30%.
- Problems occur with all three types but to different extents, and may be related to:
  - the procedure itself:
    - ablative therapy includes cyclophosphamide, busulfan and other cytotoxic and immunosuppressive drugs. Toxic effects include vomiting, cardiomyopathy, convulsions, pulmonary fibrosis, GIT mucositis and hepatic veno-occlusive disease.
    - impaired bone marrow function: bacterial, viral, fungal and pneumocystis infections may be problems in the first 4–6 months after autologous and syngeneic transplantation; immunodeficiency may be especially prolonged after allogeneic transplantation, when prolonged immunosuppressive therapy is required. Antibacterial and antiviral drugs are often given prophylactically; immunoglobulins have also been used (*see Immunoglobulins, intravenous*). Blood products are often required to restore red cell, white cell and platelet numbers. Recently, macrophage and granulocyte colony-stimulating factors have been used.
  - rejection: may require repeat transplantation.
  - graft-versus-host disease.
  - interstitial pneumonitis may occur; it may be unclear whether this is related to cytomegalovirus or other atypical infection, or directly related to radiotherapy. Mortality is up to 80%.

Boott, Francis (1792–1863). US-born London physician; qualified in Edinburgh. Read in a letter from Bigelow's father about Morton's demonstration of diethyl ether, and arranged a dental extraction by Robinson (who also administered the ether) on 19th December 1846 at his house in Gower St., London, now a nursing home and formerly the location of part of the FCAnaes examination. Informed Liston, who operated using ether 2 days later.
[James Robinson (1813–1861), English dentist]
Ellis RH (1977). Anaesthesia; 32: 197–208

Bosentan monohydrate. Endothelin receptor antagonist (both type A and type B) licensed as a treatment for pulmonary hypertension. Decreases both pulmonary and systemic BP without affecting heart rate. May cause hepatic impairment. Sitaxsentan is similar but has greater action at type A receptors and is less hepatotoxic.

Bosun warning device, *see Oxygen failure warning devices*

Botulinum toxins. Group of exotoxins responsible for botulism. Eight have been characterised (labelled A–H), each produced by a distinct strain of *Clostridium botulinum*. Types A, B and E (rarely, F and G) cause disease in humans. Types A and B have been used therapeutically in minute quantities in order to cause selective muscle weakness which may last for several months, e.g. in strabismus, blepharospasm, hemifacial spasm, torticollis, dystonias, spasmodic dysphonia and as a cosmetic procedure. Also used as a tool to investigate neurotransmitter function.

Botulism. Clinical syndrome caused by ingestion of exotoxins (botulinum toxins) produced by the anaerobic Gram-positive bacillus *Clostridium botulinum*. Exotoxin binds irreversibly to nerve endings, preventing acetylcholine release. Affects the neuromuscular junction, autonomic ganglia and parasympathetic postganglionic fibres. Classified according to the source of infection:
  - foodborne botulism: caused by ingestion of clostridium spores or exotoxin produced under anaerobic conditions (e.g. home canning).
  - wound botulism: due to contamination of surgical or other wounds. Recently seen in drug abusers injecting 'black-tar' heroin subcutaneously ('skin-popping').

- infant botulism: due to absorption of exotoxin produced within the GIT, classically after eating contaminated honey.
- adult infectious botulism: similar to the infant form but follows GIT surgery.
- inadvertent botulism: follows accidental overdose of botulinum toxin given for treatment of movement disorders (e.g. dystonia).

- Features occur within 12–72 h:
  - nausea, vomiting and abdominal pain.
  - symmetrical descending paralysis initially affecting cranial nerves, with diplopia, facial weakness, dysphagia, dysarthria, limb weakness, and respiratory difficulty.
  - autonomic disturbance: ileus, unresponsive pupils, dry mouth, urinary retention.
  - sensory deficit, mental disturbance and fever do not occur.

Diagnosed by inoculation of the patient's serum into mice which have been treated or untreated with antitoxin. Different strains of toxin may be identified. EMG studies may aid diagnosis while waiting for inoculation studies.

- Management:
  - supportive. IPPV may be necessary.
  - antitoxin to neutralise circulating exotoxin. Hypersensitivity may occur. A human botulism immunoglobulin is used for treatment of infant botulism and those allergic to the antitoxin.
  - penicillin to kill live bacilli.

Complete recovery may take months.

Caya JG, Agni R, Miller JE (2004). Arch Pathol Lab Med; 128: 653–62

See also, Biological weapons, Paralysis, acute

Bougie, *see Intubation aids*

Bourdon gauge, *see Pressure measurement*

Bovie machine, *see Diathermy*

Bowditch effect. Intrinsic regulatory mechanism of cardiac muscle in response to increased rate of stimulation. As rate increases, contractility increases.

[Henry Bowditch (1840–1911), US physiologist]

Bowel ischaemia. May affect any part of the GIT (although rarely stomach) but usually affects the large bowel. May be caused by thrombus, embolism (e.g. from mural thrombus after MI), vascular spasm, or low mesenteric perfusion with vasoconstriction (non-occlusive mesenteric ischaemia (NOMI)). May occur in patients with intra-abdominal pathology, especially following vascular surgery, or in any patient with low cardiac output. May also occur in severe intestinal obstruction. Vasoconstriction often persists after correction of the initial insult. Bowel infarction may follow as a result of reduced tissue oxygenation or reperfusion injury.

Associated with high mortality because diagnosis may be difficult, and bowel infarction may continue despite treatment. Gastric tonometry has been used to monitor GIT perfusion in critical illness.

Features include abdominal pain and distension, GIT bleeding, nausea and vomiting, tachycardia, pyrexia, leucocytosis, and metabolic acidosis. Angiography may be useful to diagnose ischaemia and differentiate its causes.

- Treatment:
  - supportive measures including antibacterial drugs, restoration of cardiac output ± vasodilator drugs.
  - intra-arterial infusion of vasodilators, e.g. papaverine 30–60 mg/h, has been used via the angiography catheter.
  - surgery to resect necrotic bowel ± remove embolus or thrombus.

Oldenberg WA, Lau LL, Rodenberg TJ, et al (2004). Arch Intern Med; 164: 1054–62

Boyle, Henry Edmund Gaskin (1875–1941). English anaesthetist, best known for the anaesthetic machine named after him. Originally introduced in 1917, it consisted of N_2O and O_2 cylinders, pressure gauges, water-sight flowmeters and ether vaporiser ('Boyle's bottle') set in a wooden case. His name is also attached to the instrument used to maintain jaw opening during tonsillectomy (Boyle–Davis gag). Boyle practised at St Bartholomew's Hospital, London, was involved in the advancement and improvement of anaesthesia in the UK, and performed much work into the use of N_2O, including under battle conditions.

[John S Davis (1824–1885), US surgeon]

Hadfield CF (1950). Br J Anaesth; 22: 107–17

Boyle's law. At constant temperature, the volume of a fixed mass of a perfect gas varies inversely with pressure.

[Robert Boyle (1627–1691), English chemist]

See also, Charles' law; Ideal gas law

Brachial artery. Continuation of the axillary artery, running from the lower border of teres minor to the antecubital fossa, where it divides into the radial and ulnar arteries. Lies at first medial, then anterior to the humerus. Around its midpoint, crossed from lateral to medial by the median nerve. Protected from the medial cubital vein in the antecubital fossa by the bicipital aponeurosis. Occasionally divides in the upper arm.

May be used for arterial cannulation, although seldom as the site of first choice because of possible distal ischaemia.

Brachial plexus. Nerve plexus supplying the arm. Arises from the ventral rami of the lower cervical and first thoracic spinal nerves, and emerges between the scalene muscles in the neck. The plexus invaginates the scalene fascia and passes down over the first rib (Fig. 24a). It accompanies the subclavian artery (which becomes the axillary artery) within a perivascular sheath of connective tissue.

- Anatomy of the scalene muscles:
  - scalenus anterior arises from the anterior tubercles of the 3rd–6th cervical transverse processes, and inserts into the scalene tubercle on the first rib.
  - scalenus medius arises from the posterior tubercles of the 2nd–6th cervical transverse processes, and inserts into the first rib behind the groove for the subclavian artery.
  - scalenus posterior is the portion of the previous muscle attached to the second rib.
- The roots lie in the interscalene groove; the trunks cross the posterior triangle of the neck; the divisions lie behind the clavicle; the cords lie in the axilla. Branches arise at different levels (Fig. 24b):
  - roots: nerves to the rhomboids, scalene muscles and serratus anterior (long thoracic nerve), and a contribution to the phrenic nerve (C5).
  - trunks: nerve to subclavius, and the suprascapular nerve (to supraspinatus and infraspinatus).
  - cords:
    - lateral:
      - lateral pectoral nerve to pectoralis major.
      - musculocutaneous nerve: passes through the belly of coracobrachialis in the upper arm, supplying

coracobrachialis, biceps and brachialis muscles and the elbow joint. Continues as the lateral cutaneous nerve of the forearm, supplying the radial surface of the forearm.
  - lateral part of the median nerve.
- medial:
  - medial pectoral nerve to pectoralis major and minor.
  - medial cutaneous nerves of the arm and forearm: supply the medial aspect of the upper arm and forearm respectively.
  - ulnar nerve.
  - medial part of median nerve.
- posterior:
  - subscapular nerves to subscapularis and teres major.
  - nerve to latissimus dorsi.
  - axillary nerve: passes posterior to the neck of the humerus. Supplies deltoid and teres minor and the shoulder joint, and continues as the upper lateral cutaneous nerve of the arm, supplying the skin of the outer shoulder.
  - radial nerve.

The plexus thus supplies the skin of the upper limb (Fig. 24c).

- Characteristic motor lesions of the plexus:
  - upper roots: 'waiter's tip' position; arm internally rotated and pronated, with wrist flexed (Erb's paralysis).
  - lower roots: claw hand (Klumpke's paralysis).

[Wilhelm Erb (1840–1921), German physician; Augusta Klumpke (1859–1927), French neurologist]

See also, Brachial plexus block; Dermatomes

Brachial plexus block. May be performed by injecting local anaesthetic solution into the fascial compartment surrounding the brachial plexus at several levels:

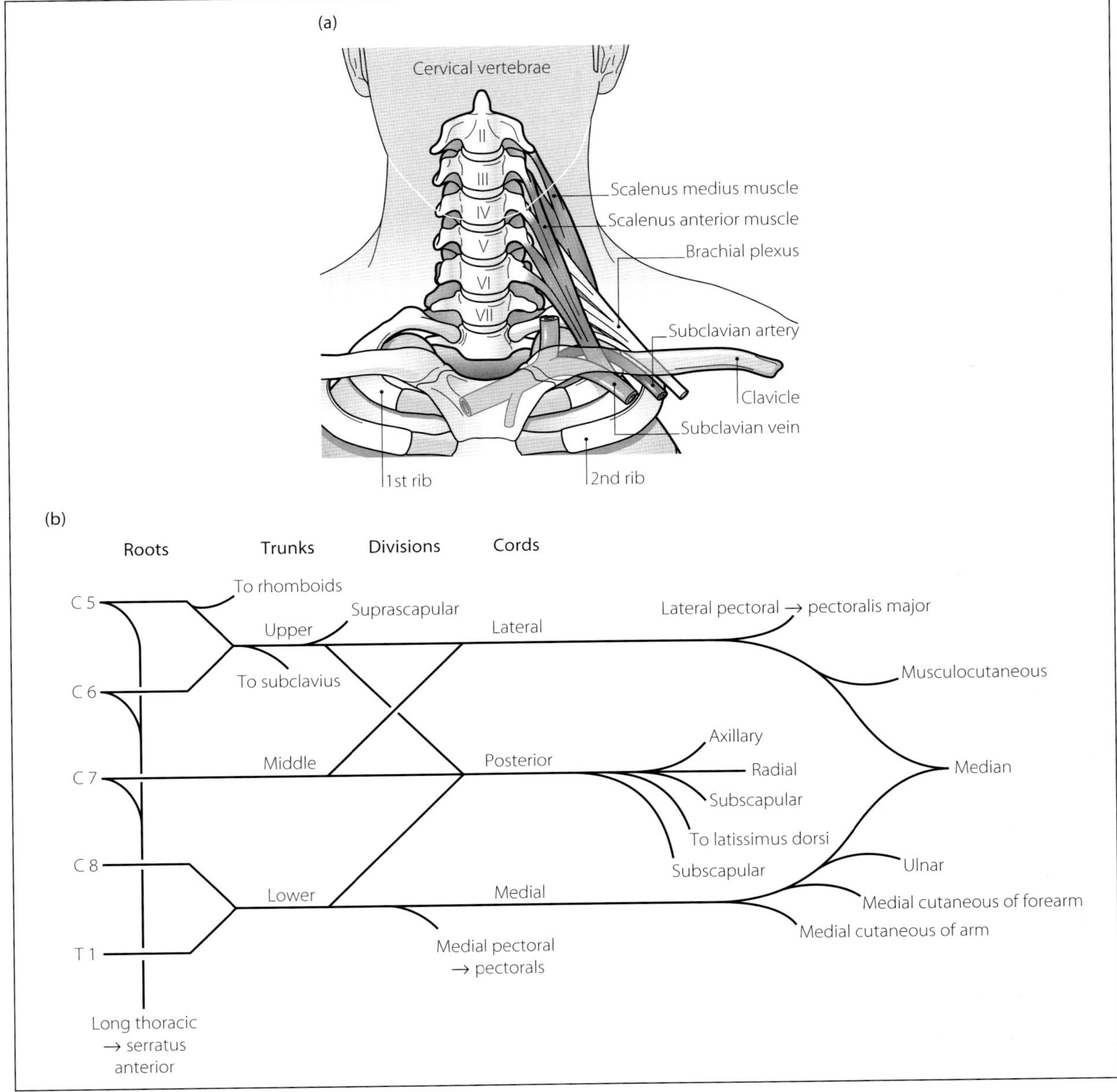

Fig. 24 (a) Relations of the upper brachial plexus. (b) Plan of the brachial plexus.

(Continued)

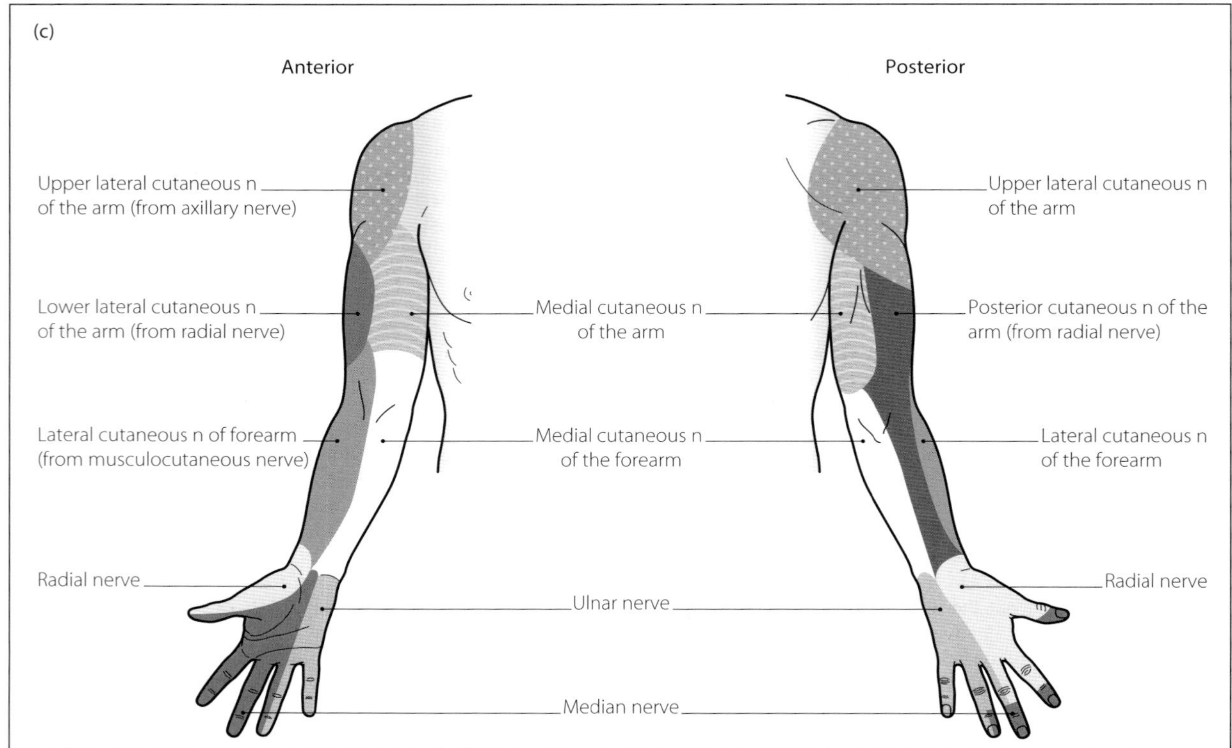

Fig. 24 Cont'd. (c) Cutaneous nerve supply of the arm

- interscalene:
  - with the patient's head turned away from the side to be blocked, a needle is inserted in the interscalene groove, lateral to the sternomastoid, and level with the cricoid cartilage. It is directed towards the transverse process of C6 (medially, caudally and posteriorly). Accidental epidural, intrathecal or intravascular injections are more likely if the needle is directed cranially.
  - 30–40 ml solution is injected when paraesthesia is produced or a click felt. If a nerve stimulator is used, contractions should be sought in the shoulder, arm or forearm.
  - produces adequate block for shoulder manipulations.
  - ulnar nerve may be 'missed'.
  - complications include phrenic nerve block, recurrent laryngeal nerve block, Horner's syndrome, inadvertent epidural or spinal block, and injection into the vertebral artery. Bilateral blocks, or blocks in patients with contralateral phrenic nerve palsy, should be avoided.
- supraclavicular:
  - with the patient's head turned away from the side to be blocked, a needle is inserted immediately posterior and lateral to the subclavian pulsation behind the mid-clavicle. In the classic technique, it is directed caudally, medially and posteriorly to the upper surface of first rib, and 'walked' along the rib until paraesthesia is produced; 8–10 ml solution are injected per division. If a nerve stimulator is used, contraction is sought in the required area to be blocked.
  - median nerve may be 'missed'.
  - complications: phrenic and recurrent laryngeal nerve blocks, Horner's syndrome, subclavian puncture, pneumothorax. Bilateral blocks should be avoided.
- subclavian perivascular:
  - with the patient's head turned away from the side to be blocked, a needle is inserted in the interscalene groove, caudal to the level of the cricoid cartilage, and cranial and posterior to a finger palpating the subclavian artery. It is directed caudally only, until paraesthesia is produced in the arm/hand, not in the shoulder (which may be caused by stimulation of the suprascapular nerve). If a nerve stimulator is used, contraction is sought in the required area to be blocked.
  - 20–30 ml solution are injected.
  - complications: as for supraclavicular block, but pneumothorax is less likely.
- axillary:
  - with the patient's head turned away, the arm abducted to 90°, and the hand under the head, a needle is inserted just above the axillary artery pulsation, as high in the axilla as possible. A click is felt as the perivascular sheath is entered.
  - 25–50 ml solution is injected, with digital pressure or a tourniquet below the injection site to encourage upward spread of solution. Careful aspiration before application of digital pressure excludes placement of the needle in the axillary vein. The arm is returned to the patient's side after injection, to avoid compression of the proximal sheath by the humeral head, or before injection if a cannula technique is used.
  - a cannula, e.g. iv type 18–20 G, may be inserted and used for repeated injection.
  - may 'miss' the musculocutaneous and axillary nerves. The former may be blocked thus:
    - upper arm: at the time of axillary block, 5–10 ml is injected above the perivascular sheath, into coracobrachialis muscle.

- elbow: 10 ml is injected in the groove between biceps tendon and brachioradialis in the antecubital fossa, and infiltrated subcutaneously around the lateral elbow.
- the intercostobrachial nerve, supplying the inner upper arm, may be blocked by superficial infiltration as the needle is withdrawn from the axillary block.
- fascial sheets within the neurovascular sheath may cause a 'patchy' block. Puncture both above and below the artery has been suggested as a remedy. Alternatively, separate identification of the different nerves with a nerve stimulator has been advocated (median: causes contraction of flexor carpi radialis; ulnar: flexor carpi ulnaris; radial: extensor muscles of hand/wrist; musculocutaneous: biceps), with the total dose divided between them. Intentional transfixion of the artery has also been described: blood is aspirated as the needle is advanced through the artery; when aspiration ceases, solution is deposited posterior to the artery.

- infraclavicular:
  - with the patient's arm abducted, a needle is inserted 2–3 cm caudal to the midpoint of a line drawn between the medial head of the clavicle and the coracoid process. The needle is advanced laterally parallel to this line and at 45° to the skin until twitches are seen in the hand (pectoral contraction indicates superficial placement of the needle, and biceps contraction may be achieved by stimulating the musculocutaneous nerve outside the plexus sheath). Has also been described with the needle directed directly posteriorly at a point 1 cm medial and 2 cm caudal to the coracoid process.
  - 30–45 ml solution is injected.
  - avoids the complications of interscalene and supraclavicular approaches, and suitable as an alternative to axillary block.
- posterior:
  - with the patient sitting or lying, and the cervical spine flexed, a needle is inserted 3 cm from the midline level with the C6–7 interspace. A loss of resistance technique or nerve stimulation has been described, with injection of 20–40 ml solution at a depth of 5–7 cm. Horner's syndrome is common; difficulty breathing may also occur and epidural and spinal blockade have been reported.

- Suitable solutions:
  - prilocaine or lidocaine 1–1.5% with adrenaline: onset within 20–30 min and lasts for 1.5–2 h.
  - bupivacaine 0.375–0.5%: onset up to 1 h; lasts for up to 12 h. Combination with 1% lidocaine speeds onset.

The area blocked is increased by using larger volumes of solution. Motor block is increased by increasing concentration, and intensity of block by increasing total dose. Although maximal safe doses have been exceeded without serious effects or high blood levels of agent, this cannot be recommended routinely. Systemic uptake of agent is greatest following interscalene block, and least following axillary block. Incidence of neurological damage is thought to be reduced by using short bevelled needles, and using a nerve stimulator rather than eliciting paraesthesia as the end-point for injection.

Bradycardia, *see Heart block; Junctional arrhythmias; Sinus bradycardia*

Bradykinin, *see Kinins*

Brain. Intracranial part of the CNS. Forms from tubular neural tissue, developing into hindbrain (rhombencephalon), midbrain (mesencephalon) and forebrain (prosencephalon):

- hindbrain:
  - medulla: continuous with the spinal cord. Communicates with the cerebellum via the inferior cerebellar peduncle. Forms the posterior part of the fourth ventricle floor. Contains the decussation of pyramidal tracts, gracile and cuneate nuclei, nuclei of cranial nerves IX, X, XI and XII, and 'vital centres', e.g. for respiration and cardiovascular homeostasis.
  - pons: communicates with the cerebellum via the middle cerebellar peduncle. Forms the anterior part of the fourth ventricle floor. Contains the nuclei of cranial nerves V, VI, VII and VIII, and pontine nuclei.
  - cerebellum: occupies the posterior cranial fossa. Consists of grey cortex covering white matter. Communicates via the medulla, pons and midbrain with the thalamus, cerebral cortex and spinal cord. Regulates posture, coordination and muscle tone. Lesions cause ipsilateral effects.
- midbrain: communicates with the cerebellum via the superior cerebellar peduncle. Contains the pineal body and cranial nerve nuclei III and IV.
- forebrain:
  - diencephalon: consists of the hypothalamus (floor of the third ventricle) with the pituitary gland below, and thalamus (lateral wall of the third ventricle). The thalamus integrates sensory pathways.
  - basal ganglia: grey matter within cerebral hemispheres. The internal capsule, containing the major ascending and descending pathways to and from the cerebral cortex, passes between the basal ganglia. They receive and relay information concerned with fine motor control.
  - cerebral cortex:
    - frontal lobes: contain motor cortices, including areas for speech and eye movement; areas for intellectual and emotional functions lie anteriorly.
    - parietal lobes: contain sensory cortices, and areas for association and integration of sensory input.
    - temporal lobes: contain auditory cortices, and areas for integration and association of auditory input and memory. Also constitutes part of the limbic system, which integrates endocrine, autonomic and motivational functions.
    - occipital lobes: contain the visual cortices, and areas for association and integration of visual sensory input.

See also, Ascending reticular activating system; Brainstem; Cerebral circulation; Cerebrospinal fluid; Motor pathways; Sensory pathways

Brainstem. Composed of midbrain, pons and medulla. Contains neurone groups involved in the control of breathing, cardiovascular homeostasis, GIT function, balance and equilibrium, and eye movement. Also integrates ascending and descending pathways between the spinal cord, cranial nerves, cerebellum and higher centres, partly via the ascending reticular activating system.

See also, Brain; Brainstem death; Breathing, control of

Brainstem death. Irreversible absence of brainstem function despite artificial maintenance of circulation and gas exchange. Clinical experience has shown that once it is diagnosed, cardiac arrest is inevitable, usually within a few days. Guidelines have been established for the withdrawal of artificial support and, where appropriate, arrangement for organ donation, when recovery is impossible. These guidelines include:

- necessary preconditions:
  - apnoeic coma (i.e. the patient is unresponsive and requiring IPPV).
  - irremediable structural brain damage caused by a disorder which can lead to brain death (e.g. subarachnoid haemorrhage, head injury, meningitis).
- necessary exclusions:
  - absence of primary hypothermia, i.e. core temperature > 35°C (n.b. secondary hypothermia often follows brainstem death).
  - absence of primary metabolic or endocrine disturbance (n.b. secondary endocrine abnormalities often follow brainstem death, e.g. diabetes insipidus, lack of thyrotropin or prolactin).
  - absence of drug intoxication, including sedatives given in ICU.
  - absence of paralysis caused by neuromuscular blocking drugs (neuromuscular blockade monitoring is useful) or neuromuscular disorders (e.g. Guillain-Barré syndrome).
  - absence of abnormal posturing (e.g. decorticate or decerebrate) or convulsions.
- necessary clinical findings:
  - absent cranial nerve reflexes:
    - pupillary light reflex.
    - corneal reflex.
    - oculovestibular reflex, i.e. no eye movement following injection of 40–60 ml icy water into the ear canal (normal response is a tonic deviation of the eyes towards the side being irrigated followed by a faster phase back towards the midline). Each ear is tested in turn, having checked that the canal is not blocked. (In the UK, testing for doll's eye movements is not used as a component of brainstem testing.)
    - gag reflex.
    - cough reflex.
  - absent motor responses within cranial nerve distribution, to any peripheral stimuli.
  - absent respiratory efforts despite arterial $P\text{CO}_2$ of 6.6 kPa (50 mmHg), and adequate oxygenation (e.g. with apnoeic oxygenation). Blood gas tensions should be measured to confirm this.

All the above requirements must be met for the diagnosis of brainstem death to be made. Two sets of tests should be performed by two doctors (registered for 5 years) who have skill in the field, one of whom is a consultant.

The tests may be carried out together or separately. No specific time interval has been recommended between testing. Although EEG, cerebral angiography and oesophageal contractility testing are performed in some centres, they are not required to make the diagnosis of brainstem death. The legal time of death is recorded as the time the first set of tests shows no activity.

Although the clinical criteria remain unchanged for paediatric patients, the interval between the two tests differs. No UK recommendations exist; therefore the US ones are usually followed for children of different ages:

- newborn to 2 months (usually performed for medicolegal reasons): interval 48 h.
- 2–12 months: 24 h.
- 1–18 years: 12 h.

Persistent vegetative state associated with absent cortical function or cortical disconnection may occur with intact brainstem reflexes. Such patients may have spontaneous respiration and may live for years without recovery, and do not satisfy the criteria for brainstem death.

Wijdicks EFM (2001). N Engl J Med; 344: 1215–21

Braun, Heinrich Friedrich Wilhelm (1862–1934). German surgeon; also practised and investigated anaesthesia. One of the pioneers of local anaesthesia, he described many local blocks, and published extensively on the subject. Introduced adrenaline to local anaesthetic solutions to prolong their action in 1902. Popularised procaine in 1905.

Breathing, control of. The exact origin of the signal for regular breathing is unknown. Brainstem centres involved in the control of breathing have been identified; their precise roles are unclear. There are three such centres:

- medullary centre:
  - dorsal neurones cause diaphragmatic contraction via contralateral phrenic nerves; they also project to ventral neurones.
  - ventral neurones cause contraction of ipsilateral accessory muscles (via vagus nerves) and intercostal muscles.
- apneustic centre in the lower pons: causes excitation of medullary inspiratory neurones. Surgical section above it causes prolonged inspiratory gasping. Vagal division in addition causes apneusis (breath held at end-inspiration).
- pneumotactic centre (nucleus parabrachialis) in the upper pons: curtails inspiration and regulates respiratory rate.

- The 'respiratory centre' comprised of these groups of neurones receives afferents from chemoreceptors and other structures:
  - chemoreceptors :
    - peripheral (aortic and carotid bodies): afferents pass via the vagus and glossopharyngeal nerves respectively. Stimulated by a fall in arterial $P\text{O}_2$, also by a rise in $P\text{CO}_2$ and hydrogen ion concentration. Their response to reduced O_2 increases markedly below 8–10 kPa (60–75 mmHg). The response to increased CO_2 is roughly linear.
    - central: present on the ventral surface of the medulla, but separate from the respiratory centre. Stimulated by a rise in hydrogen ion concentration in CSF, due to increased $P\text{CO}_2$ or metabolic acidosis.

    Hypoxaemia increases the sensitivity of the chemoreceptors to hypercapnia, and vice versa. Hypoxaemia causes direct depression of the respiratory centres, in addition to reflex stimulation. In chronic lung disease, the central chemoreceptors may not respond to increased CO_2 levels, either due to chemoreceptor 'resetting' or due to correction of CSF pH. Hypoxaemia then becomes the main drive to respiration (of importance in O_2 therapy).
  - other structures:
    - lungs:
      - pulmonary stretch receptors, involved in the Hering–Breuer and deflation reflexes.
      - juxtapulmonary capillary receptors, involved in dyspnoea due to pulmonary disease and pulmonary oedema.
      - pulmonary irritant receptors, responding to noxious stimuli.
    - proprioceptors in joints and muscles, thought to be important during exercise.
    - baroreceptors; hypertension inhibits ventilation, but this is of little clinical significance.
    - higher centres, responding to pain, fear, etc.

During anaesthesia, the responses to hypercapnia and hypoxaemia are depressed, the latter severely.

Caruana-Montaldo B, Gleeson K, Zwillich CW (2000). Chest; 117: 205–25

See also, Carbon dioxide response curve; Hypoventilation

Breathing, muscles of, *see Respiratory muscles*

Breathing systems, *see Anaesthetic breathing systems*

Breathing, work of. Equals the product of pressure change across the lung and volume of gas moved. During inspiration, most of the work of breathing is done to overcome elastic recoil of the thorax and lungs, and the resistance of the airways and non-elastic tissues (Fig. 25):

- the area enclosed by the broken line represents work done to overcome elastic forces.
- area A represents work done to overcome resistance during inspiration.
- area B represents work done to overcome resistance during expiration.

The greater the tidal volume or lung volume, the more work is required to overcome elastic recoil. The faster the flow rates, the greater the amount of work required to overcome resistance. Normally, energy is provided for expiration by potential energy stored in the stretched elastic tissues (i.e. area B lies within the broken line), but extra energy may be required in airway obstruction.

Total work of breathing is difficult to measure in spontaneous respiration. Volume may be measured with a pneumotachograph; oesophageal pressure, indicating intrapleural pressure, may be measured with an oesophageal balloon. Normally, the work of breathing accounts for less than 3% of the total body O_2 consumption at rest, but may be much higher in disease states, e.g. COPD, cardiac failure, and during exercise.

Expiratory valves in anaesthetic breathing systems increase work of expiration, particularly when not fully open. Coaxial anaesthetic breathing systems increase expiratory resistance, the Lack by virtue of its small calibre expiratory tube, and the Bain because of the high flow rate of fresh gas directed at the patient's mouth.

See also, Airway resistance; Compliance

Bretylium tosylate. Class II and III antiarrhythmic drug, originally introduced as an antihypertensive drug. Reduces sympathetic drive to the heart and prolongs the action potential. Taken up by adrenergic nerve endings, causing release of noradrenaline followed by inhibition of release. Reserved for treatment of resistant ventricular arrhythmias. Excreted largely unchanged in the urine. Difficulties with manufacture led to cessation of production in 2004.

- Dosage: 5–10 mg/kg iv, over 8–10 min (preferably 15–30 min), repeated 1–2 h later up to 30 mg/kg. Followed by 1–2 mg/min or 5–10 mg/kg 6–8 hourly. May also be given im.

Initial hypertension may be followed by severe hypotension. May cause nausea and vomiting.

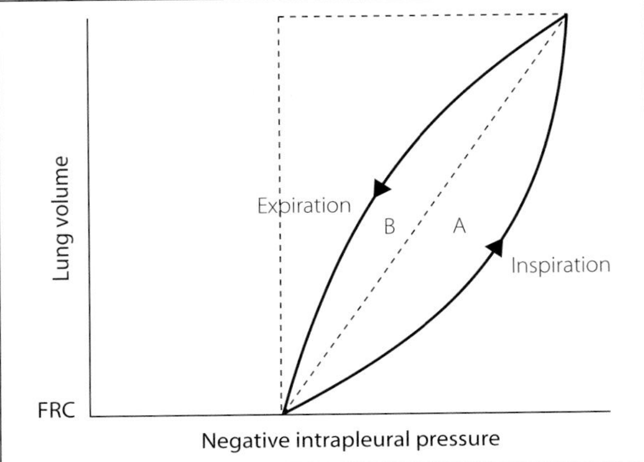

Fig. 25 Graph of intrapleural pressure against lung volume during breathing (see text)

Brewer–Luckhardt reflex. Laryngospasm in response to remote stimulation, e.g. anal or cervical dilatation.

[Nathan R Brewer and Arno B Luckhardt (1885–1957), US physiologists]

British Association for Immediate Care (BASICS). Voluntary, charitable organisation, formed in 1977, whose members provide medical assistance at the scene of an accident, medical emergency or during primary transport to hospital. Acts as the national coordinating body for schemes and individual doctors providing immediate care throughout the UK. Organises educational courses for doctors, nurses, paramedics, occupational health professionals, the emergency services, and those involved in health care at sporting and other events.

British Association of Critical Care Nurses (BACCN). Formed in 1984 from the amalgamation of various groups of UK critical care nurses. Exists to support personal and professional development of members (who include nurses, managers, educationalists, researchers and others with an interest in critical care) and to promote the art and science of critical care nursing. Its official journal is *Nursing in Critical Care*.

***British Journal of Anaesthesia*.** Second oldest journal of anaesthesia (first published in 1923), and the first to be published monthly (in 1955). Previously unassociated with any association, institution or society, it became the official journal of the College of Anaesthetists in 1990.

Spence AA (1988). Br J Anaesth; 60: 605–7

Bromethol (Tribromethanol; Avertin). CBr_3CH_2OH. Sedative drug introduced in 1927 and no longer available. Given rectally to provide deep sedation or anaesthesia, particularly in children. Also given iv. May cause cardiovascular and respiratory depression.

Bromocriptine. Dopamine receptor antagonist, used to inhibit prolactin and growth hormone secretion. Has also been used in Parkinson's disease.

- Dosage:
  - 1.0 mg orally/day, increasing up to 20–40 mg/day in endocrine disease and Parkinson's disease.
  - 2.5 mg once or twice/day for suppression of lactation postpartum.
- Side effects: nausea, vomiting, constipation, headache, dizziness, postural hypotension, confusion, dry mouth, pleural effusion, rarely retroperitoneal fibrosis. Should be avoided postpartum in pre-eclampsia, heart disease and psychiatric disorders.

Bronchial blockers, *see Endobronchial blockers*

Bronchial carcinoma. Commonest cause of death from cancer in Western men and women. Mostly associated with smoking, but also occurs following exposure to asbestos, and certain chemical and radioactive substances used in industry. Air pollution may also be a causative factor. Five-year survival in the UK is less than 10%; in the USA and certain parts of Europe it is ~15%.

- Types:
  - small cell (~20%): may arise from APUD cells, and secrete hormones. Extensive spread is usual at presentation. Extremely poor prognosis.
  - non-small cell:
    - adenocarcinoma (~40%).
    - squamous cell (~30%): most present with bronchial obstruction. Better prognosis than the other common forms.
    - large cell (~10%); particularly related to smoking.
    - others:
      - bronchiolar alveolar, carcinoid: least related to smoking.
      - carcinoma in situ.
      - others.
- Features:
  - local:
    - haemoptysis, cough, dyspnoea.
    - wheeze, stridor, chest discomfort.
    - chest infection, pleural effusion.
  - invasion of:
    - mediastinum, chest wall, etc. May cause superior vena caval obstruction, dysphagia, cardiac arrhythmias, pericardial effusion, etc.
    - vertebrae.
    - recurrent laryngeal nerve, usually on the left.
    - sympathetic trunk at C8/T1, causing Horner's syndrome.
    - brachial plexus at lung apex, causing pain and wasting in the hand/arm (with Horner's syndrome, ± rib or vertebral erosion, ± superior vena caval obstruction, = Pancoast syndrome).
  - metastases: commonly lymph nodes, bone, liver, brain.
  - other features:
    - fatigue, anorexia, weight loss, anaemia.
    - hormone secretion, e.g. causing the syndrome of inappropriate antidiuretic hormone secretion, Cushing's syndrome, hypercalcaemia due to parathyroid hormone secretion, carcinoid syndrome. Most common with small cell tumours. Thyroid and sex hormone secretion may occur.
    - sensory or motor neuropathy; cerebellar atrophy.
    - myasthenic syndrome, muscle weakness, dermatomyositis.
    - finger clubbing and hypertrophic pulmonary osteoarthropathy.

May present for bronchoscopy, mediastinoscopy or thoracic surgery. Anaesthetic considerations are related to the above features, effects of smoking and malignancy; thus preoperative assessment of respiratory, cardiovascular and neurological systems, and hormonal and metabolic status, is particularly important.

Radiotherapy is used mainly for palliative treatment of pain and obstructive lesions (e.g. superior vena caval obstruction), especially due to small cell carcinoma. Chemotherapy is also used, particularly in small cell carcinoma.

[Henry Pancoast (1875–1939), US radiologist]

See also, Polymyositis

Bronchial tree, *see Tracheobronchial tree*

Bronchiectasis. Permanent abnormal bronchial dilatation, usually suppurative. May follow pneumonia, bronchial obstruction, chronic repeated chest infections, e.g. in cystic fibrosis and immunological impairment.

- Features:
  - haemoptysis.
  - chronic cough with purulent sputum.
  - chronic respiratory insufficiency, of restrictive and/or obstructive pattern.
  - empyema, abscesses, cor pulmonale, clubbing.
  - chest X-ray: increased lung markings, patchy shadowing, thick-walled dilated bronchi.

Treatment includes antibiotic therapy, physiotherapy and postural drainage, and lung resection if disease is localised.

- Anaesthetic management:
  - preoperatively:
    - early admission for preoperative assessment, medical treatment and physiotherapy.
    - chest X-ray, arterial blood gas analysis, lung function tests as appropriate.
  - perioperatively: soiling of the unaffected lung is reduced by appropriate positioning. Double-lumen endobronchial tubes may assist surgery and allow isolation and suction of copious secretions.
  - postoperatively: adequate analgesia and physiotherapy to reduce risk of respiratory complications.

Barker AF (2002). N Engl J Med; 346: 1383–93

Bronchiolitis. Inflammation of the bronchioles; usually refers to acute infection in children but may also occur chronically in early COPD in adults. In children, respiratory syncytial virus accounts for 70% of cases, but many other viruses may also be responsible. Usually affects children under 1 year old, causing non-specific upper respiratory tract symptoms which may progress over 1–2 days to respiratory distress with diffuse crackles ± persistent wheezing. Hypoxaemia results from hypoventilation and $\dot{V}/\dot{Q}$ mismatch. May be associated with apnoea, especially in premature babies. Treatment is supportive, including humidified O_2 therapy, fluid replacement and occasionally IPPV. Ribavirin may reduce the severity of illness if given early.

Usually self-limiting, lasting under 10 days; mortality in infants admitted to hospital is about 1% if previously fit. Has been implicated in the development of subsequent asthma, although this is uncertain.

Smyth RL, Openshaw PJM (2006). Lancet; 368: 312–22

See also, Tracheobronchial tree

Bronchodilator drugs. Drugs which increase bronchial diameter.

- Postulated mechanisms of action:
  - β-adrenergic receptor agonists, e.g. salbutamol:
    - inhibit degranulation of mast cells.
    - stimulate adenylate cyclase in smooth muscle cells, leading to increased cAMP levels, thus causing reduced intracellular calcium and relaxation.
  - theophylline, aminophylline:
    - phosphodiesterase inhibitors in smooth muscle cells, increasing cAMP levels.
    - possible effect via release of catecholamines via adenosine inhibition.
    - possible effect on myosin light chains, reducing contraction.
  - anticholinergic drugs, e.g. ipratropium:
    - block cholinergic receptors, decreasing intracellular guanine monophosphate (cGMP; opposes the bronchodilating action of cAMP).
    - possible effect via reduction in intracellular calcium.

- corticosteroids:
  - anti-inflammatory action.
  - reduced capillary permeability.
  - possibly increase the effects of β-adrenergic receptor agonists.

Sodium cromoglicate and leukotriene receptor antagonists are not bronchodilators, but help to prevent bronchoconstriction by reducing inflammation.
See also, Asthma; Bronchospasm

Bronchopleural fistula. Abnormal connection between the tracheobronchial tree and pleura. Most commonly occurs 2–10 days after pneumonectomy, although it may follow trauma, chronic infection and erosion by tumour.

- Features:
  - fever, productive cough, malaise.
  - X-ray evidence of infection in the remaining lung with fall in fluid level on the affected side.
- Problems caused:
  - source of (usually) infected material in one pleural cavity, with potential contamination of the normal lung through the fistula. Repeated spillage may cause pulmonary function impairment before corrective surgery.
  - IPPV may force fresh gas through the fistula, without inflating the remaining lung. Increased pressure in the affected pleura increases the likelihood of contamination, and may impair cardiac output.
- Management:
  - chest drainage.
  - monitoring set up under local anaesthesia.
  - sitting the patient up, with affected side lowermost.
  - classical method for induction of anaesthesia: inhalational induction and intubation with a double-lumen endobronchial tube, with spontaneous ventilation. IPPV may be started once the affected side has been isolated. However, deep anaesthesia with volatile agents may cause profound cardiovascular effects, and coughing may increase contamination risk. Suggested alternatives include awake intubation under local anaesthesia, or preoxygenation, iv induction and intubation using suxamethonium (only advocated by, and for, experienced thoracic anaesthetists).
  - postoperatively, IPPV may be necessary. High frequency ventilation and differential lung ventilation have been used.

See also, Thoracic surgery

Bronchopulmonary lavage. Performed in pulmonary alveolar proteinosis, to remove accumulated lipoproteinaceous material. Has also been used in asthma and cystic fibrosis. Usually performed under general anaesthesia, and involves instillation and drainage under gravity of 20–40 litres warm buffered saline (heparin may be added) through one lumen of a double-lumen endobronchial tube, whilst ventilating via the other. The other lung is treated after a few days. Main problems are related to the pre-existing state of the patient, one-lung anaesthesia, and avoidance of soiling of the ventilated lung. Cardiopulmonary bypass has also been used.

Lavage using small volumes is sometimes used to aid diagnosis of atypical chest infections, and may be carried out via flexible bronchoscopy under local anaesthesia.

Bronchoscopy. Inspection of the tracheobronchial tree by passing an instrument down its lumen. May be:

- rigid: usually performed in the operating theatre for diagnosis of bronchial disease, removal of foreign bodies, management of haemoptysis, etc. Anaesthetic management:
  - preoperatively:
    - preoperative assessment is particularly directed at the respiratory and cardiovascular systems. Many patients will have bronchial carcinoma or other smoking-related diseases. Secretions may be improved by preoperative physiotherapy. Neck mobility and the teeth should be assessed.
    - premedication reduces awareness. The antisialagogue effects of anticholinergic drugs may be useful.
  - perioperatively:
    - iv induction of anaesthesia is usual. Inhalational induction may be indicated if airway obstruction is present, particularly in children. Neuromuscular blockade has traditionally been achieved with suxamethonium (intermittent doses or infusion), but currently one of the shorter-duration non-depolarising neuromuscular blocking drugs is more likely.
    - spraying of the larynx with lidocaine may reduce perioperative and postoperative coughing and laryngospasm.
    - ventilation: several methods may be used:
      - injector techniques; air entrainment through the bronchoscope using intermittent blasts of O_2. Automatic jet ventilators have been used for long procedures.
      - IPPV via a side arm on the bronchoscope, the proximal end of which is occluded by a window or the operator's thumb.
      - deep anaesthesia with spontaneous ventilation. Often used in children, classically using diethyl ether, then halothane, but now sevoflurane. Anaesthetic gases may be delivered via a side arm on the bronchoscope; before these 'ventilating bronchoscopes' became available, the patient breathed air and bronchoscopy was performed as anaesthesia lightened (a possible disadvantage of sevoflurane being that anaesthesia might lighten too quickly).
      - insufflation techniques, particularly apnoeic oxygenation. Suitable for short procedures only.
      - intermittent IPPV via a tracheal tube placed in the proximal end of the bronchoscope.
      - high frequency ventilation has been used.
  - monitoring as standard.
  - awareness is a particular problem, especially with jet ventilation using 100% O_2, or apnoeic oxygenation. Regular supplements or continuous infusion of iv anaesthetic agents, typically propofol, reduce the incidence, as does premedication, or the use of midazolam.
  - recovery should be in the lateral, head-down position, to encourage drainage of blood and secretions.
- fibreoptic: commonly performed for diagnostic purposes under local anaesthesia as for awake intubation, but also used by anaesthetists and intensivists during general anaesthesia and on the ICU. Uses:
  - airway management:
    - tracheal intubation in airway obstruction. Also useful for changing tracheal tubes.
    - confirmation of correct placement of tracheal/tracheostomy/endobronchial tubes. Has been used in percutaneous tracheostomy.
    - assessment of the tracheobronchial tree prior to extubation. In cases of potential postextubation airway obstruction, e.g. caused by oedema, the fibreoptic

bronchoscope can be left in situ whilst the tracheal tube is removed and the airway assessed; the tube may be resited over the bronchoscope if required.
- diagnostic:
  - chest infection, especially atypical. Washings, brushings or transbronchial/endobronchial biopsies or needle aspiration may be used. Repeated instillation of 20 ml sterile saline with subsequent aspiration (bronchoscopic alveolar lavage, BAL) may be useful in both infective and non-infective processes.
  - other lesions, e.g. tumours, tears, thermal damage, etc. May be used to investigate abnormalities on chest X-ray.
- therapeutic:
  - aspiration of sputum, aspirated material, etc. Mucolytic drugs can be instilled on to mucus plugs. BAL has been used in severe asthma.
  - removal of foreign body.
  - for haemoptysis; saline lavage may be useful for small areas of bleeding; the bronchoscope itself can be used to compress bleeding points; or it may facilitate passage of a balloon-tipped catheter into the affected segment.

- Management for bronchoscopy in the ICU:
  - coagulation studies should be performed if biopsies are planned. Electrolyte imbalance should be corrected.
  - secretions may be improved by physiotherapy. Anticholinergic drugs may reduce secretions but may also make them thick and difficult to aspirate.
  - awake patients may be managed under local anaesthesia as for awake intubation. In those with tracheal tubes, the bronchoscope may be passed through a rubber-sealed connector at the tube's proximal end and IPPV continued. Leaks may occur around the scope, especially if airway pressures are high; a swab coated in lubricant jelly wrapped around the leak may improve the seal. 5.0 mm diameter bronchoscopes require an 8.0 mm tracheal tube to ensure adequate gas flow around the bronchoscope. Passage of the bronchoscope alongside the tracheal tube has also been used, as has high frequency ventilation.
  - increased sedation and neuromuscular blockade are usually required in ventilated patients.
  - hypoxaemia may worsen during bronchoscopy, especially with increasing duration of the procedure, and may be prolonged; 100% O_2 is usually administered. Severe hypoxaemia is usually considered a contraindication.
  - arrhythmias, hypertension, coughing, bronchospasm or laryngospasm may occur during and after stimulation of the tracheobronchial tree. Topical lidocaine may reduce airway irritation. Bleeding and pneumothorax may also occur.

Plummer S, Hartley M, Vaughan RS (1998). Br J Anaesth; 80: 223–4

See also, Foreign body, inhaled; Intubation, awake

Bronchospasm. May occur during anaesthesia due to:
- surgical stimulation.
- presence of airway or tracheal tube.
- pharyngeal/laryngeal/bronchial secretions or blood.
- aspiration of gastric contents.
- anaphylactic or anaphylactoid reaction.
- pulmonary oedema.
- use of β-adrenergic receptor antagonists.

Particularly likely in smokers or in patients with asthma or COPD, and if anaesthesia is inadequate.

- Features:
  - wheezing.
  - reduced movement of reservoir bag.
  - increased expiratory time.
  - increased airway pressures.
- Must be distinguished from:
  - pneumothorax.
  - mechanical obstruction.
  - laryngospasm.
  - pulmonary oedema.
- Treatment:
  - of primary cause.
  - increased F_IO_2.
  - increased inspired concentration of volatile inhalational anaesthetic agent.
  - salbutamol 250–500 μg sc/im or 250 μg iv slowly. Delivery by nebuliser or aerosol may also be used but may be technically difficult.
  - aminophylline 3–6 mg/kg iv slowly, followed by 0.5 mg/kg/h infusion.
  - further management as for asthma.

Brown fat. Specialised adipose tissue used for heat generation because of its chemical make-up and structural composition. Of particular importance in temperature regulation in neonates. Laid down from about 22 weeks of gestation around the base of the neck, axillae, mediastinum and between the scapulae; gradually replaced by adult 'white' adipose tissue after birth, the process taking several years. Fat breakdown and thermogenesis is increased by α-adrenergic neurone activity.

BTPS. Body temperature and pressure, saturated with water vapour.

Buccal nerve block, *see Mandibular nerve blocks*

Buffer base. Blood anions which can act as bases and accept hydrogen ions. Mainly composed of bicarbonate, haemoglobin and negatively charged proteins.
See also, Acid–base balance; Buffers

Buffers. Substances which resist a change in pH by absorbing or releasing hydrogen ions when acid or base is added to the solution. In the body, buffering is one mechanism by which pH is kept relatively constant.

For the equation $HA \rightleftharpoons H^+ + A^-$, where HA = undissociated acid and A^- = anion, the equation shifts to the left if acid is added, and to the right if base is added; changes in H^+ concentration are thus minimised.

The Henderson–Hasselbalch equation describes these relationships:

$$pH = pK + \log\frac{[A^-]}{[HA]}$$

When pH equals pK of the buffer system, maximal buffering may occur, because HA and A^- exist in equal amounts.

- Body buffer systems:
  - blood:
    - carbonic acid/bicarbonate: $H_2CO_3 \rightleftharpoons H^+ + HCO_3^-$. The p$K$ is 6.1; i.e. the system is not very efficient at buffering alkaline at body pH, although it is quite efficient at buffering acid (efficiency increasing as pH falls). Since CO_2 may be eliminated via the lungs, and bicarbonate regulated via the kidneys, these mechanisms, plus the large amount of plasma bicarbonate, make this the main buffer system in the blood.
    - haemoglobin: dissociation of histidine residues gives haemoglobin six times the buffering capacity of

plasma proteins. Deoxygenated haemoglobin is a better buffer than oxygenated haemoglobin (Haldane effect).
- plasma proteins: carboxyl and amino groups dissociate to form anions; this accounts for a small amount of buffer capacity.
- phosphate: $H_2PO_4^- \rightleftharpoons H^+ + HPO_4^{2-}$. Plays a small part in buffering in the ECF.
- intracellular:
  - proteins.
  - phosphate.

See also, Acid–base balance

Bumetanide. Diuretic, similar to furosemide in its actions. 1 mg is approximately equivalent to 40 mg furosemide. Diuresis begins within minutes of an iv dose and lasts for 2 h.
- Dosage:
  - 1–5 mg orally once to thrice daily.
  - 1–2 mg iv, repeated after 20 min if required. May also be given by infusion at 1–5 mg/h.
- Side effects: as for furosemide; myalgia may also occur, especially with high doses.

BUN, *see Blood urea nitrogen*

Bundle branch block (BBB). Interruption of impulse propagation in the heart conducting system distal to the atrioventricular node. Causes are as for heart block.
- May involve right or left bundles:
  - right BBB:
    - common; usually clinically insignificant.
    - ECG findings (Fig. 26a):
      - QRS duration > 0.12 s.
      - large S wave, lead I.
      - RSR pattern, lead V_1.
    - incomplete BBB may be due to an enlarged right ventricle, e.g. due to cor pulmonale or ASD.
  - left BBB:
    - represents more widespread disease, as the left bundle is a bigger and less discrete structure, consisting of anterior and posterior fascicles. If present preoperatively, it serves as an indicator of existing heart disease.
    - ECG findings (Fig. 26b):
      - QRS duration > 0.12 s.
      - wide R waves, leads I and V_{4-6}.
    - may be due to left ventricular hypertrophy, e.g. due to hypertension or valvular heart disease.
  - hemiblock (involving individual fascicles of the left bundle):
    - left anterior hemiblock:
      - QRS may be normal or slightly widened.
      - left axis deviation > 60°.
    - left posterior hemiblock:
      - less common, because the posterior fascicle is better perfused than the anterior.
      - QRS normal or slightly widened.
      - right axis deviation > 120°.
  - bifascicular block:
    - comprised of right BBB and one hemiblock:
      - anterior:
        - right BBB ECG pattern and left axis deviation.
        - may lead to complete heart block later in life, but this is rare during anaesthesia.
      - posterior:
        - right BBB ECG pattern and right axis deviation.
        - rare.
        - at risk of developing complete heart block.
    - bifascicular block plus prolonged P–R interval (i.e. partial trifascicular block) is particularly likely to progress to complete heart block.

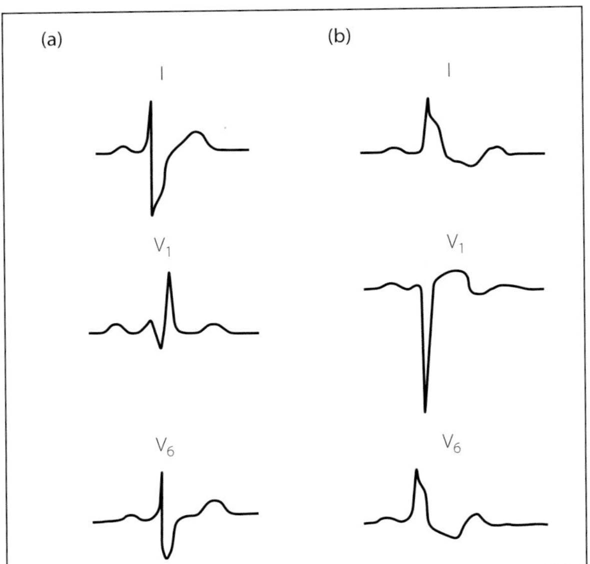

Fig. 26 ECG findings in bundle branch block: (a) right BBB; (b) left BBB

BBB itself is not a contraindication to anaesthesia, but progression to complete heart block during anaesthesia remains the main risk. Temporary perioperative cardiac pacing should be considered if BBB is associated with either a history of syncope or a prolonged P–R interval. Anaesthetic management is as for heart block.

Bungarotoxins. Snake venom neurotoxins. α-Bungarotoxin binds irreversibly to postsynaptic acetylcholine receptors at the neuromuscular junction; β-bungarotoxin acts presynaptically to block acetylcholine release. They have been used to study neuromuscular transmission.

Bupivacaine hydrochloride. Amide local anaesthetic agent, introduced in 1963. Of slower onset of action and longer duration than lidocaine, lasting 3–4 h for epidural block and up to 12 h for some nerve blocks, e.g. brachial plexus. The addition of adrenaline does not prolong the effect of bupivacaine as much as with lidocaine. 0.5% solution is equivalent to 2% lidocaine. Bupivacaine is extensively bound to tissue and plasma proteins. pK_a is 8.1. More cardiotoxic than lidocaine. Mainly metabolised by the liver, a small amount is excreted unchanged in the urine. Widely used for conduction, spinal and epidural anaesthesia. 0.25–0.5% solutions are used for most purposes. 0.75% produces more prolonged motor block when given epidurally; this concentration is contraindicated in obstetric practice because of toxicity. Contraindicated for use in IVRA. A hyperbaric 0.5% solution (with glucose 8%) exists for spinal administration (introduced 1982). Maximal safe dose: 2 mg/kg; toxic plasma levels: > 2–4 μg/ml.

The original preparation of bupivacaine is a racemic mixture of *l*- and *d*-isomers. A preparation of the single isomer *l*-bupivacaine (levobupivacaine) was developed in 1997 and is equivalent with the racemic mixture in terms of action and potency whilst having less propensity to CVS and CNS toxicity. It is available in the same concentrations as the original preparation.

See also, Isomerism; individual blocks

Buprenorphine hydrochloride. Opioid analgesic drug derived from thebaine, with partial agonist properties. Synthesised in 1968. 0.4 mg is equivalent to 10 mg morphine; it has slower onset and its effects last longer (about 8 h). May be given iv or im (0.3–0.6 mg), or sublingually (0.2–0.4 mg) 6–8 hourly. A slow-release patch (35–70 μg/h, equivalent to 0.84–1.68 mg/day) has been produced for severe chronic pain. Respiratory depression does occur, but reaches a plateau which cannot be exceeded by increasing the dose. Respiratory depression is not readily reversed by naloxone. Carries a low risk of dependence and has been used in the treatment of drug addiction.
See also, Opioid receptors

Burns. Burned patients may suffer from:
- direct thermal injury to body and airway.
- smoke inhalation, with, e.g. carbon monoxide (CO) or cyanide (CN) poisoning.
- extensive fluid loss into the dermis, into blisters and from skin surfaces.

- Management:
  - high F_IO_2 O_2 therapy. Tracheal intubation and IPPV are required in:
    - severe CO or CN poisoning. It has been suggested that CN poisoning should be assumed if there is unexplained severe metabolic acidosis, and treated accordingly.
    - upper airway obstruction. Obstruction due to oedema may develop over a few hours; thus tracheal intubation should be performed if burns to the airway are present. The latter may be indicated by burns or soot around the face and in the mouth, and are confirmed by fibreoptic bronchoscopy. Obstruction usually resolves within 2–4 days.
    - an unconscious patient.
    - respiratory failure.

    Measurement of blood gas tensions, carboxyhaemoglobin and possibly cyanide levels, should be performed. A chest X-ray is mandatory.
  - assessment of the extent of burns (rule of nines).
  - fluid replacement: many different regimens exist, using colloid, crystalloid or hypertonic solutions. Average total requirements = water 2–4 ml/kg/% burn and sodium 0.5 mmol/kg/% burn. Constant reassessment is the most important factor. Common UK regimen:
    - replacement volume (V) in ml:

$$V = \frac{\text{body weight (kg)} \times \text{\%surface area burnt}}{2}$$

      $3 \times V$ is infused in the first 12 h from the time of burn;
      $2 \times V$ in the next 12 h;
      $1 \times V$ in the next 12 h.
    - choice of fluid: colloid is thought to be best. Blood is given to keep haematocrit 35–45%. Rough guide: 1 unit per 10% burn, excluding the first 10%. Normal maintenance fluids are given in addition.
    - alternative regimen, using crystalloid:

      $2 \times$ weight $\times$ % burn in first 8 h (ml);
      $2 \times$ weight $\times$ % burn in next 16 h.

    Frequent reassessment is crucial. Urine output should be maintained at 0.5–1 ml/kg/h with osmolality 600–1000 mosmol/kg (high due to high circulating levels of vasopressin). Low urine flow with high osmolality indicates under-replacement; high flow with low osmolality indicates over-replacement, in the absence of renal failure. The fluid regimen is altered as necessary.

    Oral rehydration is acceptable in burns of up to 10% (children) to 15% (adults). Oral rehydration fluid mixtures are suitable for children. For adults, water containing 75 mmol/l sodium chloride and 15 mmol/l sodium bicarbonate has been suggested, at 2–3 times normal water intake.
  - escharotomy (incision of contracted full-thickness burn which prevents ventilation or limb perfusion) may be necessary.
  - monitoring of:
    - urine output (via catheter if > 25% burn).
    - haematocrit and plasma electrolytes.
    - respiratory function.
    - CVP.
  - analgesia: opioid infusions are often required.
  - adequate nutrition (enteral if possible via a nasogastric tube).
  - prevention of Curling ulcers, e.g. with H_2 receptor antagonists.
  - tetanus toxoid as necessary.
- Complications:
  - infection and sepsis.
  - respiratory failure and ARDS.
  - renal failure, with myoglobinuria or haemoglobinuria. Suggested by low urine osmolarity and urine/blood urea ratio < 10.
  - hypercatabolism.

Mortality is related to the extent and site of burn, and age. Recent evidence suggests that area of burn > 40%, age > 60 years, and the presence of inhalational injury are the three risk factors most strongly associated with death; absence of these risk factors is associated with 0.3% mortality; a single risk factor with 3% mortality, two risk factors with 33% mortality, and all three risk factors with 90% mortality.

- Anaesthetic considerations in patients with burns:
  - patients often require repeat anaesthetics, e.g. for change of dressings, plastic surgery, etc.
  - difficult airway and/or intubation if burns exist around the head and neck, especially if contractures develop.
  - enhanced increase in plasma potassium may follow use of suxamethonium; cardiac arrest has been reported. Most likely 3–10 weeks after the burn, but it has been reported between 9 days and 2 months. An increased number of extrajunctional acetylcholine receptors is thought to be responsible.
  - increased requirement for non-depolarising neuromuscular blocking drugs. The mechanism is unclear but may involve altered pharmacokinetics, e.g. changes in protein-binding, clearance, volume of distribution. An alternative theory suggests the release of a specific yet undiscovered substance following burns, which reduces drug interaction with the neuromuscular junction, or affects the latter directly.
  - limited venous access.
  - hypermetabolism/catabolism.
  - heat loss during prolonged surgery.
  - extensive blood loss is possible; e.g. during grafting procedures approximately 2% blood volume lost per 1% surface burn.
  - suggested techniques:
    - iv opioid analgesic drugs, traditionally combined with butyrophenones (neuroleptanaesthesia), though this is less common now.
    - inhalational analgesia with Entonox or volatile agents.
    - ketamine ± other iv agents, e.g. midazolam, propofol.
    - standard general anaesthesia.

Hettiaratchy S, Papini R (2004). BMJ; 328: 1555–7 & 329: 101–3

Burns, during anaesthesia, *see Diathermy; Electrocution and electrical burns; Explosions and fires; Laser surgery*

BURP, backward, upward and rightward pressure, *see Intubation, difficult*

Burst suppression, *see Electroencephalography*

Busulfan (Busulphan). Alkylating agent **cytotoxic drug**, given orally to treat chronic myeloid leukaemia. Causes myelosuppression which may be irreversible, and rarely **pulmonary fibrosis**. Thus important in patients presenting for **bone marrow transplantation**.

Butorphanol tartrate. **Opioid analgesic drug** with partial agonist properties, withdrawn in the UK in 1983. Similar in actions to **pentazocine**; **half-life** is about 3 h. 2–3 mg is equivalent to 10 mg **morphine**. At higher doses, it produces less respiratory depression than morphine; it also requires more **naloxone** to reverse its effects.

See also, Opioid receptors

Butyrophenones. Group of centrally acting drugs, originally described with **phenothiazines** as 'major tranquillisers' (a term no longer used). They produce a state of detachment from the environment and inhibit purposeful movement via **GABA** receptor binding. They may cause distressing inner restlessness which may be masked by outward calmness. They are powerful **antiemetic drugs**, acting as dopamine antagonists at the **chemoreceptor trigger zone**. Although some α-adrenergic blocking effect has been shown, cardiovascular effects are minimal. May cause extrapyramidal side effects, and the **neuroleptic malignant syndrome** especially after chronic usage. Used to treat psychoses (especially schizophrenia and mania), in **neuroleptanaesthesia** and as antiemetics. **Droperidol** has a faster onset of action and shorter **half-life** than **haloperidol**.

Bypass, cardiopulmonary, *see Cardiopulmonary bypass*

C

CABG, *see Coronary artery bypass graft*

Cachectin, *see Cytokines*

Cachexia, *see Malnutrition*

Caesarean section. Particular anaesthetic considerations:
- physiological changes accompanying pregnancy.
- historically, difficult tracheal intubation and aspiration of gastric contents associated with general anaesthesia (GA) have comprised the major anaesthetic causes of maternal mortality. Mortality is higher for emergency Caesarean section (CS) than for elective CS.
- aortocaval compression must be prevented by avoiding the supine position at all times.
- uterine tone is decreased by volatile anaesthetic agents.
- placental perfusion may be reduced by severe and/or prolonged hypotension and/or reduction in cardiac output.
- neonatal depression should be avoided, but maternal awareness may occur if depth of anaesthesia is inadequate.

- The usual preoperative assessment should be made, with particular attention to:
  - any predisposing cause for CS, e.g. pre-eclampsia, and other obstetric or medical conditions.
  - whether CS is elective or emergency, and whether the fetus is compromised.
  - assessment of the airway for possible difficulty with tracheal intubation.
  - maternal wish for general or regional anaesthesia, and whether epidural analgesia has been provided in labour.
  - assessment of the lumbar spine and any contraindications to regional anaesthesia.

  The decision to employ general or regional anaesthesia results from consideration of the above points.
- Regimens used to reduce the risk of aspiration pneumonitis:
  - no food by mouth. This practice has been questioned, and many centres now allow clear fluids and even certain foods (low fat and sugar content) for low risk women in labour (if not receiving opioids), although this is still controversial.
  - antacid therapy: in some centres, antacids are administered at regular intervals to all women in labour; in others, antacids are given to those considered at risk of operative delivery, or when surgery is decided upon. The clear 0.3M sodium citrate (30 ml) is preferred to the particulate magnesium trisilicate because of the latter's ability to cause chemical pneumonitis. Sodium citrate has a short duration of action, and should be given immediately before induction of anaesthesia.
  - H_2 receptor antagonists. Many different regimens have been suggested, as for antacid therapy. Women receiving pethidine (causing reduced gastric emptying) are given ranitidine or cimetidine in some centres. For elective CS, ranitidine 150 mg orally is often given the night before, and 2 h before surgery. For emergency CS, cimetidine 200 mg im has been suggested as soon as the decision to operate is made (cimetidine having a more rapid onset than ranitidine).
  - omeprazole has also been used.
  - emptying the stomach with apomorphine or a stomach tube is rarely performed because they are unpleasant and ineffective.
  - metoclopramide is often given before CS, to increase gastric emptying and increase lower oesophageal sphincter tone.

  Sedative premedication is usually avoided because of the risk of neonatal respiratory depression and difficulties over timing.
- Anaesthetic techniques:
  - all types of anaesthesia:
    - insertion of a large-bore iv cannula under local anaesthesia.
    - cross-matched blood should always be available within 30 min.
    - skilled anaesthetic assistance should always be available, as should a range of laryngoscopes, blades, tubes, and resuscitative drugs and equipment.
    - monitoring is instituted on arrival in the operating theatre.
    - aortocaval compression is reduced by positioning the patient laterally during transport to theatre and surgery.
    - ergometrine has been superseded by oxytocin following delivery because of the former's side effects, particularly hypertension and vomiting.
    - about 500 ml blood is expelled from the uterus into the circulation with delivery, and this helps offset the average blood loss at CS of 500–1500 ml (GA) or 300–700 ml (regional anaesthesia):
  - general anaesthesia:
    - preoxygenation, cricoid pressure and rapid sequence induction. An adequate 'sleep dose' of induction agent reduces risk of awareness; a 'maximal allowed dose' based on weight may be insufficient. Neonatal depression due to iv induction agents is minimal. Suxamethonium is still considered the neuromuscular blocking drug of choice by most authorities although rocuronium has been suggested as an alternative.
    - failed intubation drill if required. Difficult and failed intubation (the latter ~1:300–500) is more likely in obstetric patients than in the general population. Contributory factors include a full set of teeth, increased fat deposition, enlarged breasts, and the hand applying cricoid pressure hindering insertion of the laryngoscope blade into the mouth. Laryngeal oedema may be present in pre-eclampsia. Apnoea results in rapid hypoxaemia because of reduced FRC and increased O_2 demand.

- IPPV with 50% O_2 in N_2O is customary until delivery, but has been challenged; 33% O_2 may not be associated with neonatal hypoxaemia as originally thought.
- low concentrations of inhalational agents (up to 0.5% halothane, 1% enflurane, 0.75% isoflurane or 1.2% sevoflurane) reduce the incidence of awareness without increasing uterine atony and bleeding, or neonatal depression. Placental blood flow is thought to be maintained by vasodilatation caused by the volatile agents, and high levels of vasoconstricting catecholamines associated with awareness are avoided. Delivery of higher concentrations of volatile agents in 66% N_2O has been suggested for the first 3–5 min whilst alveolar concentrations are low, to reduce awareness.
- normocapnia (4 kPa/30 mmHg in pregnancy) is now considered ideal; severe hyperventilation may be associated with fetal hypoxaemia and acidosis due to placental vasoconstriction, impairment of O_2 transfer associated with low $P\text{CO}_2$, or reduced venous return caused by excessive IPPV.
- all neuromuscular blocking drugs cross the placenta to a very small extent, gallamine more than others. Shorter-acting drugs, e.g. vecuronium and atracurium, are usually employed, since postoperative residual paralysis associated with longer-lasting drugs has been a significant factor in some maternal deaths.
- opioid analgesic drugs are withheld until delivery of the infant, to avoid neonatal respiratory depression.
- factors increasing the likelihood of awareness include lack of premedication, reduced concentrations of N_2O and volatile agents, and withholding opioid analgesic drugs before delivery. Its incidence using low concentrations of volatile agents is less than 1%; up to 26% awareness was reported in early studies using 50% N_2O and no volatile agent.
- aspiration may also occur at the end of surgery and during recovery from anaesthesia (when the effect of sodium citrate may have worn off). Routine gastric aspiration during anaesthesia has been suggested, especially in emergency cases. Before tracheal extubation, the patient should be awake and on her side.
- advantages: usually quicker to perform in emergencies. May be used when regional techniques are inadequate or contraindicated, e.g. in coagulation disorders. Safer in hypovolaemia.
- disadvantages: risk of aspiration, difficult intubation, awareness and neonatal depression. Hypotension and reduced cardiac output may result from anaesthetic drugs and IPPV. Blood loss is greater. The mother is more sleepy and more likely to suffer pain and PONV. The risk of DVT is also thought to be increased.

▸ epidural anaesthesia (EA):
- facilities for GA should be available.
- bupivacaine 0.5% or lidocaine 2% (the latter with adrenaline 1:200 000) are most commonly used in the UK, often in combination. Addition of opioids, e.g. fentanyl, is usual (though may not be necessary if many epidural doses have been given during labour). Bicarbonate has also been added to shorten the onset time, e.g. 2 ml 8.4% added to 20 ml lidocaine or lidocaine/bupivacaine mixture, but risks precipitation if too much is added (especially to bupivacaine) or errors from mixing up to 4–5 different drugs, especially in an emergency. Commercial premixed solutions of lidocaine or bupivacaine and adrenaline have a low pH (3.5–5.5) and contain preservatives. Ropivacaine 0.5–0.75% or levobupivacaine 0.5% are also used. Adrenaline is sometimes avoided in pre-eclamptic patients because of the risk of increased placental vasoconstriction. 0.75% bupivacaine is associated with a high incidence of maternal toxic reactions, and has been withdrawn from obstetric use. Chloroprocaine is available in the USA and a small number of European countries (but not the UK); onset is rapid but so is offset. Etidocaine has also been used in the USA.
- L3–4 interspace is usually chosen (care should be taken if a higher space is used, since the actual interspace is often more cranial than that intended).
- on average, 15–20 ml solution is required for adequate blockade (from S5 to T4–6). Reliance on impairment to cold sensation or pinprick alone may be inadequate as a means of assessing the block; impairment of touch sensation has been reported to be more reliable as a predictor of intraoperative comfort. Smaller volumes may be required when epidural analgesia using concentrated solutions of local anaesthetic has been provided during labour, although low dose (mobile) epidural analgesia has been safely extended with 15–20 ml solution by slow bolus, without dangerously high blocks resulting. Smaller volumes are required for a specified level of block than in non-pregnant patients, as dilated epidural veins reduce the available volume in the epidural space.
- injection of solution in 5 ml increments at 5-minute intervals reduces the risk of hypotension and extensive blockade, e.g. due to accidental spinal injection, but increases preparatory time and total dose. Sequential positioning (e.g. on either side and sitting) between doses has been suggested as improving blockade but may not be necessary. A single injection of 15–20 ml is advocated by some as producing more rapid onset of blockade. A catheter technique is used most frequently, although injection through the epidural needle may be performed.
- opioids, e.g. diamorphine 2–4 mg and fentanyl 50–100 µg, have been given epidurally for peri- and postoperative analgesia, but maternal respiratory depression has been reported, albeit rarely.
- the incidence of hypotension may be reduced by preloading with iv fluid; traditionally 1–1.5 litres crystalloid has been used though colloid is thought to be more effective; even with preloading, hypotension may occur in up to 20–30% of cases (though the incidence varies with its definition) Aortocaval compression must be avoided at all times. Treatment includes administration of vasopressors, typically ephedrine, e.g. 3–6 mg increments iv. Prophylactic use is considered more effective, e.g. by similar boluses or 30 mg in 500 ml iv fluid adjusted as required. Animal studies have suggested that other vasoconstrictors may greatly decrease placental blood flow, although phenylephrine has become popular recently in small (25–100 µg) increments or by infusion, because it appears more effective at reducing/treating hypotension and is associated with a better neonatal acid-case profile than large doses of ephedrine (thought to be due to ephedrine's crossing the placenta to cause increased anaerobic glycolysis in the fetus via β-adrenergic stimulation).
- nausea and vomiting may be caused by hypotension and/or bradycardia.
- routine administration of O_2 by facemask has been questioned on the grounds of being ineffective and even possibly harmful to the fetus via generation of

free radicals, although evidence suggests a benefit if administered for up to 10 min.
- during surgery many women feel pressure and movement, which may be unpleasant, and all women should be warned of this possibility and of the potential requirement for general anaesthesia. Inhaled N_2O, further epidural top-ups, small doses of iv opioid drugs, e.g. fentanyl or alfentanil, iv paracetamol, and ketamine may be useful. Shoulder tip pain may result from blood tracking up to the diaphragm and may be reduced by head-up tilt. Surgery must be gentle when performing CS under regional anaesthesia, and the obstetrician should check with the anaesthetist before exteriorising the uterus or swabbing the paracolic gutters.
- advantages: the risks of GA are avoided. Onset of hypotension is usually slow and may be corrected before it becomes severe. The mother may be able to warn of aortocaval compression (e.g. feeling sick). Minimal neonatal depression occurs compared with GA. The mother is able to hold the baby soon after delivery and is not sleepy afterwards. Her partner is able to be present during the procedure. Epidural analgesia provided in labour can be extended for operative delivery. The catheter can be used for further 'top-up' during surgery if required, and for postoperative analgesia.
- disadvantages: risk of dural tap, total spinal blockade, toxic reaction to local anaesthetic agent, severe hypotension, etc. It may be slow to achieve adequate blockade with a chance of patchy block. Inability to move the legs may be disturbing.

▸ spinal anaesthesia (SA):
- general considerations as for EA.
- 0.5% bupivacaine is used in the UK; plain bupivacaine (e.g. 3 ml) produces a more variable block than heavy bupivacaine (e.g. 1.8–2.8 ml), which is the only form licensed for spinal anaesthesia. Heavy tetracaine (amethocaine) 0.5% (1.2–1.6 ml) is used in the USA.
- injection is usually at the L3–4/L4–5 interspace.
- hypotension and post-dural puncture headache are more common (reduced to under 1% if 25–27 G pencil-point needles are used). Postoperative confinement to bed is now thought not to affect the incidence of headache.
- advantages: as for EA, but of quicker onset. Blockade is more intense and not patchy. Smaller doses of local anaesthetic drug are used.
- disadvantages: single shot; i.e. may not last long enough if surgery is prolonged. Less predictable. Continuous spinal techniques allow more control over spread and duration but are technically more difficult. Risk of headache. Hypotension is of faster onset. Has been associated with poorer neonatal acid–base status, thought to be because of more rapid hypotension (if uncontrolled).

▸ combined spinal–epidural anaesthesia (CSE):
- general considerations as for EA and SA.
- allows the fast onset and dense block of SA but with the flexibility of EA. Also allows a small subarachnoid injection to be extended by epidural injection of either saline (thought to act via a volume effect) or local anaesthetic, with greater cardiovascular stability.
- usually performed at a single interspace (needle-through-needle method) or at two separate spaces.

(For contraindications, techniques, etc., see individual techniques)

CS is possible using local anaesthetic infiltration of the abdominal wall, e.g. with 0.5% lidocaine or prilocaine. Large volumes are required, with risk of toxicity. Infiltration of each layer is performed in stages. The procedure is lengthy and uncomfortable, but may be used as a last resort if other techniques are unavailable or unsuccessful. It may also be used to supplement inhalational anaesthesia following failed intubation.

[Julius Caesar (100–44 BC), Roman Emperor; said to have been born by the abdominal route; his name allegedly derived from *caedare*, to cut. An alternative suggestion is related to a law enforced under the Caesars concerning abdominal section following death in late pregnancy]

See also, Confidential Enquiries into Maternal Deaths; Fetus, effects of anaesthetic agents on; I–D interval; Induction, rapid sequence; Intubation, difficult; Intubation, failed; Obstetric analgesia and anaesthesia; U–D interval

Caffeine. Xanthine present in tea, coffee and certain soft drinks. Used as an adjunct to many oral analgesic drug preparations, although not analgesic itself. Causes CNS stimulation; traditionally thought to improve performance and mood, whilst reducing fatigue. Increases cerebral vascular resistance and decreases cerebral blood flow. Half-life is about 6 h. Has been used iv and orally for treatment of post-dural puncture headache.
- Dosage: up to 30 mg in compound oral preparations. 150–300 mg orally for post-dural puncture headache, 6–8 hourly; 250 mg iv (with 250 mg sodium benzoate).
- Side effects: as for aminophylline, especially CNS and cardiac stimulation.

Caisson disease, *see Decompression sickness*

Calcitonin. Hormone (mw 3500) secreted from the parafollicular (C) cells of the thyroid gland. Involved in calcium homeostasis; secretion is stimulated by hypercalcaemia, catecholamines and gastrin. Decreases serum calcium by inhibiting mobilisation of bone calcium, decreasing intestinal absorption and increasing renal calcium and phosphate excretion. Used therapeutically in the treatment of severe hypercalcaemia, postmenopausal osteoporosis, Paget's disease and intractable pain from bony metastases. Porcine or salmon calcitonin is most commonly used, but human preparations (20 times weaker) are available for patients with resistance or allergy to the former.
- Dosage:
  - hypercalcaemia: from 5–10 units/kg/day im/sc in 1–2 divided doses up to 400 units 6–8 hourly. Porcine/salmon calcitonin.
  - Paget's disease/intractable pain: 50–100 units/day sc/im.
- Side effects: nausea, facial flushing, urinary frequency.

[Sir James Paget (1814–1899), English surgeon]

See also, Procalcitonin

Calcium. 99% of body calcium is contained in bone; plasma calcium consists of free ionised calcium (50%) and calcium bound to proteins (mainly albumin) and other ions. The free ionised form is involved as a second messenger in many intracellular responses to chemical and electrical stimuli, e.g. neuromuscular transmission, muscle contraction, cell division and movement, and certain oxidative pathways. Also involved in coagulation. Its actions are mediated via binding to intracellular proteins, e.g. calmodulin, causing configurational changes to proteins and enzyme activation. Intracellular calcium levels are much higher than extracellular, due to relative membrane impermeability and membrane pumps employing active transport. Calcium entry via specific channels leads to direct effects, e.g. neurotransmitter release in neurones, or further calcium release from intracellular organelles, e.g. in cardiac and skeletal muscle.

Ionised calcium increases with acidosis, and decreases with alkalosis. Thus for accurate measurement, blood should be taken without a tourniquet (which causes local acidosis), and without hyper-/hypoventilation. Ionised calcium is measured in some centres, but total plasma calcium is easier to measure; normal value is 2.12–2.65 mmol/l. Varies with the plasma protein level; corrected by adding 0.02 mmol/l calcium for each g/l albumin below 40 g/l, or subtracting for each g/l above 40 g/l.

- Regulation:
  - vitamin D: group of related sterols. Cholecalciferol is formed in the skin by the action of ultraviolet light, and is converted in the liver to 25-hydroxycholecalciferol (in turn converted to 1,25-dihydroxycholecalciferol in the proximal renal tubules). Formation is increased by parathyroid hormone and decreased by hyperphosphataemia. Actions:
    - increases intestinal calcium absorption.
    - increases renal calcium reabsorption.
    - mobilises bone calcium and phosphate.
  - parathyroid hormone: secretion is increased by hypocalcaemia and hypomagnesaemia, and decreased by hypercalcaemia and hypermagnesaemia. Actions:
    - mobilises bone calcium.
    - increases renal calcium reabsorption.
    - increases renal phosphate excretion.
    - increases formation of 1,25-dihydroxycholecalciferol.
  - calcitonin: secreted by the parafollicular cells of the thyroid gland. Secretion is increased by hypercalcaemia, catecholamines and gastrin. Actions:
    - decreases intestinal absorption of dietary calcium.
    - inhibits mobilisation of bone calcium.
    - increases renal calcium and phosphate excretion.

Calcium is used clinically to treat hypocalcaemia, e.g. during rapid blood transfusion. It is also used as an inotropic drug, e.g. during cardiac surgery. Although ionised calcium concentration may be low after cardiac arrest, its use during CPR is no longer recommended unless persistent hypocalcaemia, hyperkalaemia or overdose of calcium channel blocking drugs are involved, because of adverse effects on ischaemic myocardium, and coronary and on cerebral circulations.

Calcium chloride 10% contains 6.8 mmol/10 ml and 14.7% contains 10 mmol/10 ml; calcium gluconate 10% contains 2.2–2.3 mmol/10 ml, depending on the formulation. 5–10 ml calcium chloride or 10–20 ml calcium gluconate are usually recommended by slow iv bolus. The chloride preparation is usually recommended for CPR, although equal rises in plasma calcium are produced by gluconate, if equal amounts of calcium are given. Arrhythmias and prolonged hypercalcaemia may follow the use of either.

Aguilera IM, Vaughan RS (2000). Anaesthesia; 55: 779–90

Calcium channel blocking drugs. Most common name for a group of drugs which interfere with slow channel calcium entry into cells (also called calcium ion antagonists). In the myocardium this results in depletion of ATP stores, reducing myocardial contractility and O_2 consumption. Also cause coronary and peripheral vasodilatation, increasing coronary blood flow and reducing preload, and depress the initiation and propagation of cardiac electrical impulses to varying extents. Used to treat angina, hypertension, SVT, and post-MI ischaemia.

- Classified according to pharmacological effects *in vitro* and *in vivo*:
  - class I: potent negative inotropic and chronotropic effects: verapamil: acts mainly on the myocardium and conducting system; thus used to treat supraventricular arrhythmias, angina and hypertension. Severe myocardial depression may occur, especially in combination with β-adrenergic receptor antagonists.
  - class II: peripheral effects, with minimal direct myocardial activity (although may cause reflex tachycardia):
    - nifedipine: acts mainly on coronary and systemic vascular muscle, with little myocardial depression. Used in angina and hypertension. Systemic vasodilatation may cause flushing and headache, especially for the first few days of treatment.
    - nicardipine: similar to nifedipine, but with less myocardial depression.
    - amlodipine and felodipine: similar to nifedipine and nicardipine, but with longer duration of action and therefore taken once daily.
    - isradipine, lacidipine, lercanidipine and nisoldipine: similar to nifedipine but used for hypertension only. Nisoldipine has similar effects but is used for both angina and hypertension.
    - nimodipine: particularly active on cerebral vascular smooth muscle, it is used to relieve cerebral vasospasm following subarachnoid haemorrhage.
  - class III: slight negative inotropic effects, without reflex tachycardia: diltiazem: used in angina, hypertension and tachycardias.

The above drugs act mainly on the L-type calcium (long-lasting) channels; these are more widely distributed than the T-type (transient) channels which are confined to the sinoatrial node, vascular smooth muscle and neurohormonal cells of the kidney. Mibefradil, a T-type calcium channel blocking drug, caused little reflex tachycardia or negative inotropism but was withdrawn after just a few months because of severe interactions with several other drugs. N-type calcium channels are concentrated in neural tissue and are the binding site of omega toxins produced by certain venomous spiders and cone snails. A derivative of the latter, ziconotide, has recently been introduced as a treatment for chronic pain.

Additive effects might be expected between these drugs and the volatile anaesthetic agents, all of which decrease calcium entry into cells. Reduction in cardiac output, decreased atrioventricular conduction and vasodilatation may occur to different degrees, but severe interactions are rarely a problem in practice. Non-depolarising neuromuscular blockade may be potentiated.

Overdose with calcium channel blocking agents causes hypotension, bradycardia and heart block. Traditional treatment involves iv calcium chloride, glucagon and catecholamines. Heart block is usually resistant to atropine and hypotension may not respond to inotropes or vasopressors. High dose insulin has been successful in reversing refractory hypotension.

Calcium resonium, *see Polystyrene sulphonate resins*

Calcium sensitisers. New class of inotropic drugs undergoing clinical trials for the treatment of heart failure. Act directly on the contractile proteins of myocardial muscle cells without increasing intracellular calcium, thus improving myocardial contractility without increasing myocardial

oxygen consumption or provoking arrhythmias. Examples include levosimendan and pimobendan.
Kass DA, Solaro RJ (2006). Circulation; 113: 305–15

Calorie. Unit of energy. Although not an SI unit, widely used, especially in relation to food-derived energy.

1 cal = energy required to heat 1 g water by 1°C.
1 kcal (1 Cal) = energy required to heat 1 kg water by 1°C,
= 1000 cal.
1 cal = 4.18 joules.

Calorimetry, indirect, *see Energy balance*

cAMP, *see Adenosine monophoshate, cyclic*

Campbell–Howell method, *see Carbon dioxide measurement*

Canadian Journal of Anesthesia. Official journal of the Canadian Anesthetists' Society. Launched in 1954 as the *Canadian Anaesthetists' Society Journal* until 1987. From 1987–1999 known as the *Canadian Journal of Anaesthesia*.

Candela. SI unit of luminous intensity. Definition relates to the luminous intensity of a radiating black body at the freezing point of platinum.

Cannabis. Mildly hallucinogenic drug obtained from the *cannabis sativa* plant. A mixture of at least 60 chemicals (cannabinoids) including the main psychoactive δ-9-tetrahydrocannibinol. Cannabinoid specific receptors have been identified in central and peripheral neurones (CB_1 receptors) and peripherally in the spleen and macrophages (CB_2); both types are G protein-coupled receptors.

Possible therapeutic uses include relief of symptoms in AIDS related disorders and as an antiemetic agent during chemotherapy. Also has analgesic, anticonvulsant and possibly anti-muscle spasmodic properties, hence its use in neurological disorders such as multiple sclerosis. Withdrawal symptoms are rare but chronic impairment has been reported.

Present law prohibits prescription of cannabis without a Home Office Licence and this has hampered meaningful clinical trials; there has been pressure to allow freer administration in certain chronic conditions and even to decriminalise it altogether although this is controversial. Reclassified as a Class C drug under the Misuse of Drugs Act 1971 in 2004. Nabilone is a synthetic cannabinoid used as an antiemetic in chemotherapy-induced nausea and vomiting.
Kumar RN, Chambers WA, Pertwee RG (2001). Anaesthesia; 56: 1059–68

Capacitance. Ability to retain electrical charge; defined as the charge stored by an object per voltage difference across it. The unit of capacitance is the farad (F), one farad being the capacity to store one coulomb of charge for an applied potential difference of one volt.

A capacitor comprised of conductors separated by an insulator may be charged by a potential difference across it, but will not allow direct current to flow. Its stored charge may subsequently be discharged, e.g. in defibrillation. Repeated charging and discharging induced by an alternating current results in current flow across a capacitor.
[Michael Faraday (1791–1867), English chemist]

Capacitance vessels. Comprised of venae cavae and large veins; normally only partially distended, they may expand to accommodate a large volume of blood before venous pressure is increased. Innervated by the sympathetic nervous system in the same way as the arterial system (resistance vessels), they act as a blood reservoir. 60–70% of blood volume is within the veins normally.

Capacitor, *see Capacitance*

Capillary circulation. Contains 5% of circulating blood volume, which passes from arterioles to venules via capillaries, usually within 2 s. Controlled by local autoregulatory mechanisms, and possibly by autonomic neural reflexes. Molecules and ions which readily cross the capillary walls (mainly by diffusion) include water, O_2, CO_2, glucose and urea. Hydrostatic pressure falls from about 30 mmHg (arteriolar end) to 15 mmHg (venous end) within the capillary. Direction of fluid flow across capillary walls is determined by hydrostatic and osmotic pressure gradients (Starling forces).

Capillary refill time. Time taken for capillary refill after pressure on a digit for 5 s. Normally < 2 s; prolonged in hypoperfusion and hypothermia. Should be measured with the digit at the level of the heart.

Capnography. Continuous measurement and pictorial display of CO_2 concentration (capnometry refers to measurement only). During anaesthesia, used to display end-tidal CO_2; this may be achieved using:
- spectroscopy (most commonly infra-red).
- mass spectrometer.

The equipment used must have a very short response time in order to produce a continuous display.
See also, Carbon dioxide, end-tidal; Carbon dioxide measurement

Capreomycin. Cyclic polypeptide antibacterial drug used to treat TB resistant to other therapy (especially in immunocompromised patients). Also used in other mycobacterial infections. Poorly absorbed orally, peak levels occur within 2 h of im injection. Excreted unchanged in the urine.
- Dosage: 1 g/day by deep im injection for 2–4 months, then 1 g 2–3 times weekly, reduced in renal failure.
- Side effects: renal and hepatic impairment, ocular disturbances, rashes, vertigo, tinnitus, hearing loss, blood dyscrasias, hypokalaemia, hyponatraemia, hypocalcaemia, hypomagnesaemia, neuromuscular blockade.

Capsaicin. Naturally occurring substance found in hot chilli peppers. Acts via specific neuronal membrane receptors (vanilloid receptors), mainly Aδ and C pain fibres. Initial stimulation is followed by depletion of substance P by reducing its synthesis, storage and transport. Has been applied topically for temporary relief of pain associated with neuralgias, e.g. postherpetic neuralgia, and arthritis. Should be applied 6–8 hourly. Takes 1–4 weeks to produce its effect. There may be burning on initial application.

Captopril. Angiotensin converting enzyme inhibitor, used to treat hypertension and cardiac failure (including following MI), and diabetic nephropathy. Shorter acting than enalapril; onset is within 15 min with peak effect at 30–60 min. Half-life is 2 h. Excreted renally; thus it should be avoided in renal impairment.
- Dosage: 6.25–50 mg orally, 8–12 hourly.
- Side effects: severe hypotension after the first dose, cough, taste disturbances, rash, abdominal pain, agranulocytosis, neutropenia, hyperkalaemia, renal impairment. Severe

hypotension may occur after induction of anaesthesia and in hypovolaemia.

Contraindicated in pregnancy and porphyria.

Carbamazepine. Anticonvulsant drug, used to treat all types of epilepsy except petit mal. Has fewer side effects than phenytoin, and has a greater therapeutic index. Also used for pain management, e.g. in trigeminal neuralgia, and in manic-depressive disease.

- Dosage: 100–200 mg orally in divided doses, up to 2.0 g/day, or 125–250 mg rectally in divided doses, up to 1.0 g/day. Monitoring plasma levels may help determination of optimal dosage (target levels 20–50 μmol/l).
- Side effects: dizziness, visual disturbances, GIT upset, rash, hyponatraemia, cholestatic jaundice, hepatitis, syndrome of inappropriate ADH secretion. Blood dyscrasias may occur rarely. Enzyme induction may cause reduced effects of other drugs, e.g. warfarin.

  Contraindicated in atrioventricular conduction defects and porphyria.

Carbapenems. Group of bactericidal antibacterial drugs; contain the β-lactam ring and thus impair bacterial cell wall synthesis like the penicillins. Include imipenem, meropenem and ertapenem.

Carbenoxalone sodium. Glycyrrhizinic acid derivative used to treat peptic ulcer disease (and also available in a mouthwash to treat mouth ulcers). Inhibits pepsin activity and stimulates mucus secretion. Less effective than H_2 receptor antagonists. Now only available in the UK as part of compound preparations with antacids. May cause sodium and fluid retention, headache and myopathy.

Carbetocin. Analogue of human oxytocin, licensed for prevention of uterine atony after delivery by Caesarean section under regional anaesthesia. Acts within 2 min of injection, its effects lasting over an hour.

- Dosage: 100 μg iv.
- Side effects: as for oxytocin.

Carbicarb. Experimental buffer composed of 0.3M sodium carbonate and 0.3M sodium bicarbonate, used to treat acidosis. Unlike bicarbonate, there is no net generation of CO_2; thus restoration of normal pH is not accompanied by increased arterial $P\text{CO}_2$. The problem of intracellular acidosis that occurs with bicarbonate is thus avoided.

Carbohydrates (Saccharides). Class of compounds with the general formula $C_n(H_2O)_n$, hence their name, although they are not true hydrates. n usually exceeds 3. Range in size; mono- and disaccharides (simple sugars) are most common, where n = 5 or 6 (pentoses or hexoses, e.g. glucose, sucrose). Large polysaccharides include starch, cellulose and glycogen. Metabolites often contain phosphorus. Some polysaccharides are combined with proteins, e.g. mucopolysaccharides. Act as a source of energy in food, e.g.:

$$C_6H_{12}O_6 + 6O_2 \rightarrow 6CO_2 + 6H_2O + \text{energy}$$

1 g carbohydrate yields about 17 kJ energy (4 Cal).

- Ingested carbohydrates are broken down thus:
  - mouth: salivary amylase: starch → smaller units (n up to about 8).
  - small intestine:
    - pancreatic amylase: starch as above.
    - maltase: maltose → glucose.
    - lactase: lactose → glucose + galactose.
    - sucrase: sucrose → glucose + fructose.

Hexoses and pentoses absorbed from the GIT pass to the liver for energy production, storage molecule synthesis or alternative pathways.

See also, Metabolism

Carbon dioxide (CO_2). Gas produced by oxidation of carbon containing substances, including foodstuffs. Average rate of production under basal conditions in adults is about 200 ml/min, although it varies with the energy source (*see Respiratory quotient*).

- Partial pressures of CO_2:
  - inspired: 0.03 kPa (0.2 mmHg).
  - alveolar: 5.3 kPa (40 mmHg).
  - arterial: 5.3 kPa (40 mmHg).
  - venous: 6.1 kPa (46 mmHg).
  - expired: 4 kPa (30 mmHg).

Isolated in 1757 by Black. CO_2 narcosis was used for anaesthesia in animals by Hickman in 1824. Used to stimulate respiration during anaesthesia from the early 1900s, to maintain ventilation and speed uptake of volatile agents during induction; also used to assist blind nasal tracheal intubation. Administration is now generally considered hazardous because of the adverse effects of hypercapnia; avoidance of its accidental administration during anaesthesia has been achieved in modern anaesthetic machines by removing cylinders from anaesthetic machines altogether. Manufactured by heating calcium or magnesium carbonate, producing CO_2 and calcium/magnesium oxide.

- Properties:
  - colourless gas, 1.5 times denser than air.
  - mw 44.
  - boiling point −79°C.
  - critical temperature 31°C.
  - non-flammable and non-explosive.
  - supplied in grey cylinders; pressure is 50 bar at 15°C, about 57 bar at room temperature.
- Effects: as for hypercapnia.

[Joseph Black (1728–1799), Scottish chemist]

See also, Acid–base balance; Alveolar gas transfer; Carbon dioxide absorption, in anaesthetic breathing systems; Carbon dioxide dissociation curve; Carbon dioxide, end-tidal; Carbon dioxide measurement; Carbon dioxide response curve; Carbon dioxide transport

Carbon dioxide absorption, in anaesthetic breathing systems. Investigated and described by Waters in the early 1920s, although used earlier. Exhaled gases are passed over soda lime or a similar material, e.g. baralyme, and reused. In totally closed systems, only basal O_2 requirements need be supplied; absorption may also be used with low fresh gas flows and a leak through an expiratory valve.

- Advantages:
  - less inhalational agent required, i.e. cheaper.
  - less pollution.
  - warms and humidifies inhaled gases.
- Disadvantages:
  - high flows are required initially, to ensure nitrogen washout. If N_2O is also used, risk of hypoxic gas mixtures makes an O_2 analyser mandatory.
  - failure of CO_2 absorption may be due to exhaustion of soda lime or inefficient equipment; thus capnography is required.
  - resistance and dead space may be high with some systems, and inhalation of dust is possible.
  - trichloroethylene is incompatible with soda lime.
  - chemical reactions between the volatile agent and soda lime if the latter dries out excessively (*see Soda lime*).

- Methods:
  - Waters' cannister: cylindrical drum, 8 × 12 cm, containing 1 lb (0.45 kg) soda lime. Reservoir bag at one end, facepiece with fresh gas supply and expiratory valve at the other; exhaled gases pass to and fro through it. Most efficient when tidal volume equals the contained air space (400–450 ml). Smaller cannisters are used for children. Dead space equals the volume between the patient and soda lime; it increases during use as the soda lime nearest the patient is exhausted. Efficiency is also reduced by channelling of exhaled gases through gaps in the soda lime if loosely packed and allowed to settle. Also heavy and bulky to use.
  - circle systems: first introduced by Sword in 1930. Popular because of concern about pollution and cost of inhalational agents. Soda lime cannisters are held vertically, reducing the risk of channelling.

[Brian Sword (1889–1956), US anaesthestist]

Carbon dioxide dissociation curve. Graph of blood CO_2 content against its P_{CO_2} (Fig. 27). The curve is much steeper than the oxyhaemoglobin dissociation curve, and more linear. Different curves are obtained for oxygenated and deoxygenated blood, the latter able to carry more CO_2 (Haldane effect). The area lying between the dissolved CO_2 and the oxygenated haemoglobin curves represents the CO_2 carried as bicarbonate ion in plasma and erythrocytes.

Carbon dioxide, end-tidal (P_ECO_2). Partial pressure of CO_2 measured in the final portion of exhaled gas. Approximates to alveolar P_{CO_2} in normal anaesthetised subjects; the difference is about 0.4–0.7 kPa (3–5 mmHg). The difference increases in $\dot{V}/\dot{Q}$ mismatch and increased CO_2 production. May be monitored continuously during anaesthesia (often measured and displayed as CO_2 concentration in end-tidal gas), e.g. using infra-red capnography or mass spectrometry.

- Measurement is useful for assessing adequacy of ventilation, and allows normo- or hypocapnia to be produced as required during IPPV. Measurement also aids detection of:
  - efficient cardiac massage or return of spontaneous cardiac output in CPR.
  - oesophageal intubation, since CO_2 is only present in the oesophagus and stomach in small amounts, if at all.
  - PE (including fat or air embolism): P_ECO_2 falls due to increased alveolar dead space and reduced cardiac output.
  - rebreathing.
  - disconnection.
  - MH: P_ECO_2 rises as muscle metabolism increases.
- Display of a continuous trace is more useful than values alone (Fig. 28):
  - phase 1: zero baseline during inspiration; a raised baseline indicates rebreathing.
  - phase 2: dead space gas (containing no CO_2) is followed by alveolar gas, represented by a sudden rise to a plateau. Excessive sloping of the upstroke may indicate obstruction to expiration.
  - phase 3: near-horizontal plateau indicates mixing of alveolar gas. A steep upwards slope indicates obstruction to expiration or unequal mixing, e.g. COPD.
  - phase 4: rapid fall to zero at the onset of inspiration.
  - additional features may be present:
    - superimposed regular oscillations corresponding to the heart beat.
    - small waves representing spontaneous breaths between ventilator breaths, e.g. if neuromuscular blockade is insufficient.
    - failure of baseline to return to zero indicates rebreathing of CO_2.

See also, Carbon dioxide measurement; End-tidal gas sampling

Carbon dioxide measurement. Estimation of arterial P_{CO_2}:

- direct: Severinghaus CO_2 electrode: glass pH electrode separated from arterial blood sample by a thin membrane. CO_2 diffuses into bicarbonate solution surrounding the glass electrode, lowering pH. pH is measured and displayed in terms of P_{CO_2}. Kept at 37°C, and calibrated with known mixtures of CO_2/O_2 before use. Samples are stored in ice or analysed immediately, to reduce inaccuracy due to blood cell metabolism.

  Indwelling intravascular CO_2 electrodes are available for continuous monitoring of P_{CO_2}.
- indirect:
  - from gas:
    - to obtain gas for analysis:
      - end-tidal gas sampling (end-tidal P_{CO_2} approximates to alveolar P_{CO_2} which approximates to arterial P_{CO_2}).
      - rebreathing technique of Campbell and Howell: rebreathing from a 2 litre bag containing 50% O_2

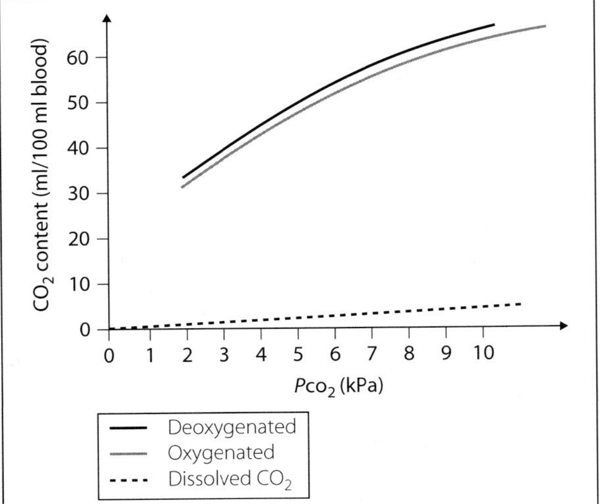

Fig. 27 Carbon dioxide dissociation curve

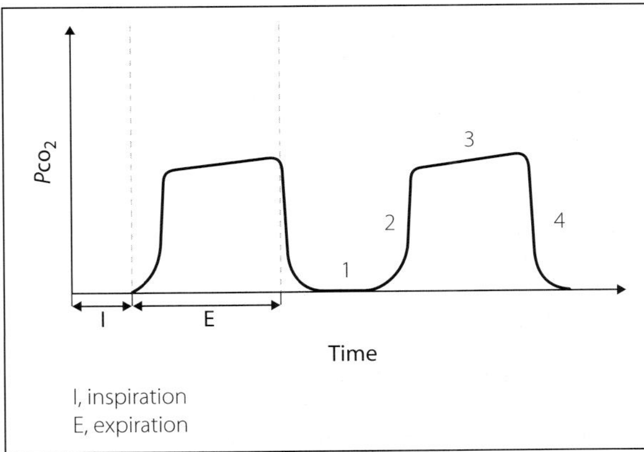

Fig. 28 Normal trace of end-tidal P_{CO_2}

for 90 s, then a further 30 s after 3 min rest. Bag $P\text{CO}_2$ then approximates to mixed venous $P\text{CO}_2$. Arterial $P\text{CO}_2$ is normally 0.8 kPa (6 mmHg) less than mixed venous $P\text{CO}_2$.
- subsequent gas analysis:
  - chemical: formation of non-gaseous compounds, with reduction of overall volume of the gas mixture (Haldane apparatus).
  - physical: capnography and mass spectrometry are most widely used. An interferometer, gas chromatography, etc. may also be used.
- from blood/tissues:
  - transcutaneous electrode: requires heating of the skin; relatively inaccurate.
  - measurement of venous $P\text{CO}_2$ and capillary $P\text{CO}_2$: inaccurate and unreliable.
  - Siggaard-Andersen nomogram: equilibration of the blood sample with gases of known CO_2.
  - van Slyke apparatus: liberation of gas from blood sample with subsequent chemical analysis.
  - fibreoptic sensors: under development.

[John W Severinghaus, San Francisco anaesthetist; EJ Moran Campbell (1925–2004), English-born Canadian physiologist; John BL Howell, Southampton physician]

Carbon dioxide narcosis. Loss of consciousness caused by severe hypercapnia, i.e. arterial $P\text{CO}_2$ exceeding approximately 25 kPa (200 mmHg). Thought to be due to a profound fall in pH of CSF (under 6.9). Increasing central depression is seen at arterial $P\text{CO}_2$ greater than 13 kPa (100 mmHg), and CSF pH under 7.1. Other features of hypercapnia may be present.

Used by Hickman in 1824 to enable painless surgery on animals.

Carbon dioxide response curve. Obtained by measuring minute ventilation at different arterial CO_2 tensions. Rebreathing from a 6 litre bag containing 50% O_2 and 7% CO_2 may be used, measuring minute ventilation and bag $P\text{CO}_2$ periodically. This is easier than increasing inspired CO_2 levels and measuring the response after equilibration at each new level. The curve may be used to indicate depression of respiratory drive (Fig. 29); increased threshold is represented by a shift of the curve to the right (1), and decreased sensitivity by depression of the slope (2). Both may follow administration of opioid and other depressant drugs, and in chronic hypercapnia; the opposite occurs in hypoxaemia.
See also, Breathing, control of

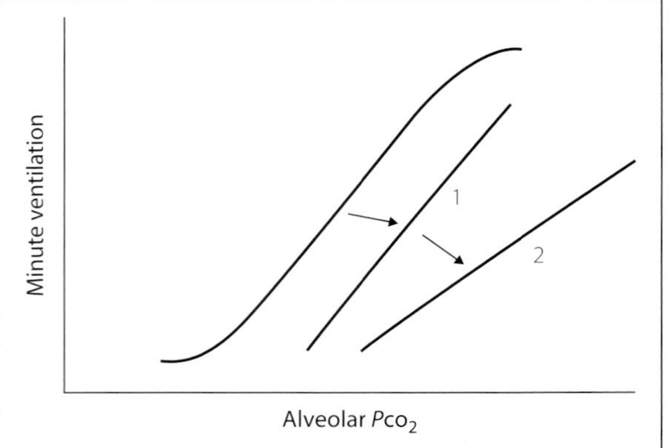

Fig. 29 Carbon dioxide response curve (see text)

Carbon dioxide transport. In arterial blood, approximately 50 ml CO_2 is carried per 100 ml blood, as:
- bicarbonate: 45 ml.
- carbonic acid: 2.5 ml.
- carbamino compounds with proteins, mainly haemoglobin: 2.5 ml.

In venous blood, 54 ml is carried per 100 ml blood, as:
- bicarbonate: 47.5 ml.
- carbonic acid: 3.0 ml.
- carbamino compounds: 3.5 ml.

CO_2 is rapidly converted by carbonic anhydrase in red cells to carbonic acid, which dissociates to bicarbonate and hydrogen ions. The former passes into plasma in exchange for chloride ions (chloride shift); the latter are buffered mainly by haemoglobin. Haemoglobin's buffering ability increases as it becomes deoxygenated, as does its ability to form carbamino groups (Haldane effect).
See also, Acid–base balance; Buffers; Carbon dioxide dissociation curve

Carbon monoxide diffusing capacity, *see Diffusing capacity*

Carbon monoxide poisoning. May result from inhalation of fumes from car exhausts, fires, heating systems, coal gas supplies, etc. Often coexists with cyanide poisoning. Although not directly toxic to the lungs, carbon monoxide (CO) binds to haemoglobin with 200–250 times the affinity of O_2, forming carboxyhaemoglobin, which dissociates very slowly. The amount of carboxyhaemoglobin formed depends on inspired CO concentration and duration of exposure.

Production of CO in circle systems has been reported under certain circumstances.

- Effects:
  - reduced capacity for O_2 transport.
  - oxyhaemoglobin dissociation curve shifted to the left.
  - inhibition of the cellular cytochrome oxidase system; tissue toxicity is proportional to the length of exposure.
  - aortic and carotid bodies do not detect hypoxia, since the arterial $P\text{O}_2$ is unaffected.
- Features:
  - non-specific if chronic, e.g. headache, weakness, dizziness, GIT disturbances, etc.
  - if acute: as above, with convulsions and coma if severe.
  - the 'cherry red' colour of carboxyhaemoglobin may be apparent.
  - O_2 saturation measured by pulse oximetry may be misleading because carboxyhaemoglobin is interpreted as oxygenated haemoglobin.
  - neurological symptoms (e.g. dystonia, ataxia, parkinsonism), personality changes and impaired memory may follow recovery from CO coma.
- Treatment:
  - O_2 therapy: speeds carboxyhaemoglobin dissociation. Tracheal intubation and IPPV may be necessary. Elimination half-life of carbon monoxide is reduced from 4 h to under 1 h with 100% O_2; it is reduced further to under 30 min with hyperbaric O_2 at 2.5–3 atm. At this pressure, dissolved O_2 alone satisfies tissue O_2 requirements. Hyperbaric O_2 has been suggested if the patient is unconscious, has arrhythmias, is pregnant or has carboxyhaemoglobin levels above 40%.
  - carboxyhaemoglobin levels correlate poorly with severity of symptoms, because of variable effects of tissue toxicity. Values often quoted:
    - 0.3–2%: normal non-smokers (some CO from pollution, some formed endogenously).

- 5–6%: normal smokers.
- 10–30%: mild symptoms common.
- above 60%: severe symptoms common.

Carbon monoxide transfer factor, *see Diffusing capacity*

Carbonic anhydrase. Zinc-containing enzyme catalysing the reaction of CO_2 and water to form carbonic acid, which rapidly dissociates to bicarbonate and hydrogen ions. Absent from plasma, but present in high concentrations in:
- red blood cells: important in buffering, CO_2 transport and O_2 transport.
- renal tubular cells: important for maintaining acid–base balance.
- gastric mucosa: important in hydrochloric acid production.
- ciliary body: involved in aqueous humour formation.

Inhibited by acetazolamide and sulphonamides.

Carboprost. Prostaglandin $F_2\alpha$ analogue, used for the induction of second trimester abortion; also used to treat postpartum haemorrhage unresponsive to conventional therapy. Given as the trometamol salt.
- Dosage: 250 μg by deep im injection repeated as required every 15–90 min, up to 2 mg. Has also been injected into the myometrium.
- Side effects: vomiting, diarrhoea, leucocytosis, fever, bronchospasm, uterine rupture.

Carboxyhaemoglobin, *see Carbon monoxide poisoning*

Carcinogenicity of anaesthetic agents, *see Environmental safety of anaesthetists; Fetus, effects of anaesthetic agents on*

Carcinoid syndrome. Results from secretion of vasoactive and other substances from certain tumours, usually found in the terminal ileum of the GIT (85%). Secreted compounds are metabolised by the liver so that symptoms are absent until hepatic metastases are present. Tumours may also arise in the lung and gonads. May be associated with neurofibromatosis.
- Features:
  - flushing, mainly of the head and neck. May be associated with vasodilatation, hypotension, wheezing, skin wheals and sweating.
  - diarrhoea, perhaps with nausea and vomiting. Typically episodic, along with flushing. Weight loss is common.
  - endocardial fibrosis involving the tricuspid and pulmonary valves may cause right-sided cardiac failure.

Symptoms are traditionally ascribed to secretion of 5-HT (diarrhoea) and kinins (flushing), but many more substances have been implicated, e.g. substance P, prostaglandins, histamine and vasoactive intestinal peptide. Diagnosis includes measurement of urinary 5-hydroxyindole acetic acid, a breakdown product of 5-HT.
- Anaesthetic management:
  - perioperative treatment with various drugs has been used to reduce hyper-/hypotensive episodes and bronchospasm:
    - somatostatin analogues, e.g. octreotide: inhibits release of inflammatory mediators and has become the first-line treatment of many authorities.
    - 5-HT antagonists: ketanserin, cyproheptadine, methysergide.
    - others include aprotinin and antihistamine drugs.
  - invasive cardiovascular monitoring and careful fluid balance.
  - use of cardiostable drugs where possible; avoidance of drugs causing histamine release.
  - suxamethonium has been claimed to increase mediator release via fasciculations but this is uncertain.
  - drugs should be prepared for treatment of bronchospasm and hyper-/hypotension.
  - admission to HDU/ICU postoperatively.

Cardiac arrest. Sudden circulatory standstill. Common cause of death in cardiovascular disease, especially ischaemic heart disease. May also be caused by PE, electrolyte disturbances, e.g. of potassium or calcium, hypoxaemia, hypercapnia, hypotension, vagal reflexes, hypothermia, anaphylactic reaction, electrocution, drugs, e.g. adrenaline, and instrumentation of the heart, e.g. percutaneous cannulation.
- Features: unconsciousness within 15–30 s, apnoea or gasping respiration, pallor, cyanosis, absent pulses. Pupillary dilatation is usual.
- May be due to:
  - VF; usually associated with myocardial ischaemia. The most common ECG finding (about 60%), with the best prognosis.
  - asystole: occurs in about 30%. More likely in exsanguination and hypoxia, especially in children. May also follow vagally mediated bradycardia.
  - electromechanical dissociation (EMD)/pulseless electrical activity (PEA). May occur in widespread myocardial damage. The least common ECG finding, with the worst prognosis, unless due to mechanical causes of circulatory collapse, e.g. PE, cardiac tamponade, pneumothorax, etc.

  Asystole and EMD/PEA may convert to VF, which eventually converts to asystole if untreated.

Only 15–20% of patients leave hospital after cardiac arrest. Up to 30–40% survival is thought to be possible if prompt CPR is instituted. Permanent brain damage is thought to occur within 4–5 min unless CPR is instituted. The prognosis is better if the patient regains consciousness within 10 min of the circulation restarting.

See also, Advanced life support, adult; Basic life support, adult; Cerebral ischaemia

Cardiac asthma. Acute pulmonary oedema resembling asthma. Both may feature dyspnoea, decreased lung compliance and widespread rhonchi, although pulmonary oedema is suggested by pink frothy sputum. Increased airway resistance may result from true bronchospasm, or from bronchial oedema.

Cardiac catheterisation. Passage of a catheter into the heart chambers for measurement of intracardiac pressures and O_2 saturations, or for injection of radiological contrast media for radiological imaging (angiocardiography). Used to investigate ischaemic heart disease, valvular heart disease and congenital heart disease; also used for treatment of lesions, e.g. balloon valvotomy, atrial septostomy (e.g. in transposition of the great arteries), percutaneous transluminal coronary angioplasty.
- Technique:
  - commonly performed under local anaesthesia except in small children, in whom general anaesthesia is required.
  - access is via a peripheral vein or artery, e.g. femoral or brachial vessels, using either a cut-down technique or percutaneous guidewire (Seldinger technique).
  - the right side of the heart is approached as for pulmonary artery catheterisation.

- the left side of the heart is approached retrogradely under X-ray control, via a peripheral artery or from the right side through the atrial septum or a defect thereof.
- Information gained:
  - pressure values, waveforms and gradients between chambers.
  - saturation values; greater than expected values on the right side indicate a left-to-right **shunt**.
  - **cardiac output** may be measured using the **Fick principle**.
  - angiocardiography: cardiac function may be assessed on cine film, or the coronary vessels filled with dye to assess patency.

Approximate normal pressures and measurements are shown in Table 8.

Cardiac compressions, *see Cardiac massage*

Cardiac cycle. Sequence of events occurring during cardiac activity; usually represented by the Wiggers' diagram which details changes in vascular pressures (especially **arterial BP**), **heart** chamber pressures, **ECG** and **phonocardiography** tracings during normal **sinus rhythm** (Fig. 30).

- Divided into five phases:
  - phase 1: atrial contraction: responsible for about 30% of ventricular filling. Some blood regurgitates into the venae cavae and pulmonary veins.
  - phase 2: isometric ventricular contraction: lasts from the closing of the tricuspid and mitral valves until ventricular pressures exceed aortic and pulmonary artery pressures, and the aortic and pulmonary valves open.
  - phase 3: ventricular ejection: most rapid at the start of systole. Lasts until the aortic and pulmonary valves close.
  - phase 4: isometric ventricular relaxation: lasts until the tricuspid and mitral valves open.
  - phase 5: passive ventricular filling: most rapid at the start of diastole.

[Carl J Wiggers (1883–1963), US physiologist]

See also, Arterial waveform; Pulse; Stroke volume; Venous waveform

Cardiac enzymes. Enzymes normally within cardiac cells; released into the blood after injury (e.g. after **MI** or cardiac contusion), thus aiding diagnosis:

- creatine kinase (CK or CPK):
  - normally < 190 iu/l.
  - rises 4–6 h after MI, peaks at 12 h, falls at 2–3 days.
  - three specific isoenzymes exist for skeletal muscle (CKMM), brain (CKBB) and myocardium (CKMB). Presence of CKMB in the plasma indicates myocardial necrosis.
- aspartate aminotransferase (AST):

Table 8 Normal pressures and O_2 saturations obtained during cardiac catheterisation

Site	Pressure (mmHg)	Saturation (%)
Right atrium	1–4	75
Right ventricle	25/4	75
Pulmonary artery	25/12	75
Left atrium	2–10	97
Left ventricle	120/10	97
Aorta	120/70	97

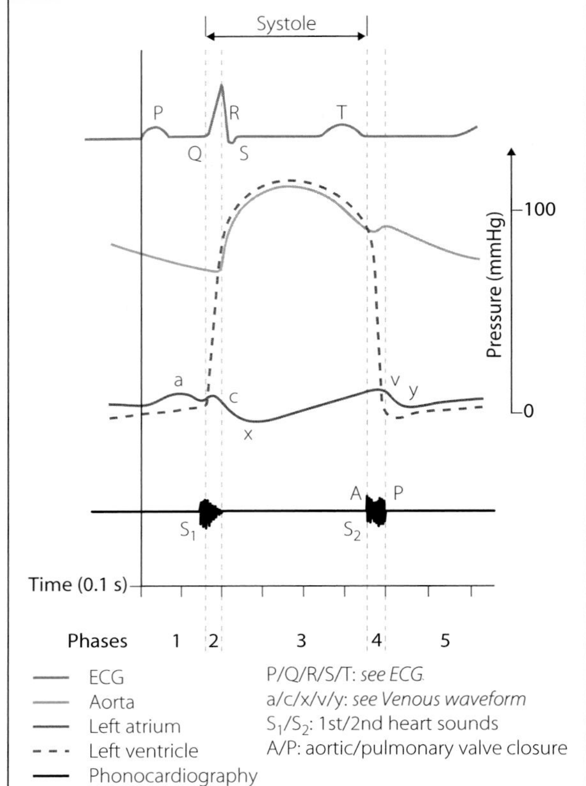

Fig. 30 Cardiac cycle

  - normally < 35 iu/l.
  - rises after 12 h, peaks at 1–2 days.
- lactic dehydrogenase (LDH):
  - normally < 300 iu/l (depends on the assay).
  - rises after 12 h, peaks at 2–3 days, falls after 5–7 days.
  - five isoenzymes exist; an increase in the level of LDH1 or the ratio of LDH1:LDH2 indicates myocardial necrosis.
- troponin I:
  - found only in cardiac muscle.
  - more sensitive and specific indicator of acute MI than CKMB.
  - normally undetectable.
  - rises after 4–8 h after MI, peaks at 12 h, falls at 5–9 days.
  - levels indicating MI depend upon the assay used by individual labs.
  - should be distinguished from troponin T, a similar marker which does not appear to be as specific for cardiac muscle damage.

Kemp M, Donovan J, Higham H, Hooper J (2004). Br J Anaesth; 93: 63–73

Cardiac failure. Usually defined as inability of the heart to produce sufficient output for the body's requirements and venous return. The diagnosis is clinical, ranging from mild symptoms on exertion only, to **cardiogenic shock**. Several terms have been used to describe different forms of cardiac failure:

- left or right ventricular failure (the most commonly used classification). The left ventricle is usually affected by general disease because its workload is much greater than that of the right.

- forward or backward failure: the former refers to failure with reduced **cardiac output**; the latter refers to increased filling pressures with oedema, etc.
- congestive cardiac failure: the term sometimes refers to backward failure, but is often reserved for left-sided failure leading to right-sided failure.
- high output failure: associated with increased **preload** and increased cardiac output.
- diastolic failure: recently recognised form in which the **ejection fraction** may be normal but ventricular filling is impaired.

- Caused by:
  - increased workload:
    - **preload**:
      - **aortic/mitral regurgitation**.
      - **ASD/VSD**.
      - severe **anaemia**, fluid overload, **hyperthyroidism**.
    - **afterload**:
      - **hypertension**.
      - pulmonary/**aortic stenosis**, hypertrophic obstructive **cardiomyopathy**.
      - **pulmonary hypertension**, **PE**.
  - reduced force of contraction:
    - **MI**, **ischaemic heart disease**.
    - cardiomyopathy.
    - **arrhythmias**.
    - **myocarditis**.
  - reduced filling:
    - tricuspid/**mitral stenosis**.
    - **cardiac tamponade**, constrictive **pericarditis** (right side).
    - reduced ventricular compliance, e.g. amyloid infiltration.
- Effects:
  - ventricular end-diastolic pressure increases, leading to compensatory mechanisms:
    - ventricular hypertrophy.
    - increased myocardial contractility (**Starling's law**).
    - neuroendocrine response: mainly increased sympathetic activity, with tachycardia, vasoconstriction and increased force of contraction. **Aldosterone**, **renin/angiotensin** and **vasopressin** activity are increased, especially in chronic failure, but mechanisms are unclear. Salt and water retention result.
  - ventricular **compliance** is reduced, leading to increased atrial pressure and atrial hypertrophy. Eventually, ventricular dilatation occurs, with higher wall tension required to produce a given pressure (**Laplace's law**).
  - **coronary blood flow** is reduced by tachycardia, raised end-diastolic pressure, and increased muscle mass.
  - left-sided failure may lead to **pulmonary oedema**, pulmonary hypertension, **$\dot{V}/\dot{Q}$ mismatch**, decreased lung compliance and right-sided failure.
  - right ventricular failure: **CVP** and **JVP** increase, with peripheral oedema and hepatic engorgement.
  - reduced peripheral blood flow leads to increased O_2 uptake and reduction of mixed venous Po_2.
  - sodium and water retention exacerbate oedema.
- Features:
  - reduced cardiac output may result in hypotension, confusion and coma.
  - left-sided failure:
    - dyspnoea, typically worse on lying flat (orthopnoea) and sometimes waking the patient at night (paroxysmal nocturnal dyspnoea).
    - peripheral shutdown, basal crepitations, left ventricular hypertrophy. Extra **heart sounds**, e.g. gallop rhythm and **heart murmurs** may be present. **Cheyne–Stokes respiration** may accompany low output.
    - acute pulmonary oedema.
  - right-sided failure:
    - raised JVP.
    - dependent oedema, e.g. ankles if ambulant, sacrum if bed-bound.
    - hepatomegaly/**ascites**; the liver may be tender.
    - right ventricular hypertrophy.
  - **chest X-ray** may reveal cardiomegaly, upper lobe blood diversion, fluid in the pulmonary fissures, **Kerley lines**, **pleural effusion** and pulmonary oedema. **ECG** may reveal ventricular hypertrophy and strain, arrhythmias, etc.
- Management:
  - general: of underlying cause, rest, sodium restriction; O_2 therapy if acute.
  - **ACE inhibitors**, often in combination with a **diuretic**.
  - diuretics: thiazide in mild failure with good renal function, otherwise a loop diuretic. **Spironolactone** may be added in low dosage to ACE inhibitor/diuretic therapy in severe, non-responsive failure.
  - **digoxin**: improves symptoms and performance but not mortality.
  - **β-adrenergic receptor antagonists** have been used in selected cases with stable, left ventricular systolic failure (carvedilol, bisoprolol and modified-release metoprolol).
  - other **vasodilator drugs**, e.g. nitrates, **angiotensin II receptor antagonists** have been used in patients unable to tolerate ACE inhibitors.
  - **inotropic drugs**: oral drugs are mostly disappointing. The most effective drugs are administered by iv infusion.
  - emergency treatment: as for pulmonary oedema and **cardiogenic shock**.
- Response to treatment (Fig. 31):
  - 1: inotropic drugs/arterial vasodilators.
  - 2: diuretics/venous vasodilators.
  - 3:
    - drug combinations, e.g. inotropes + vasodilators; often produce the greatest improvement
    - **intra-aortic counter-pulsation balloon pump**.

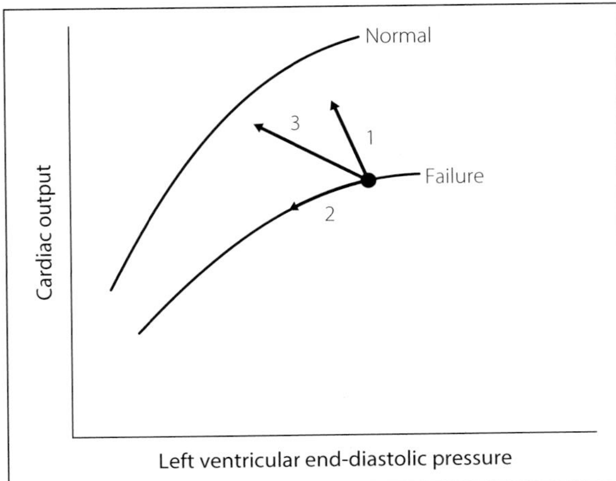

Fig. 31 Response to treatment of cardiac failure by Starling's curve (see text)

- Anaesthetic considerations:
  - cardiac failure is consistently associated with increased perioperative morbidity and mortality; it should therefore be treated preoperatively whenever possible.
  - treatment as above. Electrolyte disturbances and digoxin toxicity may occur.
  - anaesthetic drugs should be given in small doses and slowly, because:
    - arm–brain circulation time is increased.
    - increased proportion of cardiac output goes to vital organs, e.g. brain and heart; thus greater effects are seen on these organs than in normal cardiac output states.
  - danger of myocardial depression, hypoxia, arrhythmias.
  - use of epidural/spinal anaesthesia is controversial; the benefit of reduction of SVR may be offset by the risk of hypotension. Perioperative risk is not diminished.
  - general anaesthetic management is as for the underlying condition.

Jessup M, Brozena S (2003). N Engl J Med; 348: 2007–18

Cardiac glycosides. Drugs derived from plant extracts, used to treat supraventricular arrhythmias and cardiac failure (their use in the latter is controversial, since short-term benefit may not result in improved mortality). Their actions are thought to be partly due to inhibition of the sodium/potassium pump, although increased calcium mobilisation may also be involved. The drugs have long half-lives (e.g. ouabain 20 h; digoxin 36 h; digitoxin 4 days), large volumes of distribution (e.g. digoxin 700 litres) and low therapeutic index.

- Actions:
  - increase myocardial contractility and stroke volume (direct effect).
  - decrease atrioventricular conduction, sinus node discharge, and thus heart rate (indirect effect via the vagus, and direct effect).
- Side effects: as for digoxin. They are increased by hypokalaemia, hypercalcaemia and hypomagnesaemia. Toxicity is also more likely in renal failure and pulmonary disease.

Digoxin is most widely used. Ouabain is more rapidly acting.

Cardiac index (CI). Cardiac output corrected for body size, expressed in terms of body surface area:

$$CI = \frac{\text{cardiac output (l/min)}}{\text{surface area (m}^2\text{)}}$$

Normal value is 2.5–4.2 l/min/m^2.

Cardiac massage. Periodic compression of the heart or chest in order to maintain cardiac output, e.g. during CPR. Both open (internal) and closed (external) cardiac massage were developed in the late 1800s. The latter became more popular in the 1960s following clear demonstration of its value in dogs and man, and was subsequently adopted by the American Heart Association and the Resuscitation Council (UK) as method of choice.

- Closed cardiac massage:
  - with the patient supine on a rigid surface, the heel of one hand is placed on the lower third of the sternum, 1–2 fingers' breadths cranial to the notch between the xiphisternum and rib cage (excessive trauma may result if compression is applied to the xiphisternum or ribs). The other hand is placed on the first, with fingers clear of the chest. With elbows straight and shoulders vertically above the hands, regular compressions are applied, with ratio of compression:relaxation 50:50 to 60:40. The sternum should be depressed 3.5–5 cm at each compression, at a rate of 100/min.
  - efficacy is assessed by feeling the femoral or carotid pulse, although palpable peak pressures may not reflect blood flow. End-tidal CO_2 measurement has been used to assess adequacy of massage; an increase reflects improved cardiac output.
  - may produce up to 30% of normal carotid and cerebral blood flows and cardiac output. Coronary flow is low during cardiac massage, and falls rapidly when massage is stopped.
  - slightly different technique in children up to 8 years:
    - under 1 year: tips of 2 fingers placed on the sternum, one finger's breadth below a line joining the nipples. The sternum is depressed by about ⅓ of the depth of the child's chest at a rate of 100/min.
    - up to 8 years: heel of one hand placed over the lower half of the sternum, the fingers lifted to avoid applying pressure on the ribs. The sternum is depressed by about ⅓ of the depth of the child's chest at a rate of 100/min.
  - theories of mechanism (both may occur):
    - cardiac pump (as originally suggested): the heart is squeezed between sternum and vertebrae during compressions, expelling blood from the ventricles. During relaxation, blood is drawn into the chest by negative intrathoracic pressure, and the ventricles fill from the atria ('thoracic diastole'). Thought to be more important in children and when the heart is large.
    - thoracic pump: the theory arose from arterial and cardiac chamber pressure measurements during CPR, and from the phenomenon of cough-CPR. Positive intrathoracic pressure pushes blood out of heart and chest during compressions; reverse flow is prevented by cardiac and venous valves, and collapse of the thin-walled veins. During relaxation, blood is drawn into the chest by negative intrathoracic pressure.

      Intrathoracic pressures may be maximalised by synchronising compressions with IPPV breaths, with or without abdominal binding or compression ('new' CPR). Devices used to augment the thoracic pump mechanism include:
      - automatic chest compressor ('chest thumper').
      - 'active compression/decompression' device: applies suction to the chest wall between compressions to increase venous return.
      - impedance valve inserted in the ventilating system: impedes passive inspiration during the 'release' phase, thus increasing intrathoracic negative pressure and increasing venous return. During compression the extra venous return results in greater cardiac output.

      Improved blood flows and outcome have been claimed but further studies are awaited.
- Open cardiac massage:
  - increasingly used, because blood flows and cardiac output are greater than with closed massage. Also, direct vision and palpation are useful in assessing cardiac rhythm and filling, and defibrillation and intracardiac injection are easier.
  - skin and muscle are incised in an arc under the left nipple in the 4th or 5th intercostal space, stopping 2–3 cm from the sternum to avoid the internal thoracic artery. Pericardium is exposed using blunt dissection and pulling the ribs apart. The heart is squeezed from the patient's left side using the left hand, with fingers anteriorly over the right ventricle and thumb posteriorly over the left ventricle. The rate of compressions is determined by

cardiac filling. The descending aorta may be compressed with the other hand. The pericardium is opened for defibrillation or intracardiac injection. Because of the emergency nature of the procedure and the low risk of infection, sterile precautions are usually waived.
- may also be performed per abdomen through the intact diaphragm; the heart is compressed against the sternum. Minimally invasive direct cardiac massage via a small thoracostomy has recently been described.
- usually reserved for trauma, peroperative use, intra-abdominal or thoracic haemorrhage, massive PE, hypothermia, chest deformity, and ineffective closed massage.

See also, Cardiac output measurement

Cardiac output (CO). Volume of blood pumped by the heart per minute. Equals stroke volume (litres) × heart rate (beats/min). Normally about 5 l/min (0.07 litres × 70 beats/min) in a fit 70 kg man at rest; may increase up to 30 l/min, e.g. on vigorous exercise. Often corrected for body surface area (cardiac index).

Of central importance in maintaining arterial BP (equals cardiac output × SVR) and O_2 delivery to the tissues (O_2 flux).

Affected by metabolic rate (e.g. increased in pregnancy, sepsis, hyperthyroidism and exercise), drugs, and many other physiological and pathological processes which affect heart rate, preload, myocardial contractility and afterload.

- Distribution of normal CO (approximate values):
  - heart: 5%.
  - brain: 14%.
  - muscle: 20%.
  - kidneys: 22%.
  - liver: 25%.
  - rest: 14%.

(for comparisons of blood flow and oxygen consumption, see Blood flow)

- Effects of iv anaesthetic agents on CO:
  - reduced by propofol > thiopental > etomidate, mostly via decreased contractility though propofol may also cause vasodilatation and bradycardia.
  - increased by ketamine.
- Effects of inhalational anaesthetic agents on CO:
  - reduced by enflurane > halothane > isoflurane/desflurane > sevoflurane > N_2O. Proposed mechanisms include direct myocardial depression (via reduced concentration or modified activity of intracellular calcium ions during systole), inhibition of central or peripheral sympathetic nervous system outflow, and altered baroreceptor activity.
  - maintained by diethyl ether via sympathetic stimulation despite a direct myocardial depressant effect.

See also, Cardiac output measurement

Cardiac output measurement. Methods which have been used include:
- Fick principle: most commonly O_2 consumption is measured. Requires samples of mixed venous and arterial blood. Alternatively, CO_2 production may be measured, deriving arterial $P\text{CO}_2$ from end-tidal expired partial pressure. Mixed venous $P\text{CO}_2$ may be derived from analysis of expired gas collected in a closed rebreathing bag, using a mass spectrometer. Both methods are lengthy, complicated and not suitable for routine use. A new technique, NiCO, employs partial $P\text{CO}_2$ rebreathing and end-expiratory CO_2 measurement.
- dilution techniques:
  - dye dilution: a known amount of dye is injected into the pulmonary artery, and its concentration measured peripherally using a photoelectric spectrometer. Indocyanine green is used because of its low toxicity, short half-life and absorption characteristics (i.e. unaffected by changes in O_2 saturation). Semilogarithmic replotting of the data curve is required, with extrapolation of the straight line obtained to correct for recirculation of the dye (Fig. 32). Cardiac output is calculated from the injected dose, the area under the curve within the extrapolated line and its duration. Curves of short duration are produced by high cardiac output; curves of long duration are produced by low cardiac output. Data from repeated injections may be affected by previous ones.

    Lithium has also been used as an alternative to indocyanine green; it is injected via a central venous catheter and measured by a lithium-sensitive electrode incorporated into an arterial cannula, e.g. placed in the radial artery.
  - thermodilution: suitable for use in the ICU or operating theatre:
    - intermittent: 5–10 ml cold dextrose or saline is injected through the proximal port of a pulmonary artery catheter, with temperature changes measured by a thermistor at the catheter tip. Injection is usually performed at end-expiration. A plot of temperature drop against time is produced as for dye dilution but without the secondary peak. Cardiac output is calculated by a bedside computer using the Stewart–Hamilton equation; an average of at least three measurements is used. Measurement may be inaccurate in the presence of intracardiac shunts or tricuspid regurgitation, if the measured injectate volume or temperature is inaccurate, if the speed of injection varies, or if the thermistor is against a vessel wall. Repeated measurements may be made without being affected by previous ones.

      In transpulmonary thermodilution cardiac output measurement, ice-cold saline is injected via a central venous catheter and is dispersed into the intravascular area and the extravascular space during passage through the lungs. Pulse contour cardiac output derived from rapid beat-to-beat analysis of the arterial (aortic) pressure wave is calibrated with an arterial thermodilution measurement to give a continuous

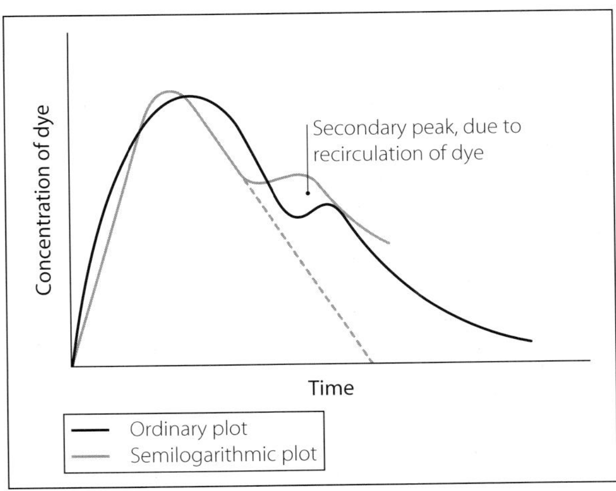

Fig. 32 Dilution technique for measuring cardiac output

indication of cardiac output. Use of an intra-arterial fibreoptic catheter and injection of cold dye allows measurement of intrathoracic blood volume and extravascular lung water. If indocyanine green is used, the intravascular dye distribution volume during the first cardiopulmonary passage equals intrathoracic blood volume; indocyanine green is extracted selectively from the blood by the liver and this can therefore be used as a liver function test. Total circulating blood volume can be calculated after complete mixing of the indocyanine green with the blood has occurred.
- continuous: employs a specially modified pulmonary artery catheter, containing a thermal filament extending 14–25 cm from its distal tip (thus lying within both the RA and the right ventricle during use) which adds an average of 7.5 W heat to the blood in a repetitive on–off sequence every 30–60 s. Changes in blood temperature are measured by a thermistor 4 cm from the catheter tip. A typical thermodilution 'washout' curve is constructed by applying a formula to cross-correlate the thermistor temperature with the thermal energy input sequence. Cardiac output is computed from the curve as above.
- PiCCO: a technique combining transpulmonary thermodilution and arterial pulse contour analysis.
- echocardiography: two-dimensional echocardiography can be used to measure the movement of the anterior and posterior ventricular walls, and ejection fraction. Derivation of stroke volume relies on the shape of the ventricular cavity being ellipsoid, which may not always be the case. Three-dimensional echocardiography may produce better results. Transoesophageal echocardiography has also been used. Alternatively, the velocity of blood in the ascending aorta may be measured using the Doppler effect, allowing estimation of the length of a column of blood passing through the aorta in unit time. This is multiplied by the cross-sectional area of the aorta to give stroke volume. Portable devices use either oesophageal or suprasternal probes, the latter being less accurate and reliable.
- cardiac catheterisation and angiography allows estimation of left ventricular volume and ejection fraction, as does radioisotope scanning.
- impedance plethysmography and induction cardiography: thought to be useful in estimating changes in individual subjects, but not useful for absolute measurements.
- aortovelography and ballistocardiography: inaccurate.
- electromagnetic flow measurement may be achieved during surgery by placing a probe around the root of the aorta, but its use is obviously limited.

Jhanji S, Dawson J, Pearse RM (2008). Anaesthesia 63: 172–81

Cardiac pacing. Repetitive electrical stimulation of cardiac activity, used to treat brady- or tachyarrhythmias.
- May be:
  - temporary:
    - transvenous; i.e. pacing wire passed via a central vein to the right ventricle under X-ray control. Usually bipolar, i.e. with two electrodes at the end of the wire; current passes from the distal to the proximal electrode, stimulating adjacent myocardium. Wires may be rigid, or flexible and balloon-tipped. Technique of insertion: as for central venous cannulation; the procedure may be technically difficult. In biventricular pacing (for heart failure) a lead is placed in the left ventricle via the coronory sinus.

    Indications include acute MI (inferior MI often requires temporary pacing; anterior often requires permanent pacing). Preoperative use should be considered in:
    - heart block: 3rd degree, sometimes 2nd degree (e.g. if Mobitz type II, associated with symptoms, or intended surgery is extensive).
    - bundle branch block, e.g. bifascicular with symptoms or P–R prolongation.
    - bradyarrhythmias.

    Technique of pacing:
    - bradyarrhythmias: once the wire is in place, the pacemaker box is set to V00 (see below) and the minimal current is determined (usually about 1–2 mA). The pacing output is set 2–3 times higher and the system changed to VVI. Failure to pace may result from disconnections, oversensing or failure to capture. The pacing box should be converted to V00 and the wire repositioned if necessary. Dual chamber pacing may be achieved using a special atrial wire in addition to the ventricular one.
    - tachyarrhythmias, e.g. SVT, atrial flutter: A00 pacing is used, stimulating via a right atrial lead. The rate is slowly increased from 60/min to the spontaneous rate, held for 30 s, and pacing stopped. If unsuccessful, pacing at 400–800/min may be used to provoke AF, which usually reverts spontaneously to sinus rhythm. VT may be treated by slow ventricular V00 pacing, atrial pacing, or ventricular pacing at 10–30% faster rate than spontaneous for 5–10 beats only (burst pacing), with defibrillation available. Advantages over cardioversion include avoidance of anaesthesia and the adverse effects of electrical shock, easier repetition if unsuccessful, and availability of pacing if bradycardia or asystole occur.
    - the pacing wire may conduct small currents directly to the heart with risk of electrocution (microshock); the metal contacts should therefore be insulated.
    - transthoracic pacing may also be used, with large surface area skin electrodes (e.g. one over the cardiac apex, one over the right scapula or clavicle) and pulse duration of up to 50 ms to reduce cutaneous nerve and muscle stimulation. Avoids complications of transvenous pacing, and quicker to perform.
    - transoesophageal pacing has also been used but is less reliable.
  - permanent: a pulse generator (pacemaker) is implanted subcutaneously. Electrodes are usually unipolar; i.e. one intracardiac electrode, with current returning to the pacemaker via the body. The heart electrode is usually endocardial, passed via a central vein; epicardial electrodes have been used.

Cardiac risk index (Goldman cardiac risk index). Scoring system for preoperative identification of patients at risk from major perioperative cardiovascular complications. Derived retrospectively in 1977 from data from 1001 patients undergoing non-cardiac surgery; analysis identified nine variables correlating with increased risk:
- third heart sound/elevated JVP: 11 points.
- MI within 6 months: 10 points.
- ventricular ectopic beats > 5/min: 7 points.
- rhythm other than sinus: 7 points.
- age > 70 years: 5 points.
- emergency operation: 4 points.
- severe aortic stenosis: 3 points.
- poor medical condition of patient: 3 points.
- abdominal or thoracic operation: 3 points.

Patients with scores above 25 points had 56% incidence of death, with 22% incidence of severe cardiovascular complications. Corresponding figures for scores below 26 points were 4% and 17% respectively, with 0.2% and 0.7% for scores less than 6.

A more recent revised cardiac risk index identifies six independent predictors of major cardiac complications following non-cardiac surgery:

- high risk surgery (intraperitoneal, intrathoracic or suprainguinal vascular surgery).
- history of ischaemic heart disease.
- history of heart failure.
- cerebrovascular disease.
- insulin dependent diabetes mellitus.
- preoperative serum creatinine > 177 μmol/l.

Relative risk for no factors is ~0.4%; for 1 factor it is ~1%, for 2 factors ~2.4% and for 3 or more factors ~5.4%.

Confirmed by other studies as having high specificity but low sensitivity; i.e. high scoring patients are high risk, but not all high risk patients are identified.

[Lee B Goldman, Boston cardiologist]

Ridley S (2003). Anaesthesia; 58: 985–91

See also, Ischaemic heart disease; Preoperative assessment

Cardiac surgery. First performed in the late 1800s and 1900s but limited by the effects of circulatory interruption. Use of hypothermia increased the range of surgery possible, but 'open' heart surgery, i.e. employing cardiopulmonary bypass (CPB) was not developed until the 1950s.

- Indications:
  - requiring CPB:
    - ischaemic heart disease, i.e. coronary artery bypass graft (CABG; but see below).
    - congenital heart disease, e.g. VSD, ASD, Fallot's tetralogy.
    - others, e.g. heart transplantation, pulmonary embolectomy for PE, chest trauma.
  - not requiring CPB: patent ductus arteriosus, aortic coarctation, pericarditis, cardiac tamponade. CABG is increasingly performed 'off-pump'.
  - percutaneous procedures, e.g. percutaneous transluminal coronary angioplasty and stent insertion, and pacemaker insertion, are usually performed under local anaesthesia. General anaesthesia is required for electrophysiological studies and insertion of implantable defibrillators.
- Preoperative assessment and management:
  - as for ischaemic and congenital heart disease. Cardiac risk index may be used for assessing risk. Cardiac failure is particularly important. Respiratory and cerebrovascular disease is common. Investigations include assessment of renal function, often liver function tests and coagulation studies. Chest X-ray, ECG, cardiac catheterisation studies and echocardiography are usual. Carotid Doppler studies may be indicated.
  - most cardiovascular drugs are continued. Oral anticoagulant drugs are usually stopped or changed to heparin.
  - premedication is traditionally heavy since anxiety is usually marked. An opioid/hyoscine mixture is often used, sometimes with benzodiazepines. Premedication is often omitted in emergency surgery. A GTN patch or β-adrenergic receptor antagonists are often used. Antibiotic prophylaxis usually includes flucloxacillin and an aminoglycoside.
- Induction and maintenance of anaesthesia:
  - preoxygenation is usually employed.
  - venous and arterial cannulation is usually performed under local anaesthesia. Central venous cannulation is often reserved until the patient is anaesthetised.
  - iv induction employs standard agents in small doses, as for ischaemic heart disease. Etomidate is commonly used. Ketamine is usually avoided. Benzodiazepines have been used.
  - standard neuromuscular blocking drugs are suitable; pancuronium is often used as it is long acting and maintains BP although it may cause tachycardia.
  - opioid analgesic drugs are used to provide a smooth induction and avoid the hypertensive response to intubation, e.g. fentanyl 5–10 μg/kg, alfentanil 30–50 μg/kg, or remifentanil 1 μg/kg followed by 0.05–2 μg/kg/min. High dose techniques, e.g. fentanyl or alfentanil up to 100–125 μg/kg have been used but lead to prolonged postoperative IPPV.
  - N_2O is often avoided because of cardiac depression, especially in combination with high dose opioids. It may also increase SVR and increase the size of air bubbles. Volatile inhalational anaesthetic agents are used in low concentrations. The choice of agent is controversial, because of myocardial depression, heart rate changes and other effects. Isoflurane is implicated in causing coronary steal, but causes little myocardial depression or sensitisation to catecholamines. It has also been suggested that volatile agents, especially sevoflurane, might protect against subsequent ischaemia.
  - TIVA with propofol is commonly used.
- Monitoring:
  - 5 lead ECG.
  - direct arterial BP measurement.
  - CVP measurement.
  - pulmonary artery catheterisation may be used in complex cases. Left-sided pressures may be measured directly via a needle during surgery.
  - transoesophageal echocardiography is increasingly used. An oesophageal Doppler probe may be used to assess perioperative myocardial workload and myocardial ischaemia.
  - temperature measurement (core and peripheral).
  - electrolyte and blood gas analysis should be readily available. Activated clotting time (ACT) may be determined in the operating theatre (*see Coagulation studies*).
  - a urinary catheter is usual unless surgery is straightforward and short.
- Pre-CPB management:
  - as for any operation.
  - stimulation during sternotomy may cause hypertension and require further analgesia.
  - after baseline ACT measurement, heparin 2–3 mg/kg (90 mg/m^2 surface area) is injected iv through a tested line (sometimes injected by the surgeon). Prostacyclin has been used but is expensive and its role is uncertain. ACT measured after 1 minute should be > 480 s or 3 times baseline; aortic and right atrial cannulation may then be performed for CPB.
- Management during CPB:
  - circulation is gradually taken over by the pump.
  - drugs are diluted by the crystalloid prime, thus iv boluses are often required, e.g. opioid, benzodiazepine, induction agent, neuromuscular blocking drug. Fentanyl may be taken up by the oxygenator membrane. Infusions may also be used, or drugs may be added to the CPB circuit. Inhalational agents may be fed to the oxygenator.
  - haemodilution occurs.
  - the place of cerebral protection is uncertain.

- hypothermia is used to reduce tissue O_2 requirements; the aorta is cross-clamped and cardioplegia used, lowering heart temperature to 10–15°C. Intentional fibrillation is sometimes used, avoiding cardioplegia. Mild hypothermia (32–35°C) is often used to provide some neuroprotection while avoiding problems of moderate (28–32°C) and profound (22–27°C) hypothermia, especially disturbed coagulation. Lower temperatures (15–20°C) are used during circulatory arrest.
- IPPV is stopped; continuous positive pressure is sometimes applied to maintain some lung expansion. Air is thought to be better than 100% O_2 because of increased atelectasis with the latter; N_2O is avoided because of the risk of air embolism.
- optimal perfusion pressure is controversial; 50 mmHg is generally thought to be the minimum. CPB details are also controversial, e.g. type of oxygenator, pulsatile/non-pulsatile flow.
- SVR decreases as haemodilution occurs; vasopressor drugs, e.g. phenylephrine or metaraminol, may be needed to maintain perfusion pressure. SVR then slowly increases due to absorbtion of the crystalloid and vasodilatation with GTN or phentolamine may be needed. Some cardiovascular drugs such as nicorandil and angiotensin converting enzyme inhibitors may exacerbate hypotension.
- ACT is checked every 30 min, with further heparin given if necessary, e.g. ¼–½ initial dose. Potassium is added as required according to plasma levels. Arterial blood gases analysis is performed at 37°C in most machines; values have been traditionally corrected to body temperature to account for increased solubility of CO_2 at low temperatures ('pH stat'), but this is now considered unnecessary and management conducted according to uncorrected values ('alpha stat'). Bicarbonate is usually not administered unless base excess exceeds 7–8. Blood is transfused to keep the haematocrit above 0.2–0.3.
- after repair of the lesion, the cross-clamp is removed and rewarming undertaken. Cardiac activity (usually VF but sometimes sinus rhythm) usually returns spontaneously. Internal defibrillation is performed at 30–32°C, and normal P_{O_2}, pH and electrolyte concentration. 20–50 J is usually used. Cardiac pacing is sometimes required; epicardial wires may be inserted prophylactically for postoperative use.
- CPB blood flow is gradually decreased as cardiac output increases. Drug boluses are given iv as before. Manual IPPV helps expel air from the pulmonary vessels. 100% O_2 or an O_2/air mixture is usually employed.

- Post-CPB and postoperative care:
  - left atrial pressure is optimised to 8–12 mmHg; vasodilators are used to accommodate CPB fluid volume.
  - a low output state may occur, especially if ventricular function was poor preoperatively and ischaemia time was prolonged. It may be improved by:
    - inotropic drugs: calcium is often used as a temporary measure but may worsen reperfusion injury. Others include dopamine, dobutamine, adrenaline and isoprenaline, more recently enoximone, milrinone and dopexamine. The choice is according to individual patient and drug characteristics, and personal preference.
    - vasodilators (often combined with inotropes).
    - correction of potassium/acid–base imbalance.
    - intra-aortic counter-pulsation balloon pump is occasionally required.
  - heparin is reversed with protamine, injected slowly to reduce side effects, especially in pulmonary hypertension. 1 mg/mg heparin is usually used, although less may be required.
  - hypertension is common if left ventricular function is good, especially in aortic valve disease. Vasodilators may be required.
  - temperature may fall as core heat is transferred to the periphery.
  - arrhythmias and heart block may occur.
  - pericardial and pleural drains are inserted before sternal closure.
  - transfer to ICU must be carefully managed because of the potential dangers from interrupted monitoring and infusions, and movement.
  - postoperative management is related to:
    - bleeding: may be surgical, or caused by consumption or dilution of platelet and coagulation factors during CPB, the effects of massive blood transfusion, or inadequate reversal of heparin. Perioperative aprotinin, antifibrinolytic drugs and desmopressin have been used to reduce blood requirements.
    - treatment of hyper-/hypotension and arrhythmias.
    - low output state as above. Cardiac tamponade may require drainage on ICU.
    - maintenance of fluid balance and urine output. The crystalloid load from CPB usually causes diuresis but pulmonary oedema may occur, especially if cardiac output is low.
    - rewarming; central/peripheral temperature difference is a useful indication.
    - maintenance of electrolyte, acid–base and blood gas balance. Hypokalaemia is common.
    - IPPV is usually continued for a few hours, sometimes overnight. Opioid/benzodiazepine boluses are commonly used for sedation. Immediate extubation after surgery is increasingly performed in appropriately selected cases. Usual criteria for weaning include cardiovascular and respiratory stability, adequate warming and perfusion, good urine output, minimal blood loss and good orientation and arousal. Impaired gas exchange may be associated with pre-existing lung disease, atelectasis, and CPB-related factors, e.g. embolisation with bubbles and platelet aggregates, complement activation, etc., especially if CPB was prolonged.
    - CNS changes: CVA occurs in less than 2% of patients undergoing open-heart surgery, but subtle changes are found in up to 60%, thought to be related to embolisation (e.g. with bubbles, aggregates, etc. during CPB) and/or inadequate perfusion. Effects may possibly be reduced by filtering the arterial inflow line.

Cardiac tamponade. Compression of the heart by fluid (e.g. blood) within the pericardium, restricting ventricular filling and reducing stroke volume and cardiac output.

Myocardial O_2 supply is reduced by hypotension, increased end-diastolic pressure, tachycardia and compression of epicardial vessels. Tamponade should be differentiated from pneumothorax and cardiac failure.

- Features:
  - dyspnoea, restlessness, oliguria, hypotension, peripheral vasoconstriction. JVP, CVP and left atrial pressure are raised, and pulsus paradoxus is present. Jugular venous distension may occur during inspiration or when pressure is applied over the liver (Kussmaul's sign). Cardiovascular collapse and death may occur, especially if acute (e.g. following chest trauma).

- ECG complexes may be small, and the heart shadow globular and enlarged on the chest X-ray. Confirmed by echocardiography.

Immediate management is pericardiocentesis; subsequently, surgery may be required.

- Anaesthetic considerations: drugs or manoeuvres which reduce venous return, heart rate or myocardial contractility should be avoided, especially with coexistent hypovolaemia. IPPV should be performed cautiously.

[Adolf Kussmaul (1822–1909), German physician]
See also, Cardiac surgery

Cardiogenic shock. Shock associated with primary cardiac pump failure. Diagnosis is suggested by acute haemodynamic changes including:
- systolic BP 30 mmHg below basal levels for more than 30 min.
- cardiac index < 2.2 l/min/m^2.
- arteriovenous oxygen difference > 5.5 ml/100 ml.
- pulmonary capillary wedge pressure (PCWP) > 15 mmHg.

Most commonly caused by acute MI affecting either right or left ventricle, but it may also follow cardiac surgery and chest trauma. Shock due to PE, cardiac tamponade, prolonged arrhythmias and acute myocarditis is sometimes included in the definition. Heart rate and SVR are usually increased to compensate for hypotension, exacerbating myocardial O_2 supply/demand imbalance. Acidosis resulting from poor perfusion further impairs myocardial contractility.

- Features:
  - as for shock.
  - increased left ventricular filling pressures and pulmonary oedema are usual. However, relative hypovolaemia may be present due to redistribution of fluid to lungs, previous fluid restriction, diuretic therapy and sweating. Right-sided failure may occur, e.g. in right ventricular infarction.
- Management:
  - as for MI including thrombolytic therapy, O_2 administration, etc. Early percutaneous transluminal coronary angioplasty may be indicated.
  - optimising left ventricular filling pressure; PCWP is a more useful guide than CVP, unless failure is predominantly right-sided. A PCWP of 18–22 mmHg is thought to be optimal for the failing heart, even though this is higher than normal. Colloid is usually employed if PCWP is low, inotropic and vasodilator drugs if PCWP is high.
  - intra-aortic counter-pulsation balloon pump and cardiac surgery may be required.

Prognosis is generally poor, especially after MI (mortality 70–90%) and without aggressive therapy.
See also, Cardiac failure

Cardioinhibitory centre (Cardioinhibitory area). Comprised of the nucleus ambiguus and adjacent neurones in the ventral medulla, with some input from the dorsal motor nucleus and nucleus of the tractus solitarius. Produces vagal 'tone', increased by baroreceptor discharge. Also receives afferents from higher centres. Impulses pass to the vasomotor centre, inhibiting it, and via the vagus nerve. Thus involved centrally in controlling arterial BP.

Cardiomyopathy. Disease of myocardium. Suggested definitions include:
- myocardial disease of unknown aetiology.
- myocardial disease not due to respiratory, coronary, or congenital heart disease, hypertension or rheumatic fever.

- May be:
  - dilated (congestive):
    - reduced contractility and ejection fraction, with ventricular dilatation.
    - causes cardiac failure, arrhythmias, angina and systemic embolism from mural thrombus.
    - prognosis is poor; death is usually within a few years of cardiac failure.
    - a similar pattern may occur with alcoholism, viral infection, cytotoxic drugs, connective tissue diseases, and metabolic and infiltrative disorders, e.g. sarcoidosis. Peripartum cardiomyopathy is defined as that occurring in the absence of other causes and in the last month (the last trimester has been suggested) of pregnancy or the first 5 months after pregnancy. It typically presents as cardiac failure and may recur in subsequent pregnancies.
    - treatment includes digoxin, diuretics, antiarrhythmic drugs, vasodilator drugs and anticoagulant drugs.
    - anaesthetic management: as for ischaemic heart disease. Myocardial depression, hypovolaemia and increased SVR are particularly hazardous.
  - hypertrophic (obstructive; HOCM):
    - familial disorder, with left ventricular hypotrophy especially affecting the upper interventricular septum, causing left ventricular outflow obstruction.
    - causes arrhythmias, syncope, angina and cardiac failure. Infective endocarditis may occur.
    - treatment includes diuretics, antiarrhythmics and β-adrenergic receptor antagonists; the last reduce force and rate of contraction, reducing outflow obstruction. Conversely, digoxin should be avoided. Anticoagulants are often used in arrhythmias. Surgery has been used to relieve obstruction.
    - anaesthetic management includes antibiotic prophylaxis as for congenital heart disease. The following especially should be avoided: increased sympathetic activity with increased contractility and tachycardia, arrhythmias, hypovolaemia and reduced SVR.
  - restrictive:
    - very rare; due to fibrosis or infiltration.
    - effects and management are as for constrictive pericarditis.

ECG is usually non-specific, showing arrhythmias, bundle branch block, ventricular hypertrophy and ischaemia. Chest X-ray may show cardiac enlargement and pulmonary oedema. Echocardiography, cardiac catheterisation and nuclear cardiology may be useful.

Davies MJ (2000). Heart; 83: 469–74

Cardioplegia. Intentional cardiac arrest caused by coronary perfusion with cold electrolyte solution, to allow cardiac surgery. After establishment of cardiopulmonary bypass, a cannula is inserted into the ascending aorta and connected to a bag of solution (traditionally at 4°C) having excluded air bubbles. After aortic cross-clamping distal to the cannula, the solution is passed under 200–300 mmHg pressure into the aortic root, closing the aortic valve and perfusing the coronary arteries. In aortic valve disease, individual coronary artery cannulation may be required. Severe coronary stenosis may require further injection of solution through the bypass graft. Asystole usually occurs after 100–200 ml, but 1 litre is used (20 ml/kg in children) in order to cool the heart to 10–12°C.

Further infusion may be required in prolonged surgery. Iced saline is placed around the heart to maintain hypothermia.

- Solutions used may contain:
  - NaCl 110–140 mmol/l: prevents excess water accumulation. May increase calcium entry if sodium concentration is too high.
  - KCl 10–20 mmol/l: causes depolarisation and cardiac arrest in diastole, reducing myocardial O_2 demand. Higher concentrations may cause arterial spasm.
  - $MgCl_2$ 16 mmol/l and $CaCl_2$ 1.2–2.2 mmol/l: reduce automatic rhythmogenicity and protect against potassium-induced damage post-bypass. Excessive calcium may cause persistent myocardial contraction (stone heart). Magnesium reduces calcium entry.
  - $NaHCO_3$ 0–10 mmol/l.
  - procaine 0–1 mmol/l: stabilises the membrane, reducing arrhythmias post-bypass.
  - other additives are more controversial, and include:
    - buffers, e.g. histidine and tromethamine: help maintain normal intracellular pH and encourage ATP generation.
    - metabolic substrates, e.g. glucose and amino acids: increase ATP generation.
    - mannitol: reduces water accumulation and may improve cardiac function.
    - free radical scavengers.
    - corticosteroids.
    - calcium channel blocking drugs.
- Other controversies:
  - use of blood instead of crystalloid: optimal osmotic, buffer and metabolic make-up but increased viscosity.
  - oxygenation of the solution.
  - use of warm solution: may cause better myocardial relaxation, with reduced membrane and protein damage associated with low temperatures.
  - continuous versus intermittent injection.

Usual solution pH is 5.5–7.8 and osmolality 285–300 mosmol/kg.

Cardiopulmonary bypass (CPB). Developed largely by Gibbon in the 1950s from animal experiments performed in 1937. Haemolysis was caused by initial disc/bubble oxygenators; improved membrane oxygenators were developed in the late 1950s. Used in cardiac surgery; similar techniques are used for extracorporeal membrane oxygenation and extracorporeal CO_2 removal in respiratory failure.

- Principles:
  - venous drainage: under gravity via a right atrial cannula or separate superior/inferior vena caval cannulae if the right atrium is opened. Blood also drains via right atrial and left heart suckers/vents to avoid pooling of blood in the operative field. Blood passes through a filter and defoaming chamber, which may be combined with a reservoir and/or oxygenator.
  - oxygenator: flat screens and rotating discs were originally used. The main types are now:
    - bubble oxygenators: tiny bubbles provide a large surface area for gas exchange. Thorough defoaming is required. Thought to increase the risk of microscopic air emboli, blood component damage and consumption of coagulation factors.
    - membrane oxygenators: hollow capillary fibres through which blood passes, with gas exchange across their walls. Flat membrane oxygenators are also available. Popular, since adverse effects are less likely. Have been used for several days without requiring replacement. Can also be used for concurrent ultrafiltration.

    Most incorporate temperature exchangers. CO_2 and O_2 are supplied independently to the oxygenator as required, e.g. 2.5% CO_2 in O_2.
  - pumps: usually rotating roller pumps using wide tubing. Rotating chambers are also used, reducing damage to blood components. Flow is traditionally non-pulsatile but pulsatile flow may provide better organ perfusion, with lower vasopressin and angiotensin levels; however, the equipment required is more complex and expensive. Pulsations may be synchronised with the ECG if the heart is pumping. Flows used vary between centres but are usually 1.0–2.4 l/min/m^2 surface area (up to 80 ml/min/kg). Lower flows are required with hypothermia.
  - arterial return: via ascending aorta (rarely, femoral artery) using a short wide cannula to reduce resistance and avoid accidental cannulation of aortic branches. The return is filtered to remove platelet aggregates, fibrin, debris, etc. 150–300 μm filters are standard; microemboli may be reduced by smaller filters but increased risk of complement activation has been suggested.
- Use:
  - disposable systems are usually employed.
  - the system is primed with 1.5–2.5 litres crystalloid usually, although colloid may be used, and rarely blood. Heparin 20 mg/l may be added. The tubing is checked for bubbles before use; flushing the system with CO_2 before priming has been suggested, to reduce bubble formation.
  - anticoagulation, introduction and termination of CPB: as for cardiac surgery.
- Complications:
  - technical, e.g. leaks, bubbles, disconnections, obstruction, coagulation, power failure, etc. Vascular damage may occur during cannulation.
  - embolisation with clot, debris, bubbles, defoaming agent, etc. Bubbles may enter via the heart cavity during surgery, especially at end of bypass. Subtle neurological changes are thought to be related to microembolisation.
  - related to surgery or anticoagulation.

[John H Gibbon (1903–1974), US surgeon]

Cardiopulmonary resuscitation (CPR). Over many centuries, numerous techniques have been tried in order to restore life; early attempts included use of heat, smoke, cold water, beating and suspension from ropes.

- Artificial ventilation was developed within the last 400 years:
  - use of bellows via the mouth or nose is attributed to Paracelsus in the early 1500s. Used via tracheal tubes in the 1700s, e.g. by Kite.
  - postural techniques, e.g. compressing the chest and abdomen from behind with the victim prone, moving the arms, or using tilting boards, etc.: used from the 1850s.
  - expired air ventilation: developed in the 1700s, although reported earlier.
- cardiac massage, external and internal, was first attempted in the late 1800s; external massage was popularised in the early 1960s.
- defibrillation was investigated in animals in the 1700s/1800s; internal defibrillation was performed in man in the 1940s and external defibrillation in the 1950s.
- CPR is divided into:
  - basic life support (BLS): traditionally without any equipment, and therefore suitable for 'lay person resuscitation'. Increasingly includes the use of simple equipment (although this has been defined as 'basic life

support with airway adjuncts'), e.g. airways, facepieces, self-inflating bags, oesophageal obturators, laryngeal mask airway.
- advanced life support: as above, plus use of specialised equipment, techniques (e.g. tracheal intubation), drugs, monitoring, etc.; usually confined to hospitals.

Regular updates on guidelines are provided by the Resuscitation Council (UK), European Resuscitation Council, International Liaison Committee on Resuscitation and the American Heart Association (*see Basic life support, adult, and Advanced life support, adult*).

See also, Brainstem death; Cardiopulmonary resuscitation, neonatal; Cardiopulmonary resuscitation, paediatric; Cough-CPR

Cardiopulmonary resuscitation, neonatal. Prompt resuscitation is important in order to prevent permanent mental or physical handicap. Neonatal cardiac arrest is almost always caused by hypoxaemia and thus prompt management of apnoea and airway obstruction is vital.

- Equipment required includes:
  - a tilting resuscitation surface, with radiant heater, clock and ECG monitor.
  - suction equipment.
  - O_2 with funnel and facepieces.
  - self-inflating bag (volume 250 ml, with pressure relief valve set at 30–35 cmH_2O).
  - pharyngeal airways (sizes 000, 00 and 0).
  - tracheal tubes: shouldered (Cole) tubes have been used, but straight-sided ones are preferable since the former may cause greater trauma to the larynx in addition to increasing resistance to flow. Suitable sizes:
    - 2.0–2.5 mm tubes for babies under 750 g weight or 26 weeks' gestation.
    - 2.5–3.0 mm for 750–2000 g or 26–34 weeks.
    - 3.0–3.5 mm for over 2000 g or 34 weeks.
  - laryngoscope, usually with straight blade (size 0–1).
  - iv cannulae including umbilical venous and arterial catheters.

Requirement for resuscitation may be anticipated from the course of pregnancy and labour and fetal monitoring. The Apgar score may also be useful.

- Basic principles are as for adult CPR, adjusted to the context of the neonate:
  - meconium present: previous guidelines have suggested early suction of the mouth and nose when the head is delivered, followed by active suction of the trachea (unless the baby is vigorous and screaming) under direct vision and avoidance of mask ventilation in case it dissipates the meconium peripherally. The risk from withholding effective ventilation during suction is now felt to outweigh any advantage, unless the mouth is full of meconium, since aspiration of meconium is likely to have already occurred by the time suction is instituted. General management is therefore as below.
  - drying and wrapping the baby. For babies < 30 weeks' gestation, placing it under a radiant heater and wrapping it with food-grade plastic wrapping is a quick and effective way of maintaining its temperature without needing to dry it.
  - early assessment of the heart rate (the most important indicator), respiratory effort and colour:
    - heart rate > 100/min and the baby is centrally pink: no further treatment required.
    - heart rate > 100/min but poor respiration and central cyanosis: tactile stimulation, facial O_2, gentle oropharyngeal suction.
    - heart rate < 100/min and poor respiration: five inspiration breaths lasting for 2–3 s, to aid lung expansion. Airway pressures should not exceed 30–35 cmH_2O. Air or oxygen is acceptable. If there is no response, adequacy of ventilation should be checked and a further 5 inspirations attempted. If still no response, tracheal intubation should be considered but this should not delay chest compressions.
  - if heart rate < 60/min despite good ventilation, cardiac massage should be instituted, with both hands encircling the chest or using two fingers (*see Cardiopulmonary resuscitation, paediatric*). Compressions should occur at 120/min, depressing the sternum 2–3 cm and with a ratio of 3:1 with breaths.
  - if heart rate < 60 after 30 s, drugs should be given:
    - adrenaline 1:10 000 may be given via the tracheal tube; 0.5 ml (preterm) or 1 ml (term).
    - umbilical venous catheterisation is usually the most accessible route for iv administration of drugs (n.b. the umbilical cord contains a single vein and two arteries).
    - initial iv drugs: adrenaline 1:10 000: 0.1 ml/kg initially, then 0.3 ml/kg, then 1 ml/kg after 4.2% bicarbonate 1–2 ml/kg (higher concentrations have been associated with intraventricular haemorrhages). The cannula should be flushed with saline after each drug.
    - others:
      - 4.5% albumin 10 ml/kg if hypovolaemia is suspected.
      - 10% dextrose 2–2.5 ml/kg if hypoglycaemia is present.
      - naloxone 10 μg/kg im, iv or sc repeated every 2–3 min or 60 μg/kg im as a single injection, if the mother has received opioids during labour.

Congenital abnormalities, e.g. diaphragmatic hernia, tracheo-oesophageal fistula, etc., should be remembered.

[Frank Cole (1918–1977), US anaesthetist]

Biarent D, Bingham R, Richmond S, et al (2006). Resuscitation; 67 Suppl 1: 97–113

See also, Pugh, Benjamin

Cardiopulmonary resuscitation, paediatric. The same principles apply as for adult CPR, but primary cardiac disease is uncommon. Sinus bradycardia progressing to asystole is more common, especially if due to hypoxaemia or haemorrhage. Thus cardiac arrest is often secondary to respiratory arrest or exsanguination, and usually represents a severe insult.

- 2005 Recommendations of the Resuscitation Council (UK), adapted from European Resuscitation Council Guidelines:
  - basic life support (BLS):
    - assess as for adults. a lone rescuer should continue for about a minute before seeking help.
    - 'ABC' of resuscitation:
      - Airway: as for adults.
      - Breathing: expired airway ventilation with 5 rescue breaths each over 1–1.5 s; mouth-to-mouth and nose if < 1 year, mouth-to-mouth otherwise. Repeated up to 5 times if required to achieve effective ventilations.
      - Circulation: up to 10 s to check for signs of circulation, then external cardiac massage at 100/min.
    - ratio for cardiac massage: breaths of 15:2 (30:2 for a lone rescuer).
  - advanced life support:
    - iv access/monitoring as for adults. An intraosseous needle may be useful if venous access is difficult (*see*

Intraosseous fluid administration). For monitoring small children via the defibrillator, it may be easier to apply the paddles to the front and back of the chest.
- asystole/pulseless electrical activity:
  - adrenaline 10 µg/kg iv (0.1 ml of 1:10 000 solution) or 100 µg/kg (1.0 ml of 1:10 000 solution) via the tracheal tube (the least satisfactory route). Repeat every 5 min.
  - BLS for a further 2 min.
- VF/VT:
  - defibrillation using 4 J/kg (one paddle below the right clavicle, the other at the left anterior axillary line).
  - BLS for further 2 min, then repeat the above.
  - repeat as necessary; after the 3rd shock give amiodarone 5 mg/kg and an immediate 4th shock. Consider treatable causes of cardiac arrest.

- Special situations: choking, electrocution, near-drowning, trauma, neonatal CPR (*see Cardiopulmonary resuscitation, neonatal*).
- Other drugs:
  - atropine: 0.02 mg/kg iv or tracheal, up to 0.6 mg.
  - bicarbonate: 1 mmol/kg iv (1 ml/kg 8.4% solution).
  - calcium chloride: 0.2 mmol/kg iv (0.3 ml/kg 10% solution).
  - glucose 10%: 1 g/kg iv (10 ml/kg).
- Fluid bolus in hypovolaemia: 10 ml/kg colloid (traditionally 4.5% albumin initially).

Biarent D, Bingham R, Richmond S, et al (2006). Resuscitation; 67 Suppl 1: 97–113

See also, Paediatric anaesthesia

Cardioversion. Restoration of sinus rhythm by application of synchronised DC current across the chest. Current delivery is synchronised to occur with the R wave of the ECG, since delivery during ventricular repolarisation may produce VF (R on T phenomenon).

- Used for:
  - AF, particularly of recent onset.
  - atrial flutter; usually successful with low energy.
  - VT, usually successful with low energy.
  - SVT.

Energy levels of 20–200 J are usually used.

Digoxin-induced arrhythmias may convert to serious ventricular arrhythmias; therefore digoxin is usually withheld for at least 24 h.

In chronic atrial arrhythmias, anticoagulation is often administered to reduce risk of systemic embolisation. Preparation of the patient, drugs and equipment, and monitoring should be as for any anaesthetic. The procedure is painful, therefore requiring brief sedation/anaesthesia. A single iv agent is commonly used, e.g. thiopental, etomidate, propofol or diazepam. Etomidate causes least myocardial depression and is perhaps preferable. Further injections may be required if repeated shocks are delivered. 100% O_2 is breathed via a facepiece.

See also, Defibrillation

Care of the critically ill surgical patient (CCrISP). Course first run by the Royal College of Surgeons of England in 1996 following funding by the Hillsborough Disaster Trust. Primarily aimed at basic surgical trainees, but open to those from other disciplines; concentrates on teaching how to identify patients at risk of serious clinical deterioration and those who are already seriously ill. Using a systematic means of patient assessment (similar to other ALS, ATLS, APLS courses, etc.), candidates are taught to manage immediate life-threatening events (e.g. airway obstruction, haemorrhage, sepsis, injury) and to organise subsequent care (monitoring, pain relief, nutrition, etc.) in the general ward, operating theatre, HDU or ICU. The course consists of lectures, workshops and simulated patient assessments which concentrate on practical, interpretative and communication skills.

[Hillsborough, Sheffield; football stadium at which 96 fans were crushed to death in 1989]

Anderson ID (1997) Br J Hosp Med; 57: 274–5

Carfentanil. Opioid analgesic drug, developed in 1974. Over 8700 times as potent as morphine, and used to immobilise large animals.

Carotid arteries. Anatomy is as follows (*see Fig. 110; Neck, cross-sectional anatomy*):
- common carotids:
  - right: arises from the brachiocephalic artery behind the sternoclavicular joint.
  - left: arises from the aortic arch medial to the left lung, vagus and phrenic nerves, then passing behind the sternoclavicular joint.
  - ascend in the neck within the carotid sheath.
  - divide level with C4 into internal and external carotids.
- internal carotid:
  - bears the carotid sinus at its origin.
  - runs firstly lateral, then behind and medial to the external carotid, with the internal jugular vein laterally and vagus and sympathetic chain posteriorly.
  - passes medial to the parotid gland, styloid process, glossopharyngeal nerve and pharyngeal branches of the vagus (with the external carotid lateral to these structures).
  - passes through the carotid canal at the base of the skull, with the internal jugular now lying posteriorly. After a tortuous path through the canal, it divides into the middle and anterior cerebral arteries.
- external carotid:
  - lies first deep, then lateral to the internal carotid, with the internal jugular posteriorly.
  - enters the parotid gland, ending behind the neck of the mandible.
  - branches, from below upwards:
    - ascending pharyngeal.
    - superior thyroid.
    - lingual.
    - facial.
    - occipital.
    - posterior auricular.
    - superficial temporal.
    - maxillary.

See also, Carotid artery surgery; Carotid body; Cerebral circulation

Carotid artery surgery. Usually endarterectomy, performed in patients with carotid stenosis. Reduces the risk of CVA by 55–70% in patients with severe stenosis (> 70% occlusion) with or without symptoms; surgery is less beneficial in lesser degrees of stenosis. The place of surgery in patients with completed CVAs or near-occlusion is uncertain. Perioperative CVA may occur in under 7% of cases; risks are greatest in the elderly (though the benefits of surgery have also been shown to be greatest in this group). Nerve injury in the neck (usually transient) may occur in up to 20% of cases. Mortality of the procedure is about 5% for symptomatic and 3–4% for asymptomatic stenoses, mostly from MI or CVA.

Mortality is greatest in older women or those with symptomatic generalised cardiovascular disease. Percutaneous carotid artery stenting has been shown to be as effective as endarterectomy in patients with severe stenosis (*see Neuroradiology*).

- Anaesthetic considerations:
  - preoperatively: poor condition of patients: atherosclerosis often affects coronary and renal, as well as cerebral, vessels. Smoking, diabetes mellitus and hypertension are common. Drug therapy may include aspirin, dipyridamole and other antiplatelet drugs.
  - perioperatively:
    - positioning of the patient and restricted access: the eyes must be protected, and the tracheal tube guarded against kinking. Lidocaine spray to the vocal cords reduces stimulation during initial positioning. Vertebrobasilar insufficiency (often together with cervical spine disease) is common and necessitates careful positioning of the neck during intubation and surgery.
    - several techniques have been tried to maintain cerebral blood flow and limit ischaemia during surgery:
      - hypothermia.
      - cerebral protection, e.g. using barbiturates. Glucose infusions have been implicated as exacerbating cerebral ischaemic damage, and are avoided.
      - hypoventilation, increasing cerebral blood flow via hypercapnia; cerebral steal may occur.
      - vasopressor drugs to maintain intraoperative BP, e.g. phenylephrine.
      - carotid shunting, bypassing the clamped section of artery.

      Choice of technique is controversial but most now advocate normocapnia and normotension; hypotension is definitely to be avoided.

      Arterial pressure may be measured distal to the atheroma, before and after carotid clamping. A shunt is usually inserted if the pressure after clamping (stump pressure; provides some indication of collateral flow) is less than 30–50% of the preclamp value.
    - the following may be used to detect cerebral ischaemia: EEG, cerebral function monitor, transcranial Doppler ultrasound, or measurement of evoked potentials and cerebral blood flow.
    - cervical plexus block allows surgery to be performed on an awake patient; if ischaemic symptoms occur following carotid artery clamping, general anaesthesia with shunt insertion may be performed.
    - direct arterial BP monitoring is mandatory, with avoidance of hypotension at all times.
    - capnography allows adjustment of IPPV to normocapnia and aids detection of air embolism.
    - manipulation of the carotid sinus may lead to bradycardia and hypotension. Infiltration of lidocaine around the sinus prevents this, but may be followed by hypertension postoperatively.
  - postoperatively:
    - patients may require HDU/ICU admission for monitoring and further care.
    - assessment of neurological function: deficit occurs in $<7\%$ of patients. The hyperperfusion syndrome is caused by increased blood flow (in vessels with poor autoregulation) following relief of stenosis. It may result in headache, convulsions and intracranial haemorrhage.
    - control of BP: hypertension is common and may be related to pain, agitation, dysfunction of carotid sinus baroreceptors or impending neurological damage. Hypotension is less common and may be associated with bradycardia.
    - airway obstruction may occur if bleeding occurs. Even after uncomplicated cases, some degree of airway narrowing is common because of oedema.

Howell SJ (2007). Br J Anaesth; 99: 119–31

Carotid body. Small (2–3 mg) structure situated above the carotid bifurcation on each side; involved in the chemical control of breathing. Contains:

- glomus cells (type I cells): thought to be inhibitory neurones. Contain dopamine.
- glial cells (type II cells).
- nerve endings: thought to be the chemoreceptors themselves.

Afferents pass via the glossopharyngeal nerve to the brainstem regulatory centres.

Rate of discharge is increased by reduced O_2 delivery (e.g. reduced arterial PO_2 or reduced cardiac output) or by impaired utilisation of O_2 (e.g. due to cyanide poisoning). Below arterial PO_2 of 13.3 kPa (100 mmHg), rate of discharge rises greatly for any further decrease. Response time is rapid enough to cause fluctuations in discharge rate with breathing. Discharge rate is also increased by a rise in arterial PCO_2, or fall in arterial pH.

Each carotid body receives 0.04 ml blood/min, equivalent to 2 l/100 g tissue/min (the highest blood flow per 100 g tissue in the body). Because of such high blood flow, dissolved O_2 alone is enough to provide the requirement for O_2; thus discharge is not increased by anaemia or carbon monoxide poisoning, where O_2 carriage by haemoglobin is reduced but arterial PO_2 is not.

See also, Breathing, control of

Carotid sinus. Dilatation of the internal carotid artery, just above the carotid bifurcation. Baroreceptors present in the walls respond to increased distension caused by raised arterial BP by increasing the rate of discharge via the carotid sinus nerve, a branch of the glossopharyngeal nerve. Resultant inhibition of the vasomotor centre and stimulation of the cardioinhibitory centre cause reduction in sympathetic tone and increase in vagal tone respectively. BP and heart rate therefore fall. The baroreceptors also respond to the rate of increase of BP. Similar baroreceptors exist in the walls of the aortic arch.

See also, Carotid sinus massage

Carotid sinus massage. Manual stimulation of the carotid sinus baroreceptors, causing reflex inhibition of the vasomotor centre and activation of the cardioinhibitory centre. Depression of sinoatrial (SA) and atrioventricular (AV) nodes results in bradycardia and may reduce myocardial contractility.

The sinus should be gently massaged below the angle of the jaw, where the carotid pulse is palpable. Concurrent ECG recording should be available. Only one side (the right is usually more effective) should be massaged at one time and for not longer than 5 s, or excessive reduction in cerebral blood flow may occur. It should be performed with care in patients with evidence of cerebrovascular disease. May restore sinus rhythm in SVT, and may aid diagnosis of other arrhythmias by slowing the ventricular rate, e.g. AF and atrial flutter. In sinus tachycardia, it causes gradual slowing of rate with speeding up when massage is stopped. May also demonstrate SA and AV node disease by causing severe bradycardia or sinus arrest.

Syncope, transient ischaemic attacks and CVA, asystole and VT are rare complications.

Carticaine, *see Articaine*

Caspofungin. Antifungal drug used for treatment of invasive aspergillosis or candida infection.
- Dosage: 70 mg by if infusion on the first day, 50 mg daily thereafter.
- Side effects: GIT upset, tachycardia, flushing, dyspnoea, electrolyte disturbances, allergic reactions.

Catabolism. Breakdown of molecules into smaller ones, usually associated with energy production.
- Includes:
  - digestion of foodstuffs as in metabolism of carbohydrate, fat and protein.
  - breakdown of body stores, e.g. in malnutrition, severe illness and the stress response to surgery. These may occur in combination on ICU because of:
    - inadequate nutrition, e.g. nil by mouth, ileus, fluid restriction, etc.
    - increased energy and O_2 consumption associated with injury, especially multiple trauma, burns, and sepsis.

  Includes breakdown of:
    - protein: causes increased urinary urea excretion and may contribute to reduced plasma albumin. Nitrogen loss may exceed 20–30 g/day, i.e. up to 5 kg body weight/week (mainly lost from muscle). Amino acids produced are used for synthesis of glucose, acute phase reactants and cell components.
    - fat: triglycerides from adipose tissue are broken down to fatty acids (used as an energy source) and glycerol (used to synthesise glucose).
    - carbohydrates: glycogen is broken down to glucose.

See also, Nutrition, total parenteral

Catecholamines. Group of substances containing catechol (benzene ring with OH groups at positions 3 and 4) and amine portions; includes naturally occurring (e.g. dopamine, adrenaline, noradrenaline) and synthetic (e.g. dobutamine, isoprenaline) compounds. Catecholamines act at adrenergic receptors in the CNS and sympathetic nervous system; although many other substances may produce similar effects, i.e. are sympathomimetic drugs, they may not be true catecholamines.

Synthesis of naturally occurring catecholamines proceeds in many steps from the amino acid phenylalanine (Fig. 33a). Formation of dopamine occurs in the cytoplasm; it is then taken up by an active process into vesicles and converted to noradrenaline.

Catecholamines are metabolised via catechol-*O*-methyl transferase (COMT) and monoamine oxidase (MAO) (Fig. 33b).

See also, Inotropic drugs

Catechol-O-methyl transferase (COMT). Enzyme present in most tissues (especially liver and kidneys) but not in nerve endings; catalyses the transfer of a methyl group from adenosylmethionine, a methionine derivative, to the 3-hydroxy group of the catechol part of catecholamines. Involved in the metabolism of circulating catecholamines and their derivatives, whilst catecholamines at nerve endings are metabolised by monoamine oxidase.

Inhibitors of COMT (e.g. entacapone) have been investigated as adjuncts to levodopa in Parkinson's disease; they block metabolism of levodopa in the peripheral circulation and thus increase the activity of levodopa.

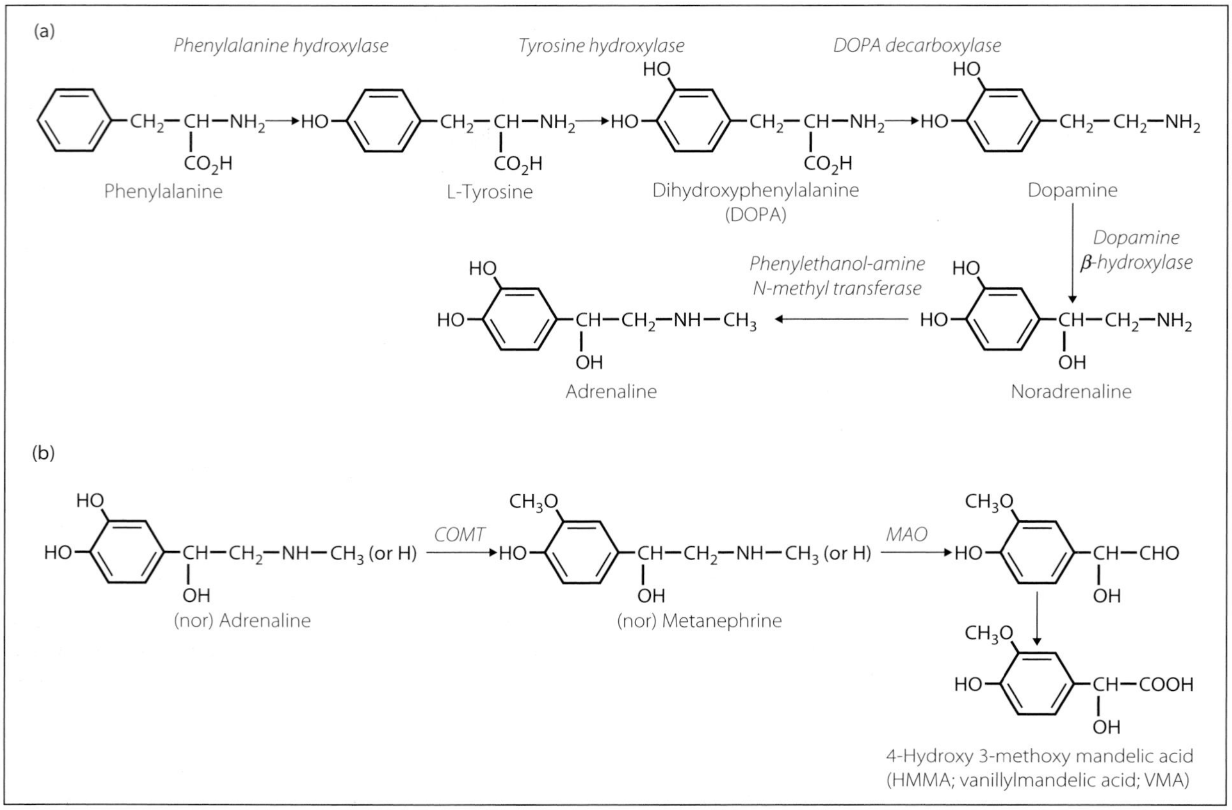

Fig. 33 (a) Catecholamine synthesis. (b) Catecholamine metabolism

Catheter mounts (Tracheal tube adaptors). Original term refers to adaptors connecting the fresh gas supply to a catheter passed through the larynx into the trachea (insufflation technique), before tracheal intubation became popular. The term now refers to adaptors connecting the tracheal tube to the end of the anaesthetic breathing system. Various connectors fit between the distal end and the tracheal tube; the proximal end should be of standard 22 mm taper. Some contain heat–moisture exchangers.

Catheter-related sepsis. Strictly, nosocomial infection involving a catheter in any site, but the term usually refers to intravascular devices (peripheral, central venous or arterial). Defined in clinical practice as isolation of the same organism from culture of both the blood and a catheter segment from a patient with symptoms and signs of bloodstream infection (preferably from a distant venepuncture), in the absence of any other septic focus. Occurs in about 5% of cases in ICU. Should be differentiated from colonisation (growth of > 15 colony forming units from a catheter segment in the absence of local or systemic infection), which occurs in about 25% of cases, and local infection (erythema, tenderness, induration and purulence within 2 cm of the skin insertion site). In all cases, organisms are thought to grow in 'biofilms' on the surface of the catheter.

- Risk factors include:
  - site of catheter: affects central lines more than arterial lines more than peripheral lines. Subclavian lines are often considered the least likely to become infected. Femoral lines are usually considered more likely than those elsewhere but this may not be so if proper care is taken during and after placement.
  - age < 1 year or > 60 years.
  - immunodeficiency or use of immunosuppressive drugs.
  - severity of underlying illness.
  - presence of other focus of infection.
  - use of cut-down to insert line.
  - use of the line for parenteral feeding.
  - length of time the line is in situ is usually cited as a risk factor, but evidence is weak if adequate attention has been paid to aseptic insertion.

Organisms involved usually come from the patient's own skin flora or from medical or nursing staff. *Staphylococcus aureus* or *epidermidis* are most commonly responsible although Gram-negative organisms may be involved. Candida may also be responsible.

- Management:
  - taking of blood cultures peripherally and via the line. Use of an endoluminal brush has been described.
  - exclusion of other sources of infection.
  - antibacterial drugs.
  - removal, and sending for culture, of the distal part of the line involved.
  - if possible, a new line should not be inserted at the same site. Changing a suspected line over a guidewire should also be avoided.
  - the following has been used for lines whose removal is considered especially undesirable (e.g. being used for long-term parenteral nutrition and poor venous access elsewhere): concomitant antibiotic (in high concentration) and fibrinolytic agent into the catheter as a 'lock', with parenteral antibacterial therapy. The line should be removed if the patient's condition has not improved after 36 h; use of the catheter may be restarted after 48 h if improvement occurs.
- Prevention:
  - use of intravascular catheters only where definitely indicated, and removal when no longer needed.
  - scrupulous aseptic technique during insertion and aftercare. Chlorhexidine appears to be more effective than 10% povidone-iodine and 70% alcohol for cleansing the skin.
  - regular replacement of catheters (e.g. every 3–7 days) is often advocated but there is little evidence supporting this.
  - daily inspection of insertion sites and regular changing of sterile dressings (24–48 h). Clear plastic dressings have been associated with increased rates of infection in some studies. Use of antimicrobial ointment or fenestrated chlorhexidene impregnated discs at the skin entry sites may also be beneficial.
  - infection rates may be decreased by the use of 'iv teams'.
  - use of a separate dedicated lumen for parenteral nutrition.
  - measures of unproven benefit include tunnelling of catheters, routine flushing, and the use of in-line filters. Catheters incorporating antibacterial or heparin-treated coatings have been claimed to reduce colonisation with organisms, especially when tunnelling is also performed.

Raad I, Hanna H, Maki D (2007). Lancet Infect Dis; 7: 645–57

See also, Central venous cannulation; Central venous cannulation, long term; Infection control; Intravenous fluid administration; Sepsis

Cauda equina syndrome. Syndrome of leg weakness, perineal sensory loss and urinary and faecal incontinence; has followed spinal anaesthesia especially if a continuous microcatheter technique has been used. Possible mechanisms of injury include:

- direct trauma from lumbar puncture, intraneural injection, trauma from the catheter or epidural haematoma.
- poor mixing of local anaesthetic, especially hyperbaric, in the CSF. This results in pooling of anaesthetic in the terminal dural sac, especially if large doses are used to extend the resultant inadequate block (local anaesthetics being directly neurotoxic in high concentrations, especially lidocaine).
- passage of the catheter into the subdural space with high local concentrations of local anaesthetic around the cauda equina.

It has been suggested that the cauda equina nerve fibres are more vulnerable to damage because they lack protective sheaths. Symptoms may appear soon after surgery and may be permanent.

See also, Transient radicular irritation syndrome

Caudal analgesia. Produced by injection of local anaesthetic agent into the sacral canal, a continuation of the epidural space. First described independently by Cathelin and Sicard in 1901, predating lumbar epidural anaesthesia. Easily performed, but with a large failure rate due to variations in sacral anatomy. Produces block of the sacral and lumbar nerve roots; thus ideal for perineal surgery. Higher blocks require greater volumes of anaesthetic solution, but are more unpredictable. Useful as a supplement to general anaesthesia, and for provision of postoperative analgesia. Catheter insertion has been performed for continuous caudal block.

- Technique:
  - usually performed with the patient in the lateral position, with the knees drawn up to the chest. The prone and knee–elbow positions may also be used.

- the sacral hiatus lies at the third point of an equilateral triangle formed with the two posterior superior iliac spines (each overlain by a skin dimple). The sacral cornua are palpable on either side of the hiatus.
- using an aseptic technique, a needle is introduced in a slightly cranial direction through the hiatus. Ordinary iv needles and cannulae are commonly used, although specific caudal needles are available.
- when the canal is entered (a click may be felt as the sacrococcygeal membrane is pierced), the needle is directed cranially, and advanced not more than 2 cm into the canal. The dura normally ends at S2, level with the posterior superior iliac spines, but may extend further.
- after aspirating to confirm absence of blood or CSF, local anaesthetic is injected, feeling for accidental subcutaneous injection with the other hand. There should be little resistance to injection with a 19–21 G needle. If the patient is awake, pain is felt if the needle tip is under the periosteum of the anterior wall of the canal. Caudal needles may bear a side hole to prevent this complication.

- Doses:
  - 20–30 ml 0.25–0.5% bupivacaine, or 1–2% lidocaine with adrenaline, in young adults, reduced in the elderly. The average volume of the sacral canal is 30–35 ml.
  - 0.5 ml/kg 0.25% bupivacaine has been used for sacrolumbar blockade in children; 1 ml/kg for upper abdominal blockade and 1.25 ml/kg for midthoracic blockade. 0.125% bupivacaine provides analgesia with less motor blockade.

Complications are as for epidural anaesthesia, but much less common. Insertion of the needle into the rectum, or presenting part of the fetus in obstetrics, has been reported.
[Fernand Cathelin (1873–1945), French surgeon; Jean-Athanase Sicard (1872–1929), French neurologist]
See also, Vertebral ligaments

Causalgia, *see Complex regional pain syndrome type 2*

Caval compression, *see Aortocaval compression*

Cave of Retzius block, *see Retzius cave block*

CAVH, Continuous arteriovenous haemofiltration, *see Haemofiltration*

CAVHD, Continuous arteriovenous haemodiafiltration, *see Haemodiafiltration*

CCF, Congestive cardiac failure, *see Cardiac failure*

CCrISP, *see Care of the critically ill surgical patient*

CCT, Central conduction time, *see Evoked potentials*

CCU, *see Coronary care unit*

Cefamandole (Cephamandole). Antibacterial drug; 2nd generation cephalosporin with wide spectrum of activity against Gram-negative and -positive bacteria. Achieves good tissue penetration including CSF. Approximately 60% protein-bound and excreted unchanged in the urine.
- Dosage: 0.5–2.0 g iv/im 4–8 hourly.
- Side effects: blood dyscrasias, hepatic impairment.

Cefazolin (Cephazolin). Antibacterial drug; 1st generation cephalosporin used to treat respiratory, urinary tract and soft tissue infections. Not recommended in meningitis as it crosses the blood–brain barrier poorly. 80% protein-bound and excreted largely unchanged in the urine.
- Dosage: 0.5–1.0 g iv/im 6–12 hourly.
- Side effects: blood dyscrasias, hepatic impairment.

Cefotaxime. Antibacterial drug; 3rd generation cephalosporin active against Gram-positive and -negative organisms including haemophilus, klebsiella, streptococcus, staphylococcus (but less so than cefuroxime), proteus, serratia, enterobacter and escherichia species. Increasingly the first choice antibiotic for bacterial meningitis in adults and children until the organism is known. Half-life is about 1 h; extensively protein-bound, it undergoes hepatic metabolism to an active metabolite, with 50–80% excreted unchanged in the urine.
- Dosage: 1–2 g 12 hourly iv/im, up to 12 g/day in 3–4 doses in severe infections.
- Side effects: phlebitis, rash, GIT upset, colitis.

Cefoxitin. Antibacterial drug; 2nd generation cephalosporin active against bowel flora including *Bacteroides fragilis*; thus sometimes used to treat intra-abdominal sepsis. Approximately 70% protein-bound, and excreted largely unchanged in the urine.
- Dosage: 1–2 g iv/im 6–12 hourly up to 12 g/day.
- Side effects: blood dyscrasias, thrombophlebitis, vertigo, GIT upset, pseudomembranous colitis, renal and hepatic impairment.

Cefpirome. 4th generation cephalosporin with good activity against Gram-positive organisms including staphylococcus. Excreted largely unchanged by the kidney; thus reduced dosage is required in renal impairment.
- Dosage: 1–2 g iv, 12 hourly.
- Side effects: headache, nausea, hepatic impairment, skin rashes, taste disorders.

Cefradine (Cephradine). Antibacterial drug; 1st generation cephalosporin similar to cefazolin. 10% protein-bound and excreted unchanged in the urine.
- Dosage: 0.5–1.0 g iv/im 6–12 hourly.
- Side effects: as for cefazolin.

Ceftazidime. Antibacterial drug; 3rd generation cephalosporin especially active against multiresistant Gram-negative bacteria and pseudomonas. Largely unmetabolised and 90% excreted in the urine.
- Dosage: 1–2 g iv/im 8–12 hourly.
- Side effects: painful im injections, diarrhoea, hepatic impairment.

Ceftriaxone. Antibacterial drug; 3rd generation cephalosporin structurally related to cefotaxime, with similar spectrum of activity although more active against enterobacter. Has the longest half-life of all the cephalosporins (5–9 h). Undergoes biliary and renal excretion.
- Dosage: 1–4 g iv/im once daily.
- Side effects: pain on injection, leucopenia, hepatic and renal impairment, precipitation (as calcium salt) in urine or gallstones.

Cefuroxime. Antibacterial drug; 2nd generation cephalosporin, most closely related to cefamandole. Has a wide spectrum of activity against both Gram-positive and -negative organisms including β-lactamase producing staphylococcus, haemophilus and some enterobacter species. Penetrates well into CSF. The only 2nd generation agent that achieves therapeutic CSF levels. Excreted unchanged in the urine.

- Dosage: 0.75–1.5 g iv/im 6–8 hourly.
- Side effects: GIT upset, rashes, rarely blood dyscrasias.

Cellulitis. Skin infection resulting in local inflammation (warmth, erythema and pain) usually with fever and leucocytosis. Lymphangitis and lymphadenitis may be present. Portals of entry of pathogens include local trauma (including insertion of iv catheters, etc.) and abrasions. More common in those with impaired lymphatic drainage and in iv drug abusers. Organisms commonly responsible include β-haemolytic streptococci and *Staphylococcus aureus*, thus guiding initial antibacterial drug therapy if microbiological identification is uncertain (e.g. phenoxymethylpenicillin with flucloxacillin, or erythromycin or co-amoxiclav alone).

Swartz MN (2004). N Engl J Med; 350: 904–12

See also, Staphylococcal infections; Streptococcal infections

CEMACH, Confidential Enquiries into Maternal and Child Health, *see Confidential Enquiries into Maternal Deaths*

CENSA, *see Confederation of European National Societies of Anaesthesiology*

Central anticholinergic syndrome. Syndrome following the use of anticholinergic drugs (especially hyoscine), thought to be due to a decrease in inhibitory acetylcholine activity in the brain. Other drugs with anticholinergic activity may cause it, including antihistamine drugs, phenothiazines, antidepressant drugs, antiparkinsonian drugs and pethidine. Has also been reported after volatile anaesthetic agents, ketamine and benzodiazepines. Reported incidence varies but has been up to 5–10% after general anaesthesia.

- Features:
  - confusion, agitation, restlessness, anxiety, amnesia, hallucinations.
  - speech disturbance, ataxia.
  - nausea, vomiting.
  - muscle incoordination.
  - convulsions, coma.
  - peripheral anticholinergic effects, e.g. tachycardia, dry mouth and skin, blurred vision, urinary retention.
- Treatment: physostigmine 0.04 mg/kg slowly iv. It usually acts within 5 min; features may recur after 1–2 h.

Central conduction time, *see Evoked potentials*

Central pain. Diffuse continuous pain, usually burning and unilateral, with or without increased sensitivity and altered sensation. Due to CNS lesions, e.g. CVA, classically (but not exclusively) involving the thalamus (thalamic syndrome). Often associated with depression. Associated signs and distribution of pain are related to the site of lesion. May be helped by phenothiazines, tricyclic antidepressant drugs and carbamazepine.

Central pontine myelinosis. Demyelination occurring within the pons. May occur in hyponatraemia although it is uncertain whether low sodium concentration itself or the rapidity of its correction is more important in its aetiology. May also occur in alcoholism, malnutrition, following diuretic therapy, and following liver transplantation. Accompanied by extrapontine demyelination in 10% of cases.

May be asymptomatic, or present with the 'locked in' syndrome, behavioural disturbances, tetraplegia, pseudobulbar palsy, convulsions or coma. Diagnosis is confirmed by MRI scanning.

Thought to be prevented by slow correction of hyponatraemia (< 12 mmol/l per 24 h), with avoidance of overcorrection.

Central venous cannulation. Cannulation of a vein within the thorax via peripheral venepuncture.

- Performed for:
  - vascular access, e.g. for dialysis, TPN, infusion of irritant or potent drugs.
  - measurement of CVP.
  - cardiac catheterisation, pulmonary artery catheterisation and transvenous cardiac pacing.

The catheter tip should ideally lie in the superior vena cava above the pericardial reflection, to reduce risk of arrhythmias and cardiac tamponade should erosion and bleeding occur. However, a tip placed too high may be associated with thrombosis.

- May be performed at different sites:
  - internal jugular vein:
    - easy to perform and reliable.
    - may cause pneumothorax or damage the common carotid artery, brachial plexus, phrenic nerve, thoracic duct (on left) or sympathetic chain.
    - uncomfortable for the patient.
  - subclavian vein:
    - more convenient and comfortable for long-term use.
    - less chance of correct placement.
    - greater chance of pneumothorax or haemothorax.
    - may damage the subclavian artery; direct pressure cannot be applied to stop bleeding.
  - external jugular vein:
    - easy to perform since the vein is more superficial than the internal jugular or subclavian veins.
    - it may be difficult to thread the catheter through the junction with the subclavian vein. A J-shaped guidewire may help.
  - femoral vein:
    - often easier than other routes, especially in obese patients.
    - avoids the pleura and lungs completely.
    - useful in superior vena caval obstruction.
    - traditionally avoided because of the risk of infection. Thromboembolism and femoral arterial puncture may also occur.
  - axillary vein:
    - since venepuncture is extrathoracic, risk of pneumothorax is reduced.
    - the axillary artery may be compressed directly if accidentally punctured.
    - may damage the medial cutaneous nerve.
  - arm vein:
    - minimal risk of serious complications.
    - threading of a 'long line' is often difficult, especially via the cephalic vein because of valves at the junction with the axillary vein. Abduction of the arm may help.
    - 50% chance of correct placement.

Air embolism, subcutaneous emphysema and sepsis are risks of all techniques. Patients should be in the head-down position for jugular and subclavian cannulation to prevent air embolism. An aseptic technique is used to avoid catheter-related sepsis. Introduction of a catheter into the heart may cause arrhythmias (therefore ECG monitoring is required) or cardiac perforation. Reintroduction of the needle into the cannula should never be performed whilst the tip is in the patient, as pieces of cannula are easily sheared off.

Endocardial damage and central vein thrombosis may also occur, especially with pulmonary artery catheters and with prolonged placement.

Successful placement is suggested by easy aspiration of non-pulsatile blood, obtaining the venous waveform, and variation of measured pressure with respiration. Placement of the catheter in the right ventricle results in excessive swinging of central venous pressure with each heartbeat. Catheter position must be checked by X-ray, and pneumothorax excluded. Correct positioning may also be confirmed during insertion by filling the cannula with saline and connecting its proximal end to the left arm lead of the ECG. As the right atrium is approached, the P waves become increasingly peaked and tall, becoming biphasic as the atrium is entered. Hand-held ultrasound devices have been used to identify the vein and recent guidelines issued by NICE support their routine use for internal jugular venous cannulation.

Taylor RW, Palagiri AV (2007). Crit Care Med; 35: 1390–6

See also: Axillary venous cannulation; Central venous cannulation, long term; Femoral venous cannulation; Subclavian venous cannulation

Central venous cannulation, long term. Usually employed for long-term TPN, administration of drugs, e.g. chemotherapy and antibiotics, and blood sampling. First developed in the 1970s. Silastic catheters (Hickman–Broviac) are usually inserted via the subclavian vein and tunnelled subcutaneously (emerging from the skin between the sternum and nipple). A Dacron cuff on the subcutaneous part incites an inflammatory reaction, providing fixation and a possible barrier to infection within 1–2 weeks. Single- and double-lumen catheters are available.

Catheters are inserted under sterile conditions via a surgical cut-down procedure, or percutaneously using the Seldinger technique. In the latter, the catheter is passed into the vein through a sheath which is split and peeled away as the catheter is advanced.

Catheters may remain in place for years if required, with regular heparinised flushing and aseptic handling.

[John W Broviac, US physician; Robert O Hickman, US paediatrician]

See also, Central venous cannulation; Nutrition, total parenteral

Central venous pressure (CVP). Pressure within the right atrium and great veins of the thorax. Measured via central venous cannulation, using a manometer or transducer. An estimate may be made by observing the distension of neck veins (JVP). CVP is usually measured with the patient lying flat, and expressed in cmH_2O above a point level with the right atrium, e.g. mid-axillary line. Normally 0–8 cmH_2O; 5–10 cmH_2O lower if the sternal angle is used as the reference point. By convention, it is measured at the end of expiration. The venous waveform may be seen on a pressure tracing, with the effects of ventilation superimposed (see below).

- Increased by:
  - raised intrathoracic pressure, e.g. IPPV, coughing. CVP normally rises in expiration during spontaneous ventilation.
  - impaired cardiac function, e.g. outlet obstruction, cardiac failure, cardiac tamponade. Primarily reflects right-sided function; thus CVP may be normal in the presence of left ventricular failure and pulmonary oedema, or raised in right-sided failure with normal left-sided function. With normal cardiac function, pressures on both sides move together. Left-sided function may be assessed by pulmonary artery catheterisation.
  - circulatory overload.
  - venoconstriction.
  - superior vena caval obstruction (the normal venous waveform may be lost).
- Decreased by:
  - reduced venous return, e.g. due to hypovolaemia, venodilatation.
  - reduced intrathoracic pressure, e.g. in inspiration during spontaneous ventilation.

Useful in indicating right ventricular preload and cardiac function; e.g. a volume challenge of 200–300 ml saline causing a persistent rise in CVP of 2–5 cmH_2O suggests poor ventricular function in a normovolaemic patient.

Also used to monitor haemorrhage, and in estimating the adequacy of volume replacement; e.g. hypovolaemia is suggested if a volume challenge of 300–500 ml saline causes an increase in CVP that is not sustained for more than 10–15 min. Serial measurements are thus more informative than single readings.

Measurement is indicated in shock, hypovolaemia, acute cardiovascular disease and major surgery.

Magder S (2006). Crit Care Med; 34: 2224–7

Cephalosporins. Semisynthetic antibacterial drugs, derived from the natural substance cephalosporin C. Bactericidal, they act by inhibiting the synthesis of bacterial cell walls. Similar in pharmacology to penicillins; cross-sensitivity in penicillin-allergic individuals is rare with 2nd–4th generation cephalosporins. The 'generation' classification is based partly on their antibacterial activity and when they were introduced (generally, successive generations have greater activity against Gram-negative organisms):

- 1st generation, e.g. cephalothin (largely replaced by cefazolin and cefradine): good activity against Gram-positive organisms including penicillinase-producing staphylococci; poor activity against enterococci and Gram-negative organisms.
- 2nd generation, e.g. cefamandole, cefuroxime: slightly less active than cephalothin against Gram-positive organisms but greater stability against enterobacteria and *Haemophilus influenzae*. The cephamycin antibacterial drugs, e.g. cefoxitin, are classified as 2nd generation although they have greater activity against anaerobes, especially *Bacteroides fragilis*.
- 3rd generation, e.g. cefotaxime, ceftriaxone: yet more stable against Gram-negative bacteria although less active against Gram-positive organisms than 1st generation drugs (but still very active against streptococci). Ceftazidime has enhanced activity against pseudomonas.
- 4th generation, e.g. cefpirome.

CEPOD, *see National Confidential Enquiry into Patient Outcome and Death*

Cerebral abscess. Collection of infected material, often encapsulated, within the brain parenchyma. More common in males, with peak incidence in the third decade. Infection often arises from local spread (e.g. following paranasal sinusitis, otitis or cerebral trauma) or metastatic spread (e.g. following bacterial endocarditis or lung abscess) when cerebral abscesses are often multiple. May also occur in cyanotic heart disease when cardiac output is no longer 'filtered' by the lungs.

- Causative organisms:
  - often multiple.

- most commonly, Gram-positive *Streptococcus milleri*, Gram-negative anaerobic bacteroides species and aerobic Gram-negative organisms such as proteus, *Escherichia coli* and pseudomonas.
- in immunocompromised patients, nocardia, actinomycetes and toxoplasma.
- Features:
  - headache, hyper- or hypothermia, nausea, neck stiffness, convulsions, coma. Focal neurological signs depend on the location of the abscess.
  - CT scan with contrast (or MRI scan) may reveal typical ring enhancement of the abscess.
  - lumbar puncture (once raised ICP has been excluded by a brain scan) may produce normal CSF unless the abscess has ruptured into the subarachnoid or ventricular spaces.
- Treatment:
  - antibacterial drugs directed against the most likely organism (must be able to penetrate the abscess wall), e.g. benzylpenicillin, metronidazole and cefotaxime if otitis/sinusitis is suspected, may be required for up to 2 years.
  - surgical drainage or excision is indicated if ICP is markedly raised or neurological function deteriorates despite antibacterial therapy.

Cerebral blood flow (CBF). Normally 14% of cardiac ouput, approximately 700 ml/min (50 ml/100 g/min). Grey matter receives about 70 ml/100 g/min whereas white matter receives about 20 ml/100 g/min. The amount of CBF is critical: if falls to 20 ml/100 g/min EEG slows; at 15 ml/100 g/min EEG is flat, and at 10 ml/100 g/min irreversible cerebral damage occurs.

- Measurement:
  - applying the Fick principle, using N_2O (Kety–Schmidt technique). Values are obtained for the whole brain; regional variations in flow are not demonstrated.
  - detection of radioactive decay over different parts of the head, following inhalation of radioactive xenon or injection of dissolved radioactive xenon into a carotid artery. Regional differences are detected.
  - regional flow may also be measured by positron emission tomography, functional MRI and Doppler probes placed extracranially.
- Affected by:
  - metabolic factors: CBF increases in metabolically active areas.
  - chemical factors:
    - arterial $P\text{CO}_2$ (Fig. 34a): hypercapnia increases CBF via cerebral vasodilatation. Hypocapnia decreases CBF; a reduction from 5.3 to 4 kPa (40 to 30 mmHg) reduces CBF by 30%. Reduction may not be sustained for more than 24–48 h of hypocapnia.
    - arterial $P\text{O}_2$ (Fig. 34a): minimal effect until $P\text{O}_2$ falls below 6.7 kPa (50 mmHg).
    - autoregulation (Fig. 34b): CBF remains constant between a MAP of 60 and 160 mmHg (limits are raised in the hypertensive patient). Autoregulation is impaired after cerebral trauma, hypoxaemia and hypercarbia.
  - temperature: hypothermia decreases cerebral metabolism which results in a decrease in CBF (a ~5% drop per °C drop in temperature).
  - neural control: sympathetic stimulation causes cerebral vasoconstriction, parasympathetic stimulation causes cerebral vasodilatation.
  - drugs: all the volatile anaesthetic agents cause dose-dependent vasodilatation and abolition of autoregulation. Hyperventilation before introduction of the agent may reduce this effect; with isoflurane, hyperventilation following introduction is effective. Ketamine also increases CBF; thiopental, etomidate, benzodiazepines and propofol reduce it. Opioid drugs cause little change if $P_a\text{CO}_2$ is kept within normal levels.

See also, Cerebral circulation; Cerebral ischaemia; Cerebral steal

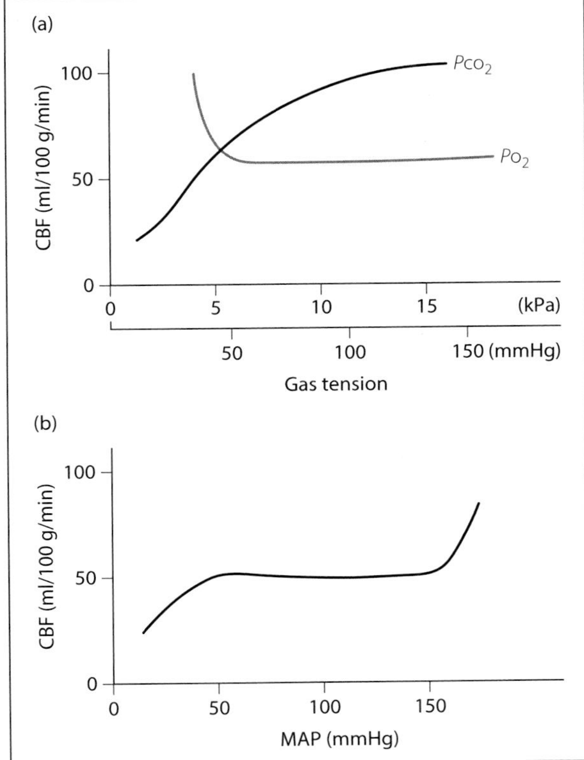

Fig. 34 Variation of cerebral blood flow with: (a) arterial $P\text{O}_2$ and $P\text{CO}_2$; (b) blood pressure

Cerebral circulation.

- Arterial supply: ⅔ via the two internal carotid arteries and ⅓ via the two vertebral arteries. These two systems are joined by the anterior and posterior communicating arteries, thus forming the anastomosis (patent in 50% of individuals) known as the circle of Willis (Fig. 35a):
  - anterior cerebral artery: supplies superior and medial parts of the cerebral hemisphere.
  - middle cerebral artery: supplies most of the lateral side of the hemisphere. Internal branches supply the internal capsule, through which most ascending and descending pathways pass. Commonly affected by CVA.
  - posterior cerebral artery: supplies the occipital lobe and the medial side of the temporal lobe.
- Venous drainage (Fig. 35b):
  - deep structures drain via the internal cerebral vein on each side; these form the midline great cerebral vein which passes back to join the inferior sagittal sinus.
  - cerebral and cerebellar cortices drain via dural sinuses:
    - superior and inferior sagittal sinuses in the midline, between the layers of dura of the falx cerebri. The superior usually drains into the right transverse sinus; the inferior via the straight sinus into the left transverse sinus.

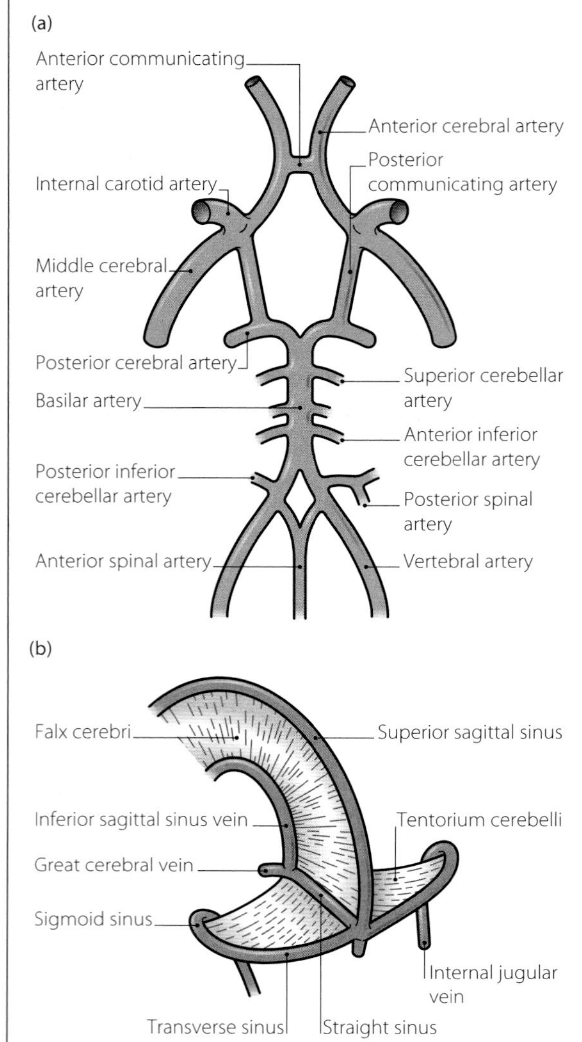

Fig. 35 Cerebral circulation: (a) arterial; (b) venous

- transverse sinuses within the tentorium cerebelli: pass via the sigmoid sinuses through the jugular foramina to become the internal jugular veins.
- cavernous sinuses on either side of the pituitary fossa: receive blood from the eyes and nearby parts of the brain, draining into the transverse sinuses and internal jugular veins.

Both arterial and venous circulations may be imaged using conventional or MRI angiography.
[Thomas Willis (1621–1675), English physician]

Cerebral function analysing monitor. Development of the cerebral function monitor which provides information about the frequency distribution of the EEG signal as well as overall activity. Thus the relative proportions of the four standard EEG waveforms are presented. Said to be more useful than the cerebral function monitor, but suffers from similar drawbacks.

Cerebral function monitor. Device adapted from the conventional EEG, e.g. for use during anaesthesia. The signal from two parietal electrodes is filtered and amplified to produce a display of average peak voltage, charted on slow-moving paper. Thus monitors overall cerebral activity. Has been used to monitor depth of anaesthesia, but unreliable, especially using volatile anaesthetic agents. Used in neurosurgery, cardiac surgery and carotid artery surgery, where trends in activity may reflect changes in cerebral perfusion. Has also been used in ICU, e.g. for head injury, poisoning and overdoses, status epilepticus.
See also, Anaesthesia, depth of

Cerebral ischaemia. Inadequate blood supply to brain. May be:
- global:
  - complete, e.g. cardiac arrest or severely raised ICP with hypotension.
  - incomplete, e.g. hypotension and cerebrovascular disease.
- focal or regional, e.g. cerebrovascular disease, emboli, local lesions, e.g. tumours; may also be complete or incomplete.

- Effects of complete ischaemia:
  - energy stores decrease and waste products accumulate.
  - anaerobic metabolism increases, with greater acidosis if a glucose source is available.
  - protein synthesis is reduced and breakdown increased; impaired cell membrane pump activity results in leak of potassium out of cells, and chloride and calcium into cells.
  - neurotransmitters accumulate as their breakdown and uptake cease, e.g. GABA and glutamate.
  - free radicals are liberated.
  - recovery is thought to be impossible after about 4–5 min, although neuronal survival may be possible experimentally after 30–60 min.

Reperfusion may be hindered by swelling, haemorrhage, etc.
- Effects of incomplete ischaemia:
  - reduced O_2 supply and waste product removal as above, but with continued glucose supply. Thus acidosis etc. is worse than if ischaemia is complete.
  - reduction in cerebral blood flow from the normal 50 ml/100 g/min causes the following:
    - 30–40 ml/100 g/min: EEG slows.
    - 20 ml/100 g/min: no spontaneous electrical activity. Lactate rises.
    - 15 ml/100 g/min: evoked potentials disappear. Anaerobic metabolism occurs and pH decreases.Ionic changes begin.
    - 10 ml/100 g/min: water accumulates. Irreversible damage occurs.

Hypoxaemia with uninterrupted blood supply is better tolerated because of continued removal of waste products despite O_2 lack.

Damage is thought to result from increased intracellular calcium levels, free radicals, arachidonic acid metabolites, or lactic acid production. Investigated lines of treatment have been directed against these (cerebral protection/resuscitation). Effects depend on duration, site and cause of ischaemia, and patient factors, e.g. age, other disease, etc. Watershed areas between the main cerebral arteries are most at risk from ischaemia, especially in the elderly, if vessels are diseased, if blood viscosity is high, etc. Chronic ischaemia may cause transient ischaemic attack, CVA or dementia. During anaesthesia, excessive hyperventilation combined with hypotension may cause ischaemia.

Zauner A, Daugherty WP, Bullock MR, Warner DS (2002). Neurosurgery; 51: 289–302

See also, Brainstem death; Cerebral circulation; Cerebral metabolism; Cerebral steal

Cerebral metabolic rate for oxygen ($CMRO_2$). Volume of O_2 consumed by the brain. Equals cerebral blood flow × arteriovenous O_2 content difference (*see Fick principle*). Normally about 50 ml/min (20% of total basal requirement), or 3.5 ml/100 g/min. Indicative of global cerebral metabolism, over 90% of which is aerobic; the relationship may not hold if O_2 or glucose supplies are reduced and alternate metabolic pathways employed.

Reduced by hypothermia (about 5% reduction per °C drop). Also reduced in old age and by certain drugs, e.g. barbiturates, benzodiazepines, volatile anaesthetic agents; increased by seizures, ketamine and possibly N_2O.

Cerebral metabolism. Glucose is the main substrate, although ketone bodies, amino acids and fats may be utilised, e.g. in starvation. 90–95% of glycolysis is aerobic, hence the requirement for a continuous supply of O_2. O_2 consumption is about 3.5 ml/100 g/min; CO_2 output is the same.

Cerebral metabolic rate for O_2 ($CMRO_2$) is used as a measure of global cerebral metabolism, and does not reflect regional variations; e.g. neuronal cells consume more O_2 than glial cells, grey matter more than white. Similar measurements may be made using glucose consumption (cerebral metabolic rate for glucose; normally about 4.5 mg/100 g/min) and lactate production (cerebral metabolic rate for lactate; normally about 2.3 mg/100 g/min).

Cerebral blood flow is closely related to cerebral metabolism.

See also, Cerebral ischaemia

Cerebral microdialysis. Method of sampling neurotransmitters or metabolites present in the ECF of the brain, e.g. glucose, pyruvate, lactate, glycerol and glutamate. First used in humans in 1990, with bedside analysers becoming available in the 2000s. Has been used to detect and measure physiological and pathophysiological chemical changes, e.g. in Parkinson's disease, cerebral ischaemia, cerebral neoplasia, subarachnoid haemorrhage and head injury. A small microdialysis catheter is placed in the brain tissue and a 'perfusion' fluid passed through it. Substances within the ECF pass into the perfusion fluid by diffusion, forming a dialysate, chemical analysis of which allows assessment of the local, as opposed to global, cerebral metabolism.

Tisdall M, Smith M (2006). Br J Anaesth; 97: 18–25

Cerebral oedema. Increased brain water content. May be:
- vasogenic: increased vascular permeability and defective blood–brain barrier, e.g. associated with inflammatory conditions, tumours, trauma. Plasma protein and fluid penetrate the brain, tracking along fibre tracts. Exacerbated by raised hydrostatic pressures.
- cytotoxic: cell damage due to cerebral ischaemia, hypoxia, encephalitis, toxins, metabolic disturbances, etc.; cells become depleted of ATP and accumulate water and sodium.
- osmotic: occurs when brain osmolality exceeds plasma osmolality, e.g. severe hyponatraemia, during haemodialysis, rapid reduction of plasma glucose in diabetic ketoacidosis.
- hydrostatic: seen in severe hypertension when fluid is forced out of cerebral capillaries.
- interstitial: in hydrocephalus the CSF may be forced from the ventricular system into white matter.
- high altitude cerebral oedema (HACE): may have similar mechanism to vasogenic cerebral oedema.

- Effects:
  - raised ICP, reduced cerebral perfusion pressure, compression of blood vessels and vital structures, papilloedema and coning.
  - increased distance for O_2 diffusion from capillaries to cells.
  - impaired consciousness, convulsions and coma.

Revealed by CT scanning.
- Management:
  - of primary cause.
  - IPPV, with hypocapnia to arterial $P\text{CO}_2$ 3.8–4.2 kPa (28–32 mmHg). The beneficial effects of hyperventilation may be reduced after 24 h. Fluid restriction to 1.5–2 l/day is usually instituted. Venous drainage is encouraged by head-up posture, good sedation/paralysis and unobstructed jugular veins, as for ICP reduction. Measures are usually carried out for 24–48 h after the insult.
  - corticosteroids are used for oedema due to mass lesions, e.g. tumour or haematoma, but are ineffective in global oedema. Dexamethasone is usually employed, e.g. 4–8 mg iv 6–8 hourly.
  - diuretics:
    - mannitol 0.25–1 g/kg iv; relies on an intact blood–brain barrier. Urea is rarely used now.
    - furosemide 10–40 mg.
  - hypertonic intravenous solutions (e.g. 7.5% saline) have been used.

Cerebral perfusion pressure (CPP). Difference between MAP and ICP; represents the pressure head available for cerebral blood flow. Normally 70–75 mmHg; critical level for cerebral ischaemia is thought to be 30–40 mmHg. In the presence of raised ICP, MAP increases in order to maintain CPP (Cushing's reflex).

Cerebral protection/resuscitation.
- Possible techniques:
  - general measures:
    - maintaining normotension and oxygenation.
    - maintaining metabolic stability and other organ function.
  - increasing or maintaining cerebral perfusion pressure:
    - nimodipine in subarachnoid haemorrhage: thought to reduce vasospasm and maintain blood flow. Of uncertain benefit in other intracranial pathology.
    - reduction of ICP, e.g. hypocapnia or mannitol.
    - haemodilution.
    - cerebral angioplasty/endovascular thrombolysis in focal ischaemia.
  - reducing metabolic rate for O_2:
    - hypothermia: used in cardiac surgery and under investigation in severe brain injury. Appears to have sustained benefit pre- and post-ischaemic injury.
    - barbiturates: thought to be beneficial in transient incomplete ischaemia only, since some electrical activity is required for $CMRO_2$ reduction. Routine use is controversial, unless for sedation or treatment of convulsions. Profound hypotension is a major side effect. Phenytoin has also been investigated.
    - isoflurane: possibly beneficial in incomplete global ischaemia; cerebral steal is possible in focal ischaemia. Efficacy has not been established in humans.
  - reducing cell damage:
    - avoidance of hyperglycaemia (thought to exacerbate the effects of ischaemia). Shown to have sustained benefits pre- and post-ischaemic injury.

- free radical scavengers including lazaroids.
- glutamate antagonists: glutamate is increased in ischaemia, and is thought to cause cell damage.
- xenon may have a neuroprotective role via its NMDA receptor antagonism.

Fukuda S, Warner DS (2007). Br J Anaesth; 99: 10–17

Cerebral salt wasting syndrome. Loss of sodium (and water) via the kidneys associated with intracranial disease (e.g. subarachnoid haemorrhage, head injury). May be mediated by excessive secretion of atrial natriuretic peptide. Results in hyponatraemia and decreased plasma volume (unlike the syndrome of inappropriate antidiuretic hormone secretion in which plasma volume is increased). Treatment is with fluid and sodium replacement.

Cerebral steal. Diversion of blood flow away from abnormal areas of brain, e.g. tumours, infarcts and ischaemic areas, secondary to vasodilatation of normal cerebral blood vessels, e.g. due to hypercapnia. Vessels supplying the abnormal areas may already be maximally dilated; vasodilatation in normal areas may thus reduce blood flow in abnormal areas, with possibly deleterious effects. The reverse may occur in hypocapnia; thus general vasoconstriction may increase blood flow to abnormal areas (inverse steal).

Cerebral venous thrombosis. Most commonly affects the superior sagittal, lateral, cavernous or straight sinuses, although cerebral veins may be involved (*see Cerebral circulation*).

- Aetiology:
  - infective:
    - local, e.g. cerebral abscess, meningitis, sinusitis, otitis.
    - systemic, e.g. endocarditis, TB, HIV infection, bacteraemia, viraemia.
  - non-infective:
    - local, e.g. head injury, neurosurgery, cerebral tumour, hyperosmolar infusion via jugular veins.
    - general, e.g. hypercoagulable coagulation disorders.

Features depend on the site but include those of raised ICP, cranial nerve palsies, and CVA. Cavernous venous thrombosis results in facial oedema and swelling of the eye.

Diagnosed clinically and by CT or MRI scanning, and cerebral angiography. MRI is now the investigation of choice.

Treatment is directed at the underlying cause; systemic heparin and direct infusion of fibrinolytic drugs have been used.

Stam J (2005). N Engl J Med; 352: 1791–8

Cerebrospinal fluid (CSF). Clear fluid bathing the CNS, providing support and protection against trauma, and helping to regulate ICP. Total volume is 100–150 ml, of which ⅓–½ is spinal.

- Production:
  - by choroid plexuses mainly in the lateral but also in the 3rd and 4th ventricles at about 500 ml/day.
  - formed by secretion, and filtration of plasma. Formation is largely independent of ICP, but removal increases with increasing pressure.
- Circulation (Fig. 36):
  - from the lateral ventricles to the 3rd ventricle via the foramina of Monro, thence to the 4th ventricle via the aqueduct.
  - leaves the 4th ventricle via the foramen of Magendie (midline posteriorly) and Luschka (laterally) to pass down to the spinal cord or up over the cerebral hemispheres.

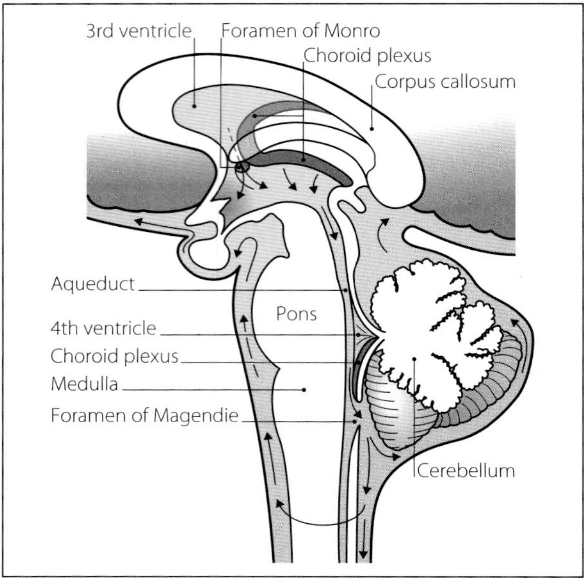

Fig. 36 Circulation of CSF

  - passes into dural venous sinuses via arachnoid villi, and possibly from spinal nerve cuffs into spinal veins.
- Normal constituents:
  - sodium: 135–145 mmol/l.
  - chloride: 115–125 mmol/l.
  - calcium: 1–1.5 mmol/l.
  - potassium: 2.5–3.5 mmol/l.
  - glucose: 2.7–4.2 mmol/l (if blood glucose normal).
  - pH: 7.3–7.5.
  - protein: 0.2–0.4 g/l.
  - urea: 1.5–6.0 mmol/l.
  - lymphocytes: 0–5 × 10^6/l.

[Alexander Monro (1733–1817), Scottish anatomist; Francois Magendie (1783–1855), French physiologist; Hubert von Luschka (1820–1875), German anatomist]

See also, Blood–brain barrier; Lumbar puncture

Cerebrovascular accident (CVA; Stroke). Third commonest cause of death in the West.

- Caused by:
  - infarction (80–85%), e.g. caused by atheroma, embolism, arteritis/arterial spasm or hypotension. If symptoms resolve within 24 h, defined as a transient ischaemic attack, although CT scanning may reveal evidence of permanent damage. Multiple small emboli may cause dementia.
  - haemorrhage, usually (60%) associated with bleeding from a small intracerebral vessel in the presence of hypertension. May also occur in patients taking anticoagulant drugs and those with intracranial aneurysms, arteriovenous malformation, etc. Subarachnoid haemorrhage usually occurs from congenital aneurysms.
- Features:
  - impaired consciousness.
  - upper and lower motor neurone lesions; distribution depends on the site and extent of the lesion, e.g. lesions may cause contralateral hemiplegia/paresis, hemisensory loss and homonymous hemianopia. Single limbs and the face may be affected. Speech disorders are common if the dominant hemisphere is affected.

- Treatment:
  - supportive: includes control of arterial BP and blood glucose levels (hyperglycaemia is associated with worse outcome). Early enteral nutrition and normothermia also improve prognosis.
  - in ischaemic stroke, outcome is improved if intravenous thrombolysis is performed within 3 h of onset of symptoms. Aspirin decreases recurrence of ischaemic episodes. Full anticoagulation has no place in treatment but low dose heparin is given to decrease the incidence of DVT and PE.
  - in haemorrhagic stroke, care is largely supportive. Large haematomas (especially in the posterior fossa) may be surgically removed.
- Anaesthetic considerations:
  - assessment for predisposing conditions, e.g. hypertension, coagulation disorders, embolic conditions, trauma, arteritis due to connective tissue diseases, infections, etc.
  - immobility, contractures, etc.: may affect drip sites, etc. Risk of DVT.
  - bulbar lesions and laryngeal incompetence, and autonomic disturbances.
  - communication difficulties.
  - massive hyperkalaemia after suxamethonium has been reported up to 6 months after CVA.
  - hyperventilation and reduction of cerebral blood flow, and hypotension, should be avoided during anaesthesia. Cerebral steal may occur.
  - confusion is common postoperatively.

Risk of CVA during anaesthesia is increased in cardiac surgery, carotid artery surgery and neurosurgery.

Treib J, Grauer MT, Woessner R, Morgenthaler M (2000). Intensive Care Med; 26: 1598–611

See also, Brain; Cerebral circulation; Cerebral ischaemia

Certoparin, *see Heparin*

Cervical plexus block. Provides analgesia of the upper cervical dermatomes; used for head and neck surgery and treatment of pain.

The plexus is formed from the anterior branches of the upper four cervical nerves, lying between the anterior and posterior tubercles of the cervical vertebral transverse processes.

- Technique:
  - the patient is placed supine, looking away from the side to be blocked, with the neck partially extended. The transverse processes of C2–4 are palpated posterior to a line between the mastoid process and transverse process of C6.
  - a fine needle is introduced perpendicular to the skin, 1–3 cm towards each transverse process in turn until contact is made or paraesthesia felt.
  - after careful aspiration 3–5 ml solution, e.g. 0.5% lidocaine with adrenaline, is injected at each level to block the deep branches. A further 3–5 ml is injected as the needle is withdrawn. The superficial branches are blocked by injecting 15–20 ml posterior to the middle of the sternomastoid muscle.

Complications include intravascular injection or puncture (e.g. vertebral artery), subarachnoid injection, sympathetic block, phrenic nerve block and recurrent laryngeal nerve block.

Cervical spine. Comprised of seven cervical vertebrae. Important in the positioning of the neck in airway management including tracheal intubation. Injury may often accompany head injury.

Popitz MD (1997). Anesth Analg; 84: 672–83

See also, Intubation, difficult; Spinal cord injury; Vertebral ligaments

CFAM, *see Cerebral function analysing monitor*

CFM, *see Cerebral function monitor*

cgs system of units. System based on the centimetre, gram and second; replaced in 1960 by the SI system based on the metre, kilogram and second.

See also, Units, SI

Charcoal, activated. Charcoal meeting certain adsorbence standards.

- Uses:
  - administered orally or via a nasogastric tube to reduce gastrointestinal absorption of certain toxic compounds (e.g. barbiturates, tricyclic antidepressant drugs) in the treatment of poisoning and overdoses. In addition to adsorbing toxins present in the stomach, it reduces blood levels by preventing enterohepatic circulation. Most effective when substances toxic in small amounts have been ingested, and within 1 h of ingestion (prehospital administration has been suggested). Adult dosage: 50–100 g 4 hourly, or 25 g 2 hourly.
  - during anaesthesia, waste gases have been passed through containers of activated charcoal (the Aldasorber) in an attempt to reduce pollution. Volatile anaesthetic agents are adsorbed, but not N_2O. The amount adsorbed is measured by weighing the container.
  - coated activated charcoal is used during haemoperfusion.

Bond GR (2002). Ann Emerg Med; 39: 273–86

Charge. Quantity of electricity. Flow of charge constitutes a current. SI unit is the coulomb.

Charles' law. At constant pressure, the volume of a fixed mass of gas is proportional to its temperature.

[Jacques Charles (1746–1823), French chemist]

See also, Boyle's law; Ideal gas law

Chassaignac's tubercle. Transverse process of C6, against which the common carotid artery may be felt and compressed. Useful landmark for stellate ganglion block.

[Charles Chassaignac (1804–1879), French surgeon]

Checking of anaesthetic equipment. Should be performed before anaesthetising any patient. The requirement for following a checklist is mandatory in many countries including the UK.

- The following should be checked before every operating theatre session (Association of Anaesthetists' guidelines):
  - anaesthetic machine:
    - check electricity supply if appropriate.
    - note any information/service labels present.
    - check the identity and attachments of all pipelines.
    - CO_2 cylinders should only be present if specifically requested. Blanking plugs should be fitted to unused yokes.
    - check the O_2 supply and reserve cylinders.
    - check the other gases are connected and that all pipeline pressure gauges read 400 kPa (4 bar).
    - check each flow valve and flowmeter throughout its whole range.
    - check the anti-hypoxic device linking the O_2 and N_2O flowmeters, and the O_2 flush.

- check the vaporisers are seated properly, filled and able to be turned on. Test the vaporiser fittings for leaks by obstructing the common gas outlet with the vaporiser turned on and off, and repeat the test immediately after changing a vaporiser (because this leak test is fairly crude, some machines have a leak testing device with a rubber bulb, to be fitted to the gas outlet and compressed; a leak is indicated by the bulb slowly filling).
- obstruct the gas outlet, ensuring that the pressure relief valve opens (if fitted).

▸ scavenging: check correct connection.

▸ anaesthetic breathing system:
- ensure correct configuration and firm attachment of connections.
- close the expiratory valve. Obstruct the distal end of the tubing to fill the reservoir bag; ensure no leaks.
- open the valve, checking the bag empties.
- coaxial breathing systems: as above, plus testing for correct attachment of the inner tubing of Bain system:
  - obstruct the distal end of the inner tube; the flowmeters should fall and pressure build up behind the obstruction.
  - close the expiratory valve and fill the bag by occluding the distal end of the outer tube. Use the O_2 flush with the tube now unobstructed: the reservoir bag should empty due to gas entrainment, unless the inner tube is detached (Pethick's test).
- circle systems: check one-way valves, bag, etc. Ensure the soda lime is properly packed and not expired.
- ventilator: check on manual settings as above, and on automatic settings with the outlet obstructed, for adequate ventilating pressures and pressure relief. Check the disconnect alarm and that alternative means of IPPV are available, e.g. self-inflating bag.

▸ ancillary equipment (before each case):
- drugs, iv fluids, etc.
- tracheal tubes, cuffs, introducers, etc., laryngoscopes (including spare), suction apparatus, tipping trolley. Check the entire breathing system including catheter mount, angle-piece, filter and connections are patent (i.e. no obstructions) before each case. Single-use equipment should be kept packaged until the point of use to avoid obstruction with solid objects.
- check all monitoring devices including O_2 analyser are functioning and have appropriate alarm limits (and for BP, an appropriate measuring frequency) set.

It is also recommended that performance of a check is recorded on each patient's anaesthetic chart, and a logbook kept with each anaesthetic machine.

[Simon L Pethick, Canadian anaesthetist]

Chelating agents.
- Examples (with the metals chelated):
  - dimercaprol (antimony, arsenic, bismuth, mercury, gold).
  - sodium calcium edetate (lead, copper, radioactive metals).
  - penicillamine (copper, lead, gold, mercury, zinc).
  - desferrioxamine (iron, aluminium).
  - trisodium edetate (calcium).

Chemical weapons. Substances used for hostile purposes, either by certain nations in 'legitimate' chemical warfare or by terrorists. The agents may be targeted at people, animals and/or plants. Usually classified according to their physiological effects:
  - toxins derived from living organisms, e.g. botulinum toxins, ricin (derived from castor bean), saxitoxin (derived from marine organisms).
  - nerve agents, e.g. acetylcholinesterase inhibitors (e.g. sarin, soman, VX gas and tabun).
  - blood agents, e.g. cyanide.
  - blistering or choking agents, e.g. mustard gas, chlorine, phosgene.
  - vomiting agents, e.g. adamsite.
  - tear gas.

Management includes specific and general supportive measures; consideration should also be directed towards protection of staff, decontamination of clinical areas and equipment, disposal of bodies and other aspects of major incidents.

White SM (2002). Br J Anaesth; 89: 306–24

See also, Biological weapons; Cyanide poisoning; Incident, major

Chemoreceptor trigger zone (CTZ). Area situated in the area postrema of the medulla, on the lateral walls of the 4th ventricle. Lies outside the blood–brain barrier; chemoreceptor cells within it are thus directly exposed to blood-borne chemicals. Stimulated by noradrenaline, dopamine, acetylcholine, 5-HT and opioid receptor agonists. Circulating emetics, e.g. opioid analgesic drugs, may cause vomiting by stimulating the CTZ, which sends efferents to the vomiting centre of the medulla. Some antiemetic drugs, e.g. phenothiazines, act by inhibiting dopamine receptors within the CTZ.

Chemoreceptors. Receptors responding to chemical stimulation, producing action potentials when triggered by certain (often specific) molecules. The precise linking mechanisms are generally unknown.
- Examples:
  - taste and smell receptors.
  - O_2, CO_2 and hydrogen ion receptors.
  - chemoreceptor trigger zone cells.

See also, Aortic bodies; Breathing, control of; Carotid bodies

Chest drainage. Removal of air or liquid from the interpleural cavity, e.g. in the management of pneumothorax, haemothorax and pleural effusions.
- Effusions and small pneumothoraces are often drained by pleural tap. Technique:
  - the patient is usually seated with shoulders flexed and arms resting on a pillow. A posterior approach is usual.
  - the needle or cannula is advanced above the upper edge of the rib (upper chest for pneumothorax; lower for effusion) to avoid the nerve and vessels in the intercostal space. Air entry is prevented by connecting the needle to a syringe at all times, and aspirating continuously during advancement.
  - a three-way tap prevents air entry during aspiration.

Wide-bore chest drains (pleural drains) are inserted for drainage of larger fluid collections and pneumothoraces. They may also be inserted prophylactically in patients with rib fractures about to undergo anaesthesia, especially involving IPPV. Sizes 20–28 FG (French Gauge: external circumference in mm; approximately 3× external diameter) are suitable for most adults although small-bore drains (10–20 FG), often inserted using a Seldinger technique, are preferred by some because they are said to be easier to insert and more comfortable, though they are more likely to block. IV cannulae may be inserted for emergency treatment of tension pneumothorax.
- Insertion (of wide-bore tubes):
  - the site chosen is usually between the 4th and 7th intercostal spaces, between the mid-axillary and anterior

axillary lines. Previous recommendations for use of the 2nd intercostal space anteriorly have lost popularity because a drain in this position tends to transfix the pectoral muscles and may interfere with ventilation. Patients may be sitting or supine.
- using aseptic technique, the skin and subcutaneous tissues are infiltrated with local anaesthetic agent, down to the periosteum of the upper surface of the chosen rib. The needle is advanced above the rib, continuing to inject local anaesthetic. Imaging should be used if aspiration fails to confirm the correct site.
- the chest wall is incised about 2 cm below the proposed site of pleural incision, cutting down on to the rib below. Blunt dissection is achieved using artery forceps, through to the pleural cavity and the tip of a finger inserted to sweep adherent lung away from the insertion site. IPPV should be temporarily halted if possible when the pleura is actually punctured, to reduce damage to the lung.
- the drain is inserted into the pleural cavity and slid into position (usually towards the apex). Although a rigid trocar has been traditionally used, this has largely been abandoned to reduce the likelihood of trauma to the lung. Blunt dissection may not be required if small-bore tubes are inserted under imaging.
- the drain is connected to an underwater seal device (see below), observing the water level for swinging/bubbling with respiration. One-way flutter valves may also be used, e.g. Heimlich valve (flattened rubber tube within a clear plastic tubing).
- a suture is inserted around the puncture site to aid sealing after removal, and dressings are applied.
- plastic tubes are most commonly employed. Most tubes have side holes to aid drainage, and a radio-opaque longitudinal line.
- chest X-ray demonstrates the position and effect of the drain.
- complications include haemorrhage, trauma to intrathoracic structures, vagally mediated bradycardia during insertion, post-expansion pulmonary oedema, disconnection or blockage of the drain, and aspiration of air or water from the seal into the chest.
- the drain is usually removed 12–24 h after cessation of air or fluid loss, often after a trial period of clamping. Chest X-ray is mandatory following removal.

- The underwater seal should have certain features (Fig. 37a):
  - tube A must be wide to minimise resistance. Its volumetric capacity should exceed half of the patient's maximal inspiratory volume or water may be aspirated into the chest during inspiration.
  - the volume of water above the end of tube B should exceed half of the patient's maximal inspiratory volume to prevent indrawing of air during inspiration.
  - the end of tube B should not be more than 5 cm below the surface of the water, or its resistance may prevent air being blown off.
  - the drain should always be at least 45 cm below the patient.
  - tube A should be temporarily clamped when the underwater seal's integrity may be disrupted, e.g. during transfer from bed to trolley, etc.
  - suction may be applied to tube C, although this is controversial. 10–20 cmH_2O suction is usually employed.
  - a three-bottle system is often used, especially after cardiac or thoracic surgery (Fig. 37b). Bottle A acts as a fluid trap, e.g. for accurate measurement of blood. Bottle B provides the underwater seal. Bottle C allows suction; the height of the water level determines the amount of suction applied before air is drawn in through tube D as a safety suction-limiting device. Modern systems incorporate all three bottles in one plastic unit.

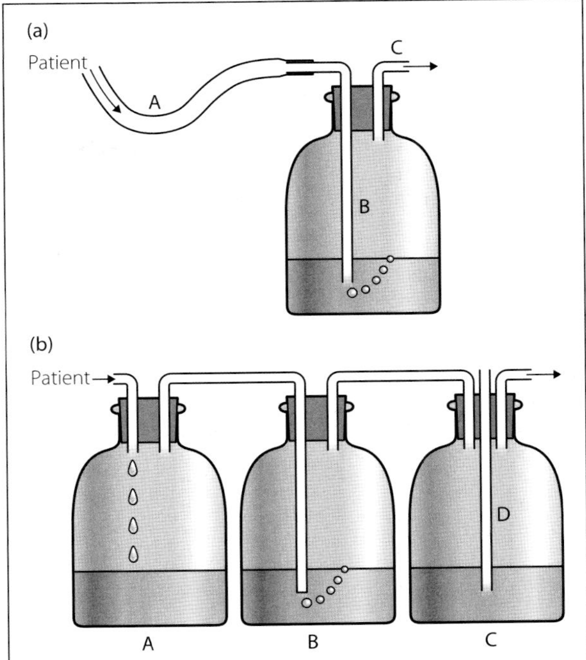

Fig. 37 Chest drainage systems: (a) one-bottle; (b) three-bottle

Laws D, Neville E, Duffy J (2003). Thorax; 58: 53–9

Chest infection. Includes tracheitis, laryngotracheobronchitis (croup), acute bronchitis, bronchiolitis, acute exacerbations of COPD and bronchiectasis and pneumonia.
- Pneumonia may be:
  - primary: specific pathogens are usually involved:
    - bacteria, e.g. *Streptococcus pneumoniae* (causing classical lobar pneumonia), *Haemophilus influenzae, Mycobacterium tuberculosis, Klebsiella pneumoniae.*
    - viruses, e.g. influenza, parainfluenza, measles. Viral bronchitis is very common and rarely severe unless coexisting disease is present.
    - others (often classified as large viruses/small bacteria), e.g. legionella, mycoplasma, rickettsia, chlamydia.
    - fungi, e.g. aspergillus.
  - opportunistic: occurs in immunodeficiency, e.g. infection with fungi, pneumocystis pneumonia (especially in HIV infection) and viruses, e.g. cytomegalovirus and herpes.
  - secondary: a respiratory tract abnormality allows usually fewer pathogenic organisms to spread, e.g. by aspiration from the GIT, upper airway, sinuses, etc. Thus bronchopneumonia may follow bronchial infection, causing patchy inflammation, collapse, consolidation and oedema. Commonly occurs in hospitalised patients, e.g. following anaesthesia, atelectasis, aspiration of gastric contents and hypoventilation. Gram-negative bacteria are commonly responsible, e.g. *Pseudomonas aeruginosa* and *Escherichia coli.*
- Features:
  - malaise, pyrexia, tachycardia. Legionnaires' disease may cause back pain and renal impairment.

- cough, sputum, haemoptysis.
- increased $\dot{V}/\dot{Q}$ mismatch and shunting causing hypoxaemia and tachypnoea.
- clinical and radiological features of consolidation and collapse, possibly leading to pleural effusion and empyema. Severe pulmonary destruction and abscess formation (suppuration) may follow, especially in staphylococcal infection.
- may lead to respiratory failure or bronchiectasis.

Microbiological diagnosis may be made on sputum culture; treatment is started according to the most likely organism. Serology or bronchial biopsy/washings may be useful in atypical cases.

- Treatment:
  - antimicrobial drugs.
  - supportive therapy; i.e. O_2 therapy, physiotherapy, etc.
- Anaesthetic/ICU relevance:
  - preoperative assessment and treatment of chest disease.
  - prevention of aspiration and reduction of atelectasis.
  - postoperatively: physiotherapy, adequate analgesia and avoidance of hypoventilation are important, especially in pre-existing chest disease.
  - risk of contamination of anaesthetic equipment by infected cases.
  - treatment of respiratory failure on ICU, or development of nosocomial pneumonia in patients receiving IPPV. The latter is a common problem and is related to impaired host defences, instrumentation of the airway and colonisation of the GIT with pathogenic organisms. Selective decontamination of the digestive tract has been used to reduce the incidence of nosocomial pneumonia (i.e. not present or incubating at the time of hospital admission) on ICU.

See also, Chest X-ray; Mycoplasma infections; Nosocomial infection; Pseudomonas infections; Streptococcal infections

Chest trauma. May be caused by road traffic accidents (RTAs), falls, assaults including stabbings and shootings, and explosions. Trauma may be:

- penetrating: in stabbing injuries, trauma tends to be localised to the track of the implement. In gunshot wounds, a small entry point may disguise major internal disruption (because of rapid dissipation of kinetic injury).
- non-penetrating:
  - blunt trauma, e.g. deceleration injury in RTAs. Damage is caused by direct impact (e.g. rib fractures, myocardial contusion) and shearing forces (e.g. aortic rupture, tracheobronchial tears).
  - blast injuries: sudden external chest and abdominal compression may cause alveolar and pulmonary vessel rupture, with oedema and haemorrhage. Further injury may result from flying objects, etc.
- Immediate life-threatening conditions:
  - severe hypoventilation caused by:
    - airway obstruction (especially likely with associated head injury).
    - pneumothorax/haemothorax.
    - flail chest.
  - reduced cardiac output caused by:
    - hypovolaemia caused by haemorrhage. Major vessel damage often accompanies fracture of the first two ribs. Aortic rupture usually occurs just beyond the left subclavian artery.
    - cardiac tamponade.
    - tension pneumothorax.
- Other conditions less immediately dangerous:
  - respiratory:
    - sternal/rib fractures.
    - tracheobronchial tears.
    - diaphragmatic rupture.
    - lung contusion.
    - aspiration of gastric contents (especially with head injury).
    - blast injury: symptoms may occur 2–3 days later. There may be associated smoke inhalation.

    $\dot{V}/\dot{Q}$ mismatch and shunt results in hypoxaemia. Ventilatory failure may also occur. Infection, ARDS, etc., may ensue.
  - cardiovascular:
    - myocardial contusion: may present as arrhythmias, cardiac failure or valve rupture.
    - damage to the coronary vessels and great vessels.
  - other injuries: head injury, vertebral and limb injuries, etc. Oesophageal rupture may occur, with risk of mediastinitis.
- Management:
  - immediate assessment and management of the above life-threatening conditions, i.e. sealing of any penetrating wound with dressings, etc., O_2 therapy, iv fluid administration. Airway patency and adequate respiratory movement should be checked. Chest percussion and auscultation may suggest pneumothorax or haemothorax. Heart sounds may be muffled in tamponade. Pulsus paradoxus may indicate tamponade or tension pneumothorax, whilst unequal pulses may suggest aortic dissection or rupture. Hypotension may occur in hypovolaemia, tamponade, tension pneumothorax and myocardial contusion.
  - subsequent assessment:
    - chest X-ray: may reveal pneumothorax, surgical emphysema, fractures, evidence of aspiration, and widened mediastinum (may represent aortic rupture, especially if associated with left haemothorax, depressed left main bronchus and oesophageal displacement to the right). Lung contusion may appear as fluffy patchy shadowing within a few hours of injury.
    - arterial blood gas analysis/pulse oximetry are especially useful.
    - ECG as a baseline. Serial ECG and cardiac enzyme changes may occur in myocardial contusion.
    - for other injuries.
  - chest drainage/pericardiocentesis as appropriate.
  - methods of analgesia include iv opioid analgesic drugs in small doses (but with risk of respiratory and cerebral depression), intercostal nerve block, interpleural analgesia, and epidural anaesthesia with local anaesthetic agent or opioids.
  - nasogastric tube to prevent gastric dilatation.
  - surgery may be required for severe haemorrhage or trauma to the aorta, diaphragm, tracheobronchial tree, oesophagus, etc.
  - physiotherapy/antibiotics. Lung contusion is exacerbated by overhydration, but hypovolaemia must be avoided.

Chest X-ray. Useful as an indication of structural abnormalities of cardiovascular and respiratory systems, but less informative about function. Often used as a screening test for unsuspected disease, e.g. preoperatively (*see Investigations, preoperative*).

- Plan for the interpretation of chest X-rays (Fig. 38):

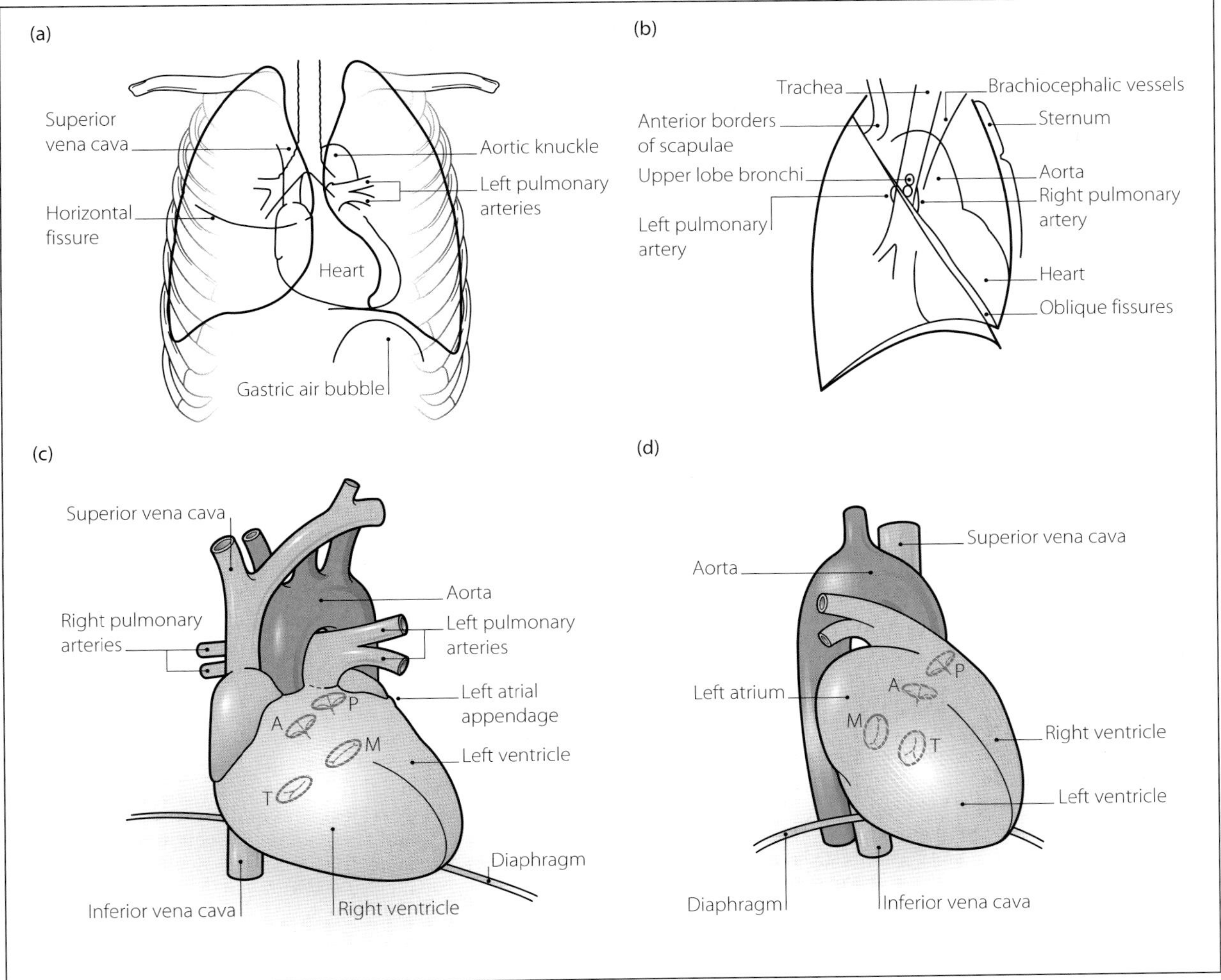

Fig. 38 Normal appearance chest X-ray: (a) PA; (b) lateral; (c) mediastinal structures, PA; (d) mediastinal structures, lateral. Position of valves: P, pulmonary; A, aortic; M, mitral; T, tricuspid

- describe the film:
  - date and patient's name.
  - orientation: i.e. right/left marker. Posteroanterior (PA): the scapulae shadows are carried laterally. Anteroposterior (AP): usually portable films, i.e. the patient is too ill to leave the ward. Assume PA unless AP is written on the film.
- describe any obvious abnormality first, otherwise continue with the plan.
- heart shadow:
  - normal width is under 50% of thoracic diameter (PA film).
  - abnormal border: may be aneurysm, chamber dilatation or overlying lesion.
  - part of border indistinct: may represent lung collapse/consolidation.
  - calcified/prosthetic valves: the aortic valve lies above a line drawn from the anterior costophrenic angle to the hilum on the lateral X-ray; the mitral valve lies below.
- upper **mediastinum** (i.e. width, aortic shadow, hila):
  - hilar enlargement may be due to pulmonary vascular or lymph node enlargement, or overlying lesion. The left hilum is usually higher than the right by 1–2 cm.
  - the carina usually overlies T4–5 on inspiration.
- lung fields:
  - upper zone (above anterior part of 2nd rib).
  - midzone (between 2nd and 4th rib).
  - lower zone (below 4th rib).
  - compare each with the other side for translucency. Look for **pneumothorax**.
  - the anterior portions of the first eight ribs are visible with normal expansion.
  - the left hemidiaphragm is usually lower than the right by 2 cm.
  - if shadowing is seen, the lesion may lie in skin, bone, lung, etc.; i.e. one cannot determine the lesion's depth from the PA/AP film alone; this requires a lateral film.
  - lung consolidation:
    - no evidence of collapse.
    - the border of the shadow with neighbouring structures is lost, aiding identification of the affected lung portion; e.g. an indistinct heart border represents consolidation anteriorly, since the heart lies anteriorly in the chest. Thus in lower lobe consolidation (posterior in the chest) the heart border remains clear.
  - lung collapse: as for consolidation, with reduced expansion on the affected side, mediastinal shift or

tracheal deviation. The collapsed portion of lung may be visible against neighbouring structures.
- pleural effusion: seen as an opacity sloping upwards and outwards at the lung base; if horizontal, it represents a gas/fluid interface.
- Kerley's lines may be present.
- upper lobe blood diversion (representing dilatation of the pulmonary vessels) occurs in left ventricular failure and left-to-right cardiac shunts. Proximal dilatation with peripheral narrowing (pruning) may represent pulmonary hypertension.
  - bones:
    - ribs (metastases, fractures, notching).
    - scapulae, vertebrae, humerus.
  - soft tissues:
    - below diaphragm.
    - above clavicles; neck.
    - axillae.
    - breasts.
    - central lines, tracheal tubes, etc.

Easily missed diagnoses to be remembered if unable to spot an abnormality include pneumothorax, dextrocardia and aortic coarctation.
See also, Thoracic inlet

Cheyne–Stokes respiration. Abnormal pattern of breathing characterised by alternating periods of hyperventilation and apnoea. Ventilation increases in depth and frequency to a peak, then decreases to apnoea. The cycle then repeats.
- Caused by:
  - central disturbance of control of breathing. Hypoventilation causes hypercapnia, which causes hyperventilation. Resultant hypocapnia causes apnoea until the arterial $P\text{CO}_2$ rises again. This pattern may occur in cerebral disease, head injury and opioid poisoning.
  - prolonged circulation between the lungs and brain. Hyperventilation continues until hypocapnia is registered by central chemoreceptors, although the CO_2 tension at the lungs is much lower. When the CO_2 content of blood arriving centrally is high enough to restart breathing, the CO_2 content of blood at the lungs is much higher, causing hyperventilation as it arrives at the chemoreceptors. This may occur with reduced cardiac output, e.g. in cardiac failure.

[John Cheyne (1777–1836), Scottish-born Irish physician; William Stokes (1804–1878), Irish physician]
See also, Breathing, control of

Chi-square analysis, *see Statistical tests*

CHI, Commission for Health Improvement, *see Healthcare Commission*

Chloral hydrate. Sedative prodrug, introduced in 1869. Metabolised to trichloroethanol, which has a half-life of 8–10 h. Causes minimal cardiovascular or respiratory depression. Gastric irritation may occur; it is less frequent with triclofos or dichloralphenazone, both of which are also metabolised to trichloroethanol.
- Dosage: 25–50 mg/kg (children) orally/rectally. 0.5–1 g (adults).

Chloramphenicol. Bacteriostatic antibacterial drug; inhibits bacterial ribosomal activity and thus protein synthesis. Has a broad spectrum of activity but because of its potential toxicity is usually reserved for life-threatening infections especially with *Haemophilus influenzae* and typhoid. Penetrates into CSF extremely well, thus often used in meningitis. 70% protein-bound, it undergoes extensive hepatic metabolism. Half-life is 4 h.
- Dosage: 50–100 mg/kg orally/iv daily in 4 divided doses.
- Side effects:
  - aplastic anaemia (often irreversible), peripheral or optic neuritis, nausea, vomiting, diarrhoea, erythema multiforme, nocturnal haemoglobinuria.
  - the 'grey baby syndrome' (cardiovascular collapse) may occur in neonates unable to metabolise the drug. Plasma concentrations should be monitored in children under 4 years old; recommended peak and trough levels are 15–25 μg/ml and < 15 μg/ml respectively.
  - may enhance the effect of warfarin.

Chloride shift (Hamburger shift). Movement of chloride ions into red blood cells as O_2 is given up and exchanged for CO_2 in the tissues. CO_2 enters the cells, is converted to carbonic acid by carbonic anhydrase, and dissociates into hydrogen ions and bicarbonate. The former are buffered by the reduced haemoglobin; the latter passes into the plasma. Chloride ions enter the cells to maintain electrical equilibrium. The reverse occurs in the lungs.
[Hartog J Hamburger (1859–1924), Dutch physiologist]

Chlormethiazole, *see Clomethiazole*

Chloroform. $CHCl_3$. Inhalational anaesthetic agent; used in 1847 by Simpson, although it had been used earlier. Rapidly became more popular than diethyl ether, and was administered to Queen Victoria during childbirth. Sweet smelling and pleasant to inhale, with similar properties to halothane including non-flammability. Given by pouring on to a towel, especially in Scotland, or by inhalers, especially in London. Risk of sudden death, usually during induction, was attributed to respiratory depression in Scotland and cardiac standstill in England. The First and Second Hyderabad Commissions in 1888 and 1889 respectively, financed by the Nizam of Hyderabad (1866–1911), concluded that sudden death by respiratory depression preceded cardiac arrest. The reverse was generally accepted over 20 years later. VF occurred most commonly. Also caused severe hepatic failure. Gradually replaced by diethyl ether by the early/mid 1900s.
Payne JP (1981). Br J Anaesth; 53: 11S–15S
For physical properties, see Inhalational anaesthetic agents

Chloroprocaine hydrochloride. Ester local anaesthetic agent, introduced in 1952. Of short onset and duration of action, with low systemic toxicity and rapid offset (after approximately 45 min). Hydrolysed by plasma cholinesterase. Used for epidural anaesthesia, particularly for Caesarean section in the USA and a few European countries but not available in the UK. Used in 2–3% solutions. Neurological deficits (after accidental intrathecal injection) and backache have followed use of preparations containing preservative. Maximal safe dose is about 15 mg/kg.

Chloroquine. Antimalarial drug, also used to treat rheumatoid arthritis. Should be used with caution in patients with hepatic or renal impairment, pregnancy and epilepsy. No longer recommended in falciparum malaria since most strains are resistant.
- Dosage:
  - treatment: 600 mg orally, then 300 mg after 6 h and 300 mg daily for 2 days.
  - for sensitive strains of severe falciparum malaria, iv therapy may be used: 10 mg base/kg iv over 8 h, then

5 mg/kg 8 hourly × 3. Oral therapy is started when possible to a total dose of 25 mg/kg.
   - prophylaxis: 300 mg once weekly 1 week before travel and for 6 weeks after returning.
- Side effects: GIT upset, headache, visual disturbance, skin and hair reactions, blood dyscrasias, psychosis, ECG changes, neuromuscular and myopathic weakness. Has a low therapeutic index and overdosage may cause rapidly developing arrhythmias and convulsions.

Chlorphenamine maleate (Chlorpheniramine). Antihistamine drug; competes with histamine at H_1 receptors. Used to treat allergic reactions, both mild, e.g. hay fever, and severe, e.g. anaphylactic reaction. Also used to treat generalised itching, e.g. in obstructive jaundice or after spinal opioids. Duration of action is up to 6 h.
- Dosage:
   - 4 mg orally 4–6 hourly.
   - 10–20 mg im, sc or iv by slow injection, up to 40 mg/day.
- Side effects:
   - drowsiness, anticholinergic effects.
   - hypotension and central nervous stimulation may follow iv injection.

Chlorpromazine hydrochloride. Phenothiazine, used as an antipsychotic and sedative drug, also in terminal disease and intractable hiccup. First used in the early 1950s, and called Largactil because of its large number of actions. Has been used before and during anaesthesia (e.g. lytic cocktail). Has powerful sedative and antiemetic properties, with anticholinergic, antidopaminergic and α-adrenergic receptor antagonist effects.
- Dosage: 25–50 mg orally or im, 8 hourly (larger doses may be required). May also be given iv (but not licensed), well diluted to avoid thrombophlebitis. Hypotension may follow parenteral injection. May be given rectally as chlorpromazine base 100 mg.
- Side effects: as for phenothiazines.

Choanal atresia. Congenital blockage of one or both nasal passages. Incidence is 1:8000 births. If bilateral, it causes severe airway obstruction from birth, since neonates are obligatory nose breathers. Respiratory distress and cyanosis are characteristically reduced during crying, when mouth breathing occurs. May be demonstrated following attempted passage of a soft catheter through the nostrils. Other congenital defects and syndromes may be associated, e.g. VSD.
- Management:
   - oropharyngeal airway insertion, with secure taping to the face.
   - puncture of membrane/bone is usually performed within a few days, and plastic tubes inserted.
- Anaesthetic management: classically, awake tracheal intubation is performed following preoxygenation, using an oral tube and throat pack; modern management and general considerations are as for any neonate. Extubation is performed awake.

Choking. Acute airway obstruction in a conscious person. There may be wheezing, coughing and obvious distress; if obstruction is complete the victim is silent. Typically the victim grips his/her throat.
- Management:
   - adults:
      - removal of material from the mouth if obvious.
      - a series of up to 5 sharp slaps between the shoulder blades, with the victim leaning well forward.
      - Heimlich manoeuvre (or upper abdominal thrusts aiming towards the diaphragm if the victim is supine) up to 5 times, then 5 back slaps, etc.
      - CPR along standard lines if required.
   - children:
      - blind sweeps with the finger inside the mouth should be avoided since objects may be pushed further down the airway.
      - up to 5 back slaps with the child prone (head lower than chest).
      - up to 5 chest thrusts in the supine position (similar technique to external cardiac massage but sharper and more vigorous; one every 3 s).
      - the mouth is checked, with expired air ventilation if apnoeic.
      - the cycle is repeated but with up to 5 abdominal thrusts instead of chest thrusts, then alternating the two in successive cycles. Abdominal thrusts should be avoided in children < 1 year since visceral rupture may occur.

Cholangitis, acute. Acute bacterial infection of the biliary tract. Varies from mild illness to acute fulminant cholangitis with a 50% mortality. Almost always associated with complete or partial biliary obstruction, e.g. caused by gallstones or surgery. May occur in critically ill patients as an unsuspected cause of SIRS.
- Features:
   - Charcot's triad: fever, abdominal pain and jaundice; occurs in 60% of cases.
   - increased bilirubin, alkaline phosphatase and transaminases in 90% of cases.
   - positive blood culture (most commonly *Escherichia coli*, enterococci, klebsiella) in 45% of cases.

Ultrasound and/or hepatobiliary scanning may confirm the diagnosis.
- Management:
   - supportive: iv fluids, O_2 therapy, analgesia, antibacterial drugs. Full ICU support may be required in fulminant cases.
   - emergency percutaneous, open or endoscopic gallbladder drainage.

[Jean M Charcot (1825–1893), Paris neurologist]

Cholecystitis, acute. Inflammation of the wall of the gallbladder. A recognised complication of critical illness, it may occur in the absence of gallstones (acalculous cholecystitis). Aetiology may include gallbladder ischaemia, biliary 'sludging' and cystic duct obstruction; contributory factors include fever, sepsis, dehydration, opioid analgesic drugs and TPN. Mortality may be 50%.
- Features:
   - fever, leucocytosis, abdominal pain/tenderness and loss of bowel sounds.
   - increased alkaline phosphatase and bilirubin in 50% of cases.
   - diagnosis is confirmed by ultrasonography and hepatobiliary scanning.
- Management:
   - broad-spectrum antibacterial drugs to cover aerobic and anaerobic organisms.
   - emergency percutaneous, endoscopic or open drainage of the gallbladder may be required if clinical deterioration continues despite antibacterial therapy.

See also, Biliary tract

Cholinergic crisis. Syndrome caused by relative overdosage of acetylcholinesterase inhibitors causing excess nicotinic (muscle weakness, fasciculation) and muscarinic (sweating, miosis, lacrimation, abdominal colic, etc.) stimulation by **acetylcholine**. May occur in **myasthenia gravis**, when differentiation from myasthenic crisis may be difficult. Administration of **edrophonium** 2 mg iv may improve myasthenic crises but worsen or have no effect on cholinergic crises. Usually treated by stopping acetylcholinesterase inhibitor therapy, giving **atropine**, and providing respiratory support if required.

Cholinergic receptors, *see Acetylcholine receptors*

Cholinesterase, plasma (Pseudocholinesterase). Circulating **enzyme**, produced by the liver, of unknown primary function but which hydrolyses **suxamethonium**, removing choline groups to produce first succinylmonocholine and then succinic acid. Also present in other tissues, e.g. brain and kidneys.

- Reduced enzyme activity causes prolonged paralysis after suxamethonium, and may be due to:
  - inherited atypical cholinesterase. Several autosomal recessive genes have been identified, using the degree of enzyme inhibition by various substances (e.g. dibucaine or fluoride) to describe the enzyme characteristics:
    - normal enzyme (designated E1u): 94% of the population are homozygotes. **Dibucaine number** (DN) is 75–85, and fluoride number (FN) 60.
    - atypical enzyme (E1a): 0.03% of the population are homozygotes, with DN 15–25 and FN 20.
    - silent gene (E1s): 0.001% of the population are homozygotes, with no plasma cholinesterase activity.
    - fluoride-resistant enzyme (E1f): 0.0001% of the population are homozygotes; DN is 65–75 but FN is 30.

    Paralysis may last 2–4 h in homozygotes for silent and atypical genes, and 1–2 h in homozygotes for the fluoride-resistant gene. In addition, heterozygotes with one normal and one abnormal gene (e.g. E1u/E1a; 5% of the population) with DN 40–60 may show prolonged paralysis of about 10–20 min. Most of these have the atypical gene. Combinations of abnormal genes comprise less than 0.01% of the population and also show slight or marked prolongation of paralysis.
  - acquired deficiency of normal cholinesterase, e.g. in **hepatic failure**, **hypoproteinaemia**, **pregnancy**, **malnutrition**, **burns**, or following **plasmapheresis**.
  - inhibition of cholinesterase by drugs, e.g. **echothiophate**, **cyclophosphamide**, **tetrahydroaminocrine**, **hexafluorenium** or phenelzine.

Plasma cholinesterase also hydrolyses other drugs, e.g. **mivacurium**, ester **local anaesthetic drugs**, **diamorphine**, **aspirin** and **propanidid**. Although **esmolol** and **remifentanil** are readily hydrolysed by non-specific cholinesterases, plasma cholinesterase itself is not thought to be important in their breakdown.

Chronic bronchitis, *see Chronic obstructive pulmonary disease*

Chronic obstructive airways disease (COAD), *see Chronic obstructive pulmonary disease.*

Chronic obstructive pulmonary disease (COPD; Chronic obstructive airways disease; COAD). Term encompassing chronic bronchitis and emphysema, which although different histologically, often coexist. The main features are lower airway obstruction, hyperinflated lungs and impaired gas exchange.

- Chronic bronchitis:
  - defined clinically by productive cough each morning for at least 3 months per year, for at least 2 successive years.
  - results from chronic bronchial irritation, e.g. by smoke, dust or fumes, causing:
    - mucosal hypersecretion.
    - mucosal oedema.
    - bronchoconstriction.
  - features: cough, dyspnoea, wheeze, tendency to develop **chest infection** causing acute exacerbations. Sufferers are typically described as 'blue bloaters' because of cyanosis and oedema.
  - **FEV_1**, expiratory flow rate and FEV/**FVC** are decreased, with increased **residual volume** and **FRC**, and **$\dot{V}/\dot{Q}$ mismatch**.
  - **hypoxaemia** and **hypercapnia** result, with possible loss of the central response to CO_2 (the mechanism is unclear). **Hypoxic pulmonary vasoconstriction** may lead to **pulmonary hypertension** with **cor pulmonale** and right ventricular failure.
- Emphysema:
  - defined histologically by dilated alveoli and/or respiratory bronchioles, often in upper areas of the lungs. Different patterns of dilatation are identified. Elastic recoil is reduced.
  - causes: as above, plus α_1-antitrypsin deficiency; the latter typically affects the lung bases.
  - features: dyspnoea. Air trapping and increased airflow resistance result from airway collapse during forceful expiration. Breath sounds are usually quiet. Sufferers are typically described as 'pink puffers' because of absent cyanosis and marked dyspnoea.
  - work of breathing is markedly increased, with hypocapnia (i.e. hyperventilation as opposed to hypoventilation as in chronic bronchitis), but only mild hypoxaemia.
  - FEV_1 is reduced and FRC increased as above.

Diffusing capacity is decreased in both conditions. **Respiratory muscle fatigue** may be a factor.

- Patients may present with **respiratory failure** requiring **non-invasive positive pressure ventilation** or **IPPV** on ICU/HDU. Main considerations:
  - the decision to intubate/ventilate is sometimes hard, since **weaning from ventilators** is often difficult or even impossible. Useful information in making the decision concerning IPPV:
    - level of normal activity and lifestyle.
    - previous admissions, whether ventilated and ease of weaning.
    - whether the current crisis represents gradual decline or an acute treatable event, e.g. infection.
  - management is as for respiratory failure. **Doxapram** may be used in an attempt to prevent the requirement for IPPV: 1.5–4 mg/min according to response, with frequent arterial blood gas analysis. IPPV via a tightly fitting mask is increasingly used for acute exacerbations of COPD. **Minitracheotomy** or **tracheostomy** may assist weaning.
- Anaesthetic management:
  - preoperatively:
    - **preoperative assessment** for exercise tolerance, bronchospasm, cor pulmonale and history of previous admissions. Patients are likely to be smokers; thus cardiovascular assessment including **ECG** is important. **Chest X-ray** may reveal a hyperexpanded chest, flattened diaphragm, narrow mediastinum, emphysematous bullae or infection. Arterial blood gas analysis and **lung function tests** may be useful.

- improvement by physiotherapy and antibiotics if infection is present, and bronchodilator drugs if there is a reversible element to airway obstruction.
- premedication: increased sensitivity to respiratory depressants, especially in chronic bronchitis, is rarely a problem. Pethidine, promethazine and atropine are often used; the latter may help prevent perioperative bronchospasm and reduce secretions, but may increase their tenacity.

- perioperatively:
  - regional techniques are often suitable; problems may include inability to lie flat, possibility of coughing, and sensitivity to sedative drugs if used.
  - general anaesthesia:
    - inhalational techniques with a facepiece are suitable for short procedures, with minimal airway manipulation.
    - if tracheal intubation is undertaken, topical or iv lidocaine may be used to reduce irritation by the tracheal tube. Tracheal suction is often required. Bronchospasm and coughing may occur. Emphysematous bullae are at risk of expansion or rupture with IPPV and N_2O. Capnography allows maintenance of expired P_{CO_2} at the patient's normal (i.e. preoperative) level.
    - drugs causing histamine release are usually avoided.
- postoperative problems include:
  - sputum retention, bronchospasm, atelectasis and infection. Physiotherapy and bronchodilator therapy are important. Respiratory failure may occur. Doxapram may be useful. Ventilation is often improved in the sitting position.
  - hypoventilation may be exacerbated by pain, depressant drugs and high F_IO_2. Adequate postoperative analgesia is vital; regional techniques are particularly useful, as excessive use of systemic opioids must be avoided. Parenteral opioids are best given by infusion or small iv increments.
  - patients with severe disease or those receiving spinal opioids should be managed on ICU/HDU.
  - elective IPPV may allow adequate gas exchange whilst depressant anaesthetic drugs are cleared. It also 'covers' the period of worst postoperative pain and allows stabilisation before weaning.

Sutherland ER, Cherniak RM (2004). N Engl J Med; 350: 2689–97

Churchill, Frederick, *see Liston, Robert*

Ciclosporin (Cyclosporin). Isomerase binding immunosuppressive drug which interferes with proliferation of activated T lymphocytes. Main use is to prevent and treat rejection following organ transplantation. Has also been used in myasthenia gravis and other autoimmune diseases. Oral administration has 30% bioavailability.

Eliminated via hepatic metabolism, its half-life assuming normal liver function is 19 h.

- Dosage: 3–5 mg/kg/day iv, followed by 12–15 mg/kg/day orally. After 1–2 weeks, the dose is reduced by 5–10% per week. Therapeutic blood levels vary between centres but should be monitored.
- Side effects:
  - reduces GFR by at least 20% in almost all patients; renal function returns to normal within 2 weeks of stopping the drug, even following prolonged use. Irreversible nephrotoxicity occurs in a minority of cardiac and renal transplant patients.
  - GIT upset, gum hyperplasia, hirsutism, hyperkalaemia, mild hepatic impairment, hypertension, tremor, occasionally convulsions and encephalopathy.
  - interacts with other drugs that cause hyperkalaemia or nephrotoxicity, and increases plasma concentrations of several drugs including diclofenac and digoxin.

Cigarette smoking, *see Smoking*

Ciliary activity. Continuous beating of the cilia of respiratory epithelial cells results in flow of thick mucus from the nose to the pharynx, and from the bronchi to the larynx. The mucus is then swallowed or expectorated. A more watery mucus layer lies between the thick layer and the epithelium, lubricating the cilia. Important in aiding removal of foreign particles, microbes, etc. and clearing of the airways. Reduced by smoking, extremes of temperature, volatile inhalational anaesthetic agents, opioid analgesic drugs and prolonged exposure to high O_2 levels. Prolonged inhalation of dry gases, anticholinergic drug administration and volatile agents may impair mucus production or flow.

Patients with inborn deficiency of cilia protein are predisposed to bronchiectasis; if associated with decreased spermatic activity, situs inversus and chronic sinusitis this constitutes Kartagener's syndrome.

[Manes Kartagener (1897–1975), Swiss physician]

Cimetidine. H_2 receptor antagonist, of faster onset and shorter-acting than ranitidine, lasting about 4 h. Half-life is 2 h; up to 5 h in renal failure.

- Dosage:
  - 400 mg orally, usually once/twice daily. Effective if given 90 min preoperatively.
  - 200 mg im or iv by infusion (may cause bradycardia and hypotension after rapid iv injection).
- Side effects:
  - gynaecomastia, rarely impotence (binds to androgen receptors).
  - hepatic enzyme inhibition (binds to microsomal cytochrome P_{450}). The actions of drugs such as warfarin, phenytoin and theophylline may be prolonged, and toxic effects seen.
  - confusion, especially in the elderly and very ill.
  - rarely, liver impairment and blood dyscrasias.

Cinchocaine hydrochloride. Amide local anaesthetic agent, synthesised in 1925. Formerly, widely used in the UK for spinal anaesthesia, in doses of 0.5–2.0 ml of 1:200 in 6% dextrose heavy solution. Now unavailable apart from compound ointments for haemorrhoids. Has been used for epidural anaesthesia (1:600 solution), infiltration and nerve blocks (1:1000–2000 with adrenaline), and surface analgesia, up to 2 mg/kg maximum. Of slower onset and duration of action than lidocaine, and more toxic.

Used to estimate plasma cholinesterase activity (dibucaine number).

Ciprofloxacin. 4-Quinolone type antibacterial drug; acts by inhibiting bacterial DNA replication. Has a broad spectrum of activity, but especially against Gram-negative bacteria including klebsiella, escherichia, salmonella, shigella, campylobacter, neisseria, pseudomonas, haemophilus and enterobacter species. Less active against Gram-positive bacteria, e.g. streptococcus and anaerobes. Also active against chlamydia and certain mycobacteria.

- Dosage:
  - 250–750 mg orally 12 hourly.
  - 200–400 mg iv over 30–60 min, 12 hourly.
- Side effects
  - GIT upset, headache, skin reactions, renal and hepatic impairment, arthralgia, tendon inflammation/damage; less commonly blood dyscrasias, haemolytic anaemia, confusion, convulsions.
  - may enhance the effects of theophyllines and warfarin.
  - difficult to administer in critically ill patients since it may block nasogastric tubes, and chelates with Ca^{2+}, Mg^{2+} and Fe^{2+}, reducing bioavailability.

Circle of Willis, *see Cerebral circulation*

Circle systems. CO_2 absorption with soda lime was used by Waters in 1923, and a circle system employing valves by Sword in 1926. Usage increased in 1930s with the introduction of cyclopropane, then declined. Interest resurged in the 1990s because of worries about volatile anaesthetic agent cost and pollution.

- Advantages:
  - cheap, since low gas flows are required.
  - reduced risk of pollution, and of explosions and fires with inflammable agents.
  - warmth and humidity of expired gases are retained, with further warming and humidification in the CO_2 absorber, although efficiency is reduced by passage through lengths of tubing.
  - spontaneous/controlled ventilation is easily performed without changing the system.
  - allows easy monitoring of O_2 uptake/CO_2 output.
- Disadvantages:
  - production of carbon monoxide has occurred when volatile agents containing the CHF_2 moiety (desflurane, enflurane or isoflurane) are passed over dry warm absorbent (especially baralyme), e.g. at the start of a Monday morning operating session following prolonged passage of dry gas through the absorber. Avoidance of allowing the absorbent to dry out has been suggested.

    Other substances which may accumulate in the circle, especially if very low fresh gas flows are used over a long time, include methane and hydrogen from bacterial activity in the patient (the former may interfere with certain gas analysers and give falsely high concentrations of volatile agents); alcohol derived from the patient; compound A and bromochlorodifluoroethylene following use of sevoflurane and halothane respectively; acetone in some starved patients; and the solvent used in orthopaedic cement. None of these has been associated with adverse clinical effects.
  - higher resistance and thus work of breathing.
  - bulky equipment.
  - slow changes in anaesthetic concentrations at low gas flows.
  - risk of hypoxic gas mixtures if N_2O is used.
  - more connections to come apart, valves to stick, etc.
- Systems used:
  - resistance is reduced by using wide-bore tubing.
  - consist of absorber, two one-way valves, adjustable pressure-limiting (APL) valve, reservoir bag, tubing to and from the patient and for fresh gas supply (FGF). Efficiency is increased by placing:
    - FGF downstream to APL valve (avoids venting of fresh gas).
    - bag and patient on opposite sides of the one-way valves (maintains circulatory gas flow).

    Examples of arrangements (Fig. 39): system A is efficient for spontaneous ventilation and IPPV; dead space gas is conserved beyond the APL valve during expiration whilst alveolar gas is flushed by FGF via the APL valve. System B is less efficient because the APL valve is further away from the patient; dead space and alveolar gases mix more before reaching it. System B is more convenient practically, however, since all components are away from the patient.
  - ready-assembled circle systems are usual now, arranged as in system B within one housing (jumbo absorber). Older systems had an on/off switch that could bypass the soda lime; to prevent the risk of this happening accidentally these are not present on newer systems.
- Use:
  - if N_2O is used, build-up of nitrogen in the system may lead to a low F_IO_2. Nitrogen is removed first from the lungs, then slowly from body tissues. A high FGF (5–7 l/min) for 7–10 min is sufficient to remove most body nitrogen; the remainder (approximately 1 litre) slowly accumulates within the system. High flows are also required to prevent excessive dilution of FGF by exhaled gas during initial uptake of FGF gases. Hourly flushing with high flows has been suggested. Reflushing is required if the circle is broken at any time. Increased N_2O concentration within the system as its uptake decreases may also contribute to low F_IO_2.
  - if only O_2 is used, hypoxic mixtures do not occur, but atelectasis and O_2 toxicity are more likely.
  - with high flow, the APL valve is open.
  - low flow is defined as equal to or under 3 l/min FGF:
    - APL valve totally closed: FGF supplies basal requirements only, i.e. 220–250 ml/min O_2.
    - APL valve slightly open, i.e. allowing a small leak: 1–3 l/min is often used as a compromise between the closed and high flow systems.
  - IPPV is achieved by hand or by switching the reservoir bag to a bellows which may be compressed intermittently by an integral ventilator (if present in the anaesthetic machine). If there is no integral ventilator, a suitable ventilator, e.g. Penlon Nuffield may be attached to the reservoir bag attachment by tubing of adequate length to prevent mixing of the driving gas (O_2) and the FGF.
  - continuous gas analysis is particularly important.
  - vaporisers:
    - out of circle (VOC):
      - usual plenum vaporisers are used on the back bar of the anaesthetic machine.

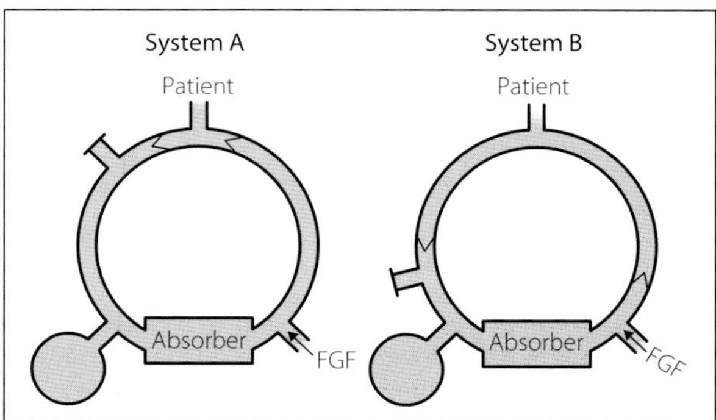

Fig. 39 Examples of circle systems (see text)

- the concentration of volatile agent within the circle is less than that delivered by the vaporiser, because of dilution by exhaled gas. The difference is highest initially, when uptake of agent is greatest, unless high FGFs are used. The time to reach equilibrium is least for insoluble agents.
- in circle (VIC):
  - low resistance vaporisers are required, e.g. Goldman's (*see Vaporisers*). Delivered concentration is related to gas flow through the vaporiser.
  - as volatile agent is present in exhaled gas entering the vaporiser, high concentrations are possible. During spontaneous ventilation, respiratory depression increases as the concentration increases, reducing gas flow through the vaporiser. Thus dangerous levels of agent are not reached. During IPPV, this feedback mechanism is absent; i.e. dangerous levels are attainable.
- liquid anaesthetic may be injected directly into the tubing.

[Brian Sword (1889–1956), US anaesthetist]

Circulation, respiration, abdomen, motor and speech scale (CRAMS scale). Trauma scale for use in adult pre-hospital triage when categorising severity of injury. Scores of 2 (normal), 1 or 0 are assigned to each of the five systems assessed. Rarely used in isolation now.
Gormican SP (1982). Ann Emerg Med; 11: 132–5

Cisapride. Prokinetic drug chemically related to metoclopramide but without antidopaminergic activity or central depressant effects. Increases lower oesophageal pressure and increases gastric emptying and intestinal motility. Acts by increasing acetylcholine release in the myenteric plexus within the gut wall. Reverses morphine-induced gastric stasis. Withdrawn from use in July 2000 because of reports of serious ventricular arrhythmias, often resulting from concomitant use of other drugs such as antifungal and antibacterial drugs.

Cisatracurium besylate. Non-depolarising neuromuscular blocking drug, one of the 10 stereoisomers of atracurium (the 1R *cis*–1′R cis isomer; makes up 15% of atracurium, contributing about 60% of its activity). Introduced in 1995, it causes minimal histamine release with cardiovascular stability. Also, although up to 70% metabolised by Hofmann elimination (cf. atracurium, 50–60%), produces about 10 times less laudanosine than atracurium after prolonged infusion, because of its greater potency and thus smaller total dosage. Initial dose: 0.1–0.2 mg/kg. Intubation is possible approximately 120 s after a dose of 0.15 mg/kg. Effects last 30–40 min. Supplementary dose: 0.03 mg/kg. Has been given by iv infusion at 0.06–0.18 mg/kg/h (1–3 μg/kg/min). Storage requirements are as for atracurium. Faster degradation occurs when diluted in Hartmann's solution and 5% dextrose than in other iv fluids.
See also, Isomerism

Citrate and citrate solutions, *see Blood storage; Sodium citrate*

CJD, *see Creutzfeldt–Jakob disease*

Clapeyron–Clausius equation. Describes the theoretical variation of SVP with temperature, depending on latent heat of vaporisation (LH). Assumes LH is independent of temperature, and that the volume of liquid is negligible compared to that of the vapour.
[Benoit-Paul Clapeyron (1799–1864), French engineer; Rudolf Clausius (1822–1888), German physicist]

Clark electrode, *see Oxygen measurement*

Clarke, William E (1818–1878). US physician; used diethyl ether to allow dental extraction in January 1842 in New York, but only reported this after Morton's demonstration in 1846.

Clarithromycin. Macrolide-type antibacterial drug derived from erythromycin and with similar mechanism of action and spectrum of activity, although more active against *Streptococcus pneumoniae* and *Staphylococcus aureus*, and with greater penetration of tissues. GIT side effects are less common than with erythromycin.

- Dosage:
  - 250–500 mg orally 12 hourly.
  - 500 mg iv 12 hourly.
- Side effects: nausea, vomiting, hepatic impairment, phlebitis, Stevens–Johnson syndrome.

Clathrates. Compounds formed by inclusion of molecules within a crystal lattice of a different substance. Formation of clathrates with water (gas hydrates) affecting brain cell membranes (as 'icebergs' within them) was suggested by Pauling and Miller in 1961 as a basis for the mechanism of action of inhalational anaesthetic agents.
Now considered incorrect since:

- for some fluorocarbons, potency is not related to clathrate formation.
- some inhalational agents do not form clathrates at body temperature and pressure.
- effects of combining different agents are not accounted for.

[Linus Pauling (1901–1994) and Stanley L Miller (1930–2007), US chemists]
See also, Anaesthesia, mechanism of

Clavulanic acid. β-Lactamase inhibitor, used in combination with amoxicillin (as co-amoxiclav) and ticarcillin in order to prevent their breakdown by penicillinase produced by *Staphylococcus aureus* and other bacteria. Has been associated with cholestatic jaundice.

Clearance. Calculated figure, representing removal of a substance from plasma or blood by passage through an organ. Defined as the volume of plasma in ml completely cleared of substance per minute; thus for the kidney it equals:

$$\frac{\text{amount of substance excreted in urine per unit time}}{\text{plasma concentration of substance}}$$

$$= \frac{\text{urinary concentration (mmol/l)} \times \text{urine volume (ml/ min)}}{\text{plasma concentration (mmol/l)}}$$

The concept is useful in comparing excretion rates of different drugs; it is also used to determine renal blood flow and GFR. If there is incomplete removal by the kidney, clearance for a substance is less than GFR. If the substance is secreted into the urine by tubular cells, clearance exceeds GFR.
See also, Pharmacokinetics

Clearance, creatinine, *see Creatinine clearance*

Clearance, free water. Volume of plasma cleared of excess water per minute. Equals urine volume (ml/min) minus osmotic clearance (ml/min). Normally negative, i.e. water

is being conserved, and hypertonic urine produced. Positive in water diuresis.
See also, Clearance, osmotic

Clearance, osmotic. Estimation of renal solute excretion. Equals

$$\frac{\text{urine osmolality (mosmol/l)} \times \text{urine volume (ml/min)}}{\text{plasma osmolality (mosmol/l)}}$$

If urine is hypotonic, urine volume exceeds osmotic clearance; if hypertonic, osmotic clearance is greater. The difference between them is free water clearance. Normally under 3 ml/min; increased by osmotic diuretics.
See also, Clearance, free water

Cleft lip and palate, *see Facial deformities, congenital*

Clindamycin. Bacteriostatic antibacterial drug, a semisynthetic derivative of lincomycin. Although active against aerobic and anaerobic Gram-positive organisms, its use is limited to the treatment of staphylococcal bone and joint infection, peritonitis and endocarditis because of its side effects (especially infection with *Clostridium difficile* and the development of pseudomembranous colitis). 95% protein-bound, it undergoes hepatic metabolism to inactive metabolites, with 20% excreted unchanged in the urine. Poor levels are attained in CSF.

- Dosage:
  - 150–450 mg orally 6 hourly.
  - 0.6–4.8 g/day in 2–4 divided doses im or by iv infusion (maximal single iv dose 1.2 g).
- Side effects: GIT upset, pseudomembranous colitis, hepatic impairment, rashes, blood dyscrasias, pain on injection, thrombophlebitis.

Clinical governance. Term denoting a particular aspect of risk management and quality assurance in which responsibility for maintaining standards of care is defined and placed with specified individuals and departments. In the NHS, the chief executive of each Trust is responsible for the care provided, although each department is expected to take steps to ensure high standards and both detect and act upon deficiencies at individual or departmental level. Requires that evidence-based medicine is in day-to-day use, that good practice and innovations are systematically disseminated and applied, and that the quality of data collected to monitor clinical care is of a high standard. Two bodies were set up in 1999 to monitor these processes: the National Institute for Clinical Excellence (NICE) and the Commission for Health Improvement (CHI), (subsequently the Healthcare Commission). The concept arose formally from political and medical reactions to well-publicised examples of inadequate care, its introduction achieving particular impetus following the high death rate after paediatric cardiac surgery in Bristol in the 1980s/early 1990s. As a result of disciplinary rulings following this case, all clinicians are now expected to monitor their own performance and undergo regular appraisal and revalidation.

Clinical trials. Performed to determine whether a treatment is useful, how it compares with other treatments, whether it affects different groups of patients differently, and how it is best given (e.g. drug dosage regimen, route, etc.).

- Setting up a trial:
  - aims of the trial are defined.
  - the number of patients is defined; ideally, the number is calculated by first defining the size of difference considered clinically important, and then the sample size required to enable such a difference to be revealed if present (i.e. power analysis). Groups should usually be of equal size if possible.
  - subjects:
    - patients with other diseases, those taking other drugs, etc. are excluded where possible.
    - controls:
      - pairs may be matched for age, sex, race, degree and duration of illness, etc. and one of each pair assigned to each treatment.
      - cross-over studies: patients act as their own controls by receiving first one treatment then another. The effect of the first treatment on the second must be excluded.
      - randomisation into groups.
      - historical controls are avoided where possible.
      - treatment is compared with no treatment, placebo or existing treatment.
  - bias is further reduced by blindness:
    - single-blind (patient is unaware of treatment identity).
    - double-blind (doctor and patient are unaware).
  - variability is reduced by using the same location, time of day, medical/nursing staff, technique, etc., for all patients.
  - approval by a Research Ethics Committee: includes qualified and lay persons. Considers whether exposure of patients to the new treatment or denial of the old treatment to controls, or vice versa, is justified, whether adequate information is given to potential participants, and whether proper consent is obtained. No patient should be worse off than if the trial were not running.
  - approval is also required from the institution (e.g. Trust Research & Development Department) and regulatory authorities if drugs or devices are involved (in the UK, the Medicines and Healthcare products Regulatory Agency; in the USA, the Food and Drug Administration).
  - data:
    - what to measure; i.e. according to defined aims.
    - objective measurements are less prone to observer bias than subjective assessment.
    - how many measurements; e.g. measurement of too many variables increases the likelihood of at least one being significantly different due to chance alone.
    - which statistical test to use, and how to express results; e.g. use of the null hypothesis or confidence intervals.
  - end-point of the trial:
    - according to the numbers studied.
    - sequential analysis: the trial stops when results attain significance.

See also, Drug development; Meta-analysis; Statistics

Clomethiazole edisylate (Chlormethiazole). Sedative drug, structurally related to vitamin B_1. Has been used for sedation and as an anticonvulsant drug, e.g. in pre-eclampsia. Traditionally used to treat acute alcohol withdrawal. No longer available for iv use because of the risk of severe CVS/RS depression and fluid overload (contained no electrolytes).

- Dosage: 1–4 capsules (equivalent to 5–20 ml elixir which contains 50 mg/ml) orally, 3–4 hourly.
- Side effects: nasal irritation, GIT upset, headache, agitation.

Clonazepam. Benzodiazepine, used mainly to treat epilepsy. Has also been used in disorders of movement, e.g. dystonias, etc., and as an adjunct to pain management. Has similar effects to diazepam. 50% protein-bound after iv injection. Metabolised in the liver and excreted in the urine. Elimination half-life is 24–48 h.

- Dosage:
  - 1–8 mg/day orally in adults, depending on response.
  - 0.25–1 mg/day in infants.
  - 0.5–1 mg diluted in water for iv injection.
- Side effects include sedation (occasionally excitation), bronchial and salivary hypersecretion, and rarely hepatic impairment and blood dyscrasias.

Clonidine hydrochloride. α-Adrenergic receptor agonist, used as an antihypertensive drug and in the prophylaxis of migraine. Licensed in the US in 1997 for use via the epidural route for pain therapy. Has also been given intrathecally. Has been used in the treatment of alcohol withdrawal in ICU patients. Acts centrally by stimulating presynaptic α_2-adrenergic receptors, causing suppression of catecholamine release (i.e. activates a negative-feedback control system). May also stimulate inhibitory postsynaptic α_1-receptors, and may have some action peripherally. Its main effect is on vasomotor centre output. Also has an analgesic and sedative action. When administered by mouth preoperatively, it reduces MAC of inhalational anaesthetic agents.

Its half-life is about 23 h. Metabolised in the liver, with about 65% excreted unchanged in the urine and 20% in the faeces.

- Dosage:
  - 150–300 μg/day orally in divided doses, up to 1.2 mg.
  - 150–300 μg by slow iv injection. Effects occur within 10 min, and last 3–7 h. Transient hypertension and bradycardia may occur.
  - 30 μg/h via epidural route, adjusted according to response (boluses of 100–300 μg have been used for acute pain although not licensed for this use). Hypotension may occur.
- Side effects: sedation, dry mouth, depression, urinary retention, reduced gastric motility. Increased sensitivity to parenteral catecholamines may occur; sudden withdrawal of clonidine may cause a severe hypertensive crisis.

Clopidogrel, *see Antiplatelet drugs*

Closing capacity. Lung volume at which airway closure occurs, mainly in the dependent parts of the lung. Equals closing volume plus residual volume. In fit young adults, closing capacity (CC) is considerably less than FRC; thus airway closure does not occur during normal quiet breathing. Airway closure occurring within FRC results in shunting.

- Measurement: inspiration of a bolus of marker gas, e.g. helium (He) at the end of maximal expiration (i.e. residual volume), followed by inspiration of air to total lung capacity (Fig. 40). Expired He concentration is measured during slow expiration: the same phases are seen as in Fowler's method (which may also be used to measure CC). Initially, dead space gas is exhaled, containing no He. Then, a mixture of dead space and alveolar gas, followed by alveolar gas. The He bolus entered the upper airways, because the lower ones were collapsed at residual volume. Thus at CC, there is a sharp rise in expired He concentration.
- Increased by:
  - age: CC = FRC in neonates and infants.
    CC = FRC in the supine position at 40 years.
    CC = FRC in the upright position at 65 years.
  - increased intrathoracic pressures, e.g. asthma.
  - smoking.

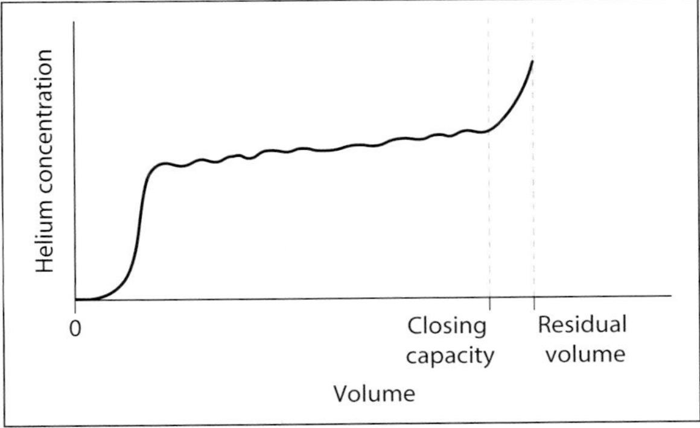

Fig. 40 Measurement of closing capacity

CC may encroach upon a FRC reduced by obesity, the supine position and anaesthesia. PEEP and CPAP may reduce airway closure.

Drummond GB, Milic-Emili J (2007). Br J Anaesth; 99: 772–4

Closing volume, *see Closing capacity*

Clostridial infections. Caused by members of the Gram-positive, spore forming, anaerobic, toxin producing bacteria of the genus *Clostridium*. Species include:

- *Cl. perfringens*: causes gas gangrene.
- *Cl. tetani*: causes tetanus.
- *Cl. botulinum*: causes botulism.
- *Cl. difficile*: the most common enteric pathogen in hospital patients (carried by about 20%), causing a range of GIT infections including mild watery diarrhoea, severe non-specific colitis and fulminant pseudomembranous colitis. Produces two toxins (A, an enterotoxin and B, a cytotoxin). Most common cause of toxin production is antibacterial drugs:
  - rarely causative (vancomycin, erythromycin, tetracyclines, gentamicin).
  - uncommonly causative (quinolones, aztreonam, imipenem, metronidazole).
  - most likely to be causative (β-lactams, clindamycin).

  Diarrhoea is initially watery, without mucus or blood. There may be a fever and leucocytosis. Onset of pseudomembranous colitis is heralded by high fever, leucocytosis and large volumes of diarrhoea containing mucus and frank blood. Diagnosed by demonstration of *Cl. difficile* toxin in stools.

  Treatment of *Cl. difficile* diarrhoea is with oral vancomycin or metronidazole. IV metronidazole may be appropriate for cases of pseudomembranous colitis. Infection control measures are required.

Clover, Joseph Thomas (1825–1882). English anaesthetist; took over from Snow as anaesthesia's pioneer after the latter's death. A medical student at University College Hospital, London, said to have been present at Liston's historic operation in 1846. Started his medical career in surgery and general practice. Devised inhalers for chloroform and later diethyl ether which delivered accurate concentrations of agent and were much copied by other practitioners. Also described the use of N_2O, alone or in combination with volatile agents. His apparatus included large capacity rubber bags, filled with N_2O or air and carried over the shoulder.

Buxton DW (1923). Br J Anaesth; 1: 55–61

C_m, *see Minimal blocking concentration*

$CMRO_2$, *see Cerebral metabolic rate for oxygen*

CMV, *see Cytomegalovirus*

COAD, Chronic obstructive airways disease, *see Chronic obstructive pulmonary disease*

Coagulation. Clot formation; follows vasospasm and platelet plug formation which cause temporary haemostasis.
- Normal sequence of events:
  - vasospasm, thought to be mediated by vasoconstrictor substances released from platelets, e.g. 5-HT and thromboxane.
  - platelet plug: platelets are attracted by collagen exposed by damaged vascular endothelium. Adherence is followed by release of 5-HT and ADP, the latter causing further aggregation.
  - clot formation: the platelet plug is bound by resultant fibrin to form the definitive clot. Clot retraction is caused by platelet contractile microfilaments. The classical explanation of the coagulation pathway involves many circulating factors in a cascade mechanism; each factor, when activated, activates the next in turn (Fig. 41). Most are produced by the liver. Nomenclature of factors is largely historical, according to the chronological order of discovery. The intrinsic pathway is initiated by exposure of blood to collagen, or *in vitro* by contact with glass, e.g. test tubes. The extrinsic pathway is initiated by substances released from damaged tissues. Each may activate the common pathway, which culminates in formation of a tight fibrin clot.

    More recently, a single pathway has been proposed, in which tissue factor (TF; a membrane glycoprotein not normally exposed on the surface of intact blood vessels) binds to circulating factor VII, resulting in a complex (VII/TF), which then activates the coagulation cascade mainly via factors IX and X (and thence the common pathway). The central role of factor VIIa is reflected in the use of its recombinant human form eptacog alpha in haemophilia and intractable haemorrhage.

Normally, the clotting mechanism is balanced by opposing reactions preventing coagulation, e.g. antithrombin III (formed from activated factor X) which inhibits active factors II, IX, X, XI and XII. Prostacyclin secreted by the vascular endothelium inhibits platelet aggregation.

Other pathways may be involved with the coagulation cascade, e.g. active factor XII leads to activation of fibrinolysis and kinin formation.

See also, Anticoagulant drugs; Coagulation disorders; Coagulation studies

Coagulation disorders. May result in impaired coagulation or hypercoagulability. The former is more common and may arise from defects in:
- blood vessels:
  - infection, e.g. meningococcal disease, sepsis.
  - metabolic disease, e.g. hepatic failure, renal failure, scurvy.
  - congenital, e.g. hereditary telangiectasia.
- platelets:
  - thrombocytopenia.
  - DIC.
  - impaired function, e.g. antiplatelet drugs.
- coagulation:
  - congenital, e.g. haemophilia, von Willebrand's disease (also associated with blood vessel and platelet defects).
  - heparin, warfarin, hepatic failure, vitamin K deficiency, DIC.
  - increased fibrinolysis.

Blood transfusion may be associated with dilution of platelets and coagulation factors by fluids and blood components deficient in them. Impaired organ function and possible DIC may contribute.

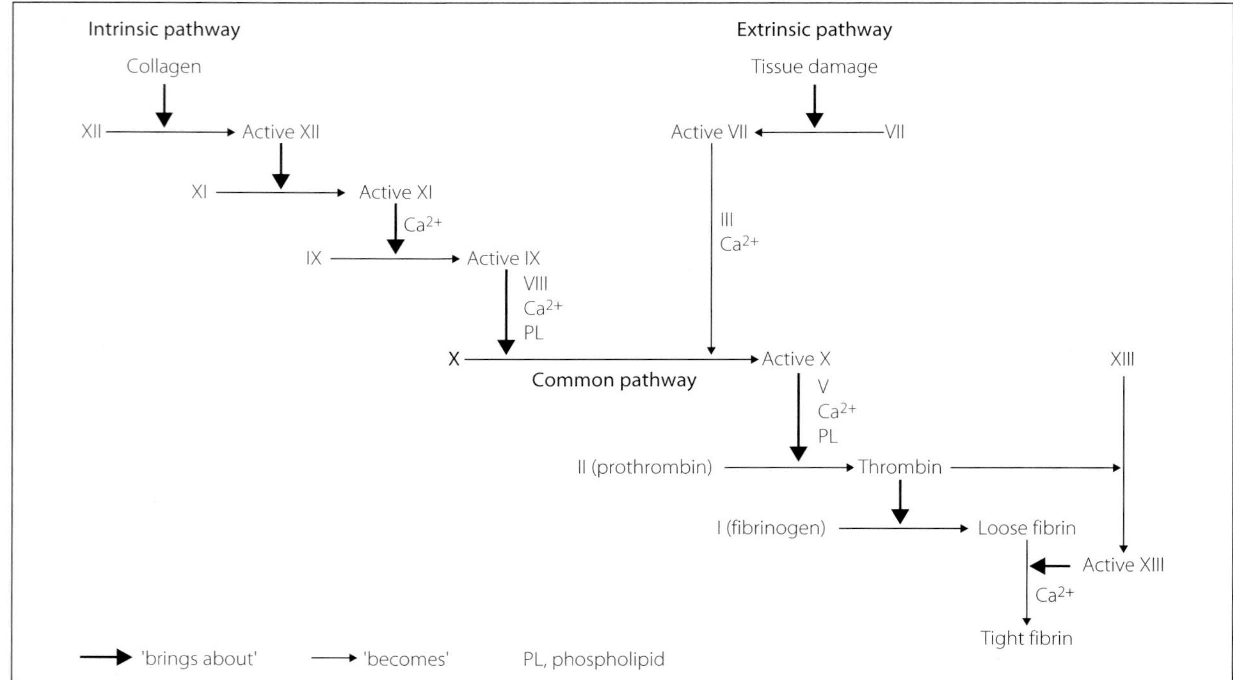

Fig. 41 Coagulation cascade

Table 9 Change in prothrombin time (PT), activated partial thromboplastin (APPT), thrombin time (TT), fibrin degradation products (FDPs), platelet count and fibrinogen levels in various coagulation disorders

Disorder	*PT*	*APPT*	*TT*	*FDPs*	*Platelets*	*Fibrinogen*
Thrombocytopenia	→	→	→	→	↓	→
DIC	↑	↑	↑	↑	↓	↓
Heparin therapy	↑	↑	↑	→	→*	→
Warfarin therapy	↑	↑	→	→	→	→
Hepatic failure	↑	↑	↑	→	→	↓
Massive blood transfusion	↑	↑	↑	→	↓	→
Primary fibrinolysis	↑	↑	↑	↑	→	↓

↑, Increase; ↓, decrease; →, no change.
*But thrombocytopenia may follow several days of heparin therapy.
Note: DIC may complicate hepatic failure and massive blood transfusion.

Diagnosed by the underlying problem, aided by coagulation studies (Table 9).

- Treatment:
  - of underlying disease.
  - replacement of defective circulatory components.

Abnormal hypercoagulability may lead to recurrent DVT and PE. It may result from:

- primary disorders:
  - protein C deficiency: protein C is a circulating anticoagulant protein; when activated by thrombin it inactivates factors V and VIII. Deficiency (the extent of which may be variable) thus results in increased tendency to form thrombosis.
  - protein S deficiency: protein S is a cofactor for protein C; deficiency also results in thrombophilia.
  - activated protein C resistance: inherited abnormality of factor V, resulting in resistance to cleavage by protein C. A particular form of factor V, factor V Leiden, is present in about 2% of Northern European individuals; the risk of thrombosis in homozygotes is estimated at up to 50%.
  - antithrombin III deficiency: may result in thrombophlebitis, thrombosis and PE.
  - others, e.g. prothrombin gene variants, deficiency of fibrinolytic components or factor XII.
- secondary to malignancy, pregnancy, diabetes mellitus, platelet and vessel wall abnormalities, hyperviscosity and venous stasis. Circulating inhibitors (lupus anticoagulant and anticardiolipin antibodies) may develop spontaneously or in patients with SLE, resulting in the antiphospholipid syndrome. In this condition, activated partial thromboplastin time may be prolonged although patients are at increased risk of thrombosis, possibly related to inhibition of factor XII activation or prostacyclin production from vascular endothelium.

[Leiden; city in Netherlands where the factor was first identified in 1993]

Martlew VJ (2000). Br J Anaesth; 85: 446–55

Coagulation studies. May test different parts of the coagulation pathways:

- whole blood coagulation:
  - whole blood clotting time: bedside test of intrinsic and common pathways (i.e. spontaneous coagulation occurring in a glass tube without external reactive substances, e.g. tissue fluid). 1 ml blood is added to each of three glass tubes, kept at body temperature. The first is tilted every 15 s until clotted, then the second, third, etc. The time until the third is clotted is normally about 9–12 min.
  - activated clotting time (ACT): bedside test; commonly used to monitor heparin anticoagulation during cardiac surgery. Similar to whole blood clotting time, but celite is added to the blood for quicker results. Automated devices are usually used to detect fibrin formation, with a small bar magnet within the test tube. The tube is placed within the device and rotated slowly; when fibrin forms in the tube, the magnet starts to rotate, thereby activating the detector. Normal value is 100–140 s. Values of 3–4 times the pre-heparin value are considered adequate during extracorporeal circulation.
- clotting factors: performed on fresh citrated plasma, with cells and platelets removed; physical activation of coagulation is avoided by using non-wettable plastic tubes. Normal plasma is used as a control:
  - prothrombin time (PT): tests the extrinsic and common pathways. Plasma then calcium is added to brain extract and phospholipid. Normal value is 11–15 s. International Normalised Ratio (INR; formerly British Ratio) is the ratio of sample time to a standard. A target ratio of 2–2.5 is used for prophylaxis of DVT with warfarin; 2–3 for treatment of DVT, PE and transient ischaemic attacks; 3–4.5 for prophylaxis of recurrent DVT or PE, and for patients with prosthetic heart valves and other arterial prostheses. A ratio of 1.5 is considered safe for surgery.
  - activated partial thromboplastin time (APTT; also partial thromboplastin time with kaolin, PTTK): tests the intrinsic and common pathways. Plasma, phospholipid and calcium are added to kaolin. Normal value is 35–40 s. A target ratio of 2–4 compared with normal plasma is used for treatment of DVT or PE with heparin. A ratio of 1.5 is considered safe for surgery.
  - mixture tests: if PT or APTT is prolonged, the patient's plasma may be mixed with normal plasma and the test repeated. If the test is normal, factor deficiency is present; if still prolonged, the sample plasma contains an inhibitor, e.g. antibody.
  - specific factor assays, e.g. factor VIII assay.
  - reptilase time (RT): snake venom is added to plasma, converting fibrinogen to fibrin. Unaffected by heparin; thus if normal but the thrombin time is prolonged, presence of heparin is suggested. A prolonged RT suggests fibrinogen deficiency.
- platelets:
  - platelet count: normally 150–400 × 10^9/l.
  - bleeding time: a standard incision is made on the forearm using a pricking device or template; a BP cuff is inflated around the upper arm to 40 mmHg. The incision is dabbed with filter paper every 30 s until the bleeding stops. Normal value is 2–9 min. Susceptible to considerable variation; therefore infrequently used.
  - commercially available devices: used as a rapid indicator of coagulation status, e.g. during liver transplantation:
    - thromb(o)elastography (TEG): fibrin strands form between an oscillating container of fresh blood and a drum within it; the movements of the drum are recorded on to paper to produce a characteristic clotting profile whose shape and dimensions represents the speed of coagulation and quality of clot.

- Sonoclot: a tubular probe oscillates up and down within the sample and the resistance to motion encountered is plotted on a graph. As the blood clots, resistance increases; it then peaks and falls as a result of clot retraction and disruption of the clot, giving a characteristic tracing ('clot signature').
- PFA-100: blood is aspirated through a microscopic hole in a membrane coated with collagen and adrenaline or ADP; the time for a platelet plug to occlude the hole completely is the 'closure time' and is related to platelet function.

- fibrinolysis:
  - fibrinogen assay: normally 1.5–4.0 g/l.
  - thrombin time (TT): tests conversion of fibrinogen to fibrin. Exogenous thrombin is added to plasma. Normal value is 10–15 s. Inhibited by fibrin degradation products resulting from fibrinolysis. Also inhibited by heparin.
  - fibrinogen degradation products; normally < 10 mg/l. D-dimer concentration is normally < 500 ng/ml.
  - plasminogen assay.
  - clot lysis times, e.g. euglobulin, precipitated from plasma by adding acid. Contains fibrinogen, plasminogen and plasminogen activator. Addition of thrombin causes clot formation; subsequent lysis depends on the amount of plasminogen activating capacity present. Whole blood clot lysis and other variants are also used.

Co-amoxiclav. Broad-spectrum antibacterial drug; a mixture of amoxicillin and clavulanic acid in varying proportion. Active against Gram-negative and -positive organisms, it is mainly used in respiratory, middle ear and urinary infections.

- Dosage: (expressed as amoxicillin):
  - 250–500 mg orally 8 hourly.
  - 1 g iv 6–8 hourly.
- Side effects: as for amoxicillin; also cholestatic jaundice, erythema multiforme and interstitial nephritis.

Coanda effect. Development of reduced pressure between a fluid jet from a nozzle and an adjacent surface, resulting in adherence of the jet to the surface. Reduced pressure results from entrainment of surrounding molecules into the turbulent jet, with those next to the surface quickly 'used up'. If the jet has two surfaces to which it might adhere, it will attach to one only, without splitting. A small signal jet across the nozzle may switch the main jet from one surface to the other; this has formed the basis of control mechanisms in fluidics, e.g. control of ventilators.

Similar behaviour of fluids has been suggested to occur beyond constrictions in blood vessels, e.g. coronary arteries, contributing to ischaemia and infarction.

The effect was originally applied to the development of jet engines.

[Henri Coanda (1885–1972), Romanian engineer]

Coarctation of aorta. Accounts for 5–10% of congenital heart disease. More common in males. May be associated with Turner's and Marfan's syndromes. Acquired coarctation is rare and usually follows chest trauma or vasculitides.

Over 95% are post-ductal, often presenting in later life. There may be associated cerebral aneurysms or a bicuspid aortic valve.

- Features:
  - hypertension, left ventricular hypertrophy and cardiac failure. BP is high in the arms, normal or low in the legs. CVA and endocarditis may occur.
  - weak femoral pulses, delayed compared with the radials.
  - systolic heart murmur; may be loudest posteriorly.
  - ECG findings include left ventricular hypertrophy.
  - characteristic chest X-ray findings:
    - double aortic knuckle ('3' sign).
    - small descending aorta.
    - rib notching; seen at the middle of the lower border of the ribs posteriorly; caused by enlarged collateral vessels.
    - left ventricular enlargement/failure.

The preductal (proximal to the ductus arteriosus) form is more severe, usually presenting in infancy with cardiac failure. Often associated with cerebral aneurysms, bicuspid aortic valve, patent ductus arteriosus, VSD, and mitral and aortic abnormalities.

Repaired surgically via left thoracotomy; more recently, balloon angioplasty and stenting of the constricted segment has been reported.

- Anaesthetic management is similar to that for thoracic aortic aneurysm, in particular:
  - preoperative treatment of hypertension and cardiac failure.
  - antibiotic prophylaxis as for congenital heart disease.
  - arterial BP should be monitored in the right arm as the left subclavian artery is usually clamped during resection.
  - complications include:
    - haemorrhage.
    - hypertension following aortic clamping, ischaemia to the spinal cord, bowel and kidneys, and acidosis and hypotension following unclamping.
  - hypertension may persist postoperatively and require treatment, especially in older patients.
  - simultaneous BP measurement in the arms and legs is often performed.

See also, Cardiac surgery

Coaxial anaesthetic breathing systems. Functionally, they are versions of Mapleson A (Lack) and D (Bain) anaesthetic breathing systems, but more convenient to use:

- Lack (Fig. 42a): the expiratory valve is at the anaesthetic machine end (cf. Magill system). Thus easier to adjust and scavenge waste gases, especially when the patient's head is covered. The patient end is also lighter. The outer tube is wider than usual to accommodate the inner tube,

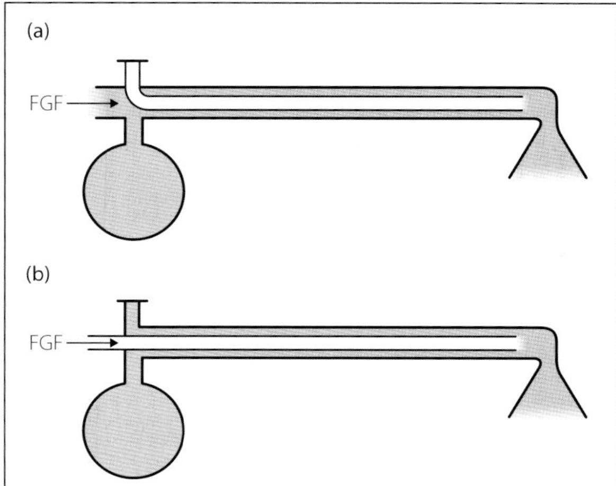

Fig. 42 Coaxial breathing systems: (a) Lack; (b) Bain

itself as wide as possible to reduce resistance to expiration. The system is therefore bulky and relatively inflexible. It has greater resistance to expiration than the Magill system. Required fresh gas flows are as for the Magill system. Parallel versions are also available, in which the inner tube is replaced by a second external tube running alongside the main tube. Both tubes are wide-bore and thus of low resistance.
- Bain (Fig. 42b): lighter and longer than the standard systems, with the expiratory valve at the machine end, allowing easy adjustment and scavenging. Some resistance to expiration results from the flow of fresh gas directed at the patient's mouth from the inner tube. Ideal fresh gas flow rates for spontaneous ventilation are controversial, as high flows cause greater resistance. Suggested values range from 100 to 250 ml/kg. May be used for IPPV using a ventilator, e.g. Penlon Nuffield attached to the reservoir bag fitting (bag removed) by a length of tubing whose volume exceeds tidal volume. Disconnection of the inner tube from the fresh gas source (resulting in the whole length of tubing becoming dead space) must be excluded before use (*see Checking of anaesthetic equipment*).

A coaxial version of the circle system is available, which connects to the inspiration and expiration ports of a standard CO_2 absorber. It is claimed that the countercurrent heat exchange mechanism, in which the expiratory gases warm the inspiratory gases as they pass in opposite directions along the coaxial tube's length, results in greater transfer of heat to the inspiratory gas than in the conventional non-coaxial circle.

[J Alistair Lack, Salisbury anaesthetist; JA Bain, Canadian anaesthetist]

Cocada. Ball of coca leaves, mixed with guano and cornstarch, thought to be chewed by South American Incas to release free cocaine base. Dribbling of saliva on to wounds then allowed relatively painless surgery.

Cocaine/cocaine hydrochloride. Ester local anaesthetic agent, the first one discovered. An alkaloid originally extracted from the leaves and bark of South American coca plants. Used in 1884 for topical analgesia of the eye (by Koller), intercostal nerve block (by Anrep), mandibular nerve block (by Halstead and Hall) and other uses including local infiltration. Now restricted to surface analgesia because of its toxicity. Commonly used as a 10% spray or paste to reduce bleeding caused by nasal intubation. Causes vasoconstriction by preventing uptake of noradrenaline by presynaptic nerve endings; also inhibits monoamine oxidase.
- Toxicity:
  - CNS stimulation: convulsions at high doses, followed by central depression and apnoea.
  - sympathetic stimulation: arrhythmias, tachycardia, hypertension and myocardial ischaemia may occur.
  - addiction may occur with chronic use. Cardiomyopathy and sudden death have been associated with chronic abuse.
- Maximal safe dose: 3 mg/kg.

Excreted mainly via the liver; a small amount is excreted unchanged in the urine.

[Richard J Hall (1856–1897), Irish-born US surgeon]

See also, Cocaine poisoning

Cocaine poisoning. Increasing problem in the developed world, especially with the production of the more addictive freebase cocaine (crack) by dissolution of the salt in alkaline solution and extraction with organic solvents (e.g. ether). Although usually of high purity, illegally obtained cocaine may contain caffeine, phencyclidine, ephedrine, amfetamines, strychnine and others.

The toxic dose depends on the individual's tolerance and route of administration but doses above 1 g are likely to be fatal. Effects are enhanced and prolonged by alcohol. Detectable in urine but serum levels are unhelpful because of a large volume of distribution and rapid metabolism.
- Clinical features:
  - CNS: euphoria, anxiety, agitation, psychosis, hallucinations, convulsions, hyperthermia, intracranial haemorrhage, coma. Status epilepticus suggests continued drug absorption (e.g. following rupture of cocaine-filled packets swallowed for smuggling purposes), intracranial haemorrhage or hyperthermia.
  - CVS: ventricular tachyarrhythmias, severe hypertension (may result in CVA or aortic dissection), myocardial infarction caused by coronary thrombosis or spasm, dilated cardiomyopathy. The actions of sympathomimetic drugs may be greatly enhanced.
  - RS: non-cardiogenic pulmonary oedema, bronchospasm, pulmonary infiltrates ('crack lung'), pulmonary haemorrhage, pneumothorax/pneumomediastinum.
  - renal: renal failure caused by renal artery spasm, hypotension or rhabdomyolysis.
- Management:
  - supportive: resuscitation, sedation, antiarrhythmic drugs, antihypertensive drugs, etc. (avoiding β-blockade alone since it may result in unopposed α-mediated severe hypertension), general management as for poisoning and overdoses.
  - laparotomy may occasionally be required to remove ingested bags of the drug.
  - general anaesthesia may be hazardous because of the risk of severe hypertension and arrhythmias following laryngoscopy and tracheal intubation.

'Cockpit drill', *see Checking of anaesthetic equipment*

Codeine phosphate. Naturally occurring opioid analgesic drug, isolated in 1832; used to relieve mild to moderate pain. Also used in diarrhoea, and to suppress the cough reflex, e.g. in terminal care. Has similar effects to morphine, but with less potency and efficacy. About 5–10% is metabolised to morphine via the cytochrome P_{450} system; in about 5–10% of the population metabolism is reduced to under 3%, resulting in reduced analgesia. The specific enzyme involved is also inhibited by a number of drugs including antidepressants.

Although classically used as an analgesic in neurosurgery, its use has been superseded by morphine. Partly excreted unchanged via the kidneys, and partly metabolised in the liver.
- Dosage: up to 60 mg orally or im; 1–1.5 mg/kg for children. Available in combination with paracetamol (8 mg, 15 mg and 30 mg with 500 mg paracetamol). Codeine should not be given iv (severe hypotension may follow).

Co-dydramol, *see Dihydrocodeine*

COELCB, *see Current-operated earth-leakage circuit breaker*

Coeliac plexus block. Sympathetic nerve block involving blockade of the coeliac ganglions, one lying on each side of L1 (aorta lying posteriorly, pancreas anteriorly and inferior vena cava laterally) and closely related to the coeliac plexus. Through them pass afferent fibres from abdominal (but not pelvic) viscera.

Performed for relief of pain from non-pelvic intra-abdominal organs, especially due to pancreatic and gastric malignancies. Has also been used in acute/chronic pancreatitis (relaxes the sphincter of Oddi) and to provide intra-abdominal analgesia during surgery. Usually performed percutaneously with the patient prone, under X-ray control. CT scanning has been used.

- Point of needle insertion: 5–10 cm from the midline, level with the spinous process of L1, below the 12th rib. A long (> 10 cm) needle is inserted at 45° to the skin, directed medially and slightly cranially. It is passed until the needle tip lies anterior to the upper part of the body of L1. 15–25 ml local anaesthetic agent is injected on each side, e.g. prilocaine or lidocaine 0.5% with adrenaline, followed by 25 ml 50% alcohol if required, e.g. on the following day if the block is successful. Flushing with saline prevents alcohol deposition during needle withdrawal. Severe hypotension may result, even after unilateral block.

[Ruggero Oddi (1845–1906), Italian surgeon]

See also, Sympathetic nervous system

Co-fluampicil. Broad-spectrum antibacterial drug; a mixture of ampicillin and flucloxacillin in equal parts.

Cognitive Behavioural Therapy (CBT). Method of examining how subjects think about themselves and their environment, and how their behaviour affects their thoughts and feelings, in order to change both aspects of their life. Focuses on identifying current patterns and problems, as opposed to the past, and developing coping strategies and skills. Particularly useful in disorders associated with anxiety and depression; has been used to complement chronic pain management.

COLD, Chronic obstructive lung disease, *see Chronic obstructive pulmonary disease*

Colistin. Antibacterial drug, also known as polymyxin E. Acts on the lipopolysaccharide and phospholipid components of Gram-negative bacterial cell walls, including pseudomonas. Not absorbed when given orally; therefore has been used in selective decontamination of the digestive tract. Rarely given iv because of its side effects.

- Dosage:
  - 1.5–3 million units orally, 8 hourly.
  - 1 million units by nebulised solution, 12 hourly (dose halved if under 40 kg).
  - 1–2 million units iv/im, 8 hourly.
- Side effects: paraesthesia, vertigo, neuromuscular blockade, renal impairment, dysarthria, visual disturbance, confusion.

Colitis, *see Bowel ischaemia; Inflammatory bowel disease; Pseudomembranous colitis*

College of Anaesthetists. Founded in 1988, replacing the Faculty of Anaesthetists, Royal College of Surgeons of England; became the Royal College of Anaesthetists in 1992. Similarly, the Faculty of Anaesthetists at the Royal College of Surgeons in Ireland became the College of Anaesthetists at the RCSI in 1998.

Mushin W (1989). Anaesthesia; 44: 291–2

Colligative properties of solutions. Those properties varying with the number, and not character, of solute particles present. Thus, as concentration increases:

- freezing point decreases.
- osmotic pressure increases.
- boiling point increases.
- vapour pressure of solvent decreases (Raoult's law).

Measurement of osmolarity/osmolality may utilise any of the above properties, since the changes produced by addition of solute are proportional to the amount added.

Colloid. Substance unable to pass through a semipermeable membrane, being a suspension of particles rather than a true solution (cf. crystalloid). The term is used to describe iv fluids which remain confined to the intravascular compartment, at least initially. More useful than crystalloids when replacing a vascular volume deficit, e.g. in haemorrhage, but of less use correcting specific water and electrolyte deficiencies, e.g. in dehydration. Also more expensive. Sometimes called plasma substitutes or plasma expanders, because the increase in plasma volume may be greater than the volume of colloid infused, due to their higher osmolality than plasma.

- Available products:
  - blood products, e.g. blood, albumin, plasma: should be used for specific blood component deficiency only, since supplies are short, and risks of blood transfusion are present. Approximate current cost per unit: red cells £120; platelets £200; fresh frozen plasma £30.
  - hydroxyethyl starch: solutions with differing degrees of substitution (40–74%) have been produced, with varying duration of action and effects on circulating volume. Incidence of severe reactions is about 1/10–16 000; cost is £10–20/500 ml.
  - gelatin derivatives. Effects last a few hours only. Severe reactions: 1/13 000 (succinylated), 1/2000 (urea linked; lower incidence with the newer formulation since 1981). Cost: £3–4/500 ml.
  - dextrans. May affect renal function and coagulation. Severe reactions: 1/4500, reduced to 1/84 000 with hapten pretreatment. Cost: £4–5/500 ml.

See also, Colloid/crystalloid controversy

Colloid/crystalloid controversy. Arises from conflicting theoretical, experimental and clinical evidence concerning the use of iv colloid or crystalloid in shock, most work concerning haemorrhage.

- Arguments in favour of:
  - colloid:
    - more logical choice for intravascular volume replacement, since a greater proportion remains in the intravascular space for longer after infusion.
    - less volume is required to restore cardiovascular parameters, e.g. BP, CVP, pulmonary artery capillary wedge pressure, etc. Thus initial resuscitation is more rapid.
    - less peripheral/pulmonary oedema follows its use for the above reasons, and also because there is less reduction of plasma oncotic pressure.
  - crystalloid:
    - expands the intravascular compartment adequately if enough is used (traditionally said to be 2–4 times the colloid requirements although more recent evidence suggests a ratio nearer 1.5:1 for the same degree of intravascular expansion).
    - in haemorrhage, fluid moves from the interstitial space into the vascular compartment and third space; this ECF depletion is better replenished by crystalloid.
    - if vascular permeability is increased, colloids will enter the interstitial space and increase interstitial oncotic pressure, thus exacerbating oedema. Crystalloids do not increase interstitial oncotic pressure to the same extent.

- peripheral oedema is usually not a problem.
- risk of allergic reactions to colloids.
- crystalloid is much cheaper than colloid.
- Difficulties in assessing fluid resuscitation:
  - infusion is usually guided by cardiovascular end-points but their relation to interstitial fluid, ECF, etc. is unclear.
  - lung water may increase markedly before gas exchange is impaired.
  - other clinical processes may be involved, e.g. cardiovascular disease, impaired gas exchange and increased vascular permeability due to sepsis, ARDS, etc. The position is even less clear than in uncomplicated haemorrhage.

In the US, crystalloid, e.g. Hartmann's solution, is widely used for iv resuscitation, whereas colloids are more commonly used in the UK. Mixtures are favoured by many, guided by the nature of the deficit.

Colloid oncotic pressure, *see Oncotic pressure*

Colton, Gardner Quincy (1814–1898). US lecturer and showman; studied medicine but never qualified. Demonstrated the exhilarating effects of N_2O inhalation for entertainment in 1844, inspiring Wells to suggest its use for dental analgesia. Said to have administered N_2O to Wells whilst the latter's tooth was painlessly removed. Left his lectures to prospect for gold, returning to N_2O and popularising its reintroduction by founding the Colton Dental Association in 1863.

Smith GB, Hirsch NP (1991). Anesth Analg; 72: 382–91

Coma. State in which the patient is totally unaware of both self and external surroundings, and unable to respond meaningfully to external stimuli. Results from gross impairment of both cerebral hemispheres, and/or the ascending reticular activating system.

- Caused by:
  - focal brain dysfunction, e.g. tumour, vascular events, demyelination, infection, head injury.
  - diffuse brain dysfunction:
    - infection, e.g. meningitis, encephalitis.
    - epilepsy.
    - hypoxia and hypercapnia.
    - drugs, poisoning and overdoses.
    - metabolic/endocrine causes, e.g. diabetic coma, hepatic or renal failure, hypothyroidism, extreme electrolyte disturbance, e.g. hyponatraemia.
    - hypotension, hypertensive crisis.
    - head injury.
    - subarachnoid haemorrhage.
    - hypothermia, hyperthermia.

Assessment of the pupils, doll's eye movements, posture and motor responses (e.g. decerebrate and decorticate postures) and respiratory pattern is especially useful. Investigations are directed towards the above causes.

Initial management includes respiratory and cardiovascular support as for CPR. In addition, longer-term management includes attention to pressure areas, mouth, skin and eyes, physiotherapy, prophylaxis against DVT, nutrition and fluid balance, and urinary catheterisation.

Stevens RD, Bhardwaj A (2006). Crit Care Med; 34: 31–41

See also, Brainstem death; Coma scales

Coma scales. Scoring systems for assessing the degree of coma in unconscious patients and charting their progress; may also give an indication of outcome.

- Include general scales, e.g. AVPU scale or a simple 1–5 scoring system:
  - 1 = fully awake.
  - 2 = conscious but drowsy.
  - 3 = unconscious but responsive to pain with purposeful movement, e.g. flexion.
  - 4 = unconscious; responds to pain with extension.
  - 5 = unconscious with no response to pain.
- Other data, e.g. from eye reflexes, are ignored; hence more complex or specific scoring systems are used, e.g.:
  - Glasgow coma scale (GCS). The FOUR (full outline of unresponsiveness score) scale uses the motor and eye opening components of the GCS but replaces the verbal score with scores for pupillary reaction and respiratory pattern, which reflect brainstem function.
  - for specific conditions, e.g. hepatic failure, subarachnoid haemorrhage.

Servadei F (2006). Lancet; 367: 548–9

Combined spinal–epidural anaesthesia (CSE). Technique in which the epidural space is located in the usual way as for epidural anaesthesia, but spinal anaesthesia is performed either alongside or, more commonly, by inserting a long spinal needle through the epidural needle to puncture the dura. The advantages of spinal anaesthesia (speed of onset, density of block) are therefore combined with those of epidural anaesthesia (flexibility, the ability to extend for intra- or postoperative analgesia); in addition the technique allows finer spinal needles to be used if a needle-through-needle method is employed, since the position of the needle's tip can be estimated more easily as it passes through the epidural space into the dura. Has been used in obstetric analgesia and anaesthesia and other types of surgery. Disadvantages include the increased cost if a long spinal needle is used, the possibility that the epidural catheter is inserted through the dural hole, inadequate block if the catheter cannot be threaded easily (with the patient in the same position for a long time), and a theoretical increased risk of infection by 'breaching the dura'. If saline is used to identify the epidural space, the appearance of clear fluid at the hub of the spinal needle may cause confusion if free flow is not obtained. Different needle systems exist to ease CSE, including epidural needles with a 'back hole' at the distal end to allow the spinal needle to pass through the epidural needle without being bent by the latter's curved tip, or double-lumen epidural needles to enable the catheter to be threaded before intrathecal injection. Various locking devices, to prevent the spinal needle from moving relative to the epidural needle once the intrathecal space has been located, are also available. The presence of microscopic metal fragments following needle-through-needle CSE has been claimed but is disputed.

In 'epidural volume expansion' (EVE), a bolus of epidural saline, injected via either the needle or catheter, is used to increase the cranial spread of a (usually small) spinal dose of local anaesthetic. The mechanism is thought to be compression of the dural sac by the epidural fluid, and has been implicated in the occasionally very high block when a spinal is performed after (inadequate) epidural anaesthesia. EVE has been claimed to produce a reliably extensive block from a smaller than usual dose of drug, whilst reducing side effects such as hypotension and motor block. However, it is not universally employed because the extra spread is usually relatively modest (a few segments only) and use of a smaller dose increases the risk of discomfort/inadequate block.

Cook TM (2000). Anaesthesia; 55: 42–64

Combitube, *see Oesophageal obturators and airways*

Commission for Health Improvement (CHI), *see Healthcare Commission.*

Committee on Safety of Medicines (CSM). Advisory body, originally set up as the Committee on Safety of Drugs in 1963 after the thalidomide disaster. Became the CSM in 1971 when the Medicines Act became law. Was the body responsible for granting certificates to new drugs before clinical trials and product licences, and for monitoring postmarketing safety. Joined with the Medicines Commission in 2005 to form the Commission on Human Medicines (CHM), a committee of the Medicines and Healthcare products Regulatory Agency, charged with advising ministers on licencing policy, taking responsibility for drug safety issues, advising on appointments related to human medicines, and hearing evidence from drug companies if licence applications are rejected.
See also, Adverse drug reactions; Drug development

Compartment syndromes. Impaired circulation and function of tissues within a fascial compartment, associated with increased pressure within the compartment. May be caused by external compression (e.g. tourniquets, limb plasters, etc.) or increased volume of intracompartmental contents (e.g. following trauma, severe exercise, prolonged immobility, bleeding or ischaemia of the underlying tissues). May lead to disruption of capillaries, leakage of intravascular fluid into the tissues, impaired perfusion, myoglobinuria (crush syndrome) and gangrene. Total ischaemia leads to irreversible muscle changes after 4 h. The forearm or lower leg is most commonly affected. Pressure within the lower leg compartments is normally under 15 mmHg when supine, and may be monitored using a simple manometer.

- Features:
  - increasing pain despite immobilisation of the limb.
  - altered sensation in dermatomes corresponding to nerves running through the compartment.
  - increased pressure within the compartment on palpation and also when measured.
  - peripheral pulses may be present.

Treatment includes release of tourniquets, dressings, plaster casts, etc.; surgical fasciotomy may be required. The abdominal compartment syndrome may occur e.g. in abdominal trauma.

Competition, drug, *see Antagonist; Dose–response curves*

Complement. Term describing a series of plasma proteins (labelled C1–C9), synthesised in the liver and involved in immunological and inflammatory reactions. Activation of the system causes a cascade, amplifying the initial stimulus.

- Pathways (Fig. 43):
  - classical (discovered first):
    - activated by immunological reactions, i.e. requires prior exposure to antigen, although it may follow prior exposure to a cross-reacting antigen.
    - antibody–antigen complex binds to C1.
    - via C4, C2 and C3, forming a complex which activates C5.
  - alternative:
    - activated by aggregated IgA, infections, or spontaneous reaction.
    - via other factors: B, D and H forming a complex activating C5.
    - may amplify itself or the classical pathway via C3b formation.

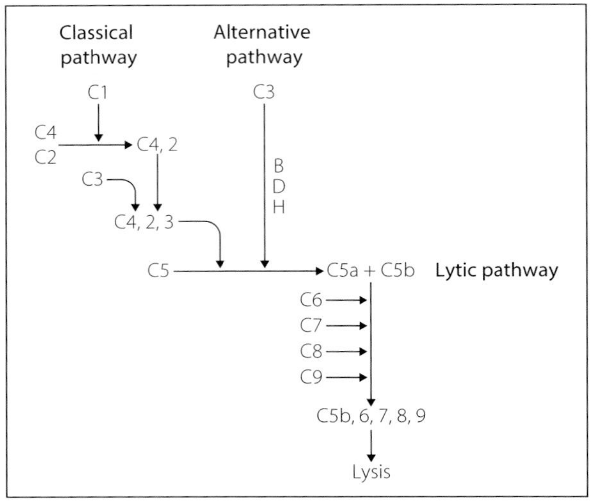

Fig. 43 Complement system

  - lytic:
    - activated by products of the above pathways, causing C5 to form C5a and C5b. The latter binds to the target membrane.
    - C5b binding in turn by C6, C7, C8 and C9.
    - the resultant complex causes membrane lysis.
- In addition, activated factors produced during all pathways may:
  - bind to mast cells and basophils, causing degranulation and release of histamine.
  - be chemotactic for phagocytes, aiding phagocytosis.
  - cause vasodilatation and increase capillary permeability.

Complement activation may be involved in many disease processes. IgM and IgG both bind complement, and are involved in hypersensitivity reactions, e.g. adverse drug reactions. Althesin could cause either classical or alternative pathway activation. Assays for individual components may assist determination of the pathways involved; e.g. low levels of C4 indicate classical pathway activation, etc.

Complex regional pain syndrome type 1 (CRPS type 1). Formerly called reflex sympathetic dystrophy, it consists of continuous pain (usually allodynia or hyperalgesia) in part of an extremity after trauma including fractures, but which does not correspond to the distribution of a single peripheral nerve. Worse with movement. Associated with sympathetic hyperactivity, with cool clammy skin; it may proceed to a pale, cold extremity with tissue atrophy and stiffness. Usually occurs within weeks of trauma, which may be mild. In Sudeck's atrophy, osteoporosis is also present. Treatment includes mobility, physiotherapy, rehabilitation and sympathetic nerve blocks, although the place of the latter is controversial.
[Paul HM Sudeck (1866–1945), German surgeon]
Raja SN, Grabow TS (2002). Anesthesiology; 96: 1254–60
See also, Complex regional pain syndrome type 2

Complex regional pain syndrome type 2 (CRPS type 2). Formerly called causalgia, it is similar to complex regional pain syndrome type 1 in all respects except there is actual nerve damage. Consists of burning pain in the distribution of the damaged peripheral nerve, most commonly median, ulnar or sciatic. May occur within a month of injury, and may radiate beyond the nerve's normal cutaneous distribution.

Exacerbated by cutaneous stimulation in the affected area, and often by emotional upset. Results from abnormal sweat and vasomotor sympathetic efferent pathways, possibly due to abnormal connections between efferent sympathetic fibres and somatic sensory fibres at the injury site. The skin of the affected limb is classically cold, moist and swollen, becoming atrophic later and leading to disuse and osteoporosis.

Treatment traditionally has included sympathetic nerve blocks but this is currently controversial.

Harden RN (2001). Br J Anaesth; 87: 99–106

See also, Complex regional pain syndrome type 1

Compliance. Volume change per unit pressure change; thus a measure of distensibility, e.g. of lungs, chest wall, heart, etc. For measurement of lung compliance, transmural pressure is required, i.e. the difference between alveolar and intrapleural pressures. The former is measured at the mouth during periods of no gas flow, e.g. with the lungs held partially inflated and a few seconds allowed for stabilisation, or using a shutter at the mouth to interrupt flow momentarily. Intrapleural pressure is measured using a balloon positioned in the lower third of the oesophagus. The resulting pressure/volume curve is approximately linear at normal tidal volumes (Fig. 44). Different curves are measured during lung inflation and deflation (hysteresis); this is thought to represent the effects of surface tension.

Human lung compliance is about 1.5–2 l/kPa (150–200 ml/cmH_2O); reduced when supine because of decreased FRC. Chest wall compliance is thought to be similar, but measurement is difficult because of the effects of respiratory muscles. Total thoracic compliance requires measurement of alveolar and ambient pressure difference, and equals about 0.85 l/kPa (85 ml/cmH_2O).

- Compliance measurements are related thus:

$$\frac{1}{\text{total thoracic}} = \frac{1}{\text{chest wall}} + \frac{1}{\text{lung}}$$

- Lung compliance is divided into two components:
  - static; i.e. alveolar ‘stretchability’; measured at steady state as above.
  - dynamic; related to airway resistance during equilibration of gases throughout the lung at end-inspiration or expiration.

  Time constant (resistance × compliance) is a reflection of combined static and dynamic compliance.

Compliance is related to body size; thus specific compliance is often referred to (compliance divided by FRC). It increases in old age and emphysema, due to destruction of elastic lung tissue. It is reduced in pulmonary fibrosis, vascular engorgement and oedema; dynamic compliance is decreased in chronic bronchitis. It is also reduced at the extremes of lung volume, as well as at the lung apices and bases in erect subjects.

See also, Breathing, work of

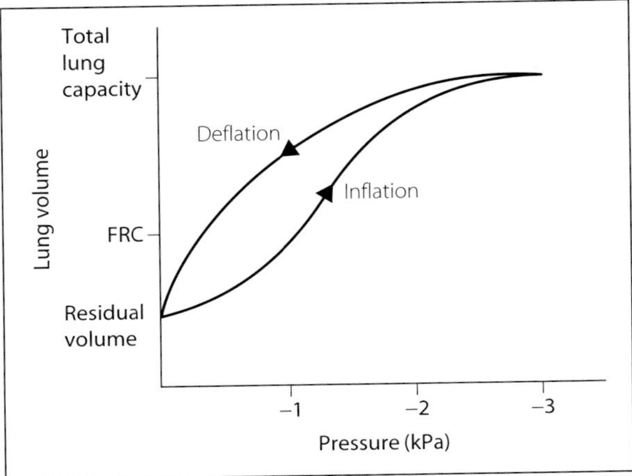

Fig. 44 Pressure/volume curve of lung

Complications of anaesthesia, *see Anaesthetic morbidity and mortality*

Compound A, Pentafluoroisopropenyl fluoromethyl ether, *see Sevoflurane*

Compressed spectral array, *see Power spectral analysis*

Computed (axial) tomography (CAT scanning; CT scanning). Imaging technique in which an X-ray source and detector are held opposite each other, with the patient midway between. The source and detector are rotated stepwise about the mid-point, thus scanning the patient from different angles. At each step, the amount of X-rays reaching the detector is measured, and the spatial arrangement of structures within the patient ‘slice’ computed and displayed on a screen. In spiral CT scanning, the X-ray tube and detector are able to rotate around the patient as the latter moves through the scanner, resulting in a helical scan from which axial slices may be reconstructed. Spiral scanning is quicker than conventional scanning and allows greater detail, especially during contrast studies. Used initially for brain scanning, now for all parts of the body. Used primarily for detection of malignancy, it has also been used to investigate ischaemic heart disease, to identify regions of MI, and for cinematographic angiography using contrast media. Spiral CT scanning is increasingly used to diagnose PE.

Patients must remain still during scanning, and may require sedation or general anaesthesia, e.g. children and patients with head injury. Choice of techniques and drugs is dictated by the patient’s condition; monitoring and maintenance of the airway are particular concerns. Management is similar to that for radiotherapy.

See also, Radiology, anaesthesia for

Computers. Commonly used in research and clinical settings, e.g.:

- data handling:
  - input of data by hand or directly from monitors, etc.
  - analysis and derivation of data, e.g. ECG analysis, cerebral function monitoring, cardiac output measurement.
  - display of information, e.g. on screen, paper, to disk, etc. Trends over different time scales, selection of data, etc. are easily produced.
  - statistical analysis and audit.
  - determining models, e.g. for pharmacokinetics, to predict drug behaviour.
- control systems:
  - gas flows, volatile agent injection into gas streams, etc.
  - closed loop systems: continuous feedback of information regarding a variable to the controlling device, which maintains steady state by adjusting an effector mechanism (e.g. computer-controlled infusion of sodium nitroprusside in the treatment of hypertension).
- decision making:
  - diagnostic.
  - teaching/training.
  - patient management, e.g. use of expert systems, risk analysis of treatment options, etc.

See also, Fuzzy logic; Internet

COMT, *see Catechol-O-methyl transferase*

Concentration effect. Phenomenon whereby increased concentration of inhalation anaesthetic agent results in earlier equilibrium of pulmonary uptake. As concentration increases, the effect of alveolar absorption of agent between breaths is reduced.

Conductance. Reciprocal of resistance. For electrical circuits, the SI unit is the siemens. The term is often used to describe the permeability of cell membranes to various ions. [Sir William Siemens (1823–1883), German-born English engineer]

Confederation of European National Societies of Anaesthesiologists (CENSA). Organisation founded in 1998, originally created as the European Regional Section of the World Federation of Societies of Anaesthesiologists. Consisted of approximately 40 national anaesthetic societies with about 40 000 members in total. Organised European congresses every 4 years (from 2000, every 2 years) and was involved in various educational projects throughout Europe. Amalgamated with the European Society of Anaesthesiologists and the European Academy of Anaesthesiology to form the European Society of Anaesthesiology in 2005.
Kettler D, Wilkinson D (2000). Eur J Anaesth; 17: 145

Confidence intervals. Range of values derived from sample data, relating the data to the actual population. 95% confidence intervals (95% CI) contain the true (population) value with a probability (*P* value) of 0.05.

When used to express the results of statistical tests, confidence intervals differ from null hypothesis testing thus:

- null hypothesis testing indicates whether a difference in data is statistically significant (i.e. unlikely to be due to chance alone); the significance is expressed as a *P* value.
- confidence intervals indicate the likely magnitude of such a difference, by giving a range within which the true value is likely to lie. By using the same units as the data, they allow estimations of clinical relevance to be made; for example, a statistically very significant result may be clinically irrelevant if the actual differences involved are very small.

Confidence intervals are wide if the sample size is small or standard deviation is large. If the 95% CI of a difference between groups do not include zero, this is equivalent to the difference having a P value < 0.05; if they include zero then $P > 0.05$.
Asai T (2002). Br J Anaesth; 89: 807–9
See also, Statistical significance

Confidential Enquiries into Maternal Deaths. Report into all maternal deaths in the UK (Scotland and Northern Ireland were excluded until 1985). Originally conducted by the Royal College of Obstetricians and Gynaecologists in the 1930s. Published initially by the Department of Health, its first report covered 1952–54. From 1999 to 2005, administered within the NICE which, in 2003, combined the project with the Confidential Enquiries into Stillbirths and Deaths in Infancy (CESDI) to form the Confidential Enquiries into Maternal and Child Health (CEMACH)). CEMACH is now an independent body, its enquiries commissioned by the National Patient Safety Agency since 2005. Details of cases are collected from a variety of sources and administered centrally by regional CEMACH offices. Information is collected from all involved staff, observing strict confidentiality. Regional and central assessors (in anaesthetics, obstetric medicine, psychiatry, general practice, pathology and midwifery) review and categorise the deaths according to cause. Causes of deaths may be:

- direct: arising directly from pregnancy or an intervention relating to it.
- indirect: resulting from disease that pre-exists or develops during pregnancy, and is aggravated by pregnancy, or from an intervention not related to the pregnancy but influenced by it.
- late: occur between 42 days and 1 year after the end of pregnancy.
- coincidental (previously fortuitous): unrelated to pregnancy.

Direct deaths have numbered ~100–130 in the last 20 years, while indirect deaths have increased from ~80–90 to ~150–160. In the last decade the main causes of death have been cardiac disease, thrombosis/thromboembolism, suicide/psychiatric disease/substance abuse, pre-eclampsia/eclampsia, haemorrhage, sepsis, amniotic fluid embolism and ectopic pregnancy. Obesity and social exclusion/poor access to services are particularly highlighted as contributing factors in the most recent reports.

Anaesthesia was a consistent direct cause of death for many years, ranking third after hypertensive disease and thromboembolism in several previous reports (Table 10). In the latest (2002–2005) report, there were six direct deaths resulting from anaesthesia but another 31 in which poor perioperative anaesthetic management may have contributed to the outcome.

Improvements in anaesthetic mortality are thought to reflect better training and facilities, and are likely to be greater than suggested by the above figures, since the number of anaesthetic procedures performed has markedly increased. Most direct and indirect anaesthetic deaths in previous reports have involved Caesarean section; common factors have been lack of senior involvement, difficulty with tracheal intubation, aspiration of gastric contents, haemorrhage and lack of ICU or HDU facilities. The need for proper training, facilities and help is repeatedly stressed. In the more recent reports, communication failures, lack of senior availability, underestimation of severity of illness by trainees, delayed resuscitation and administration of blood products, inadequate ICU/HDU facilities, drug error and the risks of

Table 10 Direct deaths attributable to anaesthesia in Confidential Enquiries into Maternal Deaths reports, 1970–2005

Period	*No.*	*Proportion*	*Rate per 100 000 maternities*
1970–72	37	10.8	1.28
1973–75	27	11.9	1.05
1976–78	27	12.4	1.21
1979–81	22	12.4	0.87
1982–84	18	13.0	0.72
1985–87	6	4.3	0.26
1988–90	4	2.8	0.17
1991–93	8	6.3	0.35
1994–96	1	0.7	0.05
1997–99	3	2.8	0.14
2000–02	6	5.7	0.30
2002–05	6	4.5	0.28

rapid iv injection of large doses of oxytocin have been highlighted.

Cooper GM, McClure JH (2008). Br J Anaesth; 100: 17–22

See also, Audit; Obstetric analgesia and anaesthesia

Confidential Enquiry into Perioperative Deaths, *see National Confidential Enquiry into Patient Outcome and Death*

Confusion in the intensive care unit. An acute confusional state is the most common form of psychiatric disorder encountered in the ICU and may form part of the syndrome of ICU psychosis. Often represents an acute reaction to a number of pathological processes that may occur in the critically ill patient. The elderly are more susceptible. Symptoms include disorientation in space and time, agitation, slow responses, slurred speech and hallucinations; often worse at night.

- Causes include:
  - systemic infection.
  - CVS disease, e.g. hypotension, MI, endocarditis.
  - RS disease, e.g. hypoxaemia, hypercapnia, chest infection.
  - CNS disease, e.g. encephalitis, meningitis, head injury, space-occupying lesions, post-ictal states.
  - drug therapy/withdrawal especially sedatives.
  - drug abuse/withdrawal, e.g. alcohol, opioids, amfetamines.
  - metabolic disorders, e.g. hypo/hyperglycaemia, hypo/hypernatraemia, hypercalcaemia.
  - hypo/hyperthermia.
  - thiamine deficiency.
  - pain, full bladder.
  - sleep deprivation.
- Management includes appropriate investigation and treatment of the underlying cause, reassurance, re-establishment of the sleep–wake cycle, and promotion of a calm environment, e.g. by reducing noise levels. Sedation may sometimes be appropriate.

Pun BT, Ely EW (2007). Chest; 132: 624–36

Confusion, postoperative. Occurs in 10–60% of patients during emergence from anaesthesia, especially in the elderly.

- Possible causes include:
  - drugs: any, especially depressant drugs, ketamine, and those associated with the central anticholinergic syndrome.
  - hypoxaemia, hypercapnia.
  - hypotension.
  - restlessness due to pain or full bladder.
  - metabolic disturbances, e.g. hypoglycaemia, hypernatraemia, hyponatraemia, acidosis, etc.
  - alcohol and benzodiazepine withdrawal.
  - sepsis.
  - intracranial problems, e.g. raised ICP, CVA, post-ictal state, etc.
  - pre-existing confusion.
  - reduced cerebral blood flow resulting from perioperative hyperventilation (especially in the elderly) has been suggested as a cause.

Confusion within a few days of surgery may be caused by any illness, e.g. sepsis, pulmonary disease, etc., especially in the elderly. Appropriate investigation, e.g. blood gas analysis, should be performed, rather than simply administering sedation, which may exacerbate the confusion. Many old patients are confused with a change of environment, i.e. hospitalisation. Long-term decreases in intellectual function are thought to be possible, particularly in the elderly.

Congenital heart disease. Incidence: up to 1% of live births; 15% survive to adulthood without treatment. May be associated with other congenital defects or syndromes.

- Simple classification:
  - acyanotic (no shunt):
    - coarctation of aorta (5–10%).
    - pulmonary and aortic stenosis (10–15% together).
  - potentially cyanotic, i.e. left-to-right shunt; may reverse if pulmonary hypertension develops (Eisenmenger's syndrome):
    - ASD (10–15%).
    - VSD (20–30%).
    - patent ductus arteriosus (10–15%).
  - cyanotic, due to:
    - right-to-left shunt:
      - Fallot's tetralogy (5–10%).
      - pulmonary atresia with septal defect.
      - tricuspid valve lesions including Ebstein's anomaly, with septal defect.
    - abnormal connections:
      - transposition of the great arteries (5%).
      - anomalous systemic or pulmonary venous drainage, the latter with right-to-left shunt.
    - mixing of systemic and pulmonary blood, e.g. single atrium or ventricle.

Has also been classified functionally as:

- obstructive: e.g. coarctation, valve stenosis.
- shunt; may be:
  - restrictive: amount of shunt is affected relatively little by changes in pulmonary or systemic vascular resistance, since the flow across the connection itself is relatively fixed, e.g. small VSD.
  - non-restrictive: amount of shunt depends largely on the relationship between pulmonary and systemic vascular resistance, since flow through the connection is variable, e.g. large VSD.
- complex, i.e. involving both obstruction and shunt, e.g. Fallot's tetralogy.

Common features include feeding difficulty, failure to thrive, cyanosis, dyspnoea, heart murmurs and cardiac failure. Patients may present soon after birth. Investigation includes echocardiography and cardiac catheterisation. Increased risk of surgery within first year of life is offset by the high mortality without surgery. Palliative procedures are sometimes performed early, with later corrective surgery, e.g.:

- pulmonary balloon valvuloplasty in pulmonary stenosis.
- shunt procedures to increase pulmonary blood flow in severe right-to-left shunt, e.g. Fallot's tetralogy. A prosthetic graft is inserted between the subclavian and pulmonary arteries (formerly involved direct anastomosis of the subclavian artery itself (Blalock–Taussig procedure)). Balloon atrial septostomy is sometimes performed in transposition of the great arteries, to allow oxygenated blood to pass from left to right sides of heart.
- pulmonary banding to reduce pulmonary blood flow and prevent pulmonary hypertension in large left-to-right shunts.

Principles of anaesthesia are as for cardiac surgery and paediatric anaesthesia. Inhalational or iv techniques are suitable. Uptake of inhalational agents is slower when right-to-left shunts exist. Ketamine is preferred by some anaesthetists. Air bubbles in iv lines are particularly hazardous in right-to-left shunts, with risk of systemic embolism. Nasal tracheal tubes are preferred when postoperative IPPV is required.

- Antibiotic prophylaxis is given for invasive procedures in patients with congenital heart disease (or prosthetic heart valves) to prevent endocarditis; UK guidelines:
  - dental (local anaesthesia):
    - amoxicillin 3 g orally 1 h preoperatively (clindamycin 600 mg instead, if allergic to penicillin).
    - if previous endocarditis, treat as below.
  - dental (general anaesthesia):
    - amoxicillin 3 g orally 4 h preoperatively, + 3 g as soon as possible postoperatively, or:
    - amoxicillin 1 g iv before induction, + 500 mg orally 6 h later.
    - if prosthetic valve or previous endocarditis: amoxicillin 1 g + gentamicin 120 mg iv before induction. Oral amoxicillin 500 mg 6 h later (if allergic to penicillin, vancomycin 1 g iv over at least 100 min + gentamicin 120 mg before induction or teicoplanin 400 mg + gentamicin 120 mg iv before induction, or clindamycin 300 mg iv + 150 mg 6 h later).
  - genitourinary/colonic surgery: as for high risk dental.

[Alfred Blalock (1899–1964), US surgeon; Helen Taussig (1898–1986), US physician]

See also, Preoperative assessment; Pulmonary valve lesions; Valvular heart disease

Congestive cardiac failure, *see Cardiac failure*

Coning. Herniation of brain structures caused by increased ICP. May be:

- supratentorial, e.g. caused by CVA, subarachnoid haemorrhage, cerebral abscess, encephalitis, neoplasm, trauma, etc. Supratentorial pressure may result in:
  - central herniation: the diencephalon is forced through the tentorial opening. Early signs include altered alertness, sighing and yawning, small pupils and conjugate roving eye movements. Appropriate motor responses give way to decorticate posture. As midbrain compression occurs, Cheyne–Stokes respiration appears, pupils become moderately dilated and decerebrate posture is seen. Medullary compression results in hypertension, bradycardia and respiratory arrhythmias (Cushing's reflex) and is a terminal event.
  - uncal herniation: usually caused by a rapidly expanding mass (e.g. traumatic haematoma) in the middle fossa or temporal lobe, which pushes the medial uncus over the edge of the tentorium. Decreased consciousness occurs late and the earliest consistent sign is a unilateral dilating pupil caused by the ipsilateral oculomotor nerve (cranial nerve III) as it is compressed against the tentorial edge. Delay in decompression at this stage results in irreversible brainstem damage.
- infratentorial: caused by posterior fossa masses. May result in:
  - upward cerebellar herniation causing midbrain compression, cerebellar infarction and hydrocephalus.
  - tonsillar herniation: the cerebellar tonsils are forced through the foramen magnum resulting in medullary compression. May follow lumbar puncture in the presence of increased ICP.

Conjoined twins. Incidence is about 1 in 200 000 births. Radiological assessment may require repeat anaesthesia. Each twin requires a separate anaesthetic team. Tracheal intubation and access may be difficult, depending on the site of union. If circulation is shared, induction of the first twin may be delayed, as anaesthetic drugs are taken up by the second twin. Induction of the second twin may thus be rapid. Blood loss at separation may be massive. Adrenal insufficiency may be present in one twin.

Thomas JM, Lopez JT (2004). Paediatr Anaesth; 14: 117–29

Connective tissue diseases. Group of diseases sharing certain features, particularly inflammation of connective tissue and features of autoimmune disease. Rheumatoid arthritis, SLE and systemic sclerosis (SS) are more common in women; polyarteritis nodosa (PN) is more common in men.

- Features may include the following:
  - autoimmune involvement: immunoglobulins may be directed against IgG (rheumatoid factors) and cell components, e.g. nuclear proteins, phospholipids, etc. Organ specific antibodies are also common, e.g. against thyroid and gastric parietal cells, smooth muscle and mitochondria. T and B cell dysfunction, immune complex deposition and complement activation may also occur. Diagnosis of specific disease is aided by the pattern of immune disturbance.
  - systemic involvement:
    - musculoskeletal: arthropathy, myopathy.
    - skin: rash, mouth ulcers. Thickening in SS, with characteristic pinched mouth.
    - renal: glomerulonephritis, vasculitis, nephrotic syndrome.
    - fever, malaise.
    - cardiovascular: pericarditis, myocarditis, conduction defects, vasculitis (affecting any organ). Raynaud's phenomenon (fingers turn white, then blue, then red on exposure to cold, stress, vibration, etc.) is common.
    - haematological: anaemia, leucopenia, thrombocytopenia. Lupus anticoagulant may be present in SLE.
    - hepatosplenomegaly.
    - central and peripheral nervous involvement, e.g. central lesions, neuropathies and psychiatric disturbances (especially with SLE).
    - pulmonary: fibrosis, pleurisy, pleural effusions and pulmonary infiltrates. Pulmonary hypertension may occur. Haemorrhage with PN.
    - Sjögren's syndrome (reduced tear and saliva formation and secretion) may occur.
    - GIT: reduced oesophageal motility, oesophagitis and risk of regurgitation, especially in SS.

Treatment includes corticosteroids and other immunosuppressive drugs. Antimalarial drugs are used in SLE.

- Anaesthetic considerations:
  - careful preoperative assessment to identify the above features, complications and drugs, with appropriate management.
  - mouth opening may be difficult in SS.
  - general management: as for rheumatoid arthritis.

Other conditions without circulating rheumatoid factors may have systemic manifestations, e.g. ankylosing spondylitis and associated conditions. Arthritis may accompany inflammatory bowel disease and intestinal infection.

[Maurice Raynaud (1834–1881), French physician; Henrik Sjögren (1899–1986), Swedish ophthalmologist]

See also, Vasculitides

Connectors, tracheal tube. Adaptors for connecting tracheal tubes to anaesthetic breathing systems (Fig. 45). Modern connectors are plastic, and 15 mm in size distally.

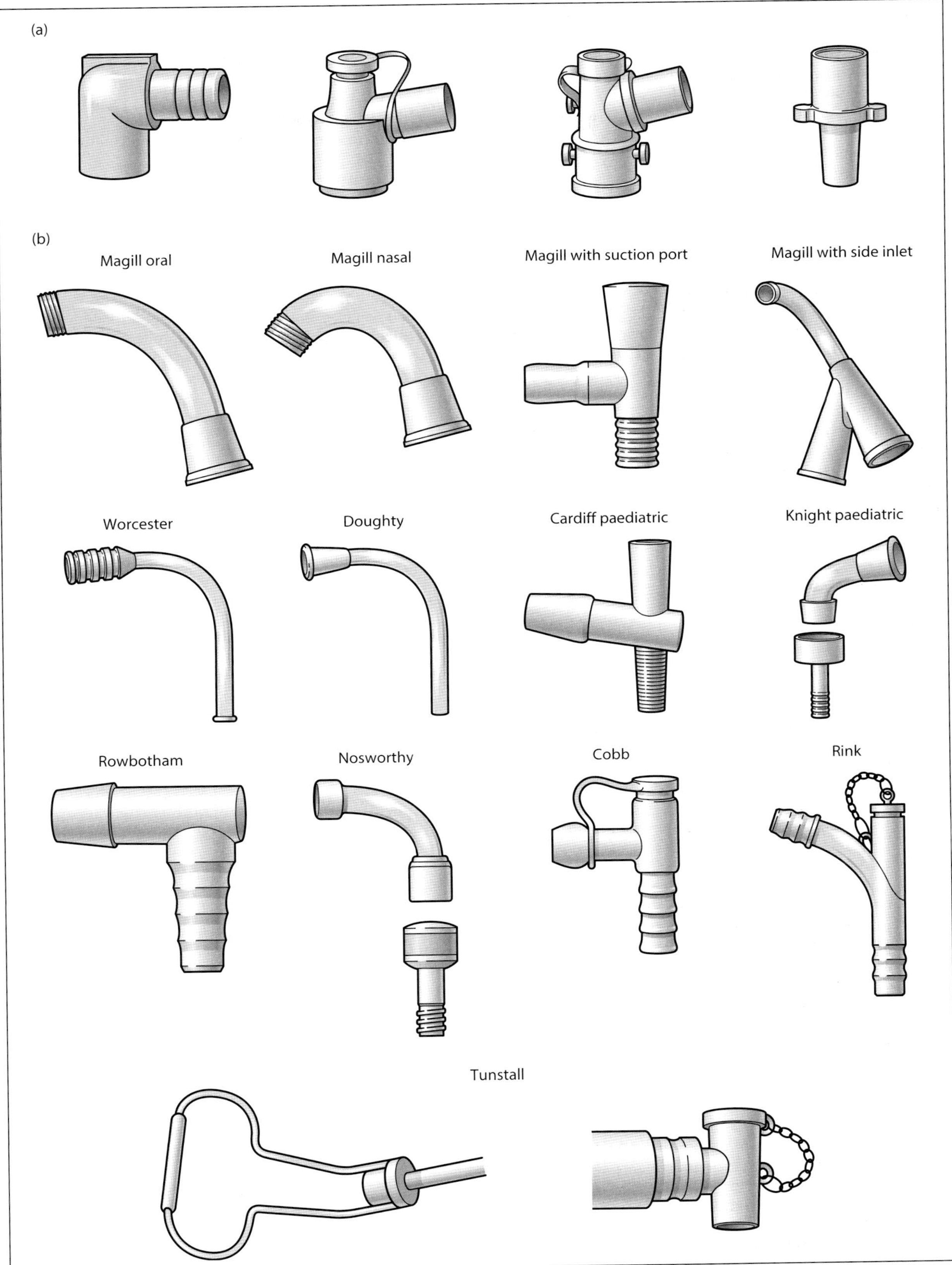

Fig. 45 Different types of tracheal tube connector: (a) plastic; (b) metal

They fit to any standardised 15/22 mm equipment, e.g. directly to breathing tubing or to catheter mounts. They may connect directly or via angle pieces, which may swivel. Some incorporate a capped port for tracheobronchial suction, insertion of fibreoptic instruments, etc.

- Other types are less widely used now, and are named after the anaesthetists who described them or where they were developed:
  - Magill: various types.
  - Rowbotham.
  - Nosworthy: pushed together and twisted to lock.
  - Cobb: allows tracheobronchial suction.
  - Rink: curved to reduce turbulence.
  - Worcester: for tonsillectomy.
  - Doughty: for tonsillectomy.
  - Cardiff paediatric: allows suction.
  - Knight paediatric: similar to Nosworthy's.
  - Tunstall: for infants; the wire portion is taped to the baby's forehead to allow fixation of nasal tubes, e.g. on ICU.

[WA Cobb (described 1943), London anaesthetist; Michael D Nosworthy, Ernest H Rink (1905–1959), Andrew G Doughty and Peter F Knight, London anaesthetists; Michael E Tunstall, Aberdeen anaesthetist]

Conn's syndrome, *see Hyperaldosteronism*

Consent for anaesthesia. Required before general and local anaesthetic techniques may be performed. Failure to obtain consent may result in a charge of battery; in addition, inadequate counselling whilst obtaining consent may result in charges of negligence.

- Consent requires:
  - adequate capacity of the patient to understand: the patient should be over 16 years (in England and Wales) and 'of sound mind', i.e. unaffected by drugs, extreme pain, etc. (this decision should be made by the treating doctor although it may be aided by consulting with colleagues). Consent on behalf of children is given by their parents or legal guardians, although this may be overruled by the courts. The 'emancipated minor' is a child under the age of majority who is able to understand and therefore make decisions about his/her treatment (though in English law he/she may consent to treatment but not refuse it ['Gillick competent']).

    If the patient lacks capacity (e.g. is unconscious) then life-saving treatment may proceed if it is felt to be in his/her 'best interests' (n.b. these may not be the same as 'medical best interests') and every attempt should be made to find out the patient's views and wishes. In England and Wales, the Mental Capacity Act 2005 laid down formal procedures for the appointment of advocates for persons lacking capacity, and also strengthens the status of advance decisions (in Scotland, advocates for incapacitous patients already had legal status).
  - disclosure of relevant information: traditionally, in the UK, doctors have used their discretion to explain risks and benefits as they feel appropriate for the patient concerned, as long as their decision is judged reasonable according to current medical opinion. In the USA, legally required 'Informed Consent' (i.e. full explanation of risks, benefits and alternatives) is judged according to what a reasonable patient would expect to have explained to him/her. Increasingly, in the UK, emphasis has shifted towards what patients want to know, rather than what doctors think they should know.
  - patient's understanding of the options and their implications.
  - voluntary decision and the time in which to make it.
- Consent may be:
  - verbal or written. The latter serves as proof of consent afterwards, but is no 'stronger' than verbal consent, which should be witnessed if possible.
  - express or implied (i.e. by allowing treatment, insertion of a cannula, etc., the patient is demonstrating consent, without having specifically expressed it).

Consent forms are now standard for surgery and the consenting process was updated in guidance issued by the UK Department of Health in 2001. A separate section for anaesthesia has been suggested, although the ability of junior surgeons (who usually obtain consent) to inform the patient adequately in this respect has led to some controversy. There is disagreement about the requirement for consent forms in other procedures; e.g. epidural analgesia in labour requires written consent only in some UK units. The Association of Anaesthetists of Great Britain & Ireland issued guidance in 2006 that did not recommend a separate anaesthetic consent form, although the importance of recording the discussion around consent was stressed.

In the ICU/emergency setting, consent for invasive interventions (e.g. tracheal intubation, venous cannulation, surgery, etc.) often cannot be obtained from the patient and similar procedures apply as above. Until the Mental Capacity Act, no person could legally give consent for another, although it has been customary to obtain 'informed assent' from the next of kin though it had no legal status.

White SM, Baldwin TJ (2003). Anaesthesia; 58: 760–74

See also, Medicolegal aspects of anaesthesia

Constipation. Common postoperatively as a result of opioid analgesic drug administration and immobility. On the ICU, may be related to lack of food, drugs (e.g. opioids), altered GIT flora and impaired neurological function, e.g. spinal cord injury. Patients should undergo rectal examination to exclude faecal impaction. Treatment is with oral or rectal laxatives and attention to any underlying cause. Manual evacuation may be required in unconscious patients.

Contamination of breathing equipment. Although hospital acquired infection is common and sometimes fatal, the role of cross-infection involving anaesthetic equipment is uncertain although a common breathing system has been implicated in the cross-infection of patients with hepatitis C. Routine treatment of anaesthetic apparatus varies between hospitals, e.g. breathing systems cleaned or sterilised after each case, daily, weekly, etc. Disposable equipment is increasingly used for convenience and cheapness. Recent guidelines have called for effective breathing system filters to be routinely placed between the patient and breathing system and in certain countries (e.g. parts of Australia) their use is mandatory.

Particularly important in ICU, immunodeficiency states, and in high risk infectious cases, e.g. HIV infection, hepatitis, chest infection, TB (equipment is sterilised after use and other precautions taken, e.g. bacterial filters).

- Methods of killing contaminating organisms:
  - disinfection: kills most organisms but not spores, etc. Achieved by:
    - pasteurisation: 30 min at 77°C. Rubber/plastic items may be distorted.
    - chemical agents:
      - formaldehyde, formalin (no longer used).
      - alcohol 70%.
      - chlorhexidine 0.1–0.5%.
      - glutaraldehyde 2%: expensive and may irritate skin.

- hypochlorite 10%: may corrode metal.
- hydrogen peroxide, phenol 0.6–2%.

Must be followed by rinsing and thorough drying.

- sterilisation: kills all organisms and spores. The term sterility assurance level (SAL) is a measure of the probability of complete sterility of the item. A SAL of 10^{-6} (i.e. probability of an organism surviving on the item following sterilisation is one in a million) is considered acceptable. Methods include:
  - dry heat, e.g. 150°C for 30 min.
  - moist heat:
    - autoclave (most common method), e.g.:
      - 30 min at 1 atm at 122°C;
      - 10 min at 1.5 atm at 126°C;
      - 3 min at 2 atm at 134°C.

      Steam is used to increase temperature. Indicator tape or tubes are used to confirm that the correct conditions are reached.
    - low temperature steam + formaldehyde.
- ethylene oxide: expensive and flammable (the latter risk is reduced by adding 80–90% fluorohydrocarbons or CO_2). Toxic and taken up by plastics; up to 2 weeks' elution time is suggested before use.
- γ-irradiation: used commercially but expensive and inconvenient for most hospital use.
- gas plasma sterilisation: new technique where equipment is exposed to a mixture of highly ionised gas and free radicals. Provides low temperature, dry sterilisation with short cycle times.

The above methods do not destroy the prion protein responsible for variant Creutzfeldt-Jakob disease; this has led to increasing interest in disposable instruments. New enzyme based agents which disrupt prion structure are under investigation.

[Louis Pasteur (1822–1895), French bacteriologist]

See also, COSHH regulations

Continuous positive airway pressure (CPAP). Application of positive airway pressure throughout all phases of spontaneous ventilation. May be achieved with various systems, applied via a tightly fitting mask or tracheal tube. In order to apply positive pressure throughout ventilation, a reservoir bag, or a fresh gas flow exceeding maximal inspiratory gas flow, must be provided. The latter may be achieved using a Venturi mixing device. Increases FRC, thereby reducing airway collapse and increasing arterial oxygenation. $F_{I}O_2$ may thus be reduced.

- Uses:
  - to aid weaning from ventilators.
  - to improve oxygenation during one-lung anaesthesia.
  - in conditions of chronic airway collapse and hypoventilation, e.g. obesity hypoventilation syndrome.
  - in acute respiratory failure to avoid tracheal intubation.
  - in neonates, e.g. in respiratory distress syndrome, bronchomalacia and tracheomalacia, especially if associated with apnoeic episodes. May be applied via nasal cannulae.
- Complications: as for PEEP, but less severe. Barotrauma and reduction in cardiac output are more likely in neonates. Some patients cannot tolerate the sensation of CPAP.

Nasal CPAP, using a tightly fitting nasal mask, is the mainstay of treatment of obstructive sleep apnoea.

Contraceptives, oral. Main anaesthetic considerations are related to the risk of venous thromboembolism which is 2–6 times as common in patients taking the combined contraceptive pill. Patients taking the combined pill containing third generation progesterones (desogestrel or gestodene) are at the greatest risk. Other risk factors, e.g. inherited hypercoagulable states, smoking, obesity, etc., increase the risk further. Although 4 weeks' discontinuation of therapy before major or leg surgery has traditionally been advocated, it has been claimed that this is based on insufficient evidence. If other risk factors exist, discontinuation of therapy (or sc heparin in view of the risk of pregnancy) has been suggested. The pill is restarted after the first period beyond a fortnight postoperatively. No extra precautions are generally thought to be necessary for minor surgery, e.g. dilatation and curettage, or with oestrogen-free therapy.

Stone J (2002). Anaesthesia; 57: 606–25

See also, Hormone replacement therapy

Contrast media, *see Radiological contrast media*

Controlled drugs (CDs). Refers to those governed by the Misuse of Drugs Act 1971 (the term is often reserved for drugs described in Schedule 2 of the Misuse of Drugs Regulations, 1985). The Association of Anaesthetists issued guidelines on the handling of CDs in the operating theatre suite in 1995; their recommendations were:

- preference for prefilled syringes or similar devices to be licensed medicinal products rather than special items produced in a licensed facility for individual patients, with medicines prepared in an unlicensed site (e.g. pharmacy) being least preferable.
- local guidelines for ordering, storage, handling and administration of CDs, including doctors' signatures in the CD register; recording in the notes the amount given; return of unopened ampoules; and disposal of unused drug (e.g. by discarding on to absorbent material before disposal).
- ability for ODPs to issue and handle CDs (along with registration of ODPs etc.).
- an end to the sharing of ampoules between patients.

See also, Abuse of anaesthetic agents

Convulsions (Fits). Usually refer to tonic–clonic epileptic seizures. They increase cerebral and whole body O_2 demand and CO_2 production, whilst airway obstruction and chest wall rigidity may result in hypoventilation. Thus hypoxaemia, acidosis, hypercapnia and increased sympathetic activity may occur. Patients may also injure themselves. Fits may be generalised or focal. Anaesthetic involvement is usually necessary when they occur perioperatively, or in status epilepticus.

- Caused by:
  - pre-existing epilepsy (i.e. a continuing susceptibility to fits; may include other causes listed below).
  - hypoxaemia.
  - metabolic, e.g. hypoglycaemia, hyponatraemia, hypocalcaemia, uraemia.
  - anaesthetic drugs:
    - diethyl ether; convulsions classically occurred postoperatively in pyrexial children given anticholinergic premedication on hot days.
    - enflurane especially following perioperative hyperventilation and hypocapnia.
    - ketamine, methohexital and doxapram in susceptible patients. Although propofol may cause myoclonic jerking, initial reports of epileptic seizures following its use are now thought to be unfounded. Similarly, etomidate may cause non-epileptic twitching.
    - local anaesthetic drugs in overdose.

- pethidine in very high or prolonged dosage. Convulsions may also follow its interaction with monoamine oxidase inhibitors.
   - other drugs, e.g. alcohol, phenothiazines, tricyclic antidepressant drugs. Several drugs in overdose (e.g. cocaine).
   - fat embolism, also clot or air embolism.
   - head injury, CVA, cerebral infections, meningitis, neurosurgery, brain tumours and other cerebral disease.
   - eclampsia.
   - pyrexia in children.
   - acute O_2 toxicity (Bert effect).
- Management:
   - protection of the airway and maintenance of oxygenation, with positioning on the side if possible. Tracheal intubation and IPPV may be required, e.g. if large amounts of depressant drugs are needed.
   - anticonvulsant drugs:
     - diazepam 5 mg increments iv up to 20 mg; may be given rectally. Midazolam 5–10 mg im has been used as an alternative when iv cannulation is impossible. Lorazepam iv 75 µg/kg is the first-line treatment for status epilepticus.
     - phenytoin iv, 15 mg/kg slowly, with ECG monitoring.
   - other drugs used in the control of seizures include paraldehyde and magnesium sulphate (in eclampsia). If seizures persist following phenytoin the patient should be treated as for status epilepticus.

Cooley, Samuel, *see Wells*

COPD, *see Chronic obstructive pulmonary disease*

Copper kettle, *see Vaporisers*

Co-proxamol, *see Dextropropoxyphene*

Cordotomy, anterolateral. Destruction of lateral spinothalamic tracts, classically in the cervical region (C1–2); used in chronic pain management. Usually performed percutaneously under X-ray control, using sedation. Electrical stimulation is used to confirm correct positioning of the needle before thermocoagulation.

Provides contralateral analgesia lasting up to 3 years; thus it is usually reserved for patients with a life expectancy below this, e.g. patients with malignancy. Descending respiratory fibres lie close to the sectioned fibres and therefore cordotomy is usually not performed in patients with respiratory disease. May damage pyramidal pathways, or cause Horner's syndrome, bladder disturbances and paraesthesiae. Complications are more likely if cordotomy is bilateral.

See also, Sensory pathways

Corning, James Leonard (1855–1923). New York neurologist; first described (and coined the term) spinal anaesthesia in 1885. He had intended to observe the effects of cocaine on the spinal cord by injecting it into the interspinal space of a dog, believing erroneously that the interspinal blood vessels communicated with those of the cord. Hindquarter paralysis and anaesthesia followed. Repeated the experiment on a human, and subsequently suggested its use in the treatment of neurological disease. Epidural anaesthesia may have been produced in some of his studies. Published the first textbook on local anaesthesia in 1886.

Coronary angioplasty, *see Percutaneous transluminal coronary angioplasty*

Coronary artery bypass graft (CABG). Performed for ischaemic heart disease unresponsive to medical treatment (including unstable angina). Saphenous vein grafts were first performed in 1967. Sections of the long saphenous vein in the leg are removed, reversed (because of valves) and anastomosed between the aorta and coronary artery distal to its obstruction. Internal thoracic (internal mammary) artery grafting was first performed in man in the 1950s but discarded until its revival in the 1970s. Following dissection from the posterior surface of the anterior thoracic cage, the artery is anastomosed to the coronary artery. Results are better than saphenous vein grafting because prolonged patency is more likely, but the incidence of perioperative bleeding is greater.

'Minimal access' coronary surgery involves internal thoracic artery grafting through tiny incisions in the left side of the chest, offering the advantages of arterial grafts to the left anterior descending coronary artery without the need for cardiopulmonary bypass although one-lung ventilation is still required. More recently, a technique of 'off-pump' CABG has been developed, in which median sternotomy is carried out enabling multiple grafts on the beating heart. Surgery requires good access (cardiac displacement), stabilisation of the heart's wall at the site of anastomoses using special devices, and the use of intracoronary shunts or strategies to limit periods of arterial occlusion. Anaesthesia is complicated by the need for cardiovascular stability, normothermia and bradycardia during anastomoses to reduce movement (bradycardia is less important with stabilising devices). Complications and costs are felt to be less than with traditional CABG but long-term randomised trials are relatively lacking.

- Life expectancy is improved following CABG in:
   - moderate/severe angina, triple vessel disease and impaired ventricular function.
   - double vessel disease including severe stenosis of the proximal left anterior descending artery.
   - severe stenosis of the left main stem coronary artery.

Life expectancy is not improved in single vessel disease or if angina is not present.

Percutaneous transluminal coronary angioplasty is an alternative but emergency CABG may be required if unsuccessful.

Anaesthesia is as for ischaemic heart disease and cardiac surgery. Combinations of aspirin, dipyridamole and full anticoagulation are used postoperatively to maintain graft patency.

Mortality is under 1% for 1–2 grafts, but increases if more grafts are anastomosed. Mortality is greater in women.

Coronary artery disease, *see Ischaemic heart disease*

Coronary blood flow. Normally approximately 5% of cardiac output, i.e. 250 ml/min or 80 ml/100 g/min. May increase up to five times in exercise. The inner 1 mm of the left ventricle obtains O_2 via diffusion from blood in the ventricular cavity; the remainder of the ventricle is supplied via epicardial vessels. The left coronary vessels are compressed by the contracting myocardium during systole; thus flow to the subendocardium occurs during diastole only. Superficial areas receive more constant flow. Atrial and right ventricular flow occurs throughout the cardiac cycle. The left ventricle is therefore most at risk from myocardial ischaemia.

- Left ventricular blood flow is related to:
   - difference between aortic end-diastolic pressure and left ventricular end-diastolic pressure.
   - duration of diastole (inversely related to heart rate).
   - patency/radius of the coronary arteries; related to:

- autoregulation: normally maintains blood flow above MAP of 60 mmHg, possibly via the action of adenine nucleotides, potassium, hydrogen ions, prostaglandins, lactic acid or CO_2 released from myocardial cells.
- autonomic neural input: has little direct influence, being overridden by the effect on SVR, myocardial contractility, etc.
- coronary stenosis/spasm and the state of collateral vessels (e.g. coronary steal).
- drugs causing vasoconstriction/dilatation.

- blood viscosity.

The oxygen extraction of the myocardium is almost 75% and therefore increased O_2 demand can only be met by increased flow and is important if ischaemia is to be prevented. Reductions in flow may be minimised by controlling the above factors. Coronary perfusion pressure and duration of diastole may be assessed by the diastolic pressure–time index.

- Measurement:
  - Fick principle using N_2O or argon. Requires coronary sinus catheterisation.
  - thermodilution techniques to estimate coronary sinus flow, thus providing an indication of left ventricular drainage.
  - nuclear cardiology may be used to indicate regional flow.

See also, Coronary circulation; Ischaemic heart disease; Myocardial metabolism

Coronary care unit (CCU). The first CCUs opened in 1961–63 and evolved from the concept that recovery from collapse following MI was possible with prompt CPR. Modern CCUs contain ECG monitoring, defibrillators, drugs and trained staff available 24 hours a day. They are used for surveillance and treatment of arrhythmias and cardiac failure, limitation of infarct size and restoration of blood flow in occluded coronary vessels using fibrinolytic drugs. Mortality from MI is thought to be reduced as a result. Now used also for patients without MI.

Anon (1988). Lancet; ii: 830–1

Coronary circulation.

- Arterial supply (Fig. 46a):
  - right coronary artery: arises from the anterior aortic sinus. Passes between the pulmonary trunk and right atrium, and runs in the right atrioventricular groove between the right atrium and ventricle. Descends the anterior surface of the heart, continuing inferiorly to anastomose with the left coronary artery. Supplies the right ventricle and sinoatrial node and, in 90% of the population, the atrioventricular node and posterior and inferior parts of the left ventricle.
  - left coronary artery: arises from the left posterior aortic sinus. Passes lateral to the pulmonary trunk and runs in the left atrioventricular groove. Supplies the anterior wall of the left ventricle and the interventricular septum via its left anterior descending branch, and the lateral wall of the left ventricle via its circumflex branch.

  The artery that supplies the posterior descending and the posterolateral arteries determines the dominant coronary artery; in 60% of the population, the right coronary artery is dominant.

- Venous drainage (Fig. 46b):
  - ⅓ via small veins directly into the right atrium (venae cordis minimae (Thebesian veins) and anterior cardiac veins).
  - ⅔ via the coronary sinus, draining into the right atrium by the opening of the inferior vena cava.

[Adam Thebesius (1686–1732), German physician]

See also, Coronary blood flow

Coronary sinus catheterisation. Performed using fluoroscopy. May be used to determine:

- coronary sinus blood flow, using a thermodilution technique.
- coronary blood flow, using the Fick principle.
- blood O_2 and lactate levels. The latter are raised in myocardial ischaemia, due to decreased uptake by myocardial tissue and increased production.

Coronary steal. Diversion of blood from poorly perfused areas of myocardium to those already adequately perfused. May be caused by vasodilator substances acting on small coronary arteries but not on larger epicardial vessels. Poorly perfused areas supplied by stenosed vessels may be

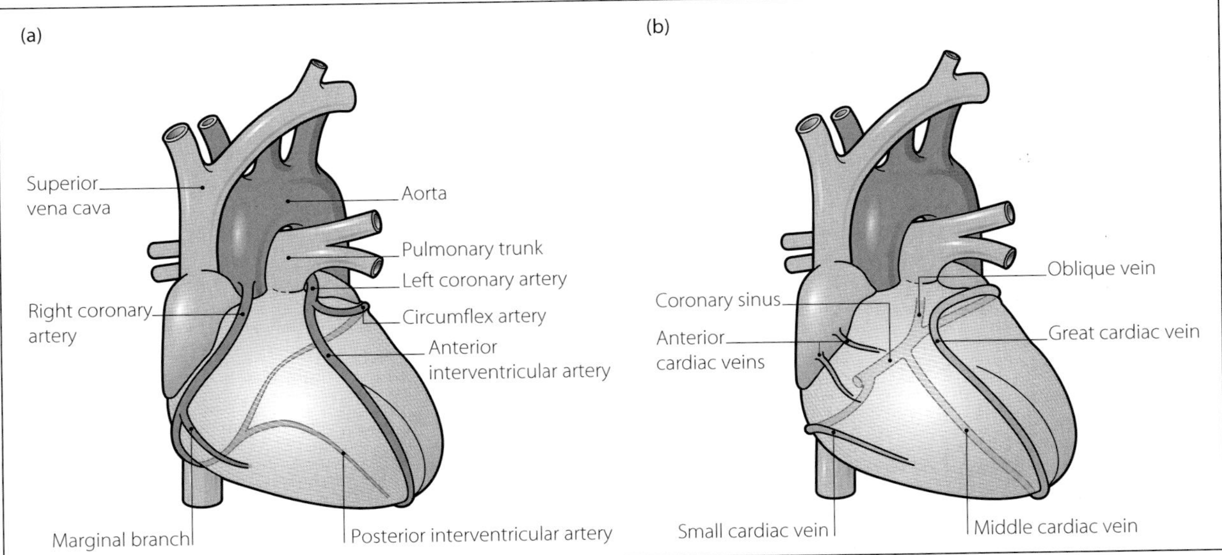

Fig. 46 Coronary circulation: (a) arterial; (b) venous

dependent on collateral vessels for blood flow. Dilatation of normal small arteries increases flow to normal areas, but the stenosed vessels are unable to dilate sufficiently, resulting in steal. Antianginal drugs, e.g. nitrates, are thought to increase collateral flow by acting predominantly on the large epicardial vessels. Adenosine, dipyridamole, papaverine and isoflurane have all been shown to cause steal. The use of isoflurane in patients with ischaemic heart disease has therefore been questioned.

Coroner. Independent judicial officer of the Crown who has a duty to investigate the circumstances of some deaths. Are barristers, solicitors or legally qualified medical practitioners, and are assisted by Coroner's Officers. Cases are referred mostly from doctors, but also from registrars of births and deaths and from other sources, e.g. police. A death should be reported if:
- its cause is unknown.
- the deceased was not seen by the certifying doctor after death or within the fortnight preceding it.
- it was violent, unnatural or suspicious.
- it may have been caused by an accident (whenever it occurred).
- it may have been caused by neglect (by self or others).
- it may have been caused by industrial disease or related to employment.
- it may have been caused by abortion.
- it occurred during an operation or before recovery from an anaesthetic.
- it may have been suicide.
- it occurred during or shortly after detention in police or prison custody.

HIV infection alone is not an indication for referral.

Following referral, the coroner may hold an inquest in a small percentage of cases; a verdict may then be issued as to the manner and cause of death.

Cor pulmonale. Right ventricular hypertrophy secondary to increased pulmonary vascular resistance due to chronic lung disease. COPD is the commonest cause, but any disease that causes chronic hypoxaemia (e.g. pulmonary fibrosis) may result in hypoxic pulmonary vasoconstriction, eventually with pulmonary vascular muscle hypertrophy and pulmonary hypertension. Right ventricular failure may ensue. PE is included in some definitions.
- Features:
  - those of the underlying disease, including cyanosis and hypoxaemia.
  - those of right-sided cardiac failure: peripheral oedema, raised JVP, hepatomegaly, 3rd heart sound.
  - of pulmonary hypertension and underlying disease on chest X-ray. The ECG may show right ventricular hypertrophy and axis deviation, peaked P waves (P pulmonale), and T wave and S–T segment changes in the right chest leads.
- Anaesthetic management:
  - as for COPD/underlying disease.
  - as for cardiac failure.
  - as for pulmonary hypertension.

Correlation, *see Statistical tests*

Corticosteroids. Group of corticosteroid hormones released from the adrenal gland. Divided into two groups according to activity:
- mineralocorticoids: mainly aldosterone. Synthetic mineralocorticoids include fludrocortisone, used for replacement therapy and in congenital adrenal hyperplasia and postural hypotension.
- glucocorticoids: mainly cortisone (hydrocortisone). The term 'corticosteroid therapy' usually refers to use of drugs with predominantly glucocorticoid activity, although most have mineralocorticoid activity too. Corticosteroids are used in adrenocortical insufficiency, and to suppress inflammatory and immunological responses, e.g. in connective tissue diseases, raised ICP due to tumours, etc., skin diseases, blood dyscrasias, allergic reactions, asthma, myasthenia gravis, and following organ transplantation. Have been used in ARDS but their efficacy is disputed. Use in severe sepsis is now thought to increase mortality.

  Prednisolone 5 mg has equivalent anti-inflammatory activity to 20 mg hydrocortisone, 4 mg methylprednisolone and 0.75 mg dexamethasone. All except hydrocortisone have little mineralocorticoid activity and are thus suitable for long-term disease suppression.
- The drugs are associated with many side effects:
  - related to mineralocorticoid activity: water and sodium retention, hypokalaemia, hypertension.
  - hyperglycaemia and diabetes mellitus, osteoporosis and pathological fractures, skeletal wasting with proximal myopathy.
  - GIT effects: dyspepsia, peptic ulcer disease.
  - mental changes: euphoria, depression.
  - spread of infection. Severe chickenpox is a particular risk.
  - decreased wound healing.
  - cataract formation.
  - growth suppression in children.
  - Cushing's syndrome may occur with high dosage.
  - adrenal suppression, due to inhibition of ACTH release. Pituitary–adrenal axis function may take 6 months to recover following withdrawal of therapy; during this time patients are unable to mount a normal cortisone response to stress (secretion increases from 25 mg/day to 300 mg/day), and may develop circulatory collapse. Patients at risk are those who have:
    - received corticosteroid therapy for longer than 2 weeks within the previous 2 months (up to 1 year has been suggested).
    - adrenocortical insufficiency, adrenalectomy, etc.

    Based on studies of normal cortisone responses following surgery, estimated amounts required are 25 mg hydrocortisone equivalent for minor surgery; 50–75 mg/day for 1–2 days for moderate surgery; and 100–150 mg/day for 2–3 days for major surgery. These estimates include current medication; thus patients already taking the required amount do not need supplementation.

See also, Stress response to surgery

Corticotropin (Corticotrophin), *see Adrenocorticotrophic hormone*

COSHH regulations (Control of Substances Hazardous to Health). Came into force in 1989 in Scotland, England and Wales, and in 1991 in Northern Ireland. The regulations were revised in 1994, 1999, and 2002. Stipulate that employers must identify and control any substances which may be hazardous to health, e.g. chemicals and micro-organisms. Important guidance is given to allow employers to assess the risk to employees, eliminate or control the risk (e.g. with protective clothing, adequate ventilation), monitor the exposure and health of employees, and provide information and training. Employees must make full use of any control measure provided. Anaesthetic implications include concerns about the environmental safety of anaesthetists, scavenging, and contamination of anaesthetic equipment.

Costs of anaesthesia. Intraoperative anaesthetic cost constitutes about 5–6% of total hospital costs whereas the total cost in intraoperative patient care is approximately 30%. Anaesthetic costs may be divided into:
- overhead costs:
  - capital equipment, e.g. ventilators, anaesthetic machines, etc. Often difficult to quantify since the life of equipment may be uncertain.
  - maintenance.
  - staff salaries, e.g. anaesthetists, anaesthetic assistants, recovery nurses, etc.
- running costs:
  - drugs, e.g. iv and inhalational anaesthetic agents, neuromuscular blocking drugs, opioids, antiemetics, iv fluids, etc.
  - piped gases (and those in cylinders).
  - consumable items, e.g. iv cannulae, tracheal tubes, airways, etc.

Estimates of the total costs of individual procedures have been made but vary widely according to the country and hospital, and the methods used for the calculations. In addition, techniques or drugs which appear more expensive may have cost savings elsewhere, e.g. by reducing postoperative complications and hospital stay. With increasing scrutiny of healthcare costs, calculations of anaesthetic costs and 'value-based anaesthetic care' may become more common and pressure applied to anaesthetic departments to reduce their costs, despite the relatively small amounts compared to those incurred by the surgeons themselves. However, it has been estimated that about half the intraoperative anaesthetic costs could be influenced by the choice of drugs and anaesthetic techniques.

Costs of intensive care. Actual costs of ICU treatment are difficult to quantify since no standardised model of costing has been validated as being applicable to all types of unit. Methods used have included dividing the total annual expenditure by the number of patients treated and the use of severity of illness and workload scoring systems. Costs have been divided into six 'cost blocks':
- capital equipment: includes depreciation, maintenance and lease charges (~6%).
- estates: includes building depreciation, water, sewage, energy and maintenance charges (~3%).
- non-clinical support: includes administration and cleaning (~8%).
- clinical support: includes physiotherapy, radiology, laboratory services, pharmacy, dietetics (~8%).
- consumables: includes drugs, fluids, nutrition, disposables (~25%).
- staff: medical, nursing, technical (~50%).

ICU costs are significantly higher in the first 24 h after admission and for patients with greater severity of illness as defined by the various scoring systems.

Co-trimoxazole. Synthetic antibacterial drug containing one part trimethoprim to five of the sulphonamide sulfamethoxazole. The former inhibits bacterial synthesis of dihydrofolic acid, whilst the latter inhibits production of tetrahydrofolic acid by dihydrofolate reductase; the combination thus inhibits bacterial nucleic acid and protein production. Previously widely used to treat exacerbations of COPD and urinary tract infections, its indications now are restricted to prophylaxis and treatment of pneumocystis pneumonia and toxoplasmosis unless specific reasons for its use exist, because of its side effect profile.
- Dosage: 960 mg–1.44 g orally/iv, 12 hourly.
- Side effects: nausea, diarrhoea, erythema multiforme, pancreatitis, hepatic impairment, blood dyscrasias.

Cough. Reflex partially under voluntary control. A deep inspiration is followed by forceful expiration against a closed glottis which is suddenly opened to allow explosive exhalation. An intrathoracic pressure of up to 40 kPa may be produced, and the speed of exhaled air may exceed 900 km/h. Solid objects, liquids and mucus are thus expelled from the airways. Afferent pathways for coughing are from the mucosa of the larynx, trachea and large bronchi via the vagus nerve and medulla, and are stimulated by physical or chemical irritants.
- Factors associated with coughing during anaesthesia include:
  - insertion of a pharyngeal airway, tracheal tube, etc. if depth of anaesthesia is inadequate.
  - introduction of inhalational anaesthetic agents at too high a concentration.
  - use of certain iv anaesthetic agents, e.g. methohexital.
  - presence/aspiration of blood, saliva, gastric contents, etc.
  - increased airway reactivity, e.g. asthma, COPD, upper respiratory tract infection, smoking.

In ICU, cough may be produced by airway manoeuvres such as tracheobronchial suctioning, especially if the carina is stimulated. Persistent coughing may cause inadequate ventilation, and excessive intrathoracic pressures may reduce cardiac output (causing 'cough syncope' in non-anaesthetised patients). Deepening of anaesthesia, increased F_IO_2 and neuromuscular blockade may be required.

The reflex is protective, helping to prevent sputum retention and atelectasis. Postoperatively, it may be reduced by:
- impaired mechanical movement, e.g. due to pain, muscle weakness, neuromuscular blockade or disease, central and peripheral nervous disorders.
- depressed cough reflex, e.g. depressant drugs, central lesions.

Opioid analgesic drugs, e.g. codeine, are sometimes used to suppress cough, e.g. in malignant disease.

Cough-CPR. Maintenance of cerebral perfusion and consciousness during severe arrhythmias, e.g. VF, by repeated coughing. Each cough increases intrathoracic pressure and expels arterial blood from the thorax; each gasp draws in venous blood. Has been successful for up to 1–2 min pending availability of a defibrillator.
See also, Cardiopulmonary resuscitation

Coulomb. Unit of charge. One coulomb is the amount of charge passing any point in a circuit in 1 s when a current of 1 ampere is flowing.
[Charles Coulomb (1738–1806), French physicist]

COX, *see Cyclo-oxygenase*

CPAP, *see Continuous positive airway pressure*

CPD/CPD-A, Citrate–phosphate–dextrose/Citrate–phosphate–dextrose–adenine, *see Blood storage*

CPEx, Cardiopulmonary exercise testing; *see Exercise testing*

CPR, *see Cardiopulmonary resuscitation*

CPX, Cardiopulmonary exercise testing; *see Exercise testing*

Crack, *see Cocaine*

CRAMS scale, *see Circulation, respiration, abdomen, motor and speech scale*

Cranial nerves. Comprised of 12 pairs, passing from the brain via foramina at the base of the skull. Convey motor and sensory fibres involved in somatic, parasympathetic (visceral) and special visceral (e.g. muscles of face and taste sensation) pathways:

- I: olfactory nerves (convey smell sensation from the nasal mucosa); pass through the cribriform plate of the ethmoid bone to the olfactory bulb.
- II: optic nerve (conveys visual sensation from the retina); passes through the optic canal and via the optic chiasma, tract and radiation to the visual cortex in the occipital lobe of the brain (*see Pupillary reflex*).
- III: oculomotor nerve (somatic motor fibres supply the extraocular muscles except superior oblique and lateral rectus; parasympathetic fibres supply the pupillary sphincter and ciliary muscles after synapsing in the ciliary ganglion). In the posterior fossa, the nerve passes from the upper midbrain between the cerebral peduncles and lies near the edge of the tentorium cerebelli (hence the early ipsilateral pupillary dilatation that occurs in acute rises of ICP, when the nerve is compressed against the edge of the tentorium (Hutchinson's pupil)). In the middle cranial fossa, it passes forwards on the lateral wall of the cavernous sinus as far as the supraorbital fissure. Before entering the fissure it divides into superior and inferior branches.
- IV: trochlear nerve (motor supply to the superior oblique muscle). Passes from the dorsum of the lower midbrain, then forwards in the lateral wall of the cavernous sinus to enter the supraorbital fissure.
- V: trigeminal nerve (sensory fibres supply the anterior dura, scalp and face, nasopharynx, nasal and oral cavities and air sinuses; motor fibres supply the muscles of mastication). The sensory nuclei are in the medulla, midbrain and pons. The nerve passes from the pons to the trigeminal ganglion lateral to the cavernous sinus, where it divides into ophthalmic, maxillary and mandibular divisions. The motor nucleus is in the pons; the root bypasses the ganglion to join the mandibular division branches.
  - ophthalmic division (V_1): branches (lacrimal, frontal and nasociliary nerves) pass via the superior orbital fissure. Associated with the ciliary ganglion.
  - maxillary division (V_2): passes via the foramen rotundum. Associated with the pterygopalatine ganglion. Branches (nasal, nasopalatine, palatine, pharyngeal, zygomatic, posterior superior alveolar and infraorbital nerves) are involved with lacrimation and sensory and sympathetic supply to the nose, nasopharynx, palate and orbit.
  - mandibular division (V_3): passes via the foramen ovale. Associated with the otic (parotid gland) and submandibular (submandibular and sublingual glands) ganglia. Sensory branches are the meningeal, buccal, auriculotemporal, inferior alveolar and lingual nerves.

  (*See Gasserian ganglion block; Mandibular nerve blocks; Maxillary nerve blocks; Ophthalmic nerve blocks.*)
- VI: abducens nerve (motor supply to the lateral rectus). Passes from the lower pons through the cavernous sinus and supraorbital fissure. Often involved in injury to the skull.
- VII: facial nerve (mixed sensory and motor nerve): passes laterally from the lower pons through the internal acoustic meatus to the geniculate ganglion. Passes through the temporal bone to emerge through the stylomastoid foramen. Runs forward to the parotid gland. Branches:
  - motor supply to the muscles of facial expression: divides within the parotid gland into temporal, zygomatic, buccal, mandibular and cervical branches from above down. Branches also pass to the digastric, stylohyoid, auricular and occipital muscles.
  - greater petrosal nerve: passes from the geniculate ganglion to the pterygopalatine ganglion and fossa, to supply the lacrimal gland.
  - chorda tympani: leaves the facial nerve before it enters the stylomastoid foramen; conveys taste sensation from the anterior ⅔ of the tongue and parasympathetic fibres to the submandibular gland.
- VIII: vestibulocochlear nerve (special somatic sensory nerve): cochlear and vestibular components are involved in hearing and balance respectively. The nerve is formed in the internal acoustic meatus and passes to nuclei in the floor of the 4th ventricle. Connects centrally with cranial nerves III, IV, VI, XI and descending pathways to the upper cervical cord.
- IX: glossopharyngeal nerve (conveys sensation from the pharynx, back of the tongue and tonsil, middle ear, carotid sinus and carotid body, taste from the posterior ⅓ of the tongue, and parasympathetic fibres to the parotid gland; provides motor supply to stylopharyngeus). Passes from the medulla through the jugular foramen, and then passes between the internal and external carotid arteries to the pharynx.
- X: vagus nerve (provides parasympathetic afferent and efferent supply to the heart, lungs, and GIT as far as the splenic flexure, motor supply to the larynx, pharynx and palate, and conveys taste sensation from the valleculae and epiglottis, and sensation from the external ear canal and eardrum). Passes from the medulla via the jugular foramen.
- XI: accessory nerve (motor supply to the sternomastoid and trapezius muscles). Arises from the upper five cervical segments of the spinal cord, passing upwards through the foramen magnum to join the smaller cranial root. Leaves the skull through the jugular foramen; the cranial root joins the vagus (to the pharynx and larynx) and the spinal root passes to the sternomastoid.
- XII: hypoglossal nerve (motor supply to all muscles of the tongue except palatoglossus). Passes from the medulla, then through the hypoglossal canal behind the carotid sheath to the tongue.

- Cranial nerves may be assessed by testing:
  - I: ability to smell substances, e.g. peppermint, cloves, etc. Irritant substances are avoided, since they may act via the Vth nerve.
  - II:
    - visual acuity using distant objects/charts.
    - visual fields, e.g. ability to discern peripheral movement whilst looking straight ahead. Size of blind spot.
    - appearance of optic discs.
    - pupillary reflex to light and accommodation.
  - III, IV, VI: full eye movements without diplopia. Results of specific lower motor neurone lesions:

- III: eye displaced downwards and outwards, pupil dilated, ptosis.
- IV: downward gaze impaired; eyeball rotated inwards by inferior rectus when attempted.
- VI: lateral gaze impaired. Upper motor neurone lesions may cause impaired conjugate movements.

- V:
  - skin sensation in each division (*see Fig. 75; Gasserian ganglion block*), e.g.:
    - ophthalmic: forehead, corneal reflex (afferent arc V, efferent pathway VII).
    - maxillary: cheek next to nose.
    - mandibular: side of jaw.
    - ability to open/close jaw against resistance.
- VII:
  - facial expression: ability to smile, show teeth, whistle, raise eyebrows, screw up eyes against resistance, blow out cheeks. Movement in the upper part of the face is preserved in upper motor neurone lesions, and lost in lower motor neurone lesions.
  - taste sensation of the anterior tongue, e.g. to salt, sugar, citric acid.
- VIII:
  - ability to hear, e.g. fingers rubbing next to the ear.
  - using a tuning fork: air conduction is lost in middle ear disease, with preservation of bone conduction (Rinne's test). Both are impaired in nerve damage. If the tuning fork is placed on the forehead, the sound is heard best on the affected side in middle ear disease, on the unaffected side in nerve disease (Weber's test).
- IX, X:
  - taste sensation of the posterior tongue.
  - soft palate elevation is equal on both sides.
  - gag reflex.
  - voice and phonation.
- XI: ability to raise shoulders, and rotate head to the side, against resistance.
- XII: protrusion of tongue in the midline (to the affected side if abnormal). Absence of wasting and ability to move from side to side.

[Sir Jonathan Hutchinson (1828–1913), English surgeon; Friedrich Rinne (1819–1868) and Friedrich Weber (1832–1891), German otologists]

'Crash induction', *see Induction, rapid sequence*

C-reactive protein (CRP). Plasma protein, so called because it reacts with the C polysaccharide of pneumococci. Complexes formed when CRP binds to saccharides of micro-organisms activate the classical complement pathway and stimulate cell-mediated cytotoxicity. Part of the acute phase response, it is synthesised in the liver in response to the cytokine interleukin-6. Plasma levels are normally under 10 mg/l but increase within 6–10 h of tissue damage. Has therefore been used to aid diagnosis of acute inflammation, e.g. infection, and to monitor the response to treatment. Although in the ICU, because of underlying critical illness, 'resting' plasma levels rarely lie within the 'normal' < 10 mg/l range (e.g. may exceed 200 mg/l), a 25% change from the previous day's value may still be used to indicate acute changes in inflammatory status.

Póvoa P (2002). Intensive Care Med; 28: 235–43

Creatinine. Basic compound formed mainly in skeletal muscle from phosphorylcreatine. The latter is formed from ATP and creatine, and is a source of ATP during exercise. Creatinine production remains fairly constant, hence the value of plasma creatinine measurement as a reflection of renal function (cf. urea, whose production varies with the amount of protein breakdown occurring). Normal value: 60–130 μmol/l; serial values are more useful indicators of renal function than single measurements. As GFR decreases, creatinine levels rise slowly up to about 200 μmol/l (GFR below 40 ml/min), rising greatly thereafter for small decreases of GFR. Thus measurement is less useful at high values, and values above 200 μmol/l represent severe renal impairment.

See also, Creatinine clearance

Creatinine clearance. Clearance of creatinine, used as an approximation for GFR. Although some creatinine is secreted by renal tubules, this source of error tends to be cancelled out by the overmeasurement of plasma creatinine at low levels. Commonly estimated, since creatinine is easily measured. Usually averaged over 24 h to reduce error from inaccurate urine volume measurement. Normal value: 90–130 ml/min.

Cremophor EL. Polyoxyethylated castor oil, formed from ethylene oxide and castor oil. Used as an emulsifying agent in preparations of certain drugs. Implicated as causing adverse drug reactions, sometimes severe, after iv injection. Has led to the withdrawal of iv induction agents, e.g. Althesin, propanidid and the original formulation of propofol, although injectable preparations of other drugs may still contain it (e.g. ciclosporin, vitamin K).

CREST syndrome, *see Systemic sclerosis*

Creutzfeldt–Jakob disease (CJD). Group of human transmissible encephalopathies caused by infectious proteins known as prions. Infection results in the formation of an abnormal form of a cellular membrane protein (prion related protein) that causes destruction of neuronal tissue and overgrowth of glial cells. At least four forms are recognised:

- sporadic (sCJD) cause is unknown, accounts for ≤ 90% of cases. Occurs in the elderly; incidence is 1 per million population/year. Dementia is prominent and death occurs within 6 months.
- familial: caused by gene mutation, accounts for ≤ 10% of cases.
- iatrogenic: identical to sCJD but due to transmission of prion protein during neurosurgical procedures, corneal grafts and administration of human growth hormone. Accounts for < 5% of cases. Kuru, a prion disease caused by ingestion of infected neural tissue during cannibalism, is seen in the Fore tribe of Papua New Guinea.
- variant (vCJD): first described in 1996 in young people. Due to ingestion of beef from cattle infected by bovine spongiform encephalopathy (BSE), since the causative agent of both vCJD and BSE is identical. The prion associated with vCJD differs from that of sCJD. Over 160 cases have been reported in the UK between 1990 and 2007, with the peak incidence in 2000.

The incubation period of the disease is variable but may be up to 40 years (e.g. with Kuru) but is considerably shorter with other forms (e.g. vCJD). Clinical features of vCJD include early psychiatric changes, sensory disturbances, ataxia, stimulus sensitive myoclonus, dystonia and dementia. Definitive diagnosis requires brain biopsy although high concentrations of prion protein are found on tonsillar biopsy.

- Anaesthetic implications:
  - high exposure rate of the population to BSE infected beef may result in an epidemic of vCJD, although the

chance of this is now felt to be small given the decline in the number of cases since 2003.

- contamination of surgical and anaesthetic instruments may result in transmission of prion protein, especially during operations on tissues with high concentrations of the abnormal protein, e.g. brain, spinal cord, tonsils, lymph nodes and lower GIT. Disposable instruments have been introduced for high risk cases and care must be taken to use disposable or sheathed laryngoscope blades in these cases. Conventional decontamination of instruments does not destroy the prion protein. Particular difficulties present for decontamination of fibreoptic instruments.

  Particular problems may also arise from the disposable instruments, e.g. for tonsillectomy in the UK in 2001; accidental extubation was reported following use of the disposable mouth gag and disposable diathermy equipment was implicated in causing troublesome bleeding – the latter resulting in at least two postoperative deaths before the requirement to use disposable equipment was withdrawn (though subsequently reintroduced).
- vCJD has been transmitted by blood transfusion and since 1998, blood products in the UK have been sourced from countries with no BSE and blood for transfusion has been leucodepleted. The Department of Health announced in 2002 that FFP for children born after 1995 (who should not have been exposed to BSE via the food chain) would be obtained from unpaid US blood donors. In 2004, after the death of a patient who possibly contracted vCJD via transfused blood, UK donors were banned from giving blood if they had received a transfusion since 1980.

[Hans G Creutzfeldt (1885–1964), German psychiatrist; Alfons M Jakob (1884–1931), German neurologist]

Farling P, Smith G (2003). Anaesthesia; 58: 627–9

Cricoid pressure (Sellick's manoeuvre). Digital pressure against the cricoid cartilage of the larynx, pushing it backwards. The oesophagus is thus compressed between the posterior aspect of the cricoid and the vertebrae behind. The cricoid cartilage is used since it forms the only complete ring of the larynx and trachea. Used to prevent passive regurgitation of gastric and oesophageal contents, e.g. during induction of anaesthesia.

The cricoid cartilage is identified level with C6, and the index finger is placed against the cartilage in the midline, with the thumb and middle finger on either side. Moderate pressure may be applied before loss of consciousness, and firmer pressure maintained until the cuff of the tracheal tube is inflated.

Estimates of the force required vary from 20 N to over 40 N (approximately corresponding to a mass of 2 kg to over 4 kg), most recent guidance suggesting 20–30 N as optimal. It must be released during active vomiting, to reduce risk of oesophageal rupture. Incorrectly performed cricoid pressure may hinder laryngoscopy either by distorting the laryngeal anatomy or flexing the neck; the latter may be prevented by the assistant's second hand being placed behind the patient's neck although this too may hinder laryngoscopy if hyperextension is produced. Cricoid pressure may also hinder placement of the laryngeal mask airway.

Also used in difficult tracheal intubation, to aid laryngoscopy.

[Brian A Sellick (1918–1996), London anaesthetist]

See also, Induction, rapid sequence

Cricothyrotomy. Puncture or incision of the cricothyroid membrane (passes between the thyroid cartilage above and the cricoid cartilage below) of the larynx. Performed to allow ventilation in airway obstruction, e.g. as a last resort following failed intubation.

With the neck extended, the cricoid cartilage is identified level with C6, and a cricothyrotomy device inserted in the midline above the cartilage. Most devices consist of a needle with or without a cannula, connected to a standard 15 mm fitting or needle hub. Aspiration of air confirms correct placement. Special tubes, introducers and guidewires are also available.

In emergencies, a wide bore needle or cannula may be used, connected to a means of ventilation in a number of different ways:

- via a 3.5 mm tracheal tube connector, or via a 2 ml syringe with its plunger removed and an 8 mm tracheal tube connector inserted in its open end: the connector attaches to a standard anaesthetic breathing system but even with 10–15 l/min O_2 fresh gas flow, flow rates through the cannula may be less than 100 ml/s and chest movement may not be seen.
- via an iv fluid giving set or a three-way tap extension, attached proximally to O_2 tubing and thence to a standard wall- or cylinder-mounted O_2 outlet. With gas flows of 10–15 l/min, up to 400 ml/s may be delivered through the cannula, usually adequate to produce visible chest movements.
- via an injector device, e.g. as used for bronchoscopy; connects directly to the needle hub. Gas flows as much as 800 ml/s may be produced through the cannula.

Exhaled gases must be free to escape, or barotrauma may result. In upper airway obstruction, further punctures may be required to allow exhalation. Incorrect cannula placement may cause severe subcutaneous emphysema. Haemorrhage may occur. The cannula should be firmly fixed in place; in the initial emergency it should be gripped firmly during attempts to ventilate the lungs to prevent its dislodgement.

Cricothyroid puncture is also performed for transtracheal injection of lidocaine, during awake intubation. The minitracheotomy device may also be used for sputum aspiration.

Crile, George Washington (1864–1943). Eminent US surgeon, a major contributor to regional anaesthesia. Described the combination of opioids, regional block and general anaesthesia in order to block separate facets of anaesthesia, calling the concept anociassociation (led to the concept of balanced anaesthesia). Also investigated the pathogenesis and treatment of shock, and described a pneumatic garment for its treatment in 1903.

Tetzlaff JE, Lautsenheiser F, Estafanous FG (2005). Reg Anesth Pain Med; 29: 600–5

Crisis resource management. Strategy for coping with critical incidents, developed initially in the airline industry (as Cockpit and then Crew resource management) as a means of dealing effectively with crises and preventing them from evolving into disasters. Has since been adapted to other high risk industries and also to anaesthesia. Consists of a number of components:

- being aware of the immediate and wider environment, e.g. knowing what equipment and staff are available; manipulating the environment as required (e.g. turning on the light in a dark operating theatre).
- applying appropriate attention to one's surroundings, including monitors.
- use of all available resources and allocating them appropriately, e.g. using cognitive aids (e.g. printed algorithms); delegating personnel according to their skills.

- planning and anticipation, e.g. rehearsing drills; mobilising resources when likely to be needed rather than when they are actually needed; calling for help early.
- effective leadership.
- effective communication, including specific and directed requests/orders (and receiving confirmation that they have been understood correctly).

Commonly forms part of training programmes involving anaesthetic simulators but can be incorporated into many risk management programmes.

Critical care. System designed to look after seriously ill patients, with levels of care allocated according to clinical need (and not to staffing levels, location, etc.). Four levels are recognised in the UK:

- level 0: patients whose needs can be met by normal ward care in an acute hospital, e.g. those requiring oral or iv bolus medication or patient controlled analgesia. Observations required less frequently than 4 h.
- level 1: patients recently discharged from a higher level of care, in need of additional and more frequent monitoring and clinical advice, or requiring critical care outreach services.
- level 2: patients requiring single organ monitoring or support (e.g. nasal CPAP), preoperative optimisation or extended postoperative care, or those with major uncorrected physiological abnormalities (e.g. increased respiratory rate, tachycardia, hypotension, decreased Glasgow Coma Score) and at risk of deterioration.
- level 3: patients requiring advanced respiratory monitoring and support e.g. IPPV (but excluding electively IPPV for < 24 h postoperatively), those requiring monitoring and support of two or more organ systems, or those with chronic impairment of one or more organ systems who require support for an acute reversible failure of another organ system (e.g. severe ischaemic heart disease and major perioperative haemorrhage).

Thus the term encompasses care provided on both ICUs and HDUs.

***Critical Care Medicine*.** Monthly journal of the Society of Critical Care Medicine. First published in 1972.

Critical damping, *see Damping*

Critical flicker-fusion test, *see Recovery testing*

Critical illness polyneuropathy. Acute sensorimotor axonopathy associated with critical illness, usually involving IPPV and sepsis and/or MODS but it may also be seen in uncomplicated respiratory failure. Usually self-limiting, its severity is related to the duration of critical illness. Of unknown aetiology, although toxic, metabolic, nutritional and vascular factors have been suggested. Clinical manifestations include muscle wasting, decreased or absent tendon reflexes and difficulty weaning from ventilators. Has been implicated in cases of severe hyperkalaemia following administration of suxamethonium. Accurate diagnosis requires electrophysiological studies which demonstrate axonal degeneration and exclude other causes such as demyelination, compression neuropathies and disorders of the neuromuscular junction (e.g. caused by prolonged treatment with neuromuscular blocking drugs).

Although complete clinical recovery usually occurs following resolution of the critical illness, electrophysiological studies may show residual axonal dysfunction.

Schweickert WD, Hall J (2007). Chest; 131: 1541–9

Critical incidents. Term derived from the aircraft industry; usually defined as any event which results in actual harm, or would do so if not actively managed. Thus includes all complications of anaesthesia/intensive care, whether or not harm is done (e.g. breathing system disconnection, irrespective of whether hypoxaemia or hypoxic brain damage occurs). In its broadest sense, the term also includes harm to medical and nursing staff, etc., e.g. back injury while lifting a patient. It has been argued that critical incidents should exclude those considered outliers of normal practice, e.g. transient hypotension following iv induction of anaesthesia, although some authorities stress the value in noting such events in order to alert anaesthetists to the possibility of more extreme occurrences subsequently.

Critical incident reporting schemes are a central part of risk management and a ready topic for audit, and have become a useful tool for assessing quality, e.g. in quality assurance. They have also been used for assessing training, e.g. as specific subjects in anaesthetic examinations or anaesthetic simulators. Wider use of critical incident reporting schemes has been suggested as a more effective means of improving service than traditional reliance on outcome studies (e.g. looking at mortality), first because serious adverse outcomes are rare and second because a proactive approach is inherently more attractive than a reactive one. A problem common to all reporting schemes is the under-reporting of incidents, although this may be improved by education and guarantees of anonymity. In addition, they may not always suggest means of improving care.

- Terms used in critical incident reporting schemes include the following:
  - latent errors: within the 'system', e.g. having two drugs presented in very similar ampoules, next to each other in the cupboard.
  - active errors: produce immediate effects.
  - human errors: those involving direct human contribution, e.g. the giving of the incorrect drug; may be caused by:
    - slips: the action is unintended, e.g. picking up the wrong syringe.
    - lapses: the action is intended but the error is related to memory, e.g. forgetting the patient is allergic to penicillin.
    - violations: e.g. not checking the drug with another person when that is the policy of the department.

In addition, human errors may be classified as knowledge-based, rule-based or skill-based.

In the UK, the National Patient Safety Agency was established in 2001 to coordinate national reporting of critical incidents and dissemination of lessons learned from them.

See also, Crisis resource management

Critical pressure. Pressure required to liquify a vapour at its critical temperature. Examples:

- O_2: 50 bar.
- N_2O: 72 bar.
- CO_2: 73 bar.

Critical temperature. Temperature above which a vapour cannot be liquified by any amount of pressure. Above this temperature, the substance is a gas; below it, the substance is a vapour. Examples:

- O_2: –118°C.
- N_2O: 36.5°C.
- CO_2: 31°C.

See also, Isotherms; Pseudocritical temperature

Critical velocity. Velocity above which laminar flow in a tube becomes turbulent.
Proportional to

$$\frac{\text{viscosity of fluid}}{\text{density of fluid} \times \text{radius of tube}}$$

thus refers to a specific fluid within a tube of specific radius.
At critical velocity, Reynolds' number is greater than 2000.

Crohn's disease, *see Inflammatory bowel disease*

Cromoglicate (Cromoglycate), *see Sodium cromoglicate*

Cross-matching, *see Blood cross-matching*

Croup (Laryngotracheobronchitis). Upper respiratory obstruction and stridor in children due to viral infection affecting the larynx, trachea and bronchi; most commonly due to parainfluenza (especially type I), respiratory syncytial and influenza viruses. The typical barking 'croupy' cough, the child's age (usually 6 months–2 years) and the gradual onset help distinguish it from epiglottitis, which is usually of more acute onset, affects children of 2–5 years, and is associated with greater systemic upset. Lateral neck X-ray helps exclude epiglottitis.
Corticosteroids (oral, parenteral or nebulised) remain the mainstay of treatment; if ineffective, nebulised adrenaline may be used in an attempt to avoid intubation: racemic solution (equal amounts of *d*- and *l*-isomers) is widely used in the USA: 0.5 ml of 2.25% solution is diluted to 4 ml in saline. In the UK, (0.4 ml) 400 µg/kg of the generally available non-racemic preparation (comprising mostly the more active *l*-isomer) has been used, up to a maximum of 5 ml (5 mg). It may be repeated after 30 min if required. ECG monitoring should be instituted and therapy stopped if the heart rate exceeds 180/min. Mucosal swelling may recur after treatment so careful monitoring is required. Helium/oxygen mixtures may provide short-term improvement.

CRP, *see C-reactive protein*

CRPS, *see Complex regional pain syndromes*

Crush syndrome. Acute oliguric renal failure following trauma usually involving impaired circulation of a limb. May occur in direct trauma and in comatose patients who lie on a limb for prolonged periods. Muscle swelling and necrosis lead to release of myoglobin with resultant myoglobinuria. Renal impairment is compounded by any associated hypotension and dehydration. Potassium is also released from the damaged muscle; severe hyperkalaemia may be fatal unless dialysis is instituted.
Hyperphosphataemia and hypocalcaemia also occur.
Gonzalez D (2005). Crit Care Med; 33: S34–41

Cryoanalgesia. Use of extreme cold to damage peripheral nerves and provide pain relief lasting up to several months. Causes axonal degeneration without epineurial or perineurial damage, allowing slow regeneration of the axon without neuritis or neuroma formation. Has been used in chronic pain management, and perioperatively to provide prolonged postoperative analgesia, e.g. applied to intercostal nerves in thoracic surgery.
See also, Cryoprobe; Refrigeration anaesthesia

Cryoprecipitate, *see Blood products*

Cryoprobe. Instrument used to freeze tissues. Compressed gas (e.g. CO_2 or N_2O) is passed through a narrow tube and allowed to expand suddenly at its tip. Work done by the gas as it expands results in a temperature drop (Joule–Thomson effect; an example of an adiabatic change) to as low as –70°C in the metal sheath of the probe. Used to destroy superficial lesions, e.g. in gynaecology and dermatology; also used in ophthalmology and to provide cryoanalgesia.

Crystalloid. Substance which, in solution, may pass through a semipermeable membrane (cf. colloid). Saline solutions, dextrose solutions and Hartmann's solution are commonly used clinically as iv fluids.
See also, Colloid/crystalloid controversy

CSE, *see Combined spinal–epidural anaesthesia*

CSF, *see Cerebrospinal fluid*

CSF filtration. Technique first used in 1991 in severe Guillain–Barré syndrome unresponsive to other therapies. Its aim is to remove cellular and soluble components known to be involved in the pathological and inflammatory processes of the underlying disorders. CSF is removed through an intrathecal catheter into a closed system via a syringe and pump and then reinjected through a filter with a pore size of 0.2 µm. Is now used in some cases of acute and chronic inflammatory demyelinating polyneuropathies, multiple sclerosis, amyotrophic lateral sclerosis and bacterial meningitis.

CSM, *see Committee on Safety of Medicines*

CT scanning, *see Computed (axial) tomography*

CTZ, *see Chemoreceptor trigger zone*

Cuffs, of tracheal tubes. Seal the trachea to avoid gas leakage and contamination with liquids from above, e.g. blood, gastric contents. Popularised by Waters and Guedel in the 1920s. Usually inflated with air following tracheal intubation, until the audible gas leak is just eliminated. The degree of distension of a pilot balloon, or measurement of cuff pressure, indicates the extent of cuff inflation.

- Main problems are related to pressure exerted by the cuff on the tracheal walls causing mucosal ischaemia:
  - may occur if capillary arteriolar pressure is exceeded (i.e. greater than about 25 mmHg). Intracuff pressures of up to 30 mmHg have been measured with high-volume low-pressure cuffs, and up to 200 mmHg with low-volume high-pressure cuffs (*see Laplace's law*). The former are therefore preferable, especially for prolonged intubation, e.g. in ICU. Hand-held cuff inflators may incorporate pressure gauges to indicate intracuff pressure during inflation.
  - intracuff pressure may increase during anaesthesia due to increased temperature or diffusion of N_2O into the cuff. Saline or N_2O mixtures have been used for cuff inflation, to avoid the latter problem. Monitoring of intracuff pressure, or intermittent deflation and inflation, has been suggested during long operations and in ICU.
  - the anterior tracheal wall is affected more than the posterior wall, since the former is less distensible due to the cartilage rings.
  - mucosal inflammation may lead to ulcer formation over cartilaginous rings; infection, tracheal dilatation and erosion of tracheal walls may follow. Tracheal stenosis may occur after extubation.

- damage is worst after prolonged use, although some degree of ciliary damage may occur within a few hours of inflation.
- damage is worse if wrinkles are formed by the cuff.

Similar problems may occur with tracheostomy tubes. Recurrent laryngeal nerve injury may be caused by a cuff inflated just below the vocal cords. Cuff placement should be 1.5–2 cm below the cords. Trauma may be caused if tracheal extubation is performed without prior deflation of the cuff. Uncuffed tracheal tubes are traditionally used for paediatric anaesthesia.

Similar considerations apply to bronchial cuffs of endobronchial tubes; bronchial rupture may follow over-vigorous inflation.

Longitudinal wrinkles in the cuff may allow seepage of secretions, etc. from the pharynx into the tracheobronchial tree; new cuffs have thus been designed in which wrinkles do not form, thereby reducing the risk of aspiration pneumonia in patients requiring chronic ventilatory support.

Filling the cuff with lidocaine (4–10%) has been described, reducing emergence phenomena such as coughing.
See also, Tracheal tubes

Cuirass ventilator, *see Intermittent negative pressure ventilation*

Curare. Dried plant extract used by South American Indians as arrow poison, containing tubocurarine (isolated in 1935) and other alkaloids. Described in Raleigh's writings in 1596. Used experimentally by Waterton and Bernard, among others, from the early/mid-1800s onwards. Used to treat tetanus and in psychiatric convulsive therapy. First used in anaesthesia by Lawen in 1912, but remained in short supply for many years. Its use became more widespread after Griffith's famous description in 1942; his supply was brought back from Ecuador by Gill.
[Sir Walter Raleigh (1552–1618), English explorer; Richard Cochran Gill (1901–1958), US explorer]

Curling ulcers. Peptic ulcers occurring after severe burns. Most common in children.
[Thomas Curling (1811–1888), English surgeon]

Current. Flow of electrical charge. Direct current describes flow of charge continuously in one direction, e.g. from a battery. Direction of flow in an alternating current changes back and forth, e.g. mains power supply. SI unit is the ampere.

Current density. Current per unit area; important in electrocution and electrical burns. A low current density, e.g. when electrical contact is over a wide area, results in little heat production; a large current density, when the area of contact is small, causes greater heat production. Thus there is no tissue damage at the site of a diathermy plate, but intense heat at the site of the probe or forceps, where area of contact is very small. Similarly, a small current delivered directly to the heart over a very small area may produce the same current density as a much larger current delivered to the whole body, and may therefore be as dangerous (microshock).

Current-operated earth-leakage circuit breaker (COELCB). Device containing equally sized coils of live and neutral wires, used in electrical circuits to prevent electrocution. The current in each wire induces magnetic flux equal and opposite to that induced by the other, so long as each wire carries the same current. Imbalance between the two currents, e.g. due to leakage of current to earth, results in unequal magnetic fluxes which do not cancel each other out. Resultant magnetic flux induces current in a third coil, causing rapid (within 5 ms) breakage of the circuit via a solenoid.

Cushing, Harvey Williams (1869–1939). US neurosurgeon, Professor of Surgery at Harvard. A pioneer in neurosurgery, he developed many techniques, including the use of diathermy, and clips for cerebral vessels. Advocated record-keeping and monitoring during anaesthesia, and investigated many aspects of neurophysiology and neuropathology, several of which bear his name. Won the Pulitzer Prize for his biography of Osler, and published many books and articles.
[Joseph Pulitzer (1847–1911), Hungarian-born US journalist; Sir William Osler (1849–1919), Canadian-born US and English physician]
Hirsch NP, Smith GB (1986). Anesth Analg; 65: 288–93

Cushing's disease. Cushing's syndrome caused by ACTH-secreting adenoma of the pituitary gland. Incidence is 2–4 per million population; 80% occur in women.

- Treatment:
  - pituitary surgery (effective in up to 80% of cases).
  - irradiation of the pituitary gland.
  - bilateral adrenalectomy in resistant cases (carries the risk of Nelson's syndrome: hyperpigmentation owing to secretion of melanocyte stimulating hormone).
  - medical treatment: metyrapone inhibits 11β-hydroxylase and reduces cortisol production. May be used before surgery, to improve the patient's condition, or after irradiation.

[Don H Nelson, US endocrinologist]
Smith M, Hirsch NP (2000). Br J Anaesth; 85: 3–14

Cushing's reflex. Hypertension with compensatory bradycardia occurring with acutely raised ICP. Due to the effect of local hypoxia and hypercapnia on the vasomotor centre as cerebral perfusion pressure falls.
See also, Cushing, Harvey Williams

Cushing's syndrome. Clinical syndrome resulting from excessive endogenous or exogenous corticosteroid levels.

- Features:
  - obesity, classically central rather than peripheral, i.e. limbs are spared ('lemon and toothpick' appearance). 'Buffalo hump' of fat behind the neck.
  - 'moon face', greasy skin, acne, hirsutism.
  - skin atrophy and poor wound healing, with increased susceptibility to infection.
  - abdominal striae.
  - osteoporosis.
  - proximal muscle weakness.
  - psychiatric disturbances.
  - hypertension.
  - hypernatraemia and hypokalaemia.
  - diabetes mellitus.
- Caused by:
  - Cushing's disease (the most common non-iatrogenic cause).
  - adrenal tumours.
  - other hormone-secreting tumours, e.g. bronchial carcinoma secreting ACTH.
  - corticosteroid therapy.
- Investigation:
  - raised urinary cortisol and 17-oxogenic corticosteroids (cortisol precursors).

- raised plasma cortisol levels; normally low at midnight, and low the morning after dexamethasone administration.
- ACTH levels are raised in Cushing's disease and ACTH-secreting tumours. Metyrapone decreases adrenal cortisol production, causing ACTH to increase: this does not occur with adrenal tumours or ACTH-secreting tumours, but does occur in Cushing's disease. The ACTH increase is measured directly, or cortisol precursors (17-oxogenic corticosteroids) are measured in the urine.

Hypertension and cardiac failure, hypernatraemia, hypokalaemia and diabetes, although not always present, may cause problems during anaesthesia. Steroid cover is required as in corticosteroid therapy. Fragile skin and veins may be easily damaged. Postoperative fluid and electrolyte balance is particularly important.

Newell-Price J, Bertagna X, Grossman A, Nieman L (2006). Lancet; 367: 1605–17

See also, Cushing, Harvey Williams

Cushing's ulcers. Peptic ulcers occurring after head injury, associated with increased gastric acid secretion.

See also, Cushing, Harvey Williams

Cut-off effect. Reduced anaesthetic potency of larger molecules in a homologous series, despite increasing lipid solubility. Possibly due to membranes' inability to accommodate molecules above a certain size.

See also, Anaesthesia, mechanism of

CVA, *see Cerebrovascular accident*

CVVH, Continuous venovenous haemofiltration, *see Haemofiltration*

CVVHD, Continuous venovenous haemodiafiltration, *see Haemodiafiltration*

Cyanide poisoning. May result from industrial accidents, self-administration, smoke inhalation, prolonged use of sodium nitroprusside, or use as a chemical weapon. Absorption may occur via stomach, skin, lungs, etc. (the latter may be rapidly fatal). Causes inhibition of the cytochrome oxidase system and other enzymes, interrupting cellular respiration. Tissues are thus unable to utilise delivered O_2 (histotoxic hypoxia). Cyanide is slowly converted to thiocyanate in the liver by the enzyme rhodanese; a small amount binds to methaemoglobin and a small amount to hydroxocobalamin.

- Features:
  - non-specific: dizziness, headache, confusion, etc. Apnoea may follow initial tachypnoea.
  - reduced arteriovenous O_2 difference, due to reduced uptake of O_2 by tissues. Metabolic acidosis with increased lactate results from tissue hypoxia.
  - convulsions and cardiorespiratory collapse may occur.
  - chronic poisoning causes peripheral neuropathy, ataxia and optic atrophy.

Measurement of plasma levels is technically difficult and may be unreliable unless performed rapidly.

- Treatment:
  - general measures as for poisoning and overdoses. O_2 therapy is particularly important. Staff must avoid self-contamination.
  - gastric lavage may be helpful.
  - dicobalt edetate 300 mg iv over 1 min, repeated if necessary. Combines with cyanide to form inert compounds. May itself cause vomiting, hypertension and tachycardia; reservation for severe cases has been suggested. Given with 50% glucose (50 ml per dose).
  - sodium thiosulphate 50%, 25 ml iv over 10 min. Converts cyanide to thiocyanate. Used together with:
    - sodium nitrite 3%, 10 ml iv over 3 min. Converts haemoglobin to methaemoglobin, which binds cyanide. More efficacious than inhaled amyl nitrite. Methaemoglobin together with carboxyhaemoglobin if present should not exceed 40% total haemoglobin.
    - hydroxocobalamin 70 mg/kg iv over 20 min. Forms cyanocobalamin with cyanide. Has been used in cyanide poisoning and to reduce nitroprusside toxicity, but not widely used in the UK.

Cyanosis. Blue discolouration of tissues due to increased amounts of reduced haemoglobin in the blood. Clinically detectable at less than 5 g/100 ml reduced haemoglobin, although this value is often quoted as the minimum. Peripheral cyanosis, e.g. of fingernails, may result from reduced peripheral circulation. Central cyanosis, typically affecting the tongue, may result from heart or lung disease, including right-to-left shunts. Methaemoglobinaemia and sulphaemoglobinaemia may also cause bluish discolouration. Cyanosis may be further mimicked by grey or blue discolouration of skin, e.g. caused by heavy metals (e.g. iron, gold and lead) or drugs (e.g. amiodarone and phenothiazines).

Cyclazocine. Obsolete opioid analgesic drug, similar to pentazocine. Produced unacceptable psychomimetic effects.

Cyclic AMP, *see Adenosine monophosphate, cyclic*

Cycling of ventilators, *see Ventilators*

Cyclizine hydrochloride/tartrate/lactate. Antiemetic drug, with antihistamine and anticholinergic actions. Available alone or combined with opioid analgesic drugs and ergotamine. Half-life is about 8 h.

- Dosage: 50 mg 4 hourly, up to 150 mg/day, orally/im/iv.
- Side effects include drowsiness and blurred vision. Painful if given iv. Rapid injection may cause tachycardia.

Cyclodextrins. Cyclic oligosaccharides, studied for their ability to encapsulate lipophilic molecules. A specific cyclodextrin, sugammadex, has been developed with optimal affinity for rocuronium, and has been shown to reverse the neuromuscular blockade produced by the latter even if given within a few minutes of paralysis. Cyclodextrins have also been studied as vehicles for drugs, e.g. propofol, in an attempt to avoid the use of emulsifiers and other carriers.

Cyclo-oxygenase (COX). Enzyme acting on arachidonic acid to produce endoperoxidases from which prostaglandins, prostacyclin and thromboxanes are formed. Exists in two forms:

- COX-1: present in many tissues; active continuously and responsible for maintenance of physiologically protective prostaglandin functions, e.g. renal blood flow, gastric mucosal protection.
- COX-2: found in few resting cells (including brain, kidney, gravid uterus); induced during inflammation especially in inflammatory cells including monocytes and macrophages.

Most NSAIDs inhibit COX-1 more than (e.g. aspirin, indometacin, naproxen, piroxicam) or the same as (e.g. ibuprofen, diclofenac) COX-2. NSAIDs which preferentially

inhibit COX-2 (e.g. parecoxib, celecoxib) have been developed in an attempt to minimise their side effects, although whilst upper GIT bleeding is less common, it may still occur, as may the other side effects of NSAIDs. The selective COX-2 inhibitor rofecoxib was withdrawn in 2004 because it was associated with an increased incidence of cardiovascular side effects, particularly MI, that was originally attributed in early studies to a cardioprotective effect of naproxen in the control group. The mechanism is thought to be unequal inhibition of prostacyclin and thromboxane synthesis.
Kam P (2000). Anaesthesia; 55: 442–9

Cyclophosphamide. Immunosuppressive and cytotoxic drug used in organ transplantation (especially bone marrow transplantation), autoimmune disease and malignancy. An alkylating agent, it binds to DNA and is toxic to both resting and dividing cells. Exerts its greatest effect on B lymphocytes, thus inhibiting antibody production. Also depresses delayed type hypersensitivity. Bioavailability is 90% after oral dosage, with peak levels at 1 h. Metabolised in the liver with a half-life of 6 h.

- Dosage: 100–300 mg/day orally or 80–300 mg/m^2/day iv.
- Side effects: nausea, vomiting, hair loss, dose-related cardiac toxicity, haemorrhagic cystitis (caused by a metabolite, acrolein), increased risk of infection and malignancy. Levels are increased by concurrent administration of allopurinol and cimetidine. May prolong suxamethonium's duration of action by decreasing cholinesterase activity.

Cyclopropane. $(CH_2)_3$. Inhalational anaesthetic agent, first used in the early 1930s. No longer available in the UK and many other countries.

Its main advantages were very rapid onset of anaesthesia (blood/gas partition coefficient 0.45) and maintenance of BP and cardiac output (largely due to sympathetic activity) despite direct myocardial depression. Extremely flammable (explosive in O_2 at 2.5–60% and in air at 2.5–10%), it also caused marked respiratory depression and reduced renal and hepatic blood flow. Commonly used for paediatric induction using 50% in O_2 (MAC of 9.2%). Supplied in orange size-B cylinders (containing 180 litres, partly as liquid) at a pressure of 5 bar.

Cycloserine. Antibacterial and antituberculous drug, used in TB resistant to first-line drugs. Contraindicated in renal impairment, epilepsy and porphyria.

- Dosage: 250–500 mg orally, 12 hourly.
- Side effects: rash, headache, dizziness, seizures, psychological changes, hepatic impairment.

Cyclosporin, *see Ciclosporin*

Cylinders. Traditionally made of molybdenum or chromium steel; newer cylinders are made of aluminium alloy and are much lighter. Composite cylinders comprise a metal (usually) liner to prevent leakage of gas, with a carbon fibre or glass fibre overwrap to provide extra strength.

Provide medical gases either directly to an output, e.g. attached to an anaesthetic machine, or from a bank of cylinders (manifold) via pipelines.

- The valve block screws into the open end of the cylinder and has the following features:
  - marked with:
    - serial number.
    - tare (weight of the empty cylinder and valve block; used for calculation of contents by weight).
    - pressure of the last hydraulic test.
    - symbol of the contained gas.
  - the valve is opened by turning a longitudinal spindle, set within a gland (stuffing box) screwed tightly into the valve block. Compression of a nylon ring around the spindle prevents leakage of gas along the spindle shaft.
  - bears the pin index system on the same face as the gas outlet.
  - a safety outlet is fitted to the valve block (USA) or between the block and cylinder neck (UK); it melts at low temperatures, allowing escape of gas in case of fire.
  - a testing collar is attached (see below).

Colour-coding (UK): shoulder colour(s) represent the predominant gas(es) in the cylinder. USA colour-coding is different. An international colouring system has been recommended, taking one of the colours from the UK system (Table 11). European standards now follow this scheme but the colours are only prescribed for the cylinders' shoulders, the suppliers being able to paint the body as they choose. A voluntary code recommends that the bodies of medical gas cylinders are painted white.

- Bodies are labelled with:
  - name and symbol of the gas.
  - volume and pressure of contained gas.
  - information and warnings about explosions and flammability where appropriate. When the gas supply is turned on suddenly, compression of the gas within the valves and pipes causes a rise in temperature. Oil or grease in the system may ignite, hence the warning against these lubricants.
- Testing:
  - every hundredth cylinder is cut into strips and tested at manufacture.

Table 11 Colour-coding of cylinders

Gas	UK: Shoulder	UK: Body	USA	Recommended international system
O_2	White	Black	Green	White
N_2O	Blue	Blue	Blue	Blue
CO_2	Grey	Grey	Grey	Grey
Entonox	White/blue quarters	Blue		
Helium	Brown	Brown	Brown	Brown
O_2 21%/helium	White/brown quarters	Black	Brown/yellow	Brown/white
Air	Black/white quarters	Grey	Yellow	Black/white

- each cylinder is tested 5-yearly to withstand high hydraulic pressures (about 200–250 bar). Cylinders are filled with water under pressure, within a water jacket. Expansion and elastic recoil of the metal are then measured.
- internal inspection with an endoscope.
- a plastic disc is placed around the valve block neck; its colour and shape are coded for the date of the last test. The year in which testing is due is stamped on the disc, and a hole punched to indicate the quarter of the year.

- Cylinder pressures:
  - O_2: 137 bar.
  - N_2O: 40 bar.
  - CO_2: 50 bar.
  - air: } 137 bar.
  - O_2/helium: } 137 bar.
  - O_2/N_2O: } 137 bar.

  (maximal values at 15°C, as marked on the cylinders)

  Modern pressure gauges are marked in kPa × 100 (1 bar = 100 kPa).

N_2O and CO_2 cylinders contain liquid; as such a cylinder empties, pressure is maintained by evaporation of liquid (although a slight drop in pressure does occur as temperature falls) until the liquid is depleted. Pressure then falls rapidly with further emptying. Gas-filled cylinders, e.g. containing O_2, provide gas whose pressure is proportional to cylinder contents.

Large Entonox cylinders contain connecting tubes from the valve block to the lower part of the cylinder, to reduce risk of hypoxic gas delivery should separation of gases occur below the pseudocritical temperature.

- Sizes of cylinders are denoted by capital letters. Usual sizes on anaesthetic machines:
  - O_2: E (contains 680 litres).
  - N_2O: E (contains 1800 litres).
  - CO_2: C (contains 450 litres).

See also, Filling ratio; Piped gas supply

Cystic fibrosis. Autosomal recessive genetic disease; the commonest lethal inherited illness in Caucasians, affecting 1 in 1500 live births. Causes impaired production of cystic fibrosis transmembrane conductance regulator (CFTR) protein, a complex channel that regulates passage of water and ions across cell membranes. Primarily affects exocrine gland function resulting in abnormally viscous secretions.

- Features:
  - repeated respiratory infection, usually by staphylococcus and pseudomonas, leading to bronchiectasis, pulmonary fibrosis and eventually pulmonary hypertension and cor pulmonale. Nasal polyps are common. Pneumothorax may occur. $\dot{V}/\dot{Q}$ mismatch, restrictive and obstructive defects and increased residual capacity often result in hypoxaemia. Arterial P_{CO_2} is usually reduced unless lung disease is severe. Laryngospasm and coughing are common during anaesthesia.
  - pancreatic insufficiency with malabsorption and intestinal obstruction (e.g. meconium ileus in the newborn). Diabetes mellitus is more common than in normal patients. Obstructive jaundice may occur.
  - renal impairment and amyloidosis may occur.

Survival beyond the 2nd and 3rd decade is now common with intensive physiotherapy, antibiotic therapy and pancreatic supplementation. Heart–lung and lung transplantation is increasingly being performed since the disease seems not to recur in transplanted lungs.

- Anaesthetic management:
  - careful preoperative assessment and continuation of physiotherapy, etc. Coagulation may be impaired. Opioid premedication is usually avoided. Anticholinergic drugs may increase secretion viscosity but are commonly used to reduce the incidence of bradycardia; they may be given on induction.
  - regional techniques where appropriate.
  - inhalational induction is prolonged because of $\dot{V}/\dot{Q}$ mismatch. Ketamine increases bronchial secretions.
  - usual technique: tracheal intubation and IPPV, with tracheobronchial suction as required. Extubation is performed awake. Humidification of gases is important.
  - careful fluid balance to avoid dehydration.
  - postoperative observation, physiotherapy, analgesia and humidified O_2 administration are important.

Davies JC, Alton EWFW, Bush A (2007). Br Med J; 335: 1255–9

Cystic hygroma. Congenital multiloculated cystic mass arising from the jugular lymph sac, the embryonic precursor of part of the thoracic duct. Contains lymph; characteristically transilluminates very well. Usually presents soon after birth. Sometimes sclerosant treatment is used; surgery is difficult because of widespread cystic tissue throughout neck. The tongue and pharynx may be involved. Main anaesthetic problems are related to airway obstruction and difficult intubation. Manual IPPV via a facepiece may be impossible; therefore spontaneous ventilation is usually maintained until intubation is achieved.

See also, Intubation, difficult

Cytochrome oxidase system. Series of iron-containing enzymes within mitochondrial inner membranes. Electron transport from oxidised nicotinamide adenine dinucleotide (NADH) or succinate proceeds via sequential cytochromes, the iron component becoming alternately reduced and oxidised as the electron is passed to the next in line. Their structure and arrangement within the membrane is thought to be crucial to their function. Electron flow is coupled to ATP formation; 3 molecules of ATP are formed per 1 of NADH and 2 ATP per 1 of succinate. Cytochrome oxidase itself is the cytochrome binding to molecular O_2 to form water, and is inhibited in cyanide poisoning and carbon monoxide poisoning.

Similar enzymes exist in other membranes, e.g. cytochrome P_{450} isoenzymes ('p' for pigment, 450 nm for enzymes' absorption peak); found in smooth endoplasmic reticulum (microsomal portion of centrifuged cellular material); these are responsible for phase I metabolism of many drugs. Genetic polymorphism of the various enzymes partly explains individuals' differing metabolism of drugs.

Chang GWM, Kam PCA (1999). Anaesthesia; 54: 42–50

Cytokines. Protein mediators released by many cells including monocytes, lymphocytes, macrophages, mast cells and endothelial cells. Involved in regulating the activity, growth and differentiation of many different cells of the immune and haemopoietic systems. The cytokines tumour necrosis factor-α (TNFα; cachectin), interleukin (IL)-1 and IL-6 are thought to be central to the pathophysiology of SIRS and sepsis in ICU; TNFα and IL-1 produce the systemic and metabolic features of SIRS, whilst IL-6 causes the acute phase protein response. All three are released following stimulation by endotoxin and other stimuli. In sepsis, high blood concentrations of IL-6 especially have been associated with poor outcome. Therapies for sepsis have been developed, directed against the actions of IL-1 and TNFα, e.g. using antibodies or antagonists, although encouraging results in animal experiments have generally not been reproduced in humans. Anti-TNFα therapies are now established in rheumatoid arthritis.

Other cytokines include additional interleukins, and interferons. Interferon-γ (IFNγ) interacts with other cytokines and has itself been investigated as a target for immunological blockade in sepsis.

Cytomegalovirus (CMV). Herpes group virus usually acquired subclinically during childhood; by age of 50 years, 50% of individuals have anti-CMV antibodies. May be transmitted by blood transfusion, hence the requirement for screening before transfusion to at risk groups. May cause major morbidity and mortality during pregnancy (resulting in cytomegalic inclusion disease: small infant with jaundice, hepatosplenomegaly, microcephaly, mental retardation) and in patients with immunodeficiency (clinical features include fever, interstitial pneumonia, enteritis, hepatitis, carditis, chorioretinitis, leucopenia and thrombocytopenia). Treatment includes antiviral drugs such as ganciclovir or foscarnet sodium.

Cytotoxic drugs. Used in the treatment of malignancy and as immunosuppressive drugs. All may cause nausea and vomiting and bone marrow suppression; most are teratogenic and require careful preparation by trained personnel. Extravasation of iv drugs may cause severe tissue necrosis. Some have side effects of particular anaesthetic/ICU relevance:

- alkylating agents (act by damaging DNA and impairing cell division): cyclophosphamide may prolong the effect of suxamethonium; busulfan may cause pulmonary fibrosis. Chlorambucil may rarely cause severe skin reactions.
- cytotoxic antibiotics: doxorubicin may cause cardiomyopathy; bleomycin may cause pulmonary fibrosis.
- antimetabolites: methotrexate may cause pneumonitis.
- vinca alkaloids: vincristine and vinblastine may cause autonomic and peripheral neuropathy.
- others: cisplatin may cause nephrotoxicity, ototoxicity and peripheral neuropathy; procarbazine has monoamine oxidase inhibitor effects; azathioprine may cause hepatic impairment, nephritis and rarely pneumonitis.

O_2 therapy has been implicated in exacerbating the pulmonary fibrosis caused by cytotoxic drugs.

Specific guidelines (issued by the Committee on the Review of Medicines) exist for the handling of cytotoxic drugs. These include the necessity for trained staff to administer drugs, designated areas for drug reconstitution, protective clothing, eye protection, safe disposal of waste material and avoidance of handling cytotoxics by pregnant staff.

Accidental intrathecal (instead of intravenous) injection of vincristine during combination chemotherapy almost inevitably results in death; in the UK, anaesthetists have been involved in such errors. Totally incompatible intrathecal/intravenous connections have been called for as a result.

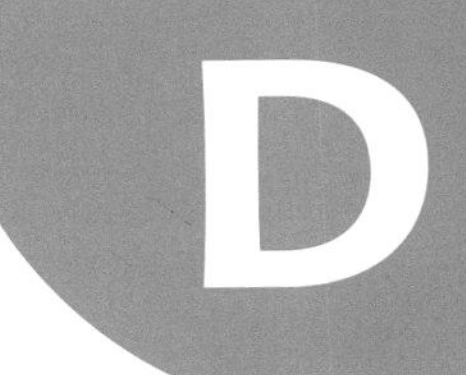

δ wave, *see Wolff–Parkinson–White syndrome*

DA examination (Diploma in Anaesthetics). First specialist examination in anaesthetics; first held in 1935 in London. Originally intended for anaesthetists with at least 2 years' experience of 2000 anaesthetics, later reduced to 1 year's residence in an approved hospital. A two-part examination was introduced in 1947, in order to ensure anaesthetists' equal footing with other specialists prior to establishment of the NHS. This examination became the FFARCS examination in 1953; the single-part DA remained separate until 1984, when the DA (UK) became the first part of the new three-part FFARCS. Phased out in 1996 with the introduction of the new FRCA examination.

Dalfopristin, *see Quinupristin*

Dalteparin sodium, *see Heparin*

Dalton's law. The pressure exerted by a fixed amount of a gas in a mixture equals the pressure it would exert if alone; thus the pressure exerted by a mixture of gases equals the sum of the partial pressures exerted by each gas.
[John Dalton (1766–1844), English chemist]

Damping. Progressive diminution of amplitude of oscillations in a resonant system, caused by dissipation of stored energy. Important in recording systems, e.g. direct arterial BP measurement. In the latter, damping mainly arises from viscous drag of fluid in the cannula and connecting tubing, compression of entrapped air bubbles, blood clots within the system and kinking. Excess damping causes a flattened trace which may be distorted (phase shift). The degree of damping is described by the damping factor (D); if a sudden change is imposed on a system, $D = 1$ if no overshoot of the trace occurs (critical damping; Fig. 47a). A marked overshoot followed by many oscillations occurs if $D \ll 1$ (Fig. 47b), and an excessively delayed response occurs if $D \gg 1$ (Fig. 47c). Optimal damping is 0.6–0.7 of critical damping, and produces the fastest response without excessive oscillations. D depends on the properties of the liquid within the system and the dimensions of the cannula and tubing.

Danaparoid sodium. Heparinoid mixture, containing no heparin, used for the prophylaxis of deep vein thrombosis. Has also been used for parenteral anticoagulation instead of heparin when the latter has induced thrombocytopenia.

- Dosage:
  - prophylaxis: 750 units 12 hourly for 7–10 days.
  - parenteral anticoagulation: 1250–3750 units (depending on body weight) iv, followed by 800 units over 2 h, 600 units over 2 h, then 200 units/h for 5 days.
- Side effects: as for heparin. Contains sulphite, which may trigger bronchospasm and hypotension in susceptible patients. Anti-Xa activity should be monitored in renal impairment or obese patients.

Dandy–Walker syndrome, *see Hydrocephalus*

Dantrolene sodium. Hydantoin skeletal muscle relaxant which acts by binding to the ryanodine receptor and limits entry of calcium into myocytes. Used to treat spastic muscle spasm and MH.

- Dosage:
  - 25–400 mg orally daily for muscle spasm.
  - 1 mg/kg iv for treatment of MH, repeated up to 10 mg/kg. The solution is irritant with pH 9–10, and is best infused into a large vein. Presented in bottles of 20 mg orange powder with 3 g mannitol and sodium hydroxide, each requiring mixing with 60 ml water. Thus preparation is lengthy. Once prepared, the solution lasts 6 h at 15–30°C. Dry powder has a shelf-life of 9 months.
- Side effects: hepatotoxicity has occurred after prolonged oral use; muscle weakness and sedation may follow iv injection. The high pH of the iv solution (9–10) may cause venous thrombosis following prolonged infusion, and tissue necrosis following extravasation.

Krause T, Gerbershagen MU, Fiege M, et al (2004). Anaesthesia; 59: 364–73

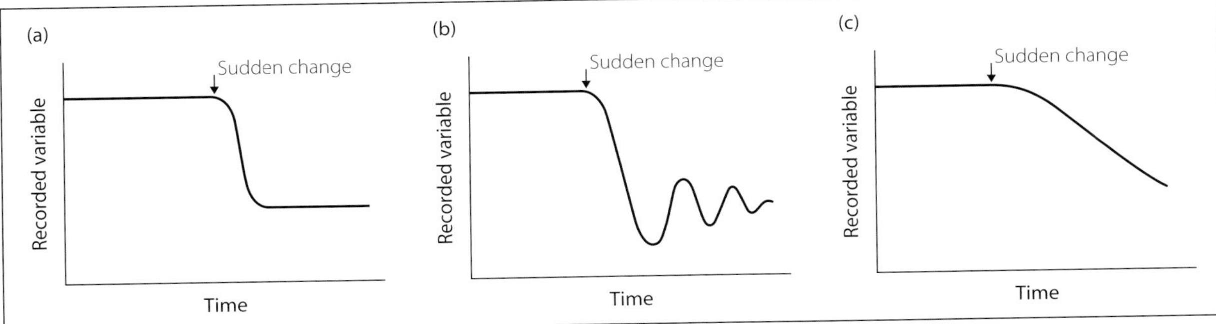

Fig. 47 Damping: (a) $D = 1$; (b) $D \ll 1$; (c) $D \gg 1$

Darrow's solution. Solution designed for iv fluid replacement in children suffering from gastroenteritis. Composed of sodium 122 mmol/l, chloride 104 mmol/l, lactate 53 mmol/l and potassium 35 mmol/l.
[Daniel Darrow (1895–1965), US paediatrician]

Data. In statistics, a series of observations or measurements.
- Data may be:
  - continuous; e.g. length in metres. The difference between 2 m and 3 m is the same as that between 35 and 36 m. Although they may be treated in the same way, there are two types of continuous data:
    - ratio: includes zero value, e.g. plasma drug concentration. 10 mmol/l is half of 20 mmol/l (i.e. the ratio of two measurements holds meaning).
    - interval: does not include zero, e.g. Celsius temperature scale (the 'zero' is an arbitrary point in the scale; thus 10°C does not represent half as much heat as 20°C). The Kelvin scale is a ratio scale since 0 K does represent absence of heat and thus 10 K represents half as much heat as 20 K.

    If normally distributed, continuous data are described by the mean and standard deviation as indicators of central tendency and scatter respectively (described as for ordinal data if not normally distributed).
  - categorical (non-continuous):
    - ordinal, e.g. ASA physical status. The difference between scores of 2 and 3 does not equal that between scores of 4 and 5, and a score of 4 is not 'twice as unfit' as a score of 2. Ordinal data are described by the median and percentiles (plus range).
    - nominal, e.g. diagnosis, hair colour. May be dichotomous, e.g. male/female; alive/dead. Nominal data are described by the mode and a list of possible categories.

Different kinds of data require different statistical tests for correct analyses and comparisons: parametric tests for normally distributed data (most continuous data), and non-parametric tests for non-normally distributed data (categorical and some continuous data). The latter may often be 'normalised' by mathematical transformation, allowing application of the more sensitive parametric tests.
See also, Clinical trials; Statistical frequency distributions

Davenport diagram. Graph of plasma bicarbonate concentration against pH, useful in interpreting and explaining disturbances of acid–base balance. Different lines may be drawn for different arterial $P\text{CO}_2$ values, but for each line, bicarbonate falls as pH falls, and increases as pH increases (Fig. 48).

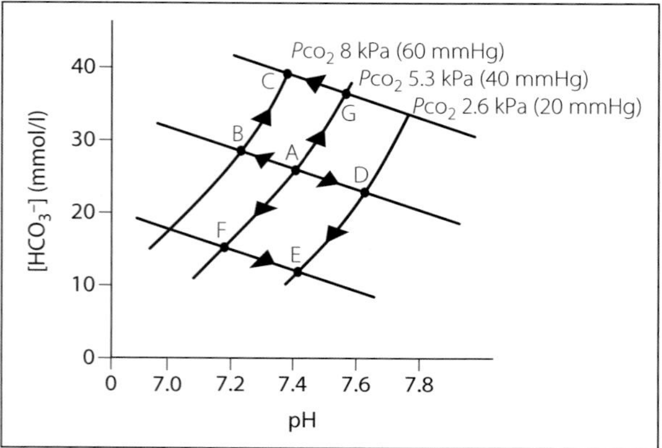

Fig. 48 Davenport diagram (see text)

- Can be used to demonstrate what happens in various acid–base disorders:
  - line BAD represents part of the titration curve for blood.
  - point A represents normal plasma.
  - point B represents respiratory acidosis; i.e. a rise in arterial $P\text{CO}_2$, reducing pH and increasing bicarbonate. In order to return pH towards normal, compensatory mechanisms increase bicarbonate; i.e. move towards point C.
  - point D represents respiratory alkalosis; compensation results in a move towards point E.
  - point F represents metabolic acidosis; respiratory compensation (hyperventilation with a fall in arterial $P\text{CO}_2$) causes a move towards point E.
  - point G represents metabolic alkalosis; compensatory hypoventilation causes a move towards point C.

The same relationship may be displayed in different ways, e.g. the Siggaard-Andersen nomogram, which contains more information and is more useful clinically.
[Horace W Davenport (1912–2005), US physiologist]

Davy, Sir Humphrey (1778–1829). Cornish-born scientist, inventor of the miner's safety lamp. Discovered sodium, potassium, calcium and barium. Suggested the use of N_2O (which he named 'laughing gas') for analgesia in 1799, whilst director of the Medical Pneumatic Institution in Bristol. Later became President of the Royal Society.

Day-case surgery. Surgery in which the patient presents to hospital and returns home on the day of operation. Increasingly performed, as it has many advantages over traditional inpatient surgery:
  - minimal psychological upheaval for the patient, especially children.
  - reduced requirement for nursing and medical supervision and hospital services, and thus cheaper.
  - allows large number of patients to be treated.
  - reduced risk of hospital-acquired infection.

Standards of anaesthetic and surgical care and equipment (including preoperative preparation, monitoring and recovery facilities) should be as for inpatient surgery. Consultant surgical and anaesthetic supervision is considered mandatory.
- Patients may be managed within:
  - separate dedicated day-case units within hospitals: provide geographical, staffing and some political independence from the main hospital, but require access to hospital facilities if needed, e.g. X-ray, laboratories, wards, ICU, etc.
  - traditional inpatient lists.
  - completely separate units, without a nearby hospital.
- Patient selection: traditional rigid criteria, e.g. relating to age, ASA physical status, weight, are now generally considered unnecessary, three main criteria being:
  - social situation, e.g. willing patient, access to a telephone, responsible adult to collect the patient and stay at home for 24 hours, etc.
  - medical condition: patient should be fully fit or any chronic disease should be stable/controlled.
  - planned procedure: low risk of complications, which should be mild; mild expected pain/PONV. Operations expected to last less than 60 min are preferable. Operations previously considered unsuitable are increasingly performed on an outpatient basis, e.g. tonsillectomy, laparoscopic cholecystectomy.

Patients must be informed of the requirements for fasting, home arrangements, etc. The use of information leaflets is widely recommended.

- Anaesthetic technique:
  - patients are fully assessed preoperatively (often using a questionnaire). Anaesthetic outpatient clinics have been used. Time of last oral intake is checked.
  - premedication is usually omitted, although short-acting drugs, e.g. temazepam, are sometimes used.
  - general principles are as for any anaesthetic, but rapid recovery is particularly desirable. Thus short-acting drugs are usually used, e.g. propofol, fentanyl, alfentanil. Sevoflurane and desflurane are commonly selected volatile agents because of their low blood gas solubility and rapid recovery. Tracheal intubation is acceptable but is usually avoided if possible. Suxamethonium is often avoided since muscle pains are more likely in ambulant patients.
  - regional techniques may be suitable (often combined with general anaesthesia to provide postoperative analgesia). Epidural and spinal anaesthesia have been successfully performed, although uncommonly in the UK.
  - facilities for admission to an inpatient ward must be available in case of excessive bleeding or other complications (required in under 5% of cases).
- Postoperative assessment must be performed before discharge; the following are usually required:
  - full orientation and responsiveness.
  - ability to walk, dress and drink.
  - adequately controlled pain.
  - controlled bleeding and swelling.
  - stable vital signs.

Written and verbal instructions are given to the patient, not to take depressant drugs or alcohol, or indulge in potentially dangerous activities (e.g. operating machinery, driving, frying food, etc.), usually for 24 h; 48 h has been suggested. These instructions may not always be followed.

Smith I, Cooke T, Jackson I, Fitzpatrick R (2006). Anaesthesia; 61: 1191–9

DDAVP, D-Amino-8-D-arginine-vasopressin, *see Desmopressin*

D-dimer, *see Fibrin degradation products*

Dead space. Volume of inspired air that takes no part in gas exchange. Divided into:
  - anatomical dead space: mouth, nose, pharynx and large airways not lined with respiratory epithelium. Measured by Fowler's method.
  - alveolar dead space: ventilated lung normally contributing to gas exchange, but not doing so because of impaired perfusion. Thus represents one extreme of $\dot{V}/\dot{Q}$ mismatch.

Physiological dead space equals anatomical plus alveolar dead space. It is measured using the Bohr equation. Assessment may be useful in monitoring $\dot{V}/\dot{Q}$ mismatch in patients with extensive respiratory disease, especially when combined with estimation of shunt fraction. Normally equals 2–3 ml/kg; i.e. 30% of normal tidal volume. In rapid shallow breathing, alveolar ventilation is reduced despite a normal minute ventilation, because a greater proportion of tidal volume is dead space.
- Increased by:
  - increased lung volumes.
  - bronchodilatation.
  - extension of neck.
  - PE/air embolism.
  - old age.
  - hypotension.
  - haemorrhage.
  - pulmonary disease.
  - general anaesthesia and IPPV.
  - atropine and hyoscine.
  - apparatus (see below).
- Decreased by:
  - tracheal intubation and tracheostomy.
  - supine position.

Apparatus dead space represents 'wasted' fresh gas within anaesthetic tubing, etc. Minimal lengths of tubing should lie between the fresh gas inlet of a T-piece and the patient, especially in children, whose tidal volumes are small. Facepieces and their connections may considerably increase dead space.

Death. Anaesthetists and intensivists may face a number of issues surrounding the death of patients:
  - practical:
    - mortality/survival prediction and allocation of resources; triage.
    - relief of symptoms, e.g. pain management, palliative care.
    - CPR.
    - diagnosis of brainstem death.
    - organ donation.
  - ethical:
    - informed consent before treatments (i.e. the risk of death).
    - withdrawing treatment or resisting heroic surgery when the outlook is hopeless.
    - advance decisions.
    - do not attempt resuscitation orders.
    - euthanasia.
  - medicolegal:
    - reporting of deaths to the coroner.
    - claims of negligence or manslaughter.
  - psychological:
    - adequate preparation and support of patients, relatives and staff.
    - counselling of staff after a patient's death, especially when unexpected.
    - organisational/educational: audit; surveys of ICU and anaesthetic morbidity and mortality; risk management, etc.

See also, Ethics; Medicolegal aspects of anaesthesia

Debrisoquine sulphate. Antihypertensive drug, acting by preventing noradrenaline release from postganglionic adrenergic neurones. Similar in effects to guanethidine, but does not deplete noradrenaline stores.

Decamethonium dibromide/diiodide. Depolarising neuromuscular blocking drug, introduced in 1948. Blockade lasts 15–20 min. No longer in use in the UK.

Decerebrate posture. Abnormal posture resulting from bilateral midbrain or pontine lesions. Composed of internal rotation and hyperextension of all limbs, with hyperextension of neck and spine, and absent righting reflexes. Similar posturing may be seen in severe structural brain damage or coning.

See also, Decorticate posture

Declamping syndrome, *see Aortic aneurysm, abdominal*

Decompression sickness (Caisson disease) Syndrome following rapid passage from a high atmospheric pressure

environment to one of lower atmospheric pressure, e.g. surfacing after underwater diving, especially if followed by air transport at high altitude. Caused by formation of nitrogen bubbles as the gas comes out of solution, which it does readily because of its low solubility. Bubbles may embolise to or form in various tissues, giving rise to widespread symptoms in: the joints ('the bends'); the CNS ('the staggers'); the skin ('the creeps'); the lungs ('the chokes'). Treated by immediate recompression.
[Caisson: pressurised watertight chamber used for construction work in deep water]

Decontamination of breathing equipment, *see Contamination of breathing equipment*

Decorticate posture. Abnormal posture resulting from lesions of the cerebral cortex, with preservation of basal ganglia and brainstem function. Composed of leg extension, internal rotation and plantar flexion, with moderate arm flexion. Passive rotation of the head to one side causes extension of the ipsilateral arm, with full flexion of the contralateral arm, due to intact tonic neck reflexes. The contralateral leg may flex. Occurs in severe structural brain damage.
See also, Decerebrate posture

Decrement, *see Fade*

Decubitus ulcers (Pressure sores). May result from a number of factors:
- inadequate peripheral circulation, e.g. peripheral vascular disease, use of vasopressor drugs.
- hypotension.
- malnutrition including mineral deficiency, etc.
- predisposing conditions, e.g. diabetes mellitus, immunodeficiency, etc.
- reduced sensation.
- diarrhoea or urinary incontinence.
- poor support of limbs, etc. with infrequent turning.

All may coexist in critically ill patients. May cause pain or be a source of infection. Prevention includes regular inspection of pressure points and turning, support of pressure points to spread the weight of the body over a wider area, attention to nutrition, etc. and use of devices such as air mattresses which vary the pressure points continuously. Once present, ulcers are managed by raising the affected limb/area, regular dressings and cleaning; more recently, a small amount of negative pressure has been applied to the area to aid healing. Erosions may also occur if tubes, etc. are allowed to exert undue pressure, e.g. around the mouth/nose.
Keller BP, Wille J, van Ramshorst B, van der Werken C (2002). Intensive Care Med; 28: 1379–88

Deep vein thrombosis (DVT). Thrombus formation in the deep veins, usually of the leg and pelvis. A common postoperative complication, especially following major joint replacement, colorectal surgery and surgery for cancer. The true incidence is unknown but may exceed 50% in high risk patients. Carries high risk of PE. May rarely cause systemic embolisation via a patent foramen ovale (present in 30% of the population at autopsy).

- Triad of predisposing factors described by Virchow in 1856:
  - venous stasis, e.g. low cardiac output (e.g. cardiac failure, MI, dehydration), pelvic venous obstruction, prolonged immobility.
  - vessel wall damage, e.g. direct trauma, inflammation, varicosities, infiltration.
  - increased blood coagulability, e.g. trauma, malignancy, pregnancy, oestrogen or antifibrinolytic administration, hereditary hypercoagulability, possibly smoking (*see Coagulation disorders*).

More common in old age, sepsis and obesity. Increased risk after surgery is thought to be related to increased platelet adhesiveness and activation of the coagulation cascade caused by tissue trauma, exacerbated by possible venous damage and pre-, peri- and postoperative immobility.

Clinical diagnosis is unreliable but suggested by tenderness, swelling and increased temperature of the calf, and pain on passive dorsiflexion of the foot (Homans' sign). The upper leg may also be involved. Accompanying superficial thrombophlebitis may be absent. Investigations include Doppler ultrasound, impedance plethysmography, thermography, uptake of radiolabelled fibrinogen or platelets, and venography. The last procedure is most reliable. Measurement of FDPs especially D-dimer has also been used, a normal level excluding DVT.

Treated by systemic anticoagulation with heparin 500–1500 units/h iv titrated to a partial thromboplastin time of 2–4 × control. Low mw heparins are increasingly used since they can be given sc once a day in fixed doses based on patients' weight, without needing laboratory monitoring. This tends to offset the increased drug cost. In addition, haemorrhagic complications are less frequent than with unfractionated heparin. Low mw heparins have thus been used to treat DVT without admission to hospital in certain patients. Warfarin is administered orally, and heparin discontinued when a prothrombin time of 2–3 × normal is achieved. Long-term interruption of leg blood flow may not be prevented, and prevention of PE has never been proven. Initial bed rest, leg elevation and analgesia are also prescribed although there is no evidence that these measures affect outcome. Optimal duration of warfarin therapy is controversial but the usual duration ranges from 6 weeks to 6 months, depending on underlying risk factors. Surgical removal of thrombus has been performed, but reaccumulation usually occurs, possibly due to vessel wall damage. Use of fibrinolytic drugs is controversial.

- Prophylaxis should be considered for all but minor surgery, and in patients immobile in ICUs. Methods used:
  - reduction of stasis:
    - heel cushion to prevent pressure on calf veins and a cushion under the knees to prevent hyperextension leading to popliteal vein occlusion.
    - elevation of legs.
    - intermittent pneumatic compression of the legs.
    - graduated compression stockings.
    - electrical stimulation of leg muscles.
    - encouragement of postoperative leg exercises and early mobility.
  - reduction of intravascular coagulation:
    - fibrinolytic drugs: not shown to prevent DVT.
    - antiplatelet drugs: have been shown to prevent DVT and PE.
    - heparin and warfarin anticoagulation: effective but with risk of haemorrhage. Low dose heparin is widely used (5000 units sc 2 h preoperatively then 8–12 hourly) and has been shown to be effective in reducing DVT and fatal PE. Low mw heparin reduces DVT without haemorrhagic side effects (*for doses, see Heparin*). Dihydroergotamine has been used together with heparin, and is thought to reduce the incidence further, possibly via venous vasoconstriction.
    - discontinuation of oral contraceptives preoperatively.
    - epidural/spinal anaesthesia is thought to be associated with increased fibrinolysis and reduced risk of DVT.

Low dose heparin and compression stockings are most commonly used.

[Rudolph LW Virchow (1821–1902), German pathologist; John Homans (1877–1954), US surgeon]

Kyrle PA, Eichinger S (2005). Lancet: 365: 1163–74

See also, Coagulation studies

Defibrillation. Application of an electric current across the heart, to convert (ventricular) fibrillation to sinus rhythm. Use of electricity was described in the late 1700s/early 1800s, but modern use arose from experiments in the 1930s–1950s, largely by Kouwenhoven. The first successful resuscitation of a patient from VF was by Claude Beck in 1947. Direct current is more effective and less damaging than alternating current.

Modern defibrillators contain a capacitor, with potential difference between its plates of 5000–8000 V (Fig. 49a). Stored charge is released during discharge; the energy released is proportional to the potential difference. An inductor controls the shape and duration of the delivered electrical pulse. With traditional monophasic defibrillation up to 400 J is used for external defibrillation (360 J actually delivered to the patient because of internal energy loss), and 20–50 J for internal defibrillation. The current pulse (up to 30 A) causes synchronous contraction of the heart muscle, thus allowing sinus rhythm to occur following a refractory period. Modern devices deliver lower energy biphasic waveforms, which are more effective at terminating VF; current is delivered in one direction followed immediately by a second current in the opposite direction (Fig. 49b). More sophisticated developments include the ability to measure and correct for the transthoracic impedance by varying the shock delivered.

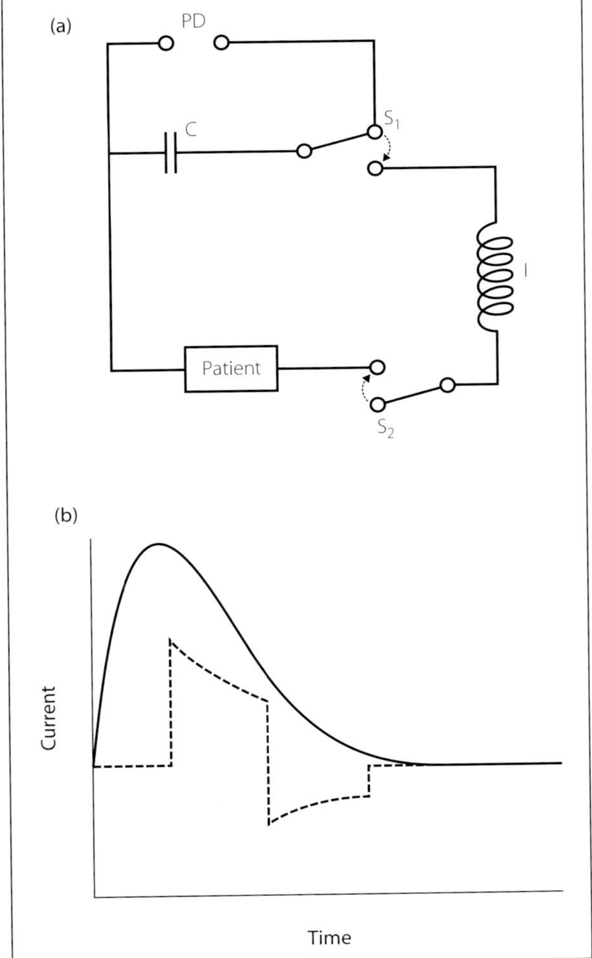

Fig. 49 Defibrillator. (a) Circuit diagram for basic model. PD, potential difference (5000–8000 V); C, capacitor; S1 and S2, switches; I, inductor. (b) Comparison of currents delivered by monophasic (solid) and biphasic (dashed) types (n.b. the latter varies in current strength and duration according to settings and/or measured transthoracic impedance)

Firm application of large paddles (one to the right of the sternum , the other over the lower left ribs in the anterior axillary line – taking care to avoid any implanted devices) using conductive jelly or pads increases efficiency. Forces of 8 kg in adults and 5 kg in children 1–8 years old are recommended. The paddles may also be placed on the front and back of the chest. Self-adhesive pads are now preferred. Thoracic impedance is reduced by the first shock, so a second discharge at the same setting will deliver greater energy to the heart. Leaving the paddles applied to the chest between shocks has been suggested, in order to improve contact (and thus reduce impedance) and to reduce the time required to apply repeated shocks. With monophasic defibrillation, the energy level has been increased over the first 2–3 shocks in an attempt to improve efficacy; this is no longer recommended routinely because there is little evidence to support it. For children, 2–4 J/kg is used. Lower energy levels are used in cardioversion. Repeated shocks may result in myocardial damage. Electrocution of members of the resuscitation team has occurred; all personnel should stand clear during discharge. Disconnection of the patient's oxygen supply and moving it 1 m from his/her chest during defibrillation is recommended, in order to avoid the risk of explosion from sparks in the presence of high-concentration O_2. Self-adhesive pads may produce fewer sparks than paddles.

Automatic external defibrillators (AEDs) identify life-threatening arrhythmias and deliver shocks, completely automatically or with the operator's approval. Their impact on resuscitation by non-medical staff has yet to be determined.

Implantable cardioverter defibrillators (ICDs) are used for recurrent VF/VT or predisposing conditions (*see Defibrillators, implantable cardioverter*)

[William Kouwenhoven (1886–1975), US engineer; Claude S Beck (1894–1971) US thoracic surgeon]

See also, individual arrhythmias; Cardiac pacing; Cardiopulmonary resuscitation

Defibrillators, implantable cardioverter. Specialised pacemakers that are designed to detect and treat potentially life-threatening arrhythmias. Have similar principles to pacemakers but are described by a different coding system (Table 12). Depending on the potential danger to the patient,

Table 12 North American Society of Pacing and Electrophysiology/British Pacing and Electrophysiology Group generic implantable defibrillator code

Position 1: chamber shocked	*Position 2: chamber paced*	*Position 3: monitoring modality*	*Position 4: anti-bradycardic chamber paced*
0 = None	0 = None	E = ECG	0 = None
A = Atrium	A = Atrium	H = Haemodynamic	A = Atrium
V = Ventricle	V = Ventricle		V = Ventricle
D = Dual	D = Dual		D = Dual

they generally respond with antitachycardia pacing, a low-energy synchronised shock (< 5 J), or a high-energy unsynchronised shock. Anaesthetic management for insertion is similar to that for pacemakers.
Allen M (2006). Anaesthesia; 61: 883–90

Deflation reflex. Stimulation of inspiration by lung deflation, initiated by pulmonary stretch receptors. Of uncertain significance in humans.
See also, Hering–Breuer reflex

Degrees of freedom. In statistics, the number of observations in a sample that can vary independently of other observations. For n observations, each observation may be compared with $n - 1$ others; i.e. degrees of freedom $= n - 1$. For chi-squared analysis, it equals the product of (number of rows − 1) and (number of columns − 1).

Dehydration. Reflects loss of water from ECF, alone or with intracellular fluid (ICF) depletion. Sodium is usually lost concurrently, giving rise to hypernatraemia or hyponatraemia, depending on the relative degrees of loss. If ECF osmolality rises, water passes from ICF into ECF by osmosis. A predominant water loss is shared by both ICF and ECF; water and sodium loss is borne mainly by ECF if osmolality is not greatly affected. Thus fever, lack of intake, diabetes insipidus, osmotic diuresis, etc. (mainly water loss) may be tolerated for longer periods than severe vomiting, diarrhoea, intestinal obstruction, diuretic therapy, etc. (water and sodium loss), although reduced water intake often accompanies the latter conditions.

The physiological response to dehydration includes increased thirst, vasopressin secretion and renin/angiotensin system activation, and CVS compensation for hypovolaemia via osmoreceptor and baroreceptor mechanisms.

Children are particularly prone to dehydration, as they exchange a greater proportion of body water each day.

- Clinical features are related to the extent of water loss:
  - 5% of body weight: thirst, dry mouth.
  - 5–10% of body weight: decreased intraocular pressure, peripheral perfusion and skin turgor, oliguria, orthostatic hypotension. JVP/CVP are reduced.
  - 10–15%: shock, coma.

Blood urea and haematocrit are increased, and urine has high osmolality (over 300 mosmol/kg) and low sodium content (under 10 mmol/l).

Treatment includes iv fluid administration: dextrose solutions are favoured for combinations of ICF and ECF losses and electrolyte solutions for ECF losses alone. Dehydration should be corrected preoperatively.
See also, Fluid balance; Fluids, body

Delirium tremens (DTs). Condition seen following alcohol withdrawal in chronic heavy drinkers. Occurs in about 5% of cases. Thought to be caused by reduction in both inhibitory $GABA_A$ activity and presynaptic sympathetic inhibition; hypomagnesaemia and hypocalcaemia may contribute to CNS hyperexcitability. Characterised by:

- tremor, agitation.
- confusion, disorientation, hallucinations (usually visual).
- sweating, tachycardia, hypertension.
- dehydration.

Usually occurs 2–3 days after withdrawal of alcohol, and lasts 3–4 days. May thus occur perioperatively.

Treatment includes rehydration (usually with glucose containing solutions since hypoglycaemia is common), correction of electrolyte imbalance and sedation. Benzodiazepines are the agents of choice, although carbamazepine and phenobarbital have also been used. Prevention is important and is achieved with the same drugs.
Kosten TR, O'Connor PG (2003). N Engl J Med; 348: 1786–95

Demand valves. Valves which allow self-administration of inhalational anaesthetic agents; they may form part of intermittent flow anaesthetic machines, or be used to administer Entonox. The standard Entonox valve was developed from underwater breathing apparatus, and contains a two-stage pressure regulator within one unit which fits directly to the cylinder. The first stage regulator is similar to those on anaesthetic machines. At the second stage, gas flow is prevented by a rod which seals the valve. The patient's inspiratory effort moves a sensing diaphragm and tilts the rod, opening the valve. Very small negative pressures are required to produce gas flow of up to 300 l/min. An expiratory valve is attached to the mask/mouthpiece elbow piece. A safety (overpressure) valve is also incorporated. Other demand valves for use with Entonox have the second stage (demand) regulator attached to the patient's mask.

Demeclocycline hydrochloride. Tetracycline, used as an antibacterial drug and to treat the syndrome of inappropriate ADH secretion (SIADH), possibly by blocking the renal action of vasopressin.

- Dosage:
  - infection: 150 mg 6 hourly, or 300 mg 12 hourly, orally.
  - SIADH: 600–1200 mg/day in divided doses, orally.
- Side effects: as for tetracycline.

Demyelinating diseases. Non-specific group of disorders, with abnormality of the axonal myelin sheath as the predominant feature. Defective myelin may be present at birth (dysmyelinating) or may arise in areas of previously normal myelin (demyelinating). Multiple (disseminated) sclerosis (MS) is the commonest of the latter and is considered below; others include postimmunisation or parainfectious encephalomyelitis.

Aetiology of MS is unknown but is probably multifactorial, involving climatic, geographical, genetic, viral and immune factors. Plaques of demyelination occur throughout the CNS, with preservation of axon continuity. Optic nerve, brainstem and spinal cord are particularly affected, with sparing of peripheral nerves. Neurological lesions are separated temporally and spatially, producing a variable clinical picture. Common presentations include limb weakness, spasticity, hyperreflexia, visual disturbances, paraesthesia and incoordination. Progression is variable with relapses associated with trauma, infection, stress and rise in body temperature.

Diagnosed clinically, supported by gadolinium enhanced MRI findings and the presence of oligoclonal IgG bands in the CSF. Evoked potential testing may support the diagnosis.

Treatment is supportive, but may include corticosteroids. Interferon beta has been shown to decrease the relapse rate in relapsing remitting MS. Hyperbaric O_2 therapy has been advocated but results are disappointing.

Anaesthetic implications are unclear, since effects of stress, surgery and anaesthesia cannot be separated from the spontaneity of new lesion formation. Thus case reports are often conflicting in their conclusions. Increases in body temperature should be avoided; avoidance of anticholinergic drugs has been suggested. An abnormal response to neuromuscular blocking drugs, including hyperkalaemia following suxamethonium, has been suggested but without direct evidence. Prolonged muscle spasms may occur, but epilepsy is rare. Increased tendency to DVT has been suggested. Impairment of respiratory and autonomic control has been reported. Although not contraindicated, epidural or spinal anaesthesia has been avoided for medicolegal reasons, although it is increasingly used as the preferred method of obstetric analgesia and anaesthesia.

Denervation hypersensitivity. Increased sensitivity of denervated skeletal muscle to acetylcholine. Develops approximately 4–5 days after denervation, and is due to proliferation of extrajunctional acetylcholine receptors over the entire muscle membrane, instead of being restricted to the neuromuscular junction. Thought to be the mechanism underlying the exaggerated hyperkalaemic response to suxamethonium seen after peripheral nerve injuries. Its cause is unclear. Also occurs in smooth muscle.

Density. For a substance, defined as its mass per unit volume. Relative density (specific gravity) is the mass of any volume of substance divided by the mass of the same volume of water.

Dental nerve blocks, *see Mandibular nerve blocks; Maxillary nerve blocks*

Dental surgery. Anaesthesia may be required for tooth extraction, conservative dental surgery or faciomaxillary surgery.

- For outpatient ambulatory surgery, the following may be used:
  - mandibular and maxillary nerve blocks.
  - relative analgesia.
  - iv sedation, e.g. Jorgensen technique and variants.
  - inhalational anaesthetic agents, including N_2O and/or volatile agents. Traditionally administered from intermittent flow anaesthetic machines, using nasal inhalers, although continuous flow machines are increasingly used. Quantiflex apparatus is also used. Occupational exposure to N_2O is a hazard, especially in small dental surgeries.
  - iv anaesthetic agents.

The use of general anaesthesia for dental surgery is declining, with local anaesthetic techniques becoming more common, especially for conservative dentistry. General anaesthesia is usually indicated for patients who have learning difficulties or are extremely nervous, children, those undergoing multiple extractions, and those with local infection (infiltration is less effective, and may spread infection). Following high-profile (though infrequent) deaths in the dental chair in the UK, general anaesthetics are now performed by anaesthetists within hospitals.

- General anaesthetic principles are as for day-case surgery; main problems:
  - high proportion of children, usually anxious and unpremedicated.
  - shared airway as for ENT surgery. Airway obstruction, mouth breathing during nasally administered anaesthesia, airway soiling and breath-holding may occur. Traditionally, anaesthesia is administered using a nasal inhaler (mask-like device held over the nose from behind the patient's head). Cuffed nasal airways have also been used.
  - arrhythmias are common, especially when halothane is used.
- Controversy has existed over the best position of the patient:
  - supine: the most familiar position for anaesthetists, and hypotension and reduced cerebral blood flow are less likely.
  - sitting: the most familiar position for dentists, with less risk of airway contamination with blood, teeth, etc. and possibly less risk of regurgitation and aspiration.

Fears over 'fainting' during anaesthesia are opposed by lack of increased mortality when the sitting position is used. The reclining position, with the foot of the chair/table raised, has been suggested as a compromise.

Mouth packs are usually employed to prevent mouth breathing, soak up blood, and prevent airway soiling. They should be placed under the tongue, pushing the tongue back to seal the mouth from the airway. Mouth gags or props are often used to hold the mouth open; the former are often held by the anaesthetist from behind the patient's head.

Dental surgery is performed on an inpatient surgery basis if airway obstruction, cardiac or respiratory disease, coagulation disorders or extreme obesity are present. Nasotracheal intubation is usually performed, and a throat pack placed. Arrhythmias may occur, although the incidence is reduced with the use of IPPV. Use of concentrated adrenaline solutions by dentists is still common, e.g. 1:80 000, despite anaesthetists' objections.

Depolarising neuromuscular blockade (Phase I block). Follows depolarisation of the neuromuscular junction postsynaptic membrane via activation of its acetylcholine receptors, but with only slow repolarisation. Effect of depolarisation of presynaptic receptors is unclear, but may be partially responsible for the fasciculation seen. Suxamethonium is the most commonly used and widely available drug; previously used drugs include decamethonium and suxethonium.

- Features of depolarising blockade:
  - may be preceded by fasciculation.
  - does not exhibit fade or post-tetanic potentiation.
  - increased by acetylcholinesterase inhibitors.
  - potentiated by respiratory alkalosis, hypothermia, hyperkalaemia and hypermagnesaemia.
  - antagonised by non-depolarising neuromuscular blocking drugs.
  - development of dual block with excessive dosage of drug.

See also, Neuromuscular blockade monitoring; Non-depolarising neuromuscular blockade

Dermatomes. Lateral walls of somites (segmental units appearing longitudinally early in embryonic development), which form the skin and subcutaneous tissues. Cutaneous sensation retains the somatic distribution, corresponding to segmental spinal levels. Thus areas of skin are supplied by particular spinal nerves; useful in determining the extent of regional anaesthetic blocks and localising neurological lesions (Fig. 50).

See also, Myotomes

Dermatomyositis, *see Polymyositis*

Desensitisation block, *see Dual block*

Desferrioxamine mesylate. Chelating agent used in the treatment of aluminium and iron poisoning.

- Dosage: 15 mg/kg/h iv to a maximum of 80 mg/kg/24 h. Also given by sc infusion in chronic iron overload, e.g. associated with haemochromatosis or repeated blood transfusions: 20–50 mg/kg/day given over 8–12 h, 3–7 times per week.

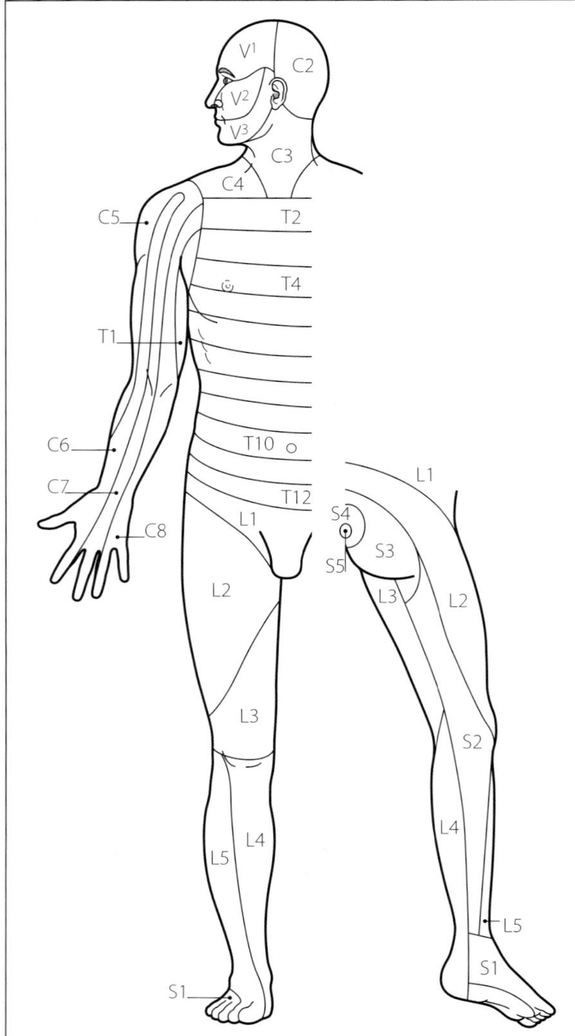

Fig. 50 Dermatomal nerve supply

- Side effects: anaphylaxis, hypotension, tachycardia, thrombocytopenia, visual and hearing loss.

Desflurane. 1-Fluoro-2,2,2-trifluoroethyl difluoromethyl ether. Inhalational anaesthetic agent, synthesised in the 1960s but only introduced in the UK in 1994. Chemical structure is the same as isoflurane, but with the chlorine atom replaced by fluorine (Fig. 51).

- Properties:
  - colourless liquid with slightly pungent vapour.
  - mw 168.
  - boiling point 23°C.
  - SVP at 20°C 88 kPa (673 mmHg).
  - partition coefficients:
    - blood/gas 0.42.
    - oil/gas 19.
  - MAC 5–7% in adults; 7.2–10.7% in children.
  - non-flammable, non-corrosive.
  - supplied in liquid form with no additive.
  - May react with dry soda lime to produce carbon monoxide (*see Circle systems*).
- Effects:
  - CNS:
    - rapid induction (although limited by its irritant properties) and recovery. Pain and restlessness may occur postoperatively if adequate analgesia is not provided, since excretion is so rapid.
    - EEG changes as for isoflurane.
    - may increase cerebral blood flow although the response of cerebral vessels to CO_2 is preserved.
    - ICP may increase due to imbalance between the production and absorption of CSF.
    - reduces $CMRO_2$ as for isoflurane.
    - has poor analgesic properties.
  - RS:
    - causes airway irritation; not recommended for induction of anaesthesia in children since respiratory complications (e.g. laryngospasm, breath-holding, cough, apnoea) are common and may be severe, especially if used with N_2O.
    - respiratory depressant, with increased rate and decreased tidal volume.
  - CVS:
    - vasodilatation and hypotension may occur, similar to that with isoflurane. May cause tachycardia and hypertension via sympathetic stimulation, especially if high concentrations are introduced rapidly.
    - coronary steal is not thought to occur; myocardial ischaemia may occur if sympathetic stimulation is excessive.
    - arrhythmias uncommon as for isoflurane. Little myocardial sensitisation to catecholamines.
    - renal and hepatic blood flow generally preserved.
  - other:
    - dose-dependent uterine relaxation.
    - skeletal muscle relaxation; non-depolarising neuromuscular blockade may be potentiated.
    - may precipitate MH.

Only 0.02% metabolised.

2–6% is usually adequate for maintenance of anaesthesia, with higher concentrations for induction. Uptake and excretion are rapid because of its low blood gas solubility; thus it has been suggested as the agent of choice in day-case surgery although this is controversial. Although more expensive than isoflurane, the difference in cost is much reduced at low flows and because equilibrium is reached more rapidly than for isoflurane and less drug is required to maintain anaesthesia once equilibrium is reached, thus making it economical for longer operations.

Supplied with a specific adaptor already fitted on the bottle. A special vaporiser is used because of desflurane's low boiling point.

```
      F   H        F
      |   |        |
  F — C — C — O — C — H
      |   |        |
      F   F        F
```

Fig. 51 Structure of desflurane

Desmopressin (D-amino-8-D-arginine-vasopressin; DDAVP). Analogue of vasopressin, with a longer lasting antidiuretic effect but minimal vasoconstrictor actions. Used to diagnose and treat non-nephrogenic diabetes insipidus. May also be used to increase factor VIII and von Willebrand factor levels by 2–4 times in mild haemophilia or von Willebrand's disease. Has also been used to improve platelet function in renal failure and to reduce blood loss in cardiac surgery.

- Dosage:
  - diabetes insipidus: 10–20 μg once/twice daily, intranasally; 100–200 μg 8 hourly, orally; or 1–4 μg/day iv/sc/im.
  - to increase factor VIII levels: 0.4 μg/kg in 50 ml saline iv 1 h preoperatively, repeated at 4 and 24 h.
- Side effects: fluid retention, hyponatraemia, pallor, abdominal cramps, and angina in susceptible patients.

Dew point. Temperature at which ambient air is saturated with water vapour. As air of a certain water content cools, e.g. when it is in contact with a cold surface, condensation occurs when the dew point is reached (e.g. misting on the surface of spectacles on entering a warm room from the cold). This process may be used to measure humidity.

Dexamethasone. Corticosteroid with high glucocorticoid but minimal mineralocorticoid activity and long duration of action, thus used where sustained activity is required but when water retention would be harmful, e.g. cerebral oedema. Also used to reduce oedema following dental surgery, in congenital adrenal hyperplasia and in the diagnosis of Cushing's disease. Has been used to prevent nausea and vomiting associated with surgery and chemotherapy, and to mature fetal lungs in premature labour.

- Dosage:
  - 0.5–10 mg daily, orally.
  - 0.5–20 mg iv (10 mg followed by 4 mg 6 hourly in cerebral oedema).
- Side effects: as for corticosteroids.

Dexmedetomidine hydrochloride. Selective α-adrenergic receptor agonist, with about 1300–1600 times the affinity for α_2-receptors as for α_1. Rapidly distributed after iv injection (half-life about 6 min) with an elimination half-life of 2–2.5 h. Volume of distribution is about 1.3 l/kg. 94% protein-bound. Inactivated mainly to glucuronides with 80–90% excreted in the urine. Has similar effects to clonidine but more predictable and easier to titrate, e.g. for sedation in ICU. Approved in the USA in 1999, it is unavailable in the UK.

- Dosage: 1 μg/kg iv over 10–15 min then 0.2–0.7 μg/kg/min.
- Side effects: as for clonidine. May cause hypertension at high doses via peripheral vasoconstriction. May also reduce renal blood flow. Has little direct effect on respiration.

Dextrans. Group of branched polysaccharides of 200 000 glucose units, derived from the action of bacteria (*Leuconostoc mesenteroides*) on sucrose. Partial hydrolysis produces molecules of average mw 40 000, 70 000 and 110 000 (dextrans 40, 70 and 110 respectively). Dextran 40 is used to promote peripheral blood flow, e.g. in arterial insufficiency and in prophylaxis of DVT. Dextrans 70 and 110 are used mainly for plasma expansion; the latter is now rarely used and is unavailable in the UK. Dextrans increase peripheral blood flow by reducing viscosity, and may coat both endothelium and cellular elements of blood, reducing their interaction. They impair platelet adhesiveness, possibly impair factor VIII activity, and may have anti-inflammatory properties.

Size of dextran molecules determines the degree of plasma expansion produced and the molecules' circulation time. Half-life ranges from 15 min for small molecules, to several days for larger ones. Major route of excretion is via the kidneys.

Supplied in 5% dextrose or 0.9% saline, as 6% (dextrans 70 and 110) or 10% (dextran 40) solutions. Dextran 70 is also supplied as a 6% solution in hypertonic saline (7.5%); 250 ml given over 2–5 min should be followed immediately by isotonic fluids.

- Side effects:
  - renal failure caused by tubular obstruction by dextran casts; mainly occurs with dextran 40 when used in hypovolaemia; concurrent water and electrolyte administration should be provided.
  - anaphylactic reactions: thought to result from previous cross-immunisation against bacterial antigens. Its incidence is reduced from 1:4500 to 1:84 000 by pretreatment with 3 g dextran 1 (mw 1000), to occupy and block antigen binding sites of circulating antibodies to dextran.
  - interference with blood cross-matching.
  - bleeding tendency. Initial administration should be limited to 500–1000 ml, and the total amount administered restricted to 10 (dextran 40) and 20 (dextran 70) ml/kg/day.
  - osmotic diuresis.

Dextrans have also been used locally to prolong the action of local anaesthetic agents, possibly by trapping the latter molecules within large macromolecules in the tissues. Inconsistent results have been reported.

See also, Colloids

Dextromoramide tartrate. Opioid analgesic drug, related to methadone. Introduced in 1956. Less sedating, and shorter acting (duration 2–3 h) than morphine, but with similar effects.

- Dosage: 5–20 mg orally.

Dextropropoxyphene hydrochloride/napsilate. Opioid analgesic drug, related to methadone. Prepared in 1953. Has weak properties alone, but powerful when combined with paracetamol (as co-proxamol). Overdose of this combination is particularly dangerous; initial respiratory depression and coma (due to dextropropoxyphene) may be treated correctly but later liver failure (due to paracetamol poisoning) may occur if appropriate prophylaxis is not undertaken. Concerns over safety, even at or just above normal doses, led to co-proxamol's phased withdrawal in the UK beginning in 2005.

Dextrose solutions. IV fluids available as 5, 10, 20, 25 and 50% solutions in water (50, 100, 200, 250 and 500 g/l respectively). Once administered, the glucose is metabolised by red blood cells, and the water distributed to all body fluid compartments. Thus used in hypoglycaemia, and to replace water losses. Also used with insulin to treat acute hyperkalaemia.

Excess administration, e.g. perioperatively, may result in hyponatraemia. Solutions of higher concentrations are increasingly hypertonic, acidic and viscous; they may cause thrombophlebitis if infused peripherally. Osmolality of 5% dextrose solution is 278 mosmol/kg; of 10% solution 523 mosmol/kg. pH of 5% solution is approximately 4.0. May cause haemolysis of stored erythrocytes when infused iv before stored blood without first flushing the line with saline, presumably because the dextrose is taken up and metabolised by the cells to leave a hypo-osmotic solution.

See also, Fluids, body; Intravenous fluid administration

Dezocine. Synthetic opioid analgesic drug, available in the USA but not in the UK. Comparable in potency, onset and duration of action to morphine. Has some opioid receptor antagonist activity, less than that of nalorphine but greater than that of pentazocine. Administered im or iv in doses of 2.5–20 mg.

Diabetes insipidus. Polyuria and polydipsia associated with reduced vasopressin activity, either because secretion by the pituitary gland is reduced (cranial) or the kidneys are unresponsive (nephrogenic):
- cranial: occurs in head injury, neurosurgery (especially post-pituitary surgery), intracranial tumours, etc. Rarely familial.
- nephrogenic: caused by drugs, e.g. lithium, demeclocycline and gentamicin; a rare X-linked recessive form may also occur.

Characterised by inappropriate passage of large volumes of dilute urine, with raised plasma osmolality. Patients cannot concentrate their urine in response to water deprivation. The two types are distinguished by their response to administered vasopressin.
- Treatment:
  - cranial: desmopressin (synthetic vasopressin analogue) 10–20 μg once/twice daily, intranasally; 100–200 μg 8 hourly, orally; or 1–4 μg/day iv/sc/im.
  - nephrogenic: thiazide diuretics.

Anaesthetic considerations are related to impaired fluid balance with hypovolaemia, dehydration, hypernatraemia and other electrolyte imbalance. Careful attention to fluid balance, with regular monitoring of urine and plasma osmolality and electrolytes, is required.

Diabetes mellitus. Disorder of glucose metabolism characterised by relative or total lack of insulin. This results in lipolysis, gluconeogenesis and glycogenolysis, with hepatic conversion of fatty acids to ketone bodies, and hyperglycaemia. The resultant glycosuria causes an osmotic diuresis, with polyuria, polydipsia and excessive sodium and potassium loss.

Affects up to 3% of the population; over 80% are over 80 years old and 50% are likely to require surgery.
- May be:
  - primary: thought to be related to genetic, infective and immunological factors, but the aetiology is unclear.
  - secondary:
    - pancreatic disease, e.g. pancreatitis, malignancy.
    - insulin antagonism, e.g. corticosteroids, Cushing's syndrome, acromegaly, phaeochromocytoma.
    - drugs, e.g. thiazide diuretics.

Classically divided into type I (insulin-dependent; IDDM), presenting in children or young adults, and type II (non-insulin-dependent; NIDDM), presenting in adults (and occasionally children) who are usually obese. Type I, an autoimmune condition possibly triggered by environmental factors on a background of genetic predisposition, is treated with insulin. Type II is treated with diet control, oral hypoglycaemic drugs (sulphonylureas, biguanides, acarbose, thiazolidinediones and meglitinides), a combination of oral hypoglycaemic drugs and insulin, or insulin alone. Resistance to insulin has been shown in type II. The World Health Organization suggests that diabetes should be diagnosed if one of the following applies:
- symptoms + plasma glucose concentration > 11.1 mmol/l.
- two fasting glucose concentrations > 7.0 mmol/l.
- two random glucose concentrations > 11.1 mmol/l if the patient is asymptomatic.

The oral glucose tolerance test is not required for most patients.
- Complications:
  - renal impairment, caused by glomerulosclerosis, vascular insufficiency, infection and papillary necrosis.
  - arteriosclerosis causing ischaemic heart disease, peripheral vascular insufficiency, and cerebrovascular disease with increased risk of CVA. Microvascular involvement may cause cardiac failure and impaired ventricular function. Hypertension is more common than in non-diabetic subjects.
  - autonomic and peripheral neuropathy, the latter sensory or motor. Single nerves may also be affected, including cranial nerves.
  - retinopathy and cataract formation.
  - skin: collagen thickening, blisters, necrobiosis lipoidica.
  - increased susceptibility to infection and delayed wound healing.
  - diabetic coma.
  - syndrome of stiff joints may occur: suggested by the 'prayer sign' (inability to press the palmar surfaces of the index fingers fully flat against one another when pressing the palms together). Has been associated with difficult tracheal intubation and reduced compliance of the epidural space.
- Anaesthetic management is related to the above complications and to the perioperative control of blood sugar. Mortality and morbidity is increased when compared with non-diabetic patients.

  Patients should be fully assessed for fitness and diabetic control, and scheduled for surgery at the beginning of the operating list. The aim is to avoid hyperglycaemia, ketoacidosis, hypoglycaemia and electrolyte imbalance:
  - NIDDM patients: for minor surgery, careful monitoring of blood sugar levels is usually all that is required. Chlorpropamide is withheld for 48 h before surgery; shorter-acting sulphonylureas and biguanides are withheld on the morning of surgery. A glucose level < 12 mmol/l is traditionally thought to be acceptable although tighter control (aiming for the same levels as in IDDM) has been suggested. Patients are treated as for IDDM when undergoing major surgery. Oral medication is restarted when eating postoperatively.
  - IDDM: patients are starved preoperatively, with morning insulin omitted. They should receive insulin and dextrose iv throughout the perioperative period, to avoid hyper- and hypoglycaemia and maintain plasma glucose between 6 and 10 mmol/l. Dextrose and insulin infusions should be through the same iv cannula, to reduce risk of accidental overdose of one infusion should the other infusion cease running. Several regimens have been successfully used:
    - Alberti regimen: 1000 ml 10% dextrose + 10 units soluble insulin + 10 mmol potassium infused at 100 ml/h. The infusion is changed to contain more or less insulin according to regular testing with glucose reagent sticks. The preoperative insulin regimen is restarted when the patient is drinking and eating normally.
    - the total daily insulin requirement is divided by four, adding the result to 500 ml 5% dextrose + 5–10 mmol potassium. The bag is infused at 100 ml/h, with regular checking of blood glucose levels.
    - 5% dextrose + 5–10 mmol potassium is infused at 100 ml/h, with insulin infused via a syringe pump, adjusted according to a sliding scale.

    Preoperative conversion to soluble insulin therapy has been used.

Since the symptoms of hypoglycaemia are masked by general anaesthesia, regular perioperative monitoring of plasma glucose is required. Administration of lactate containing solutions is usually avoided for fear of increasing plasma glucose levels although the actual increase is likely to be small.

Modern anaesthetic agents have minimal effects on diabetic control (cf. diethyl ether), but regional techniques are often preferred because they interfere less with oral intake. Insulin requirements may be increased after major surgery as part of the stress response to surgery.

Emergency surgery is particularly hazardous, especially if diabetes is poorly controlled. Adequate resuscitation must be performed, with treatment of ketoacidosis if present. Hyperglycaemia may present with abdominal pain, and abdominal surgery may reveal no abnormality.

Pregnancy may precipitate or worsen diabetes, and close medical supervision is required. During labour, regimens usually involve iv infusions of 5% dextrose, e.g. 500 ml/8 h, with iv insulin rate adjusted according to regular stick testing. Epidural anaesthesia is usually suggested, since it reduces acidosis in labour and allows Caesarean section if indicated.

[K George MM Alberti, Newcastle physician]

Robertshaw HJ, Hall GM (2006). Anaesthesia; 61: 1187–90

Diabetic coma. Coma in diabetes mellitus may be caused by:

- hypoglycaemia: caused by excessive antidiabetic therapy, excessive exertion or decreased food intake. Treatment includes iv glucose; iv/im glucagon may occasionally be useful.
- ketoacidosis: more common in insulin-dependent diabetics. Mortality is 6–10%, highest in old age. Often precipitated by other illness, e.g. infection and MI, since insulin requirements are increased. May develop insidiously.
  - features:
    - of dehydration, e.g. hypotension, tachycardia, etc.
    - of acidosis, e.g. hyperventilation.
    - vomiting, diarrhoea, abdominal pain; the last may simulate an acute surgical emergency, requiring careful review of the diagnosis.
    - smell of acetone on the breath.
  - management:
    - measurement of urea and electrolytes, glucose, arterial blood gases, full blood count. Ketone stick tests are available. Chest X-ray and blood cultures, etc.
    - general management: O_2, nasogastric tube (gastric dilatation is common), urinary catheter, CVP measurement, ECG and clinical monitoring, etc. Antibiotics are administered if infection is suspected. Prophylactic heparin is usually suggested for high risk patients.
    - fluid therapy: guided by CVP measurement; up to 6–8 litres may be required. Suitable starting regimen: 1 litre of 0.9% saline over 30 min, then hourly for 2 h, then 2 hourly, then 2–4 hourly. This is changed to 5% dextrose when blood glucose is 10–15 mmol/l (180–270 mg/dl). Hypotonic saline is used in hyperosmolar coma as below.
    - potassium supplementation is required despite any initial hyperkalaemia, since the body potassium deficit will be revealed once tissue uptake is stimulated by insulin. Suitable starting regimen: 10–20 mmol in the first litre of fluid; 10–40 mmol thereafter depending on the plasma potassium after 1 h (repeated every few hours).
    - insulin is preferably given iv, e.g. 6 units as a bolus, then 6 units/h (0.1 units/kg/h in children) until plasma glucose is 10–15 mmol/l; 2–4 units/h thereafter. Glucose is monitored hourly; a reduction of 3–5 mmol/l/h (55–90 mg/dl) is aimed for. Insulin may also be given im: 20 units initially followed by 6 units hourly; then 2 hourly when glucose is 10–15 mmol/l. Insulin is given sc when food is taken orally.
    - bicarbonate therapy is given if pH is under 7.0–7.1. Administration is guided by base excess.
    - hypophosphataemia may require replacement, e.g. with potassium phosphate. 5–20 mmol/h has been suggested.
- hyperosmolar non-ketotic coma: usually occurs in elderly patients. Typically of slow onset with polyuria and progressive dehydration. Blood glucose levels and osmolality are very high, with little or no ketonuria. Treatment includes small doses of insulin and 0.45% saline administered slowly iv. Cerebral oedema and convulsions may occur if rehydration is too rapid.
- lactic acidosis: usually occurs in elderly patients taking biguanides. Blood glucose may be normal, with little or no ketonuria.

Clinical distinction between different types of diabetic coma is unreliable. Features aiding the diagnosis are shown in Table 13.

Diagnostic peritoneal lavage, *see Peritoneal lavage*

Dialysis. Term referring to the artificial removal of water and solutes from the blood. Indications include renal failure and severe cardiac failure unresponsive to diuretic therapy; may also remove drugs from the circulation in poisoning and overdoses although only effective for smaller, non-protein-bound, water-soluble molecules. Many variants exist but they may be classified into:

- peritoneal dialysis.
- intermittent haemodialysis.
- continuous haemofiltration/haemodiafiltration.

All techniques rely on the passage of water and solutes across a semipermeable membrane; this passage may be manipulated by altering the hydrostatic or osmotic gradients across the membrane to optimise removal. In haemoperfusion, unwanted molecules (including lipid soluble protein-bound ones) are adsorbed on to activated charcoal or an ion exchange resin, thus involving a different principle from that of dialysis. Both dialysis and adsorption techniques have been used to remove circulating toxins in hepatic failure, such techniques usually being termed liver dialysis.

Diamorphine hydrochloride (Diacetylmorphine; Heroin). Opioid analgesic drug, introduced in 1898; said to cause less constipation, nausea and hypotension than morphine, but more likely to cause addiction. Also suppresses coughing to a greater extent. More soluble than morphine, thus smaller volumes of injectant are required. Rapidly hydrolysed by plasma cholinesterase to 6-monoacetylmorphine (responsible for the rapid onset of action) which is then slowly metabolised to morphine in the liver. Unavailable in the USA, Australia and parts of Europe (e.g. Germany) because of its reputation as a drug of addiction, although there is no evidence that medical use increases its abuse.

Table 13 Features of different types of diabetic coma

Type	Blood glucose (mmol/l)	Dehydration	Ketones
Hypoglycaemia	<2	0	0
Ketoacidosis	>14	+++	++
Hyperosmolar non-ketotic	>14	+++	0
Lactic acidosis	Variable	+	0 to +

- Dosage: 5 mg is equivalent to 10 mg morphine. It may be given im, iv, sc, orally, epidurally (1–5 mg) or intrathecally (100–300 µg); has also been shown to be effective when given intranasally.

See also, Spinal opioids

Diaphragm. Fibromuscular sheet separating the thorax from the abdomen. The main respiratory muscle, it flattens and descends vertically during inspiration, expanding the thoracic cavity. During expiration, it relaxes; in forced expiration, contraction of the anterior abdominal muscles pushes the diaphragm upwards.

- Consists of (Fig. 52):
  - central tendon, attached to the pericardium above.
  - peripheral muscular part. Attachments:
    - posteriorly via the medial and lateral lumbosacral arches (arcuate ligaments), to fascia covering psoas and quadratus lumborum muscles respectively. The right and left crura attach to vertebrae L1–3 and L1–2 respectively; between them lies the median lumbosacral arch (median arcuate ligament).
    - to the lower six ribs and costal cartilages anteriorly, and xiphisternum medially.
- Has three main openings which transmit the following structures:
  - inferior vena cava and right phrenic nerve at the level of T8.
  - oesophagus, vagus and gastric nerves and branches of the left gastric vessels at the level of T10.
  - aorta, thoracic duct and azygos vein at the level of T12.

The diaphragm is also pierced by the left phrenic nerve and splanchnic nerves.

The sympathetic chain passes behind the medial lumbosacral arch.

- Nerve supply: from C3–5 via the phrenic nerves, with some sensory supply to the periphery via the lower intercostal nerves.
- Development:
  - originally in the neck; descends during development, retaining its cervical nerve supply.
  - formed from:
    - oesophageal mesentery dorsally.
    - right and left pleuroperitoneal membranes laterally.
    - septum transversum anteriorly (forming the central tendon).
    - small peripheral contribution from body wall.

  Defects in development may produce diaphragmatic herniae.

See also, Hiatus hernia

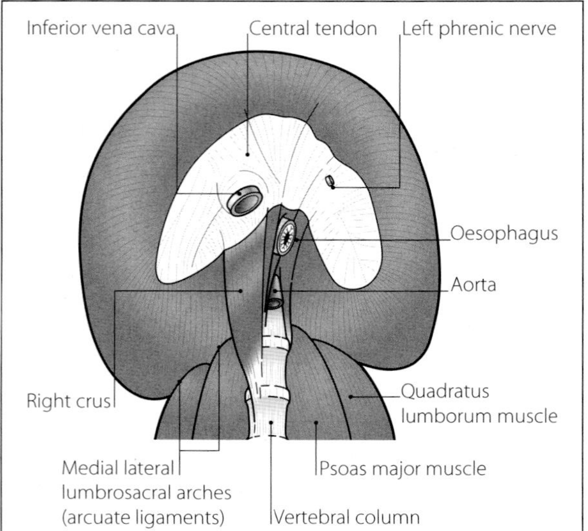

Fig. 52 Inferior aspect of diaphragm

Diaphragmatic herniae. Herniation of abdominal viscera through the diaphragm into the thorax. Congenital herniae occur in approximately 1 in 4000 live births (1 in 2500 of all births), are often familial, and are caused by failure of fusion of the various components of the diaphragm, e.g.:

- foramen of Bochdalek: through a defective pleuroperitoneal membrane, usually left-sided. The most common form (80%).
- foramen of Morgagni: between xiphoid and costal origins; more common on the right side.
- through the central tendon or oesophageal hiatus.

Usually diagnosed during routine antenatal ultrasound. Other congenital defects may be present (e.g. cardiac anomalies found in 50%).

Causes respiratory distress, cyanosis, scaphoid abdomen and bowel sounds audible in the thorax. Diagnosed clinically and by X-ray. The lung on the affected side is often hypoplastic, with decreased compliance and increased pulmonary vascular resistance (PVR). Arterial hypoxaemia reflects immature lung tissue and reduced ventilation caused by presence of thoracic bowel, and persistent fetal circulation caused by the raised PVR. PVR is further increased by hypoxic pulmonary vasoconstriction.

Immediate management includes gastric decompression, improving oxygenation and decreasing PVR. IPPV by facepiece may increase gastric distension and should be avoided. IPPV is best performed using a tracheal tube, avoiding excessive inflation pressures since pneumothorax may easily occur. PVR may be reduced by avoiding hypocapnia and hypothermia, treating acidosis, and infusing vasodilator drugs centrally, e.g. sodium nitroprusside 1–2 µg/kg/min, prostacyclin 5–10 ng/kg/min.

Anaesthesia for surgical correction is as for paediatric anaesthesia. N_2O is avoided because of distension of thoracic bowel. Excessive inflation of the hypoplastic lung at the end of the procedure should be avoided, since pneumothorax may occur. Abdominal closure may be difficult once the bowel is returned to the abdomen; postoperative IPPV may be required. The hypoplastic lung slowly re-expands, usually within a few days/weeks.

Surgery is usually delayed in severe cases, until respiratory stability is achieved. High frequency ventilation and extracorporeal membrane oxygenation have been used. Mortality is high if pneumothorax occurs and lung compliance is low.

Acquired acute herniae may follow blunt or penetrating trauma or surgery. They may impair ventilation, or only cause symptoms if strangulation or obstruction occurs. Hiatus hernia is gradual in onset.

[Giovanni B Morgagni (1682–1771), Italian anatomist; Victor A Bochdalek (1801–1883), Czech anatomist]

Brown RA, Bösenberg AT (2007). Pediatr Anesth; 17: 713–9

See also, Cardiopulmonary resuscitation, neonatal

Diarrhoea. Common problem in the ICU which contributes to increased mortality; may result in dehydration and skin excoriation, and is upsetting to the patient, relatives and staff. There are many causes including:

- infection (most often *Cl. difficile*, but occasionally salmonella and campylobacter species).
- inflammatory bowel disease.
- malabsorption.
- bowel ischaemia.
- drugs (e.g. antibacterial drugs).
- enteral nutrition.

Spurious diarrhoea may occur in severe constipation. Non-infectious diarrhoea tends to occur without blood or mucus. Stools usually return to normal after the causal agent is removed.

Management includes appropriate investigation (stool cultures and microscopy, sigmoidoscopy; more invasive endoscopy or imaging may be required) and maintenance of fluid and electrolyte balance. Probiotic agents may be useful. Specific causes are managed accordingly. Symptomatic treatment, e.g. with codeine or loperamide, may be indicated although they are generally avoided in children and in infective diarrhoea.

See also, Clostridial infections

Diastole, *see Cardiac cycle; Diastolic interval*

Diastolic blood pressure. Lowest arterial BP during diastole. Represents the pressure head for coronary blood flow, but otherwise generally thought to be less important than systolic blood pressure and MAP, although it contributes to the latter.

Diastolic BP has been used to guide therapy in hypertension, treatment usually being advocated if it exceeds 90 mmHg, but this is controversial.

Diastolic interval. Duration of diastole. Shortened when heart rate is increased; e.g. equals about 0.62 s at 65 beats/min, but only 0.14 s at 200 beats/min.

Short diastolic intervals reduce coronary blood flow and ventricular filling.

Diastolic pressure time index (DPTI). Area between tracings of left ventricular pressure and aortic root pressure during diastole (*see Fig. 60; Endocardial viability ratio*). Represents the pressure head and time available for coronary blood flow; used to calculate endocardial viability ratio.

See also, Cardiac cycle

Diathermy (Bovie machine). Device first described in 1928, used to coagulate blood vessels, and cut and destroy tissues during surgery, by the heating effect of an electric current passed through them. Alternating current with a frequency of 0.5–1 MHz is used; a sine wave pattern is employed for cutting and a damped or pulsed sine wave pattern for coagulation. Effects on skeletal and cardiac muscle are negligible at these high frequencies. The current density is kept high at the site of intended damage by using small electrodes at this site, e.g. forceps tips.

- Diathermy may be:
  - unipolar:
    - forceps, etc. act as one electrode;
    - large plate strapped to the patient's leg acts as the other electrode, often at earth potential. Current density at this site is low because of the large area of tissue through which current passes; thus little heating occurs.
  - bipolar: current is passed across tissue held between the two tips of one pair of forceps. The power used is small and the current dispersal through other tissues is negligible; thus used for more delicate surgery, e.g. eye surgery and neurosurgery. No plate electrode is required.
- Hazards:
  - interference with monitoring equipment, especially with the old spark gap diathermy machines; interference is less likely with modern solid state machines.
  - incorrect attachment of the plate may cause burns, e.g. if contact is only made over a small surface area.
  - burns may occur if the surgeon activates the diathermy accidentally, or if the forceps are touching the patient or lying on saline- or blood-soaked drapes. When not used, the forceps should be kept in a protective non-conducting holder. An audible buzzer warns that the device is operating.
  - if the plate electrode is earthed, and connections are faulty, current may take other routes to reach earth. Thus current may flow through any earthed metal conductor the patient touches, e.g. drip stands, ECG leads, etc., causing burns at the site of contact. In addition, the mains (50 Hz) current may flow through the system. A capacitor within the circuit will prevent the latter, whilst allowing the diathermy current to flow. Risks from flow of current to earth are reduced if the circuit is completely isolated from earth ('floating'), since current will no longer take these other routes.
  - may act as an ignition source of flammable substances, e.g. anaesthetic agents, bowel gases, alcohol skin preps.
  - may interfere with pacemaker function.

[William T Bovie (1882–1958), US biophysicist]

See also, Cardiac pacing; Electrocution and electrical burns; Explosions and fires

Diazepam. Benzodiazepine, widely used for sedation, anxiolysis and as an anticonvulsant drug. Has been used for premedication, and to supplement or induce anaesthesia. Insoluble in water; original preparations caused pain on injection and thrombophlebitis. These are rare with emulsions of diazepam in soya bean oil. Effects on the nervous system are via the limbic system and polysynaptic spinal pathways. Propagation of epileptiform waves is suppressed.

Injection iv may cause respiratory depression, especially in the elderly. Reduced cardiac output and vasodilatation may occur with large doses. Drowsiness and confusion, especially in the elderly, may persist for several hours after large iv doses. Absorption after im injection is unreliable and the injection is painful.

Half-life is 20–70 h, with formation of active metabolites including nordiazepam (half-life up to 120 h), desmethyldiazepam, oxazepam and temazepam. Thus repeated doses, e.g. in ICU, may lead to delayed recovery.

- Dosage:
  - 10–30 mg orally for premedication (0.5 mg/kg in children, up to 10 mg).
  - 5–10 mg iv for sedation or anticonvulsant effect, repeated as necessary. Rectal administration is also effective.

Diazoxide. Vasodilator drug, used for emergency treatment of severe hypertension. Acts directly on blood vessel walls by activating potassium channels. Previously indicated in hypertensive crisis, but the risk from sudden reduction in BP has resulted in its indication for iv use being restricted to severe hypertension associated with renal disease. Increases blood glucose level by increasing catecholamine levels and by reducing insulin release; may be used orally to treat chronic hypoglycaemia (previously used iv to treat acute hypoglycaemia).

- Dosage: 1–3 mg/kg (up to 150 mg) iv for hypertension, repeated after 5–15 min if required. MI and CVA have followed larger doses. Quickly bound to plasma proteins, therefore must be given rapidly. For hypoglycaemia, 5 mg/kg/day orally.

- Side effects: tachycardia, hyperglycaemia, fluid retention.

Dibucaine, *see Cinchocaine*

Dibucaine number. Degree of inhibition of plasma cholinesterase by dibucaine (cinchocaine). Sample plasma is added to a benzoylcholine solution, and breakdown of the latter is observed using measurement of light absorption. This is repeated using plasma pretreated with a 10^{-5} molar solution of dibucaine; the percentage inhibition of benzoylcholine breakdown by the enzyme is the dibucaine number. Abnormal variants of cholinesterase are inhibited to lesser degrees, with dibucaine numbers less than the normal 75–85%. Thus useful in the analysis and typing of different abnormal variants, which may give rise to prolonged paralysis following suxamethonium administration.

Similar testing may be performed using inhibition by fluoride, chloride, suxamethonium itself and other compounds.

DIC, *see Disseminated intravascular coagulation*

Dichloroacetate, *see Sodium dichloroacetate*

Dichlorphenamide. Carbonic anhydrase inhibitor, used to treat glaucoma but also to stimulate respiration, possibly by lowering CSF pH. Actions are similar to those of acetazolamide, but longer lasting. Has been used to assist weaning in ICU. 100–200 are given orally, followed by 100 mg 12 hourly.

Diclofenac sodium. NSAID, available for parenteral use. Has been used for postoperative analgesia, thus reducing requirements for opioids. Also used for renal colic and other painful conditions. May also be given enterally. Extensively (> 99%) protein-bound in plasma; half-life is 1–2 h. 60% excreted via urine, the rest passing into the faeces.

- Dosage:
  - 1 mg/kg im up to 75 mg, as a single dose or once/twice daily for up to 2 days. Should be given by deep intragluteal injection. Doses should alternate between left and right sides.
  - 75 mg iv, repeated after 4–6 h, for up to 2 days. For prevention of postoperative pain, 25–50 mg iv over 15–60 min, then 5 mg/h for up to 2 days. Should be diluted immediately before use with 100–500 ml 0.9% saline or 5% glucose, which should then be buffered with 0.5 ml 8.4% or 1 ml 4.2% sodium bicarbonate solution. A new preparation can be given (75 mg) without buffering or diluting.
  - 75–150 mg/day orally/rectally in divided doses (1–3 mg/kg in children). Available in a variety of suppositories, from 12.5 mg to 100 mg. A case involving a misplaced diclofenac suppository inserted vaginally and subsequent claims of rape have led to recommendations that all planned suppository insertions should be discussed beforehand with the patient.
- Side effects: as for NSAIDs. Should be used with caution in renal impairment and asthma. Muscle damage after im injection has been indicated by increased plasma creatine kinase levels. Sterile abscesses have occurred after superficial injection.

Dicobalt edetate, *see Cyanide poisoning*

Dicrotic notch, *see Arterial waveform*

Diethyl ether. $C_2H_5OC_2H_5$. Inhalational anaesthetic agent, first prepared in 1540. Paracelsus described its effects on chickens in the same year. Produced by heating concentrated sulphuric acid with ethanol. First used for anaesthesia in 1842 by Clarke and Long, who did not publish their work until later. Introduced publicly by Morton in the USA in 1846; used in London by Boott and in Dumfries in the same year. Classically given by open-drop techniques, and more recently using a draw-over technique (e.g. using the EMO vaporiser), or by standard plenum vaporiser. Inspired concentrations of up to 20% may be required during induction of anaesthesia.

No longer generally available in the UK, although widely considered one of the safest inhalational agents, largely because respiratory depression is late and precedes cardiovascular depression. Still used worldwide, because of its safety and low cost.

Its many disadvantages include flammability, high blood/gas partition coefficient resulting in slow uptake and recovery, respiratory irritation causing coughing and laryngospasm, stimulation of salivary secretions, high incidence of nausea and vomiting, and occurrence of convulsions postoperatively, typically associated with pyrexia and atropine administration. Sympathetic stimulation maintains BP with low incidence of arrhythmias, but hyperglycaemia may occur.

Has been used in severe asthma because of its bronchodilator properties.

10–15% metabolised to alcohol, acetaldehyde and acetic acid.

Differential lung ventilation (DLV). Performed when the requirements of each lung are so different that conventional IPPV cannot maintain adequate gas exchange, e.g. because the poor compliance of one lung diverts the delivered tidal volume to the other, more compliant, lung. Thus reserved for when lung pathology is unilateral or much worse on one side, e.g. following aspiration of gastric contents or irritant substances, unilateral pneumonia, bronchopleural fistula, etc. May be performed using two conventional ventilators, each connected to one lumen of a double-lumen endobronchial tube. The settings of each (including the ventilatory mode) are adjusted independently in order to achieve adequate lung expansion and gas exchange; synchronised inflation/deflation is usually not necessary although sideways motion of the mediastinum (if one lung inflates just as the other deflates) may cause haemodynamic disturbance in susceptible patients. In some circumstances, it may be possible to ventilate the better lung, whilst applying only CPAP to the diseased one.

Difficult intubation, *see Intubation, difficult*

Diffusing capacity (Transfer factor). Volume of a substance (usually carbon monoxide (CO)) transferred across the alveoli per minute per unit alveolar partial pressure. CO is used because it is rapidly taken up by haemoglobin in the blood; thus its transfer from alveoli to blood is limited mainly by diffusion across the alveolar membrane.

- Measurement:
  - a single breath of gas containing 0.3% CO and 10% helium is held for 10–20 s. Initial alveolar partial pressure of CO is derived by measuring the dilution of helium that has occurred. Expired partial pressure of CO is measured.

- continuous breathing of gas containing 0.3% CO, for up to a minute. Rate of uptake of CO is measured when steady state is reached.
- Normal value: 17–25 ml/min/mmHg.

Reduction in pulmonary diseases, e.g. pulmonary fibrosis, has been traditionally attributed to increased alveolar membrane thickness. However, $\dot{V}/\dot{Q}$ mismatch may be more important than alveolar thickening in these conditions. Also reduced when alveolar membrane area is reduced, e.g. after pneumonectomy (corrected by calculation of diffusing coefficient: diffusing capacity per litre of available lung volume).

The term 'transfer factor' is sometimes used because the measurement refers to overall measurement of gas transfer, which may be affected by ventilation, perfusion and diffusion defects distributed unevenly throughout the lung. Correlation with clinical examination is not always reliable for these reasons.

Jensen RL, Crapo RO (2003). Respir Care; 48: 777–82

Diffusion. Movement of a substance from an area of high concentration to one of low concentration, resulting from spontaneous random movement of its constituent particles. May occur across membranes, e.g. from alveoli to bloodstream.

- Rate of diffusion across a membrane is proportional to:
  - available area of membrane.
  - concentration gradient across the membrane (Fick's law).
  - $\frac{1}{\sqrt{\text{mw of the substance}}}$ (Graham's law).

For diffusion of a gas across a membrane into a liquid, e.g. across the alveolar membrane, concentration gradient is proportional to the pressure gradient, and is maintained if the gas is soluble in the liquid; i.e. rate of diffusion is proportional to solubility.

Diffusion hypoxia, *see Fink effect*

Digital nerve block. Each digit is supplied by two palmar and two dorsal digital nerves. A fine needle is introduced from the dorsal side of the base of the digit, and 2–3 ml local anaesthetic agent (without adrenaline) injected on each side, between bone and skin.

Digoxin. Most widely used cardiac glycoside, used to treat supraventricular arrhythmias, e.g. AF, atrial flutter and SVT. Described and investigated by Withering in 1785 in his *Account of the Foxglove*. Slows atrioventricular conduction and increases myocardial contractility. No longer recommended as a standard treatment of cardiac failure as it increases morbidity and mortality. Volume of distribution is large (700 litres) and half-life long (36 h); elimination is therefore lengthy after termination of treatment. Dosage must be reduced in renal impairment and in the elderly. Therapeutic plasma levels: 1–2 ng/ml (blood is taken 1 h after an iv dose, 8 h after an oral dose).

Contraindicated in Wolff–Parkinson–White syndrome, since atrioventricular block may encourage conduction through accessory pathways with resultant arrhythmia.

- Dosage:
  - loading dose for rapid digitalisation:
    - 1.0–1.5 mg orally in divided doses over 24 h (250–500 μg/day if less urgent).
    - 0.75–1.0 mg iv over at least 2 h. Fast injection may cause vasoconstriction and coronary ischaemia. IM injection is painful and unreliable.
  - maintenance: 62.5–500 μg daily (usual range 125–250 μg).
- Side effects and toxicity:
  - more common in hypokalaemia, hypercalcaemia or hypomagnesaemia.
  - nausea, vomiting, diarrhoea.
  - headache, malaise, confusion. Impaired colour vision (typically for yellow) is an early symptom.
  - any cardiac arrhythmia may occur; bradycardia, heart block, and ventricular ectopics including bi- and trigemini are commonest.
  - ECG findings:
    - prolonged P–R interval and heart block.
    - T wave inversion.
    - S–T segment depression (the 'reverse tick').
  - arrhythmias should be treated as appropriate, if severe. Potassium replacement may be required. Cardioversion may result in severe arrhythmias, and should be avoided. Phenytoin is particularly useful in ventricular arrhythmias. Digoxin-specific antibody fragments are available for use in severe toxicity.

[William Withering (1741–1799), English physician]

Dihydrocodeine tartrate. Opioid analgesic drug, of similar potency to codeine. Prepared in 1911. Causes fewer side effects than morphine or pethidine at equivalent analgesic doses. Also has a marked antitussive effect. Commonly used in combination with paracetamol as co-dydramol (500 mg/10 mg per tablet).

- Dosage: 30 mg orally or up to 50 mg sc/im, 4–6 hourly; 0.5–1 mg/kg in children.

Diltiazem hydrochloride. Class III calcium channel blocking drug and Class IV antiarrhythmic drug, used to treat angina and hypertension, especially when β_2-adrenergic receptor antagonists are contraindicated or ineffective. Causes vasodilatation and prolonged atrioventricular nodal conduction. Causes less myocardial depression than verapamil but may cause severe bradycardia. After single oral dosage, 90% absorbed but bioavailability is only 45% because of extensive first-pass metabolism. About 65% excreted via the GIT. An iv preparation is available in the USA for treatment of atrial fibrillation, atrial flutter and SVT.

- Dosage:
  - 60–120 mg 8 hourly, orally (90–180 mg 12 hourly, or 120–360 mg once daily, for sustained-release preparations).
  - 0.25 mg/kg iv over 2 min, followed by 0.35 mg/kg over 2 min then 5–15 mg/h if required.
- Side effects: bradycardia, hypotension, malaise, headache, GIT disturbances, rarely impaired liver function.

Dilution techniques. Used for measuring body compartment volumes. A known quantity of tracer substance is introduced into the space to be measured, and its concentration measured after complete mixing:

$$C_1 \times V_1 = C_2 \times (V_1 + V_2)$$

where C_1 = initial concentration of indicator
C_2 = final concentration of indicator
V_1 = volume of indicator
V_2 = volume to be measured.

The technique may be used to measure volume of blood, plasma, ECF, etc. Tracer substances include dyes and radioisotopes; the latter may be injected as radioactive ions or attached to proteins, red blood cells, etc. Gaseous markers may be used to study lung volumes, e.g. helium to measure FRC.

The principle may be extended for cardiac output measurement, where radioisotope, dye or ice-cold crystalloid solution is injected as a bolus proximal to the right ventricle, and its concentration measured distally, e.g. radial or pulmonary artery. A concentration–time curve is plotted to enable calculation of cardiac output. A double indicator dilution technique has been used to measure extravascular lung water.

Dimercaprol (BAL; British Anti-Lewisite). Chelating agent used in the treatment of heavy metal poisoning, especially antimony, arsenic, bismuth, mercury and gold. Following im injection, peak levels occur within 1 h with elimination in 4 h. Contraindicated in liver disease and glucose 6-phosphate dehydrogenase deficiency.
- Dosage: 2.5–3.0 mg/kg im 4 hourly for 2 days, 6–12 hourly on day 3 and 12–24 hourly thereafter.
- Side effects: haemolytic anaemia, transient hypertension and tachycardia, agitation, paraesthesia, headache, tremor, nausea and vomiting, erythema and pain on injection. Contains peanut oil as a solvent.

Dimethyl tubocurarine chloride/bromide. Non-depolarising neuromuscular blocking drug, derived from tubocurarine; introduced in 1948. More potent and longer-lasting (up to 2 h) than tubocurarine, and with less ganglion blockade and histamine release; i.e. more cardiostable. No longer used in the UK, although has been popular in the USA as metocurine. Excreted almost exclusively via the urine.
- Intubating dose: 0.2–0.4 mg/kg; acts within 3–5 min.

Dinoprost/dinoprostone, *see Prostaglandins*

2,3-Diphosphoglycerate (2,3-DPG). Substance formed within red blood cells from phosphoglyceraldehyde, produced during glycolysis. Binds strongly to the β chains of deoxygenated haemoglobin, reducing O_2 binding and shifting the oxyhaemoglobin dissociation curve to the right; i.e. favours O_2 liberation to the tissues. Binds poorly to the γ chains of fetal haemoglobin.
- Levels are increased by:
  - anaemia.
  - alkalosis.
  - chronic hypoxaemia, e.g. in cyanotic heart disease.
  - high altitude.
  - exercise.
  - pregnancy.
  - hyperthyroidism.
  - hyperphosphataemia.
  - certain red cell enzyme abnormalities.
- Levels are decreased by:
  - acidosis, e.g. in stored blood; requires 12–24 h for levels to be restored.
  - hypophosphataemia.
  - hypothyroidism.
  - hypopituitarism.

Diphtheria. Infection caused by *Corynebacterium diphtheriae*, a Gram-positive rod. Now rare in the Western world, due to immunisation, but formerly a major cause of death, particularly in children.
- Features:
  - symptoms of upper respiratory infection.
  - increasing malaise and fever. Diphtheria toxin may affect CNS, heart and other organs. Cranial nerve palsies, visual disturbances, and cardiac failure with conduction defects and arrhythmias may occur.
  - a thick exudative membrane may form across the posterior pharynx/larynx, causing complete obstruction.
- Treatment:
  - as for airway obstruction.
  - antitoxin administration.
  - iv benzylpenicillin.

Dipipanone hydrochloride. Opioid analgesic drug, similar to methadone and dextromoramide. Prepared in 1950. Available in the UK for oral use as tablets of 10 mg combined with cyclizine 30 mg.
- Dosage: up to 3 tablets 6 hourly. Anticholinergic effects of cyclizine may limit its use.

Dipyridamole. Antiplatelet drug, used to prevent arterial thrombus formation, e.g. on prosthetic heart valves. Modifies platelet aggregation, adhesion and survival. Also given iv for stress testing during diagnostic cardiac imaging; causes marked vasodilatation. May cause coronary steal.
- Dosage: 100–150 mg orally, 6–8 hourly (slow-release: 200 mg 12 hourly).
- Side effects: may be hazardous in severe coronary and aortic stenosis due to its vasodilating effects. Nausea, vomiting and headache may also occur.

Disaster, major, *see Incident, major*

Disequilibrium syndrome. Syndrome comprising nausea, vomiting, headache, restlessness, visual disturbances, tremor, coma and convulsions, associated with dialysis. More common in patients with pre-existing intracranial pathology or severe acidosis or uraemia. The cause is uncertain, although increased brain water is suggested by CT scanning. Rapid changes in osmolality or CSF pH have been suggested. Reduced by gradual institution of dialysis, especially if plasma urea is very high, and by careful management of sodium balance. Management is supportive.

Disinfection of breathing equipment, *see Contamination of breathing equipment*

Disodium pamidronate, *see Bisphosphonates*

Disopyramide phosphate. Class Ia antiarrhythmic drug, used to treat ventricular and supraventricular arrhythmias. Half-life is 7 h.
- Dosage:
  - 2 mg/kg up to 150 mg iv over at least 5 min, followed by 0.4 mg/kg/h infusion or 200 mg 8 hourly orally; maximum 300 mg in the first hour and 800 mg/day.
  - 300–800 mg/day orally in divided doses.
- Side effects: myocardial depression, hypotension, anticholinergic effects, e.g. urinary retention, atrioventricular block.

Disseminated intravascular coagulation (DIC). Pathological activation of coagulation by a disease process, leading to fibrin clot formation, consumption of platelets and coagulation factors (I, II and XIII), and secondary fibrinolysis. May be precipitated by shock, sepsis, haemolysis, malignancy, trauma, burns, major surgery, PE, extracorporeal circulation, and obstetric conditions, e.g. pre-eclampsia, amniotic fluid embolism, intrauterine death and placental abruption.
- Effects:
  - may occur chronically, with little clinical abnormality.
  - bruising, bleeding from wounds, venepuncture sites, GIT, lung, urinary tract and uteroplacental bed.

- capillary microthrombosis may cause multiple organ failure.
- shock, acidosis and hypoxaemia may occur.

Haematological investigation may reveal low titres of fibrinogen, coagulation factors and antithrombin III, thrombocytopenia, high titres of fibrin degradation products and prolonged prothrombin, partial thromboplastin and thrombin times.

- Treatment:
  - directed at underlying causes.
  - supportive.
  - administration of fresh frozen plasma, platelets and possibly cryoprecipitate.
  - the role of heparin is still unclear, but it should be considered if initial therapy does not improve the patient's condition. Heparin has been used mainly in the treatment of chronic DIC without major coagulopathy.
  - administration of activated protein C should be considered in sepsis related DIC.

Levi M (2007). Crit Care Med; 35: 2191–5

See also, Blood products; Coagulation disorders; Coagulation studies

Disseminated sclerosis, *see Demyelinating diseases*

Dissociation curves, *see Carbon dioxide dissociation curve; Oxyhaemoglobin dissociation curve*

Dissociative anaesthesia, *see Ketamine*

Distigmine bromide. Acetylcholinesterase inhibitor, used in urinary retention and intestinal atony, and very rarely, myasthenia gravis (duration of action is up to 24 h; thus risk of accumulation and cholinergic crisis is greater than with shorter acting drugs).

- Dosage: 5–20 mg daily, orally.
- Side effects: as for neostigmine.

Distribution curves, statistical, *see Statistical frequency distributions*

Disulfiram. Drug used as an adjunct to the treatment of alcoholism; inhibits the metabolism of alcohol by alcohol dehydrogenase with increased production of acetaldehyde, the latter causing unpleasant effects (flushing, headache, palpitations, nausea and vomiting) when alcohol is ingested. Arrhythmias and hypotension may follow large intakes of alcohol. Similar but lesser reactions may occur in patients taking metronidazole who ingest alcohol.

- Dosage: 800 mg initially, reducing over 5 days to 100–200 mg/day, orally.
- Side effects: drowsiness, nausea, vomiting, psychosis, peripheral neuritis, hepatic impairment. Causes enzyme inhibition, thus enhancing the actions of many drugs including tricyclic antidepressants, benzodiazepines, warfarin, theophylline and phenytoin.

Diuresis, forced, *see Forced diuresis*

Diuretics. Drugs increasing the rate of urine production by the kidney.

- Divided into:
  - thiazide diuretics: act at the proximal part of the distal convoluted tubule of the nephron, and also at the proximal tubule. Have low ceilings of action; i.e. maximal effects are produced by small doses. May cause hypokalaemia, hypomagnesaemia, hyperuricaemia, hyperglycaemia and hypercholesterolaemia.
  - osmotic diuretics, e.g. mannitol: increase renal blood flow by plasma expansion, then draw water into the renal tubules by an osmotic effect. Other small molecules which are filtered but not reabsorbed may have similar osmotic diuretic actions, e.g. glucose, urea and sucrose.
  - potassium sparing diuretics, e.g. triamterene, amiloride, spironolactone: act at the distal convoluted tubule, where most potassium is normally lost; spironolactone acts by aldosterone inhibition. May cause hyperkalaemia and hyponatraemia.
  - loop diuretics, e.g. furosemide, bumetanide, etacrynic acid: act at the ascending loop of Henle. More potent, with high ceilings of action. Immediate benefit in fluid overload/cardiac failure is thought to be due to vasodilatation. May cause hypokalaemia, hyperuricaemia, hypomagnesaemia and hyperglycaemia. Damage to 8th cranial nerve may occur following rapid iv injection and with concurrent aminoglycoside therapy.
  - other substances causing diuresis:
    - mercurials: no longer used. Reduce sodium and chloride reabsorption at several sites. Hypochloraemic acidosis is common.
    - carbonic anhydrase inhibitors, e.g. acetazolamide.
    - xanthines, e.g. aminophylline: reduce sodium excretion and increases GFR.
    - dopamine: increases renal blood flow and GFR; also reduces sodium absorption.
    - water and ethanol: inhibit vasopressin secretion.
    - acidifying salts, e.g. ammonium chloride: increase hydrogen ion and sodium excretion.
    - demeclocycline: blocks the action of vasopressin on the distal tubule and collecting duct; used in the syndrome of inappropriate ADH secretion.

Anaesthesia for patients taking diuretics: hypovolaemia and electrolyte disturbances are possible, especially in the elderly. Hypokalaemia may represent severe body potassium depletion; conversely potassium supplements and potassium sparing diuretics may cause hyperkalaemia. Severe hyponatraemia may follow treatment with potassium sparing diuretics. Combinations of different types of diuretic tend to be synergistic.

[Friedrich GJ Henle (1809–1885), German anatomist]

Diving reflex. Decreased respiration, vagal bradycardia and splanchnic and muscle bed vasoconstriction following immersion of the face in water. Cerebral and cardiac circulations are preserved. Occurs in mammals, birds and reptiles; it has been suggested that it may aid survival in man, e.g. in boating and skiing accidents.

Divinyl ether. Inhalational anaesthetic agent, introduced in 1933 and no longer used. Similar in potency and explosiveness to diethyl ether, but less irritant. Liver damage resulted from prolonged use. Combined 1:4 with ether as Vinesthene Anaesthetic Mixture.

DLV, *see Differential lung ventilation*

DNAR orders, *see Do not attempt resuscitation orders*

DNR orders, Do not resuscitate orders, *see Do not attempt resuscitation orders*

$\dot{D}O_2$, *see Oxygen delivery*

Do not attempt resuscitation orders (DNAR orders; Do not resuscitate orders; DNR orders). Instructions in a patient's records that CPR is not to be performed, should cardiorespiratory arrest occur. Generally reserved for patients in whom quality of life is currently so poor, or the chances of success so low, that active resuscitation is not indicated. Although previously often written without consultation with the patients or the patients' relatives, respect for patients' autonomy and views, and those of their relatives, has led to full and open discussion being preferred. Surveys have shown that patients are mostly appreciative of being included in these discussions. DNAR/DNR orders are often suspended perioperatively, since the fact that surgery is taking place implies that active treatment is worthwhile; also the results of resuscitation during anaesthesia are often better than those of CPR on the wards.

Any discussion and decision regarding DNAR/DNR orders should be clearly documented and, more importantly, all staff must be made aware of any changes in DNAR/DNR status. In the USA, the ASA has issued guidelines for anaesthetic management of patients with DNAR/DNR orders. Hospitals may offer specific forms to be signed by the patient or other legally responsible person. In the UK, matters are less formalised.

See also, Advance decisions; Ethics

Dobutamine hydrochloride. Synthetic catecholamine, used as an inotropic drug, e.g. after cardiac surgery, and in septic or cardiogenic shock. Stimulates β_1-adrenergic receptors, with weak stimulation of β_2 and α receptors. Does not affect dopamine receptors. Increases myocardial contractility, with less increase in myocardial O_2 consumption than other catecholamines. Causes less tachycardia than dopamine or isoprenaline, probably because of a reduced effect on the sinoatrial node, and less activation of the baroreceptor reflex. Reduces left ventricular end-diastolic pressure if raised.

Plasma half-life is about 2 min. Excreted via the urine. Supplied as a solution for dilution with saline or 5% dextrose prior to use.

- Usual dosage: 2.5–10 μg/kg/min by infusion; higher rates may be required.
- Side effects: tachycardia and ventricular arrhythmias at high doses.

Dog bites, *see Bites and stings*

Dolasetron mesilate. 5-HT_3 receptor antagonist, licensed as an antiemetic drug in postoperative and chemotherapy-induced nausea and vomiting. Similar to ondansetron.

- Dosage:
  - PONV: 50 mg orally or 12.5 mg over 30 s iv.
  - nausea/vomiting following chemotherapy: 200 mg orally or 100 mg infused iv 30–60 min before treatment, for up to 4 days.

Doll's eye movements (Oculocephalic reflex). Reflex elicited in unconscious patients by quickly turning the patient's head to one side and holding it there. The eyes move to the right when the head is turned to the left, and vice versa; i.e. they continue to point in the original position in relation to the body, as if fixed on a distant object. They then move to the midposition. The reflex involves bilateral vestibular apparatus and nerves, brainstem, and oculomotor nerves; it is therefore absent in brainstem death or dysfunction. Normally absent because of cerebral activity influencing eye movement; i.e. it becomes apparent if cerebral activity is suppressed or interrupted.

Domperidone maleate. Antiemetic and prokinetic drug related to metoclopramide, and with similar actions. Crosses the blood–brain barrier only slowly, thus less likely to cause sedation and dystonic reactions than other antiemetic drugs. No longer available for iv use, because of associated ventricular arrhythmias.

- Dosage:
  - 10–20 mg 4–8 hourly, orally.
  - 30–60 mg 4–8 hourly, rectally.

Donepezil, *see Acetylcholinesterase inhibitors*

Donnan effect (Gibbs–Donnan effect). Effect of charged particles on one side of a membrane on the distribution of other charged particles, when the former cannot diffuse through the membrane but the latter can. For example, intracellular proteins (negatively charged) are confined within the cell. The distribution of potassium ions (positively charged) and chloride ions (negatively charged) on either side of the membrane is therefore affected by the electrical gradient produced by the proteins, as well as their own concentration gradients. There is a fixed ratio between the concentration of diffusible ions on one side of the membrane and the concentration of those on the other. This ratio is the same for all the ions distributed about a particular membrane under the same conditions.

[Frederick Donnan (1870–1956), English chemist; Josiah Gibbs (1839–1903), US physicist]

Dopamine. Naturally occurring catecholamine and neurotransmitter, found in postganglionic sympathetic nerve endings and the adrenal medulla. A precursor of adrenaline and noradrenaline. Used as an inotropic drug, e.g. in cardiogenic or septic shock. Also used to maintain urine output when renal function is compromised. However, its ability to confer 'renal protection' has been questioned, with any effect on renal function being attributed to increased cardiac output. Uncertainty about its benefits and reports of bowel hypoperfusion have led to diminishing use of low dose ('renal') dopamine in ICU.

Supplied as the hydrochloride in a concentrated solution for dilution in saline or 5% dextrose, or as a ready-made iv solution in dextrose. Inactivated by alkali.

- Effects depend on the dose used:
  - up to 5 μg/kg/min: traditionally believed to stimulate dopamine receptors, causing renal and mesenteric vasodilatation and increasing renal blood flow, GFR, urine output and sodium excretion. However, it is now thought that these so-called 'renal effects' of dopamine are actually a non-specific response to increased cardiac output.
  - 5–15 μg/kg/min: stimulates β_1-adrenergic receptors; myocardial contractility, cardiac output, BP and O_2 consumption are increased. Pulmonary capillary wedge pressure may paradoxically increase, possibly because of increased venous return secondary to venoconstriction. Some α_2-stimulation also occurs.
  - over 15 μg/kg/min: stimulates α_1-receptors, causing peripheral vasoconstriction.

Rapidly taken up by tissues and metabolised by dopamine β-hydroxylase and monoamine oxidase pathways, with renal excretion of metabolites. Plasma half-life is about 1 min. Dosage must be reduced if the patient is taking monoamine oxidase inhibitors.

- Side effects: tachycardia and ventricular arrhythmias are common at higher doses. Severe tissue necrosis may follow peripheral extravasation; it should thus be administered into a large vein (preferably central). May cause gastric stasis and suppress release of oxytocin and other pituitary hormones. Has also been implicated in reducing T cell responsiveness and reducing GIT oxygenation via shunting of blood at mucosal level.

Dopamine receptors. Found peripherally and in the CNS. Subdivided into:
- central:
  - D_1 receptors: G protein-coupled receptor associated excitatory receptors with uncertain function. Stimulation results in increased intracellular cAMP. D_5 dopamine receptors are related.
  - D_2 receptors: G protein-coupled receptor associated inhibitory receptors found in pathways involving the basal ganglia and hypothalamus, concerned with coordination of movement, behaviour and inhibition of prolactin release. Also present in the chemoreceptor trigger zone where stimulation results in vomiting, and in the spinal cord. Butyrophenones are the classical antagonists; others include phenothiazines and metoclopramide. Bromocriptine is an agonist.
  - D_3 receptors: present in the brain especially limbic system. Function is uncertain.
- peripheral:
  - DA_1 receptors: postsynaptic; thought to be analogous to central D_1 receptors. Stimulation causes vasodilatation in renal and mesenteric vascular beds.
  - DA_2 receptors: presynaptic; stimulation inhibits noradrenaline release via negative feedback. Inhibition of cAMP formation may be involved. May also be present at cholinergic nerve endings. Inhibited by butyrophenones, i.e. thought to be analogous to central D_2 receptors.

Further subclasses of dopamine receptors may also exist.
Girault J, Greengard P (2004). Arch Neurol; 61: 641–4

Dopexamine hydrochloride. Analogue of dopamine, used as an inotropic drug in cardiac failure, e.g. after cardiac surgery. Stimulates peripheral dopamine receptors and β_2-adrenergic receptors, with indirect stimulation of β_1-adrenergic receptors via inhibition of neuronal reuptake of catecholamines. Causes peripheral (including renal) vasodilatation with reduced BP and increased cardiac output. 40% bound to red blood cells.
- Dosage: 0.5–6.0 μg/kg/min.
- Side effects include tachycardia (usually mild) and arrhythmias, nausea, vomiting and tremor.

Doppler effect. Increase in observed frequency of a signal when the signal source approaches the observer, and decrease when the source moves away. For example, the wavefronts in front of a moving car horn will be closer together than when the horn is stationary, because when each wavefront is emitted, the horn moves forward before emitting another. Similarly, the wavefronts behind the horn are further apart. To the observer, the tone of the horn changes from higher-pitched to lower-pitched as the horn approaches and passes, although the actual frequency emitted has not changed.

The principle is used clinically to determine velocities and flow rates of moving substances, e.g. in cardiac output measurement. An ultrasound beam may be directed along the path of flow; the sound waves reflect from the surfaces of the blood cells as they approach or move away. Analysis of the reflected frequencies allows determination of velocity of flow. Doppler probes contain both emitter and detector in the probe tip.

May also be used to detect arterial wall movement in arterial BP measurement; onset of movement occurs at systolic pressure, and cessation at diastolic pressure, as the cuff is deflated from high pressure. The ultrasonic beam is directed across the artery.
[Christian Doppler (1803–1853), Austrian physicist]
See also, Transcranial Doppler ultrasound

Dorsal column stimulation. Technique used in intractable pain management. Has been performed percutaneously using a wire electrode connected to an external power source, but an implantable system is usually employed. Electrodes may be placed at open laminectomy, or inserted into the epidural space through a needle. The electrodes are placed above the highest level of the pain, and connected to a subcutaneous inductance coil, usually on the abdominal wall, by insulated wires. The patient applies an external power source over the coil for pain relief. Implantable power sources may be used. The term 'spinal cord stimulation' has been suggested as being more appropriate since the exact site of stimulation in a particular case is not clear.
Oakley JC, Prager JP (2002). Spine; 27: 2574–83

Dorsal root entry zone procedure (DREZ procedure). Production of destructive lesions in the DREZ; has been used for severe chronic pain states including postherpetic neuralgia, deafferentation pain (anaesthesia dolorosa, pain associated with CVA and neurological injury), facial trauma, atypical facial pain, and migraine/cluster headache; it has also been used in severe cancer pain. Thought to interrupt the site of integration of pain pathways via the lateral spinothalamic and spinoreticulothalamic tracts. A small electrode is inserted into the spinal cord at each level of the pain and radiofrequency lesions induced in order to destroy the abnormally active dorsal horn neurones.

Dorsalis pedis artery. Continuation of the anterior tibial artery, itself a branch of the popliteal artery. Passes along the dorsum of the foot to the space between the 1st and 2nd metatarsal bones, where it enters the sole of the foot to anastomose with the lateral plantar artery. May be used as a site for arterial cannulation, lateral to extensor hallucis longus tendon with the foot flexed. Cannulation may be difficult in peripheral vascular disease.

Dose–response curves. Curves describing the relationship between dose of a drug or other physiological agent and the resultant response. A logarithmic scale is usually used for the abscissa. The classic curve is sigmoid-shaped, with increasing response as dose is increased until a plateau is reached (Fig. 53).
- Different curves are characterised by their:
  - position on the abscissa (related to potency).
  - maximal height (efficacy).
  - slope (influenced by the number of receptors that must be activated before a drug has an effect).

Drugs A and B are both agonists, but A is more potent. Drug C is less efficacious and is therefore a partial agonist. Addition of a competitive antagonist, D, to A shifts the curve to the right (i.e. reduced potency) but without altering its height (i.e. same efficacy). A non-competitive antagonist, E, shifts the curve to the right, reduces its height and alters its slope.

The curves are affected by individual variability in response, related to differences in pharmacokinetics and

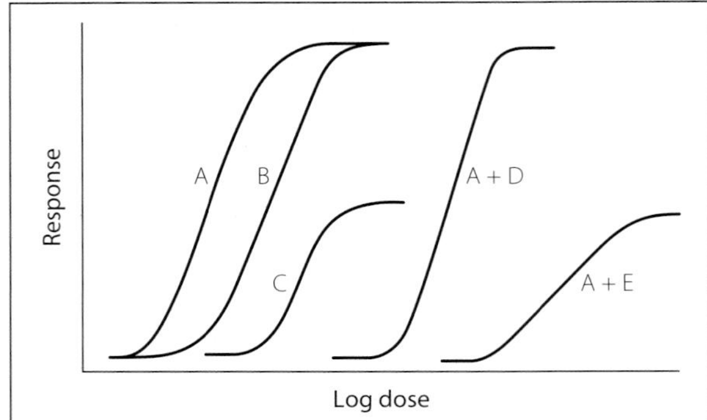

Fig. 53 Dose–response curves (see text)

pharmacodynamics. The dose of drug required to produce a certain response in a given percentage of the population (n%) is described as the effective dose, ED_n.
See also, Receptor theory

Dosulepin hydrochloride (Dothiepin). Tricyclic antidepressant drug, similar to amitriptyline. Used in endogenous depression and in chronic pain management.

- Dosage: 50–75 mg at night, orally, increased up to 225 mg/day. 25–50 mg is used in pain management.
- Side effects: as for amitriptyline.

Double-blind studies, *see Clinical trials*

Double-lumen tubes, *see Endobronchial tubes*

Down's syndrome. Syndrome resulting from presence of an extra chromosome 21 (hence the term trisomy 21). Usually due to non-dysjunction of chromosomes during germ cell formation, and rarely due to translocation in parental cells. Incidence is ~1:700 overall, increasing with maternal age. 45% of patients live to 60 years.

- Features:
  - round head and face, slanting eyes with prominent and wide epicanthic folds. Ears are low set; the mouth is small with a large tongue.
  - broad short hands, with a single transverse palmar crease; the gap between first and second toes is large.
  - congenital heart disease is common, especially ASD and VSD, Fallot's tetralogy and patent ductus arteriosus.
  - duodenal atresia and other congenital abnormalities are common as is gastro-oesophageal reflux.
  - acute myeloid leukaemia is common.
  - hypotonicity.
  - learning difficulties (IQ 20–60). Dementia is common as is postoperative agitation.
  - hypothyroidism and insulin dependent diabetes mellitus are common.
- Anaesthetic problems:
  - cardiac abnormalities.
  - airway difficulties, including difficult tracheal intubation due to macroglossia and subglottic stensosis; obstructive sleep apnoea occurs in 50–75%. Excessive secretions are common.
  - hypotonia.
  - atlantoaxial subluxation and instability.

[John Down (1828–1896), English physician]

Doxacurium chloride. Non-depolarising neuromuscular blocking drug, introduced into the USA in 1991. Has similar features to pancuronium, but without cardiovascular effects. Dosage range: 25–80 μg/kg; intubation may be performed 4–6 min after the initial dose. Effects last 1–3 h, depending on dosage. Excreted unchanged via the kidneys and liver. Causes histamine release only at much higher doses than required clinically. Has been suggested for prolonged surgery where cardiovascular stability is required, e.g. neurosurgery or cardiac surgery.

Doxapram hydrochloride. Analeptic drug, used for its respiratory stimulant properties. Acts on peripheral chemoreceptors, increasing tidal volume more than respiratory rate. May be administered by infusion in ventilatory failure in patients with COPD, in an attempt to avoid the need for IPPV. Also used in postoperative respiratory depression, without reversing opioid-induced analgesia. Has been used routinely to reduce postoperative pulmonary complications, especially in at-risk patients. Half-life is 2–4 h.

- Dosage:
  - 1–1.5 mg/kg iv over 30 s; repeated hourly.
  - 1.5–4 mg/min by infusion, according to response. Steady-state plasma levels are produced by:
    - 4 mg/min for 15 min,
    - 3 mg/min for 15 min,
    - 2 mg/min for 30 min,
    - 1.5 mg/min thereafter.
- Side effects: hypertension, tachycardia (resulting from vasomotor stimulation), restlessness, confusion, dizziness, sweating, nausea, salivation. Convulsions may occur with high doses.

Contraindicated in coronary artery disease, severe hypertension, thyrotoxicosis, asthma and epilepsy. Effects are said to be potentiated by monoamine oxidase inhibitors.

2,3-DPG, *see 2,3-Diphosphoglycerate*

DPL, Diagnostic peritoneal lavage, *see Peritoneal lavage*

Draw-over techniques. Anaesthesia in which the patient's inspiratory effort draws room air (with or without added O_2) over a volatile agent with each breath. More sophisticated, but similar to, open-drop techniques. There should be minimal resistance in the breathing system and vaporiser. Incorporation of bellows or a self-inflating bag into the breathing system allows IPPV, and provides a reservoir if continuous flow of O_2 is added. Non-rebreathing valves prevent exhalation back into the vaporiser; a unidirectional valve is necessary upstream of the bellows or bag, if used, to allow IPPV (Fig. 54).

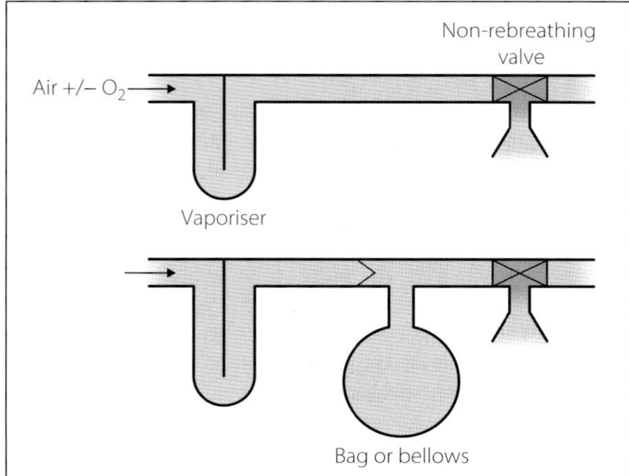

Fig. 54 Draw-over systems

- Uses:
  - shortage of compressed gas supplies, e.g. battlefields, accident sites, developing countries.
  - inhalational analgesia in obstetrics (no longer used).

Dreaming, *see Awareness*

Dressler's syndrome, *see Myocardial infarction*

DREZ, *see Dorsal root entry zone procedure*

Droperidol. Butyrophenone, discontinued in the UK in 2001 because of cases of prolonged Q–T interval. Previously used as an antipsychotic drug in psychiatry, as an antiemetic drug, for premedication and for neuroleptanaesthesia, in doses of 5–20 mg. A powerful dopamine antagonist, related to haloperidol but of shorter duration of action (6–12 h; cf. haloperidol 24–48 h). Typically caused apparent outward sedation but internal distress.

Drotrecogin alfa (alpha). Recombinant form of activated protein C, a plasma protein that inhibits prothrombinase and factor X-ase complexes via blocking the activated forms of coagulation factors V and VIII. Has been recommended by NICE in the treatment of severe sepsis that has resulted in failure of more than two major organs, in patients already receiving optimal ICU support. Costs ~£5000 per patient.
- Dosage: 24 μg/kg/h given as a continuous iv infusion for 96 h.
- Contraindicated in patients at risk of haemorrhage, its main side effect.

Drowning, *see Near-drowning*

Drug absorption, distribution, metabolism and excretion, *see Pharmacokinetics*

Drug addiction, *see Substance abuse*

Drug development. New drugs or indications for old drugs may arise from:
  - incidental observation, e.g. antiplatelet action of aspirin.
  - modification of the structure of known natural substances, e.g. H_2 receptor antagonists.
  - modification of existing drugs, e.g. opioid analgesics.
  - screening of natural compounds.
  - computer-assisted modelling of new molecules.
- Stages of development:
  - identification of the substance.
  - *in vitro* studies.
  - animal studies:
    - effects, interactions, pharmacokinetics, etc.
    - toxicology: acute/chronic (usually up to 2 years) effects, therapeutic index; use of different animals, routes, doses, etc. Includes histological/biochemical effects on organs, bacterial mutagenicity, teratogenicity, carcinogenicity, and effects on fertility.

      Doubts have been expressed over the humanity of animal experiments and problems caused by possible species differences (e.g. thalidomide was free of teratogenicity in mice and rats but had devastating effects in humans). In the UK, a Home Office licence is required in order to conduct animal studies.
  - chemical details, e.g. formulation, manufacture, quality, storage, etc.
  - human studies:
    - phase I (clinical pharmacology): 20–50 subjects, usually healthy volunteers. Pharmacokinetic and pharmacodynamic effects, safety, etc.
    - phase II (clinical investigation): 50–300 patients. Further information as above, plus effective dose ranges and regimens.
    - phase III (formal clinical trials): 250–1000+ patients. Comparison with other treatments. Frequent side effects are noted.
    - phase IV (postmarketing surveillance): 2000–10 000+ patients. Rare side effects are noted, e.g. oculomucocutaneous syndrome following oral practolol therapy. Techniques used:
      - cohort studies: large numbers are observed over long periods, noting side effects when they occur. May detect rare effects (less than 1:500), but costly and difficult to organise. May examine specific groups, e.g. the elderly, previously excluded.
      - case control studies: records of patients with a suspected side effect are analysed for previous drug exposure. Easier and cheaper than cohort studies, but less precise and more susceptible to bias. May detect side effects with frequency up to 1:500. Prove association, not causation; give relative risk.
      - voluntary reporting (yellow card system in UK). Specific anaesthetic cards are available.
      - general statistics, e.g. recording sudden changes in disease incidence, etc.

Statutory regulatory bodies are concerned with drug development from the animal study stage onwards: the Committee on Safety of Medicines in the UK, the Food and Drug Administration in the USA (the European Medicines Evaluation Agency coordinates such activities in Europe). A product licence is granted after phase III trials, and reviewed every 5 years in the UK. Financial costs of new drug development are considerable and often prohibitive.

Drug interactions. Common cause of morbidity and mortality, especially in hospital, although some interactions are beneficial.
- May be:
  - pharmacokinetic:
    - outside the body, e.g. precipitation of thiopental/atracurium mixture.
    - at site of absorption, e.g. effect of opioids and metoclopramide on gastric emptying, use of vasoconstrictors to delay local anaesthetic drug absorption, second gas effect.
    - affecting distribution, e.g. displacement of warfarin from protein-binding sites by salicylates.
    - affecting metabolism, e.g. peripheral conversion of levodopa to dopamine inhibition by concurrently administered carbidopa, enzyme induction/inhibition, e.g. by cimetidine (inhibition) or barbiturates (induction).
    - affecting elimination, e.g. decreased penicillin excretion caused by probenecid.
  - pharmacodynamic:
    - additive:
      - summation: net effect equals the sum of individual drug effects.
      - synergism: net effect exceeds the sum of individual effects.
      - potentiation: one drug increases the effect of another. Examples: decreased requirement for anaesthetic agents when opioids and other sedatives are used,

and the increase in non-depolarising neuromuscular blockade caused by aminoglycosides and phenytoin.
- antagonism: may be competitive, physiological, etc.
- indirect effects, e.g. hypokalaemia induced by diuretics increases digoxin toxicity; pethidine interaction with monoamine oxidase inhibitors; sensitisation of the myocardium to catecholamines by halothane.

See also, Dose–response curves

Drug labels, *see Syringe labels*

Dual block (Phase II block). Phenomenon seen when large amounts of suxamethonium or related drugs are administered, in which features of non-depolarising neuromuscular blockade gradually replace those of depolarising neuromuscular blockade. More commonly seen with concurrent administration of acetylcholinesterase inhibitors and in myasthenia gravis.

Typically, tachyphylaxis to suxamethonium develops after administration of 400–500 mg by infusion or repeated doses, although individual variation is wide. This is followed by non-depolarising neuromuscular blockade which may be reversed by neostigmine, although reversal is inconsistent. In doubtful cases, edrophonium 10 mg has been suggested as a test; the block worsens if depolarising, reverses if non-depolarising. Use of nerve stimulators has largely superseded this test.

Has also been termed desensitisation block, and sometimes subdivided into different phases. The mechanism is unclear; depolarisation is thought not to persist despite continued presence of the drug. Pre- or postjunctional receptor modulation may be involved.

See also, Neuromuscular blockade monitoring

Ductus arteriosus, patent (Arterial duct). Accounts for 10–15% of congenital heart disease. The duct normally closes within a few days of birth; bradykinin, prostaglandins and a rise in Po_2 are thought to be involved, although the precise mechanism is unclear. If it remains open, significant left-to-right shunt may occur.

- Features:
  - neonates/infants: cardiac failure, respiratory failure.
  - older patients:
    - may be symptomless; cardiac failure or bacterial endocarditis may occur.
    - signs: continuous murmur heard at the left sternal edge, louder on expiration; may be systolic only, if the shunt is large. A pulmonary regurgitant murmur may be present.
    - pulmonary plethora and cardiomegaly on chest X-ray.
  - pulmonary hypertension may develop when older.
- Treatment:
  - medical (neonates): indometacin 200 μg/kg iv, then two doses of 100 μg/kg (up to 8 h old), 200 μg/kg (2–7 days old) or 250 μg/kg (over 7 days old) at 12–24 h intervals.
  - surgical: ligation/division of duct; left thoracotomy is usually performed. Haemorrhage, recurrent laryngeal nerve or thoracic duct damage may occur. Postoperative IPPV may be required, especially in babies.
- Anaesthesia: as for congenital heart disease.

Prostaglandin E_1 may be used to prevent ductal closure in babies with congenital heart disease awaiting surgery, e.g. permitting right-to-left shunting to allow perfusion of the legs in severe aortic coarctation, or left-to-right shunting to allow pulmonary perfusion in severe Fallot's tetralogy.

See also, Fetal circulation

Dumfries, Scotland. Site of the first use of diethyl ether for surgery in the UK by Scott, on December 19th 1846, although Liston's use 2 days later is more famous. News of Morton's demonstration in Boston had travelled to Dumfries with Fraser, ship's surgeon aboard the Royal Mail steamship Acadia, which had reached Liverpool from America 3 days previously.

[William Scott (1820–1887) and William Fraser (1819–1863), Scottish surgeons]

Martin LV (2004). Anaesthesia; 59: 180–7

Dumping valve. Device preventing application of excessive negative pressure to patients' airways, used in scavenging systems and some breathing attachments. Usually opens at −0.5 cmH_2O, allowing air to be drawn in.

Dural tap. Accidental puncture of the dura whilst performing epidural anaesthesia; the term usually refers to puncture by the epidural needle, although the epidural catheter may rarely enter the subarachnoid space, especially if there has been a partial dural tear during insertion. Important because it may interfere with the planned anaesthetic technique and because of the risk of post-dural puncture headache. Said to occur in 1% of cases in UK hospitals, although most authorities believe this is too high, with an incidence of 0.5% or less being attainable with good training.

- Predisposing factors:
  - unfamiliar equipment, e.g. sharper or blunter needles than one is used to.
  - faulty equipment, e.g. blocked needles, sticking syringes.
  - inexperienced operator.
  - use of air instead of saline for loss of resistance has been implicated but there is no good evidence that this is true.
- Diagnosis is usually obvious since a stream of CSF flows from the needle hub, although flow may be slow and lead to confusion if saline has been used. Testing the fluid for pH (CSF > 7), temperature (CSF is warm), glucose and protein content (CSF contains both) will reliably distinguish saline from CSF.
- Management options:
  - remove needle/catheter and abandon the procedure.
  - convert the block into single-shot or continuous spinal anaesthesia (the presence of a subarachnoid catheter has been suggested as causing inflammation of the dural edges, leading to more rapid healing and closure of the hole with a reduced incidence of severe headache, although strong evidence for this is lacking).
  - resite the catheter in an adjacent interspace:
    - cautious administration of test dose and subsequent doses (fractionated injection may be safer, as partial subarachnoid injection may occur).
    - 1 litre saline may be given over 12–24 h through the catheter to reduce the incidence of post-dural puncture headache. 50–60 ml boluses of saline over 10–20 min have also been used. Avoid dehydration. Use of laxatives has been suggested as a means of reducing straining; abdominal binders have also been suggested as reducing the incidence of headache but neither method is commonly used.
    - in obstetrics, instrumental delivery has been suggested to avoid straining during the second stage of labour, but this is controversial.
    - prophylactic blood patch via the epidural catheter at the end of the case/labour is controversial since it may be less successful than one performed later; it also exposes patients to a treatment that not all will require.

- inform the patient and nursing/midwifery staff.
- management of headache if it occurs (*see Post-dural puncture headache*).

Post-dural puncture headache may rarely occur without suspected dural puncture.

Durrans's sign. Increased rate and depth of breathing following rapid injection of solution into the epidural space. More common in unconscious patients.
[Sidney F Durrans, Dorset anaesthetist]
See also, Epidural anaesthesia

DVT, *see Deep vein thrombosis*

Dye dilution cardiac output measurement, *see Cardiac output measurement*

Dyne. Unit of force in the cgs system of units. 1 dyne is the force required to accelerate a mass of 1 gram by 1 centimetre per second per second. 1 newton = 100 000 dyne.

Dynorphins. Endogenous opioid peptides; dynorphin 1–8 (8 amino acids) is found in the CNS, especially hypothalamus and posterior pituitary; dynorphin 1–17 (17 amino acids) is found in the duodenum. Thought to be involved as neurotransmitters, possibly in pain pathways; more active at κ than at μ opioid receptors.

Dysaesthesia. Abnormal unpleasant sensation, whether spontaneous or evoked; e.g. hyperalgesia, allodynia.

Dysequilibrium syndrome, *see Disequilibrium syndrome*

Dyspnoea. Feeling of breathlessness. Mechanism is unclear, but thought to be associated with the medullary interaction between abnormal respiratory drive and the motor output to respiratory muscles. Activity of chest wall and pulmonary vagal receptors, and chemoreceptors, is also involved.

- May occur in:
  - increased respiratory drive, e.g. due to hypoxaemia, hypercapnia, acidosis, pulmonary receptor activity.
  - increased work of breathing.
  - impaired neuromuscular function of respiratory muscles.

Dyspnoea related to exercise tolerance is useful as a means of assessing respiratory/cardiovascular function, e.g. during preoperative assessment. Certain patterns are characteristically associated with certain disease processes, e.g. orthopnoea (left ventricular failure, also severe restrictive lung disease) or paroxysmal nocturnal dyspnoea (left ventricular failure).
Consensus statement (1999). Am J Respir Crit Care Med; 159: 321–40
See also, Breathing, control of

Dyspnoeic index. Difference between maximal voluntary ventilation and maximum minute ventilation reached during exercise, as a percentage of maximal voluntary ventilation. Has been used to try to relate the subjective feeling of breathlessness to an objective measure of cardiorespiratory function.

Dysrhythmias, *see Arrhythmias*

Dystonic reaction. Acute side effect of dopamine antagonist drugs, e.g. many antiemetic drugs. May follow oral therapy, but particularly common after parenteral administration. More common after phenothiazine administration, e.g. prochlorperazine and perphenazine, than after metoclopramide, but the latter is especially likely to cause it in children and young women.

Consists of involuntary muscle contraction, especially involving the face. Oculogyric crisis (involuntary conjugate deviation of the eyes, usually upwards) may also occur.

- Treatment: diazepam 5–10 mg iv; benzatropine 1–2 mg iv/im; procyclidine 5–10 mg iv/im.

Dystrophia myotonica. Most common of the myotonic syndromes with prevalence of 1 in 20. Multisystem disease, inherited as an autosomal dominant trait with patients presenting at 15–35 years old.

- Features:
  - myotonia (increase in muscle tone following contraction). Exacerbated by cold.
  - cardiomyopathy and conduction defects.
  - respiratory muscle weakness and poor central control of respiration; may lead to respiratory failure.
  - central and obstructive sleep apnoea.
  - cognitive defects.
  - cataracts, frontal balding, sternomastoid and temporal muscle wasting, ptosis.
  - weakness of forearm and calf muscles.
  - testicular atrophy.
  - thyroid and adrenal impairment.
  - poor bulbar function and delayed gastric emptying.
- Anaesthetic problems:
  - related to poor cardiorespiratory reserve.
  - increased risk of aspiration of gastric contents.
  - undue sensitivity to iv anaesthetic agents, opioids and non-depolarising neuromuscular blocking drugs.
  - suxamethonium and acetylcholinesterase inhibitors may cause prolonged muscle contraction which may hinder laryngoscopy and ventilation.

Russell SH, Hirsch NP (1994). Br J Anaesth; 72: 210–16
See also, Myotonia congenita

E

Ear, nose and throat surgery (ENT surgery). Anaesthetic considerations:

- preoperatively:
  - most patients are young; many are children. Older patients with known or suspected tumours are more likely to have airway problems, and to be smokers/alcohol drinkers.
  - airway obstruction may be present. Potential difficulty with intubation should be considered. Teeth, caps, etc. are particularly at risk if rigid endoscopy is planned. Tracheostomy or cricothyrotomy may be performed under local anaesthesia preoperatively.
  - specific problems include bleeding tonsil, inhaled foreign body, epiglottitis and peritonsillar abscess.
  - premedication is according to preference; specifically it may act as an adjunct to the subsequent anaesthetic technique, e.g. hypotensive anaesthesia. Reduction of secretions is helpful for procedures involving the mouth, nose and throat.
- perioperatively:
  - induction as for paediatric anaesthesia, difficult airway, etc. Smooth induction is particularly desirable, to reduce bleeding.
  - shared airway: a tracheal tube is traditionally used for most procedures, with a throat pack if bleeding or debris is anticipated. Preformed tubes are useful. Special connectors are available. Oral intubation is suitable for most procedures including laryngectomy and tonsillectomy. A small diameter (5 mm) tube, passed orally or nasally, is usually suitable for microlaryngoscopy. Nasal intubation is usually performed for major surgery involving the face and mouth. The nasal cavity may be prepared with local anaesthetic solutions. Cocaine paste or spray or Moffett's solution is traditionally used to reduce nasal bleeding (*see Nose*). Laryngoscopy or bronchoscopy may be performed using injector techniques. Lidocaine spray to the vocal cords is usually omitted if postoperative aspiration of blood is possible.
  - increasingly, the laryngeal mask airway is being used as an alternative to tracheal intubation, even in cases traditionally managed with the latter, e.g. tonsillectomy. Minor ear operations, e.g. myringotomy/grommets, may be performed under mask anaesthesia.
  - access to the airway is restricted, therefore monitoring is particularly important. Coaxial anaesthetic breathing systems are convenient and light. Obstruction of the tracheal tube is possible, especially during tonsillectomy if a mouth gag is used.
  - advantages and disadvantages of spontaneous ventilation versus IPPV are controversial. Neuromuscular blockade is often avoided in parotid surgery, to allow direct stimulation and identification of facial nerve branches during dissection. Spontaneous ventilation, or IPPV using opioids, a volatile agent and induced hypocapnia, may be employed in this case.
  - N_2O is often avoided in middle ear surgery, because of expansion of gas-filled cavities; O_2/nitrogen or O_2/air mixtures are used instead.
  - surgery around the neck may risk damage to the laryngeal nerves (*see Hyperthryoidism*). Surgery around the face may risk damage to branches of the facial nerve. Absence of neuromuscular blockade may be requested by the surgeon in order to allow identification of nerves by electrical stimulation.
  - hypotensive anaesthesia is sometimes used, especially for major reconstructive surgery, laryngectomy, mastoidectomy and middle ear surgery.
  - thoracotomy is occasionally required, e.g. mobilisation of the stomach for anastomosis.
  - laser surgery is common, especially for laryngeal surgery.
  - blood loss should be monitored carefully especially in children, e.g. during tonsillectomy.
  - adrenaline solutions are often used by the surgeon.
  - if used, the throat pack must be removed before the patient wakes. The pharynx may be inspected to ensure absence of bleeding and blood clot, especially behind the soft palate ('coroner's clot').
  - tracheal extubation is performed with the patient deeply anaesthetised or awake (but not in between, because of the risk of laryngospasm) and in the head-down, lateral position to reduce airway soiling.
- postoperatively: as for any surgery. Major procedures may require ICU/IPPV postoperatively.

See also, Intubation, difficult; Mandibular nerve blocks; Maxillary nerve blocks

Early warning scores. Simple scoring systems used to aid identification of critically ill patients or those at risk of further clinical deterioration. Several different systems have been described, employing different groups of physiological parameters, e.g. systolic BP, heart rate, respiratory rate, temperature, neurological status and urine output, which are weighted on the basis of their deviation from a 'normal' range. Early warning schemes may be used to 'trigger' calls for assistance from the patient's primary team, a medical emergency team, an outreach team or others. In the UK, the modified early warning score is most commonly used.

Cuthbertson BH, Smith GB (2007). Br J Anaesth; 98: 704–6

See also, Acute life-threatening events – recognition and treatment

Earth-leakage circuit-breaker, *see Current-operated earth-leakage circuit-breaker*

East–Freeman automatic vent, *see Ventilators*

Eaton–Lambert syndrome, *see Myasthenic syndrome*

Ebstein's anomaly. Congenital heart defect characterised by:
- abnormal origin of tricuspid valve cusps, which arise from the right ventricle below the atrioventricular ring.
- abnormally thin right ventricle.
- ASD is usually present.

May lead to arrhythmias, conduction defects, right ventricular failure and cyanosis. Surgery may be indicated in severe cases.
[Wilhelm Ebstein (1836–1912), German physician]
See also, Congenital heart disease; Tricuspid valve lesions

$ECCO_2R$, *see Extracorporeal carbon dioxide removal*

ECF, *see Extracellular fluid*

ECG, *see Electrocardiography*

Echocardiography. Cardiac imaging using reflection of ultrasound pulses from interfaces between tissue planes. A single beam may be studied as it passes through the heart, displaying movement of tissue planes over time, usually recorded on moving paper (M mode). Alternatively, beams are directed in different directions from the same point, covering a sector of tissue; a moving cross-section may then be displayed on a screen. Analysis of the frequencies of reflected pulses may provide information about the velocity of moving structures and blood flow (Doppler effect); flow characteristics may be colour-coded and superimposed on sector images. The passage of injected saline may be studied as it travels through the heart, probably due to entrainment of small air bubbles.

Useful in diagnosing and quantifying valvular heart disease, congenital heart disease, myocardial and pericardial disease, and in assessing myocardial function. Techniques for the latter involve measurement of left ventricular dimensions and provide information about the:
- fractional systolic shortening of internal ventricular diameter, and rate of shortening.
- change in ventricular cavity area and wall thickness.

Has been used to estimate ejection fraction and cardiac output. Doppler techniques may be used to estimate pressure gradients across valves, the gradient being related to the difference in velocities across the stenosis. Abnormalities of ventricular wall movement occur in the early stages of myocardial ischaemia, before ECG changes occur.

Transoesophageal echocardiography gives a good view of much of the heart, and has been used perioperatively and in ICU to monitor left ventricular function.

Eclampsia. Convulsions caused by hypertensive disease of pregnancy (pre-eclampsia).
- Carries risk of:
  - complications of pre-eclampsia, especially coagulopathy.
  - cerebral oedema/haemorrhage, coma, death.
  - aspiration of gastric contents, cardiac failure, pulmonary oedema.
  - fetal death.

Incidence is 2–3 cases per 10 000 births in the UK, accounting for about 10% of maternal deaths. Occurs antepartum in 45% of cases, intrapartum in 20%, and postpartum in 35% (usually under 2–4 days postpartum but eclampsia has been reported up to 2–3 weeks afterwards). Only 40% of cases have hypertension and proteinuria in the preceding week, and in many cases premonitory signs of headache, photophobia, hyperreflexia, etc. do not precede convulsions, which may recur if untreated. Mortality is almost 2% in the UK, usually from CVA.
- Treatment:
  - O_2 administration. Tracheal intubation and IPPV may be required; the former may be difficult because of airway oedema.
  - anticonvulsant drugs; traditionally, diazepam and phenytoin have been used in the UK but evidence now strongly supports magnesium sulphate as being more effective for reducing recurrent convulsions and maternal/fetal complications. Thiopental is suitable in resistant cases; tracheal intubation is required.
  - head-down, left lateral position, if the trachea is unprotected.
  - lowering of BP as for pre-eclampsia.
  - delivery of the fetus.
  - admission to ICU may be required.

Sibai BM (2005). Obstet Gynecol; 105: 402–10

ECMO, *see Extracorporeal membrane oxygenation*

Ecothiopate iodide. Organophosphorus compound, used as eye drops to treat severe glaucoma. Plasma cholinesterase levels may be reduced for 3–4 weeks following its use, prolonging the action of suxamethonium.

Ecstasy, *see Methylenedioxymethylamphetamine*

ECT, *see Electroconvulsive therapy*

Ectopic beats, *see Atrial ectopic beats; Junctional arrhythmias; Ventricular ectopic beats*

ED_{50}, *see Therapeutic ratio/index*

Edema, *see Oedema*

Edetate, *see Cyanide poisoning; Sodium calcium edetate*

EDRF, Endothelium-derived relaxing factor, *see Nitric oxide*

Edrophonium chloride. Acetylcholinesterase inhibitor, used to reverse non-depolarising neuromuscular blockade, and in the diagnosis of myasthenia gravis and dual block. Has also been used to treat SVT. Binds reversibly to acetylcholinesterase, with duration of action about 5 min after a single dose. Of faster onset than neostigmine, and with fewer muscarinic side effects.
- Dosage:
  - reversal of neuromuscular blockade: 1 mg/kg iv with atropine.
  - diagnosis of myasthenia gravis: 2 mg iv, followed by 8 mg iv, if no adverse reaction has occurred. Improvement in muscle strength occurs in myasthenia gravis.
  - differentiation between myasthenic and cholinergic crises: 2 mg iv, 1 h after the last dose of cholinergic drug. Increased muscle strength occurs in myasthenic crisis; worsening of weakness in cholinergic crisis.
  - diagnosis of dual block: 10 mg iv; causes transient improvement in muscle power.
  - treatment of SVT: 5–20 mg iv.
- Side effects: bradycardia, hypotension, nausea, vomiting, diarrhoea, abdominal cramps, increased salivation, muscle fasciculation. Convulsions and bronchospasm may also occur. The ECG should always be monitored when edrophonium is administered, and atropine must always be available.

EEG, *see Electroencephalography*

Efficacy. Maximal effect attainable by a drug; e.g. morphine is more efficacious than codeine.
See also, Dose–response curves; Potency

EGTA, Esophageal gastric tube airway, *see Oesophageal obturators and airways*

Eicosanoids. Collective term used for products of arachidonic acid metabolism. Include:
- prostanoids: produced by the cyclo-oxygenase pathway, i.e. prostaglandins, prostacyclin and thromboxanes.
- leukotrienes produced by the lipoxygenase pathways.

Eisenmenger's syndrome. Right-to-left cardiac shunt developing after long-standing left-to-right shunt, because of increased pulmonary vascular resistance and pulmonary hypertension secondary to the increased pulmonary blood flow. Once it occurs, prognosis is poor, since pulmonary hypertension is not affected by surgical correction of the shunt. May follow any left-to-right shunt, although the original description referred to VSD. May occur late in ASD and patent ductus arteriosus.
- Features:
  - dyspnoea, effort syncope, angina, haemoptysis.
  - supraventricular arrhythmias, right ventricular failure, features of pulmonary hypertension.

Anaesthesia is tolerated badly; any drop in peripheral resistance increases the shunt with worsening hypoxaemia, which in turn further increases pulmonary vascular resistance. Factors which decrease pulmonary blood flow also exacerbate the right-to-left shunt, e.g. IPPV. Risk of systemic air embolism following iv injection of bubbles is high.

Pregnancy is also tolerated badly; maternal mortality is 30–50%. Very cautious epidural anaesthesia has been suggested if pregnancy progresses to term.

Heart–lung transplantation is the only definitive treatment once established.

[Victor Eisenmenger (1864–1932), German physician]

Ejection fraction. Left ventricular stroke volume as a fraction of end-diastolic volume.

$$\text{Equals: } \frac{\text{end-diastolic volume} - \text{end systolic volume}}{\text{end diastolic volume}} \times 100\%$$

Useful as an indication of the heart's ability to eject stroke volume. Measured using nuclear cardiology, echocardiography, pulmonary artery catheterisation or contrast angiography. Normally greater than 60%. May also be determined for the right ventricle.

Ejector flowmeter. Device used for scavenging from anaesthetic breathing systems. O_2 or air passing through the ejector causes entrainment of waste gases by the Venturi principle. The rate of removal is adjusted using a flowmeter until it equals the rate of fresh gas supply. Several litres of driving gas may be required per minute, at a pressure of at least 1 bar.

EKG, *see Electrocardiography*

Elastance. Reciprocal of compliance. Total elastance for lungs + chest wall is approximately 10 cmH_2O/l.

Elbow, nerve blocks. Used for minor surgery to the hand and lateral side of the arm.
- The following nerves are blocked (Fig. 55):
  - median (C5–T1): lies immediately medial to the brachial artery in the antecubital fossa. A needle is inserted with the elbow extended, level with the epicondyles, to approximately 5 mm, and 5 ml local anaesthetic agent injected. Subcutaneous infiltration blocks cutaneous branches.
  - radial (C5–T1): lies in the antecubital fossa in the groove between biceps tendon medially and brachioradialis muscle laterally. A needle is inserted level with the epicondyles with the elbow extended, and directed proximally and laterally to contact the lateral epicondyle. 2–4 ml solution is injected, and a further 5 ml during withdrawal to skin. This is repeated with the needle directed more proximally.
  - lateral cutaneous nerve of the forearm (C5–7): lies alongside the radial nerve. It is a continuation of the musculoskeletal nerve of the brachial plexus. May be blocked by subcutaneous infiltration between biceps and brachioradialis, using the same puncture site as for the radial nerve.
  - ulnar (C6–T1): passes through the ulnar groove behind the medial humeral epicondyle. With the elbow flexed to 90°, a fine needle is inserted 1–2 cm proximal to the groove, pointing distally. At 1–2 cm depth, 2–5 ml solution is injected. Neuritis may follow injection into the nerve, or block within the ulnar groove.

See also, Brachial plexus block; Wrist, nerve blocks

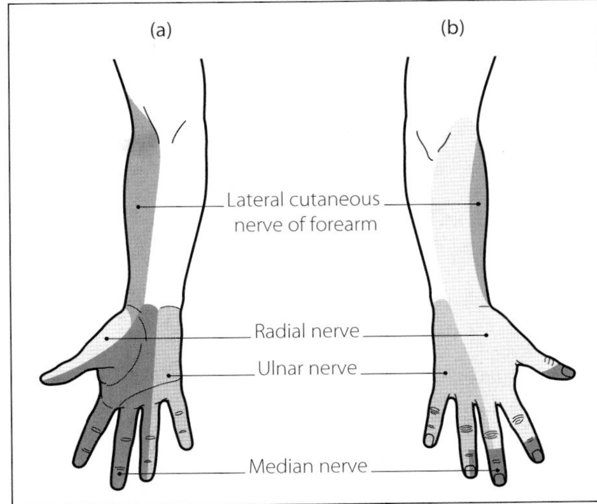

Fig. 55 Cutaneous distribution of nerves blocked at the elbow: (a) anterior; (b) posterior

Elderly, anaesthesia for. Becoming increasingly common as the population ages. Mortality and morbidity are higher in older patients.
- Anaesthetic considerations, compared with younger patients:
  - CVS:
    - ischaemic heart disease is likely, with reduced ventricular compliance and contractility, and cardiac output.
    - decreased blood flow to vital organs, e.g. kidneys, liver, etc.
    - cerebrovascular insufficiency is common.
    - widespread atherosclerosis with a more rigid arterial system. Hypertension is common.
    - veins are more tortuous and thickened, but more prone to damage; venepuncture is more difficult.
    - DVT is more common.

- RS:
  - increased closing capacity, therefore more airway collapse with resultant increase in alveolar–arterial O_2 difference. Normal alveolar Po_2 is approximately:

$$13.3 - \frac{\text{age}}{30} \text{ kPa } (100 - \frac{\text{age}}{4} \text{ mmHg})$$

  - decreased response to hypercapnia and hypoxaemia.
  - greater incidence of atelectasis, PE and chest infection postoperatively.
- pharmacology:
  - increased sensitivity to many drugs, especially CNS depressants.
  - drug distribution, metabolism and elimination are altered. A greater proportion of body weight is fat, due to a decrease in total body water. Plasma proteins are reduced with altered drug binding.
  - half-lives of many drugs are increased.
- metabolic:
  - metabolic rate is lower.
  - impaired renal function, thought to be due to decreased renal blood flow; suggested decrease in GFR is 1% per year over 20.
  - fluid balance is more critical. Dehydration is common following trauma and illness.
  - diabetes mellitus and malnutrition are more common.
- nervous system:
  - cerebrovascular disease is common.
  - confusion is more likely, and may be caused by hypoxia, drugs, hospitalisation, any illness, and possibly peroperative hyperventilation.
  - impaired hearing and memory are common.
- other considerations:
  - heat loss during anaesthesia is more likely due to impairment of both central control and compensatory mechanisms.
  - hiatus hernia is more common, with risk of regurgitation and aspiration.
  - systemic diseases and multiple drug therapy are more common.
  - cervical spondylosis is common, with reduced neck movement. Pain from arthritis may cause great discomfort, e.g. during local anaesthetic techniques. Ligaments are often calcified and tough.

In general, patients are frailer, with greater likelihood of perioperative complications and slower healing. Attention to detail, e.g. fluid balance, is more important than with younger patients, since physiological reserves are less. Smaller doses of most agents are required, and arm–brain circulation time is prolonged.

Warming blankets, adequate humidification, and appropriate monitoring, e.g. of urine output, should be provided. Postoperative O_2 therapy should be instituted immediately and possibly continued for 1–3 days, since hypoxia may readily occur.

The ‘physiological age’ of the patient is usually more relevant than their chronological age: e.g. fit 90-year-olds may present less risk than frail 70-year-olds.

Electrical anaesthesia. Induction of unconsciousness by passing high frequency alternating current across the head. Has been used in experimental animals and in human studies. Current has also been passed across the spinal cord to produce more local effects.

Electrical symbols. Used to denote components of electrical circuits. Specific symbols are also used on electrical equipment to indicate the safety features or other characteristics or instructions (Fig. 56).
See also, Electrocution and electrical burns

Electroacupuncture, *see Acupuncture*

Electrocardiography (ECG). Recording and display of cardiac electrical activity. First performed through the intact chest in 1887. Used for investigation of cardiac disease, particularly ischaemic heart disease and arrhythmias, also for monitoring cardiac rhythm.

Standard modern ECG recordings are obtained from different combinations of chest and limb leads, each set recording from a different direction, and providing information about a different part of the heart:
- standard leads:
  - I: between right arm and left arm.
  - II: between left leg and right arm.
  - III: between left leg and left arm.
- augmented unipolar leads (reference electrode is obtained by connecting all three):
  - aVR: right arm.
  - aVL: left arm.
  - aVF: left leg.
- unipolar chest leads (reference electrode is formed by the combined aV leads):
  - V_1: 4th intercostal space, right sternal edge.
  - V_2: 4th intercostal space, left sternal edge.
  - V_3: midway between V_2 and V_4.
  - V_4: 5th intercostal space, left midclavicular line.
  - V_5: 5th intercostal space, left anterior axillary line.
  - V_6: 5th intercostal space, left midaxillary line.

The display is recorded on to an oscilloscope or moving paper. Frequency range is 0.5–80 Hz. Magnitude of deflection is proportional to the amount of heart muscle, but reduced by passage through the chest. High skin resistance is reduced by cleaning with alcohol and skin abrasion. Electrodes are usually silver/silver chloride with chloride conducting gel, to reduce generation of potentials in the electrode by the recorded potential, and reduce impedance variability. Electrodes of differing compounds may generate potential by a battery-like effect. Interference may result from muscle activity, radiofrequency waves from diathermy and other equipment, and inductance by electrical equipment.

The leads may be represented on the chest and heart as in Figure 57a. Thus abnormalities of the inferior portion of the heart will be demonstrated in the inferior leads (i.e. aVF, II and III), and abnormalities of the anterolateral heart in aVL, I, II, etc. V_{1-2} demonstrate electrical activity from the right side of the heart, V_{3-4} from the septum and front, and V_{5-6} from the left side. Atrial activity may be investigated using an oesophageal lead.

Depolarisation towards a lead (or repolarisation away) results in a positive deflection; depolarisation away (or repolarisation towards) causes negative deflection. Thus in the normal ECG recording, polarity of deflection varies in the different leads.

- Plan for the interpretation of standard ECG, with normal values (Fig. 57b):
  - patient’s name, date, etc.
  - usual speed of recording is 25 mm/s; usual calibration is 1 mV/cm.
  - rate: heart rate in beats/min is calculated by dividing the number of 5 mm squares between successive QRS complexes into 300.

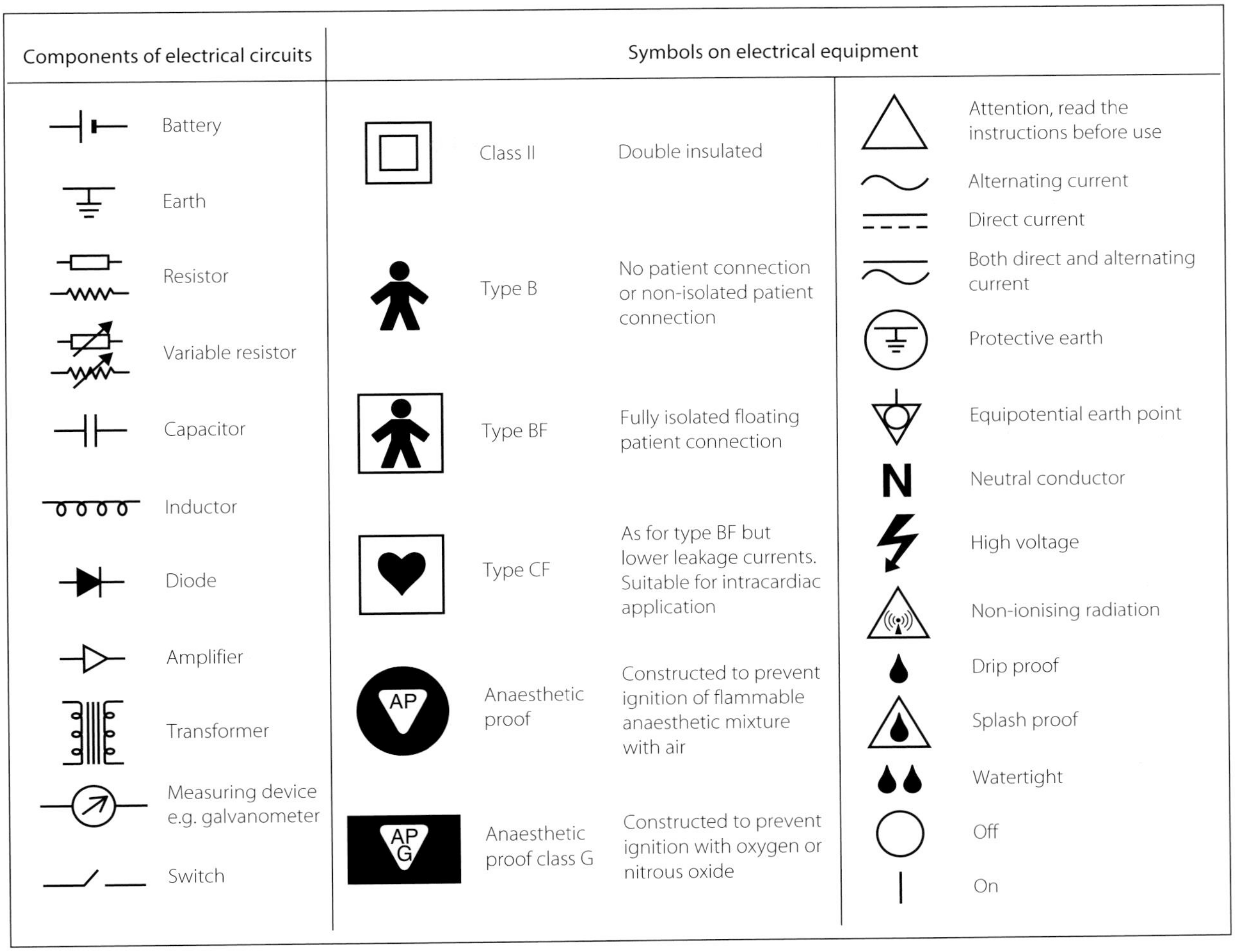

Components of electrical circuits
Battery
Earth
Resistor
Variable resistor
Capacitor
Inductor
Diode
Amplifier
Transformer
Measuring device e.g. galvanometer
Switch
Symbols on electrical equipment
Class II
Double insulated
Type B
No patient connection or non-isolated patient connection
Type BF
Fully isolated floating patient connection
Type CF
As for type BF but lower leakage currents. Suitable for intracardiac application
AP
Anaesthetic proof
Constructed to prevent ignition of flammable anaesthetic mixture with air
AP G
Anaesthetic proof class G
Constructed to prevent ignition with oxygen or nitrous oxide
Attention, read the instructions before use
Alternating current
Direct current
Both direct and alternating current
Protective earth
Equipotential earth point
N
Neutral conductor
High voltage
Non-ionising radiation
Drip proof
Splash proof
Watertight
Off
On

Fig. 56 Electrical symbols

(a)
aVR
aVL
1
2
3
4
5
6
I
V leads
III
aVF
II
(b)
R
P
T
U
Q
S
PR
QRS
ST
QT
(c)
aVR
−90º
aVL
±180º
0º
I
III
+90º
II
aVF

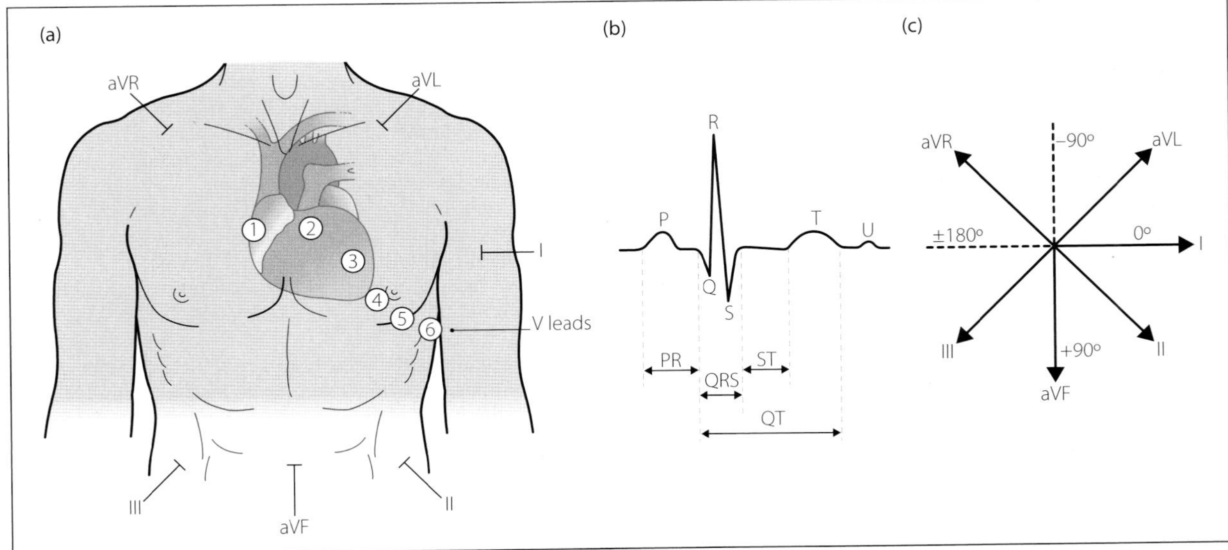

Fig. 57 The ECG: (a) arrangement of leads; (b) normal ECG; (c) electric axis

- rhythm:
  - regular or irregular. An irregular rhythm may be regularly (e.g. missing every third QRS) or irregularly irregular (e.g. completely random in AF).
  - presence/absence of P waves, flutter waves in atrial flutter, ventricular ectopic beats, pacing spikes, etc.
- axis: summation of electrical potentials from the standard and aV leads, plotted as vectors. The normal axis lies between $-30°$ and $+90°$ (Fig. 57c).

  Simple method of determination: since leads I and aVF are at right angles to each other, they can be used alone; e.g. if the QRS deflection is positive in both, the axis lies between 0 and 90°. If I is positive and aVF negative, the axis lies between 0 and $-90°$, etc.

  Left axis deviation ($< 30°$) may occur in:
  - normal subjects (especially if pregnant), ascites, etc.
  - left bundle branch block, left anterior hemiblock.
  - left ventricular hypertrophy.

  Right axis deviation ($> 90°$) may occur in:
  - normal subjects.
  - right ventricular hypertrophy.
  - right bundle branch block, left posterior hemiblock.
- P wave (atrial depolarisation):
  - positive in I, II, and V_{4-6}; negative in aVR, since depolarisation moves downwards and to the left.
  - height < 2.5 mm.
  - width < 3 mm.
  - shape.
- P–R interval: normally 0.12–0.2 s (3–5 mm squares).
- QRS complex (ventricular depolarisation):
  - usually positive in I, II and V_{4-6}; negative in aVR and V_{1-2}, since depolarisation moves downwards and to the left. Progresses smoothly across the chest leads, e.g. stepwise increase in height from V_1 to V_4; either increases or decreases in V_{5-6}.
  - duration is 0.04–0.12 s (1–3 mm squares).
  - amplitude in I+II+III > 5 mm. Left ventricular hypertrophy exists if the R wave in V_6 + S wave in $V_1 > 35$ mm. In right ventricular hypertrophy the R:S ratio > 1 in V_{1-2}.
  - shape; presence of Q waves.
  - extra waves, e.g. J and δ waves in hypothermia and Wolff–Parkinson–White syndrome respectively.
- S–T segment:
  - level within 1 mm of baseline.
  - shape.
- T wave (ventricular repolarisation):
  - orientation as for QRS complexes.
  - height < 5 mm.
  - shape.
- Q–T interval: corrected Q–T=

  $$\left(\frac{\text{measured Q} - \text{T}}{\sqrt{\text{cycle length}}}\right) \quad \text{Normal range } 0.35 - 0.43 \text{ s}$$
- U wave.

During anaesthesia/intensive care, lead II is often selected for continuous monitoring. Many simple ECG monitors only use three leads, as rate and rhythm are usually sufficient information. Myocardial ischaemia usually affects the left ventricle, and may be detected by various versions of V_5, e.g. CM_5 lead configuration (central manubrium V_5), which looks at the left ventricle:

- right arm electrode in suprasternal notch.
- left arm electrode over apex of heart (V_5 position).
- left leg electrode on left shoulder or leg serves as ground.

Other lead configurations are also used, e.g. CH_5, CC_5 and CS_5, with right arm electrode on the patient's head, right side of chest and subscapular regions respectively. The CB_5 configuration with electrode over the right scapula is better for demonstrating arrhythmias.

24-hour ambulatory ECG monitoring is performed for assessing arrhythmias and their therapy, and detecting myocardial ischaemia. Some devices run continuously whilst others are activated by the patient when they experience symptoms. The compressed recording is expanded by speeding up the playback and areas of interest viewed and analysed (usually automatically) before printing. 24-hour tapes have been used to investigate arrhythmias and ischaemia perioperatively.

See also, Cardiac cycle; Heart block: His bundle electrography; Myocardial infarction

Electroconvulsive therapy (ECT). Passage of electric current, usually alternating, across the skull to produce convulsions; used to treat severe depressive psychosis. 30–45 J is usually given over 0.5–1.5 s; it may also be given as repeated ultrashort bursts. Usually given in courses over a few weeks. First used in the late 1930s.

Brief general anaesthesia is required; partial muscle relaxation is usually provided, to allow assessment of resultant convulsions whilst reducing the risk of vertebral fractures and other trauma.

- Anaesthetic considerations:
  - preoperatively:
    - patients should be prepared, starved and investigated as for any anaesthetic procedure. Particular care is required if cardiovascular disease or intracranial pathology coexists.
    - concurrent drug therapy may include antidepressant drugs including monoamine oxidase inhibitors, lithium, etc.
    - premedication is usually omitted.
  - perioperatively:
    - monitoring is required as for any procedure.
    - a single 'minimal sleep dose' of iv agent is usually given. Methohexital was often considered the drug of choice because of its short action and convulsant properties. Propofol is commonly used, although it results in a shorter duration of seizure; it is not known whether this affects the efficacy of ECT.
    - suxamethonium 0.5 mg/kg is commonly given, although smaller doses have been used.
    - a soft mouth guard is inserted to protect the teeth and gums.
    - the lungs are ventilated with O_2 by facepiece after induction of anaesthesia, since seizure threshold is reduced by hypocapnia. Oxygenation is usually continued during and after the convulsions although the need for the former has been questioned.
    - intense parasympathetic discharge may follow passage of current, and may be followed by increased sympathetic activity. Atropine should always be available; routine administration has been suggested.
  - recovery facilities: as normal. Confusion may follow.

Ding Z, White PF (2002). Anesth Analg; 94: 1351–64

Electrocution and electrical burns. Hazard of using electrical equipment; during anaesthesia, malfunction or improper use of diathermy, monitoring equipment, infusion devices, etc. may cause sudden cardiac arrest or unnoticed burns.

Current flows between opposite poles for direct current, or from live wire to earth for alternating current, e.g. mains power. Mains voltage is 240 V at 50 Hz in the UK and 110 V at 60 Hz in the USA. Current flows via the path of least resistance; if this path includes a person, e.g. patient or doctor via earthed equipment, ECG lead, floor, etc., electrocution occurs.

- Effects:
  - heat production due to high resistance of tissues. Amount of heat is related to current density. May produce burns at sites of current entry/departure.
  - nerve and muscle stimulation; e.g. effect of current across chest (approximate values):
    - 1 mA: tingling.
    - 5 mA: pain.
    - 15 mA: tonic muscle contraction, i.e. 'can't let go' threshold.
    - 50 mA: respiratory arrest.
    - 100 mA: VF.
    - $>$ 5 A: tonic contraction of the myocardium (utilised in defibrillation).

  Magnitude of current depends on the resistance to flow, which is reduced if contacts are wet or have large surface area. Current density at the myocardium is important; thus 100 μA is sufficient to cause VF if delivered directly to the heart (microshock). Other important factors include:
    - frequency of alternating current: 50–60 Hz is particularly dangerous but cheap to provide.
    - timing of shock (e.g. R on T phenomenon).
- Methods of protection:
  - regular checking and maintenance of electrical equipment.
  - use of batteries only (impractical).
  - connection of equipment casing to earth (defined as class I equipment). Accidental contact between the live wire and casing then causes a large current to flow to earth, with melting of protective fuses and breakage of the circuit. Fuses are made of thin wire which melts at certain current loads; they serve to protect equipment in case of faults, but do not melt quickly enough to prevent dangerous currents flowing. Fuses are usually placed in live and neutral wires and mains plug.
  - double insulation of all conducting wires within equipment (class II).
  - use of isolated circuits, e.g. in diathermy, ECG, etc.: patients are not connected directly to earth via plates and electrodes, but via transformers within each piece of apparatus. Current thus cannot reach earth through the patient if contact with a live supply occurs. Class III equipment uses internal transformers to reduce voltage, e.g. to under 24 V. Internal transformers are cheaper and more practical than large external transformers, e.g. one for an operating suite.
  - reduction of stray leakage currents, e.g. due to drops in potential along the length of conductors, caused by capacitance between casing and innards or inductance. Leakage currents may be sufficient to produce microshock. Earth conductors are connected to each other to reduce differences between them. Current-operated earth-leakage circuit breakers may be used. Standards for leakage currents are defined, e.g. 10 μA maximum from the casing or delivered to the patient for intracardiac equipment; 100–500 μA for other equipment, depending on usage.
  - reduction of the risk of microshock by avoiding conducting solutions, e.g. saline in intracardiac lines such as CVP manometers. Needle electrodes are also avoided, since their resistance is low.
  - electrical equipment, plugs, etc. should not be placed on the floor where solutions may fall on them.

Medical electrical equipment is marked with the appropriate electrical symbols to indicate its level of safety features (see Fig. 56, p. 185).

Electroencephalography (EEG). Recording of electrical activity of the brain. Signals from different combinations of 20–22 scalp electrodes are presented as 16 continuous traces on paper sheets. Shape, distribution, incidence and symmetry of waves are analysed to give information about underlying brain activity, in conjunction with clinical details. Concealed abnormalities may be revealed during hyperventilation.

- Different rhythms:
  - alpha: normal 8–10 Hz waves. Prominent at the parieto-occipital area at rest with the eyes shut.
  - beta: normal 13–30 Hz waves. Prominent over the frontal area.
  - delta: abnormal 4 Hz waves; may be normal in children and during sleep.
  - theta: 4–8 Hz waves; sometimes abnormal.

As age increases, infantile beta activity is slowly replaced by adult alpha activity. Characteristic patterns occur in normal sleep. During anaesthesia, alpha rhythms become depressed, and are replaced by high frequency rhythms. Slow rhythms may reappear at deeper levels of anaesthesia, followed by periods of little or no activity separated by bursts of activity (burst suppression). The pattern differs with different agents used. Large amounts of paper are produced, making its perioperative use awkward. There may be electrical interference, and interpretation is difficult. Modified forms of EEG have therefore been developed, e.g. cerebral function monitor, cerebral function analysing monitor, power spectral analysis. Used to investigate intracranial activity in, e.g. head injury, epilepsy, cerebrovascular disease, coma, encephalopathies, surgery, etc. Similar principles are involved in measuring evoked potentials.

See also, Anaesthesia, depth of

Electrolyte. Compound which dissociates in solution to produce ions, allowing conduction of electricity; also refers to the ions themselves. Sodium, potassium, calcium, magnesium and hydrogen ions are the most important cations in the body; chloride and bicarbonate ions the most important anions.

See also, Fluids, body; Intravenous fluids

Electrolyte imbalance, *see individual disorders*

Electrolyte solutions, *see Intravenous fluids*

Electromagnetic flow measurement. Relies on the principle that a moving conductor within a magnetic field induces current which is proportional to the rate of movement (Faraday's law). Relationship of movement, field and current is described by Fleming's right-hand rule, with thumb, forefinger and middle finger of the right hand extended at mutual right angles (e.g. forefinger pointing forward, thumb upward and middle finger medially). If the forefinger points in the direction of the field, and thumb in the direction of movement, the middle finger will point in the direction of the induced current.

Electromagnets within a semicircular probe are placed around an artery, and the moving blood is the conductor. The potential difference between the walls of the vessel is measured and average velocity of blood flow determined. Alternating current is used for magnetic field generation, to avoid the effect of induction of current in the detector electrode circuit.

[Michael Faraday (1791–1867), English chemist; Sir John Fleming (1849–1945), English electrical engineer]

Electromechanical dissociation (EMD). Term used to describe a cardiac state in which organised electrical depolarisation occurs throughout the myocardium, but there is no synchronous shortening of the myocardial fibres and mechanical contractions are absent. Part of the spectrum of pulseless electrical activity, though the latter also includes mechanical contractions too weak to produce a detectable cardiac output.
See also, Cardiac arrest

Electromyography (EMG). Method of investigating neuromuscular function. Involves recording of spontaneous or evoked electrical activity from skeletal muscle; usually combined with nerve conduction studies which measure the velocity of nerve conduction following stimulation at different sites along a nerve pathway. Thus useful in distinguishing between disorders of muscle, isolated or generalised nerve disease or lesions, and disorders affecting the neuromuscular junction.

In anaesthesia, it has been used to determine frontalis muscle tone to monitor depth of anaesthesia. Also used in neuromuscular blockade monitoring; nerve stimulation and muscle action potential recording are achieved using surface skin electrodes, although needle electrodes have been used. Less convenient than devices measuring mechanical muscle response, it may detect electrical activity when mechanical contraction is undetectable.

Is also used to investigate critical illness polyneuropathy and the neuromuscular function of the eye, bladder, GIT, etc.
See also, Anaesthesia, depth of

Electron capture detector. Device used in the analysis of gas mixtures that have been separated by, for example, gas chromatography; particularly useful in detecting halogenated compounds. Electrons within an ionisation chamber pass from cathode to anode, but are 'captured' by the halogenated substance blown through the chamber. The current passing across the chamber is therefore reduced, depending on how many electrons are captured. Used to quantify the amount of known substances, not to identify unknown ones.
See also, Gas analysis

Eltanolone (3α-hydroxy-5β-pregnan-20-one). Steroid metabolite of progesterone; its CNS properties were first described in the 1950s. Has been studied as an iv anaesthetic agent. When formulated in a soya bean emulsion it produces smooth rapid onset of anaesthesia of short duration, with greater respiratory and cardiovascular stability and higher therapeutic ratio than thiopental and propofol. Rash and urticaria have been reported, especially in children.

Embryo, *see Environmental safety of anaesthetists; Fetus, effect of anaesthetic agents on*

EMD, *see Electromechanical dissociation*

Emergence phenomena. Usually consist of agitation and confusion, with laryngospasm, breath-holding, etc.; may be equivalent to the second stage of anaesthesia seen on induction, or be due to other causes of confusion, including the central anticholinergic syndrome and dystonic reactions. Hallucinations and frightening dreams are common after ketamine.

Emergency surgery. Usually refers to surgery occurring within 24 h of admission or diagnosis; i.e. includes those cases where surgery follows resuscitation, and those where surgery and resuscitation proceed simultaneously (e.g. ruptured aortic aneurysm).

- Problems may be related to:
  - inadequate preparation of patients for surgery:
  - full stomach, i.e. risk of aspiration of gastric contents.
  - untreated pre-existing disease, electrolyte imbalance, etc.
  - appropriate investigations and cross-matching of blood not performed or not ready.
  - the presenting complaint:
    - haemorrhage and hypovolaemia.
    - intestinal obstruction/intra-abdominal pathology: dehydration and hypovolaemia, electrolyte imbalance, etc. Further risk of aspiration due to delayed gastric emptying and vomiting/haematemesis.
    - trauma: haemorrhage, head injury, chest trauma, etc.
    - airway obstruction/inhaled foreign body.
    - related to specialist surgery, e.g. cardiac surgery, neurosurgery.

The balance between the need for preoperative treatment and urgency of surgery is sometimes difficult, but inadequate preoperative correction of fluid and electrolyte disturbance is consistently associated with increased perioperative mortality. Treatment of cardiac failure is also important whenever possible. Careful preoperative assessment and discussion with the surgeon is vital. Anaesthetic management is as for routine surgery but with the above considerations. Thus smaller doses of drugs than usual are given initially. Rapid sequence induction is usually employed. Measures against heat loss are important. Invasive monitoring and postoperative HDU/ICU and IPPV should be considered.

Regional techniques are particularly useful for limb surgery, but epidural/spinal anaesthesia is hazardous if hypovolaemia is present.
See also, specific procedures; Anaesthetic morbidity and mortality

Emesis, *see Vomiting*

Emetic drugs. Given to empty the stomach, e.g. following poisoning, or preoperatively to reduce risk of aspiration pneumonitis. Now rarely used, because of poor efficacy and the risk of causing aspiration; particularly dangerous after ingestion of corrosive or petroleum derivatives, or in unconscious patients. Include apomorphine and ipecacuanha; copper sulphate and sodium chloride are no longer used.

EMG, *see Electromyography*

EMLA cream (Eutectic mixture of local anaesthetics). Mixture of prilocaine base 2.5% and lidocaine base 2.5% as an oil–water emulsion. The melting point of each local anaesthetic agent is lowered by the presence of the other; the resultant mixture is effective in providing analgesia of the skin 60–90 min after topical application and covering with an occlusive dressing. May continue to be released from skin depots even after removal of surface cream. Particularly useful in children. May produce blanching of the skin; increases in methaemoglobin have been reported several hours after application.

Uses described include analgesia for venepuncture, venous and arterial cannulation, lumbar puncture, epidural injection, superficial skin surgery and relief of tourniquet pain during IVRA.

EMMV, Extended mandatory minute ventilation, *see Mandatory minute ventilation*

EMO inhaler, *see Vaporisers*

Emphysema, *see Chronic obstructive pulmonary disease*

Emphysema, subcutaneous. Presence of gas in subcutaneous tissues.
May be caused by:
- trauma, including surgery (hence the term 'surgical emphysema'); gas arises from the atmosphere, viscera or air sinuses.
- pneumothorax or rupture of a viscus, e.g. oesophagus.
- barotrauma.
- infection with gas-producing organisms, e.g. gas gangrene.
- rarely, deliberate self-injection of subcutaneous air in disordered mental states.

Often palpable under the skin, and may be visible on X-ray. The gas is slowly absorbed once the cause is treated. Multiple skin puncture has been performed to allow escape of gas, and high F_IO_2 suggested to increase absorption (O_2 being more soluble than nitrogen), but the value of these measures is unknown.

Empyema. Collection of pus within the pleural cavity. A complication of chest trauma (especially if haemothorax was present), pneumonia, chest drainage, thoracic surgery and subdiaphragmatic abscess. Clinical features include pyrexia, chest pain and productive cough. Chest X-ray features are those of a pleural effusion; if encapsulated it may resemble a pulmonary cyst. Diagnosis is confirmed by imaging and aspiration of pus. Treatment depends on aetiology but includes antibacterial drugs, drainage by intercostal tube (sometimes requiring ultrasound or CT scan guidance) or surgery. May rarely lead to bronchopleural fistula.

Enalapril maleate. Angiotensin converting enzyme inhibitor, used to treat hypertension and cardiac failure (including following MI). A prodrug, it is converted to enalaprilat by hepatic metabolism. Longer acting than captopril, with onset of action within 2 h; half-life is up to 35 h via active metabolites.
- Dosage: 2.5–40 mg daily, orally.
- Side effects: hypotension following the first dose or following induction of anaesthesia, cough, dizziness, weakness, nausea, diarrhoea, rash, renal impairment.

Encephalitis. Infection, usually viral, affecting the cerebral hemispheres. If signs of meningitis coexist the term encephalomyelitis or meningoencephalitis is used. Viruses gain entry to the CNS through peripheral nerves or following viraemia. Classified into sporadic acute, epidemic acute and postinfectious forms. Clinical features include headache, fever, neck stiffness, lethargy, confusion, coma, encephalopathy, focal neurological signs and epilepsy. May affect the brainstem, mimicking brainstem death.

May be mimicked by meningitis and cerebral abscess. Investigations include CSF examination (mild increase in protein, lymphocytosis, normal glucose), CT and MRI scanning, EEG and viral titres/cultures from blood and CSF. Treatment is largely supportive, with tracheal intubation and IPPV for patients with depressed consciousness. Aciclovir should be given to all cases of acute viral encephalitis since herpes simplex infections are common.
Steiner I, Budka H, Chaudhuri A, et al (2005). Eur J Neurol; 12: 331–43

Encephalopathy. Term denoting diffuse disorder of cerebral function with or without focal neurological deficit. Usually results in delirium, stupor and coma. Aetiology is as for coma.

Endobronchial blockers (Bronchial blockers). Used in thoracic surgery to isolate a portion of lung, e.g. to avoid air leaks during IPPV or prevent contamination of normal lung with secretions, pus, blood, etc. Less often used now, except for paediatric surgery, endobronchial tubes being more popular and versatile. Usually inserted under direct vision via a bronchoscope before tracheal intubation, although they may be passed blindly through a tracheal tube.
- Examples:
  - Magill (1943): long red rubber catheter with a distal inflatable balloon, inserted using a wire stilette.
  - Vernon Thompson (1943): similar to Magill's, with separate channels for suction and cuff inflation (with water); inserted using a stilette. A nylon mesh covers the balloon to aid grip and reduce risk of damage during surgery.
  - Fogarty catheter: available in different sizes: 5–14 mm balloon diameter. Originally described for percutaneous arterial embolectomy.
  - combined with a tracheal tube:
    - Macintosh–Leatherdale (1955; Fig. 58): tracheal and blocker components, each with a separate cuff. The blocker component passes into the left main bronchus, with a narrow suction port opening at the tip. Resembles an endobronchial tube at first glance. Designed for surgery on the left lung.

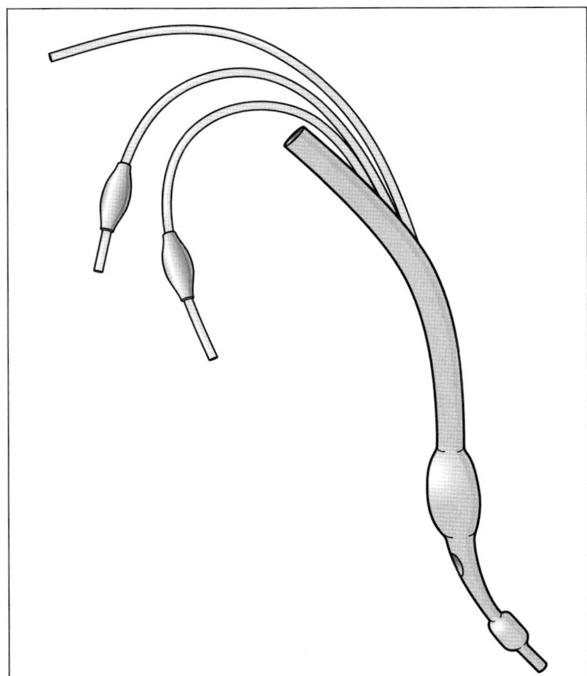

Fig. 58 Macintosh–Leatherdale endobronchial blocker

- plastic tracheal tubes incorporating an advanceable blocker are also available.
- combined with an endobronchial tube: Vellacott (1954) and Green (1958): both are designed to be passed into the right main bronchus, blocking the right upper lobe bronchus with left lung ventilation via an opening between tracheal and bronchial cuffs. The former tube has one bronchial cuff; the latter has two (one on either side of the right upper lobe bronchus) with a suction catheter opening between them and a carinal hook. Placed using a bronchoscope.

[Vernon C Thompson, London surgeon; Thomas J Fogarty, US surgeon; Robert AL Leatherdale, Dorset anaesthetist; William N Vellacott, Worcester anaesthetist; Ronald A Green, London anaesthetist]

Endobronchial tubes. Used in thoracic surgery to allow sleeve resection of the bronchus, or to isolate infected lung or potential air leak, e.g. in bronchopleural fistula or emphysematous lung cysts. Other pulmonary surgery, e.g. pneumonectomy/lobectomy, pleural, aortic, oesophageal and mediastinal surgery, is possible with conventional tracheal tubes, although surgery may be made easier by collapsing one lung. Also used in ICU in patients with severe, unilateral lung injury or bronchopleural fistula. Risks of one-lung anaesthesia should be considered before choosing their use.

- Examples:
  - single-lumen (Fig. 59a); usually mounted over a bronchoscope for insertion:
    - Magill (1936) and others: for left or right bronchial placement.
    - Gordon–Green (1955): passed into the right main bronchus. Has tracheal and bronchial cuffs, the latter with a slit to allow ventilation of the right upper bronchus. Has a carinal hook. Designed for surgery on the left lung.
    - Macintosh–Leatherdale (1955): passed blindly into the left main bronchus. Bears tracheal and bronchial cuffs, with a suction port opening between them. Designed for surgery on the right lung.
    - Brompton–Pallister (1959): passed into the left main bronchus, with tracheal cuff and two bronchial cuffs in case one is damaged. The second bronchial cuff has no pilot balloon. Designed for sleeve resection of the right upper bronchus.
  - double-lumen (Fig. 59b): all have cuffed endobronchial portions and tracheal cuffs. The endobronchial portions are curved to the left or right as appropriate; the oropharyngeal parts are concave anteriorly. They are passed blindly. Most are made of red rubber. The main problem of right-sided tubes is related to the short length of the right main bronchus before giving off the upper lobe bronchus.
    - Carlens (1950): passed into the left main bronchus. One lumen runs anterior to the other. A carinal hook aids correct placement but may hinder passage through the glottis. Designed for differential bronchospirometry. Available in sizes 35–41 FG.
    - Bryce-Smith (1959): similar to Carlens's, but with longer bronchial portion and fenestrated tracheal opening. Has no carinal hook.
    - Bryce-Smith–Salt (1960): right-sided version of the Bryce-Smith tube. The bronchial portion and cuff are slotted to allow ventilation of the right upper bronchus.
    - White (1960): right-sided version of the Carlens tube. Has a small slit in the bronchial portion and bronchial cuff.
    - Robertshaw (1962): the lumina are side by side and wider than in the others, with reduced resistance. Left- and right-sided versions are available, the latter with a slotted bronchial cuff. Available in large, medium and small sizes.
    - plastic disposable tubes, with thinner walls and low-pressure cuffs. Left- and right-sided tubes are available; the latter's cuff is deflected around a slot for the right upper bronchus.

  Left-sided tubes are usually preferred, even for right-sided surgery, because of the risk of inadequate ventilation of the right upper lobe if incorrectly positioned. Right-sided tubes are often preferred if the left main bronchus is compressed by aortic aneurysm, to prevent traumatic haemorrhage.
- Insertion:
  - as for tracheal tubes initially, with the bronchial curve concave anteriorly to aid passage through the pharynx.
  - rotated 90° when the tip is through the larynx, to direct the endobronchial part to the appropriate side. The Carlens tube must be rotated 180°, so that the hook passes through the anterior part of the glottis, before further rotation by 90°.
  - connected to the breathing system via a double catheter mount, each lumen connected via a capped connector and rubber tubing. Cuff inflation:
    - the tracheal cuff is inflated until the air leak stops; both sides of the chest are checked for ventilation.
    - the catheter mount to the tracheal lumen is clamped, and the tracheal lumen opened to air.
    - the lung is inflated via the bronchial lumen only, inflating the bronchial cuff until no air leak is heard from the tracheal lumen. Only the selected side of the chest should now move.
    - the tracheal lumen is reconnected and both sides of the chest are checked as before.
    - both lungs should now be able to be ventilated separately, by inflating via one lumen only and opening the other to air.

Fibreoptic endoscopy is the best way of checking correct positioning, since clinical assessment may not be reliable; it is especially useful with right-sided tubes. It may also be used to check for cuff herniation causing tube or bronchial obstruction.

Complications are as for tracheal intubation (*see Intubation, complications of*). Bronchial rupture may occur if excessive volumes are used for cuff inflation. Incorrect positioning, or movement during positioning of the patient, may result in uneven ventilation and impaired gas exchange.

[Eric Carlens (1914–2000), Swedish otolaryngologist; Wally Gordon, English surgeon; Ronald A Green and William K Pallister (1926–2008), London anaesthetists; Robert AL Leatherdale, Dorset anaesthetist; Roger Bryce-Smith (1918–2006), Oxford anaesthetist; George MJ White, Middlesbrough anaesthetist; Frank L Robertshaw (1918–1991), Manchester anaesthetist; Richard H Salt (1911–1995), Oxford anaesthetic technician]

See also, Tracheobronchial tree

Endocardial viability ratio (EVR). Ratio of diastolic pressure time index to tension time index, obtained by recording left ventricular and aortic root pressure tracings (Fig. 60). May indicate myocardial O_2 supply/demand ratio and likelihood of myocardial ischaemia (thought to be likely when the ratio is under 0.7).

Endocarditis, infective. Infective inflammation of the endocardial lining of the heart and valves, most commonly

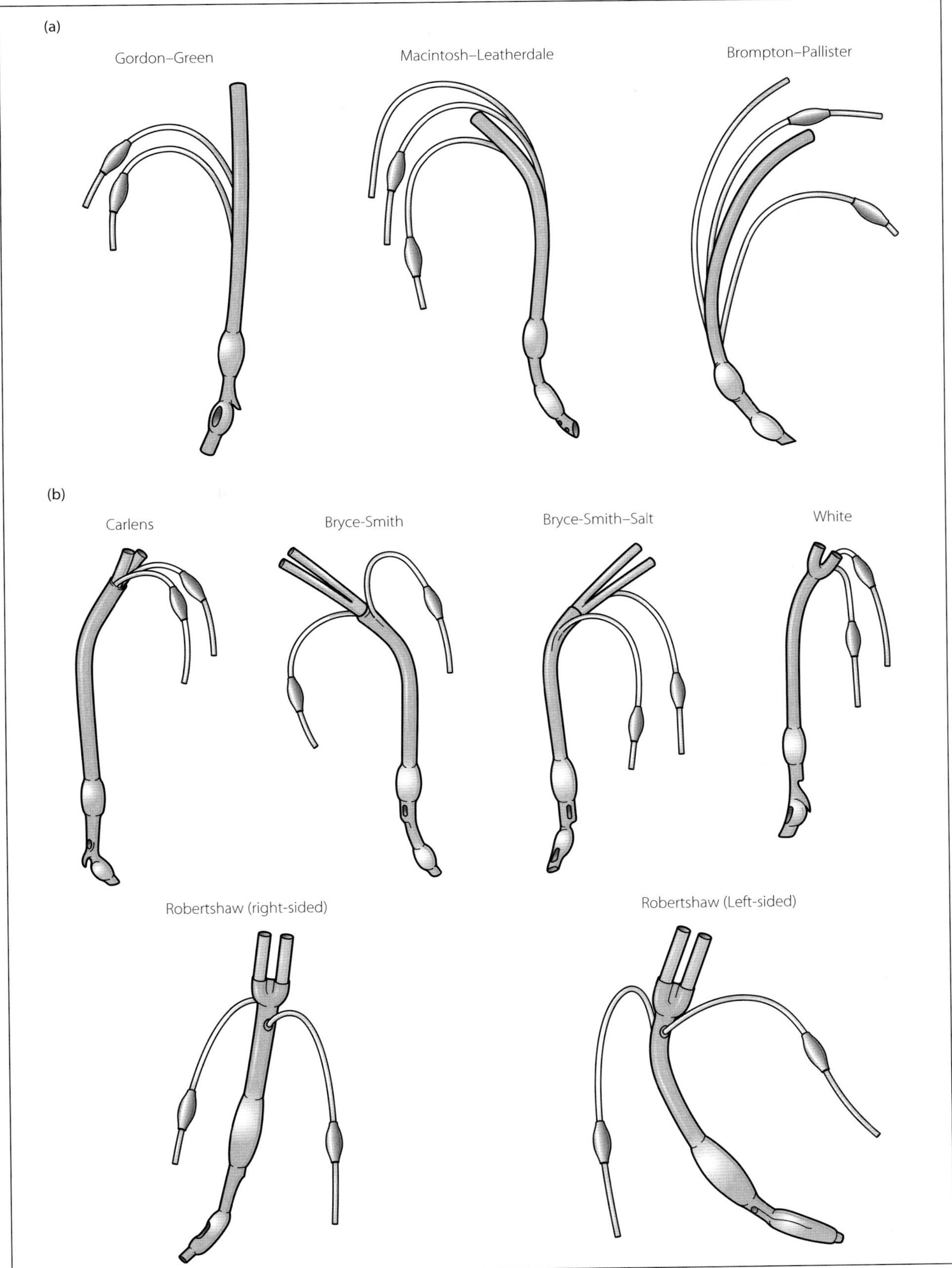

Fig. 59 Endobronchial tubes: (a) single-lumen; (b) double lumen

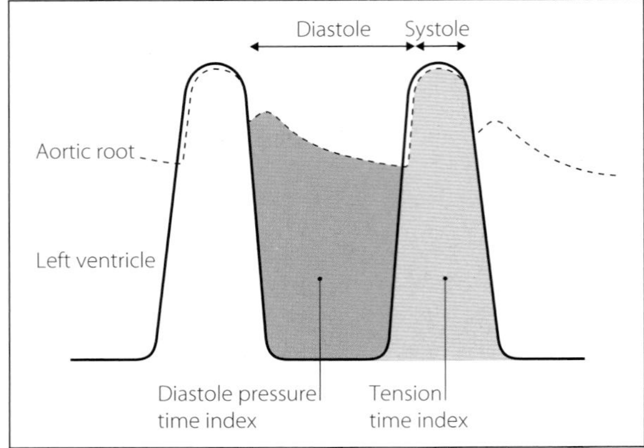

Fig. 60 Left ventricular and aortic root pressure tracings

the aortic valve (previously the mitral valve). Commonly associated with abnormal valves, e.g. rheumatic, degenerative or prosthetic valves, or congenital heart disease, but approximately 50% of cases involve normal valves. Men are twice as commonly affected. Results in tissue destruction and vegetations of platelets, macrophages and organisms, with systemic embolisation. Systemic immune complex deposition may also occur. Overall mortality is ~40%.

- Traditionally divided into acute and subacute, although definitions are imprecise:
  - acute:
    - usually due to virulent organisms, e.g. *Streptococcus pneumoniae, Staphylococcus aureus.*
    - presents early with rapid progression to death unless early aggressive treatment is instituted.
  - subacute:
    - usually due to *Streptococcus viridans.*
    - underlying structural heart disease is usual.
    - chronic malaise and slow course of disease is typical.

  Infection with atypical organisms, e.g. fungi and staphylococci, is more common in iv drug abusers.
- Features:
  - fever (90%), malaise, weight loss, night sweats, anaemia.
  - heart murmurs (85%), cardiac failure, valve lesions.
  - peripheral embolisation/vasculitic phenomena, e.g. splinter haemorrhages in nail beds, conjunctivae and retina (Roth spots), painful fingertip swellings (Osler's nodes), painless haemorrhagic lesions on palms and soles (Janeway lesions), kidneys (causing haematuria), CNS (causing CVA), etc. Splenomegaly and clubbing may occur.
- Diagnosis:
  - blood cultures (positive in 90% of cases). Can be taken even when temperature is normal since the bacteraemia is constant.
  - serological testing is performed if cultures are negative (e.g. if the patient is already on antibiotics).
  - tissue culture of skin lesions may be helpful.
  - echocardiography (initially transthoracic then transoesophageal if the former is negative).

Treatment is supportive with antimicrobial therapy depending on the infecting organism. Treatment usually lasts 4–6 weeks. Cardiac valve replacement is necessary in ~50%; indications include CVS instability associated with valve destruction, persistent fever despite prolonged antimicrobial therapy, presence of highly resistant organisms, prosthetic valve involvement and large vegetations with embolic potential. Prophylaxis in structural disease is as for congenital heart disease.

[Sir William Osler (1849–1919), Canadian-born US and English physician; Moritz Roth (1849–1914), Swiss physician; Theodore Caldwell Janeway (1872–1917), US physician]

Beynon RP, Bahl VK, Prendergast BD (2006). Br Med J; 333: 334–9

Endocrine disorders, *see individual diseases*

Endomorphins. Endogenous opioid peptides for μ opioid receptors. Produce spinal and supraspinal analgesia experimentally; have been found in the human brain although their role is uncertain.

Endorphins. Endogenous opioid peptides derived from β-lipotropin, found in the CNS, especially the anterior pituitary and hypothalamus. β-Endorphin (31 amino acids) is the most potent endogenous opioid, active mainly at μ and δ opioid receptors. Derived from pro-opiomelanocortin (99 amino acids), from which ACTH is derived. Thought to be involved in central pain pathways, emotion, etc. May also be involved in haemorrhagic and septic shock; thought to reduce SVR, cardiac output and BP, while decreasing GIT motility and sympathetic activity and enhancing parasympathetic activity. This may explain why naloxone sometimes improves cardiovascular parameters in shock.

Endothelin. Vasoconstrictor peptide derived from vascular endothelium, thought to be important in regulation of basal vascular tone and BP. Produced from an inactive precursor, it acts at specific endothelin receptors to cause vasoconstriction (type A receptors). Type B receptor activation may also result in production of nitric oxide and prostacyclin. May be involved in local blood flow and in various cardiovascular disorders, notably cardiac failure and pulmonary hypertension. Endothelin receptor antagonists such as bosentan (which antagonises both A and B receptors) have been investigated as possible treatments for these.

Endothelium-derived relaxing factor, *see Nitric oxide*

Endotoxins. Lipopolysaccharides (LPS) present on the surface of Gram-negative bacteria. LPS consists of: a lipid chain (lipid A), responsible for the biological effects; a core polysaccharide; and oligosaccharide side chains which are specific to each strain. Released when the bacteria die, and extremely toxic, probably via release and activation of many inflammatory substances including cytokines. Endotoxaemia may be involved in the aetiology of sepsis, although it may occur in the absence of infection, and proven Gram-negative sepsis may not be accompanied by endotoxaemia. Passage of GIT organisms or their endotoxins into the bloodstream across a leaking gut wall has been suggested to occur in critical illness. Attempts have been made to prevent endotoxaemia by killing GIT organisms (selective decontamination of the digestive tract), and to treat established endotoxaemia with anti-endotoxin antibodies.

Wendel M, Paul R, Heller AR (2007). Intensive Care Med; 33: 25–35

See also, Bacterial translocation

Endotracheal tubes, *see Tracheal tubes*

End-plate potentials. Depolarisation potentials produced at the postsynaptic motor end-plate of the neuromuscular

junction by binding of acetylcholine (ACh) to receptors. Their size and duration depend on the amount of ACh released, the number of ACh receptors free and the activity of acetylcholinesterase. Miniature end-plate potentials (under 1 mV) are thought to be produced by random release of ACh from single vesicles (quantal theory), and are too small to initiate muscle contraction. Simultaneous release of ACh from many vesicles follows arrival of a nerve impulse at the synapse; the resultant large end-plate potential causes depolarisation of adjacent muscle membrane, and muscle contraction.
See also, Neuromuscular transmission

End-tidal gas sampling. Gives the approximate composition of alveolar gas, unless major $\dot{V}/\dot{Q}$ mismatch exists or tidal volume is very small. Useful for estimating alveolar and hence arterial $P\text{CO}_2$, for monitoring adequacy of ventilation, etc. Alveolar concentrations of inhalational anaesthetic agents may also be monitored. May also indicate extent and rate of uptake of inhalational agents, if expired and inspired concentrations are compared, and the state of O_2 supply/demand. On-line multiple gas monitors are now routine, providing breath-by-breath measurements. Since the gas sampled by these is not strictly end-tidal, the sampling line being placed some distance away from the patient's airway, the term 'end-expiratory' is more accurately applied. Mixing of end-expiratory gas with fresh gas may lead to inaccuracy, especially if samples are taken between the breathing system filter and the anaesthetic machine.
See also, Carbon dioxide, end-tidal; Gas analysis

Energy. Capacity to perform work, whether mechanical, chemical, electrical, etc. Kinetic energy is the energy of a body due to its motion; potential energy is the energy of a body due to its state or position. Thus a body on a table has potential energy due to the effect of gravity; when it falls, this is converted to kinetic energy. Similarly, the potential energy of a stretched spring is converted to kinetic energy as it recoils. The law of conservation of energy states that energy cannot be destroyed or created, but only converted to other forms of energy, e.g. heat, light, sound, etc. Molecules within a body have potential energy due to their chemical composition and forces between them, and kinetic energy due to their movement. SI unit is the joule, although the Calorie (Cal; equals 1000 cal) is widely used for dietary energy estimations.

Energy is liberated in the body by breakdown of chemical bonds within foodstuffs, e.g. approximately 4 Cal/g carbohydrate and protein, 9 Cal/g fat, 7 Cal/g alcohol. It may be stored in high phosphate bonds, e.g. in ATP, and in other compounds, e.g. glycogen.
See also, Basal metabolic rate; Energy balance; Metabolism

Energy balance. Difference between Calorie intake and energy output. If intake is less than expenditure, energy balance is negative and endogenous food stores are utilised; if it is greater, balance is positive and the individual gains weight. Many critically ill patients (e.g. those with trauma, sepsis) have increased catabolism and glycogenolysis, insulin resistance with resultant lipolysis and increased basal metabolic rate. In order to provide adequate nutrition in these patients, it is important to estimate energy expenditure, e.g. with indirect calorimetry using bedside devices ('metabolic carts'). This allows measurement of O_2 and CO_2 exchange and thus respiratory exchange ratio; however such techniques are not widely used because of inaccuracies related to gas leaks from the patient/ventilator circuit and the effect of water vapour.

Normal subjects require about 25 Cal/kg/day; most critically ill patients require about 25–40 Cal/kg/day.
See also, Nitrogen balance

Enflurane. 2-Chloro-1,1,2-trifluoroethyl difluoromethyl ether (Fig. 61). Inhalational anaesthetic agent, introduced in 1966.
- Properties:
  - colourless volatile liquid with ether-like smell; vapour is 7.5 times denser than air.
  - mw 184.5.
  - boiling point 56.5°C.
  - SVP at 20°C 24 kPa (175 mmHg).
  - partition coefficients:
    - blood/gas 1.9.
    - oil/gas 98.
  - MAC 1.7% (middle age); 1.9% (young adults); 2.4–2.5% in children/teenagers.
  - non-flammable and non-corrosive. Stable without additives and unaffected by light.
- Effects:
  - CNS:
    - smooth and rapid induction and recovery.
    - epileptiform EEG activity may occur especially at doses >2 MAC, particularly with coexisting hypocapnia. Convulsions may occur postoperatively.
    - increased cerebral blood flow but reduced intraocular pressure.
    - has weak analgesic properties.
  - RS:
    - depresses airway reflexes less than halothane and therefore tracheal intubation is more difficult when the patient is breathing spontaneously.
    - causes greater respiratory depression than halothane or isoflurane; an increased respiratory rate is common, with decreased tidal volume.
    - bronchodilatation.
  - CVS:
    - causes greater myocardial depression than halothane. SVR is reduced, with compensatory tachycardia. Hypotension is common.
    - causes fewer arrhythmias than halothane, and less sensitisation of the myocardium to catecholamines.
  - other:
    - dose dependent uterine relaxation.
    - nausea and vomiting are uncommon.
    - muscular relaxation and potentiation of non-depolarising neuromuscular blocking drugs is greater than that seen with halothane or isoflurane.
    - may precipitate MH.

About 2% metabolised, the rest excreted via the lungs. Although fluoride ions may be produced by metabolism, toxic levels are usually not reached, although they have been reported in obese patients after prolonged anaesthesia. Patients with pre-existing renal impairment or receiving other nephrotoxic drugs or enzyme-inducing drugs, e.g. isoniazid, are also thought to be at risk.

```
   Cl      F         F
     \     |         |
H —  C  —  C  — O —  C — H
     /     |         |
   F       F         F
```

Fig. 61 Structure of enflurane

Hepatitis has been reported following enflurane; cross-sensitivity with halothane has been suggested but this is disputed.

Inspired concentrations of 1–3% are usually adequate for anaesthesia, with higher concentrations for induction.

Enkephalins. Endogenous opioid peptides, found in the CNS, especially:

- periaqueductal grey matter.
- periventricular grey matter.
- limbic system.
- medullary raphe nucleus.
- spinal cord, especially laminae II and III (substantia gelatinosa) of the dorsal horn.

Methionine enkephalin and leucine enkephalin (each 5 amino acids) are derived from proenkephalin; they are thought to be involved as neurotransmitters in pain pathways, e.g. gate control. Active mainly at δ opioid receptors.
See also, Endorphins

Enoxaparin, *see Heparin*

Enoximone. Selective phosphodiesterase inhibitor unrelated to catecholamines or cardiac glycosides. Used as an inotropic drug. Increases cardiac contractility and stroke volume without much tachycardia, and without increasing myocardial O_2 demand. Also causes vasodilatation, reducing both preload and afterload, and decreases left and right ventricular filling pressures. BP may fall.

Acts directly on cardiac muscle. Adrenergic and other receptors are thought to be uninvolved.

Has been used in cardiogenic or other types of shock, after cardiac surgery, and in patients awaiting heart transplants. Parenteral preparation contains alcohol, propylene glycol and sodium hydroxide (pH 12). Crystal formation may occur with glass syringes, etc. and if mixed with other drugs and dextrose solutions.

Undergoes hepatic metabolism to partially active metabolites, excreted renally.

- Dosage: 90 μg/kg/min over 10–30 min iv, followed by continuous or intermittent infusion of 5–20 μg/kg/min, up to 24 mg/kg/day.
- Side effects: hypotension, nausea and vomiting, insomnia, headache.

ENT surgery, *see Ear, nose and throat surgery*

Enteral nutrition, *see Nutrition, enteral*

Entonox. Trade name for gaseous N_2O/O_2 50:50 mixture, supplied in cylinders at a pressure of 137 bar. Cylinders are coloured blue with blue/white quartered shoulders. May also be supplied by pipeline. Formed by bubbling O_2 through liquid N_2O (Poynting effect).

Cylinders must be kept above −7°C (pseudocritical temperature) to prevent liquefaction of the N_2O (a process called lamination). If this occurs and gas is drawn from the top of the cylinder, O_2 will be delivered first, followed by almost pure N_2O. In the large cylinders used for connection to a pipeline system via a manifold, gas is therefore drawn first from the bottom of the cylinder by a tube; should liquefaction of N_2O now occur, N_2O containing about 20% O_2 is delivered first. Warming and repeated inversion of the cylinders will reconstitute the gaseous mixture.

Widely used for inhalational analgesia for trauma and minor procedures, e.g. physiotherapy or change of dressings; most commonly used with a demand valve for self-administration. Onset of analgesia is rapid, with minimal cardiovascular, respiratory or neurological side effects. Should unconsciousness occur, the patient drops the mask and recovery rapidly occurs. Caution is required if the patient has an undrained pneumothorax, as N_2O may increase its size.

Also widely used in the UK for inhalational analgesia during labour, although there is little evidence that pain scores are reduced.

Continuous use, e.g. in ICU, has declined because of interaction of N_2O with the methionine synthase system.
See also, Obstetric analgesia and anaesthesia

Envenomation, *see Bites and stings*

Environmental safety of anaesthetists. Hazards faced may be due to:

- inhalational agents: fears were expressed especially in the 1960s because of reported high incidence of lymphoid tumours in anaesthetists. Chronic exposure to low concentrations of volatile agent was thought to be responsible, hence attempts to remove excesses from the immediate atmosphere by adsorption or scavenging. Such an association is not supported by subsequent studies, and effects of breathing small amounts of volatile agents are thought to be minimal, if any. Effects of N_2O are now considered potentially more harmful; increased incidence of spontaneous abortion and possibly congenital malformation in theatre workers or their spouses is suspected but has never been conclusively proven. This may be via methionine synthase inhibition.

  Effect on performance is controversial; there is no conclusive evidence that the low atmospheric concentrations measured are deleterious. Any risks are reduced by testing apparatus for leaks, scavenging, avoiding spillage and monitoring contamination levels. The Health and Safety Commission in the UK set occupational exposure standards at a maximum of 100 ppm N_2O, 50 ppm enflurane/isoflurane and 10 ppm halothane (each over an 8-hour period) in 1996. In the USA, the National Institute for Occupational Safety and Health has recommended an 8-hour time-weighted average limit of 2 ppm for halogenated anaesthetic agents in general (0.5 ppm together with exposure to N_2O).
- infection, e.g. with hepatitis or HIV infection. Risks are reduced by immunisation against hepatitis B, wearing of gloves and goggles, avoidance of needles wherever possible, and careful disposal of any contaminated equipment. Needles should never be resheathed by holding their cover in one's hand. Devices for safe handling of used needles (e.g. non-removable caps or cannulae/syringes with self-retracting needles) became mandatory in the USA in 2001. In case of accidental needlestick injuries:
  - wash with soap and water.
  - encourage bleeding.
  - send patient's and victim's sera for testing for hepatitis, with immunoglobulin therapy if appropriate. Testing for HIV infection requires informed patient consent and counselling. Triple therapy with zidovudine and other anti-HIV agents is usually recommended as soon as possible after needlestick injury.

  Risk of infection after accidental exposure of healthcare workers is thought to be about 0.3% for HIV (needlestick; higher risk after conjunctival inoculation), 3% for hepatitis C and up to 30% for hepatitis B. Risk is affected by the number of viral particles inoculated and the route.

Other more contagious infections: deaths were reported following exposure to patients infected with severe acute respiratory syndrome.
- risk of electrocution and burns, explosions and fires, radiation exposure, back injury, stress and fatigue, etc. Access to addictive drugs makes abuse of anaesthetic agents easier. Alcohol abuse is common among doctors. Increased risk of suicide is suspected but not proven.
- personal injury during interhospital transfer of patients.

Similar concerns exist for staff on the ICU.
See also, Contamination of anaesthetic equipment; COSHH regulations

Enzyme. Protein accelerating the chemical reaction of a substance (the substrate) but remaining unchanged itself, i.e. a catalyst. May be highly specific for a substrate. Sensitive to pH and temperature.
- Classified according to the reaction catalysed:
  - oxidoreductases: oxidation/reduction, e.g. metabolism of many drugs.
  - transferases: transfer of groups between molecules, e.g. transaminases.
  - hydrolases: hydrolytic cleavage or reverse, e.g. acetylcholinesterase.
  - lysases: cleavage of C–C, C–N, etc. without oxidation, reduction or hydrolysis, e.g. decarboxylases.
  - isomerases: intramolecular rearrangements, e.g. mutases.
  - ligases: reactions involving high energy bonds, e.g. ATP, and formation of C–C, C–N, etc.

Reactions involve formation of intermediate structures, with formation of reaction products and reformation of enzyme.
See also, Enzyme induction/inhibition; Michaelis–Menten kinetics

Enzyme induction/inhibition. Certain drugs may alter the activity of enzymes involved in their metabolism, most importantly in the liver. Induction involves an increase in the amount of enzyme, caused by increased synthesis or decreased breakdown. It is usually related to the duration and extent of drug exposure. The cytochrome P_{450} system is often involved. Inhibition involves a reduction in the amount of enzyme or impairment of its activity.
- May affect metabolism of the original drug and other drugs, leading to drug interactions, e.g.:
  - enzyme induction:
    - barbiturates increase metabolism of warfarin, phenytoin and chlorpromazine.
    - phenytoin increases metabolism of digitoxin, thyroxine, vecuronium, pancuronium and tricyclic antidepressants.
    - alcohol increases metabolism of warfarin, barbiturates and phenytoin.
    - smoking increases metabolism of vecuronium, pancuronium, morphine, aminophylline, chlorpromazine and phenobarbital.
  - enzyme inhibition:
    - ecothiopate reduces metabolism of suxamethonium.
    - metronidazole reduces metabolism of acetaldehyde produced by alcohol metabolism.
    - cimetidine reduces metabolism of lidocaine, morphine, pethidine, labetalol, propranolol and nifedipine.

Sweeney BP, Bromilow J (2006). Anaesthesia; 61: 159–77

EOA, Esophageal obturator airway, *see Oesophageal obturators and airways*

Ephedrine hydrochloride. Sympathomimetic and vasopressor drug, mainly used to treat hypotension (especially in spinal and epidural anaesthesia). Sometimes used in the treatment of bronchospasm and autonomic neuropathy.
- Actions:
  - directly stimulates α- and β-adrenergic receptors.
  - releases noradrenaline from nerve endings.
  - inhibits monoamine oxidase.
- Effects:
  - increased cardiac rate, force of contraction and BP.
  - vasoconstriction.
  - bronchodilatation.
  - central arousal and pupillary dilatation.
  - increased sphincter tone.
  - placental and uterine blood flow are maintained; thus it has been traditionally considered the agent of choice in obstetric regional anaesthesia.
- Dosage:
  - 3–6 mg repeated as required up to 30 mg.
  - 15–60 mg orally/im, 8 hourly.

Tachyphylaxis occurs with repeated administration. May cause restlessness and palpitations in overdose.

Epibatidine. Substance related to nicotine, isolated from an Ecuadorian frog; found experimentally to produce analgesia with a potency up to 1000 times that of morphine via a non-opioid pathway (may act via nicotinic receptors). Toxic effects include hypertension, apnoea and convulsions, hence the search for safer related molecules.

Epidural anaesthesia. Strictly, refers to loss of sensation adequate to allow surgical procedures, the term 'epidural analgesia' referring to provision of pain relief, e.g. during labour; in practice the former term is often applied to both situations. Can be divided anatomically into cervical, thoracic, lumbar and caudal. Involves the placement of local anaesthetic agent into the epidural space. Caudal analgesia was first performed in 1901; lumbar blockade was performed by Pages in 1921 and popularised by Dogliotti in the 1920s–1930s, although it was probably introduced by Corning following his initial experiments. Continuous catheter techniques were introduced in the late 1940s.

Following injection, local anaesthetic may act at epidural, paravertebral or subarachnoid nerve roots, or directly at the spinal cord. Systemic effects may also occur.

Indications are as for spinal anaesthesia; main advantages are avoidance of dural puncture, and those related to catheter technique, i.e. allows control over onset, extent and duration of blockade. Thus used for peri- and postoperative analgesia, analgesia following chest trauma, obstetric analgesia and anaesthesia, and treatment of intractable pain. However, blockade is less intense than spinal anaesthesia, with greater chance of missed segments, and the dose of drug injected is potentially dangerous if incorrectly placed.

Opioid analgesic drugs may be injected into the epidural space to provide analgesia.
(*For anatomy, path taken by needle, etc., see Epidural space.*)
- Technique (lumbar block):
  - performed with the patient sitting or lying. Preparation of patient, avoidance of spillage of cleansing solution, etc., is as for spinal anaesthesia. Full aseptic technique including sterile gown is usual in the UK, especially when a catheter is inserted.
  - median/paramedian approaches are used as for spinal anaesthesia. Easier catheter insertion, with less risk of dural or vascular puncture, is claimed for the latter

approach. It may also be easier in the elderly, particularly if back flexion is difficult or the ligaments are calcified.
- after deep and superficial infiltration with local anaesthetic, the skin is punctured with a lancet, to avoid pushing a skin plug into the tissues.
- 16–19 G Tuohy needles are usually employed, especially for catheter insertion. The curved blunt tip reduces the risk of dural puncture and facilitates catheter direction (Fig. 62). The needle is usually marked at 1 cm intervals (Lee markings), and may be winged. The Crawford needle (straight-tipped with an oblique bevel) is sometimes used. The stilette is removed when the needle tip is gripped by the interspinous ligament (*see Vertebral ligaments*). Less damage to the longitudinal ligamentous fibres has been claimed if the needle is inserted with the bevel facing laterally; the needle may then be rotated 90° once the space is entered. However, insertion with the bevel facing cranially has also been advocated, since this avoids the possible risk of dural puncture during rotation of the needle.
- the epidural space is identified by using tests of the negative pressure that is usually present therein, e.g. hanging drop technique, bubble indicator placed at needle hub, collapsing balloons (e.g. Macintosh's) or drums, etc., or by the 'loss of resistance' technique:
  - a low-resistance syringe, e.g. glass, is attached to the needle (after checking first to ensure a smooth action). It may be filled with:
    - saline: minimal 'give' when compressed, thus easier to judge resistance to injection. May be confused with CSF if dural puncture occurs (differentiated by detection of glucose/protein in CSF but not in saline, using reagent strips).
    - air: avoids confusion with CSF but compressible in the syringe, i.e. 'bounces'; judgement of loss of resistance is therefore harder. Neckache is common; it is thought to be caused by small air emboli (may be detected by sensitive Doppler ultrasound). Pneumocephalus has been reported.
    - local anaesthetic: may be less painful during insertion, but risks iv or subarachnoid injection.
  - continuous pressure is applied to the plunger as the needle is advanced, until a sudden 'give' is felt. Alternatively, pressure is applied intermittently after each (small) advance of the needle. The former technique is thought to be more likely to push the dura away from the needle when the epidural space is entered. In either case, the operator's other hand controls advancement, e.g. by placing the back of the hand against the patient's back and gripping the needle firmly between thumb and fingers.
  - high resistance to injection is encountered whilst the needle tip is in the ligamentum flavum; sudden loss of resistance with easy injection occurs when the epidural space is entered.

  More recently, syringe devices with spring-loaded plungers have been described; when the epidural space is entered the plunger automatically moves within the barrel.
- injection of a test dose through the needle is controversial and rarely performed, especially if a catheter is to be inserted.
- injection through the needle may be 'single shot' or fractionated; faster onset and higher block are claimed for the former but better control and safety claimed for the latter.
- catheter technique:
  - a 16–18 G catheter is inserted through the needle and directed usually upwards within the epidural space. Incidence of bloody tap is thought to be reduced if saline is injected before the catheter is inserted. If insertion is difficult, injection of 5–10 ml saline or slight straightening of the legs may help. The catheter should never be pulled back through the needle, as its tip may be sheared off. Smaller needles are available for children.
  - the needle is removed over the catheter. 2–5 cm of the latter is usually left in the space; too little may increase risk of its falling out; too much may increase risk of inadequate block, e.g. by passing through an intervertebral foramen. After observation for CSF or blood drainage, the catheter is fixed to the patient's back.
  - catheter types:
    - single end hole: thought to be more likely to obstruct, and to produce incomplete blockade, e.g. if the tip is near an intervertebral foramen.
    - closed end with (usually three) side holes The most common type in the UK. May account for development of extensive blockade, e.g. if the distal hole is located in the subarachnoid space and the proximal hole is in the epidural space. Solution injected slowly is thought to leave via the proximal hole with epidural block as expected; rapid injection may produce subarachnoid injection. Similar events may occur with iv placement of the tip.
  - a 0.2 µm filter is attached to the proximal end of the catheter to reduce bacterial contamination and injection of fragments from ampoules, etc.
  - test doses of 2–3 ml local anaesthetic (or bigger volumes if low concentrations are used) are commonly used to detect accidental subarachnoid or intravascular placement of the catheter, although the use of test doses is controversial.
  - single or fractionated injections are controversial as above.
  - assessment and management of blockade: as for spinal anaesthesia.
- Thoracic block:
  - especially useful for postoperative analgesia and pain relief following trauma. Allows selective blockade of required thoracic segments with sparing of lower segments.
  - general principles are as above. The paramedian approach is usually employed, since thoracic spinous processes are angled more steeply caudally, making the median approach difficult. The negative pressure is

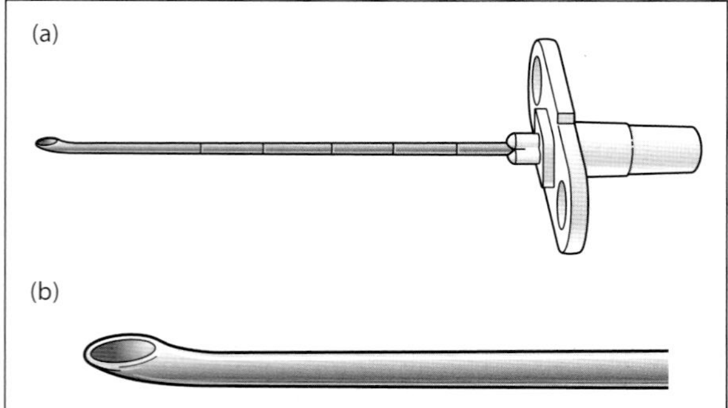

Fig. 62 (a) Winged Tuohy needle. (b) Detail of tip

of greatest magnitude in the thoracic region; this may aid identification of the epidural space.
- the needle is inserted lateral to the interspace below that to be blocked, and directed slightly medially to encounter the lamina. It is then walked off cranially to enter the ligamentum flavum.
- a catheter technique is almost always used.

- Cervical block: has been performed for pain therapy, and for carotid artery, thyroid and arm surgery. General principles are as above.
- Solutions used:
  - bupivacaine, levobupivacaine or ropivacaine 0.25–0.75%, and lidocaine 1–2%, are most commonly used in the UK. Onset with bupivacaine is about 15–30 min; effects last about 1.5–2.5 h. Lower concentrations of bupivacaine (≤ 0.1%), especially combined with opioids, e.g. fentanyl 2–4 μg/ml, are commonly used to provide analgesia whilst allowing mobility, particularly in obstetrics and for postoperative analgesia (*see Spinal opioids*). Infusions (≤ 15–20 ml/h) or boluses (≤ 20 ml) may be used; the former are especially common postoperatively since the duration of action is shorter than with concentrated solutions. Onset with lidocaine is about 5–15 min; effects last about 1–1.5 h if 1: 200 000 adrenaline is added. The more concentrated solutions are used if muscle relaxation is required. Carbonated/pH-adjusted solutions produce faster onset of denser blockade.
  - lumbar blockade: 10–30 ml is usually adequate. Rough guide: 1.5 ml/segment to be blocked, including sacral segments; 1.0 ml/segment if over 50 years or in pregnancy; 0.75 ml/segment if over 80 years.

    Reduction of requirement with age is thought to be due to decreased leakage, e.g. through intervertebral foramina. The above scheme does not take into account body size or site of injection/catheter insertion.

    Effect of gravity: the dependent side tends to experience faster and denser block.
  - thoracic block: 3–5 ml is used to block 2–4 segments at the required level.
  - cervical block: 6–8 ml is usually used.
  - tachyphylaxis is common; it may be related to local pH changes but the precise mechanism is unclear.
- Effects: similar to spinal anaesthesia, but block (and hypotension) are slower in onset. Density of block and muscle relaxation are less, with greater incidence of incomplete block.
- Contraindications: as for spinal anaesthesia.
- Complications:
  - related to insertion of needle/catheter:
    - trauma:
      - local bruising/pain.
      - neurological damage is rare, although restriction of the technique to awake patients has been suggested, especially for thoracic or cervical block. This suggestion is controversial.
    - bloody tap: if bleeding occurs through the needle, it should be withdrawn and a different space used. If blood is obtained through the catheter (vigorous aspiration is avoided as it may collapse the veins), withdrawal of the catheter 1 cm following saline flushing may be performed. If blood is still obtained when flushed, and when the open end is held below the level of the patient, a different space should be used. If no further flow of blood occurs, the catheter may be fixed. Subsequent injection of local anaesthetic is performed with care in case the catheter still lies (at least partially) within a vein.
    - epidural haematoma: as for spinal anaesthesia. Epidural catheters have been placed safely in patients undergoing subsequent anticoagulant therapy.
    - dural tap: usually obvious if caused by the epidural needle, as CSF flows back. Puncture by the epidural catheter may be harder to detect; flow of CSF may not be obvious, especially if saline was used to identify the epidural space.
    - shearing of the catheter tip: should be documented and the patient informed. Thought not to have adverse effects.
    - knotting of the catheter is possible if excessive lengths are inserted.
  - following injection of drug:
    - hypotension as for spinal anaesthesia. A further contribution may be made by systemic absorption of local anaesthetic agent.
    - iv injection of local anaesthetic.
    - extensive blockade:
      - accidental spinal blockade (subarachnoid): onset is usually within a few minutes. May lead to total spinal block if a large amount of drug is injected, with rapidly ascending motor and sensory blockade, respiratory paralysis and central apnoea, cranial nerve involvement with fixed dilated pupils, and loss of consciousness. Management includes oxygenation with tracheal intubation and IPPV, and cardiovascular support. Recovery without adverse effects is usual if hypoxaemia and hypotension are avoided.
      - subdural blockade: piercing by the catheter of the dura but not arachnoid. Onset is typically within 20–30 min; blockade may be unilateral and include cranial nerve lesions. The arachnoid may rupture if large volumes are injected, leading to high or total spinal block.
      - unexplained, with correct epidural placement of the catheter. Partial subarachnoid or subdural catheter placement is thought to be responsible for the many patchy blocks encountered in practice. Catheter migration may occur during prolonged blockade, e.g. in obstetrics.
      - isolated cranial nerve palsies, e.g. 5th and 6th, and Horner's syndrome, have been reported.

      Extensive blocks may develop after top-up injections during apparently normal epidural blocks.
    - incomplete blockade: missed segments/unilateral block. Management: as for obstetric analgesia and anaesthesia.
    - nerve damage due to injection of incorrect drugs/solutions. In addition, preservatives in certain preparations of local anaesthetics are suspected as causing damage, as are skin cleansing solutions.
    - shivering.
    - prolonged blockade: uncommon; has lasted up to 8–12 h after the last injection.
    - anterior spinal artery syndrome: thought to be related to severe hypotension, not to the technique itself.
    - adverse drug reactions to agents used: rare.
  - late:
    - arachnoiditis, cauda equina syndrome.
    - abscess formation/meningitis: thought to be rare if aseptic techniques are used.

[Fidel Pages (1886–1923), Spanish surgeon; Achilles Dogliotti (1897–1966), Italian surgeon; Edward B Tuohy (1908–1959), US anaesthetist; John Alfred Lee (1906–1989), Southend anaesthetist; Oral B Crawford, US anaesthetist]

Epidural opioids, *see Spinal opioids*

Epidural space. Continuous space within the vertebral column, extending from the foramen magnum to the sacrococcygeal membrane of the sacral canal. The vertebral canal becomes triangular in cross-section in the lumbar region, its base anterior; the epidural space is that part external to the spinal dura. It is very narrow anteriorly, and up to 5 mm wide posteriorly.

- Boundaries:
  - internal: dura mater of the spinal cord (at the foramen magnum, reflected back as the periosteal lining of the vertebral canal).
  - external:
    - posteriorly: ligamenta flava, and periosteum lining the vertebral laminae.
    - anteriorly: posterior longitudinal ligament.
    - laterally: intervertebral foramina, and periosteum lining the vertebral pedicles. The space may extend through the intervertebral foramina into the paravertebral spaces.

Contains epidural fat, epidural veins (Batson's plexus), lymphatics and spinal nerve roots. Connective tissue layers have been demonstrated by radiology and endoscopy within the epidural space, in some cases (rarely) dividing it into right and left portions.

- Pressure in the epidural space is found to be negative in most cases, occasionally positive. Postulated explanations include:
  - artefactual or transient negative pressure:
    - anterior dimpling of the dura by the needle.
    - anterior indentation of the ligamentum flavum by the needle, followed by its sudden posterior recoil when punctured.
    - back flexion causing stretching of the dural sac, and/or squeezing out of CSF.
  - true negative pressure:
    - transmitted negative intrapleural pressure via thoracic paravertebral spaces.
    - relative overgrowth of the vertebral canal compared with the dural sac.
    - true positive pressure: bulging of dura due to pressure of CSF.
- Passage taken by an epidural needle when entering the epidural space (median approach):
  - 1: skin.
  - 2: subcutaneous tissues.
  - 3: supraspinous ligament (along the tips of spinous processes from C7 to sacrum).
  - 4: interspinous ligament (between spinous processes of adjacent vertebrae).
  - 5: ligamentum flavum (between laminae of adjacent vertebrae).
  - 6: epidural space.

The normal distance between the skin and the epidural space varies between 2 and 9 cm.
For the lateral approach: 1, 2, 5, 6.
See also, Epidural anaesthesia; Vertebrae; Vertebral ligaments

Epidural volume expansion, *see Combined spinal–epidural anaesthesia*

Epiglottis, *see Larynx*

Epiglottitis. Infection caused by *Haemophilus influenzae* type b in over 50% of cases; causes enlargement of the epiglottis with upper airway obstruction. Historically most common in children aged 2–5 years but may also occur in adults (usually aged 20–40 years); the incidence in the UK has fallen since a specific vaccine was introduced. Classically follows an acute course, with fever, marked systemic upset, stridor and adoption of the sitting position with jaw thrust forward and with open drooling mouth. These features, plus absence of cough, help distinguish it from croup. Epiglottitis may progress to complete airway obstruction, which may be provoked by pharyngeal examination, iv cannulation, etc. Although lateral X-rays of the neck may reveal epiglottic enlargement, they may also provoke obstruction, and clinical assessment is sufficient in severe cases. Pulmonary oedema may occur if obstruction is severe.

- Management:
  - assessment:
    - general state: exhaustion, toxaemia, etc.
    - respiratory distress: stridor, use of accessory respiratory muscles including flaring of the nostrils, intercostal and suprasternal recession, tachypnoea, cyanosis.
  - experienced anaesthetic, paediatric and ENT help should be sought.
  - humidified O_2 administration.
  - nebulised adrenaline (0.4 ml/kg (400 μg/kg) of a 1:1000 racemic solution to a maximum of 5 ml (5 mg)).
  - iv fluids and antibacterial drugs are required, although iv cannulation should not be attempted before relief of the airway obstruction. Chloramphenicol or ampicillin is traditionally used.
  - anaesthesia is as for airway obstruction, classically inhalational induction using halothane or more recently, sevoflurane, in O_2 with the patient sitting until tracheal intubation is possible. Induction is usually slow. Apparatus for difficult intubation plus facilities for urgent tracheostomy must be available. Atropine may be given once an iv cannula is sited. An oral tracheal tube is passed initially, and is changed for a nasal tube to allow better fixation and comfort.
  - intubation is usually required for under 24 h. Spontaneous ventilation is usually acceptable. Humidification is essential. Sedation may not be required, but care must be taken to avoid accidental self-extubation.
  - extubation is performed when the clinical condition has improved, and a leak is present around the tube. Extubation may be performed under inhalational anaesthesia but this may not be necessary.

See also, Paediatric anaesthesia

Epilepsy. Tendency to epileptic seizures, associated with paroxysmal discharge of cerebral neurones.

- Traditionally classified into:
  - generalised:
    - grand mal (tonic–clonic convulsions): tonic (sustained muscle contraction) followed by clonic (jerking) phases lasting about 30 s, each with loss of consciousness. May be preceded by prodromal symptoms hours or days before, and an aura minutes before.
    - petit mal (absence seizures): characterised by 3 Hz synchronised spikes on the EEG. Rarely associated with loss of consciousness and clonic movements.
  - partial (focal):
    - may occur with or without loss of consciousness.
    - classic presentations:
      - temporal: associated with auditory, visual or olfactory hallucinations and emotional or mood changes.

- Jacksonian: clonic movements spreading from an extremity, e.g. single digit, to involve the whole body.

Definition of disease is difficult because certain stimuli will induce convulsions in normal subjects, e.g. hypoxia. Usually idiopathic, especially in childhood; intracranial lesions must be excluded in adults presenting with a single seizure. Pyrexia is a common cause in children; other causes are as for convulsions.

Treatment is with anticonvulsant drugs, and is directed at any underlying cause.

- Anaesthetic considerations:
  - preoperative assessment: frequency of seizures, date of last seizure, drug therapy (including measurement of blood levels where appropriate), etc. Identification of cause if known.
  - therapy is maintained up to surgery; benzodiazepines are often used for premedication because of their anticonvulsant activity.
  - anaesthetic drugs associated with convulsions are avoided, e.g. enflurane, ketamine. Although propofol may activate the EEG at low concentrations and has been implicated in convulsions, it has also been used successfully to treat status epilepticus. Thiopental, halothane and isoflurane are known to have anticonvulsant properties and are therefore the traditional drugs of choice. Doxapram is avoided. Hypocapnia lowers the threshold to epileptiform activity.
  - regional techniques are not contraindicated, but are often avoided for fear of reduced convulsive threshold to local anaesthetic agents, and risk of convulsions during the procedure.
  - anticonvulsant therapy is restarted as soon as possible postoperatively.

[John Hughlings Jackson (1835–1911), English neurologist]

Epinephrine, *see Adrenaline*

Epistaxis. Nasal bleeding. May occur from:
- veins of the nasal septum (younger patients).
- arterial anastomoses of the lower part of the nasal septum (Little area), especially in older patients. May be associated with hypertension.

Usually follows trauma, but predisposing conditions include bleeding disorders, hereditary telangiectasia and raised venous pressure. Bleeding may be caused by nasal intubation or passage of a nasal airway, especially if a vasoconstrictor, e.g. cocaine, is not used first.

Usually managed by nasal packing but may require ligation of the maxillary or anterior ethmoidal arteries, the former via the neck or oral route, the latter from the front of the nose.

Anaesthetic management is similar to that of the bleeding tonsil (*see Tonsil, bleeding*).

[James L Little (1836–1885), US surgeon]

EPLS, *see European Paediatric Life Support*

Epoprostenol, *see Prostacyclin*

EPSP, Excitatory postsynaptic potential, *see Synaptic transmission*

Eptacog alpha. Recombinant activated coagulation factor VII (factor VIIa). Prohaemostatic agent that activates the coagulation cascade mainly via factors IX and X. Used for patients with complicated coagulation disorders, both pre-existing (e.g. certain types of haemophilia) and acquired, e.g. after major surgery or trauma. Because of the difficulty studying the latter group, most experience is limited to case series and anecdotal reports and this, along with the high cost of the preparation (~£500 per mg), makes its use controversial. Associated with a 1–2% incidence of thrombotic complications, adding to the controversy.
- Dosage: up to 120 μg/kg iv over 3–5 min, repeated 2–6 hourly (n.b. not currently licensed for use in coagulopathy related to trauma/surgery).
- Side effects: hypersensitivity, arterial and venous thrombosis.

Levi M, Peters M, Buller HR (2005). Crit Care Med; 33: 883–90

Eptifibatide. Antiplatelet drug, used in unstable angina or non-Q wave MI. Acts by reversibly inhibiting activation of the glycoprotein IIb/IIIa complex on the surface of platelets.
- Dosage: 180 μg/kg iv followed by 2 μg/kg/min for up to 72 h (96 h if percutaneous coronary intervention performed).
- Side effects are related to increased bleeding. Platelet function takes up to 2–4 h to return to normal after discontinuation of therapy.

Equivalence. Amount of a substance divided by its valence. Equivalent weight (gram equivalent) is the weight of substance combining with or chemically equivalent to 8 g O_2, or 1 g hydrogen.

Electrical equivalence is the number of moles of ionised substance divided by valence.

Erg. cgs system unit of work. 1 erg = work done by a force of 1 dyne acting through a distance of 1 centimetre.

Ergometrine maleate. Uterine muscle stimulant, used to reduce postpartum or postabortion uterine bleeding. Uterine contraction occurs 5 min after im injection and 1 min after iv injection; it lasts up to an hour. Slowly being replaced by synthetic oxytocin because of its adverse effects (nausea, vomiting, and vasoconstriction causing a marked rise in BP and CVP; the latter is exacerbated by autotransfusion of blood from the uterus, and lasts up to several hours). Hazardous therefore in patients with cardiovascular disease, particularly pre-eclampsia. Despite this, it is often given routinely combined with oxytocin at the end of the second stage of labour. An aggravating role of ergometrine-induced vasoconstriction has been suggested in aspiration pneumonitis. Has been used as a vasopressor, e.g. in spinal anaesthesia.
- Dosage: 0.1–0.5 mg im/iv; 0.5–1.0 mg orally.

See also, Uterus

Errors. In statistics, may lead to incorrect conclusions because of inadequate test design and analysis, too small a sample size or inaccurate data collection. May be:
- type I (α; false positive): acceptance of a result as not due to chance when it is. Represented by the *P* value (probability); a value of 0.05 is usually accepted as the maximum acceptable.
- type II (β; false negative): rejection of a result as due to chance when it is not. A value of 0.2 is usually considered the maximum acceptable.

It is thus easier to demonstrate a non-significant result than a significant one. As the required *P* value is made smaller, the risk of rejecting a real result (i.e. type II error) increases. Errors may limit the usefulness of an investigation, e.g. blood test, described by its sensitivity, specificity and predictive value.

Ertapenem. Broad spectrum carbapenem and antibacterial drug, active against Gram-positive organisms and anaerobes, but not against pseudomonas or acinetobacter species, unlike imipenem or meropenem.

- Dosage: 1 g iv once daily
- Side effects: as for imipenem.

Erythrocytes (Red blood cells). Biconcave discs, about 2 μm thick and 8 μm in diameter. Produced by red bone marrow. Contain haemoglobin, maintained in an appropriate state for O_2 transport (i.e. containing iron in the reduced state, and with generation of 2,3-DPG). Also have an integral role in carbon dioxide transport. Maintenance of structural integrity and osmotic stability is via membrane pumps; the main energy source is aerobic glycolysis.

Circulating lifespan is about 120 days; they are removed by the reticuloendothelial system and broken down, with salvage and reuse of iron and amino acids from haemoglobin.

- Normal laboratory findings (adult):
  - red cell count (RBC): 4.5–6.0 × 10^{12}/l blood (male); 4.0–5.2 × 10^{12}/l blood (female).
  - reticulocyte count: under 2% of red cells. Increased in red cell loss from haemolysis or haemorrhage, signifying a normal bone marrow response. Also increased in treatment of deficiency anaemias.
  - mean corpuscle volume (MCV): 80–100 fl. Decreased in iron deficiency or defective haemoglobin synthesis. Increased when reticulocyte count is increased, or due to megaloblastic cell formation (e.g. vitamin B_{12}/folate deficiency). Also increased in alcoholism.
  - mean corpuscle haemoglobin (MCH): 26–34 pg.
  - mean corpuscle haemoglobin concentration (MCHC): 32–36 g/dl. Decreased in iron deficiency or defective haemoglobin synthesis.
  - erythrocyte sedimentation rate (ESR): < 10 mm/h. Measure of the rate at which red cells settle when a column of blood is left for 1 h. High values indicate reduced settling. Increased in many inflammatory and infective diseases, malignancy, old age and pregnancy.

Examination of the peripheral blood film gives information about haematological disease, e.g. abnormally shaped erythrocytes (sickle cell anaemia, hereditary spherocytosis, target cells in impaired haemoglobin production or liver disease, etc.).

See also, Erythropoiesis

Erythromycin. Macrolide type antibacterial drug with similar spectrum to penicillin; thus a useful alternative in penicillin allergy. Especially useful in respiratory infections (including Legionnaires' disease and mycoplasma infections) and staphylococcal infections. Also promotes GIT activity via stimulation of GIT motilin receptors; has been successfully used as a prokinetic drug in ileus (given iv or via nasogastric tube).

- Dosage:
  - 250 mg–1 g orally, 6 hourly.
  - 50 mg/kg/day by iv infusion or in divided doses 6 hourly.
- Side effects: nausea, vomiting, abdominal pain, diarrhoea, rash, reversible hearing loss, arrhythmias, pain on iv injection.

Erythropoiesis. Formation of erythrocytes, usually restricted to the vertebrae, sternum, ribs, upper long bones and iliac crests in adults. Requires iron, vitamin B_{12} and folate, and possibly other vitamins and minerals. Stepwise differentiation from stem cells includes haemoglobin synthesis and nuclear extrusion to form reticulocytes, taking about 7 days. Stimulated by erythropoietin.

Erythropoietin. Glycoprotein hormone secreted mainly by the kidneys, but also by the liver. Secretion is increased by haemorrhage and hypoxia (possibly via prostaglandin synthesis), and inhibited by increased numbers of circulating erythrocytes. Causes increased erythropoiesis. Erythropoietin receptors have also been found in the CNS and are thought to be involved in neuronal development. Infusion of erythropoietin produced by recombinant genetic engineering has been used to treat anaemia in renal failure, but treatment is very expensive. It has also been used to increase the yield of blood collected for autologous blood transfusion, e.g. 300 U/kg thrice weekly, reducing to 100 U/kg after 2 weeks. The first dose given iv produces higher levels; subsequent sc dosage produces a more sustained effect. Red cell aplasia has been reported following its sc use in renal failure.

Escape beats. On the ECG, complexes arising from sites other than the sinoatrial node, when the latter does not discharge (i.e. sinus arrest or severe bradycardia). Distinct from ectopic beats, which arise prematurely in the cardiac cycle.

Esmolol hydrochloride. Cardioselective β-adrenergic receptor antagonist, with no intrinsic sympathomimetic activity. Hydrolysed by red blood and other esterases, with a half-life of 9 min. Used to treat AF, atrial flutter and SVT, and during anaesthesia to prevent/treat tachycardia, e.g. associated with tracheal intubation. Has been used in hypotensive anaesthesia.

- Dosage:
  - SVT, etc.: 500 μg/kg/min loading dose iv for 1 min, then 50 μg/kg/min maintenance for 4 min. If the response is inadequate, the loading dose may be repeated and the maintenance dose increased to 100 μg/kg/min, and so on until a maintenance dose of 200 μg/kg/min is reached.
  - perioperative use: 0.5–1.0 mg/kg iv over 15–30 s, followed by 50–300 μg/kg/min infusion.
- Side effects: bradycardia, hypotension, sweating, nausea, confusion, thrombophlebitis, pain on injection. Bronchospasm may occur in susceptible patients.

Esophagus, *see Oesophagus*

ESR, Erythrocyte sedimentation rate, *see Erythrocytes*

Etamsylate (Ethamsylate). Haemostatic drug, thought to reduce bleeding by correcting abnormal platelet adhesion. Does not affect fibrinolysis. Has been used to prevent and treat periventricular haemorrhage in premature babies (12.5 mg/kg 6 hourly im/iv).

Ethambutol hydrochloride. Antituberculous drug added to triple therapy (isoniazid, rifampicin, pyrazinamide) if resistance is suspected.

- Dosage: 25 mg/kg orally daily for 2 months, then 15 mg/kg daily for 6 months.
- Side effects: visual disturbances, peripheral neuritis, rash, thrombocytopenia. Requires monitoring of plasma levels (peak 2–6 mg/l; trough < 1 mg/l).

Ethamsylate, *see Etamsylate*

Ethanol, *see Alcohols*

Ethanol poisoning, see Alcohol poisoning

Ether, *see Diethyl ether*

Ethics. System of moral behaviour; often translated into medical practice by reference to four basic principles:
- autonomy: the right of a fully informed individual to choose a course of action (or inaction).
- beneficence: the obligation to do good; may not necessarily lie in preserving life if that life is of such poor quality (e.g. because of pain or severe disability) that it is considered less beneficial for the patient than death itself.
- non-maleficence: the obligation to avoid doing harm (primum non nocere). Difficulties may arise if beneficial medical interventions also cause harm (recognised in the doctrine of 'double effect'), e.g. administration of morphine to a terminally ill patient to relieve pain even though it may hasten death.
- justice: the right to receive what is deserved. Although easy in certain circumstances (e.g. requirement for dialysis in acute renal failure), other situations may be less clear (e.g. liver transplantation in chronic alcoholism). Overlaps with equity (fairness), manifested in arguments over rationing of health care.

The principles underlying ethical practice are not mutually exclusive and may even oppose one another, e.g. withholding blood from a Jehovah's Witness respects his/her autonomy whilst not practising beneficence/non-maleficence.

The above approach ('principlism') is favoured by many because it is relatively simple and easy to understand, though there are many other systems for judging the moral value of medical decisions, such as consequentialism (judgement according to the outcomes of decisions) and rights-based approaches.
- Anaesthetic/ICU implications include:
  - informed consent.
  - patients' rights to confidentiality including non-disclosure of records without permission although the doctor has statutory duties which may override this (e.g. reporting of notifiable diseases, births and deaths, etc.).
  - HIV infection: there is a moral duty to treat infected patients as well as taking steps to protect oneself. A doctor who has reason to believe that he/she is infected has a duty to seek advice and testing.
  - the duty to seek Research Ethics Committee approval and informed consent for research.
  - the duty to protect patients from sick and incompetent medical colleagues (*see Sick Doctor Scheme*).
  - do not attempt resuscitation orders and advance decisions.
  - admission criteria for, and rationing of, intensive care.
  - withholding or withdrawal of treatment (including surgery) in cases of medical futility.
  - management of terminal and palliative care.
  - euthanasia.

Waisel DB, Truog RD (1997). Anesthesiology; 87: 411–17

Ethmoidal nerve block, anterior, *see Ophthalmic nerve blocks*

Ethoheptazine citrate. Analgesic drug, used for mild/moderate pain. Combined with meprobamate, a sedative muscular antispasmodic, and aspirin.
- Dosage: 75–150 mg 8 hourly, orally.
- Side effects are largely related to meprobamate and include drowsiness and hypersensitivity.

Ethosuximide. Anticonvulsant drug used in petit mal epilepsy and myoclonic seizures. Thought to block T-type calcium channels in thalamic neurones.
- Dosage: 500 mg–1.5 g orally, daily. Therapeutic plasma concentration 40–100 mg/l.
- Side effects: GIT disturbance, drowsiness, psychiatric disturbance, rash, hepatic and renal impairment, blood dyscrasias.

Ethyl alcohol, *see Alcohol poisoning; Alcohol withdrawal; Alcoholism; Alcohols*

Ethyl chloride. Inhalational anaesthetic agent, first described in 1848; popular in the 1920s particularly for induction of anaesthesia because of its rapid action. Extremely volatile (boiling point 13°C) and difficult to control; also inflammable. Now used solely for its cooling action when sprayed on to skin, to cause anaesthesia before minor procedures or to test the extent of regional blockade.

Ethylene. Inhalational anaesthetic agent, used clinically in 1923. A gas of similar blood/gas solubility to N_2O, but more potent. Also extremely explosive and unpleasant to breathe. Cylinder body and shoulder are coloured violet.

Ethylene glycol poisoning, *see Alcohol poisoning*

Ethylene oxide, *see Contamination of breathing equipment*

Etidocaine hydrochloride. Local anaesthetic agent introduced in 1972, derived from lidocaine. Onset is rapid, and duration of action is similar to that of bupivacaine. Produces motor blockade which may exceed sensory blockade. Used in 1–1.5% solutions. Maximal safe dose is 2 mg/kg. Not available in the UK.

Etomidate. IV anaesthetic agent, introduced in 1973. A carboxylated imidazole (five-membered ring containing three carbon atoms and two nitrogen atoms) compound (Fig. 63), presented in 35% propylene glycol; pH is 8.1. 75% bound to plasma proteins after injection.
- Effects:
  - induction:
    - rapid onset of sleep, lasting up to 8 min after a single dose.
    - muscle movements are common; reduced by use of opioids.
    - pain is common when injected into small veins; reduced by mixing with 1–2 ml 1% lidocaine. Thrombosis is rare.
  - CVS/RS:
    - causes less hypotension than thiopental; thus often used in shocked patients, the elderly and those with cardiovascular disease.
    - respiratory depression is less than with thiopental.

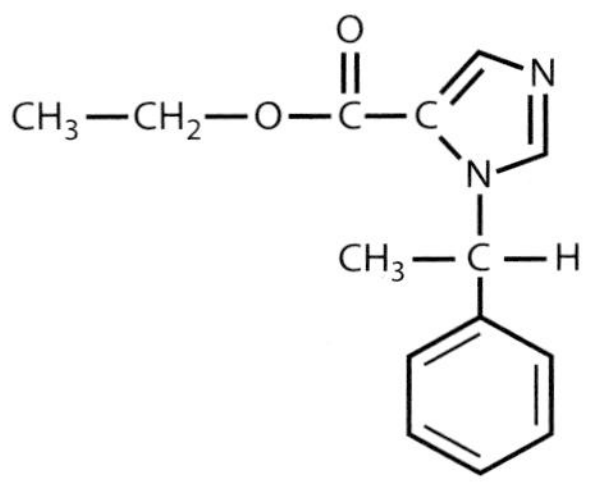

$CH_3—CH_2—O—C(=O)—C$ (imidazole ring, N-substituted with $CH_3—C—H$ bearing a phenyl ring)

Fig. 63 Structure of etomidate

- CNS:
  - not analgesic.
  - not associated with epileptiform discharges.
  - reduces cerebral blood flow and intraocular pressure.
- other:
  - increases the incidence of PONV.
  - does not cause histamine release.

● Metabolism:
- rapidly metabolised by plasma esterases and liver enzymes; elimination half-life is about 70 min. Largely excreted via the urine. Not cumulative.
- interferes with adrenal corticosteroid synthesis by inhibiting 11-β-hydroxylase and 17-α-hydroxylase. IV infusion for sedation on ICU has been implicated as increasing mortality; it is now contraindicated for this purpose. Following a single induction dose, the rise in plasma cortisol normally seen after surgery is delayed for up to 6 h. The significance of this is disputed.

● Dose: 0.2–0.3 mg/kg.

Etorphine hydrochloride. Analogue of thebaine, a naturally occurring opioid. 400 times as potent as morphine. Used to immobilise large animals.

European Academy of Anaesthesiology (EAA). Founded in 1978 to improve standards, training and research in anaesthesia. Organises the European Diploma in Anaesthesiology and Intensive Care. Amalgamated with the European Society of Anaesthesiologists and the Confederation of European National Societies of Anaesthesiologists to form the European Society of Anaesthesiology in 2005.
Thomson D (1995). Acta Anaesth Scand; 39: 442–4
See also, European Federation of Anaesthesiologists

European Board of Anaesthesiology (EBA). Governing body for specialist anaesthetic training within the European Union, under the auspices of the European Union of Medical Specialties which was founded in 1958. Works with the various anaesthetic bodies in member states.
Scherpereel P (1995). Acta Anaesth Scand; 39: 438–9

European Diploma in Intensive Care Medicine (EDIC). Organised by the European Society of Intensive Care Medicine since 1989. Consists of an English written (multiple choice) examination and an oral/clinical one (usually in the country and language of the examinee), together with a requirement for a basic medical specialty and 2 years' intensive care medicine training.

European Diploma of Anaesthesiology and Intensive Care (EDAIC). Examination held since 2005 by the European Society of Anaesthesiology, having taken over this function from the European Academy of Anaesthesiology which ran it from 1984. Consists of two multilingual parts (written and oral), each covering basic science and clinical topics. Pass rates are in the order of 60% and 80% respectively. There is also an optional in-training assessment part.
Zorab JSM (1995). Acta Anaesth Scand; 39: 579–81

European Federation of Anaesthesiologists (EFA). Umbrella organisation formed in 2001 to coordinate the activities of and encourage cooperation between the European Academy of Anaesthesiology, European Society of Anaesthesiologists and Confederation of European National Societies of Anaesthesiology. Adopted the *European Journal of Anaesthesiology* as its official journal.

European Journal of Anaesthesiology. Established in 1984. The official journal of the European Society of Anaesthesiology, having been the official journal of the European Academy of Anaesthesiology, the European Society of Anaesthesiologists, the Confederation of European National Societies of Anaesthesiology, Fondation Européenne d'Enseignement en Anaesthésiologie and European Union of Medical Specialties (since 1999) and the European Federation of Anaesthesiologists (since 2001).

European Medicines Evaluation Agency (EMEA). Body established in 1995 to regulate the introduction and investigation of new drugs throughout Europe, and to ease communication between the various national regulatory bodies. Thus acts as a link between the Committee on Safety of Medicines in the UK and similar bodies in other countries.
Herxheimer A (1996). BMJ; 312: 394

European Paediatric Life Support (EPLS). Course based on the Paediatric Advanced Life Support (PALS) course, aiming to replace the latter in Europe.

European Resuscitation Council (ERC). Formed in 1989 with a mandate to produce guidelines and recommendations appropriate to Europe for the practice of basic and advanced cardiopulmonary and cerebral resuscitation. Composed of elected representatives from the participating European countries. Held its first major international conference in 1992. Regularly produces guidelines regarding basic and advanced CPR. Has *Resuscitation* as its official journal.
See also, Resuscitation Council (UK); International Liaison Committee on Resuscitation

European Society of Anaesthesiologists (ESA). Founded in 1993 as an alternative body promoting continuous education and research in anaesthesia. Its first Annual Congress was held in 1993. Amalgamated with the Confederation of European National Societies of Anaesthesiologists and the European Academy of Anaesthesiology to form the European Society of Anaesthesiology in 2005.
Andreen M (1995). Acta Anaesth Scand; 39: 440–1

European Society of Anaesthesiology (ESA). Formed in 2005 by the amalgamated of the European Society of Anaesthesiologists, the European Academy of Anaesthesiology and the Confederation of European National Societies of Anaesthesiologists. Seeks to provide all the educational and regulatory activities of the three component organisations. Adopted the *European Journal of Anaesthesiology* as its official journal. Representation of different nationalities within the organisation is via individual members (who are all eligible to join the ESA's various committees) and the National Anaesthesia Societies Committee (NASC).
Priebe HJ (2005). Eur J Anaesth; 22: 1–3

European Society of Intensive Care Medicine (ESICM). Founded in 1982 in Geneva to advance knowledge, research and education in intensive care medicine, and subsequently to improve facilities for intensive care medicine in Europe. Holds an annual congress, organises the European Diploma in Intensive Care Medicine and administers several multicentre and multinational surveys, e.g. the European Consortium for Intensive Care Data (ECICD). Also administers the educational programme PACT. *Intensive Care Medicine* is its official journal.

European Society of Paediatric and Neonatal Intensive Care (ESPNIC). Founded and based in Brussels to advance and promote paediatric and neonatal intensive care. Has medical and nursing branches. Holds an annual congress and has *Intensive Care Medicine* as its official journal.

European Union of Medical Specialties (Union Européenne des Médecins Spécialistes; UEMS), *see European Board of Anaesthesiology*

Euthanasia. Intentional ending of a patient's life for his or her benefit, e.g. to relieve intolerable and incurable suffering. May be voluntary if administered to a competent person in response to their informed request, or non-voluntary if administered to an incompetent person. Distinction is also made between active euthanasia in which medical intervention hastens death, and passive euthanasia in which life-sustaining treatment is withheld or withdrawn (e.g. enteral feeding). Assisted suicide differs in that the physician provides the mechanism for death but the patient administers the lethal agent. Euthanasia remains illegal throughout the world except in the Netherlands, where it was legalised in 2000 with formal guidelines laid down for its use, and Belgium, where it was legalised in 2002, again with strict guidelines. Doctor-assisted suicide is legal in the Netherlands, Belgium, Oregon (USA) and Australia's Northern Territories. In Switzerland, assisted suicide has been legal since 1941 and does not require the involvement of a physician.

Emanuel EJ (2002). Arch Intern Med; 162: 142–52

EVE, Epidural volume expansion, *see Combined spinal–epidural anaesthesia*

Evoked potentials (EPs). Electrical activity recorded from the CNS or peripherally following repetitive peripheral or central stimulation. Used to investigate demyelinating disease, neuropathies and brain tumours, and in monitoring of head injury and coma. Also used to monitor and investigate depth of anaesthesia or CNS integrity during surgery.

Requires complex equipment to increase recording sensitivity and reduce interference. Recorded potentials are small (usually 1–2 μV) compared with background electrical activity (over 100 μV); the signal is amplified and (random) background activity averaged out using computer averaging. Filters reduce noise. Displayed as a plot of voltage against time; a stimulation spike occurs within 1 ms, followed by a composite pattern representing potentials from near and distant structures along the conduction pathway, depending on the sites of stimulation and recording. Upward peaks represent negative potentials by convention. Latency is the time between the stimulation spike and the first major peak; amplitude is the height from this peak to the following trough.

- Different types:
  - sensory EPs:
    - somatosensory (SEPs):
      - stimulation of the posterior tibial or median nerves, using supramaximal stimulation. Direct spinal cord stimulation may be performed to monitor cord integrity during spinal surgery.
      - recording from:
        - scalp EEG electrodes, e.g. one over the sensory area appropriate to the site of stimulus plus a reference electrode elsewhere. May also examine transmission between different sites along the conduction pathway, e.g. central conduction time (CCT) between activity at the level of C5 to cortical activity.

          In general, most anaesthetic agents increase latency and decrease amplitude (etomidate consistently increases amplitude) in a dose-related manner. Amplitude increases following tracheal intubation or skin incision, suggesting SEPs represent level of arousal rather than anaesthetic depth itself. The technique has also been used to monitor function during craniotomy, e.g. measuring CCT: impaired conduction may represent physical damage, hypoxia or ischaemia.
        - epidural space in spinal surgery; e.g. bipolar electrodes placed via an epidural needle at the lower cervical level. Electrodes may also be placed in the subdural space if the dura is opened. Skin/vertebral recording is less reliable.

          Anaesthetic agents have small effects; the technique is useful for investigating spinal conduction at any anaesthetic depth. Each side is tested individually; amplitude reduction greater than 50% during surgery is likely to indicate postoperative neurological deficit. Used for surgery for kyphoscoliosis, tumours, vascular lesions, etc., also for surgery of the brachial plexus, aortic arch, etc.
    - auditory (AEPs):
      - stimulation of the 8th cranial nerves bilaterally using headphones emitting clicks, usually at 6–10 Hz.
      - recording from scalp electrodes, e.g. vertex, mastoid, and reference on the forehead.
      - recorded pattern represents brainstem, and early and late cortical responses. Brainstem EPs are little affected by anaesthetics; early cortical EPs are most consistently affected as for SEPs.
    - visual (VEPs):
      - stimulation of optic nerves using swimming goggles incorporating light-emitting diodes; 2 Hz is usually employed.
      - recording from the occiput.
      - thought to be less reliable than SEPs or AEPs, but have been used to monitor function during surgery for lesions involving the optic nerve and chiasma, pituitary gland, etc.
  - motor EPs:
    - stimulation of the scalp using large voltages, or the motor cortex directly. Induction of potential using magnetic fields has been used.
    - recording from the median or posterior tibial nerve, or EMG of limb muscles. Very sensitive to anaesthetic agents, thus less suitable for monitoring anaesthetic depth. Recording from the epidural space is thought to be less affected by anaesthetics, and has been used for spinal surgery.

Kumar A, Bhattacharya A, Makhija N (2000). Anaesthesia; 55: 225–41

See also, Anaesthesia, depth of

Exercise. Produces physiological changes which increase oxygen flux and removal of waste products from active tissues:

- cardiovascular:
  - increased cardiac output mainly due to increased heart rate (to a maximum rate of about 195 beats/min in adults). Stroke volume increases slightly in normal individuals although it can double in trained athletes. The increase in cardiac output starts before exercise due to cortical activation of the sympathetic nervous system. Following initiation of exercise, CVS reflexes are activated following stimulation of muscle mechanoreceptors, baroreceptors and joint receptors.

- BP increases (systolic > diastolic), reflecting increased cardiac output despite decreased SVR due to vasodilatation in exercising muscles.
- increased venous return due to increased skeletal muscle pump activity and thoracic pump action.
- blood flow is diverted to skin and actively contracting muscles at the expense of renal and splanchnic blood flow. Muscle blood flow may increase 30-fold as a result of accumulation of local metabolites (e.g. K^+, lactic acid), a decrease in arterial PO_2 and an increase in PCO_2. Arteriovenous O_2 difference may increase 3-fold due to a shift of the oxyhaemoglobin dissociation curve to the right secondary to the acidosis, raised temperature in muscles and raised 2,3-DPG levels found during exercise.
- coronary blood flow may increase up to five times the resting level.

- respiratory:
  - increased minute ventilation due to increase in respiratory rate and tidal volume. The increase is proportional to the rise in oxygen demand and is due to cortical stimulation and afferent impulses from proprioceptors in muscles, tendons and joints.
  - pulmonary blood flow increases up to 6-fold. Thus oxygen uptake by the lungs can reach values of 4000 ml/min.
  - CO_2 excretion can reach values of 8000 ml/min.
- temperature regulation: the enormous amount of heat produced is dissipated by increased sweating, skin vasodilation and heat loss through expired air.

If severe exercise continues, exhaustion follows; BP falls, cutaneous vasoconstriction occurs, body temperature rises and accumulation of lactic acid and CO_2 results in increasing acidosis. Muscle cramps and fatigue occur. Exertional myoglobinuria may be seen.

Exercise testing. Most commonly, involves ECG recording while performing exercise, e.g. using a treadmill or bicycle, with workload increased in steps.

Testing is used to help diagnose obscure chest pain or breathlessness, and to indicate prognosis in ischaemic heart disease, especially following MI. S–T depression is the most significant sign during exercise, but other changes, e.g. S–T elevation, Q waves, etc., may occur. Chest pain, hypotension and arrhythmias may also be provoked. Testing may be combined with other measurements, e.g. arterial BP, respiratory rate, tidal volume, O_2 consumption, CO_2 output, arterial blood gases and cardiac output. Reduced ejection fraction (e.g. demonstrated by echocardiography) or cardiac output may suggest reversible ischaemia which may persist after cessation of exercise (myocardial stunning).

Inotropic drugs e.g. dobutamine have been used to provoke similar changes to those caused by exercise (dobutamine stress test).

Traditionally, the patient's own exercise tolerance, e.g. distance able to be walked or stairs climbed, has been used as a general indicator of cardiorespiratory function. More recently, formal cardiopulmonary exercise testing has been used to predict outcome from major surgery, using the work at which maximal O_2 consumption is reached, or the work at which anaerobic energy metabolism (anaerobic threshold) starts, as markers of cardiopulmonary reserve.

Albouaini K, Egred M, Alahmar A, Wright DJ (2007). Heart; 93: 1285–92

Exomphalos, *see Gastroschisis and exomphalos*

Exotoxins. High mw, heat labile and antigenic proteins produced by micro-organisms. Although some bacteria produce only one significant kind of exotoxin (e.g. clostridia), others produce several (e.g. streptococci and staphylococci). Exotoxins and endotoxins contribute to the pathogenesis of SIRS. Some have been used clinically, e.g. botulinum toxins.

Expert systems. Computerised systems consisting of databases of knowledge and rules which are connected to the user via an interface. The latter takes data from the database and delivers inferences to the user. A facility for adding knowledge to the database allows the system to 'learn' continually. Expert systems may be:

- diagnostic, e.g. for interpretation of arterial blood gases, etc.
- therapeutic, e.g. for providing optimal ventilator settings, etc.

Expiratory flow rate, *see Forced expiratory flow rate*

Expiratory pause, *see Inspiratory:expiratory ratio*

Expiratory reserve volume (ERV). FRC minus residual volume. Normally 1–1.2 litres. Reduced ERV is usually the cause of reduced FRC.
See also, Lung volumes

Expiratory valve, *see Adjustable pressure-limiting valve*

Expired air ventilation. Forms part of CPR. Said to be referred to in the Bible (2 Kings 4: 34–5). Reported in the 1700s and 1800s, but only became medically accepted practice in the 1950s, following demonstration that it was effective in apnoea during anaesthesia. Adequate oxygenation may be maintained with expired air of O_2 concentration 15–16%. Oxygenation is improved by the operator's inspiring O_2 between ventilations.

Having cleared the airway of food, dentures, etc., and with the patient supine, the neck is extended and the jaw held forward. In adults, the nose is pinched closed and the operator's mouth placed firmly over that of the patient (mouth-to-mouth respiration). Slow deep exhalations are made whilst observing the patient's chest for expansion. Passive exhalation is allowed. May also be performed through the patient's nose (mouth-to-nose respiration). In children, the operator's mouth is placed over the patient's nose and mouth.

Regurgitation of gastric contents may occur during expired air ventilation; this may be reduced by application of cricoid pressure if another person is available.

Various devices, some with valves, are available for avoidance of direct mouth-to-mouth contact, to improve aesthetic acceptability and reduce risk of cross-contamination; most hinder efficient ventilation. The Brook airway has a flange to cover the victim's mouth, a one-way valve and pharyngeal airway incorporated, but is now less widely used. An anaesthetic facepiece is suitable; specially designed facepieces which incorporate a one-way valve are available. Expired air ventilation may be performed through a correctly placed tracheal tube.

[Morris Brook (1911–1967), Canadian life-support instructor]

Explosions, *see Burns; Chest trauma; Explosions and fires; Incident, major; Smoke inhalation; Trauma*

Explosions and fires. Occur when a substance combines with O_2 or another oxidising agent, with release of energy.

Activation energy is required to start the process, with utilisation of energy produced to maintain combustion. If the reaction proceeds very fast, large amounts of heat, light and sound are given out, i.e. an explosion occurs. Speed of reaction is greatest for stoichiometric mixtures.

- The following are required for explosions to occur:
  - combustible substance:
    - anaesthetic agents, e.g. cyclopropane, diethyl ether. C–C bonds are susceptible to breakdown; C–F bonds are resistant, hence the non-flammability of modern inhalation anaesthetic agents.
    - alcohol used to clean skin.
    - gases, e.g. methane and hydrogen in the patient's GIT.
    - grease/oil in anaesthetic pressure gauges (*see Adiabatic change*).
  - gas to support combustion: O_2 is standard in most anaesthetic techniques. N_2O breaks down to O_2 and nitrogen with heat, producing further energy; thus reactions may be more vigorous with N_2O than with O_2 alone.
  - energy source: About 1 μJ is required for most reactions with O_2; about 100 μJ with air. Sources include:
    - sparks from:
      - build-up of static electricity.
      - electrical equipment, e.g. diathermy, monitors, switches, etc.
    - naked flames, cigarettes, hot wires, diathermy, light sources, etc.
    - lasers (*see Laser surgery*).

May result in burns, direct trauma, smoke inhalation, etc. Although uncommon now with modern techniques, explosions and fires continue to be reported.

- Precautions during anaesthesia include:
  - avoidance of flammable agents. If used, a zone of risk has been defined.
  - antistatic precautions, e.g. conductive rubber, floor, etc.
  - checking and maintenance of all electrical equipment. Use of spark-free switches.
  - use of air instead of N_2O.
  - use of circle systems.
  - air conditioning and scavenging, to reduce levels of anaesthetic agents. Sparks are reduced by maintaining relative humidity above 50%, and temperature above 20°C.

Fire-fighting equipment should be present in every operating department.

Non-combustion explosions may occur if cylinders are faulty or internal pressure excessively high.

Macdonald AG (1994). Br J Anaesth; 72: 710–22 and 73: 847–56

See also, Ignition temperature

Exponential process. One in which the rate of change of a variable at any one time depends on the value of the variable at that time.

- Different types:
  - exponential decay (negative exponential), e.g. lung deflation after a breath, radioactive decay, washout curves (Fig. 64a). Similar curves are obtained in phamacokinetics, in which several curves may be superimposed. For exponential decay:

$$y = ab^{-cx}$$

where c = a constant,
a = y at time zero,
x = time,
b = a particular base, usually e (2.718) because mathematical manipulations are easier. The equation now becomes:

$$y = ae^{-x/\tau}$$

where τ = time constant (time taken for completion of the process at the initial rate of change). At time τ:

$$y = ae^{-1}$$

Thus y at time τ = 1/e of its original value, = 36.8%. The duration of the process is also indicated by half-life (time taken for original value to fall by half; Fig. 64b).

  - build-up exponential (wash-in curve), e.g. lung inflation with a constant-pressure generator ventilator, or uptake of inhalational anaesthetic agents (Fig. 64c).
  - positive exponential (breakaway function), e.g. growth of bacteria (Fig. 64d).

Plotted on semi-logarithmic paper, exponential processes assume straight lines, e.g. used in the analysis of washout curves.

Extended mandatory minute ventilation, *see Mandatory minute ventilation*

External jugular venous cannulation. The external jugular vein passes posteriorly over the sternomastoid muscle from the angle of the jaw and joins the subclavian vein behind the midpoint of the clavicle (*see Fig. 84; Internal jugular venous cannulation*). It is often visible and thus easier to locate than the internal jugular vein, although valves may hinder cannulation and misplacement is common. In some individuals the vessel is not a distinct structure but is replaced by a venous plexus. The technique of cannulation involves placing the patient slightly head down with the arms by the side and the head turned to the contralateral side. After cleansing the skin, the skin is punctured well above the clavicle and the needle advanced immediately over the vein at about 20° to the frontal plane. A J-wire may help the catheter negotiate the valves at the junction with the subclavian vein.

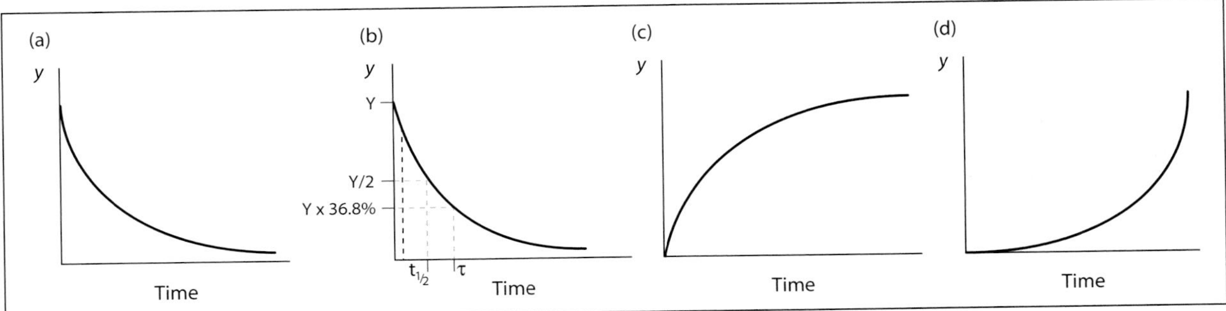

Fig. 64 Types of exponential processes: (a) and (b) exponential decay; (c) exponential build-up; (d) positive exponential

Extracellular fluid (ECF). Body fluid compartment; volume is about 14 litres (20% of body weight). Consists of interstitial fluid and plasma. Transcellular fluid (approximately 1 litre, comprised of CSF, synovial fluid, etc.) and fluid within dense connective tissue, bone, etc., are usually excluded from the definition since these fluids are not readily exchangeable.

Measurement by dilution techniques is difficult because of eventual exchange with the above compartments, and because the substance used must remain extracellular. Substances used include inulin labelled with carbon-14, mannitol, sucrose, chloride-36 ions, bromide-82 ions, sulphate and thiosulphate. Slightly different values are obtained for each.

Compositions of plasma and interstitial fluid are different (*see Fluids, body*).
See also, Dehydration; Fluid balance

Extracorporeal carbon dioxide removal ($ECCO_2R$). Method of respiratory support for extremely hypoxaemic patients. CO_2 is removed via a venovenous extracorporeal circuit and oxygenation is maintained by either apnoeic oxygenation or IPPV at very slow rates (1–4 breaths/min). The extracorporeal circuit runs at only 1 /min; thus lung ischaemia is less likely than with extracorporeal membrane oxygenation. Initial human studies showed improved survival rates compared with conventional IPPV.

Practical considerations and complications are as for cardiopulmonary bypass.

Extracorporeal circulation, *see Cardiopulmonary bypass; Extracorporeal carbon dioxide removal; Extracorporeal membrane oxygenation; Haemodiafiltration; Haemodialysis; Haemofiltration; Haemoperfusion; Plasmapheresis; Ultrafiltration*

Extracorporeal membrane oxygenation (ECMO). Method of respiratory support for extremely hypoxaemic patients. An arteriovenous extracorporeal circuit provides oxygenation and removal of CO_2 from anticoagulated blood. Very successful in neonates, e.g. with respiratory distress syndrome, but results are less clear in adults, in whom it is used mainly for temporary support prior to lung transplantation. Removal of a large proportion of the cardiac output by the arteriovenous circuit may exacerbate lung ischaemia.

Practical considerations and complications are as for cardiopulmonary bypass.

Extracorporeal shock wave lithotripsy. Introduced in the early 1980s for fragmentation of renal calculi. Has been used more recently for gallstones. Shock waves generated by the underwater discharge of a spark plug (18–24 000 V) are focused on the calculus by a computer-controlled reflector, with the patient suspended in a waterbath on a hydraulic supportive cradle. At the interface between tissue fluid and calculus, energy released from the shock wave fragments the stone. Approximately 1000–2000 shocks are required to disintegrate an average stone, taking about 30–60 min. Shocks are triggered by the ECG R wave to avoid arrhythmias. Contraindications include cardiac pacemakers unless reprogrammed (timing may be modified), aortic calcification, pregnancy and presence of orthopaedic prostheses.

Energy may be released at any interface and cause pain, e.g. at water/skin interfaces; therefore anaesthesia is required. General and regional techniques have been used. High frequency ventilation has been used, since diaphragmatic movement is reduced. Air bubbles following loss of resistance techniques using air in epidural anaesthesia have been suggested as causing neurological damage. Other anaesthetic considerations are related to positioning, temperature control, inaccessibility of the patient and monitoring, effects of immersion (increased CVP and pulmonary artery pressure), and requests for pharmacological intervention to increase heart rate and thus rate of discharge. IV fluid administration is usually required to produce a good diuresis, to wash away calculi fragments. Renal bleeding may occur if coagulation is impaired.

Plasma lactic dehydrogenase concentrations may be increased postoperatively. PONV is common.

The newest lithotriptors do not require immersion of the patient in water; the pain produced is less and sedation ± local anaesthesia may be suitable.

Extraction ratio (ER). Measure of the amount of removal of drug by an organ, e.g. liver:

$$ER = \frac{C_i - C_o}{C_i}$$

where C_i = drug concentration in blood entering the organ,
C_o = drug concentration in blood leaving the organ.

Drugs with high ER (approaching unity), e.g. lidocaine and propranolol, undergo significant first-pass metabolism in the liver after oral administration. The rate of elimination is thus dependent on hepatic blood flow as well as hepatic function, and is sensitive to enzyme induction/inhibition.

Drugs with low ER include diazepam, digoxin and phenytoin.

Extradural (epidural) haemorrhage. Haemorrhage between the periosteum and dura.

- May be:
  - intracranial: may occur from meningeal vessels (classically the middle meningeal artery), dural sinuses, or fractured bone. Features are as for head injury; typically depressed consciousness, contralateral hemiparesis and ipsilateral pupillary dilatation follow a lucid interval of a few hours after recovery from relatively minor trauma. Management: as for head injury, with urgent evacuation of the clot.
  - spinal: may occur spontaneously in patients with impaired coagulation, or following lumbar puncture, and spinal or epidural anaesthesia. Marked haemorrhage with haematoma formation may cause spinal cord/nerve compression, which may be masked by regional blockade.

Extravascular lung water (EVLW). Volume of water contained within the pulmonary interstitium and alveolar space. Usually 4–5 ml/kg. Measurement of EVLW has attracted attention as a possible means of detecting pulmonary oedema before it becomes apparent, although its usefulness in clinical practice is controversial. Controlled by Starling forces and integrity of the pulmonary capillary and alveolar epithelium. Disruption of the former (e.g. by left ventricular failure) or the latter (e.g. in acute lung injury) may result in increased EVLW.

Measured by the double indicator dilution technique in which cold indocyanine dye is injected into the right atrium. The dye is contained within the intravascular space and its dilution curve allows calculation of the intravascular compartment. In contrast, the heat (measured by a thermistor fed into the aorta) from the solution is dissipated into the surrounding lung tissue and its dilution curve represents the sum of the intravascular and extravascular compartments.

Subtraction of the curves allows calculation of the EVLW. Other methods of assessing EVLW include chest X-ray, CT and MRI scanning and positron emission tomography techniques.

See also, Cardiac output measurement; Dilution techniques

Extubation, tracheal. Problems that may occur include the following:

- cardiovascular response: similar to that on tracheal intubation but usually of reduced magnitude.
- coughing and laryngospasm: the latter is especially likely to occur at light planes of anaesthesia and in children.
- regurgitation and aspiration of gastric contents.
- airway obstruction.
- laryngeal trauma caused by the cuff if still inflated.

At the end of anaesthesia, tracheal extubation is traditionally performed with the patient either deeply anaesthetised or awake. Whilst the former avoids complications such as coughing, hypertension, etc., the latter option allows return of the patient's respiratory and laryngeal reflexes and is safer in those at risk of aspiration (in whom extubation should be performed in the lateral position) or airway obstruction. Extubation should be preceded by suction to the pharynx and larynx, preferably under direct vision, to remove secretions, etc., which might otherwise be inhaled. Secretions are particularly marked in unpremedicated patients and following neostigmine. Inflation of the lungs with O_2 immediately before and during extubation provides an O_2 reserve in case of laryngospasm and helps expel sputum, etc. from the larynx. Facilities for reintubation should be available. In patients in whom reintubation is predicted to be difficult, a bougie, fibrescope or airway exchange catheter may be placed into the trachea before extubation.

Similar considerations apply to patients in ICU after successful weaning from ventilators.

Eye, anatomy, *see Cranial nerves; Orbit; Skull*

Eye care. Important during both anaesthesia and intensive care since the eye is at risk for a number of reasons:

- the cornea is susceptible to hypoxia since it is usually covered by the eyelid when unconscious, thus preventing diffusion of O_2 from the atmosphere. General hypoxaemia may thus lead to corneal oedema which in turn may cause sloughing and corneal abrasion.
- rarely, postoperative blindness (in one or both eyes) has been reported in patients with normal preoperative vision. Ischaemic optic neuropathy associated with perioperative hypotension, anaemia, facial oedema and direct or indirect pressure on the eyes has been suggested as a cause.
- normal protective mechanisms (blink reflex, and the upturning of the eye and complete closure of the lids during normal sleep) are obtunded by anaesthesia.
- direct damage may be caused by anaesthetic equipment, etc. especially during procedures involving the head and neck, e.g. intubation.
- inhalational agents may be irritant to the cornea.
- tear production is impaired by anaesthesia, especially after 1–2 h duration; resultant drying out may lead to corneal abrasion.
- lasers are increasingly used in surgery, especially around the head and neck.

Paraffin-based ointments reduce the incidence of abrasions but may impair vision for up to several hours. Methylcellulose or saline drops may also be efficacious but require regular administration (e.g. hourly). Taping of the eyes is the simplest method of preventing corneal abrasions although many anaesthetists do this only if the eyes do not close completely.

Suresh P, Mercieca F, Morton A, Tullo AB (2000). Intensive Care Med; 26: 162–6

Eye, penetrating injury. Anaesthetic considerations:

- as for any intraocular ophthalmic surgery.
- risk of expulsion of intraocular contents should intraocular pressure (IOP) rise.
- may present as an acute emergency following trauma, for eye or other surgery, i.e. with risk of aspiration of gastric contents.

- Management:
  - preoperatively:
    - general assessment, particularly of airway and risk of difficult intubation.
    - delaying surgery should be considered if possible, to allow gastric emptying. Risk of aspiration pneumonitis may be reduced by metoclopramide, H_2 receptor antagonists, etc.
  - perioperatively: choice to be made, if surgery cannot wait:
    - to risk the rise in IOP caused by suxamethonium whilst performing rapid sequence induction. Risks may be reduced by:
      - pressure bandage to the eye.
      - methods used to reduce the rise in IOP, although not always reliable:
        - 'generous' dose of induction agent, or a supplementary dose before intubation, especially using propofol.
        - iv β-adrenergic receptor antagonists, lidocaine, opioids, acetazolamide, and non-depolarising neuromuscular blocking drug pretreatment have been studied, with mixed results.

      Some centres have reported that use of suxamethonium need not result in loss of intraocular contents.
    - to use alternative means of achieving tracheal intubation (although laryngoscopy and intubation themselves raise IOP):
      - modified rapid sequence induction, using vecuronium, atracurium or rocuronium. Injection of the neuromuscular blocking drug before injection of the induction agent has been advocated, though intubating conditions may be suboptimal and with increased risk if intubation fails. The priming principle has been used.
      - inhalational induction/awake intubation: however, coughing and straining increases IOP.
      - the above may be combined with measures to reduce risk from aspiration.

The decision is controversial; i.e. 'to save the eye or the lungs'. The individual patient's medical condition and severity of injury, and the skill of the anaesthetist, should be carefully considered before deciding on the most appropriate technique. Ultimately, safe tracheal intubation must take precedence over protection of the eye. Other drugs known to increase IOP, e.g. ketamine, should be avoided.

F wave, *see Atrial flutter*.

Facepieces. The traditional black antistatic rubber anaesthetic masks, with soft edges or inflatable rims, have largely been replaced by clear, disposable, plastic masks, especially in ICU and during CPR. Ideally, they should have minimal dead space and make an airtight seal with the patient's face. Some are malleable to improve fit. Damage may be caused to eyes, nose and face if excessive pressure is used. Dead space may be measured using water, and may be up to 200 ml if the elbow attachment is included. Paediatric facepieces may be small versions of adult ones, or may be specially designed to minimise dead space, e.g. Rendell-Baker's (anatomically moulded to fit the face).
[Leslie Rendell-Baker, Californian anaesthetist]
See also, Open-drop techniques

Facet joint injection. Injection of the posterior facets of the intervertebral joints, performed in patients with mechanical low back pain not associated with leg symptoms or signs of root irritation/compression. The posterior primary ramus of each spinal nerve divides into lateral and medial branches; the latter supplies the lower portion of the facet joint capsule at that spinal level and the upper portion of the capsule below. Thus two posterior primary rami must be blocked to anaesthetise one facet joint.

With the patient prone, the joint is located using image intensification radiography, and a needle inserted under local anaesthesia. It is walked medially and superiorly off the transverse process of the vertebra to reach the angle where the lateral edge of the facet joint meets the superomedial aspect of the transverse process. Local anaesthetic agent may be injected, or longer-lasting relief obtained by destroying the facet joint nerve using radiofrequency rhizolysis.
Cohen SP, Raja SN (2007). Anesthesiology; 106: 591–614

Facial deformities, congenital. Patients may present for radiological assessment and corrective cosmetic surgery.
- Anaesthetic considerations are usually related to:
  - airway difficulties including difficult intubation.
  - other congenital abnormalities, e.g. CVS, renal, CNS, etc.
  - general problems of paediatric anaesthesia and plastic surgery, e.g. fluid balance, heat and blood loss during prolonged procedures. Topical vasoconstrictors may be used to reduce bleeding.
  - repeat anaesthetics.
- Common conditions:
  - cleft lip and palate: incidence is about 1 in 600; it may involve the lip only (right, left or bilateral), palate only, or combinations thereof. Other abnormalities are present in up to 15% of cases. Swallowing abnormalities may be present, with risk of aspiration pneumonitis. Surgery for cleft lip is usually performed at 3–6 months, for cleft palate at 6–12 months.

    Induction of anaesthesia is as for standard paediatric anaesthesia, but tracheal intubation may be difficult if the laryngoscope blade slips into the cleft. To prevent this the cleft may be packed with gauze or the Oxford blade used. Preformed or rigid tracheal tubes are usually employed, with a throat pack. Further surgery may be required in later years.
  - mandibular hypoplasia: e.g. in Pierre Robin syndrome (macroglossia, cleft palate and cardiac defects) and Treacher Collins syndrome (choanal atresia, downwards sloping eyes, deafness, low-set ears and cardiac defects). The small mandible leaves little room for the tongue, the larynx appearing anterior. Intubation may be extremely difficult; deep inhalational anaesthesia, awake or blind nasal intubation, cricothyrotomy and tracheostomy have been employed.
  - hypertelorism (increased distance between the eyes): associated with many other abnormalities or syndromes, including airway abnormalities. Corrective surgery may include mandibular or maxillary osteotomies, craniotomy and multiple rib grafts, and is often prolonged with much haemorrhage.
  - other deformities which may produce airway problems include macroglossia, cystic hygroma and branchial cyst. Raised ICP may occur with hydrocephalus and craniosynostosis (premature closure of the cranial sutures).

[Edward Treacher Collins (1862–1919), English ophthalmologist; Pierre Robin (1867–1950), French paediatrician]
Nargozian C (2004). Pediatr Anaesth; 14: 53–9
See also, Intubation, difficult

Facial nerve block. Performed to prevent blepharospasm during ophthalmic surgery, e.g. with retrobulbar block.
- Methods:
  - local anaesthetic infiltration between muscle and bone along the lateral and inferior margins of the orbit.
  - injection of 5 ml solution over the condyloid process of the mandible, just anterior to the ear and below the zygoma.

Facial trauma. Anaesthetic and resuscitative considerations are related to the presence of other trauma (especially to head, chest and neck), alcohol ingestion, risk of aspiration of gastric contents, possible airway obstruction and difficult tracheal intubation, and postoperative management of the airway.
- Classification of facial injuries:
  - maxillary fractures: often more serious, and associated with significant head injury. Classified by Le Fort after dropping heavy objects on to the faces of cadavers:
    - I: transverse fractures of mid-lower maxilla.
    - II: triangular fracture from top of the nose to base of the maxilla.
    - III: severe fractures, with disruption of facial bones from the skull. Cribriform plate disruption and CSF leak are common.
  - zygomatic fractures: may hinder mouth opening.
  - nasal fractures: may require reduction under anaesthesia; tracheal intubation and insertion of a throat pack

should always be performed in case of epistaxis, even though reduction is usually quick.

- Anaesthetic management:
  - preoperatively:
    - assessment for the above factors. Airway obstruction and major haemorrhage are more likely with bilateral fractures.
    - gastric contents include food or drink (including alcohol), swallowed blood, etc. Fractures rarely require immediate surgery; thus a period of preoperative starvation is usually possible.
    - the patient should be warned about postoperative inability to open the mouth if the jaw is wired.
    - premedication is according to preference. Opioid premedication is usually withheld if inhalational induction of anaesthesia is planned or head injury suspected.
  - perioperatively:
    - rapid sequence induction may be necessary. Other techniques may be required if airway obstruction or cervical instability is present (e.g. awake fibreoptic tracheal intubation, tracheostomy).
    - nasal tracheal intubation is usually required. Oral intubation may be performed first to secure the airway.
    - procedures often involve wiring of jaw segments together, and splinting of the mandible to the upper jaw. Silk threads are sometimes used. Plates may be applied, with wiring 1–2 days later.
  - postoperatively:
    - tracheal extubation (if appropriate) should be performed when the patient is awake and in the lateral position. If severe oedema is anticipated, the tracheal tube is left in place postoperatively until swelling has subsided. Oral suction may be impossible.
    - the tracheal tube may be withdrawn into the pharynx to act as a nasal airway or an airway exchange catheter placed.
    - postoperative care should be on HDU/ICU, since the airway must be closely watched for obstruction, bleeding, etc. Wire cutters should be next to the patient at all times.

[René Le Fort (1829–1893), French surgeon]

See also, Dental surgery; Faciomaxillary surgery; Induction, rapid sequence; Intubation, difficult

Facilitation, post-tetanic, *see Post-tetanic potentiation*

Faciomaxillary surgery. Anaesthesia may be required for elective surgery (e.g. for facial deformities, tumours) or because of facial trauma, infection or airway obstruction. General considerations are as for ENT, plastic and dental surgery, in particular problems of access, protection of the airway (perioperatively) and the potential for long and bloody surgery. Bradycardia may occur during procedures around the face (*see Oculocardiac reflex*).

Faculty of Anaesthetists, Royal College of Surgeons of England. Founded in 1948 at the request of the Association of Anaesthetists, in order to manage the academic side of anaesthesia whilst the latter body concentrated on general and political aspects. Organised and regulated the FFARCS examination, training of junior anaesthetists, etc., until it became the College of Anaesthetists in 1988 and thence the Royal College of Anaesthetists in 1992. The corresponding Faculty in Ireland was founded in 1959, becoming a College in 1998.

Faculty of Pain Medicine, Royal College of Anaesthetists. Established in 2007, to promote education, training and excellence in the delivery and management of pain medicine.

Justins DM (2008). Brit J Anaesth; 101: 4–7

Fade. Gradual decrease (decrement) in strength of muscle contraction during tetanic stimulation, exaggerated in non-depolarising neuromuscular blockade. Thought to be caused partly by inadequate mobilisation of acetylcholine in presynaptic nerve endings at the neuromuscular junction compared with the rate of release. Block of prejunctional acetylcholine receptors, which normally increase mobilisation by a positive feedback mechanism, is thought to be involved during neuromuscular blockade. Thus patterns of fade are different with different blocking drugs, reflecting their different affinities for prejunctional receptors (e.g. greater with tubocurarine than with pancuronium).

Feldman S (1993). Anaesthesia; 48: 1–2

Failed intubation, *see Intubation, failed*

Fallot's tetralogy. Commonest cause of cyanotic heart disease (65%), accounting for 5–10% of congenital heart disease.

- Consists of:
  - VSD.
  - pulmonary stenosis (ranges from subvalvular stenosis to pulmonary atresia).
  - overriding aorta.
  - right ventricular hypertrophy.

Blood flow from right ventricle to pulmonary artery is reduced, with shunting through the VSD and aortopulmonary collaterals.

- Features:
  - hypoxaemia and cyanosis, usually from birth, with secondary polycythaemia. Dyspnoea occurs on effort.
  - acute exacerbations of shunt are traditionally blamed on infundibular spasm; increased pulmonary vascular resistance secondary to hypoxia has also been suggested. Features include worsening cyanosis, syncope and metabolic acidosis. Squatting is classically described in children; thought to increase SVR and encourage pulmonary blood flow.
  - supraventricular arrhythmias; right heart failure in adults.
  - a loud pulmonary murmur suggests mild stenosis. A large VSD may be unaccompanied by a murmur.

Corrective surgery is usually performed within the first year of life. The VSD and right ventricular outflow are repaired with patches; right ventricular pressure measurement indicates whether there has been adequate relief of obstruction. Shunt procedures are performed for palliation if marked polycythaemia or pulmonary arterial hypoplasia is present.

- Anaesthetic management:
  - as for congenital heart disease, VSD, cardiac surgery, paediatric anaesthesia.
  - infundibular spasm is provoked by fear, anxiety, etc. and may be treated with β-adrenergic receptor antagonists. Sedative premedication is often given.
  - avoidance of air bubbles in iv injectate, because of the risk of systemic embolisation.
  - peripheral vasodilatation worsens shunt and cyanosis. Vasopressor drugs, e.g. phenylephrine, may be used to increase SVR and pulmonary blood flow.

[Etienne-Louis Fallot (1850–1911), French physician]

False negative/false positive, *see Errors*

Familial periodic paralysis. Rare group of autosomal dominant myopathies due to defects in ion channels in skeletal muscle; characterised by episodes of extreme weakness, often precipitated by extremes of temperature, physical activity, stress and large carbohydrate loads. Although traditionally classified into hypo- or hyperkalaemic variants, the condition may be associated with normal plasma potassium levels. Diagnosis may be difficult, but exercise EMG has a high level of sensitivity; detection of known gene mutations can be helpful. Treatment depends on type of disease but includes the use of carbonic anhydrase inhibitors (e.g. acetazolamide), oral potassium supplements (for hypokalaemic variant) and thiazide diuretics (for hyperkalaemic variant).

Careful use of neuromuscular blocking drugs is required, with close monitoring of perioperative potassium levels. Arrhythmias may accompany potassium changes. Glucose-containing intravenous fluids should be avoided in the hyperkalaemic form of the disease. Susceptibility to MH has been suggested but is thought to be unlikely.

Fascia iliaca compartment block. Injection of local anaesthetic solution behind the fascia iliaca into a compartment between the iliacus and psoas muscles, through which run the femoral, lateral cutaneous, genitofemoral and obturator nerves. A needle is inserted 0.5 cm caudal to the junction of the lateral third of the inguinal ligament with the medial two-thirds. A click or 'give' (the latter if continuous pressure is applied to the plunger of the syringe) is felt as the needle passes through the fascia lata, followed by a second click or 'give' as the fascia iliaca is pierced; 20–30 ml local anaesthetic solution (e.g. 0.25% bupivacaine) is then injected. Distal pressure is advocated to encourage cranial extension of the solution. The swelling in the groin may similarly be massaged to encourage spread.

Dalens B, Vanneuville G, Tanguy A (1989). Anesth Analg; 69: 705–13

See also, individual nerve blocks

Fascicular block, *see Bundle branch block*

Fasciculation. Visible contraction of skeletal muscle fibre fasciculi, seen following use of suxamethonium and other depolarising neuromuscular blocking drugs. Possible damage to fibres is suggested by increased serum myoglobin and creatine kinase following suxamethonium; it may also be partly responsible for the raised potassium that occurs. Possibly related to post-suxamethonium myalgia, since measures to reduce the latter often reduce visible fasciculation.

Also occurs in motor neurone disease, spinal motor neurone lesions, and rarely in myopathies. Muscle fibre fibrillation, e.g. occurring after denervation injury, is invisible.

Fasciitis, necrotising, *see Necrotising fasciitis*

Fat, brown, *see Brown fat*

Fat embolism. Dispersion of fat droplets into the circulation, usually following major trauma. Has also been reported in acute pancreatitis, burns, diabetes mellitus, joint reconstruction (possibly related to use of methylmethacrylate cement), cardiopulmonary bypass, liposuction, bone marrow harvest and bone marrow transplantation and parenteral infusion of lipids. Post-mortem evidence of fat embolism is found in 90% of fatal trauma cases. The mechanical (infloating) theory proposes that fat liberated from fractured bone enters the venous system and impacts in pulmonary capillaries resulting in pulmonary dysfunction. Systemic embolism may occur via pulmonary arteriovenous shunts or a patent foramen ovale. The biochemical theory suggests that free fatty acids released following trauma react with pneumocytes and the subsequent inflammatory response causes pulmonary dysfunction, possibly mediated via an increase in plasma lipase. The two theories may not be mutually exclusive.

The fat embolism syndrome occurs after less than 10% of trauma cases, typically 12–36 h after long bone fractures. The incidence is thought to be reduced by early fixation of fractures.

- Features:
  - confusion, restlessness, coma, convulsions, cerebral infarction.
  - dyspnoea, cough, haemoptysis. Hypoxaemia is almost inevitable. Pulmonary hypertension and pulmonary oedema may occur. Typically, gives a 'snowstorm' appearance on the chest X-ray, but radiography may be normal. May contribute to development of ARDS.
  - petechial rash, typically affecting the trunk, pharynx, axillae and conjunctivae.
  - tachycardia, hypotension, pyrexia.
  - platelets are reduced in 50%; hypocalcaemia is also common. Coagulation disorders may occur.
  - fat droplets may be detected in cells obtained by bronchopulmonary lavage in 70% of cases. The presence of fat droplets in the urine is a non-specific finding following trauma. Retinal examination may reveal intravascular fat globules.
- Management:
  - O_2 therapy; IPPV may be required.
  - supportive therapy. Fluid restriction has been advocated for reducing lung water.
  - corticosteroids have been shown to reduce mortality.
  - heparin, aprotinin, aspirin, clofibrate, prostacyclin, dextran and alcohol infusion have all been tried, without conclusive benefit.

Prognosis is unpredictable and unrelated to severity. Mortality is 10–20%.

Mellor A, Soni N (2001). Anaesthesia; 56: 145–54

Fats (Lipids). Four main classes are present in plasma and cells:

- triglycerides:
  - composed of glycerol and fatty acids. Formed in the GIT, liver and adipose tissue.
  - the main source of dietary fat; digested in the small bowel. Initially emulsified by bile salts and broken down to monoglycerides, free fatty acids (FFAs) and glycerol by lipases within the GIT. Undigested triglycerides are only minimally absorbed but glycerol and FFAs are taken up readily. Short-chain fatty acids pass directly into the portal vein and circulate as FFAs; long-chain FFAs (over 10–12 carbon atoms) are reconstituted with glycerol to reform triglycerides prior to incorporation into chylomicrons.
  - endogenous triglycerides are synthesised in the liver and secreted as very low-density lipoproteins (VLDLs). These are hydrolysed in the blood by lipoprotein lipase; the FFAs released are taken up by tissues for resynthesis of triglycerides or remain free in the plasma. During starvation, intracellular hormone-sensitive lipase breaks down adipose triglycerides to FFAs and glycerol (increased by β-adrenergic stimulation; decreased by insulin).
- sterols:
  - include corticosteroids, bile salts and cholesterol (from which the former two are derived).

- plasma cholesterol is esterified with fatty acids, or circulates within low-density, high-density and intermediate-density lipoproteins (LDLs, HDLs and IDLs respectively) and VLDLs, especially the first. Unesterified cholesterol forms a major component of cell membranes.
- cholesterol is either synthesised, mainly in the liver, or absorbed from the GIT and delivered to the liver in chylomicrons.

▸ phospholipids:
- mainly synthesised in the liver or small intestine mucosa.
- circulate in the plasma in lipoproteins and constitute important cellular components, but not part of the depot fats. Present in myelin and cell membranes.

▸ fatty acids:
- may be saturated (no double bonds between carbon atoms) or unsaturated (variable number of double bonds). Deficiency of certain polyunsaturated fatty acids may impair capillary, hepatic, immune and GIT function, hence they are termed essential. A change in intake from omega-6 to omega-3 essential fatty acids (the latter found in fish oils and plant oils) has been suggested as reducing production of inflammatory mediators and thereby various cardiovascular and inflammatory disorders.
- esterified with triglycerides, cholesterol or phospholipids, or bound to circulating albumin as FFAs.
- FFAs are used as an energy source by most tissues.

Lipoproteins are classified according to their size: chylomicrons 80–500 nm; VLDLs 30–80 nm; IDLs 25–40 nm; LDLs 20 nm; HDLs 7.5–10 nm. LDLs and IDLs are formed from VLDLs; HDLs are formed in the liver. High levels of cholesterol, LDLs and VLDLs are associated with ischaemic heart disease, although the role of each is controversial. HDLs may be protective.

Fazadinium bromide. Obsolete non-depolarising neuromuscular blocking drug, first used in 1972. Rapidly acting, thus initially suggested as an alternative to suxamethonium. Lasts for 40–60 min, causes marked vagal blockade, and contraindicated in renal failure.

FDA, *see Food and Drug Administration*

FDP, *see Fibrin degradation products*

FEEA, *see Fondation Européenne d'Enseignement en Anaesthésiologie*

Felypressin. Synthetic analogue of vasopressin, used as a locally acting vasoconstrictor. Has minimal effects on the myocardium, therefore safer than adrenaline when used during inhalational anaesthesia. Available in combination with prilocaine for local infiltration.

Femoral artery. Continuation of the external iliac artery; enters the thigh below the inguinal ligament midway between the anterior superior iliac spine and symphysis pubis, where it lies between the femoral vein medially and femoral nerve laterally. Descends through the femoral triangle and enters (and runs in) the subsartorial canal. Ends by piercing adductor magnus 10 cm above the knee joint where it becomes the popliteal artery.

May be cannulated for arterial BP measurement, dialysis and use of the intra-aortic counter-pulsation balloon pump as well as providing access for angiography.

Femoral nerve block. Useful as an adjunct to general anaesthesia for operations involving the anterior thigh and medial lower leg. May be combined with sciatic nerve block and/or obturator nerve block for more extensive surgery, but dangerously large amounts of solution may be required. Has been used for analgesia in leg and thigh fractures.

- Anatomy:
  - the femoral nerve (L2–4) arises from the lumbar plexus, passing under the inguinal ligament to enter the femoral triangle lateral to the femoral artery. Divides into terminal branches within 3–6 cm.
  - supplies muscles of the anterior thigh, hip and knee joints. Also supplies skin of the anterior thigh and knee, and medial lower leg and foot via the saphenous branch (Fig. 65).
- Block:
  - the femoral artery is palpated below the mid-inguinal point (i.e. halfway between the superior anterior iliac spine and pubic tubercle); the femoral vein lies medially and the nerve laterally.
  - a needle is introduced through a wheal 1–2 cm lateral to the pulsation, and directed slightly cranially, to a depth of 3–4 cm. A nerve stimulator may be used to aid location of the nerve, looking for contraction of the quadriceps muscle.
  - after aspiration to exclude arterial puncture, 10–15 ml local anaesthetic agent is injected. A further 5–10 ml is

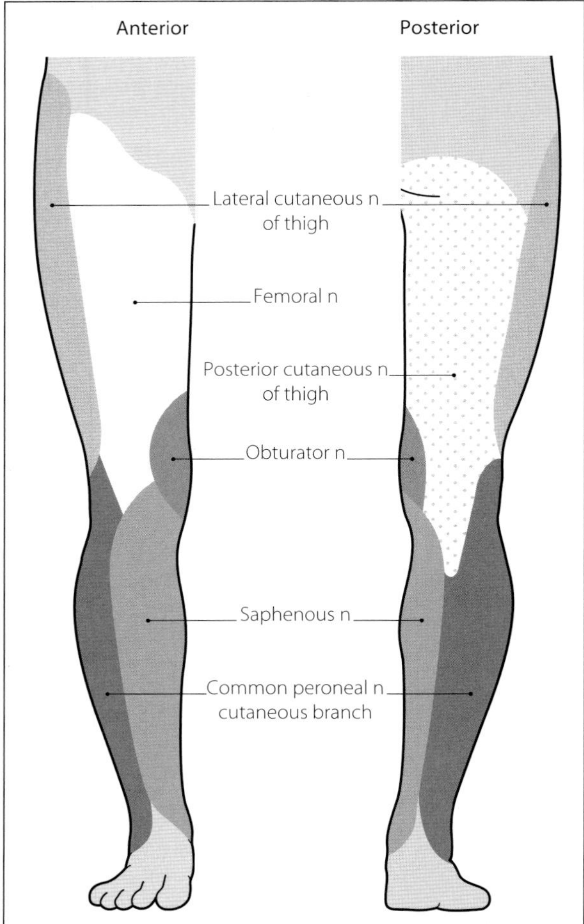

Fig. 65 Nerve supply of leg (for nerve supply of ankle and foot, see Fig. 10 Ankle, nerve blocks)

- injected in a fan laterally as the needle is withdrawn, in case cutaneous branches arise higher than normal.
- injection of 30–40 ml solution at the initial site, with distal compression, has been claimed to force solution cranially to the lumbar plexus, lying between psoas and quadratus lumborum muscles (three-in-one block). In fact, a continuous femoral 'sheath' probably does not exist as a separate entity; the 'three-in-one block' is thought to represent combined femoral and lateral cutaneous nerve blocks below the inguinal ligament as a result of non-specific overspill. Fascia iliaca compartment block is a more reliable and anatomically sound method of producing block of the three nerves.

Femoral triangle. Compartment of the anterior upper thigh; its borders are the inguinal ligament superomedially, the medial border of adductor longus medially and the medial border of sartorius laterally (Fig. 66). Its floor is formed by adductor longus, pectineus, psoas and iliacus muscles, and its roof by the fascia lata of the thigh. Contains the femoral artery, vein and canal within the femoral sheath; the femoral nerve and lateral cutaneous nerve of the thigh lie laterally.

Femoral venous cannulation. The femoral vein is the continuation of the popliteal vein and accompanies the femoral artery in the femoral triangle, ending medial to the latter at the inguinal ligament where it becomes the external iliac vein. Following skin cleansing, the patient's leg is extended and slightly abducted at the hip. The femoral vein lies 1–1.5 cm medial to the femoral artery, 2–3 cm below the inguinal ligament. The needle is inserted here and advanced at an angle of 45–60° to the frontal plane. When venous blood is aspirated, the syringe is lowered to lie flat on the skin. A Seldinger technique is usually employed thereafter.

May be performed for central venous cannulation; traditionally avoided if other routes are available because of fears of infection or thrombosis. May be useful in superior vena caval obstruction.

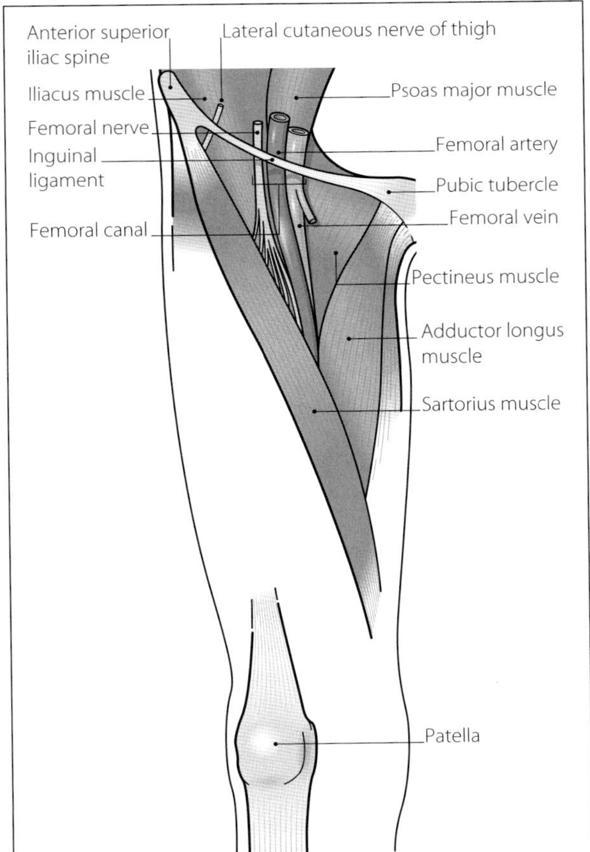

Fig. 66 Right femoral triangle (n.b. The spermatic cord emerging through the external inguinal ring superolateral to the pubic tubercle is not shown)

Fenoldopam mesylate. Selective D_1-dopamine receptor agonist, introduced in the USA in 1998 as an iv vasodilator drug. Also has mild α_2-adrenergic agonist properties. Causes increased renal blood flow, diuresis and sodium excretion. Given as an infusion, its short half-life of 5 min results in rapid offset of action. Metabolised in the liver to inactive compounds.

Fenoterol hydrobromide. β-Adrenergic receptor agonist, used as a bronchodilator drug. Similar in action to salbutamol and terbutaline but less β_2 selective. Now only available in the UK as part of a compound aerosol formulation.

- Dosage: 200–400 μg by aerosol inhalation 1–3 times daily.
- Side effects: as for salbutamol.

Fentanyl citrate. Synthetic opioid analgesic drug, derived from pethidine. Developed in 1960. 100 times as potent as morphine. Mainly used during anaesthesia; has also been used for induction in high doses, for premedication and sedation, e.g. on ICU. Also available in transdermal patches for chronic cancer pain. Onset of action is within 1–2 min after iv injection; peak effect is within 4–5 min. Duration of action is about 20 min, limited by redistribution initially as plasma clearance is less than for morphine. Postoperative respiratory depression is possible if large doses are used, especially if opioid premedication and other depressant drugs are used. Causes minimal histamine release or cardiovascular changes, although bradycardia has been reported.

- Dosage:
  - for premedication: 50–100 μg im (rarely used).
  - to obtund the pressor response to laryngoscopy: 7–10 μg/kg.
  - during anaesthesia: 1–3 μg/kg with spontaneous ventilation; 5–10 μg/kg with IPPV. Up to 100 μg/kg has been used for cardiac surgery. Muscular rigidity and hypotension are more common after high dosage. Has been used in neuroleptanaesthesia.
  - by infusion: 1–5 μg/kg/h, e.g. for sedation.
  - 25, 50, 75 or 100 μg/h transdermal patch placed on the chest or upper arm and replaced (using a different site) every 72 h. A patch employing iontophoresis has been developed for postoperative patient-controlled analgesia; containing ~10 mg fentanyl in total it incorporates a compact electronic controller, activated by pressing a small button twice within 3 s. Delivers 40 μg over 10 min, ≤ 80 doses in total or for ≤ 24 h. A blinking light indicates the number of doses given.

Commonly used for epidural and spinal anaesthesia (*see Spinal opioids*)

Fetal circulation. Oxygenated blood from the placenta passes through the single umbilical vein and enters the inferior vena cava, about 50% bypassing the liver via the ductus venosus. Most of it is diverted through the foramen ovale into the left atrium, passing to the brain via the carotid arteries

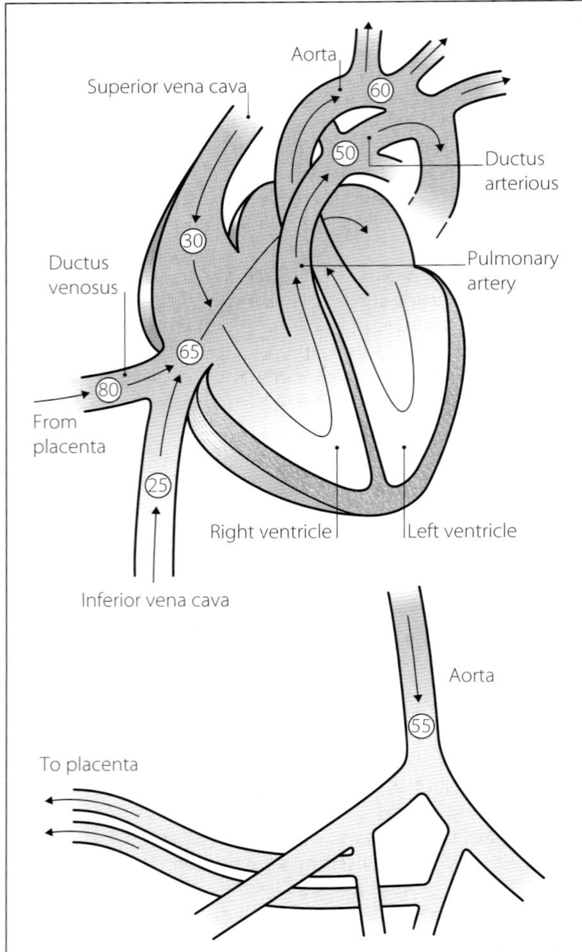

Fig. 67 Diagram of fetal circulation, Arrows denote flow of blood. Figures refer to the approximate oxygen saturation

(Fig. 67). Deoxygenated blood from the brain enters the right atrium via the superior vena cava, and passes through the tricuspid valve to the right ventricle. Because the resistance of the pulmonary vessels within the collapsed lungs is high, the blood passes from the pulmonary artery trunk through the ductus arteriosus to enter the aortic arch downstream from the origin of the carotid arteries. Thus relatively O_2-rich blood is conserved for the brain, and the rest of the body is perfused with the less oxygenated blood. Deoxygenated blood reaches the placenta via the two umbilical arteries, arising from the internal iliac arteries; they receive about 60% of cardiac output.

- Approximate values:
  - umbilical vein:
    - Po_2 4 kPa (30 mmHg).
    - Pco_2 6 kPa (45 mmHg).
    - pH 7.2
  - umbilical artery:
    - Po_2 2 kPa (15 mmHg).
    - Pco_2 7 kPa (53 mmHg).

At birth, placental blood flow ceases, and peripheral resistance increases. Lung expansion lowers pulmonary vascular resistance, both directly and via reduction of hypoxic pulmonary vasoconstriction. Thus pulmonary and right heart pressures fall, and aortic and left heart pressures rise. Pulmonary blood flow increases and flow through the ductus arteriosus and foramen ovale ceases. The ductus arteriosus usually closes within 48 h due to the high Po_2. Pulmonary artery pressure, pulmonary vascular resistance and pulmonary blood flow approach adult values by 4–6 weeks.

Neonates may revert to persistent fetal circulation, with decreased pulmonary blood flow and right-to-left shunt through the ductus arteriosus, foramen ovale or both. This may occur if pulmonary vascular resistance is increased, e.g. by hypoxia, hypothermia, hypercapnia, acidosis, polycythaemia, etc. It may occur during surgery if anaesthesia is too light or if the patient 'bucks' on the tracheal tube. Right-to-left shunt increases with worsening hypoxia and further reflex vasoconstriction. Ductal shunting may be demonstrated clinically by measuring O_2 saturation (e.g. by pulse oximetry) in the arm and leg simultaneously; a large difference (higher saturation in the arm) represents significant ductal blood flow (i.e. pulmonary artery pressure exceeds aortic pressure). If the right ventricle fails, right atrial pressure exceeds left atrial pressure, increasing shunt through the foramen ovale.

Treatment of persistent fetal circulation includes O_2 therapy, correction of acidosis, hypercapnia and hypothermia, and inotropes and fluid administration. Drugs which lower pulmonary vascular resistance, e.g. tolazoline, isoprenaline, etc. may be given. Extracorporeal membrane oxygenation has been used.

See also, Ductus arteriosus, patent

Fetal haemoglobin. Consists of two α chains and two γ chains, the latter differing from β chains by 37 amino acids. Binds 2,3-DPG less avidly than haemoglobin A (adult), thus shifting the oxyhaemoglobin dissociation curve to the left (P_{50} is 2.4 kPa (18 mmHg)) and favouring O_2 transfer from mother to fetus. At the low fetal Po_2, it gives up more O_2 to the tissues than adult haemoglobin would, because its dissociation curve is steeper in this part. Forms 80% of circulating haemoglobin at birth; replaced by haemoglobin A normally within 3–5 months. May persist in the haemoglobinopathies.

A variety of embryonic haemoglobins are present up to 2–3 months of gestation.

Fetal monitoring. Methods include:

- presence of meconium in amniotic fluid: usually represents fetal compromise, and presents risk of meconium aspiration on delivery.
- heart rate, especially related to uterine contractions. May be performed intermittently using a trumpet-shaped stethoscope (Pinard) or portable ultrasound machine, or with a cardiotocograph (CTG), a machine that measures both heart rate by external ultrasonography or fetal scalp electrode, and contractions by external transducer or intrauterine probe:
  - normal baseline heart rate is 110–160/min, with beat to beat variability of 5–25/min, related to autonomic activity. Increased baseline and reduced variability may be related to compromise, although they may also be caused by administration of depressant drugs to the mother, maternal pyrexia, etc.
  - accelerations are usually related to reactivity and well-being.
  - decelerations; usual significance:
    - early (type I), i.e. with contractions: vagally mediated, due to head compression.
    - late (type II), i.e. after contractions: represent hypoxia, although not always with acidosis.
    - variable: usually due to cord compression; they may indicate compromise if severe.

  Prolonged decelerations are more sinister, and may represent severe fetal compromise.

Recent NICE guidelines describe the CTG according to the baseline rate, variability, accelerations and decelerations as being 'reassuring' (all four are normal), 'non-reassuring' (one of the four is abnormal) or 'pathological' (two or more of the four are abnormal or one is severely abnormal). Predictive value of cardiotocography is poor in low risk patients, hence some controversy surrounds its routine use. Combination with fetal electrocardiography (ST waveform analysis) is thought to increase its sensitivity.

Signs of fetal compromise may be related to treatable conditions, e.g. uterine hypertonicity associated with excessive oxytocin administration, maternal hypotension, etc. Aortocaval compression should always be considered, especially if regional analgesia has been provided.

- fetal blood sample: pH under 7.2 represents severe acidosis. May be measured serially to observe trends.
- fetal scalp oximetry, EEG, ECG and continuous pH measurement have been investigated but are not routinely available.

Post delivery, cord blood gas analysis (pH represents degree of acidosis at time of delivery), Apgar scoring, time to sustained respiration and neurobehavioural testing of neonates may be assessed; these may be useful prognostically.
[Adolphe Pinard (1844–1934), French obstetrician]

Fetus, effects of anaesthetic drugs on. The fetus is usually defined as such from the fourth month of gestation, or when the embryo becomes recognisably human. Most major organ structures develop earlier than this.

- Main anaesthetic considerations:
  - effect of anaesthetic drugs on fetal development and spontaneous abortion:
    - animal studies suggest increased fetal loss and abnormalities following prolonged exposure to high concentrations of volatile agents and N_2O.
    - human studies have produced conflicting results. It is generally accepted that general anaesthesia should be avoided where possible during pregnancy, particularly during the first trimester.
    - N_2O has been implicated (but not proven) as increasing the incidence of spontaneous abortion in health workers chronically exposed; current opinion holds that its use is not contraindicated in pregnant patients.
    - new drugs should be avoided during early pregnancy, until more information becomes available.
  - effect of anaesthetic drugs given during labour on the neonate:
    - indirect effects:
      - reduced uteroplacental blood flow, e.g. due to oxytocin, etc., or hypotension following regional blockade or general anaesthesia.
      - maternal hypoxia, e.g. due to drug-induced respiratory depression, total spinal block, convulsions, etc.
      - increased maternal catecholamine levels during general anaesthesia with awareness; uteroplacental vasoconstriction and fetal acidosis may result. Levels are reduced in labour following epidural block; this is thought to reduce fetal acidosis.
    - direct effects:
      - related to fetal plasma levels, affected by:
        - uteroplacental blood flow.
        - placental, maternal and fetal protein concentrations and drug binding. For example, diazepam binds to albumin and is extensively transferred to the fetus; bupivacaine binds to α_1-acid glycoprotein (present in lower concentrations in the fetus) and is transferred to a lesser extent.
        - peak maternal plasma drug levels and their duration.
        - diffusion of drug across the placenta, depending on membrane thickness, molecular size and shape, degree of ionisation and lipid solubility.
        - reduced fetal hepatic and renal function. Most drugs bypass the fetal liver via the ductus venosus.
        - umbilical vein drug levels: reduced by dilution with blood from the rest of the body. Thus umbilical vein levels may not reflect fetal levels.
        - fetal hypoxia and acidosis: cause trapping of basic drugs, e.g. opioids and local anaesthetic agents, and increase blood flow to vital centres, e.g. brain. Thus brain levels may be increased.
      - specific drugs:
        - opioid analgesic drugs:
          - fetal respiratory and neurobehavioural depression are well recognised.
          - fetal opioid levels are increased by acidosis. Peak levels occur 2–5 h after im pethidine, 6 minutes after iv injection.
          - half-life in the fetus is prolonged; e.g. pethidine: up to 20 hours; that of norpethidine is longer.
          - naloxone crosses the placenta easily, but its administration is usually reserved for the fetus.
        - iv anaesthetic agents:
          - all cross the placenta rapidly, but have usually redistributed by the time of delivery. Thiopental selectively accumulates in fetal liver.
          - neurobehavioural depression has been shown following their use, although the effect is small.
        - inhalational anaesthetic agents:
          - at low inspired concentrations, any effect is small.
          - benefits of their use include uteroplacental vasodilatation and prevention of maternal awareness.
        - neuromuscular blocking drugs:
          - very little transfer follows normal use.
          - gallamine and alcuronium cross the placenta to a slightly greater extent than the others.
        - local anaesthetic agents:
          - transfer varies according to dose, site of injection (e.g. high fetal levels following paracervical block), use of vasoconstrictors and different plasma protein-binding characteristics of the fetus and mother for certain drugs; e.g. umbilical vein/maternal blood levels:
            - prilocaine: > 1.
            - lidocaine: 0.5.
            - bupivacaine: 0.3.
            - etidocaine: 0.2.
          - subtle neurobehavioural effects have been shown; initial fears about adverse effects of lidocaine compared with bupivacaine are now thought to be unfounded.
          - fetal methaemoglobinaemia may follow excessive doses of prilocaine.
          - procaine and 2-chloroprocaine are metabolised by esterases in maternal and fetal plasma.
        - others, e.g. benzodiazepines, phenothiazines, etc.:
          - all cross the placenta to some extent.
          - diazepam is more strongly bound to fetal than to maternal protein, and has been associated with neonatal hypotonia and hypothermia. Umbilical vein/maternal blood ratio is 2.0.

- all drugs that may cause central effects, and therefore cross the blood–brain barrier, may cross the placenta to similar extents, e.g. atropine, propranolol, etc.

Littleford J (2004). Can J Anesth; 51: 586–609

See also, Environmental safety of anaesthetists; Fetal monitoring; Neurobehavioural testing of neonates

FEV$_1$, *see Forced expiratory volume*

Fever, *see Pyrexia*

FFARCS examination (Fellowship of the Faculty of Anaesthetists at the Royal College of Surgeons of England). First held in 1953; became the FCAnaes examination in 1989 following the founding of the College of Anaesthetists and the FRCA examination upon granting of a Royal charter to the College in 1992. The Irish equivalent exam (FFARCSI) was first held in 1961.

FFP, Fresh frozen plasma, *see Blood products*

Fibreoptic instruments. First use of a fibreoptic instrument (choledochoscope) for tracheal intubation was in 1967 by Murphy. Fibreoptic bronchoscopes were introduced in 1968. Flexible fibreoptic intubating bronchoscopes of down to 3–4 mm diameter are now widely available.

- Features:
  - rely on total internal reflection of light within bundles of glass fibres, about 20 μm diameter.
  - each fibre is encased in glass of different refractive index, the interface acting as the reflective surface.
  - fibres are lubricated and flexible; the instrument's tip can be flexed using controls at the proximal end.
  - each instrument contains bundles for passage of light for illumination, and bundles for passage of the image back to the proximal end. The arrangement of the image-bearing bundles is identical at each end of the instrument (coherent), allowing accurate spatial representation of the object.
  - a lens at each end allows focusing. A camera may be attached to the eyepiece at the proximal end, improving ease of use by allowing the operator and others to observe the view on a screen. With improved miniaturisation it is now possible to place a small video chip directly at the distal end of the instrument, so that there is no need for fragile optical bundles to be contained within its shaft (which now contains electrical wires carrying the digital image instead).
  - may contain channels for suction, passage of gas, liquid, forceps, etc.
  - very delicate instruments; easily damaged, e.g. by teeth, etc. Careful cleaning is required; passage of disinfectant into the 'scope may disrupt lubrication between fibres.
- Apart from diagnostic (e.g. biopsy) and therapeutic (e.g. removal of secretions and foreign bodies) use, they have been used for:
  - tracheal intubation, with the patient awake or anaesthetised. Especially useful in cases of known difficult intubation. The endoscope may be passed through a tracheal tube, and then guided via the mouth or nose into the larynx. Lidocaine may be sprayed through a side port. The tube is passed over the 'scope into the trachea. Alternatively, the 'scope and tube are passed together, the former protruding a short distance from the latter. May also be guided through various airways that act as conduits. Has been used to place endobronchial tubes.
  - checking the position of tracheal or endobronchial tubes, etc. Particularly useful for endobronchial tubes. Has been used to aid placement of percutaneous tracheostomy. May be passed through special connectors with rubber ports, thus allowing undisturbed delivery of O_2 and anaesthetic gases.
  - assessment/diagnosis, sputum clearance and lavage e.g. during/after thoracic surgery or in ICU.

Considerable practice is required to achieve adequate skill in their use, which has been suggested as being desirable during all anaesthetists' training but widely acknowledged as being too difficult for most UK units to achieve.

Rigid laryngoscopes incorporating fibreoptic channels may also be used for tracheal intubation.

Fibreoptic sensors have also been used for clinical measurement of, e.g. pressure, flow and chemical concentrations.

[Peter Murphy, US anaesthetist]

See also, Intubation, awake; Intubation, difficult; Intubation, endobronchial; Intubation, tracheal

Fibrin degradation products (FDPs). Products of fibrin breakdown by plasmin; thus blood levels reflect the rate of fibrinolysis (e.g. increased levels occur in DIC). Half-life is about 9 h. May inhibit clot formation by competing for fibrin polymerisation sites. Also interfere with platelet function and thrombin; thus excess fibrinolysis may impair further coagulation. May possibly damage vascular endothelium.

Non-specific testing for FDPs has been replaced in many centres by testing for the D-dimer portion of fibrin, which is released only during fibrinolysis and is not present on fibrinogen nor released during the latter's breakdown.

Measurement of FDPs and especially D-dimer has been used to aid diagnosis of DVT, a normal value excluding the presence of thrombosis.

Normal levels: < 10 mg/l (FDPs); < 500 ng/ml (D-dimer).

See also, Coagulation studies

Fibrinogen, *see Coagulation*

Fibrinolysis. Dissolution of fibrin; occurs following clot formation allowing blood vessel remodelling, and also after wound healing. Fibrinolytic and coagulation pathways are in equilibrium normally, each composed of a series of plasma precursor molecules.

Plasminogen, a globulin, is activated to form plasmin, a fibrinolytic enzyme. Activation involves clotting factors XII and XI, kallikrein and kinins, and leucocyte products. Activation of tissue plasminogen is caused by products released by endothelial cells. Plasminogen activators and plasminogen itself bind to fibrin, with plasmin formation thus localised to the site of fibrin formation. Fibrin is degraded to fibrin degradation products, with complement and platelet activation. Fibrinolysis may be decreased by stress, including surgery; effects are greatest 2–3 days postoperatively. It may be increased by fibrinolytic drugs, and following DIC as a response to the large amount of fibrin formed. Also increased by venous occlusion, catecholamines, and possibly epidural and spinal anaesthesia. Primary fibrinolysis may occur in certain malignancies.

Fibrinolytic drugs. Drugs causing fibrinolysis by activating plasminogen. Used iv and intra-arterially to prevent thrombosis, and to break up established thrombi, e.g. PE. Have been shown to reduce mortality in acute MI when given iv within 24 h, especially within 6 h. Are also being investigated in some forms of CVA. Streptokinase acts by binding to plasminogen, the resultant complex activating other plasminogen molecules. Allergic reactions are common. Urokinase cleaves a specific peptide bond in plasminogen, converting it to plasmin; it is used mainly for thrombolysis in the eye and arteriovenous shunts. Tissue-type plasminogen activator (alteplase), reteplase and tenecteplase bind to fibrin and activate plasminogen, converting it to plasmin; like streptokinase, they are used as thrombolytics in MI. The major side effect is systemic and intracerebral haemorrhage; nausea, vomiting and back pain may also occur.

Fibrocystic disease, *see Cystic fibrosis*

Fibronectin. Glycoprotein, involved in the removal of intravascular debris and foreign substances via interaction with circulating leucocytes, enabling the opsonisation process. May become depleted in critical illness, especially trauma and sepsis; resultant impairment of opsonisation is thought to contribute to organ microperfusion and MODS. Monitoring of fibronectin levels has been suggested as an additional method of following progress in critical illness. Present in cryoprecipitate; replacement has been used therapeutically but with conflicting results.

Fick principle. Blood flow to an organ in unit time =

$$\frac{\text{amount of a marker substance taken up by the organ in that time}}{\text{concentration difference of the substance in the vessels supplying and draining the organ}}$$

The amount of a substance given up by an organ can also be used, e.g. CO_2 (see below).

May be used to determine blood flow to individual organs, e.g. cerebral blood flow (Kety–Schmidt technique) or renal blood flow.

May also be used to determine cardiac output, using O_2 or CO_2 as the substance measured, and the heart as the organ concerned:

- Using O_2: cardiac output

$$= \frac{O_2 \text{ consumption (ml/min)}}{\text{arterial} - \text{mixed venous } O_2 \text{ concentration (ml/l)}}$$

substituting normal values:

$$= \frac{250 \text{ ml/min}}{200 - 150 \text{ ml/l}}$$

$$= 5 \text{ l/min}$$

- Using CO_2: cardiac output

$$= \frac{CO_2 \text{ output (ml/min)}}{\text{mixed venous} - \text{arterial } CO_2 \text{ concentration (ml/l)}}$$

substituting normal values:

$$= \frac{200}{540 - 500 \text{ ml/l}}$$

$$= 5 \text{ l/min}$$

[Adolf Fick (1829–1901), German physiologist]

Fick's law of diffusion. Rate of diffusion across a membrane is proportional to the concentration gradient across that membrane.
See also, Fick principle

Filgrastim, *see Granulocyte colony-stimulating factor*

Filling ratio. Extent to which cylinders are underfilled with liquid substances. The presence of gas above the liquid reduces the pressure increase caused by any temperature rise, reducing the risk of pressure build-up and rupture. Defined as the weight of substance contained in the cylinder, divided by the weight of water it could contain.

- Applicable to substances at temperatures below their critical temperatures, e.g.:
  - N_2O:
    - 0.75 (temperate climate).
    - 0.67 (tropical climate).
  - CO_2: as for N_2O.
  - cyclopropane:
    - 0.51 (temperate climate).
    - 0.48 (tropical climate).

Filters, breathing system. Devices for reducing contamination of breathing equipment. Although the importance of breathing system contamination is disputed, cases of hepatitis C transmission have supported the increasing use of filters as routine. Traditionally, filters have been used to provide humidification as well as filter airborne particles and may be of three types:

- 1st generation hygroscopic devices: water-absorbing sponge with limited filtering properties although an efficient humidifier.
- 2nd generation hygroscopic devices: sponge combined with electrolet membrane; smaller pores and thus more efficient filtering properties. Less efficient and high resistance when wet.
- hydrophobic devices: actually repel water molecules, e.g. by using resin-coated ceramic fibres. The pores are very small, necessitating a large sheet to reduce resistance, folded in pleats. Very efficient even when wet.

Can be placed anywhere in the breathing system although most commonly placed between the patient and the system itself; require changing between cases. All devices increase both dead space and resistance to spontaneous ventilation.

Filtration fraction. Ratio of GFR to renal plasma flow (RPF). As RPF falls, GFR remains fairly constant because of efferent arteriolar constriction, causing filtration fraction to rise. Normally 0.16–0.2.

Fink effect. Reduced alveolar concentration of a gas resulting from its dilution by another gas leaving the bloodstream and entering the alveoli. Analogous but opposite to the second gas effect. Originally described (as 'diffusion anoxia') in 1955 as the underlying cause of hypoxaemia seen at the end of anaesthesia, when N_2O leaving the bloodstream dilutes alveolar O_2. Since recognised as having little clinical importance, the effect of hypoventilation and $\dot{V}/\dot{Q}$ mismatch being much more important.
[Bernard Raymond Fink (1914–2000), Seattle anaesthetist]

F_IO_2. Fractional inspired concentration of O_2. By convention, expressed as a decimalised fraction, e.g. 0.21, 0.5, although previously expressed as a percentage.

First-pass metabolism. Metabolism of a substance once absorbed, reducing the amount of substance before it reaches systemic circulation. Active metabolites may be formed. Most commonly refers to metabolism by the liver following oral administration of drugs, e.g. propranolol, morphine, lidocaine and GTN (i.e. drugs with a high extraction ratio). Drugs may be given by alternative routes to bypass the liver, e.g. parenterally, sublingually or rectally. May also occur in the intestinal mucosa following oral administration of e.g. methyldopa, chlorpromazine, midazolam and isoprenaline, and in the bronchial mucosa following inhalation of isoprenaline.

Flail chest. Disruption of chest wall integrity, where a portion of the thoracic cage becomes detached from the bony structure of the rest. The flail segment no longer moves outwards on inspiration, but is free to be drawn inwards by negative intrathoracic pressure; it is pushed out during expiration whilst the rest of the thorax contracts. Occurs in severe chest trauma with multiple fractures involving several ribs with or without the sternum. May also result from surgery.

- Features:
  - hypoventilation, with reduced tidal volume and vital capacity. Pendulluft is now thought not to occur; mediastinal shift results in air entry to both lungs, although overall hypoventilation may be severe. Hypoventilation is further exacerbated by pain. Ability to cough is reduced due to mechanical impairment and pain.
  - underlying lung contusion/atelectasis/pneumothorax with resultant shunt and $\dot{V}/\dot{Q}$ mismatch; thought to be more important than hypoventilation.
  - associated injuries, e.g. to mediastinum, head, abdomen, etc.
  - mediastinal shift may affect cardiac output.
- Management is as for chest trauma, i.e.:
  - O_2 administration.
  - analgesia (e.g. systemic opioids/intercostal nerve block/epidural analgesia).
  - treatment of hypovolaemia and associated injuries.
  - chest drainage if required.
  - physiotherapy.
  - nasogastric drainage helps prevent gastric dilatation.
  - if arterial blood gases are acceptable, no further treatment may be required. Improved oxygenation and chest wall splinting may be achieved by CPAP.
  - tracheal intubation and IPPV. May be continued until the underlying lung improves or surgical fixation of the flail segment (i.e. up to several weeks). IMV has been used.
  - surgical fixation of rib fractures is preferred by some surgeons.

Flame ionisation detector. Device used in analysis of gas mixtures, separated, e.g. by gas chromatography. A potential difference is applied across a flame of hydrogen gas burning in air. Addition of organic vapour to the gas stream causes a change in current flow across the flame, the amount of change proportional to the amount of substance present. Used only to quantify the amount of a known substance, not to identify unknown ones.
See also, Gas analysis

Flammability. Ability to support combustion. Dependent on molecular structure; e.g. C–C bonds readily break down with heat and O_2 to form carbon monoxide/dioxide, whereas C–F bonds are resistant. Flammability limits refer to concentrations of a substance which will support combustion; e.g.:
- cyclopropane:
  - 2.5–60% in O_2.
  - 2.5–10% in air.
  - 1.5–30% in N_2O.
- diethyl ether:
  - 2–82% in O_2.
  - 2–35% in air.
  - 1.5–24% in N_2O.

Ranges for explosive mixtures occur within these limits, especially with high O_2 concentration. The stoichiometric mixture lies within the explosive range. Flammability is greater in N_2O than in O_2, because the former decomposes to produce O_2 with release of energy. Addition of water vapour reduces flammability.

Modern, non-flammable agents will ignite only at higher concentrations than occur during anaesthesia, and require much greater amounts of energy to initiate ignition (activation energy).
See also, Explosions and fires

Flash-point. Lowest temperature at which a saturated vapour of a liquid ignites when exposed to a flame, in the presence of one or more other gas(es).

Flecainide acetate. Class Ic antiarrhythmic drug. Slows impulse conduction by blocking sodium channels and thus increasing action potential duration (in both the conducting system and myocardial cells). Used for severe VT and extrasystoles, and SVT, especially those involving accessory pathways (e.g. Wolff– Parkinson–White syndrome).
- Dosage:
  - 2 mg/kg up to 150 mg, over 10–30 min iv.
  - by infusion: 1.5 mg/kg/h for 1 h; 0.1–0.25 mg/kg/h thereafter.
  - 100–400 mg orally.
- Side effects:
  - giddiness, visual disturbances, corneal deposits.
  - myocardial depression (minor), proarrhythmias.
  - resistance to endocardial pacing.
  - increased plasma levels in hepatic/renal failure (levels should be monitored).
  - has been associated with increased risk of cardiac arrest after MI, therefore reserved for life-threatening arrhythmias.

Flow. Amount of fluid moving per unit time. Flow through a tube may be:
- laminar: flow is smooth and without eddies. Molecules at the tube's edges move more slowly; those at the centre more rapidly (Fig. 68a)

  laminar flow =

  $$\frac{\text{pressure gradient along tube} \times \text{radius}^4 \times \pi}{\text{tube length} \times \text{viscosity of fluid} \times 8}$$

  (Hagen–Poiseuille equation).
- turbulent (Fig. 68b): caused when the tube is unevenly shaped, or when the fluid flows through an orifice, around sharp edges, etc. Also occurs from laminar flow when flow velocity is too fast, exceeding the critical velocity.

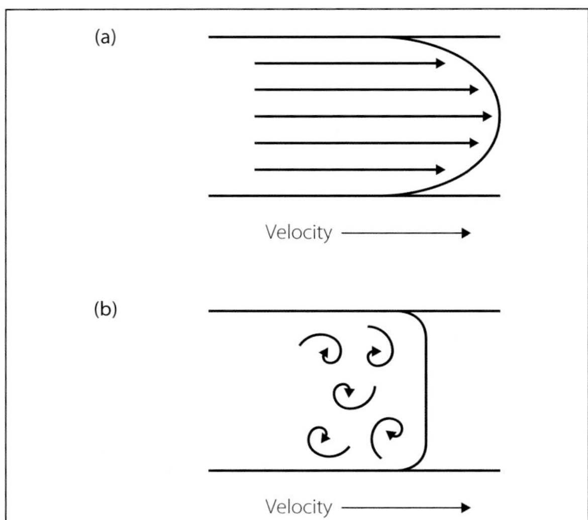

Fig. 68 Flow profiles: (a) laminar with parabolic profile; (b) turbulent with flat profile

Reynolds' number describes the relationship between tube and fluid characteristics and velocity at which turbulent flow occurs. Turbulent flow is proportional to:
- radius^2.
- $\sqrt{}$pressure gradient.
- 1/length.
- 1/density of fluid.

Flow in the airways and blood vessels is a mixture of laminar and turbulent, but behaves approximately according to the above principles.

- Measurement:
  - gas: flowmeters.
  - liquid: dilution techniques, electromagnetic flow measurement, Fick principle. Similar flowmeters to those used for gases may also be used.
  - measurement of volume over a certain time.

Flow-directed balloon-tipped pulmonary artery catheters, *see Pulmonary artery catheterisation*

Flow generators, *see Ventilators*

Flowmasta, *see Ventilators*

Flowmeters. Devices for measuring flow. Usually refer to measurement of gas flow, e.g. from cylinders and anaesthetic machines, or in breathing systems.

- May be:
  - constant orifice, variable pressure. Since flow through an orifice is proportional to the pressure difference across it, flow may be deduced by measuring the pressure difference across a fixed orifice. In the first two examples, only the downstream pressure is measured, since the pressure upstream of the orifice is constant:
    - simple pressure gauge downstream from the outlet of an O_2 cylinder. The gauge may be calibrated directly for flow, e.g. litres/min.
    - water depression flowmeter. The pressure is measured with a simple water manometer.
    - pneumotachograph. Pressure is measured electronically using transducers.
  - constant pressure, variable orifice. If the pressure across a variable orifice remains constant, the size of the orifice depends on the gas flow. Examples:
    - Rotameter, simple ball flowmeter and dry bobbin flowmeter. The size of the orifice is determined by the height of the bobbin in its tube: the greater the height, the larger the orifice. In the rotameter and ball flowmeter, the tube is of tapered bore, being wider at the top than at the bottom. The dry bobbin flowmeter tube is of uniform diameter, with small holes arranged longitudinally. The variability of the effective orifice size is provided by the number of holes below the bobbin, i.e. the bobbin's height.
    - Heidbrink flowmeter. The 'bobbin' is extended vertically to form a rod; its bottom end sits in a tapered tube whilst its top end lies opposite a linear scale above the tapered part. It functions in a similar way to the rotameter, but without rotating.
    - peak-flow meters.
  - variable pressure, variable orifice. In the watersight flowmeter, gas passes through a tube with holes along its length, immersed into water. At low gas flows, gas bubbles from the upper holes only; at higher flow rates, from the lower holes as well. The holes are marked with according flow rates. Orifice variability results from the different number of holes through which gas may pass; pressure variability arises because pressure is higher at greater depth of water.
  - constant pressure, constant orifice. Bubble flowmeters may be used for calibration at low flow rates. Gas passes along a uniform tube, carrying a thin soap film with it. Flow is deduced by measuring the velocity of the film along the tube using a timer.
- Other flowmeters include:
  - thermistor flowmeter: the cooling effect of a gas stream on a thermistor varies with flow rate.
  - ultrasonic flowmeter: turbulent eddies are formed around a rod in the gas path. The frequency of oscillation of the eddies, measured by Doppler probe, is proportional to flow rate. Alternatively, ultrasound beams may be projected diagonally across the gas, and transit time measured.

Flow can also be determined by measuring the volume of gas per unit time, e.g. using a respirometer.
[Jay A Heidbrink (1875–1957), US anaesthetist]

Flow–volume loops. Curves resulting from simultaneous measurement and plotting of air flow and lung volume during a maximal forced expiration. If residual volume is known, lung volume may be determined by measuring expired volume. Characteristic loops are obtained in certain conditions, although the loops obtained in practice are rarely as easily distinguishable (Fig. 69).

Much of the information from studying forced expiration may be obtained from flow–volume loops, e.g. forced expiratory flow rate, forced expiratory volume, and peak expiratory flow rate.
See also, Lung function tests

Flucloxacillin. Penicillinase-resistant penicillin used to treat staphylococcal infections. Peak levels occur within an hour of administration. 90% protein-bound; although metabolised in the liver, 50% appears unchanged in the urine.

- Dosage:
  - 250 mg orally/im 6 hourly.
  - 250 mg–2.0 g slowly iv, 6 hourly.
- Side effects: as for benzylpenicillin. Acute cholestatic jaundice may occur even after stopping therapy.

Fluconazole. Triazole antifungal drug used to treat local and systemic candidiasis and cryptococcal infection (including meningitis) especially associated with HIV infection. Well absorbed orally, with peak levels within 6 h. Elimination half-life 30 h.

- Dosage: 50–400 mg orally/iv daily.
- Side effects: nausea, vomiting, rashes, allergic reactions, toxic epidermal necrolysis, hepatic impairment. May increase blood levels of the antihistamines terfenadine and astemizole, resulting in prolonged Q–T syndrome and fatal ventricular arrhythmias including torsades de pointes.

Flucytosine. Intravenous antifungal drug used in systemic yeast infections; often used together with amphotericin with which it is synergistic. Resistance may occur.

- Dosage: 50 mg/kg iv over 20–40 min, 6 hourly, usually for no more than 7 days (prolonged therapy needed for cryptococcal infection). Trough plasma levels of 25–50 mg/l (200–400 μmol/l) are optimal.
- Side effects: nausea, vomiting, diarrhoea, rashes, confusion, hepatitis, blood dyscrasias. Weekly blood counts are required in prolonged treatment.

Fludrocortisone acetate. Mineralocorticoid used for replacement therapy in adrenocortical insufficiency and in

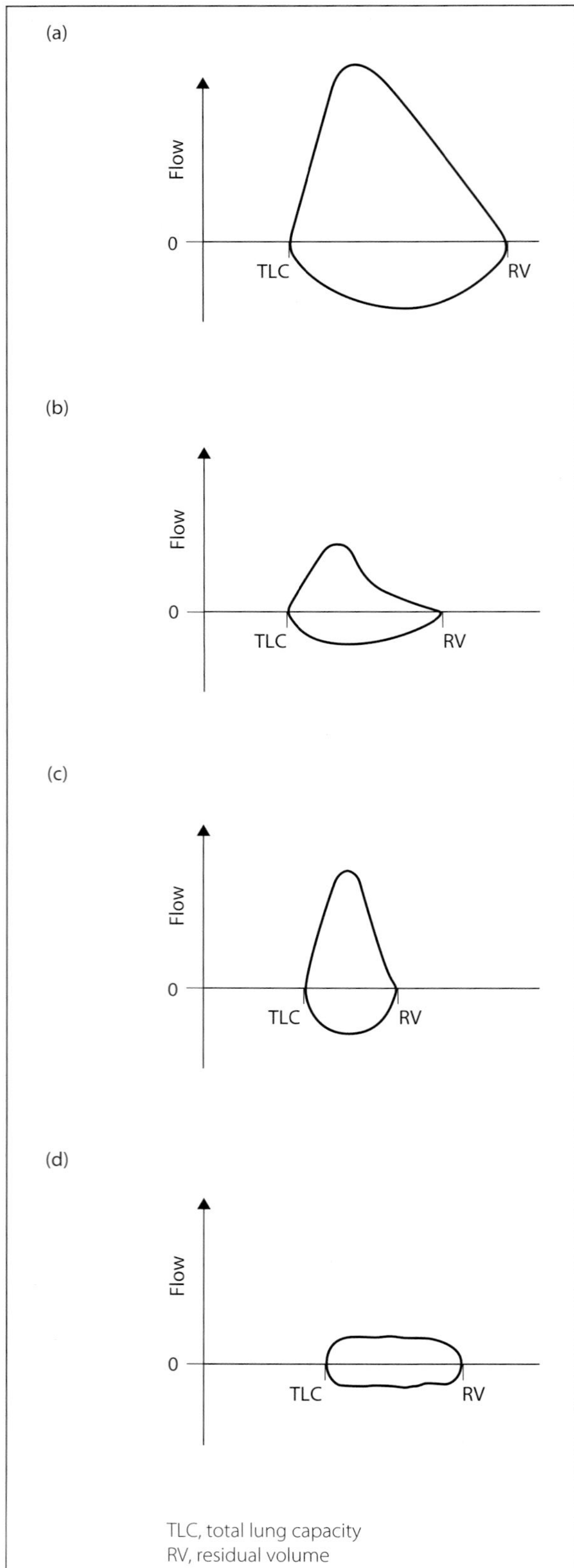

Fig. 69 Characteristic flow–volume loops: (a) normal; (b) obstructive lung disease; (c) restrictive lung disease; (d) tracheal/laryngeal obstruction

congenital adrenal hyperplasia and postural hypotension associated with autonomic neuropathy. Has similar actions to aldosterone; also has mild hydrocortisone-like actions.

- Dosage: 50–300 μg/day, orally.
- Side effects: hypertension, sodium and water retention, hypokalaemia. May also produce glucocorticoid effects.

Fluid. Form of matter whose shape is continuously changed when subjected to a shearing force, i.e. gas or liquid. Continuous shearing force results in flow; resistance to flow is proportional to viscosity. For a Newtonian fluid, e.g. water, viscosity is constant for different shear rates and flows; for a non-Newtonian fluid (e.g. blood), it varies with shear rates and flows. [Sir Isaac Newton (1642–1727), English scientist]
See also, Fluidics

Fluid balance. Normal approximate fluid intake of a 70 kg adult:

1500 ml liquid
750 ml in food
250 ml from metabolism within the body.
total: 2500 ml

Normal output:

1500 ml urine
100 ml in faeces
900 ml insensible water loss.
total: 2500 ml

Loss in sweat is normally negligible but may exceed several litres in hot environments. Insensible losses are also increased in high temperatures. About 5% of body water is exchanged per day in adults, 15% in infants; hence the increased risk of dehydration in the latter.

Balance is normally regulated to maintain ECF volume and osmolality; changes are detected by baroreceptors and osmoreceptors, with resultant compensatory mechanisms:
 - water intake is regulated by thirst; increased by hypovolaemia and hyperosmolality.
 - cardiovascular compensation for hypovolaemia.
 - urinary output is regulated by vasopressin, atrial natriuretic peptide and the renin/angiotensin system.
- Fluid balance may be disturbed in patients presenting for anaesthesia, perioperatively and in ICU:
 - reduced intake, e.g. coma, dysphagia, nausea, nil by mouth instructions.
 - increased intake, e.g. excessive iv administration.
 - redistribution, e.g. to third space.
 - reduced output, e.g. syndrome of inappropriate antidiuretic hormone secretion.
 - increased output, e.g. sweating, polyuria, vomiting, diarrhoea.

Routine administration of iv fluids perioperatively is controversial; excessive dextrose administration may lead to hyperglycaemia and hyponatraemia, whilst excessive salt solution administration may cause peripheral and pulmonary oedema. Improved recovery has been claimed following fluid administration (especially containing dextrose) during minor surgery compared with no fluids. The colloid/crystalloid controversy adds to the confused picture.

- IV fluid administration should be guided by the following:
 - maintenance requirements: 40 ml/kg/day (1.6 ml/kg/h). Requirements are greater in paediatric anaesthesia.
 - replacement of blood loss (*see Haemorrhage*).

- third space losses: with perioperative evaporative losses, approximately 10–15 ml/kg/h during major abdominal surgery.
- other losses, e.g. nasogastric aspirate.

Careful attention to fluid balance is required in all perioperative and critically ill patients to prevent complications, e.g. hypernatraemia, hyponatraemia, dehydration, renal failure, etc. Therapy is guided by CVP, urine output, BP, pulse and electrolyte balance. Body weight is a useful supplement to fluid intake/output charts.

See also, Fluids, body

Fluid therapy, *see Intravenous fluids*

Fluidics. Technology of operating control systems by utilising flow characteristics of gases or liquids. Has been used in control mechanisms of ventilators, e.g. employing the Coanda effect. The direction of a jet of gas in a valve may be switched by 'signal' jets of driving gas across the main jet. Combinations of signal jets allow complex manipulation of the valve output, without moving parts.

Pneumatic spool valves may contain moving shuttles, driven by gas from either end. The valve chamber is divided into segments by seals through which the shuttle passes; the valve output depends on the lining up of ports and channels in the shuttle and valve wall. The output may be used to drive cylinders, which may be driven from either end.

Fluids, body. Approximately 60% of male body weight is water; 50–55% in females (greater proportion of fat). Total body water may be measured using a dilution technique with deuterium oxide (heavy water). Its main constituent compartments are intracellular fluid (ICF), ECF, plasma and interstitial fluid (Fig. 70). Approximately 1 litre is contained within the GIT, CSF, etc. (transcellular fluid).

In neonates, ECF exceeds 30% (but plasma is still 5%), and ICF is less than 40%. These differences are greatest in premature babies, when ECF exceeds ICF. During childhood, the adult situation slowly develops.

Composition of fluid compartments is shown in Table 14.

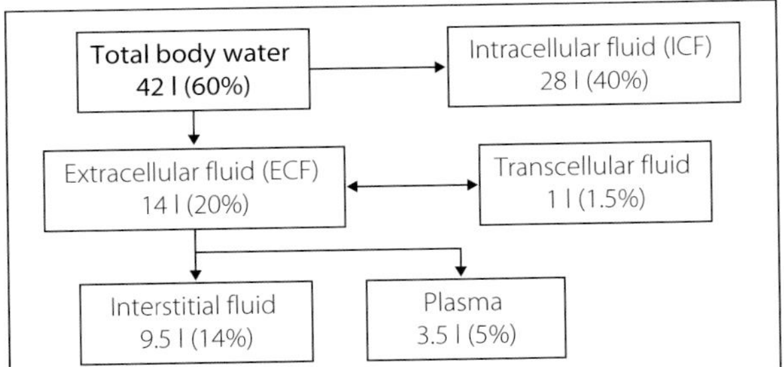

Fig. 70 Composition of body fluids, with volumes for an average 70 kg man (% body weight)

- Main methods of movement of ions and molecules between compartments:
  - diffusion.
  - facilitated diffusion: carrier molecules transport substances from high to low concentrations, requiring no energy.
  - active transport.
  - filtration.

Movement of substances is also affected by other substances, e.g. Donnan effect.

Water moves across membranes from solutions of low concentrations to those of high concentrations (osmosis). Depending on their constitution, different iv fluids will fill certain compartments more than others.

See also, Blood volume; Fluid balance

Flumazenil. Benzodiazepine antagonist, structurally related to midazolam and introduced in 1987. A competetive inhibitor of benzodiazepines at the central $GABA_A$/benzodiazepine receptor complex. Has been used to reverse excessive sedation due to benzodiazepines, e.g. following attempted suicide, prolonged sedation with benzodiazepines in ICU, and iatrogenic overdose. Benzodiazepine metabolism is unaffected. 50% protein-bound.

- Dosage: 0.2 mg iv, repeated slowly as necessary up to 1–2 mg. May also be given by infusion (0.1–0.4 mg/h).
- Side effects: nausea, vomiting, dizziness, headache, confusion, pulmonary oedema. Has caused excessive excitement and convulsions, especially in patients maintained on long-term benzodiazepines, e.g. for epilepsy. Because of its short half-life (less than 1 h), its effects may wear off with recurrence of sedation.

Fluoride ions. Nephrotoxic ions implicated in the high output renal failure seen following methoxyflurane administration. Evidence for their role:

- degree of renal impairment is proportional to plasma concentration:
  - subclinical evidence of renal impairment occurs above 50 μmol/l.
  - polyuria, decreased urinary osmolality and increased plasma sodium and osmolality occur above 80–100 μmol/l.
- infusion of fluoride ions into rats produces similar renal effects.

Mechanism of renal damage is unclear but may involve impairment of both renal Na/K/ATPase systems and vasopressin action.

- Levels are highest after methoxyflurane, but may be raised after other halogenated volatile agents:
  - methoxyflurane: 50–60 μmol/l after 2.5 MAC hours; 90–120 μmol/l after 5 MAC hours.
  - enflurane: up to 30 μmol/l after prolonged use (over 9 h). Plasma levels are highest in obese patients. Enzyme induction with isoniazid is thought to increase levels.

Table 14 Approximate composition of body fluid compartments (mmol/l)

Compartment	*Na^+*	*K^+*	*HCO_3^-*	*Cl^-*	*Ca^{2+}*	*Mg^{2+}*	*SO_4^{2-}*	*$HPO_4^{2-} + PO_4^{3-}$*
Intracellular fluid	10	150	10	3	3	30	20	100
Interstitial fluid	140	5	30	110	5	3	1	2
Plasma	140	5	28	110	5	3	1	2

- isoflurane: under 5 μmol/l even after prolonged surgery. Levels of up to 90 μmol/l have been reported after several days' use for sedation in ICU.
- halothane: minimal production of fluoride ions.
- sevoflurane: up to 40 μmol/l after prolonged surgery (unaffected by obesity).
- desflurane: minimal production of fluoride ions.

Fluotec vaporiser, *see Vaporisers*

Flupirtine maleate. Non-opioid centrally acting analgesic drug, recently investigated. Thought to act via central adrenergic pathway stimulation, although the precise mechanism is unclear. Also causes muscular relaxation via enhancement of GABA-mediated spinal inhibition.

Flurbiprofen. NSAID available for oral and pr administration; has been used for postoperative analgesia.
- Dosage: 50–100 mg 4–6 hourly up to 300 mg/day (100 mg suppositories available).
- Side effects: as for NSAIDs.

Fluroxene (Trifluoroethyl vinyl ether). Inhalational anaesthetic agent, introduced in 1954. The first fluorine containing volatile agent, now unavailable. Explosive, possibly mutagenic, and toxic to experimental animals due to biotransformation to trifluoroethanol.

Flying squad, obstetric. Mobile team including anaesthetist, obstetrician and midwife; first suggested in 1929, and organised in Glasgow in 1933. The usual problems of obstetric anaesthesia and neonatal resuscitation are compounded by the abnormal location, limitation of facilities, requirement for portable equipment, and lack of patient preparation. Commonest emergency is postpartum haemorrhage caused by retained placenta. Use of a flying squad has declined as the number of home deliveries has decreased. The above problems have led many units to withdraw anaesthetic cover from such squads, with emphasis on rapid transfer of the patient to hospital.
See also, Cardiopulmonary resuscitation, neonatal; Obstetric analgesia and anaesthesia

Foetal, *see Fetal*

Fomepizole (4-Methylpyrazole). Competitive inhibitor of alcohol dehydrogenase, available on a named patient basis for methanol or ethylene glycol poisoning. A loading dose of 15 mg/kg iv over 30 min is followed by 10 mg/kg every 12 h for 4 doses, then 15 mg/kg every 12 h until methanol or ethylene glycol concentrations are $<$ 4–6 mmol/l, and the patient is asymptomatic with normal pH. Undergoes hepatic metabolism and excreted in the urine.
See also, Alcohol poisoning

Fondaparinux sodium. Synthetic sulphated pentasaccharide derived from the factor Xa-binding moiety of unfractionated heparin. Inhibits factor Xa and indicated as an alternative to heparin for preventing postoperative DVT (currently licensed for orthopaedic surgery only). Given as a single daily sc injection of 2.5 mg for 5–9 days, the first dose 6 h after wound closure.

Fondation Européenne d'Enseignement en Anaesthésiologie (Foundation for European Education in Anaesthesiology; FEEA). Organisation founded in 1986 (with financial support from the European Union) to provide Continuous Medical Education in anaesthesiology throughout Europe. Acts in agreement with national anaesthetic societies and organises courses throughout Europe and, more recently, South America.
Scherpereel P (2000). Eur J Anaesthesiol; 17: 75–6

Food and Drug Administration (FDA). US body, involved in testing new drugs and reviewing test results. Also controls imports, and regulates foods and cosmetics. Companies must apply to the FDA before initiating clinical trials. Evolved after World War II from the 1938 Food, Drug and Cosmetics Act, restricting labelling and advertising of drugs; amended in 1968 to require that drugs be shown to be efficacious as well as safe. Thus enforces laws enacted by the US Congress. Previously, the Pure Food and Drugs Act of 1906 and subsequent amendments attempted to prevent improper labelling and fraudulent claims by manufacturers.
See also, Committee on Safety of Medicines

Foot, nerve blocks, *see Ankle, nerve blocks; Digital nerve block*

Force. That which changes a body's state of rest or motion. SI unit of force is the newton.

Forced diuresis. Method of increasing renal excretion of certain drugs using iv fluids or diuretics to increase urinary volume. Sometimes used in poisoning and overdoses. Further drug removal is achieved by manipulating urinary pH, thereby 'trapping' the ionised fraction of the drug and preventing its diffusion back into the bloodstream, since charged molecules diffuse poorly across biological membranes.
- Forced alkaline diuresis:
  - used in poisoning with acid drugs, e.g. salicylates and barbiturates.
  - 500 ml/h of the following fluids are administered in rotation:
    - 500 ml 1.26% sodium bicarbonate.
    - 500 ml 5% dextrose.
    - 500 ml 0.9% saline.
  - CVP, urine output and pH, blood gases and plasma electrolytes (especially potassium) must be closely monitored. Infusion rate is reduced in the elderly.
- Forced acid diuresis:
  - used in poisoning with alkaline drugs, e.g. amfetamines, phencyclidines.
  - 1000 ml/h of the following fluids are administered in rotation:
    - 500 ml 5% dextrose + 1.5 g ammonium chloride.
    - 500 ml 5% dextrose.
    - 500 ml 0.9% saline.
  - monitoring as above.

Severe metabolic upset and circulatory overload may occur. The technique is rarely used now, since it has been superseded by haemodialysis and haemofiltration.

Forced expiration. Means of investigating lung function, from which may be measured: forced expiratory flow rate ($FEF_{25-75\%}$), FEV, FVC and peak expiratory flow rate. Other suggested measurements exclude the first 200 ml of expiration, or analyse the flow rate at 50% of vital capacity.

Flow–volume loops and data from spirometers (e.g. the Vitalograph) may be analysed (Fig. 71). Repetition following bronchodilator therapy may indicate the extent of reversible airway obstruction.

At lung volumes of up to 60% of vital capacity, maximal expiratory flow rate is independent of effort; increasing effort

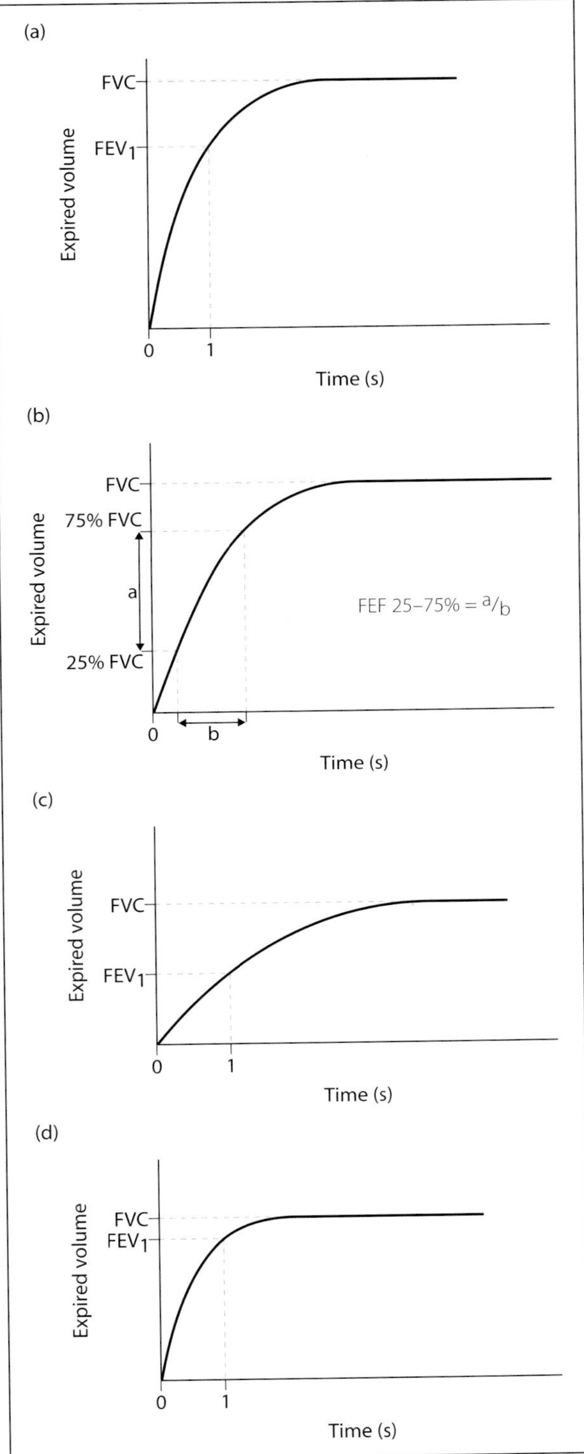

Fig. 71 Typical forced expiratory patterns: (a) normal; (b) showing calculation of FEF (25–75%); (c) obstructive lung disease; (d) restrictive lung disease

raises intrathoracic pressure, increasing the pressure difference across the airways, and leading to airway collapse.
See also, Lung function tests

Forced expiratory flow rate ($FEF_{25-75\%}$). Average flow rate measured at between 25% and 75% of forced maximal expired volume (Fig. 71). Usually changes with **forced expiratory volume**, but has wider spread of normal values.
See also, Forced expiration; Lung function tests; Peak expiratory flow rate

Forced expiratory volume (FEV). Volume of gas forcibly exhaled from full inspiration, in a set period of time (normally 1 s; the volume is then called FEV_1). Normally 80% of **FVC**, which may be measured at the same time using a **spirometer**. Reduced in obstructive lung disease, as is the FEV_1/FVC ratio. In restrictive disease, FEV_1 may be normal, but FVC is reduced.

Easier and more comfortable to measure than **maximal voluntary ventilation**.
See also, Forced expiration; Lung function tests

Forced vital capacity (FVC). **Vital capacity** measured when expiration is forced. Closure of some airways may occur when intrathoracic pressure is high, causing air-trapping. FVC thus may be less than 'true' vital capacity. Reduced in restrictive disease, the supine position, the elderly, muscle weakness, abdominal swelling, pain, and when premature airway closing occurs during forced expiration, e.g. emphysema.
See also, Forced expiration; Lung function tests; Lung volumes

Forceps. Many varieties may be used by anaesthetists, e.g. (Fig. 72):
- **Magill**'s forceps: introduced originally in 1920 to assist placement of gum-elastic bougies for insufflation anaesthesia. Used to guide tracheal tubes into the larynx, or nasogastric tubes into the oesophagus, under direct vision. May damage the tracheal tube cuff if grasped. Also used to place pharyngeal packs or to remove foreign bodies. The operator's hand is held out of the line of vision by the angled handles. Adult and paediatric sizes are available, as are single-use versions. Many modifications have been described.
- Krause's forceps: used to hold local anaesthetic soaked pledgets in the piriform fossae for blocking the superior laryngeal nerves for awake intubation. They bear a spring catch and spiked jaws.
- several tongue forceps exist; formerly used to pull the tongue forward to relieve airway obstruction, but now more likely to be used for fixing tubing, drapes, etc.

[Herman Krause (1848–1921), German laryngologist; Berkley GA Moynihan (1865–1936), English surgeon]
See also, Mouth gags

Foreign body, inhaled. Most common in children. May obstruct upper or lower airways. Should be considered in any child with **stridor** or persistent cough and chest infections. Most small objects lodge in the right main bronchus, because of its more vertical angle of origin and greater width. Organic matter, e.g. peanuts, may cause intense bronchial inflammatory reactions within a few hours, with oedema and possibly bronchial obstruction. **Bronchiectasis** may be a late complication. Other features may include:
- distal **atelectasis**.
- distal air-trapping if the object acts as a ball-valve. Chest X-ray in expiration may reveal unilateral overinflation.
- features of **airway obstruction**.
- infection.

- Removal is via rigid **bronchoscopy**. Anaesthetic management:

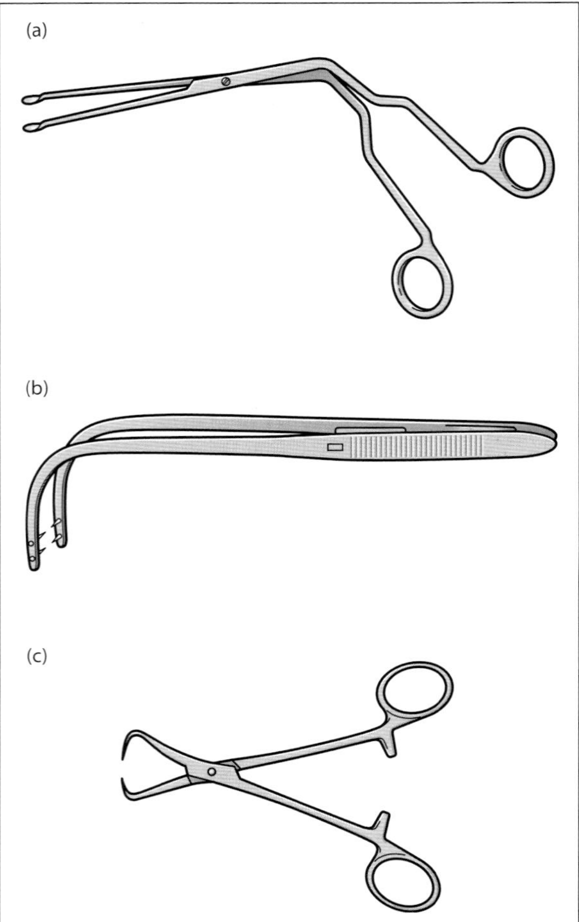

Fig. 72 Types of forceps used in anaesthesia: (a) Magill; (b) Krause; (c) Moynihan tongue forceps

- preoperatively:
  - assessment for severity of airway obstruction.
  - premedication with atropine. Sedative drugs are suggested by some as being helpful; by others as being a hindrance.
- perioperatively:
  - an experienced anaesthetist's presence is mandatory.
  - classically, an inhalational induction is performed, using halothane (more recently, sevoflurane) in O_2. N_2O is avoided in case of distal air-trapping, and to raise F_IO_2. Induction may be slow.
  - iv induction is preferred by some.
  - lidocaine spray to the vocal cords may reduce risk of peri- and postoperative laryngospasm.
  - classically, spontaneous ventilation is employed using ether, with bronchoscopy performed as anaesthesia lightens. Halothane or sevoflurane is most commonly used now. Avoidance of IPPV is usually advocated, to reduce risk of blowing the object further distally. In practice, adequate depth of anaesthesia and oxygenation may be difficult to maintain with spontaneous ventilation, without excessive hypercapnia.
- postoperatively:
  - close monitoring is required in case of bronchospasm or laryngospasm.
  - humidified O_2 administration by mask.

Forward failure, *see Cardiac failure*

Foscarnet sodium. Antiviral drug, reserved for treatment of cytomegalovirus retinitis in AIDS, when ganciclovir is contraindicated because of its toxicity or when herpes simplex virus infections are unresponsive to aciclovir.
- Dosage: 20 mg/kg iv over 30 min then 20–120 mg/kg daily according to renal function. For resistant herpes simplex virus infections, 40 mg/kg 8 hourly for 2–3 weeks.
- Side effects: nausea, renal failure, GIT upset, hypocalcaemia, convulsions.

Fosphenytoin sodium. Water-soluble prodrug, completely converted to phenytoin after parenteral administration, with a conversion half-life of 15 min. Useful in treating acute partial and generalised tonic–clonic seizures. Particularly appropriate in management of status epilepticus. 1.5 mg of fosphenytoin is equivalent to 1 mg of phenytoin. Can be administered iv or im with good absorption. Following its administration, monitoring of phenytoin levels is not recommended until conversion to phenytoin is complete (i.e. within 2 h after iv infusion and 4 h after im injection).
- Side effects: paraesthesia, hypotension, nystagmus, ataxia, skin reactions, pruritus. Severe hypotension and arrhythmias including heart block, VF and asystole have been described following its use; monitoring of ECG, BP, pulse rate and respiratory function is recommended for 30 min after the end of the infusion.

Fourier analysis. Mathematical breakdown of waveforms into simple sine wave constituents. Any complex waveform consists of sine waves of different frequencies: the slowest (fundamental) frequency and harmonics thereof. Used in analysis and reconstruction of waveforms, e.g. transmission of electrical signals. The higher the frequencies analysed, the more accurate the reproduction.
[Baron Jean-Baptiste Fourier (1768–1830), French mathematician]

Fournier's gangrene, *see Necrotising fasciitis*

Fowler's method (Single breath nitrogen washout). Method of investigation of lung volumes, described in 1948. The subject breathes air normally, and takes a maximal breath of O_2 (i.e. to vital capacity) from the end of normal expiration (i.e. FRC). Exhaled nitrogen concentration is measured during maximal slow expiration (i.e. to residual volume), and plotted against volume of expired gas. A rapid-response nitrogen meter is required.
- Four phases are described (Fig. 73):
  - phase 1: O_2 from the conducting airways (anatomical dead space), containing no nitrogen.
  - phase 2: mixture of dead space gas and alveolar gas.
  - phase 3: alveolar gas, containing the nitrogen present in the alveoli before the O_2 breath started. There is a slight upward slope normally, increased in lung disease.
  - phase 4: at closing capacity, lower alveoli and airways collapse, thus the exhaled gas comes from upper airways only. At the onset of the O_2 inspiration, the upper airways were already considerably expanded (with nitrogen-containing air) compared with lower ones, since most ventilation is of upper lung regions at normal tidal volume. Most of the inspired O_2 therefore entered the lower alveoli, since they started off smaller. When they collapse, nitrogen-rich gas from the upper alveoli is exhaled, giving rise to phase 4.

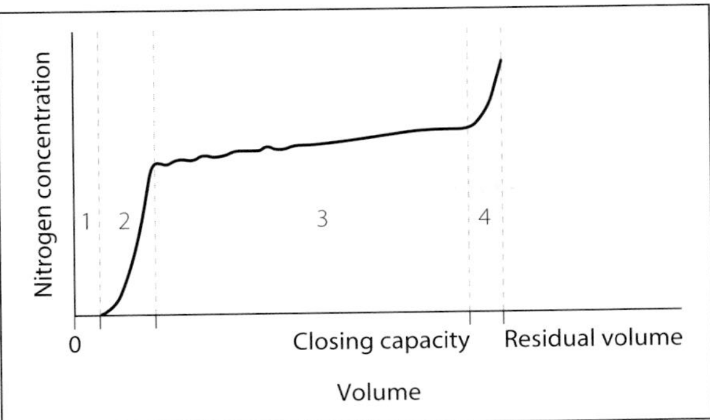

Fig. 73 Fowler's method of estimating anatomical dead space and closing capacity (see text)

Anatomical dead space is measured to the mid-point of phase 2.

CO_2 measurement may be used in a similar way, using capnography.

[Ward S Fowler, US physiologist]

Fractional shortening, *see Left ventricular fractional shortening*

Frankenhauser's plexus block, *see Paracervical block*

FRC, *see Functional residual capacity*

FRCA examination (Fellowship of the Royal College of Anaesthetists). Predated by the FFARCS examination (1953–89) and the FCAnaes examination (1989–92). Since 1985 (as the FFARCS examination) it consisted of three parts: I, relating to the fundamentals of clinical anaesthesia; II, relating to the basic sciences; III, relating to the practice of anaesthesia as a whole. Replaced in 1996 by a two-part examination: the Primary relating to basic sciences and clinical safety; and the Final relating to applied basic sciences and the practice of anaesthesia/intensive care. Recent pass rates are in the order of 40–50% for each part.

Free radicals. Atoms or molecules with unpaired electrons, i.e. only one within an orbital. Produced as intermediaries during stages of certain biological reactions, e.g. involving reduction of molecular O_2 to oxide ions, with production of oxygen-derived free radicals (OFRs) including superoxide ($O^{\cdot}{}_2{}^{-}$), hydroxyl ($OH^{\cdot}$) and hydroperoxy ($HO^{\cdot}{}_2$) radicals, the latter two being particularly reactive. Hydrogen peroxide is involved in formation of many OFRs. Thought to be involved in normal phagocyte function and host defence; released into phagosomes to destroy bacteria, etc. May also be produced by radiation and certain chemicals, and increased production has been implicated in many disease processes including pulmonary O_2 toxicity, halothane hepatitis, ARDS, paracetamol poisoning, burns, carcinogenesis and bowel ischaemia. Defence mechanisms against normal free radical formation may be overwhelmed, resulting in oxidation of tissues, especially cell membrane lipids, proteins, nucleic acids and extracellular matrix. Reactions with free radicals may liberate further free radicals, with further injury, etc.

Defence mechanisms include the enzymes superoxide dismutase (SOD) and catalase, and antioxidants (free radical scavengers), e.g. glutathione and vitamin E. Increasing these substances indirectly, or administering them directly, may reduce tissue injury in some experimental models, especially involving O_2 toxicity, but extrapolation to clinical use is unclear.

Free water clearance, *see Clearance, free water*

Freud, Sigmund (1856–1939). Austrian neurologist and psychiatrist, the inventor of psychoanalysis. Postulated that cocaine might be a treatment for morphine addiction, and a stimulant for psychoneurotic patients. Investigated the drug with his friend Koller, who introduced it as the first local anaesthetic drug. Fled from Vienna to London in 1938 to escape the Nazis.

Friedreich's ataxia. Hereditary (autosomal recessive) condition consisting of progressive degeneration of spinocerebellar and pyramidal tracts and dorsal root ganglia, mainly affecting the legs. Onset is in childhood or teens.

- Features:
  - upper motor neurone weakness, with upgoing plantar reflexes (if present).
  - ataxia, dysarthria and nystagmus.
  - impaired joint position, vibration and touch sense. Reflexes may be absent.
  - kyphoscoliosis and pes cavus.
  - cardiomyopathy in over 50% of patients, with risk of cardiac failure and arrhythmias.
- Anaesthesic precautions:
  - preoperative assessment of neurological, cardiovascular and respiratory systems.
    - cautious use of neuromuscular blocking drugs.
    - risk of respiratory insufficiency postoperatively; physiotherapy, O_2 therapy and adequate analgesia are required.

Other rarer, hereditary ataxias also exist.

[Nikolaus Friedreich (1825–1882), German neurologist]

Frontal nerve block, *see Ophthalmic nerve blocks*

Frusemide, *see Furosemide*

Fuel cell, *see Oxygen measurement*

Fuller's earth. Soft clay-like substance which contains silica and clay minerals and found naturally in many parts of the world. Used for pressing and cleaning cloths and fleeces ('fulling') and in the purification of oils. Used as an adsorbent in paraquat poisoning.

Functional imaging. The study of changes in cerebral haemodynamic and metabolic status in response to external stimuli. Techniques include positron emission tomography which provides maps of regional blood flow and oxygenation, functional MRI which produces high resolution oxygenation maps, and near infra-red spectroscopy which provides a continuous measure of tissue oxygenation.

Functional residual capacity (FRC). Lung volume, the sum of residual volume and expiratory reserve volume. Normally 2.5–3.0 litres for an average male.

- Measurement:
  - helium dilution: breathing of air with a known concentration of helium from a spirometer, starting from the end of normal expiration. CO_2 is absorbed using soda lime, and O_2 replaced as it is used. The helium distributes between spirometer, tubing and the subject's lungs, with minimal uptake by the bloodstream. After

equilibrium is reached, the new concentration of helium is measured:

total amount of helium in the system

= initial concentration × volume of apparatus

= new concentration × volume of (apparatus + lungs)

- nitrogen washout: the subject breathes 100% O_2 from end of normal expiration, and total volume of expired gas over several minutes is analysed for nitrogen content. This amount of nitrogen was originally contained in the FRC to give a concentration of 79%; thus FRC may be calculated.
- body plethysmograph.

The helium dilution and nitrogen washout techniques do not include collapsed portions of lung, or those with poor air entry (if not enough time is allowed for equilibration). Measurements using the body plethysmograph include these areas, which may not participate in gas exchange. Comparison of the tests may indicate the degree of airway collapse/hypoventilation.

- FRC is important because hypoxaemia may result if it is reduced:
  - if closing capacity (CC) exceeds FRC, airway closure occurs with quiet breathing, with $\dot{V}/\dot{Q}$ mismatch. Hypoxaemia of old age is thought to result from this, since CC rises with age.
  - FRC serves as an O_2 reserve; thus a reduced FRC holds less O_2, e.g. should airway obstruction occur. The FRC O_2 store helps prevent large swings in arterial $P\text{O}_2$ during respiration.

  Reduced FRC may also reduce lung compliance and increase pulmonary vascular resistance.
- Reduced by:
  - supine position.
  - obesity.
  - pregnancy.
  - anaesthesia, even with IPPV (mechanism is unknown, but thought to involve decreased muscle tone and shift of thoracic and peripheral blood to the abdomen).
  - restrictive lung disease, e.g. pulmonary fibrosis; it may also be reduced in pulmonary oedema, infection, atelectasis, ARDS, etc.
- Increased by:
  - PEEP and CPAP.
  - increased airway resistance, e.g. asthma.
  - exercise due to sustained inspiratory muscle tone.

Fungal infection in the ICU. The incidence of nosocomial infection involving fungi is increasing in ICU practice, related to increased use of antibiotics and immunodeficiency (either present before the presenting illness or acquired during it). Immunosuppressed patients may also present with fungal infection acquired outside hospital. *Candida albicans* is most commonly involved but other candida species, *Torulopsis glabrata* and other normal gut commensals may also be involved. Risk factors for pathogenic colonisation include prolonged antibacterial therapy, severe illness, presence of intravascular and urinary catheters, TPN and immunosuppression. Diagnosis may be difficult since blood cultures may be negative even with severe fungal infection; however, it has been suggested that clinically significant infection exists if fungus is obtained from multiple sites. Treatment is with antifungal drugs, especially amphotericin, fluconazole and flucytosine, although whether to treat patients with evidence of fungal colonisation is controversial.

Furosemide (Frusemide). Loop diuretic, derived from sulphonamides. Decreases renal sodium and water reabsorption, with potassium loss. IV injection causes vasodilatation, with diuresis within 30 min.

- Dosage:
  - depends on renal function and response: 5–10 mg may cause considerable diuresis given orally or iv (less than 4 mg/min) to healthy patients. Up to 500 mg may be given in severe renal impairment.
  - suitable starting dose in fluid retention or cardiac failure: 0.5–1.0 mg/kg.
  - often given as an infusion, e.g. on ICU: 1–4 mg/h, although recent evidence suggests that renal failure is not prevented by this strategy.
- Side effects:
  - ototoxicity, especially after rapid iv injection.
  - hypokalaemia.
  - raised creatinine, urea and uric acid may occur.
  - rash, thrombocytopenia and leucopenia rarely.

Fusidic acid (Sodium fusidate). Steroidal antibacterial drug, chemically related to the cephalosporins. Used to treat penicillin-resistant staphylococcal infections, especially endocarditis and osteomyelitis (achieves high levels in bone). Well absorbed from the GIT and metabolised in the liver to inactive metabolites. Half-life 5–6 h; 98% protein-bound.

- Dosage: 0.5–1.0 g orally or iv, 8 hourly.
- Side effects include nausea, vomiting, rashes, jaundice (with high doses).

Fuzzy logic. Method of describing and controlling systems in which various qualities are described in terms of degrees, rather than absolutes, e.g. varying shades of grey instead of merely black and white. Allows finer control than yes/no systems since even if the latter are made more discerning by defining many divisions (e.g. black, very dark grey, dark grey, medium grey, etc.) there will always be a 'step' between adjacent ones. In fuzzy logic, each division (or shade, above) overlaps its neighbours, and thus any point may be defined according to the extent to which it 'belongs' to each shade. Has been used in various systems, e.g. control of iv infusions.

Grant P, Naesh O (2005). J R Soc Med; 98: 7–9

FVC, *see Forced vital capacity*

G protein-coupled receptors (GPCRs). Large family of transmembrane receptors which bind a wide variety of ligands including neurotransmitters and hormones. The target receptors of many drugs including adrenergic, dopamine, opioid, 5-HT and histamine agents. The receptor consists of seven membrane-spanning helices bound on the inner surface of the membrane to a G protein, so-called because they bind guanine diphosphate (GDP) and triphosphate (GTP). G proteins consist of three subunits: Gα, Gβ and Gγ. In the inactive state, Gα has GDP on its binding site (Fig. 74a). Activation of the GPCR by a ligand causes an allosteric change in the Gα subunit resulting in the displacement of GDP and replacement by GTP; the Gβ and Gγ subunits dissociate from the complex (Fig. 74b). The activated Gα subunit in turn activates an effector molecule, e.g. adenylate cyclase (*see Fig. 5; Adenosine monophosphate, cyclic*). Activated Gα is a GTPase which rapidly reconverts GTP to GDP, thus restoring the G protein to its inactive state.

Many types of Gα subunit exist, including:

- $G\alpha_s$: stimulates adenylate cyclase increasing levels of cAMP in the cell, e.g. β-adrenergic agonists and glucagon are $G\alpha_s$ coupled.
- $G\alpha_i$: inhibits adenylate cyclase, e.g. α_2-adrenergic receptor agonists are $G\alpha_i$ coupled.
- $G\alpha_q$: activates phospholipases C generating inositol triphosphate (IP_3), e.g. α_1-adrenergic receptor agonists are $G\alpha_q$ coupled.

In addition to their coupling to second messenger systems, G proteins can also be directly coupled to ion channels. They have been investigated as possible sites for interaction with anaesthetic agents.

Hollmann MW, Danja Strumper D, Herroeder S, Durieux ME (2005). Anesthesiology; 103: 1066–88

See also, Receptor theory

G proteins, *see G protein-coupled receptors*

G6PD deficiency, *see Glucose 6-phosphate dehydrogenase deficiency*

GABA, *see γ-Aminobutyric acid*

Gabapentin. Oral anticonvulsant drug, also used in chronic pain management. In epilepsy, used mainly as add-on therapy for partial seizures. Although structurally related to GABA, it is thought to act by blocking voltage-gated calcium channels in the CNS. May also be useful as an adjunct for postoperative pain relief. Peak plasma levels occur within 2–3 h of administration, with half-life of 5–7 h. Excreted renally.

- Dosage: 300 mg orally on the first day; 12 hourly then 8 hourly on successive days then adjusted gradually according to response up to 800 mg 8 hourly.
- Side effects include sedation, dizziness, ataxia, nystagmus, tremor, diplopia, nausea, convulsions, cough.

Kong VKF, Irwin MG (2007). Br J Anaesth; 99: 775–86

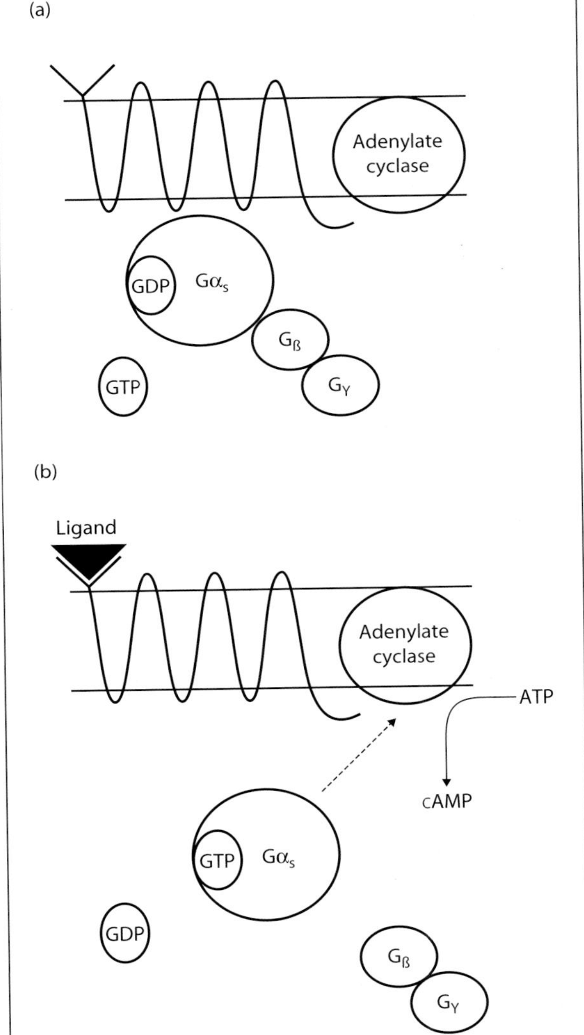

Fig. 74 G protein-coupled receptor in (a) inactive and (b) activated states (see text)

Gabexate mesilate. Synthetic serine protease inhibitor; has been studied as a protective and therapeutic agent in pancreatitis, as a neuroprotective agent in spinal cord injury, and as a treatment for DIC.

Gag reflex. Elevation and constriction of the pharynx following stimulation of the posterior pharyngeal wall. The afferent pathway is via the glossopharyngeal nerve; the efferent is via the vagus. Elevation of the soft palate when it is touched relies on afferent fibres in the maxillary division of the trigeminal nerve; often the two reflexes are elicited together. The gag reflex is abolished following local anaesthesia and lesions of the pharynx, lesions involving the vagal nuclei in the medulla, and deep anaesthesia or coma. Absence of the gag reflex may indicate that the airway is at risk, e.g. from aspiration of vomitus. The reflex is assessed as part of testing for brainstem death.

Gain, electrical. Ratio of output signal amplitude to input signal amplitude. Thus a measure of amplification of signal, e.g. in monitoring equipment. May be specified as voltage, current or power gain; expressed as a simple ratio, or for power gain, also expressed as logarithm (base 10) of the ratio (in bels or decibels).
[Alexander Bell (1847–1922), Scottish-born US inventor]

Gallamine triethiodide. Medium-acting non-depolarising neuromuscular blocking drug, first used in 1948; no longer available in the UK because of its anticholinergic action causing marked tachycardia, its ability to cross the placenta, and its reliance on renal excretion.

Galvanic skin response (Skin conductance response; Sympathogalvanic response). Test of sympathetic afferent, efferent and spinal interconnecting pathways, used to assess the effects of sympathetic nerve blocks. Has also been used to assess other regional blocks in which sympathetic blockade occurs, e.g. epidural anaesthesia, brachial plexus block. Skin electrodes are placed on dorsal and ventral surfaces of the hand/foot, with a reference electrode elsewhere. Opposite sides of the body are normally compared. The output is displayed on an oscilloscope (e.g. ECG machine); a steady line results. With intact sympathetic pathways, pinching the skin causes altered skin conductance via changes in sweat gland secretion, displayed as a deflection lasting under 5 s. Deflection is abolished by successful blockade. The response may be diminished by use of atropine, repeated testing and in the elderly.

Preblockade size of deflection has also been used to assess suitability for subsequent sympathetic block.

Changes in skin potential may also be measured.

Ganciclovir. Antiviral drug, related to aciclovir but more active against cytomegalovirus and more toxic, thus reserved for severe infections and to prevent infection during immunosuppression following organ transplantation. Valganciclovir, a prodrug, is available for oral use.

- Dosage: 5 mg/kg iv 12 hourly for 2–3 weeks (treatment) or 1–2 weeks (prophylaxis), followed by 5 mg/kg daily.
- Side effects: many, including blood dyscrasias, rash, hepatorenal impairment, GIT upset, arrhythmias, coma. Contraindicated in pregnancy. May cause severe myelosuppression in combination with zidovudine.

Ganglion blocking drugs. Nicotinic acetylcholine receptor antagonists acting at autonomic ganglia. The first antihypertensive drugs, now rarely used because of widespread side effects caused by sympathetic blockade (postural and exertional hypotension, decreased sweating) and parasympathetic blockade (constipation, urinary retention, impotence, dry mouth, blurring of vision). May first stimulate then block receptors (e.g. nicotine) or exhibit competitive antagonism (e.g. hexamethonium, pentolinium, trimetaphan). None is generally available in the UK.

Because of the similarity between neuromuscular and ganglionic nicotinic receptors, ganglion blockers (e.g. hexamethonium) may cause neuromuscular blockade, and neuromuscular blocking drugs (e.g. tubocurarine) may cause ganglionic blockade.

Gangrene. Death and decay of body tissues; usually a consequence of ischaemia ± bacterial decomposition but may be caused by micro-organisms in well-perfused tissue (e.g. gas gangrene). Traditionally a clinical diagnosis, thus described according to the causative insult and clinical appearances even though some of the terms are now obsolete: traumatic gangrene (resulting from direct injury); gas gangrene (associated with gas formation within the tissues); Fournier's gangrene (affecting the perineum); wet gangrene (associated with venous congestion and oedema); dry gangrene (affected tissue is blackened and shrunken). Many terms have been superseded by more specific ones, e.g. necrotising fasciitis.
[Jean A Fournier (1832–1914), Paris dermatologist]

Gas. Form of matter whose constituent molecules or atoms are constantly moving, and whose mean positions are far apart. Tends to expand in all directions, and diffuse and mix with other gases. Governed by the gas laws under ideal circumstances. Formed by a liquid above its critical temperature. The constituent particles are sufficiently far apart for the forces (e.g. Van der Waals forces) between them to be almost negligible, unless the gas is compressed. Pressure exerted by a gas is proportional to the number of collisions of atoms/molecules against the container's walls.
See also, Boyle's law; Charles' law; Ideal gas law

Gas analysis. Possible methods:

- chemical:
  - gas reacts chemically with other substances to form non-gaseous compounds, with reduction of overall volume (e.g. Haldane apparatus) or pressure (e.g. van Slyke apparatus). Alternatively, the reaction results in emission of light which is measured by a photodetector (e.g. chemiluminescence nitric oxide analysis (NO + ozone producing O_2 + NO_2 + light).
  - electrochemical: gas reacts with other substances, the number of electrons transferred during the reaction being proportional to the concentration of gas in the sample. Used in nitric oxide analysers (NO being converted to NO_2).
- physical:
  - spectroscopy.
  - adsorption of vapours on to surfaces:
    - rubber strips, e.g. in the Dräger Narkotest. Tension of the strips is reduced by volatile agents; the extent is proportional to their concentration. Temperature compensated with a bimetallic strip. Adjustable for use with different agents and in the presence of N_2O, to which it is also sensitive. Has a slow response; now rarely used.
    - silicone polymer coating a vibrating quartz crystal, e.g. in the Engström Emma. Change in frequency of vibration (caused by passing current through the crystal) is proportional to the concentration of volatile agent, which may be specified.
  - interferometer: a light beam is split and passed through two chambers, one for reference and the other for samples. The beams are delayed to different extents; thus the emergent beams are out of phase. The resultant interference pattern is visualised through a telescope, and is displaced when gas is drawn into the sample chamber. Degree of change is related to

the sample concentration. Used for calibration, e.g. of vaporisers, not for perioperative monitoring.
- mass spectrometry.
- gas chromatography and detectors, e.g. katharometer, flame ionisation detector, electron capture detector.
- fuel cell, and paramagnetic and polarographic analysers, used for O_2 measurement.
- other methods, e.g. depending on different viscosities of gases, or velocity of sound through gases, are rarely used now.

[Heinrich Dräger (1847–1917), German engineer; Carl-Gunnar Engström (1912–1987), Swedish physician]
See also, Carbon dioxide measurement

Gas chromatography. Technique used for gas analysis. The sample mixture is injected into a stream of inert carrier gas, e.g. nitrogen, helium or argon (mobile phase), which passes through a column of silica–alumina particles coated in oil or wax (stationary phase). Separation of the sample component gases occurs along the column's length, depending on their relative solubilities in the two phases. Temperature of the column is carefully controlled, e.g. in an oven. Liquids may also be analysed. Suitable detectors, e.g. katharometer, flame ionisation detector or electron capture detector, are required.

Gas flow. Principles of flow are as for any fluid. Clinical applications:
- flow is turbulent in the upper airway, trachea and bronchi, especially during forceful breathing; i.e. gas viscosity is more important than density. Thus in upper airway obstruction, flow is increased if low density gas is used, e.g. helium–oxygen mixture.
- flow is laminar in small bronchioles; i.e. viscosity is important; although tube radius is very small, velocity is also very low. Helium has traditionally been considered of no use in improving gas flow in asthma, primarily a disease of small airways, but some evidence suggests that helium–oxygen may be useful in severe asthma, suggesting an element of turbulent flow.
- flow may be mostly laminar during quiet breathing, with turbulence at branches in the trachea and bronchi. Turbulence is more likely at mid-inspiration/expiration, when flow rate is highest (e.g. up to 50 l/min).

  Turbulence usually occurs in anaesthetic breathing systems during peak flow, especially if sharp-angled bends are present, e.g. at connections between components. Turbulence is more likely with narrow tubing and tubes.
- other applications include the Venturi principle, fluidics, flow–volume loops and flowmeters.

See also, Airway resistance

Gas gangrene. Infection due to clostridium species, usually *Cl. perfringens* (formerly *welchii*), a spore-forming Gram-positive anaerobic bacillus found in soil and faeces. Classically associated with deep war wounds, especially those contaminated with dirt or foreign bodies, but may follow any trauma, e.g. surgery. The incubation period is under 4 days, usually under 1 day.

The organism produces gas within tissues, often detectable clinically as subcutaneous emphysema. Local spread is rapid, with oedema, pain and tissue necrosis; endotoxin production causes generalised debilitation and toxaemia.

Prevented by cleansing of wounds and excision of dead tissue. Penicillin is effective prophylaxis. In established infection, penicillin therapy and surgical excision of all affected tissue are required. Hyperbaric O_2 therapy has been used to increase local tissue O_2 content; antitoxin therapy is more controversial.
See also, Clostridial infections; Oxygen, hyperbaric

Gas laws, *see Avogadro's hypothesis; Boyle's law; Charles' law; Dalton's law; Henry's law; Ideal gas law*

Gas transport, *see Carbon dioxide transport; Oxygen transport*

Gasp reflex. Production of a deep slow breath following a large positive pressure inflation of the lungs. Originally described in cats and dogs, but may be seen in newborn babies; during neonatal resuscitation, it may occur within primary apnoea. A similar response may also be seen after opioid administration in anaesthetised patients.

Head's paradoxical reflex, although similar, is produced under different experimental circumstances.
See also, Cardiopulmonary resuscitation, neonatal

Gasserian ganglion block. Block of the trigeminal ganglion which lies medially in the middle cranial fossa within a dural reflection (Meckel's cave), lateral to the internal carotid artery and cavernous sinus. Results in anaesthesia of the face, forehead, and anterior scalp (Fig. 75). Used mainly for treatment of trigeminal neuralgia, but also for surgery to the face.
- Technique:
  - with the patient supine and looking straight ahead, a 22 G 10 cm needle is introduced 3 cm lateral to the angle of the mouth, level with the second upper molar. Aiming at the pupil from the front, and the midpoint of the zygoma from the side, it is inserted until it contacts bone (greater wing of sphenoid, anterior to the foramen ovale). It is redirected posteriorly 1–1.5 cm deeper, passing through the foramen (paraesthesia radiating to the distribution of the appropriate branch). Electrical stimulation of the needle and X-ray imaging may be used to confirm correct positioning.

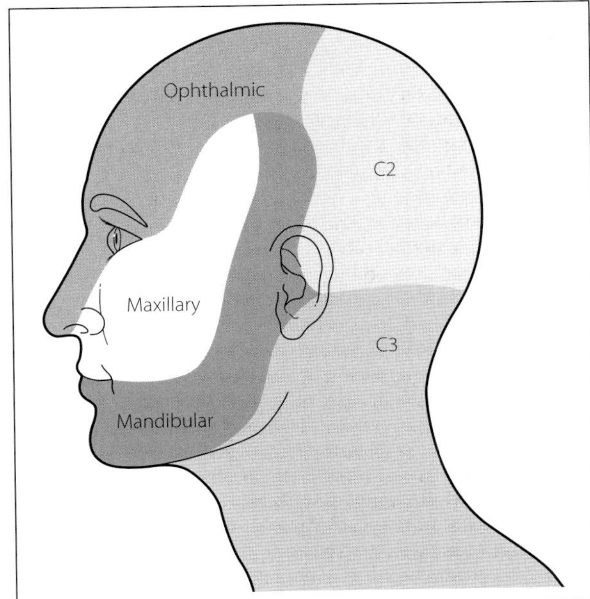

Fig. 75 Innervation of the face

- after careful aspiration, 1–2 ml solution, e.g. 1% lidocaine, is injected. Alcohol injection or thermocoagulation may follow if ablative therapy is required. Accidental subarachnoid injection may occur.

May be painful; general anaesthesia or sedation may be employed, with waking up or reversal to confirm paraesthesia, followed by resedation for ablation. Propofol or a midazolam/flumazenil combination has been used.

[Johann Gasser (1723–1765), Austrian anatomist; Johann Meckel (1714–1774), German anatomist]

See also, Mandibular nerve block; Maxillary nerve block; Ophthalmic nerve block

Gastric contents. Anaesthetic importance:
- absorption of orally administered drugs; e.g. related to gastric emptying, pH, and drug interactions within the stomach.
- aspiration of gastric contents; severity of aspiration pneumonitis is related to the pH and volume of aspirate, although the particulate nature of the aspirate is also important.

- Gastric secretion is increased by:
  - presence of food in the mouth (vagal reflex).
  - anger, stress.
  - presence of food in the stomach (local reflex).
  - protein meal, via duodenal gastrin secretion.
  - hypoglycaemia.
  - alcohol, caffeine.
- Gastric secretion and acidity are decreased by:
  - vagotomy.
  - H_2 receptor antagonists.
  - proton pump inhibitors.
  - drinking water.

Gastric acidity is decreased by antacids.

Gastric volume is related to gastric emptying and intake. Volume is reduced by H_2 antagonists and protein pump inhibitors, but increased by antacids.

Ng A, Smith G (2001). Anesth Analg; 93: 494–513

Gastric emptying. Normally results from peristaltic waves of contraction passing through the cardia, antrum, pylorus and duodenum, occurring up to three times/minute after a meal. Small amounts of liquid traverse the pylorus, which closes as the contraction wave reaches it, redirecting most of the propelled (solid) material back into the proximal stomach for further mixing. Thus liquids leave faster than solids. Carbohydrates leave faster than proteins and fats are slowest, via inhibitory feedback mechanisms involving duodenal hormone secretion.

- Slowed by:
  - lying down.
  - anxiety, fear, pain, etc.
  - mechanical obstruction and duodenal distension.
  - labour (little effect unless opioids given).
  - drugs, e.g. opioid analgesic drugs, anticholinergic drugs, alcohol, dopamine.
- Increased by:
  - gastric distension.
  - drugs, e.g. metoclopramide, domperidone (opioid-induced gastric stasis is not reversed; cf. cisapride).

Rate of emptying is important because of the risks of nausea, vomiting, regurgitation and aspiration of gastric contents. Emptying also affects absorption of orally administered drugs. Traditionally, 4–6 h starvation is usually required preoperatively in all but life-threatening emergencies, depending on the nature of the food/drink; gastric emptying is assumed to be complete in this time. However, gastric contents may be considerable, particularly after solid food. Small volumes of water (150 ml) given 2–3 h preoperatively have been shown to reduce the volume and acidity of gastric contents. Recent guidelines call for withholding of all solid food on the day of surgery, unrestricted clear fluids (i.e. possible to read print through) up to 3 h preoperatively, and consideration of H_2 receptor antagonists for patients at risk.

- Measurement:
  - measurement of plasma levels of orally administered substance, e.g. paracetamol (absorbed from the small intestine, not from the stomach).
  - serial nasogastric aspiration, with measurement of orally administered marker substance.
  - measurement of impedance across the lower chest/upper abdomen; alters as composition of tissues, i.e. gastric contents, changes.
  - oral administration of radioisotope, with measurement of radioactivity over the stomach.
  - ultrasound imaging.
  - X-ray imaging following oral contrast medium.

Emptying can be aided by naso- or orogastric aspiration. The latter is more efficient, using a wide bore tube with multiple holes and lumina, but is unpleasant and rarely used now. Emetic drugs are also rarely used.

Ng A, Smith G (2001). Anesth Analg; 93: 494–513

Gastric intramucosal pH, *see Gastric tonometry*

Gastric lavage. Performed for removal of drugs, poisons, etc. following poisoning and overdose; traditionally recommended up to 4 hours after ingestion (longer if gastric emptying is delayed, e.g. by anticholinergic drugs, aspirin), or at any time if the patient is unconscious. Involves passage of a wide bore orogastric tube, with aspiration to ensure the trachea has not been entered inadvertently. 300–600 ml warm water is introduced and allowed to drain under gravity; this is repeated until the aspirate is clear. Pulmonary aspiration may occur; the patient should be placed in the head-down lateral position with suction available. Tracheal intubation is required if laryngeal reflexes are absent. Lavage should not be performed if petroleum derivatives have been ingested, since pulmonary aspiration is particularly hazardous. Oesophageal/gastric perforation is also likely if caustic substances have been ingested. Now considered to have a very limited role.

Gastric tonometry. Method of indirect measurement of gastric intramucosal pH, which is used as an indicator of gastric (and therefore GIT) mucosal O_2 delivery and consumption. Intramucosal acidosis may thus indicate impaired GIT O_2 delivery or impaired utilisation, and has been proposed as a more sensitive indicator of poor splanchnic perfusion and mortality, and guide to vasoactive drug therapy in the ICU or during major surgery, than traditional markers.

A tonometer incorporating a saline-filled balloon is placed via the oesophagus into the stomach, and luminal $P\text{CO}_2$ (which approximates to intramucosal $P\text{CO}_2$) determined by measuring $P\text{CO}_2$ in the saline. A gas-filled balloon has also been used, with recirculation of gas into and out of the balloon with continuous measurement of $P\text{CO}_2$ at the distal end of the system. H_2 receptor antagonists eliminate the effect of gastric acid combining with pancreatic bicarbonate to produce CO_2, and increase sensitivity. Direct measurement is also possible but involves mucosal trauma and is less reliable. Arterial bicarbonate concentration is measured simultaneously and approximates to mucosal concentration, allowing calculation of intramucosal pH (pH_i).

Although enthusiastically supported by some, gastric tonometry has not found widespread acceptance into clinical practice, partly because of cost, unfamiliarity with the technique and poor specificity.
Kolkman JJ, Otte JA, Groeneveld ABJ (2000). Br J Anaesth; 84: 74–86

Gastrointestinal haemorrhage. May arise from any part of the GIT, although most acute bleeds are caused by gastric or duodenal ulcers or erosions. May result in the need for one or more of resuscitation, surgery or ICU management. Mortality is 5–10% (higher in certain conditions, e.g. 30% in oesophageal varices). Features range from obvious gross haematemesis to vomiting of small amounts of 'coffee grounds' (blood altered by gastric acid) or the passage of melaena.

- Main considerations:
  - of the underlying cause, e.g. oesophageal varices associated with alcoholism; NSAID-induced ulceration associated with arthritic disease; the possibility of coagulation disorders; systemic effects of malignancy.
  - haemorrhage and hypovolaemia generally.
  - presence of a full stomach and the risk of aspiration of gastric contents.
  - difficulty securing the airway whilst there is copious haematemesis.
- Management:
  - resuscitation, O_2, etc.
  - endoscopy to identify the bleeding site; performed as soon as the patient has been stabilised. It may be possible to treat certain lesions via this route, e.g. with adrenaline injection of bleeding points (0.5–1.0 ml of 1:10 000). Other investigations may be useful, e.g. radionuclear imaging or conventional angiography (it may be possible to embolise bleeding vessels once identified).
  - specific management, e.g. oesophageal varices.
  - medical management as for peptic ulcer disease.
  - surgery.

GIT haemorrhage associated with stress ulcers may occur in critically ill patients on the ICU, placing a severe stress on an already compromised CVS.

Gastro-oesophageal reflux. Normally prevented by the lower oesophageal sphincter and anatomical arrangement of the oesophagus and stomach. Common in, but not exclusive to, hiatus hernia and obesity. May cause burning retrosternal pain, especially on stooping/lying. Regurgitation of bitter fluid into the mouth may also occur. Associated oesophagitis may cause pain after meals, especially if spicy. Medical treatment is as for peptic ulcer disease/hiatus hernia; it includes losing weight and avoidance of provocative postures. Anaesthetic management is as for hiatus hernia.
Ng A, Smith G (2001). Anesth Analg; 93: 494–513

Gastro-oesophageal sphincter, *see Lower oesophageal sphincter*

Gastroschisis and exomphalos. Congenital malformations of the abdominal wall, associated with protrusion of abdominal contents:
  - gastroschisis: abdominal wall defect, not associated with the midline or umbilicus. Incidence is 1:30 000.
  - exomphalos: midline defect, related to the umbilicus. Incidence is 1:5–10 000.
- Associated with:
  - prematurity.
  - other congenital abnormalities, e.g. cardiac defects (especially VSD), other GIT malformations and genitourinary abnormalities.
- Initial problems:
  - damage to exposed organs.
  - fluid and electrolyte balance.
  - heat loss.
  - infection.
- Treatment:
  - the bowel is covered with a dry towel/plastic bag.
  - primary surgical closure is preferable to delayed closure if possible.
- Anaesthetic considerations: as for paediatric anaesthesia plus the above considerations. In addition:
  - N_2O diffuses into the bowel, increasing its size, and is avoided.
  - abdominal closure may be difficult, with increased intra-abdominal pressure. Postoperative IPPV may be necessary. Staged closure may be performed using a Silastic pouch if adverse effects of primary closure are excessive.
  - postoperative nutrition and prevention/treatment of infection are important.

Gate control theory of pain. Proposed in 1965 by Melzack and Wall to account for the influence of psychological and physiological variables on pain transmission. Suggests that impulses flow from periphery to brain through a 'gate' at spinal level, the opening or closure of which is influenced by other neural pathways. Pain is felt when impulse flow exceeds a certain critical level. The gate is closed by descending and large ascending (Aβ) fibres and opened by small ascending (C) fibres. It is thought to be located in the substantia gelatinosa (SG), laminae II and III of the dorsal horn; interneurones project to target cells which then project cranially. The theory has been modified since conception to account for expanding experimental and clinical evidence of neurotransmitter and receptor involvement (Fig. 76):
  - C fibres from deep receptors (e.g. chemical damage) project to SG cells, probably via substance P ('pushes' gate open). Cranial projection is via spinoreticular fibres.
  - Aβ fibres (activated by e.g. high frequency, low amplitude TENS) inhibit the above synapse presynaptically;

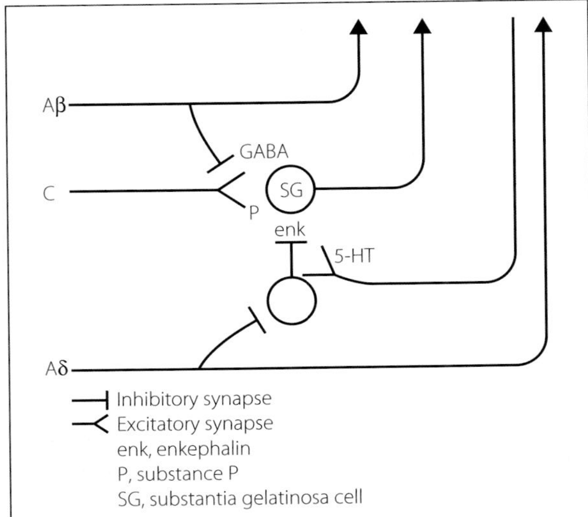

Fig. 76 Gate control theory of pain

GABA is thought to be the neurotransmitter (closes gate). The Aβ fibres also project cranially.

- Aδ fibres from superficial receptors (e.g. temperature, pinprick, acupuncture, low frequency TENS) project cranially, via spinothalamic fibres. Cause 5-HT-mediated descending pathways to close the gate via enkephalin-secreting interneurones acting on target cells.

  Descending fibres are also affected by mood, emotion, etc.

  Aδ fibres also project directly on to interneurones inhibiting enkephalin secretion (i.e. opens gate).

[Patrick D Wall (1925–2001), English neuroscientist; Ronald Melzack, Montreal psychologist]

Dickenson AH (2002). Br J Anaesth; 88: 755–7

See also, Sensory pathways

Gauge. Measure of thickness/width; applied in medicine to cannulae, needles, catheters, etc. Common systems include wire gauges used for needles and cannulae and the French Gauge (Charrière), originally applied to urinary catheters and which equals external circumference in mm (approximately 3 × external diameter).

[Joseph FB Charrière (1803–1876), Paris instrument-maker]

Gay-Lussac's law, *see Charles' law*

GCSF, *see Granulocyte colony-stimulating factor*

Gelatin solutions. Colloid solutions derived from animal gelatin, a derivative of collagen. Commonly used forms contain urea-linked (Haemaccel) or succinylated (Gelofusine) gelatin components (Table 15); average mw is about 35 000. Used clinically as plasma substitutes, e.g. in haemorrhage and shock. Cheaper than albumin solutions and starch solutions, but with shorter half-life (about 4 h). Only 1% metabolised with no accumulation in reticuloendothelial system. Allergic (anaphylactoid) reactions have followed rapid infusion, especially of Haemaccel (said to be reduced in its current form); usually mild but occasionally severe. The incidence of reactions is less than 0.15%.

Renal function and blood cross-matching are unaffected. Gelatin solutions may interfere with platelet function and coagulation (via reduction in von Willebrand factor activity) and restriction of their administration in major haemorrhage has been suggested, although this is controversial. The calcium in Haemaccel may coagulate stored blood if infused through the same giving set without first flushing with saline.

Table 15 Components of gelatin solutions

Solution	Gelatin (g/l)	Sodium (mmol/l)	Chloride (mmol/l)	Calcium (mmol/l)	Potassium (mmol/l)
Haemaccel	35 urea-linked	145	145	6.26	5.1
Gelofusine	40 succinylated	154	125	0.4	0.4

Gelofusine, *see Gelatin solutions*

Gender differences and anaesthesia. Many factors may contribute to differences between men's and women's responses to anaesthetic and analgesic drugs, for example:

- pharmacokinetics:
  - absorption and drug binding: some differences but little evidence relating to anaesthetic drugs. Alcohol is absorbed more rapidly in women because it is broken down less in the gastric mucosa than in men.
  - distribution: greater fat:water ratio in women; thus volume of distribution of water-soluble drugs, e.g. vecuronium, is reduced, and of fat-soluble drugs, e.g. diazepam, is increased. It has been suggested that women recover more quickly after propofol anaesthesia than men.
  - metabolism: e.g. greater metabolism of morphine to the active 6-glucuronide than the antagonistic 3-glucuronide in women, compared to men. Other differences may relate to sex-specific isoenzyme systems but experimental results are often conflicting.
  - excretion: renal excretion is affected by body weight and composition.
- pharmacodynamics: women are thought to be more susceptible to the analgesic effects of opioid analgesic drugs and neuromuscular blocking drugs and although different pharmacokinetics may contribute, pharmacodynamic factors have also been suggested. Reduced sensitivity and earlier waking of women after propofol may also be a pharmacodynamic phenomenon.

Further differences may result from cyclical changes in body fluid and hormonal status during the menstrual cycle (e.g. PONV may be affected by phase of menstrual cycle). There are also significant effects of pregnancy. Psychological factors and the reported greater incidence of adverse effects in women may also contribute to apparent differences between the sexes.

Pleym H, Spigset O, Kharasch ED, Dale O (2003). Acta Anaesthesiol Scand; 47: 241–59

Genetics. Some variations in the human genetic code have functional effects, e.g. pharmacogenetics or the quantity of a protein produced in response to activation of gene transcription. Genetic variation may also affect disease predisposition and severity of illness as well as response to therapy. A new technique, genetic profiling, may allow individual risk to be more accurately assessed and perhaps specific treatments or drugs to be tailored to patients, e.g. on ICU. Potentially of use in disorders such as severe sepsis and ARDS.

Genitofemoral nerve block, *see Inguinal hernia field block*

Gentamicin. Broad-spectrum aminoglycoside; active as an antibacterial drug, especially against Gram-negative organisms, but poorly active against haemolytic streptococci, haemophilus and anaerobes; thus usually given with a penicillin ± metronidazole when given without definite microbiological diagnosis. Under 10% protein-bound and excreted renally, with plasma half-life of 2–3 h in normal renal function.

- Dosage: 1–1.5 mg/kg slowly iv or im, 8 hourly. Less frequent administration is required in renal impairment. One-hour (peak) plasma levels should not exceed 10 mg/l; trough levels should not exceed 2 mg/l. A single iv dose of 5–7 /kg over 30–60 min provides an equally good response to traditional dosage, with fewer complications (including renal impairment). Monitoring is also easier.
- Side effects: as for aminoglycosides.

Geriatric patient, *see Elderly, anaesthesia for*

GFR, *see Glomerular filtration rate*

GHBA, *see γ-Hydroxybutyric acid*

Gland/gland nut, *see Cylinders*

Glasgow coma scale (GCS). Scoring system originally suggested for assessment of patients with head injury; now widely applied to other causes of coma (though more useful in the former than the latter). Originally described for adults, it has been modified for use in infants. A maximum of 15 points may be scored (Table 16), expressed as a total or, more usefully, separated into the three categories (e.g. 'M_3, V_2, E_2' gives more information than 'GCS 7'). Changes in scores over time are more useful than single values.

Teasdale G, Jennett B (1974). Lancet; ii: 81–3

See also, Coma scales; Trauma scales

Glaucoma. Damage to the eye associated with raised intraocular pressure (IOP).

- Anaesthetic considerations:
  - related to IOP:
    - avoidance of drugs which raise IOP, e.g. ketamine. Systemic atropine is safe; topical use may cause mydriasis and obstruction of drainage of aqueous humour.
    - IOP increases following tracheal intubation and extubation.
    - avoidance of trauma to the eye, steep head-down position, coughing, straining, etc., which may increase IOP.
    - IOP may be reduced by specific measures, e.g. iv mannitol, acetazolamide, etc.
  - related to concurrent drug therapy:
    - timolol drops and related drugs: systemic absorption and β-blockade may occur.
    - ecothiopate drops: may prolong suxamethonium's action.
    - pilocarpine and physostigmine drops: systemic absorption and bradycardia may occur.
    - acetazolamide: electrolyte imbalance may occur.
    - cannabis may be used by patients with glaucoma although evidence that it lowers IOP is scanty.

Glomerular filtration rate (GFR). Volume (ml) of plasma filtered by the kidneys per minute. Normally 120 ml/min (173 l/day).

- Depends on:
  - effective glomerular surface area: reduced by contraction of mesangial cells within the glomerulus, e.g. in response to angiotensin II, vasopressin, noradrenaline, leukotrienes, histamine and certain prostaglandins. Dopamine and atrial natriuretic peptide cause relaxation.
  - permeability of the capillary wall, basement membrane and glomerular epithelium. Dependent on size (molecules under 4–8 nm pass through relatively easily), protein-binding and charge (filtration of cations is favoured over that of anions because of the negative charge of the glomerular wall). Increased in certain diseases.
  - hydrostatic gradient across the capillary walls. Affected by:
    - renal blood flow and capillary vascular tone (e.g. noradrenaline constricts the afferent arterioles predominantly, whilst angiotensin II constricts the efferent arterioles). Autoregulation is thought to involve afferent arteriolar vascular tone.
    - ureteric obstruction/renal oedema.
  - osmotic gradient: rarely clinically important.

Measured by iv infusion of a substance which is freely filtered and neither reabsorbed nor secreted by the renal tubules. It must also be non-toxic, not metabolised and have no effect on GFR. At steady state, the clearance of the substance is calculated. The volume of plasma cleared per minute then equals the volume filtered per minute i.e.:

$$\text{GFR} = \frac{\text{urine concentration} \times \text{urinary volume/min}}{\text{plasma concentration}}$$

Inulin, a carbohydrate derived from plant tubers, is usually used. Radioactive chromium-labelled EDTA may also be used.

Provides an indication of renal function, but is difficult to measure routinely. Creatinine clearance approximates to GFR, and is commonly measured instead. Creatinine is actually secreted by the renal tubules to a small degree, but measurement of plasma levels overestimates by a small amount, tending to cancel any error.

More recently, the MDRD equation (Modification of Diet in Renal Disease Study Group) has been developed that allows an estimated value (eGFR) to be calculated from the serum creatinine concentration, adjusted for sex (creatinine concentration lower in women), age (creatinine concentration lower in older people), and race (creatinine concentration higher in African–Americans than Caucasians). The eGFR is more accurate than a 24-h urine collection for creatinine

Table 16 Glasgow coma scale for adults and infants

Glasgow coma scale for adults			Glasgow coma scale for infants		
Activity	*Best response*	*Scale*	*Activity*	*Best response*	*Scale*
Motor	Obeys commands	6	Motor	Obeys commands	6
	Localises pain	5		Localises pain	5
	Withdraws from pain	4		Withdraws from pain	4
	Flexes in response to pain	3		Flexes in response to pain	3
	Extends in response to pain	2		Extends in response to pain	2
	No response	1		No response	1
Verbal	Fully orientated	5	Verbal	Coos or babbles	5
	Confused	4		Irritable cries	4
	Inappropriate words	3		Cries to painful stimuli	3
	Incomprehensible sounds	2		Moans to painful stimuli	2
	No response	1		None	1
Eye opening	Eyes open spontaneously	4	Eye opening	Spontaneous	4
	Eyes open to command	3		To speech	3
	Eyes open in response to pain	2		To pain	2
	Eyes remain closed	1		None	1

clearance but is not applicable to the extremes of age or body size, muscle disease, vegetarian diet or pregnancy.
See also, Nephron; Renin/angiotensin system

Glomerulonephritis. Renal disease of usually unknown aetiology, but often involving renal immune complex deposition or antibodies against glomerular basement membrane. Histological classification is unrelated to clinical presentation, which may include:
- oliguria, salt and water retention, hypervolaemia and hypertension due to impaired glomerular filtration (nephritic syndrome). Classically follows streptococcal infection.
- proteinuria, causing hypoproteinaemia and marked oedema if severe (nephrotic syndrome).
- others: hypertension, haematuria, loin pain, renal failure (acute and chronic).

- Anaesthetic considerations:
  - impaired renal function.
  - oedema and hypoproteinaemia.
  - hypertension.
  - drug therapy: may include antihypertensive drugs and corticosteroids.

Couser WG (1999). Lancet; 353: 1509–15
See also, Goodpasture's syndrome

Glomus tumours. Rare tumours arising from glomus bodies (arteriovenous anastomoses adjacent to blood vessels, richly innervated and thought to be involved with regulating local blood flow). More common in the limbs, but may arise from the glomus jugulare (tympanic body) in the upper jugular bulb. The latter may extend into the cerebellum and brainstem, middle ear, internal jugular vein or laterally into the neck. Thus associated with neurological lesions, including of lower cranial nerves. May rarely secrete catecholamines or 5-HT. Anaesthetic concerns include excessive length of surgery and blood loss, and those of neurosurgery.
Jensen NF (1994). Anesth Analg; 78: 112–19

Glossopharyngeal nerve block. Used to supplement topical anaesthesia and/or superior laryngeal nerve block, e.g. in awake intubation. Also used for tonsillectomy and glossopharyngeal neuralgia. Acute airway obstruction has followed its use for awake intubation and post-tonsillectomy analgesia.
- Techniques:
  - internal:
    - posterior: having applied topical anaesthesia to the tongue, it is depressed and an angled needle inserted behind the middle of the posterior tonsillar pillar, to 1 cm depth. After aspiration, 3 ml local anaesthetic agent is injected. Blocks the sensory pharyngeal, lingual and tonsillar branches, and the motor branch to stylopharyngeus. Carotid puncture is more likely using this approach than with the anterior.
    - anterior: after topical anaesthesia, the tongue is displaced away from the side to be blocked, revealing a gutter between the tongue and the teeth. A needle is inserted 0.25–0.5 cm at the posterior end of the gutter, and 2 ml local anaesthetic injected. Blocks the lingual branch primarily.
  - external: 5–6 ml solution is injected just behind and deep to the styloid process, found 2–4 cm deep, midway between the tip of the mastoid process and angle of the jaw. Internal carotid and jugular vessels lie very close.

Glossopharyngeal neuralgia. Recurrent, sudden, stabbing pain in the distribution of the glossopharyngeal nerve. May result from nerve compression by vertebral or posterior inferior cerebellar arteries, local musculoskeletal anomalies, or trauma. May be relieved by topical local anaesthetic to oropharyngeal trigger areas. Treatment includes glossopharyngeal nerve block using local anaesthetic at weekly intervals; alcohol injection or surgical resection of the glossopharyngeal rootlets may be required.

Glottis, *see Larynx*

Glucagon. Hormone secreted by the A (α) cells of pancreatic islets. Acts on the glucagon receptor (a G protein-coupled receptor), resulting in hepatic adenylate cyclase stimulation, leading to glycogen breakdown and release of glucose, hence its emergency use in hypoglycaemia. Also increases hepatic glucose formation from amino acids, and breakdown of fats to form ketone bodies. Stimulates secretion of growth hormone, insulin and somatostatin. Has inotropic and chronotropic actions on the heart, unrelated to adrenergic receptors. Thought to increase calcium transport into myocardial cells, possibly via adenylate cyclase activation; it has been used in the treatment of β-adrenergic receptor antagonist poisoning. Half-life is less than 10 min.

Secretion is increased by β-adrenergic stimulation, stress, exercise, amino acids, gastrin, cholecystokinin and starvation. It is decreased by hyperglycaemia, somatostatin, ketone bodies, fatty acids, insulin and α-adrenergic stimulation.
- Dosage:
  - hypoglycaemia: 0.5–1 mg sc/im/iv.
  - β-receptor antagonist overdose: 50–150 μg/kg iv.

Glucocorticoids. Hormones secreted by the adrenal cortex; consist mainly of cortisol and corticosterone. Thought to act via interaction with cellular nuclear proteins, with alteration of enzyme synthesis and cell function. Secretion is increased by ACTH.
- Actions:
  - increased glycogen and protein breakdown, and glucose synthesis, with increased blood glucose levels.
  - required for efficient functioning of catecholamines on metabolism, bronchi and CVS, also for correct movement of fluid across the vascular endothelium and fluid balance. This may explain the hypotension seen in adrenocortical insufficiency.
  - required for efficient muscle contraction and nerve conduction; also involved in inflammatory/immunological responses.
  - mild aldosterone-like activity.

Large doses of glucocorticoids suppress inflammation, and are used in many inflammatory and immunological diseases.
See also, Adrenal gland; Corticosteroids

Glucose. Carbohydrate, of central importance as an energy source within the body.
- Main metabolic pathways (Fig. 77):
  - production:
    - from breakdown of carbohydrate foodstuffs.
    - from glycogen stores, or other endogenous molecules (e.g. protein, fats) via intermediate steps in glucose metabolism; occurs in the liver during starvation, exercise, etc. Produces glucose 6-phosphate, which is converted by hepatic glucose 6-phosphatase to glucose which enters the bloodstream. Other tissues, e.g. muscle, lack this enzyme, and glucose 6-phosphate is catabolised directly via the glycolytic pathway.

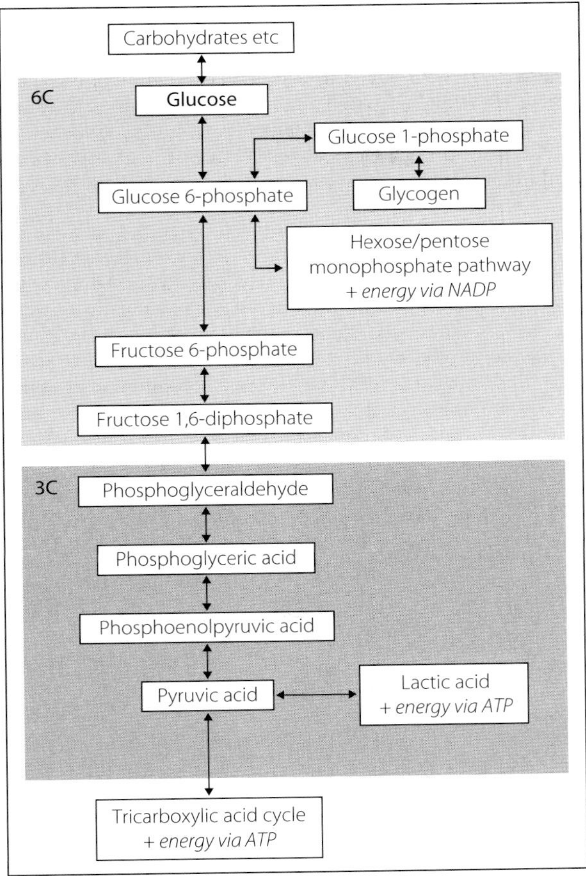

Fig. 77 Main metabolic pathways of glucose

- uptake:
  - from the GIT via carrier-assisted transport, i.e. as part of an active transport mechanism for sodium ions. Thus indirectly utilises energy.
  - from the bloodstream into cells by the action of insulin.
- utilisation for energy production: via conversion into glucose 6-phosphate and subsequent breakdown (glycolysis).
- conversion to glycogen via glucose 6-phosphate and glucose 1-phosphate.
- hexose/pentose monophosphate shunt: alternative energy producing pathway from glucose 6-phosphate, with reduction of nicotinamide adenine dinucleotide phosphate (NADP).
- conversion to fats and proteins.

Fasting plasma levels are maintained at 4–6 mmol/l (72–108 mg/dl) by the action of various hormones mainly on the liver; e.g. insulin decreases blood glucose, whilst glucagon, catecholamines, growth hormone, glucocorticoids and thyroid hormones increase it.

Filtered and reabsorbed in the proximal tubules of the kidneys; renal capacity for reabsorption is exceeded above plasma levels of about 10 mmol/l (180 mg/dl). Congenital inability to reabsorb glucose results in renal glycosuria at normal plasma levels. The renal threshold may also be reduced in pregnancy and tubular damage.

See also, Catabolism; Diabetes mellitus; Metabolism; Nutrition

Glucose–insulin–potassium infusion. Infusion regimen used in an attempt to reduce the size of MI, increase cardiac output and reduce arrhythmias. First used in the 1960s but abandoned because of doubts over its efficacy; more recent evidence has suggested a reduction in mortality. Thought to reduce plasma free fatty acid levels, reducing myocardial energy and O_2 requirements; it possibly augments anaerobic metabolism by increasing ATP supply. Regimens vary but most involve 25–50 units insulin and 40–50 mmol potassium added to 500 ml of 25–50% glucose, infused iv at 100 ml/h. Glucose/insulin infusion has also been used in hyponatraemia due to the 'sick cell syndrome'; it supposedly restores ionic balance.

Glucose 6-phosphate dehydrogenase deficiency (G6PD deficiency). Sex-linked inherited disorder of red blood cell metabolism, common in Mediterranean, African, Middle Eastern and South-East Asian populations. Impairs the hexose monophosphate shunt of glucose metabolism, required for cell protection against products of oxidation. Results in haemolysis, which may be chronic or associated with acute illness (especially typhoid and viral hepatitis infection), drugs (e.g. antimalarials, sulphonamides, aspirin and related drugs, methylthioninium chloride (methylene blue)), and ingestion of broad beans (favism). Reduction of methaemoglobin is impaired, thus avoidance of prilocaine has been suggested.

Chronic haemolysis is also associated with other inborn errors of metabolism, e.g. pyruvate kinase deficiency.

Glucose reagent sticks. Plastic strips bearing reagents, used to measure glucose concentration, e.g. in blood or urine. Glucose is converted by glucose oxidase to gluconic acid and hydrogen peroxide, the latter oxidising a dye to produce a colour change. Accuracy is increased by using reflectance colorimeters to quantify the colour change, and may be reduced by use of alcohol swabs for cleaning the skin. They are less accurate at lower (hypoglycaemic) glucose levels. Useful as a bedside test, and for home monitoring of glucose levels.

Glucose tolerance test. Investigation used in the diagnosis of diabetes mellitus. Involves administration of glucose either orally or iv, usually the former. 1.75 g/kg is given orally up to 75 g, in at least 250 ml water. Blood glucose normally rises from fasting levels to a peak at 10–60 min, declining thereafter. Fasting and 2 h levels are used for diagnosis:

- venous plasma glucose under 7.8 mmol/l (140 mg/dl) fasting and at 2 h: normal.
- venous plasma glucose over 11.1 mmol/l (200 mg/dl) at 2 h: diabetic.
- intermediate values: 'impaired glucose tolerance'.

Diabetes is usually diagnosed on random and fasting blood sugar estimations alone. The tolerance test is mainly used to investigate diabetes in pregnancy, although there is disagreement about the cut-offs and definitions used.

α-Glucosidase inhibitors. Saccharide hypoglycaemic drugs which compete with saccharidases in the small intestine, thus slowing the breakdown of poly- and disaccharides to monosaccharides in the gut. Used alone or in combination with other drugs to improve glycaemic control, especially postprandial hyperglycaemia. Include acarbose, miglitol and voglibose.

Glue-sniffing, *see Solvent abuse*

Glutamate. Amino acid, active as an excitatory neurotransmitter throughout the CNS, especially brain. Released presynaptically, it activates various specific receptors:

- AMPA (α-amino-3-hydroxy-5-methyl-4-isoxazolepropionate) receptors: involved in rapid neurotransmission.
- kainate (a neurotoxin) receptors: similar effects to those of AMPA receptors.
- NMDA receptors: slower response; thought to be involved in longer-term responses including modulation of pain responses and survival after ischaemia.
- others, linked to G receptor-coupled proteins: less clearly understood.

Manipulation of glutamate pathways is currently an active area of research since it is thought to be involved in pain perception, wakefulness and memory, post-injury or ischaemia neurotoxicity (via glutamate-mediated intracellular calcium accumulation) and spinal cord neurotransmission. It may also have a role in anaesthesia itself.

Glutamine, *see Amino acids; Glutamate*

Glyceryl trinitrate (GTN; Nitroglycerin). Vasodilator drug, used to treat myocardial ischaemia and cardiac failure, and to lower BP, e.g. in severe hypertension and hypotensive anaesthesia. Acts via nitric oxide release to affect vascular smooth muscle (mainly venous), lowering preload and reducing SVR and pulmonary vascular resistance. Also increases coronary blood flow. A cutaneous slow-release patch may be applied preoperatively in patients with ischaemic heart disease, and these have also been applied to sites of iv fluid administration, reducing infusion failure by up to 60%. Has also been used to reduce uterine contraction, e.g. in premature rupture of membranes (cutaneous patch) or as an acute tocolytic drug (iv or sublingual).

- Dosage:
  - sublingually 0.3–1.0 mg, repeated as required. Lasts about 20–30 min. Available as 0.3 mg or 0.5 mg tablets; also as a 0.4 mg/dose spray.
  - orally as slow-release tablets: 2.6–6.4 mg, 8–12 hourly.
  - cutaneously: 5–10 mg/day applied to the chest; 5 mg 3–4 hourly to infusion sites.
  - iv: 0.2–5 μg/kg/min. Effects occur within 2–5 min and last 5–10 min after stopping the infusion. Some preparations contain 30–50% propylene glycol and alcohol. GTN is adsorbed on to PVC; polyethylene and rigid plastic/glass infusion sets are acceptable.
- Side effects: headache, flushing, hypotension, tachycardia.

Tachyphylaxis is common.

Glycine. Amino acid, thought to be active as an inhibitory neurotransmitter at spinal interneurones. Increases membrane chloride conductance, causing postsynaptic hyperpolarisation. May also be involved in inhibitory pathways within the ascending reticular activating system. Used as an irrigating solution for TURP. Systemic absorption is thought possibly to be associated with CNS symptoms, e.g. transient blindness, either via central inhibitory pathways or conversion to ammonia.

Glycogen. Storage form of glucose; consists of glucose molecules linked together into a branched polymer. Found mainly in liver and skeletal muscle, and formed from glucose 1-phosphate, derived from glucose 6-phosphate. Glycogenolysis provides glucose for glycolysis, and is increased by adrenaline via liver β-receptors (via cAMP) and α-receptors (via intracellular calcium). Defects in the various storage and breakdown pathways result in the glycogen storage disorders.

Glycogen storage disorders. Inborn errors of metabolism affecting glycogen and glucose metabolism. All are rare, and almost all are autosomal recessive. Classified according to the deficient enzyme and the site of abnormal glycogen storage; 12 types have been described. Common to most are hypoglycaemia and acidosis with hepatomegaly; cardiac, mental and renal impairment may also occur.

- The following are of particular concern:
  - type I: von Gierke's disease: glucose 6-phosphatase deficiency; i.e. cannot convert glucose to glycogen. Hypoglycaemia, acidosis, mental and growth retardation, hepatomegaly, platelet dysfunction and renal impairment may occur, with death within early childhood.
  - type II: Pompe's disease: glycogen is deposited in skeletal, cardiac and smooth muscle. Cardiac failure and generalised muscle weakness are common. The tongue may be enlarged. Enzyme replacement therapy is under investigation.
  - type V: McArdle's disease: skeletal muscle phosphorylase deficiency, impairing glycogenolysis. Muscle weakness and myoglobinuria may occur, the latter, etc. following suxamethonium. Muscle atrophy may follow use of tourniquets for surgery. Hypoglycaemia and acidosis are common.

[Edgar von Gierke (1877–1945), German pathologist; Joannes C Pompe (1901–1945), Dutch pathologist; Brian McArdle (1911–2002), English physician]

Glycolysis. Breakdown of glucose (6 carbon atoms) to pyruvic acid or lactate (3 carbon atoms). Each step in the pathway (*see Fig. 77; Glucose*) is catalysed by a specific enzyme. Energy released during the process is utilised by production of ATP. The reactions occur anaerobically, with a net gain of 2 moles of ATP per mole glucose. Under aerobic conditions, pyruvic acid enters the tricarboxylic acid cycle with a net gain of 36 more moles of ATP. Anaerobic energy production is less efficient; formation of lactate from pyruvate limits ATP production to 2 moles per mole glucose. This may occur in exercising muscle and red blood cells.

Passage of glucose into muscle and fat cells is increased by insulin, with increased glycolysis; most other cell membranes are relatively permeable to glucose. In the liver, glucose 6-phosphatase levels control the rate of glycolysis; insulin causes increased levels and starvation decreased levels.

Other pathways may branch from the glycolytic pathway, e.g. the hexose monophosphate shunt from glucose 6-phosphate in red blood cells. Protein and fat derivatives may enter the glycolytic chain and glycogen may be broken down to glucose 6-phosphate via glucose 1-phosphate.

Glycopeptides. Group of antibacterial drugs; include vancomycin and teicoplanin. Both are true antibiotics since they are derived from micro-organisms. Have bactericidal activity against aerobic and anaerobic Gram-positive organisms including meticillin-resistant *Staphylococcus aureus*.

Glycoprotein IIb/IIIa inhibitors, *see Antiplatelet drugs*

Glycopyrronium bromide (Glycopyrrolate). Anticholinergic drug, used as premedication and pre- and perioperatively to prevent or treat bradycardia. Also used to prevent muscarinic effects of acetylcholinesterase inhibitors used to reverse neuromuscular blockade. A quaternary ammonium compound; therefore has minimal central effects, as opposed to atropine and hyoscine. Also less likely to cause tachycardia, mydriasis and blurred vision, but markedly reduces sweat and salivary gland activity. Its action persists for longer than that of atropine, reducing postoperative bradycardia. Dry mouth may persist postoperatively.

- Dosage:
  - 4–5 μg/kg im/iv.
  - with acetylcholinesterase inhibitors: 10–15 μg/kg.

'Golden hour'. Period following trauma in which active intervention is thought to be crucial in preventing the development of severe organ (especially brain) injury or death, and hence improving outcome. The concept has arisen from the observation that many trauma victims die shortly after the insult; many of the survivors have evidence of persisting brain injury; and experimental brain injury may be considerably exacerbated by subsequent aggravating factors such as hypoxaemia and hypotension (and these two factors in particular are common after severe trauma). Similar considerations are likely to apply to other organs although to less dramatic or significant extents.

Recognition of the importance of the first hour or so after trauma has fuelled the debate on whether it is better to resuscitate and stabilise victims at the scene of the accident before transfer to a hospital, or take them at once ('scoop and run'). The former approach is now generally accepted as being preferable in most cases for the above reasons, although controlled studies are rare and there are situations in which 'scoop and run' is favoured, e.g. penetrating cardiac trauma. In practice, the emphasis is on maintenance of oxygenation, stabilisation of major fractures and control of external haemorrhage before as rapid a transfer as possible.
See also, Head injury; Transportation of critically ill patients

Goldman cardiac risk index, *see Cardiac risk index*

Goldman constant-field equation. Describes the relationship between sodium, potassium and chloride ions, and membrane permeability to each:

$$V = \frac{RT}{F}\ln\frac{P_{K^+}[K_o{}^+] + P_{Na^+}[Na_o{}^+] + P_{Cl^-}[Cl_i{}^-]}{P_{K^+}[K_i{}^+] + P_{Na^+}[Na_i{}^+] + P_{Cl^-}[Cl_o{}^-]}$$

Where V = membrane potential
R = gas constant
F = Faraday constant
$P_{K^+}, P_{Na^+}, P_{Cl^-}$ = permeability to potassium, sodium and chloride respectively
$[K_o{}^+]$, $[Na_o{}^+]$, $[Cl_o{}^-]$ = outside concentration of ions
$[K_i{}^+]$, $[Na_i{}^+]$, $[Cl_i{}^-]$ = inside concentration of ions.

[David E Goldman (1910–1998), US physiologist; Michael Faraday (1791–1867), English chemist]

Goodpasture's syndrome. Combination of glomerulonephritis, rapidly progressive pulmonary haemorrhage and antibodies against glomerular basement membrane (the first two may also occur without these antibodies, e.g. in systemic vasculitides and connective tissue disease, and strictly, do not constitute Goodpasture's syndrome). The antibodies react against a specific antigen present in the basement membrane and also in the alveolar membrane, hence the association. Often follows an upper respiratory tract infection or exposure to certain chemicals (e.g. following glue sniffing), presumably via formation of new antigenic molecules resulting in autoantibody formation. Usually responds well to aggressive immunosuppressive therapy if treated early (i.e. before significant renal impairment). Plasmapheresis has been used.
[Ernest W. Goodpasture (1886–1960), US pathologist]

Graft-versus-host disease (GVHD). Condition affecting recipients of organ or tissue transplants in which donor inflammatory cells recognise host cells as being 'foreign' and mount an inflammatory response against them. Particularly problematic and aggressive when the transplanted cells are immunologically active, e.g. bone marrow transplantation; acute GVHD typically occurs within 2–3 months of transplantation and may result in skin rash, hepatic impairment, diarrhoea and death. A chronic form may also occur, again affecting mainly the skin, liver and GIT. Occurs to some extent in up to two-thirds of bone marrow recipients. Thought to be caused by transplanted T lymphocytes, GVHD may be prevented by various immunosuppressive drugs (and anti-T-cell antibodies) and removal of T cells from donor marrow preparations, e.g. with radiation treatment. Activation of cytokines and other inflammatory mediators is also thought to be involved. Treatment is with immunosuppressive drugs (typically ciclosporin and prednisolone) although the response may be poor unless started early. If survived, GVHD may protect against subsequent relapse of leukaemia. GVHD has also been described after intestinal, heart–lung and liver transplantation. A form has also followed blood transfusion, especially in immunocompromised recipients or when first degree relatives donate blood (involves close mismatch of leucocyte antigen haplotypes). Typically occurs up to a month post-transfusion; features are similar to those above.
Bacigalupo A (2007). Br J Haematol; 137: 87–98

Graham's law. Rate of diffusion of a gas is inversely proportional to the square root of its mw.
[Thomas Graham (1805–1869), Scottish chemist]

Gram-negative/positive bacteria, *see Bacteria*

Granisetron hydrochloride. 5-HT_3 receptor antagonist, licensed as an antiemetic drug in postoperative and radio-/chemotherapy-induced nausea and vomiting. Similar to ondansetron.

- Dosage:
  - PONV: 1 mg slowly iv, repeated up to 2 /day.
  - nausea/vomiting following radiotherapy or chemotherapy: 1–2 mg orally, followed by 2 mg/day in 1–2 doses, or 3 mg iv (diluted in 15 ml saline over 30 s or as iv infusion over 5 min), repeated up to twice in 24 h. A maximum of 9 mg/day should be given by any route.

Granulocyte colony-stimulating factor. Substance used to stimulate neutrophil production especially in febrile neutropenic patients receiving chemotherapy. Has also been studied as a possible treatment of MODS, SIRS and sepsis. Various recombinant human preparations are available:
  - filgrastim (unglycosylated G-CSF) and lenograstim (glycosylated G-CSF): similar effects on neutrophils. Side effects include musculoskeletal pain, hypotension, allergic reactions, hepatosplenomegaly, hepatic impairment.
  - molgramostim (GM-CSF): stimulates production of all granulocytes and macrophages. Has more side effects than the above preparations.

Gravity suit, *see Antigravity suit*

Greener, Hannah (1832–1848). Fifteen-year-old girl, traditionally accepted as being the first recorded death under anaesthesia although this is probably not the case (see below). She was having a toenail removed under open chloroform anaesthesia in Newcastle in January 1848, when she suddenly collapsed and died, despite attempted revival with brandy.

A report published in England in March 1848 referred to the death in July 1847 of a 55-year-old man, Alexis Montigny,

in Auxerre, France. He died during removal of a breast tumour under ether anaesthesia, possibly because of airway obstruction ± aspiration or pulmonary oedema. Other reports from 1847 described early postoperative deaths associated with ether anaesthesia although the causes are unclear.
Knight PR, Bacon D (2002). Anesthesiology; 96: 1250–3

Griffith, Harold Randall (1894–1985). Canadian anaesthetist in Montreal; famous for the use of curare in anaesthesia in 1942. None of the patients described apparently required respiratory assistance. Active in many other areas of anaesthetic research, including the properties of cyclopropane. Of world renown, he received many honours and medals.
Seldon TH (1986). Anesth Analg; 65: 1051–3

Growth hormone. Polypeptide hormone released from the anterior pituitary gland. Release is increased by:
- hypoglycaemia, sleep and exercise.
- stress; i.e. produced as part of the stress response to surgery.
- protein meal and glucagon.
- dopamine receptor agonists.

Growth hormone-releasing and inhibiting hormones (the latter is somatostatin) are released by the hypothalamus; growth hormone release is inhibited by growth hormone itself.
- Effects:
  - increased skeletal growth and cell division.
  - increased protein synthesis, lipolysis and gluconeogenesis (anti-insulin effect). Oversecretion causes gigantism before puberty, acromegaly thereafter.

G-suit, *see Antigravity suit*

GTN, *see Glyceryl trinitrate*

GTT, *see Glucose tolerance test*

Guanethidine monosulphate. Antihypertensive drug, depleting adrenergic neurones of noradrenaline and preventing its release. Rarely used for hypertension now, but sometimes useful in complex regional pain syndromes type 1 and 2 (formerly reflex sympathetic dystrophy and causalgia respectively); e.g. 10–25 mg in 20 ml saline injected iv into the exsanguinated arm (30–40 mg in 40 ml for leg), and the tourniquet kept inflated for 10–20 min. Close cardiovascular observation is required afterwards; hypotension may be delayed. A small amount of lidocaine is sometimes added. The procedure may be repeated, e.g. on alternate days for a number of weeks, often with long-lasting results.

May cause diarrhoea and postural hypotension.

Guedel, Arthur Ernest (1883–1956). US anaesthetist, practising in Indiana, then California. Considered a pioneer of modern anaesthesia; published extensively on many subjects, including tracheal tube cuffs, divinyl ether, cyclopropane, his pharyngeal airway (*see Airways*), and a classic description of the stages of anaesthesia. Received many honours and medals.
Baskett TF (2004). Resuscitation; 63: 3–5

Guillain–Barré syndrome (Acute inflammatory/postinfection polyneuropathy). Neuropathy described in 1916, although previously reported by Landry in 1859. Incidence is 1–2 per 100 000, affecting all ages. 50–60% of cases follow viral illness within the preceding month; up to 10% follow vaccination or surgery. A diarrhoeal illness involving campylobacter is a common association.

The mechanism of the disease is unclear, but it involves lymphocytic infiltration and demyelination of spinal and cranial nerves and nerve roots, with axonal damage if severe. Autonomic nerves are sometimes affected. Pyramidal or cerebellar impairment is rare. Immune involvement is suggested by animal experimental models, detection of antineuronal antibodies, and the response to immunoglobulin therapy and plasmapheresis.
- Features:
  - weakness, usually bilateral and symmetrical; typically ascending from the legs but it may affect any region first. Bulbar involvement may occur. May develop over 1–2 days to 2–3 weeks; 90% of patients are maximally affected within 3–4 weeks. Areflexia occurs. 30% require respiratory support. Recovery takes from several weeks to months, and up to years if axonal damage has occurred. 10–15% are left with residual disability; 5% relapse.
  - sensory disturbance: paraesthesia occurs in 50%, usually with glove and stocking distribution. Reduced touch, sensation and joint position sense may also occur. Pain may occur, e.g. in the calves and back.
  - features of autonomic disturbance include hypotension or hypertension, tachycardia, arrhythmias, ileus and urinary retention.

Diagnosed by history/clinical features. CSF protein is raised (without an increase in white cell count) in over 90% of patients after a few days. Nerve conduction studies help differentiate demyelination from axonal damage.

The differential diagnosis is extensive and includes myasthenia gravis, poliomyelitis, porphyria, lead and solvent poisoning, botulism, and other causes of peripheral neuropathy.
- Management:
  - supportive:
    - careful turning/nursing care/physiotherapy.
    - heparin prophylaxis against DVT.
    - adequate nutrition.
    - prompt treatment of infection, e.g. urinary, respiratory, etc.
    - treatment of cardiovascular abnormalities as appropriate.
    - respiratory: close monitoring, usually of vital capacity; 15 ml/kg is usually taken as the minimum before IPPV is instituted, together with other features of respiratory failure. Sedation is rarely required. Tracheal intubation is also required if laryngeal reflexes are impaired. Tracheostomy is often necessary since prolonged respiratory support may be required.
  - immunoglobulin therapy is now usually the specific treatment of choice: 0.4 g/kg/day iv over 3–5 days (*see Immunoglobulins, intravenous*).
  - plasmapheresis: most beneficial if performed within the first 2 weeks, and before ventilatory support is required. It is usually performed daily for 4–5 days.
  - corticosteroids have been shown to have no role.
  - CSF filtration has been used in severe, resistant cases.

[Georges Guillain (1876–1961), Jean A Barré (1880–1967) and Octave Landry (1826–1865), French neurologists]
Hughes RA, Cornblath DR (2005). Lancet; 366: 1653–66

GVHD, *see Graft-versus-host disease*

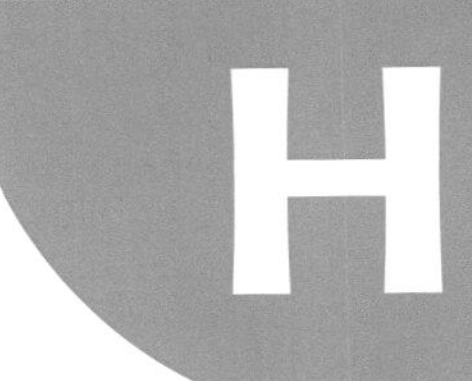

H_2 receptor antagonists. Act by competitive inhibition of H_2 histamine receptors. Used to reduce histamine-mediated gastric acid secretion, e.g. in peptic ulcer disease, gastro-oesophageal reflux, to reduce risk from aspiration of gastric contents, and to reduce gastric/duodenal bleeding in patients in ICU. Their widespread routine use in critically ill patients is reducing because they may increase the risk of nosocomial chest infections. Have also been used with antihistamine drugs to reduce the severity of adverse drug reactions and other allergic responses involving histamine.

- Drugs include:
  - cimetidine: introduced first. Cheapest, but with more side effects. Inhibits hepatic microsomal enzymes.
  - ranitidine: fewer side effects than cimetidine and does not cause hepatic enzyme inhibition. Longer duration of action.
  - nizatidine: similar to ranitidine.
  - famotidine: similar to ranitidine. Available for oral use only. Half-life is 2–3 h and duration of action about 10 h.

Haemaccel, *see Gelatin solutions*

Haematocrit (Hct). Total red cell volume as a proportion of blood volume; expressed as a fraction of unity (formerly expressed as a percentage). Slightly higher in venous blood than in arterial blood, because of entry of chloride ions (chloride shift) into red cells with accompanying water entry by osmosis. An easily measured index of O_2 carrying ability of the blood, assuming normal red cell haemoglobin concentration. Normal values: 0.4–0.54 (male); 0.37–0.47 (female). Reduced Hct of 0.3–0.35 (haemodilution) is thought to be beneficial for tissue O_2 delivery, e.g. in severely ill patients, because of reduced blood viscosity and increased flow; a value below this level is thought to be undesirable because of reduced O_2-carrying capacity despite increased blood flow.

- Useful as a guide to adequate fluid replacement therapy, e.g.:
  - blood loss: indicates relative need for red cells/colloid.
  - plasma loss, e.g. burns: plasma deficit may be determined:

    fall in plasma volume (%) =

$$100 \times \left[1 - \left(\frac{1 - \text{new Hct}}{\text{new Hct}} \times \frac{\text{original Hct}}{1 - \text{original Hct}}\right)\right]$$

See also, Investigations, preoperative

Haemoconcentration. Increase in haematocrit and haemoglobin concentration following dehydration or plasma loss. Degree of haemoconcentration may indicate the extent of fluid deficiency. Does not occur initially after haemorrhage, since red cells and plasma are lost together; compensatory mechanisms restoring blood volume cause subsequent haemodilution. In prolonged severe 'irreversible' shock, however, fluid leaves the capillaries with resulting haemoconcentration.

Haemodiafiltration. Modification of continuous arteriovenous or venovenous haemofiltration (CAVHD or CVVHD respectively) in order to improve efficiency and solute clearance rate. Circuitry and other aspects are identical to those for haemofiltration except that 1–2 l/h of dialysate fluid is allowed to run countercurrent to the blood flow on the filtrate side of the haemofilter (Fig. 78). Solute is cleared by a combination of diffusion and convection.

Haemodialysis. Dialytic technique for removal of solutes and water from blood by their passage across a semipermeable membrane into dialysis fluid (dialysate). Indications include renal failure, fluid overload and pulmonary oedema, electrolyte disturbances, severe acidosis and some cases of drug poisoning and overdoses.

- Principles:
  - vascular access: usually via a: 'single needle' single lumen catheter (through which blood is withdrawn into the dialyser and then returned to the patient in an alternating cycle); double-lumen central venous catheter (or two single ones); silastic arteriovenous shunt connecting adjacent vessels, e.g. radial artery/cephalic vein (Scribner shunt); or permanent arteriovenous fistula (*see Shunt procedures*).
  - passage of blood via an extracorporeal circuit to a semipermeable cellophane membrane or hollow fibre system. Traditional cellulose based membranes may be associated with complement activation and subsequent inflammatory cascade; thus newer synthetic membranes (e.g. polyacrylonitrile, polysulphone) are increasingly used although more expensive. Dialysate may be passed on the other side of the membrane, usually in a countercurrent fashion. Blood flow is usually 150–300 ml/min. The following are exchanged:
    - solutes: pass by diffusion from blood to dialysate, depending on the concentration gradient, size (mw) of solute, membrane porosity and duration of dialysis. Thus fluids of different composition may be used to remove different amounts of solute as required. Most dialysis fluids contain sodium, chloride, calcium, magnesium, acetate or bicarbonate (as an alkali source; bicarbonate itself cannot be added directly since it may precipitate calcium and magnesium) and variable amounts of glucose and potassium. Solutes may also pass across the membrane by applying a hydrostatic pressure across the membrane thereby removing water (ultrafiltration); solutes that can pass through the membrane pores are swept along with the water (solvent drag).
    - water: removed by ultrafiltration. The amount of water extracted depends on the magnitude of the pressure gradient; positive pressure may be applied to the blood side of the membrane, or negative pressure to the dialysate side.
  - anticoagulation of the extracorporeal circuit is required, e.g. with heparin or prostacyclin infused into the line

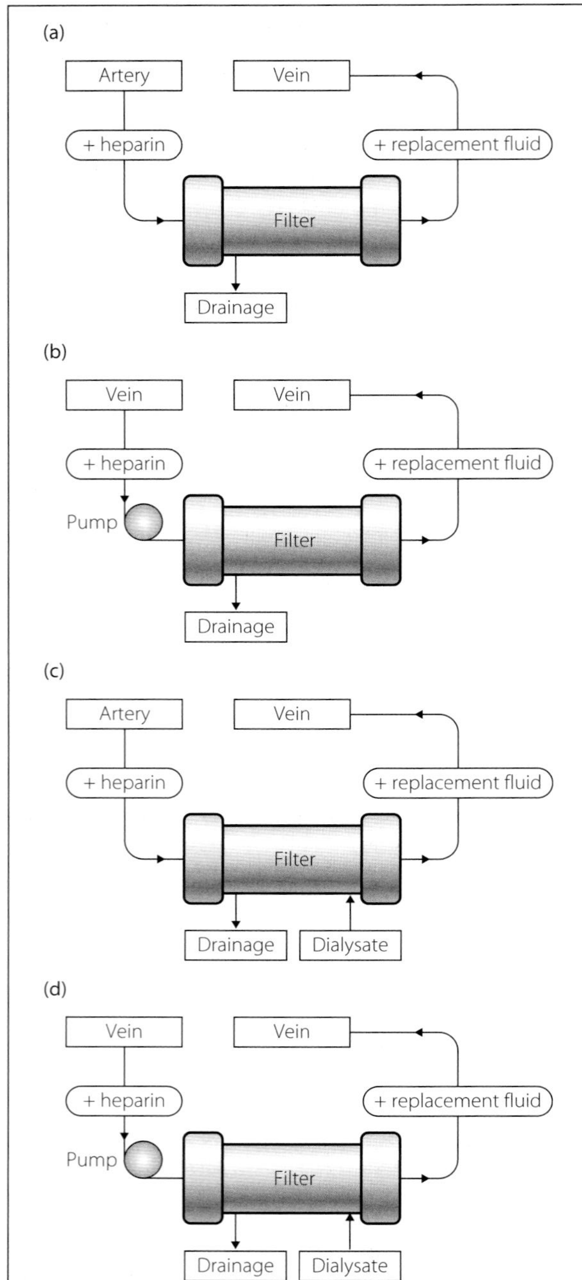

Fig. 78 Circuits used for (a) continuous arteriovenous haemofiltration (CAVH); (b) continuous venovenous haemofiltration (CVVH); (c) continuous arteriovenous haemodiafiltration (CAVHD); (d) continuous venovenous haemodiafiltration (CVVHD). Replacement fluid is often given pre-filter (termed pre-dilution) in order to prolong life of the filter

upstream to the dialysis machine. Control of coagulation with infusion of protamine to the downstream line has been used but may be difficult.
- return of blood to the patient.

Performed intermittently, e.g. for 4–6 h daily/weekly as required.

- Complications:
  - technical, e.g. related to vascular access and bleeding, air embolism, clotting within the circuit. Modern machines usually incorporate alarms and monitors for air bubbles.
  - hypotension: may be related to hypovolaemia, disequilibrium syndrome or acetate in the dialysate (thought to cause vasodilatation and cardiac depression; replacement with bicarbonate has been suggested although it is more complex to achieve).
  - hypoxaemia: mechanism is unclear.
  - electrolyte and acid–base disturbances.
  - increased rate of removal of many therapeutic drugs including salicylates, phenobarbital, disopyramide, methyldopa, lithium, theophylline, and many antibacterial drugs.

[Belding H Scribner (1921–2003), Seattle nephrologist]
See also, Dialysis; Haemodiafiltration; Haemofiltration

Haemodilution. Lowering of haematocrit and haemoglobin concentration due to fluid shift, retention or administration. May follow compensatory restoration of blood volume after haemorrhage, or iv fluid therapy with only partial replacement of red cell losses. Also occurs as a physiological process in pregnancy. Reduction of haematocrit lowers blood viscosity and increases blood flow, although O_2 content falls. Optimal haematocrit following acute blood loss is thought to be about 0.3; in addition to improved tissue blood flow, hazards of blood transfusion and risk of DVT are reduced. Animal studies of cerebral ischaemia have suggested reduced infarct size if early haemodilution is achieved, although human evidence is lacking.

Haemofiltration. Common form of renal replacement therapy used in the ICU. First described in 1977; its main benefit over haemodialysis is cardiovascular stability. Initially described as continuous arteriovenous haemofiltration (CAVH; Fig. 78a) using an extracorporeal circuit via a surgically performed arteriovenous shunt (*see Shunt procedures*) or using large bore arterial and venous cannulae. Blood flow through the circuit relied upon the arterial–venous pressure difference. Now more frequently employs a continuous venovenous circuit (CVVH; Fig. 78b) using a large bore double lumen venous cannula and a peristaltic roller pump which incorporates monitors to detect air embolism and extremes of circuit pressure. Blood is pumped at 100–200 ml/min. Anticoagulation of the extracorporeal circuit, but not the patient, is achieved using heparin (200–1000 U/h) or prostacyclin (2–10 ng/kg/min) administered pre-filter. Anticoagulation is not usually necessary if the patient has a coagulopathy.

Both CAVH and CVVH rely on the passage of blood through a filter containing a highly permeable membrane (polysulphone, polyamide or polyacrylonitrile; surface area 0.6–1.0 m^2) which acts as an artificial glomerulus. Ultrafiltration occurs by virtue of the hydrostatic pressure gradient between the blood and ultrafiltrate sides of filter; solute removal occurs because of convection. Water and solutes lost from the plasma are replaced by haemofiltration fluid containing water and essential electrolytes. Ultrafiltration can be slow and titrated to the patient response. Replacement fluid is infused into the 'arterial' limb of the circuit (pre-dilution) or, more usually, into the 'venous' limb after the filter (post-dilution). Predilution may be useful when there is a high filtrate removal rate (> 10 l/day) or a high haematocrit (> 35%) as it decreases viscosity and subsequent clotting in the circuit. However, predilution decreases the efficiency of the system as the blood being filtered contains a lower concentration of waste products.

Both CAVH and CVVH require an exchange of 12–20 l/day to achieve adequate solute clearance. Filtration can be increased by applying a negative pressure to the filtrate side of the filter or by increasing the distance between the filter and filtrate collecting chamber. In haemodiafiltration, dialysate fluid is passed through the filter to improve efficiency and solute clearance rate (Fig. 78c and 78d).

Complications are related to the extracorporeal circuit and vascular access (air embolism, clotting, haemorrhage, complement activation, infection), ultrafiltration (hypovolaemia), electrolyte loss (hyponatraemia, hypocalcaemia), hypothermia, metabolic alkalosis (use of large volumes of lactate-rich replacement fluid) and removal of therapeutic drugs, including parenteral nutrition.

It has been suggested that CAVH and CVVH have a blood purification effect in sepsis by removing molecules such as cytokines, although this is controversial.

See also, Haemodialysis; Renal failure

Haemoglobin (Hb). Red-coloured pigment in erythrocytes, composed of:

- globin: four polypeptide subunits, in two pairs. Different types of haemoglobin contain different types of polypeptide:
  - Hb A (adult): two α chains, two β chains.
  - Hb A_2 (usually 2–3%): two α chains, two δ chains.
  - Hb F (fetal): two α chains, two γ chains.

  There are 141 amino acid residues in α chains; 146 in β, δ and γ chains.

  Fetal Hb is normally replaced by Hb A within 6 months of birth, unless polypeptide chain production is abnormal, e.g.:
  - thalassaemia: reduced synthesis of normal chains.
  - haemoglobinopathies, e.g. sickle cell anaemia: abnormal β chains are synthesised.
- haem: porphyrin derivative containing iron in the ferrous (Fe^{2+}) state. One haem moiety, containing one iron atom, is conjugated to each polypeptide. Oxidation of the iron to the ferric (Fe^{3+}) state forms methaemoglobin.
- Reactions of Hb:
  - the iron atom in each haem moiety, remaining in the ferrous state but sharing one of its electrons, can reversibly bind one O_2 molecule, forming oxyhaemoglobin. Thus each Hb molecule can bind four O_2 molecules. In its deoxygenated form, the Hb molecule exists in a 'taut' configuration. Binding of one O_2 molecule breaks salt linkages between α- and β-globin chains and produces a more 'relaxed' configuration. This results in increased affinity for further binding (cooperativity), resulting in the sigmoid shaped oxyhaemoglobin dissociation curve. Affinity is reduced by increasing $P\text{CO}_2$ (Bohr effect), acidity, temperature and amount of 2,3-DPG present. Fetal Hb has greater affinity for O_2 than has adult Hb.
  - CO_2 may bind reversibly to amino groups of the polypeptide chains, forming carbamino compounds ($RNH_2 + CO_2 \rightarrow RNHCO_2H$). Deoxygenated Hb reacts in this way more than oxygenated (Haldane effect).
  - imidazole groups of histidine residues act as buffers in the blood. A large buffering capacity results from the many histidine residues contained in Hb, and the large amount of Hb in the blood. Deoxygenated Hb is a weaker acid and better buffer than oxygenated.
  - others:
    - with carbon monoxide, forming carboxyhaemoglobin.
    - formation of methaemoglobin.
    - causing sulphaemoglobinaemia.
    - prolonged exposure to raised glucose levels in diabetes mellitus, forming glycosylated Hb.

Normal blood Hb concentration is 13–17 g/dl (men), 12–16 g/dl (women).

Hb is split into globin and haem portions when erythrocytes are destroyed. The iron is extracted and reused, the porphyrin ring opened to form biliverdin. The latter is converted to bilirubin and excreted via bile.

Hsia CC (1998). N Engl J Med; 338: 239–47

See also, Anaemia; Carbon dioxide transport; Carbon monoxide poisoning; Methaemoglobinaemia; Myoglobin; Oxygen transport; Polycythaemia

Haemoglobinopathies. Disorders of abnormal haemoglobin production (cf. thalassaemias: impaired production of normal haemoglobin). Over 300 variants have been described, mostly due to single amino acid substitutions. Originally named after letters of the alphabet, then after the place of origin of the first patient described. Most are clinically insignificant, but some may lead to acute or chronic haemolysis, and some are associated with impaired O_2 binding and secondary polycythaemia. Sickle cell anaemia is the most important; it may be combined with other abnormalities, e.g. haemoglobin C. The latter on its own may cause mild haemolytic anaemia and splenomegaly.

Haemolysis. Abnormal destruction of erythrocytes. Normal red cell survival is about 120 days; bone marrow compensation may restore red cell volume if the lifespan is shortened. Anaemia may result if haemolysis is excessive, bone marrow abnormal, or iron, etc. deficient. Haemolysis may result in jaundice, decreased haptoglobin concentration (see below) and reticulocytosis.

- Caused by:
  - genetic red cell abnormalities:
    - membrane abnormalities, e.g. hereditary spherocytosis, elliptocytosis.
    - haemoglobinopathies, thalassaemia.
    - enzyme deficiencies, e.g. glucose 6-phosphate dehydrogenase deficiency.
  - acquired disorders:
    - immune:
      - autoimmune:
        - primary.
        - secondary to:
          - connective tissue diseases.
          - malignancy.
          - infection, e.g. viral, mycoplasma.
          - drugs, e.g. penicillins, methyldopa, rifampicin, sulphonamides.
      - incompatible blood transfusion (including rhesus blood group incompatibility).

      Antibodies bound to red blood cells may be detected by the direct Coombs' test; those circulating in the blood may be detected by the indirect Coombs' test.
    - non-immune:
      - infection, e.g. malaria, generalised sepsis.
      - drugs, e.g. sulphonamides, phenacetin.
      - renal and hepatic failure.
      - hypersplenism.
      - trauma, e.g. prosthetic heart valves, extracorporeal circuits. Also associated with red cell damage following contact with vasculitic endothelium (e.g. haemolytic-uraemic syndrome).
      - paroxysmal nocturnal haemoglobinuria.
- Haemolysis may be:
  - extravascular: most common type; involves sequestration of red cells from the circulation.
  - intravascular, e.g. haemolytic-uraemic syndromes, paroxysmal nocturnal haemoglobinuria, incompatible blood transfusion. In the last example, renal damage

results from immune complex and red cell stroma deposition. Haemoglobin is released into the plasma and binds to haptoglobulin; the resultant complex is rapidly removed by the liver. Thus the amount of plasma haptoglobulin is inversely related to the degree of haemolysis. If haemolysis is severe, free haemoglobin may appear in glomerular filtrate; if proximal tubular reabsorption is exceeded, haemoglobinuria and haemosiderinuria may result.

[Robin RA Coombs (1921–2006), Cambridge immunologist]

Haemolytic-uraemic syndrome. Acquired condition involving thrombocytopenia, a microangiopathic haemolytic anaemia and endothelial injury to the renal vasculature leading to acute renal failure. Usually occurs in children, especially following diarrhoea or upper respiratory infection, but may occur in adults. May occur in cancer, infections and during chemotherapy administration. Closely related to thrombotic thrombocytopenic purpura, but neurological features such as CVA which characterise the latter are uncommon. A similar condition may occur postpartum or in women taking the contraceptive pill.

Treatment is mainly supportive. Although heparin and prostacyclin have been used, their benefit is unproven. Plasmapheresis and immunosuppressive drugs have also been used.

See also, Haemolysis

Haemoperfusion. Removal of toxic substances from plasma by adsorption on to special filters, e.g. amberlite resin, activated charcoal granules coated in acrylic gel or cellulose. Performed in poisoning and overdoses, and hepatic failure. Modern devices are extremely efficient; complete removal of toxin from the body is limited by tissue binding. Thus haemoperfusion is most effective for poisons with small volumes of distribution, e.g. barbiturates, disopyramide, theophylline, meprobamate and methaqualone; these are rarely taken in overdose. Tricyclic antidepressants are not removed. Requires vascular cannulation (e.g. femoral vein), extracorporeal circuit and heparinisation. Blood flow of 100–200 ml/min is employed, continued for several hours according to the clinical condition or plasma toxin levels.

Complications: as for dialysis. Thrombocytopenia was common with earlier adsorption columns.

Haemophilia. Coagulation disorder with an incidence (type A) of 1:5000–10 000, inherited as a sex-linked recessive defect. Thus affects males, although female carriers may exhibit mild disease. Female homozygotes virtually always die *in utero*. Results in deficiency of factor VIII (haemophilia A) or IX (haemophilia B; Christmas disease; one-tenth as common), leading to increased bleeding into muscles, joints and internal organs. The intrinsic coagulation pathway is slowed, with activated partial thromboplastin time prolonged and bleeding time normal. Specific factor VIII/IX assay reveals reduced activity, and von Willebrand factor assay is normal.

- Intensive care/anaesthetic considerations:
  - risk of haemorrhage:
    - spontaneous bleeding may occur at factor VIII levels below 5%; prolonged bleeding may follow surgery or trauma at 5–15%. At 15–35%, bleeding is likely only if surgery or trauma is major; it is unlikely if levels exceed 35%, but over 50% is suggested for surgery where possible.
    - factor VIII is given as a concentrate (preferred), as cryoprecipitate, or as fresh frozen plasma, with haematological advice and monitoring of blood levels. Half-life is 8–12 h; adequate levels are required for at least a week postoperatively. About 15% of patients have circulating antibodies to factor VIII or IX, making control more difficult; eptacog alpha may be useful in such cases.

      Desmopressin 0.4 μg/kg iv may transiently increase levels of factor VIII by 3–6 times in mild cases, and tranexamic acid 1 g orally may also be given.
    - im injections are avoided.
    - care should be taken with any invasive procedure including venesection or arterial blood sampling.
    - NSAIDs and antiplatelet drugs should be avoided.
  - high risk of HIV infection in haemophiliacs given pooled factor VIII before the availability of recombinant factor VIII in the mid/late 1980s and of recombinant factor IX in 1997.

[Stephen Christmas (1947–1993); name of British patient in whom the disease was first described]

See also, Coagulation studies; von Willebrand's disease

Haemorrhage. Physiological effects of acute haemorrhage:
  - blood volume is reduced, leading to reduced venous return and cardiac output.
  - arterial BP falls, with activation of the baroreceptor reflex, reduced parasympathetic activity and increased sympathetic activity. Tachycardia, peripheral arterial vasoconstriction (to skin, viscera and kidneys) and venous constriction restore BP, initially. Classified in ATLS guidelines into four classes:
    - I: up to 15% of blood volume lost (usually little physiological change).
    - II: 15–30% lost (tachycardia, peripheral vasoconstriction, postural hypotension).
    - III: 30–40% lost (hypotension, mental confusion, maximum tachycardia).
    - IV: > 40% lost (cardiovascular collapse and shock).

    Bradycardia and hypotension may occur with over 20–30% of loss; it is thought to be vagally mediated, due to cardiac afferent C-fibre discharge caused by ventricular distortion and underfilling.
  - increased vasopressin secretion and renin/angiotensin system activity causes vasoconstriction, sodium and water retention and thirst.
  - catecholamine and corticosteroid secretion increase as part of the stress response.
  - increased movement of interstitial fluid to the intravascular compartment and third space.
- Long-term effects:
  - increased 2,3-DPG production, increasing tissue O_2 delivery.
  - increased plasma protein synthesis.
  - increased erythropoietin secretion and erythropoiesis.

  Volume restoration takes 1–3 days after moderate haemorrhage, with reduction of haematocrit and plasma protein concentration.
- Features: as for hypovolaemia.
- Management:
  - local pressure over bleeding points/pressure points, supine position, raising the feet, O_2 therapy, military antishock trousers, etc., specific haemostatic measures.
  - large bore intravenous cannulae and iv fluid administration:
    - cross-matched blood is best (but some benefit in cardiac output and tissue flow is derived from haemodilution).

- O Rhesus-negative blood is used in life-threatening haemorrhage, but ABO compatible blood should be used if available.
- colloid maintains intravascular expansion for longer than crystalloid.
- crystalloid: saline is more effective than dextrose.
- CVP and urine output measurement are useful for monitoring volume replacement.

See also, Blood loss, perioperative; Blood transfusion; Colloid/crystalloid controversy

Haemostasis, *see Coagulation*

HAFOE, High air-flow oxygen enrichment, *see Oxygen therapy*

Hagen–Poiseuille equation. For laminar flow of a fluid of viscosity η through a tube of length L and radius r, with pressure gradient P across the length of the tube:

$$\text{Flow} = \frac{Pr^4 \pi}{8 \eta L}$$

Originally derived by observing flow of liquid through rigid cylinders of different dimensions, with different driving pressures. Applied to blood flow through blood vessels, and gas flow through breathing systems and airways, although these tubes are neither rigid nor perfect cylinders.
[Jean Poiseuille (1797–1869), French physiologist; Gotthilf HL Hagen (1797–1884), German engineer]

Haldane apparatus. Burette for measuring gas volumes before and after removal of CO_2 by reaction with potassium hydroxide. The volume percentage of CO_2 in the original gas mixture may thus be determined. Similar determination of O_2 concentration may be performed, using pyrogallol as the absorbant.
[John Haldane (1860–1936), Scottish-born English physiologist]
See also, Carbon dioxide measurement; Gas analysis

Haldane effect. Increased capacity of deoxygenated blood for CO_2 transport compared with oxygenated blood.

- Results from:
  - increased binding of reduced haemoglobin to CO_2, forming carbamino groups (accounts for 70% of the effect).
  - increased buffering ability of reduced haemoglobin, allowing more CO_2 to be transported as bicarbonate.

See also, Haldane apparatus

Half-life ($t_{1/2}$). In an exponential process, the time taken for the variable to reach half its original value. Remains constant, whatever its starting point; thus indicates the rate of such a process, usually a decay.

- Examples:
  - radioactive half-life (time taken for half the original number of atoms to disintegrate).
  - drug half-life (time taken for drug concentration to fall by half, whether resulting from redistribution, elimination, etc.).

In pharmacokinetics, context-sensitive half-life refers to the time for plasma concentration of a drug to decrease by 50% after terminating an iv infusion which has maintained steady-state plasma concentration. For example, for propofol it is approximately 20 min after 2 hours' infusion, 30 min after 6 hours' infusion and 50 min after 9 hours' infusion. Corresponding figures for midazolam and alfentanil are in the order of 40 min, 70 min and 80 min; for fentanyl: 40 min, 4 h and 5 h. Ultra-short acting drugs are less affected by 'context' (i.e. duration of infusion); for example for remifentanil it is approximately 3 min irrespective of the duration of the infusion.
See also, Time constant

Hall, Richard, *see Halsted, William Stewart*

Haloperidol. Butyrophenone antipsychotic/neuroleptic agent. Acts by blocking central dopamine receptors. Also acts on cholinergic, serotonergic, histaminergic and α-adrenergic receptors. Has tranquillising effects without impairing consciousness. Useful in the treatment of schizophrenia; has also been used to sedate psychotic patients in ICU. Half-life is approximately 20 h.

- Dosage:
  - 1.5–5.0 mg orally, 8–12 hourly; up to 100 mg may be needed in severe schizophrenia.
  - 2–10 mg im, 4–8 hourly, depending on the response, up to 18 mg. A depot preparation, haloperidol decanoate, is given by deep im injection for long-term therapy in psychoses (50–300 mg 4 weekly).
- Side effects include extrapyramidal symptoms (parkinsonism, dystonia, restlessness and tardive dyskinesia); can trigger the neuroleptic malignant syndrome. Other side effects are similar to those of chlorpromazine, but with less sedation and fewer antimuscarinic effects.

Halothane. 2-Bromo-2-chloro-1,1,1-trifluoroethane (Fig. 79). Inhalational anaesthetic agent, introduced in 1956. Its use rapidly spread because of its greater potency, ease of use, non-irritability and non-inflammability compared with diethyl ether and cyclopropane. Fears over liver damage on repeated administration (halothane hepatitis) and introduction of newer agents (especially sevoflurane, which has replaced halothane as many anaesthetists' agent of choice for airway obstruction) have led to a decline in its use and it was discontinued in the UK in 2007.

- Properties:
  - colourless liquid; vapour has characteristic pleasant smell and is 6.8 times denser than air.
  - mw 197.
  - boiling point 50°C.
  - SVP at 20°C 32 kPa (243 mmHg).
  - partition coefficients:
    - blood/gas 2.5.
    - oil/gas 225.
  - MAC 0.76%.
  - non-flammable.
  - adsorbed on to rubber.
  - may corrode aluminium, tin and certain alloys when moist.
  - supplied in liquid form with thymol 0.01%; decomposes slightly in light.
- Effects:
  - CNS:
    - smooth rapid induction, with rapid recovery.
    - anticonvulsant action.

```
   F        Br
    \      /
F — C  —  C — H
    /      \
   F        Cl
```

Fig. 79 Structure of halothane

- increases cerebral blood flow but reduces intraocular pressure.
- poor analgesic properties.

- RS:
  - non-irritant. Pharyngeal, laryngeal and cough reflexes are abolished early, hence its value in difficult airways.
  - respiratory depressant, with increased respiratory rate and reduced tidal volume.
  - bronchodilatation and inhibition of secretions.
- CVS:
  - myocardial depression possibly via reduction of intracellular calcium mobilisation, and bradycardia via increased vagal tone. Has ganglion blocking and central vasomotor depressant actions. Hypotension is common.
  - myocardial O_2 demand decreases.
  - slight vasodilatation only.
  - arrhythmias are common, e.g. bradycardia, nodal rhythm, ventricular ectopics/bigemini.
  - sensitises the myocardium to catecholamines, e.g. endogenous or injected adrenaline.
- other:
  - dose-dependent uterine relaxation.
  - nausea/vomiting is uncommon. GIT motility is decreased.
  - skeletal muscle relaxation; non-depolarising neuromuscular blocking drugs may be potentiated. Shivering is common during recovery.
  - may precipitate MH.

Up to 20% is metabolised in the liver, usually via oxidative pathways. Reduction is thought to be more likely under hypoxic conditions, and may be important in the development of hepatitis. Metabolites include bromine, chlorine and trifluoroacetic acid; negligible amounts of fluoride ions are produced. Repeated administration after recent use may result in hepatitis.

0.5–2.0% is usually adequate for maintenance of anaesthesia, with higher concentrations for induction. Tracheal intubation may be performed easily with spontaneous respiration, under halothane anaesthesia.

See also, Vaporisers

Halothane hepatitis. Hepatitis following halothane exposure; first reported in 1958. Incidence and characteristics are controversial and difficult to study, because of its rarity and other causes of hepatic impairment after surgery. In the USA, the National Halothane Study (1969) reported 850 000 hepatitis cases occurring within 6 weeks of anaesthesia, 250 000 of whom had received halothane. Only nine cases were unexplained by other causes; seven of these had received halothane. Studies since then do support the existence of the condition. Its incidence is 1:6000 to 1:30 000, although mild hepatic dysfunction as indicated by deranged liver function tests may occur in up to 20% of patients receiving halothane. Hepatitis is more common following repeated use, especially in rapid succession, although the safe time interval is not known. It may be more common in middle-aged women and in obese patients. There may be a genetic predisposition. Incidence is unrelated to pre-existing liver disease. It has been shown to occur in children although less commonly than in adults.

Most patients are thought to be unharmed by repeated administration; some show mild impairment of liver function and a few progress to hepatic failure, with poor prognosis.

- Main theories of mechanism:
  - a toxic metabolite of halothane causes direct liver damage. Supported by the need in certain animal models for increased halothane metabolism via enzyme induction (e.g. with barbiturate pretreatment) before hepatitis occurs. Hypoxia is also required, suggesting involvement of reductive metabolism (normally oxidative metabolism occurs). However, the theory is not supported by similar hepatotoxicity following enflurane and isoflurane under similar circumstances, despite their low metabolism. Also, reductive metabolites themselves are not hepatotoxic, and other factors may increase toxicity without increasing metabolism, e.g. fasting, or high doses for short periods.
  - immune reaction to halothane or hepatocytes altered by halothane. Suggested by finding increased autoimmune antibodies in affected patients' sera. Antibodies reacting with rabbit halothane-altered hepatocyte membrane determinants are found in 75% of affected patients, and may be used as a diagnostic test. Immune reaction to a metabolite may be involved; trifluoroacetyl halide has been implicated.
  - hepatic O_2 supply reduced by cardiovascular effects of halothane, causing ischaemic necrosis. Enzyme induction caused by barbiturates increases O_2 demand, exacerbating supply/demand imbalance. Although hypoxia is thought to contribute to hepatitis, this theory is not considered the most important.

Much experimental work has been performed in animals, with interspecies variation; extrapolation to humans is difficult.

- The Committee on Safety of Medicines in 1986 recommended avoidance of halothane following:
  - history of previous exposure and adverse reactions.
  - previous exposure within 3 months unless the indications are felt clinically overriding.
  - history of unexplained jaundice/pyrexia after previous exposure to halothane.

This recommendation led to much controversy amongst UK anaesthetists, some supporting the routine use of alternative agents and some defending halothane as the best drug for most anaesthetics, and worried that it might eventually be withdrawn. Hepatitis has followed exposure to enflurane and isoflurane, but their repeated use is generally felt to be safe. However, it is possible that binding of halothane metabolites to hepatocytes predisposes to subsequent hepatitis following exposure to the other agents.

Mikatti NE, Healy TEJ (1997). Eur J Anaesth; 14: 7–14

'Halothane shakes', *see Shivering, postoperative*

Halsted, William Stewart (1852–1922). US surgeon, considered the founder of local anaesthetic nerve blocks with Hall and others in New York from 1884, using cocaine (although Anrep had performed intercostal blocks previously). He and Hall described blocks of most of the nerves of the face, head and limbs, experimenting on each other and becoming cocaine addicts in the process. Highly regarded for his surgical skills, becoming Professor at Baltimore. Trained Cushing. Also introduced rubber gloves into surgery.
[Richard J Hall (1856–1897), Irish-born US surgeon]

Hamburger shift, *see Chloride shift*

Hanging drop technique. Method of identifying the epidural space, e.g. during epidural or spinal anaesthesia. A drop of saline is placed at the hub of a needle which is advanced towards the epidural space; when the space has been entered the drop is drawn into the needle by the negative pressure within the space. Not always reliable, since negative pressure is not always present.

Haptoglobin. Alpha-globulin synthesised by the liver, which binds free haemoglobin in the blood. Normal serum level is 0.3–1.9 g/l; this usually binds 100–140 mg free haemoglobin per 100 ml plasma. Haptoglobin–haemoglobin complex is rapidly removed from the circulation by the reticuloendothelial system; if the liver is unable to produce new haptoglobin quickly enough the plasma haptoglobin level falls. Although the reduction in haptoglobin is used mainly as a sensitive indicator of intravascular haemolysis, it may also occur if haemolysis is extravascular.

Haptoglobin is an acute phase protein, but may also be raised in carcinoma, inflammatory disease and after trauma or surgery.

See also, Acute phase response

Harmonics. Related sine waveforms; the frequency of each is a multiple of the fundamental frequency of the first harmonic, the slowest component of the series. Complex waveforms may be produced by adding higher harmonics to the first (fundamental) harmonic (Fourier analysis). Monitoring equipment must be able to reproduce harmonics of high enough frequency for the signal recorded; e.g. up to the 10th harmonic for many recorders. More harmonics are required for more complex waveforms with higher frequencies, increasing the required frequency response of the monitor concerned, e.g. ECG 0.5–80 Hz, EEG 1–60 Hz, EMG 2–1200 Hz.

Harnesses. Used to secure breathing attachments or facepieces to the patient. May damage soft tissues around the face, and airway obstruction may still occur.

- Examples:
  - Clausen harness: triangular back placed behind the head, with straps at each corner for attachment to hooks around the facepiece.
  - Connell harness: square back placed behind the head, with attachments at each end for the sides of the facepiece.
  - Hudson harness (for dental surgery): long strap for fixation of the catheter mount from the nasotracheal tube; binds around the patient's forehead.

Formerly widely used during anaesthesia, the Clausen or Connell harnesses (or their disposable silicone/rubber equivalents) are also used for mask IPPV or CPAP.

[RJ Clausen (1890–1966), English anaesthetist; Karl Connell (1873–1941), US surgeon; Maurice WP Hudson (1901–1992), London anaesthetist]

Hartmann's solution (Ringer's lactate; Compound sodium lactate). IV fluid containing sodium 131 mmol/l, potassium 5 mmol/l, calcium 2 mmol/l, chloride 111 mmol/l and lactate 29 mmol/l. pH is 5–7. Originally formulated from Ringer's solution to allow fluid replacement and treatment of metabolic acidosis in sick children, using an isotonic solution containing more sodium than chloride. Lactate is metabolised to bicarbonate within a few hours, and the hazards of bicarbonate administration avoided. Now widely used as the crystalloid of choice for ECF replacement, since it closely resembles this fluid in make-up; however, its advantage over saline solutions for routine use has been questioned.

Often avoided in patients with renal failure because of the risk of hyperkalaemia, in sick patients or those with hepatic failure because of the risk of lactic acidosis, and in diabetics because of the risk of lactate metabolism to glucose (although the actual increase in blood glucose concentration is likely to be small). Has been associated with clotting of stored blood transfused through a blood warmer without first flushing the line with saline, presumably because of the calcium content.

[Alexis Hartmann (1898–1964), US paediatrician]

Lee JA (1981). Anaesthesia; 36:1115–21

Hayek oscillator, *see Intermittent negative pressure ventilation*

Hb, *see Haemoglobin*

HBE, *see His bundle electrography*

Hct, *see Haematocrit*

HDU, *see High dependency unit*

Head injury. Common cause of morbidity and mortality in trauma, especially in young males; it should be suspected in all trauma cases especially those involving the chest and neck. Divided into closed or penetrating (the latter having a worse outcome), whilst brain injury can be divided into:

- that occurring at time of injury (primary) and which cannot be influenced by treatment. Injury results from deceleration of the brain inside the bony skull, lacerations from bony prominences on the base of the skull, shearing effects, rotational forces and the 'cheese-cutter' effect of blood vessels. Effects range from macroscopic contusions to diffuse axonal injury. Injury may be on the side of the injury or opposite (contrecoup).
- that resulting from potentially preventable or treatable causes (e.g. hypoxaemia, hypotension, hypercapnia, perhaps associated with other injuries). Compression due to cerebral oedema or intracerebral, intraventricular, epidural or subdural haemorrhage can be included here although the first two are usually associated with direct brain injury.

- Features:
  - external signs of head injury, e.g. bruising, lacerations, etc. Cervical spine fractures or serious ligamentous injuries should be assumed until proven otherwise. Chest trauma is common. Other injuries may be present.
  - impaired consciousness and amnesia. Often associated with alcohol or other cause of coma. Brainstem death may occur.
  - pupils: the 3rd cranial nerve on the side of an expanding cerebral lesion is stretched over the edge of the tentorium cerebelli, causing ipsilateral dilatation and absence of the light reflex with the consensual light reflex preserved. Eventually, the contralateral pupil is also affected.
  - bradycardia and hypertension may occur (Cushing's reflex), and irregular respiration as compression continues.
  - hemiparesis/hemiplegia, upward plantar reflexes. Cranial nerve involvement may reflect the site of injury; e.g. 1–6 in anterior fossa, 7–8 in middle fossa and 9–10 in posterior fossa injuries. Other CNS signs are often variable.
  - other:
    - infection.
    - Cushing's ulcers.
    - convulsions.
    - disturbance of CSF dynamics, causing CSF leak (rhinorrhea or otorrhoea) or hydrocephalus.
    - respiratory, e.g. aspiration pneumonitis, infection, PE, pulmonary oedema, ARDS, etc.

- diabetes insipidus or syndrome of inappropriate antidiuretic hormone secretion, cerebral salt wasting syndrome.
- DIC.

- Management:
  - as for coma and trauma, i.e. CPR: O_2 administration, airway, breathing, circulation, etc. The Glasgow coma scale is widely used for assessment although the simpler AVPU scale is also commonly used. Continuous reassessment is important.
  - opioid analgesic drugs should be avoided in spontaneously breathing patients, because of the risk of central and respiratory depression and their effects on the pupils; codeine is traditionally used, as these effects are held to be less, but this may represent codeine's lesser potency.
  - cervical spine and skull X-rays to identify fractures, and CT scanning to identify haemorrhage, oedema, etc. Ultrasound has been used to identify midline shift, before subsequent CT scanning.
  - Criteria for skull X-ray:
    - unconsciousness or amnesia at any time.
    - neurological signs.
    - CSF/blood from nose or ear.
    - serious scalp injury.
    - difficulty in assessment, e.g. confusion, alcohol, etc.
  - Criteria for CT scan:
    - deterioration in conscious level, pupillary signs or other observations.
    - focal neurological signs.
    - fractured skull and confusion.
    - continuing unconsciousness.
  - Criteria for consulting a neurosurgeon:
    - fractured skull with confusion or worse impairment of conscious level, focal neurology or convulsions.
    - coma persisting after resuscitation (i.e. Glasgow coma score < 8).
    - deterioration in conscious level or the development of other neurological signs.
    - persistent confusion, even without a skull fracture.
    - compound depressed skull fracture.
    - suspected base of skull fracture.

    Transfer for CT scan requires tracheal intubation if conscious level is depressed, i.e. GCS ≤ 8.
  - if injury is severe, tracheal intubation and IPPV are performed, traditionally maintaining arterial $P\text{CO}_2$ at about 4–4.5 kPa to reduce ICP and cerebral oedema. During intubation, steps should be taken to prevent aspiration of gastric contents or worsening of any associated cervical spine injury. Continued hyperventilation is less often employed now as it is recognised that in head injury cerebral blood flow may already be reduced and aggressive hyperventilation may result in excessive cerebral vasoconstriction and cerebral ischaemia; $P\text{CO}_2$ is therefore acutely lowered by hyperventilation only to offset any acute increases in ICP. Other indications for IPPV include:
    - hypoxaemia.
    - respiratory irregularity, hypo- or hyperventilation.
    - uncontrolled convulsions, raised ICP or hyperthermia.
    - extensor or flexor posturing.

    Other measures to prevent a high ICP and reduce cerebral O_2 requirements include:
    - heavy sedation + neuromuscular blockade (the latter has been implicated in increased mortality but this is controversial as the evidence is weak). Thiopental coma or other forms of cerebral protection/resuscitation are sometimes employed although controversial.
    - head-up tilt of about 15°.
    - use of diuretics including mannitol, although dehydration *per se* is now generally felt to be less beneficial than maintaining cerebral perfusion pressure with inotropes if necessary. Recent evidence (CRASH trial: corticosteroid randomisation after significant head injury) suggests that corticosteroids may increase mortality.
    - hyperglycaemia may worsen outcome and tight glycaemic control should be instituted.
    - prophylactic use of anticonvulsant drugs is controversial but is common if craniotomy is required or if the cerebral perfusion pressure falls.
    - whole body cooling may lower ICP but does not improve outcome; however, hyperthermia does worsen brain injury and should be treated aggressively.
  - in some ICUs, ICP monitoring is undertaken and cerebral perfusion pressure calculated. EEG and related monitoring, evoked potentials, transcranial Doppler ultrasound and jugular bulb catheterisation have been used to follow progress.
  - other drug therapy includes antibiotic cover for CSF leaks (traditionally a sulphonamide although prophylaxis is less frequently used now) and H_2 receptor antagonists.

Surgery may be required for associated injuries, elevation of depressed fractures or evacuation of intracranial haemorrhage; the latter may require burr holes or craniotomy.

- Anaesthesia for patients with head injuries: as for neurosurgery and emergency surgery. In particular:
  - other injuries may be present.
  - regional techniques are often difficult, especially if the patient is confused. Sedation is dangerous. Burr holes may be drilled under local anaesthesia.
  - spontaneous ventilation must be avoided, even for minor procedures, since a small increase in cerebral blood flow and intracranial volume may cause a catastrophic rise in ICP. All patients should be managed as if ICP is raised.

Moppett IK (2007). Br J Anaesth; 99: 18–31 and Helmy A, Vizcaychipi M, Gupta AK (2007). Br J Anaesth; 99: 32–42

See also, Cerebral metabolic rate for oxygen; Coning; Faciomaxillary surgery

Head's paradoxical reflex. Sustained diaphragmatic contraction, followed by shallow respiration, following a small passive lung inflation. Seen only in rabbits, and following cooling and partial rewarming of the vagi. Significance is unknown.

Widdicombe J (2004). J Physiol; 559: 1–2.

[Sir Henry Head (1861–1940), English neurologist]

See also, Gasp reflex

Health and safety issues, *see COSHH regulations; Environmental safety of anaesthetists; Scavenging*

Healthcare Commission. Independent organisation, formed in 2003–4 from the Commission for Health Improvement (CHI) which was established in 1999 with the aims of improving the quality of patient care in the NHS by assessing all NHS organisations at regular intervals and publishing its findings, investigating serious failures, checking that the NHS follows national guidelines and advising on best practice in clinical governance. The new Commission continues with the functions of CHI but has also taken over certain functions of the Audit Commission (audits NHS organisations and evaluates their cost-effectiveness) and the National Care Standards Commission (regulates independent hospitals and care homes), and is responsible for publishing annual ratings of all NHS organisations in England and an annual report to Parliament on the state of health care. It also assesses complaints and the promotion of public health.

Due to be replaced (along with the Commission for Social Care Inspection and the Mental Health Act Commission) by the Quality Care Commission, a new body, in ~2009.

Heart. Develops from a single tube which doubles up forming primitive atrium and ventricle; divided by septa into left and right sides (*see Atrial septal defect; Ventricular septal defect*). The primitive arterial outlet (truncus arteriosus) splits spirally to form the aorta and pulmonary trunk; the venous inlet (truncus venosus) absorbs into the smooth-walled part of the right atrium.

- Surface anatomy:
  - right border: from 3rd to 6th right costal cartilages, 1–1.5 cm from the left sternal edge.
  - left border: from 2nd left costal cartilage, 1–1.5 cm from the left sternal edge, to the apex beat (usually at the 5th left intercostal space in the midclavicular line).
  - upper limit: level with the angle of Louis (T4–5).
  - base: level with the xiphisternum (T8–9).

The left border is composed mainly of left ventricle, the right border mainly of right atrium, and the base mainly of right ventricle as on the chest X-ray. Weighs about 300 g. Encased within pericardium.

- Chambers:
  - right atrium:
    - bears the auricular appendage (remnant of the original atrium).
    - receives superior and inferior venae cavae, and coronary sinus.
  - right ventricle:
    - crescent-shaped in cross-section, due to bulging of the left ventricle.
    - tendinous cords from the interventricular septum and papillary muscles attach to the tricuspid valve.
    - pulmonary valve: comprised of three cusps.
  - left atrium: receives four non-valved pulmonary veins.
  - left ventricle:
    - thick walled.
    - the two-cusped mitral valve is anchored with tendinous cords as for the tricuspid valve. The anterior cusp is bigger than the posterior.
    - aortic valve: comprised of three semilunar cusps, one anterior and two posterior.
- Blood supply: *see Coronary circulation*
- Nerve supply: from vagus and sympathetic nervous system from upper thoracic and cervical ganglia; mainly T1–4. The cardiac plexus receives branches from both components of the autonomic nervous system.

[Antoine Louis (1723–1792), French surgeon]

See also, Action potential; Atrial . . . ; Cardiac . . . ; Coronary . . . ; Heart . . . ; Left ventricular . . . ; Myocardial . . . ; Ventricular . . .

Heart, artificial. Device used to replace or assist the heart in end-stage disease when heart transplantation is unavailable, or following cardiac surgery. Permanent replacement is not feasible at present, but temporary support is increasingly used as a short-term measure.

- Types:
  - ventricular assist devices:
  - assist either or both ventricles.
  - roller or centrifugal pumps provide non-pulsatile flow; pneumatic pumps provide pulsatile flow. Newer devices involve a spinning 'impeller' within a conduit, drawing blood in a continuous stream from the left ventricular apex and delivering it to the descending aorta.
  - permanent devices: pneumatically or electrically powered, with an external power source.

Main problems are related to infection, thromboembolism, and reliability and flexibility of the devices.

Boehmer JP, Popjes E (2006). Crit Care Med; 34 (Suppl): S268–77

Heart block. Usually refers to atrioventricular (AV) block, i.e. interruption of impulse propagation between atria and ventricles. Bundle branch block refers to interruption distal to the atrioventricular node.

- Classification:
  - 1st degree (Fig. 80a): delay at the AV node; block is never complete:
    - P–R interval > 0.2 s at normal heart rate.
    - usually clinically insignificant.
    - caused by:
      - ageing.
      - ischaemic heart disease.
      - increased vagal tone.
      - drugs, e.g. halothane, digoxin.
      - cardiomyopathy, myocarditis, etc.
  - 2nd degree: occasional complete block. May be:
    - Mobitz type I (Wenckebach phenomenon) (Fig. 80b):
      - AV delay; P–R interval lengthens with successive P waves until complete AV block occurs, and no QRS complex follows the P wave. The cycle then repeats.
      - usually due to AV conduction delay.
      - rarely proceeds to complete heart block.
    - Mobitz type II (Fig. 80c):
      - sudden block below the AV node; i.e. P–R interval may be normal. May occur regularly, e.g. every third complex.

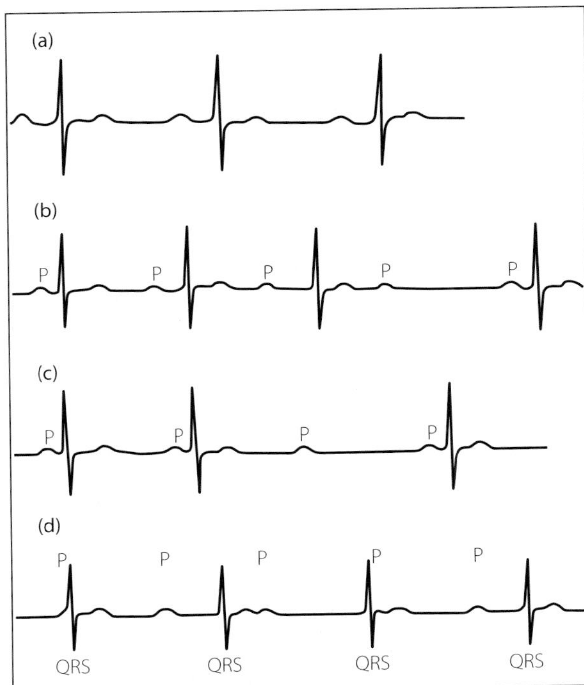

Fig. 80 Heart block: (a) 1st degree; (b) 2nd degree, Mobitz I; (c) 2nd degree, Mobitz II; (d) 3rd degree

- at risk of developing complete heart block, particularly if it occurs regularly.
- 3rd degree (Fig. 80d): complete heart block, at the AV node or below (the latter is trifascicular block. If incomplete, it may appear as bifascicular block with P–R prolongation):
  - ECG demonstrates independent atrial and ventricular activity, the latter arising from an ectopic site. The ventricular rate is usually slow, especially if the ectopic site is far from the AV node (wide QRS complexes; rate < 45/min).
  - clinical findings:
    - hypotension is common.
    - wide pulse pressure (large stroke volume).
    - cannon waves in the JVP.
    - escape ventricular arrhythmias may occur.
  - caused by:
    - old age.
    - ischaemic heart disease.
    - myocarditis/cardiomyopathy.
    - cardiac surgery.
    - increased vagal tone.
    - β-adrenergic antagonists, digoxin.
    - hyperkalaemia.
    - congenital abnormality.

For patients undergoing surgery who have pre-existing complete heart block or predisposing conditions, a pacing wire should be inserted preoperatively. Drugs decreasing AV conduction, e.g. β-receptor antagonists and halothane, should be avoided. Isoprenaline 0.02–0.2 μg/kg/min may be used to increase ventricular rate in complete heart block, and should be available, as should a back-up pacing box. Cardiac output should be maintained where possible. Antiarrhythmic drugs suppressing ventricular activity should be avoided.
[Karl Wenckebach (1848–1904), Dutch physician; Woldemar Mobitz (1889–1951), German cardiologist]
See also, Pacemakers

Heart, conducting system. Composed of:
- sinoatrial node: at the junction of the superior vena cava and right atrium. Normally discharges more rapidly than the rest of the heart, thus setting the rate of contraction, although all cardiac muscle is capable of originating electrical impulses spontaneously.
- atrioventricular node (AV node): lies in the atrial septum, above the coronary sinus opening. Normally the only means of conduction between atria and ventricles.
- bundle of His (or Kent): divides into left and right bundle branches above the interventricular septum, passing down on either side subendocardially:
  - the left bundle branch divides into anterior and posterior fascicles.
  - Purkinje fibres spread from the ends of bundle branches/fascicles to the rest of the ventricles.

Impulses pass from node to node through normal atrial muscle, then via specialised cardiac muscle cells, insulated from the rest of the myocardium by connective tissue sheaths. Conduction through each of the following takes about 0.1 s:
- atria.
- AV node.
- bundle of His/Purkinje system.

Vagal and sympathetic innervation is directed to both nodes; conduction through the AV node is slowed by the former and speeded by the latter.

Ventricular depolarisation begins at the heart's apex and spreads outwards and upwards, encouraging upward expulsion of blood from the ventricles.

Interruption of impulse conduction may result in bundle branch block and heart block.
[Wilhelm His (1863–1934), German anatomist; Albert Kent (1863–1958), English physiologist and radiologist; Johannes von Purkinje (1787–1869), Czech physiologist]

Heart failure, *see Cardiac failure*

Heart–lung transplantation. First performed in 1968 but with poor results; outcomes have steadily improved since the 1980s. In the UK ~50 are performed each year, with 1-year survival ~85%. Isolated lung transplantation initially produced poor results but interest has increased more recently.
- Indications: usually pulmonary hypertension or Eisenmenger's syndrome. Has been performed for pulmonary fibrosis, cystic fibrosis, emphysema, etc.
- Donor:
  - as for heart transplantation, with normal chest X-ray, minimal sputum and no history of aspiration or pulmonary oedema. Arterial $P\text{O}_2$ should exceed 13.3 kPa (100 mmHg) with $F_I\text{O}_2$ 0.4.
  - the heart and lungs are placed into a bag and immersed in cold electrolyte solution, with IPPV at low rates and perfusion of the coronary arteries with donor blood. Whole body transfer using cardiopulmonary bypass has also been used.
- Recipient:
  - immunosuppression and general management as for heart transplantation.
  - the trachea is divided above the carina. Damage to vagi, phrenic and recurrent laryngeal nerves is possible.
  - PEEP and inotropes are usually required; isoprenaline is particularly useful because of its ability to reduce pulmonary vascular resistance. Pulmonary oedema and sputum retention are common. The cough reflex is destroyed and ciliary activity impaired.
  - weaning from IPPV is as for cardiac surgery.
  - lung rejection may occur without heart rejection, and may be difficult to detect. Graft-versus-host disease may also occur.

Heart murmurs. General principles:
- caused by turbulent flow of blood, including abnormal flow through a normal valve or normal flow though an abnormal valve or orifice.
- systolic murmurs may be physiological; diastolic murmurs are always pathological.
- stenotic murmurs are harsh and usually immediate; regurgitant murmurs are soft and usually follow a pause.
- low murmurs are heard best with the stethoscope bell, high pitched ones with the diaphragm.
- left-sided murmurs are heard best in expiration; right-sided ones best in inspiration.
- murmurs radiate usually in the direction of turbulent flow.
- when auscultating the heart, murmurs are best described by:
  - time of occurrence.
  - site and radiation.
  - character including relation to respiration. Loudness is usually expressed as a score of 1–5: 1 = only just audible; 5 = audible without a stethoscope.
  - associated heart sounds.

- Classification:
  - systolic:
    - pansystolic:
      - VSD.
      - mitral regurgitation.
      - tricuspid regurgitation.
    - ejection:
      - aortic stenosis or sclerosis.
      - pulmonary stenosis.
      - ASD.
  - diastolic:
    - mitral stenosis.
    - aortic regurgitation.
  - continuous:
    - patent ductus arteriosus.

(n.b. Venous hum: due to kinking of major neck veins, especially in children. Abolished by pressure on the neck.)
See also, Cardiac cycle; Preoperative assessment; Pulmonary valve lesions; Tricuspid valve lesions

Heart rate. Normal range in adults is usually defined as 60–100 beats/min, but it may be less than 50/min in fit young subjects, and increase up to 200/min on exercise. Rate is about 100/min in the heart denervated of sympathetic and parasympathetic innervation. In children, heart rate decreases with age from 110–160/min during infancy, reaching adult values at about 12 years.

- Rate is increased by:
  - sympathetic activity, e.g. secondary to hypotension, hypoxaemia, hypercapnia, pain, fear, anger, exercise, inspiration.
  - hormones, e.g. catecholamines, thyroxine.
  - infection and fever.
  - Bainbridge reflex.
  - drugs, e.g. salbutamol.
- Rate is decreased by:
  - parasympathetic activity via the vagus nerve, e.g. secondary to the baroreceptor reflex, fear, pain, raised ICP, expiration.
  - hypoxaemia.
  - drugs, e.g. neostigmine, β-adrenergic receptor antagonists.

Critically ill children often respond to handling, tracheobronchial suction, hypoxaemia and acidosis with a profound bradycardia; this may be an ominous sign.
See also, Arrhythmias; Pacemaker cells; Sinus arrhythmia; Sinus bradycardia; Sinus rhythm; Sinus tachycardia

Heart sounds. The first sound is due to closure of the tricuspid and mitral valves; it lasts 0.15 s with frequency 25–45 Hz. The second is due to closure of the aortic and pulmonary valves; it lasts 0.12 s with frequency 50 Hz. Valve opening is normally silent.

- Intensity:
  - quiet in obese or well-built subjects.
  - 2nd sound is quiet in aortic stenosis, since valve mobility is reduced.
  - 1st sound is quiet in mitral regurgitation, since valve closure is incomplete.
  - 1st sound is increased in mitral stenosis, since the valve is kept open right up to systole by increased left atrial pressure, instead of gradual closure at end of diastole.
- Splitting of the second sound:
  - heard at the left sternal edge.
  - the aortic component normally precedes the pulmonary component, since left ventricular contraction is faster than that of the right.
  - increased in inspiration, when right ventricular contraction is delayed by increased preload. Fixed in ASD; reversed in left bundle branch block and severe aortic stenosis, when left ventricular contraction is markedly delayed.
- Extra sounds:
  - 3rd heart sound (thought to be due to ventricular filling). Occurs shortly after the 2nd sound. May occur in normal subjects, also in reduced ventricular compliance/increased volume, e.g. in cardiac failure, mitral regurgitation, VSD.
  - 4th heart sound (thought to be due to atrial contraction under pressure with forceful ventricular distension). Occurs shortly before the 1st sound. May occur in aortic stenosis, pulmonary stenosis, hypertension.
  - gallop rhythm: all four sounds, e.g. cardiac failure.
  - others, e.g. the late ejection click of aortic stenosis, the late systolic click of mitral valve prolapse, and the early diastolic opening snap of mitral stenosis.
  - heart murmurs.

See also, Cardiac cycle; Preoperative assessment

Heart transplantation. First performed in humans in 1967 by Barnard. Initial problems were infection and rejection. Interest resurged in the late 1970s with the introduction of ciclosporin, leading to establishment of centres worldwide.

- Indications: mostly end-stage ischaemic heart disease and cardiomyopathy; also congenital heart disease, valvular disease and others.
- Contraindications include age over 50 years, insulin-dependent diabetes mellitus, active infection, and recent PE/MI; these contraindications have been relaxed as expertise increases and chances of survival improve.
- Donor:
  - normal past medical history/examination and ECG. A short period of cardiac arrest, and minimal requirements for inotropic support are acceptable. Age should be under 40. ABO compatibility with the recipient is required.
  - initial management including heparin and cardioplegia is as for cardiac surgery. The heart is placed in cold crystalloid solution and both the atria opened; it is transported in ice.
- Recipient:
  - most patients are prepared for the possibility of emergency transplantation. By definition, they are in poor general health, i.e. high risk.
  - immunosuppressive drugs include ciclosporin, corticosteroids, azathioprine and antithymocyte immunoglobulin.
  - all iv lines, tracheal tube, laryngoscope, tubing, etc., are sterile to reduce infection, with gown and gloves worn.
  - general management is as for cardiac surgery. After cardiopulmonary bypass and aortic cross-clamping, the ventricles are removed, leaving most of the atria. The atria and aortas are anastomosed. The donor heart may also be piggy-backed next to the original heart, anastomosing left atria, aortas, pulmonary arteries and venae cavae.
  - inotropes are usually required for over 24 h. The denervated heart rate is usually faster than that of the innervated heart, with no response to indirectly acting drugs, e.g. atropine. Directly acting drugs, e.g. isoprenaline, are used. The rate responds slowly to circulating catecholamines.

Postoperative care is as routine, but barrier nursing is required.

- regular endocardial biopsy via the right internal jugular vein is performed to detect rejection, e.g. weekly, then monthly for 3 months, then 6 monthly.
- late complications include cardiac allograft vasculopathy (obliterative vasculopathy which leads to late allograft failure).

For anaesthesia in a heart recipient, aseptic techniques are used, and directly acting cardiovascular drugs as above. Otherwise, management is as for any high risk cardiac case.

90% of recipients return to full activity and 40% to work 1 year after transplantation. However, current demand for hearts for transplantation exceeds supply. Cardiac denervation during transplantation means that many patients (about 90%) do not suffer angina. Xenotransplantation is an exciting potential development, but at present, concerns have been raised about its safety.

[Christian N Barnard (1922–2001), South African surgeon]

See also, Heart–lung transplantation

Heat. Form of **energy** associated with movement of molecules, atoms and smaller structural units; it moves from one site to another owing to a **temperature** difference between them.

- Heat is transferred by:
  - radiation: especially from bright shiny bodies to dark matt bodies.
  - convection: as air next to a warm body is warmed, it expands and becomes less dense, rising and being replaced by colder air.
  - evaporation: heat is transferred to liquid molecules, providing the energy required to break the bonds between them in forming a vapour.
  - conduction: especially via good conductors of heat, e.g. metals.

All these routes may be important in **heat loss during anaesthesia**.

See also, Temperature regulation

Heat capacity. Quantity of **heat** required to raise the **temperature** of a mass by 1 K (J/K). Specific heat capacity (C) is the quantity of heat required to raise the temperature of unit mass of substance by 1 K (J/kg/K). The total heat capacity of an object may be calculated from knowledge of the mass and values for C of its constituent parts.

- Examples of C:
  - human tissues, including blood: 3.5 kJ/kg/K.
  - water: 4.18 kJ/kg/K (1 Cal/kg/°C).

For a gas, C_p is specific heat capacity at constant pressure, and C_v is specific heat capacity at constant volume. C_p–C_v equals the work done in expansion of the gas. For an ideal gas, $C_p - C_v = R$ (**universal gas constant**).

Since gases are much less dense than liquids, the energy required to heat unit volume is much less. Thus little energy is expended in heating inspired air (although significant energy is expended humidifying it).

See also, Latent heat

Heat loss, during anaesthesia. Prevention is important because of the adverse effects of **hypothermia** and the increased postoperative O_2 consumption (up to 10 times) caused by **shivering**. In addition, the duration of action of neuromuscular blocking drugs is prolonged and drug excretion delayed. Particularly important in **neonates** and children, and in the **elderly**, because of reduced reserves.

- Temperature may fall by several °C during prolonged surgery, via:
  - increased loss of **heat**:
    - radiation (accounts for 40–50% of loss): increased if the patient is uncovered and surrounded by cold objects. Also increased by vasodilatation.
    - convection (15%): increased if the patient is uncovered.
    - evaporation (30–35%): increased if a body cavity is opened, e.g. abdomen, especially if environmental humidity is low. Heat loss via evaporation in the trachea and airways may be considerable if inspired gases are unhumidified.
    - conduction (3%): usually a less important route; increased by use of cold irrigating solutions, etc.
  - reduced heat production and impaired **temperature regulation**. The latter may be peripheral (e.g. vasodilatation, shivering and impaired piloerection) or central (central effects of drugs).
- Prevention:
  - identification of high risk patients:
    - elderly.
    - children.
    - severely ill patients with malnutrition.
    - prolonged surgery.
    - major blood loss.
    - open body cavity.
    - **sickle cell anaemia**.
  - **temperature measurement** during anaesthesia.
  - covering during transfer to the operating suite.
  - maintenance of ambient temperature at 22–24°C and **humidity** about 50% (compromise between patient temperature and staff comfort).
  - covering with drapes, reflective garments and head coverings (especially children).
  - warming of all skin cleansing solutions and iv fluids.
  - **humidification** of inspired gases.
  - warming blankets, e.g. using heated water or air.
  - warming of the bed, etc. postoperatively.

Sessler DI (2008). Anesthesiology; 109: 318–38

Heat of vaporisation, *see Latent heat*

Heat–moisture exchanger (HME; Swedish nose; hygroscopic condenser). Passive humidifier device. Positioned between the breathing tubing and the facepiece, tracheal/tracheostomy tube or other airway device. Contains material (e.g. sponges, paper or metal gauze) which acts as a screen and which can absorb large amounts of water. As expired gas passes through, water vapour condenses on the filter screen which also gains heat. The water and heat are given up when dry cool inspiratory gas passes through in the next phase of breathing. HMEs may be disposable or refillable. Light and cheap; with up to 90% efficiency for modern devices. Second generation devices have some bacterial filtering properties conferred by an electret membrane (the molecules' polarity is aligned to increase filtering efficiency) but at the expense of increased resistance to flow and reduced efficacy if wet. Newer hydrophobic filters are efficient humidifiers as well as being protective against bacterial and viral transmission, even when wet. All devices increase dead space and may also increase resistance to spontaneous ventilation. Blockage and inadequate ventilation have occurred when HMEs have been used with heated humidifiers and drug nebulisers, or in the presence of copious secretions.

Ward B, Park GR (2000). Clin Intensive Care; 11: 169–76

See also, Filters, breathing system; Humidification

Heatstroke, *see Hyperthermia*

Heavy metal poisoning. Poisoning as a result of ingestion or inhalation of fumes of lead, mercury, arsenic, cadmium, bismuth, aluminium, antimony, chromium, cobalt, copper, gold, manganese, nickel, thallium, vanadium or zinc. Renal, hepatic, neurological and gastrointestinal damage are common following ingestion; acute lung injury often follows inhalation of fumes. Antidotes (chelating agents) include dimercaprol (for antimony, arsenic, bismuth, gold, mercury, thallium and lead), penicillamine (copper and lead), ascorbic acid (chromium), succimer (arsenic, mercury), unithiol (arsenic, mercury, nickel) and sodium calcium edetate (lead, manganese, zinc).

Hedonal. Obsolete anaesthetic agent, one of the first to be used iv (1905); also used rectally and orally. Poorly water soluble, requiring large volumes of injectate. Of very slow onset and prolonged duration of action.

Heidbrink valve, *see Adjustable pressure-limiting valve*

Heimlich manoeuvre. Method of relieving choking caused by a foreign body using rapid compression of the upper abdomen. The resultant rise in intrathoracic pressure expels the object from the upper airway. The operator stands behind the subject with hands clenched over the subject's epigastrium, the operator's arms passing under the subject's. A sharp thrust is delivered inwards and upwards. A similar manoeuvre may be performed with the subject lying. Compression of the lower chest has been found to be as effective. Clearance of one's own airway by falling forwards on to the back of a chair has been reported.
[Henry J Heimlich, US surgeon]

Heimlich valve. Disposable device used in the treatment of pneumothorax. Consists of a flattened rubber tube within a clear plastic tube; attached to a thoracostomy tube, it allows the venting of air from within the chest and prevents the ingress of air. May block/malfunction if blood passes through valve. Useful during the prehospital phase of resuscitation or during interhospital transfer. Now infrequently used since the introduction of plastic underwater seal bottles and portable, disposable bag/valve assemblies.
See also, Chest drainage

Helium. Inert gas, present in natural gas and to a lesser extent in air. Less dense than nitrogen. Thus, if flow is turbulent, greater flow of a helium/O_2 mixture will occur than of a nitrogen/O_2 mixture, as turbulent flow depends on fluid density (and density of 21% O_2 in helium is 34% of that of 21% O_2 in nitrogen). Used therefore to increase alveolar O_2 supply in upper airway obstruction. Of less use in lower airway obstruction, e.g. asthma, because most peripheral flow is laminar and therefore depends on viscosity, which is greater for helium/O_2 mixtures than for nitrogen/O_2. However, some benefit may occur where flow is turbulent.

Supplied in cylinders with brown shoulders and body, at 137 bar. Also available with 21% O_2, in brown-bodied cylinders with brown and white quartered shoulders, at the same pressure.

Has also been used to investigate small airway resistance to flow, by comparing flow–volume loops breathing air and helium/O_2. The two curves are more similar in small airway obstruction than in normal lungs.

Because of its very low solubility, helium is also used in measurement of lung volumes.
Harris PD, Barnes R (2008). Anaesthesia; 63: 284–93

HELLP syndrome (Syndrome of haemolysis, elevated liver function tests and low platelets). Condition first recognised in 1982; thought to represent part of the spectrum of pre-eclampsia characterised primarily by abnormal blood tests rather than hypertension, proteinuria and oedema (although they may occur). HELLP syndrome is associated with significant maternal morbidity, including DIC, placental abruption, acute renal failure, pulmonary oedema and hepatic rupture. General principles of management are as for pre-eclampsia; in addition plasma exchange, administration of fresh frozen plasma and prostacyclin have been used.
Sibai BM (2004). Obstet Gynecol; 103: 981–91

Hemicholinium. Synthetic compound which blocks choline transport into cholinergic nerve endings. Thus reduces acetylcholine synthesis and storage. Used in experimental pharmacology.

Hemo..., *see Haemo...*

Henderson–Hasselbalch equation. Equation describing the relationship between concentrations of dissociated and undissociated acid or base, dissociation constant and pH. Originally described in relation to any buffer system; now often specifically applied to the bicarbonate buffer system.

For the reaction of CO_2 with water to form carbonic acid, which dissociates to form bicarbonate and hydrogen ions:

$$CO_2 + H_2O \rightleftharpoons H_2CO_3 \rightleftharpoons H^+ + HCO_3^-$$

The dissociation constant K_a for the dissociation of H_2CO_3 then equals

$$\frac{[H^+][HCO_3^-]}{[H_2CO_3]}$$

Taking logarithms of both sides:

$$\log K_a = \log[H^+] + \log\frac{[HCO_3^-]}{[H_2CO_3]}$$

$$\text{therefore} - \log\ pH = -\log\ K_a + \log\frac{[HCO_3^-]}{[H_2CO_3]}$$

$$\text{or, } pH = pK_a + \log\frac{[HCO_3^-]}{[H_2CO_3]}$$

Since $[H_2CO_3]$ is related to $[CO_2]$ by the original reaction, and $[CO_2]$ is related to $P\text{CO}_2$ and a solubility factor (0.03 mmol/l/mmHg, or 0.23 mmol/l/kPa),

$$pH = pK_a + \log\frac{[HCO_3^-]}{P\text{CO}_2 \times 0.03}$$

with $P\text{CO}_2$ measured in mmHg

$$\text{or } pK_a + \log\frac{[HCO_3^-]}{P\text{CO}_2 \times 0.23}$$

with $P\text{CO}_2$ measured in kPa.

Describes what happens to pH, $P\text{CO}_2$ and $[HCO_3^-]$ in various acid–base disturbances.

Maximal efficiency of a buffering system occurs at pH values close to its pK_a. pK_a for carbonic acid/bicarbonate is 6.1 at body temperature; its importance arises from the ability to excrete CO_2 via the lungs.
[Lawrence Henderson (1878–1942), US biochemist; Karl Hasselbalch (1874–1962), Danish physiologist]
See also, Acid–base balance

Henry's law. Amount of gas dissolved in a solvent is proportional to its partial pressure above the solvent, at constant temperature.
[William Henry (1744–1836), English chemist]

Heparin sodium/calcium. Anticoagulant drug, used to prevent and treat thromboembolism. Has also been used in DIC. Discovered in 1916. A mucopolysaccharide, derived from animal lung and intestine. Strongly acidic and electronegative, binding strongly to proteins and amines.

- Actions:
  - accelerates the action of antithrombin III, a naturally occurring inhibitor of activated coagulation factors XII, XI, IX, X and thrombin.
  - inhibits platelet aggregation by fibrin.
  - activates lipoprotein lipase, involved in fat transport.
  - thought to be involved in immunological/inflammatory reactions, possibly via binding to histamine and 5-HT. Contained within mast cells.

Fast onset but short acting, with half-life of about 90 min; therefore most effectively given by iv infusion (heparin sodium). Effects persist for 4–6 h. Effects are monitored by measuring the activated partial thromboplastin time (APTT), although thrombin and clotting times are also prolonged. In low dosage, acts by preventing spontaneous activation of factor X in hypercoagulable states (e.g. postoperatively), without affecting the ability to form clots when required. Thus given sc to prevent DVT, although there may be individual variation in effect.

Low mw heparins inhibit factor X preferentially and thus cause fewer systemic anticoagulation effects, with less effect on platelet function. Also have longer half-lives. They have been suggested as causing fewer haemorrhagic effects than unfractionated heparin, when given for prophylaxis. Several low mw heparins exist, with varying properties according to the particular preparation (e.g. ratio of anti-X to anti-II activity).

- Dosage:
  - unfractionated heparin:
    - prophylaxis of DVT: 5000 units sc 2 h preoperatively, then 8–12 hourly until the patient is walking.
    - treatment of thrombosis: 5000 units iv, then 1000–2000 units/h (14–28 units/kg/h) by infusion, or 5000–10 000 units iv 4 hourly by bolus. APPT is kept at 1.5–2.5 times normal. Oral anticoagulation is usually commenced at the same time as heparin.
    - during arterial surgery, 100 units/kg iv; for cardiac surgery, 300 units/kg. Also used to anticoagulate extracorporeal circuits, e.g. cardiopulmonary bypass, haemofiltration.
  - low mw heparin:
    - prophylaxis of DVT:
      - dalteparin sodium: 2500 units sc 1–2 h preoperatively (repeated after 12 h in high risk patients), followed by 2500 units once daily (5000 units if high risk) for 5 days.
      - enoxaparin: 2000 units (20 mg) sc 1–2 h preoperatively (4000 units (40 mg) 12 h preoperatively in high risk patients), followed by 2000 units once daily (4000 units if high risk) for 7–10 days.
      - tinzaparin: 3500 units sc 2 h preoperatively (4500 units 12 h preoperatively in high risk patients), followed by 3500 units once daily (4500 units if high risk) for 7–10 days.
      - bemiparin sodium: 2500 units sc 2 h preoperatively or 6 h postoperatively, followed by 2500 units once daily (3500 units if high risk) for 7–10 days.
    - treatment of thrombosis: may be more effective than unfractionated heparin and does not require laboratory adjustment of dosage. Treatment should be continued for at least 5–6 days, during which time oral anticoagulants should also be given:
      - dalteparin: 200 units/kg once daily (100 units/kg 12 hourly in patients at risk of haemorrhage) (maximal daily dose 18 000 units).
      - enoxaparin 150 units/kg (1.5 mg/kg) 12 hourly.
      - tinzaparin 175 units/kg once daily.
      - bemiparin: 115 units/kg once daily for 5–9 days.

  Higher doses are required in pregnancy.
- Side effects:
  - increased bleeding: cessation of infusion is usually adequate; protamine may be given but only partially reverses low mw heparin.
  - thrombocytopenia: antibody-mediated condition occurring in up to 3% of cases, typically 5–10 days after starting therapy. May be associated with increased tendency to thrombosis. Heparinoids and hirudins are alternatives should this occur.
  - hypersensitivity.
  - osteoporosis following prolonged use.
  - inhibition of aldosterone secretion has been described and regular monitoring of plasma potassium concentration is recommended if the duration of therapy exceeds 7 days.

Side effects are less frequent with low mw heparins than with unfractionated heparin.

See also, Coagulation studies

Heparinoids. Derivatives of heparin; heteropolysaccharides consisting of straight chains with different degree of sulphation. Danaparoid is the only preparation licensed for use in the UK.

Hepatic failure. May follow:
  - chronic disease and cirrhosis:
    - chronic autoimmune hepatitis.
    - chronic viral hepatitis.
    - drugs, e.g. methyldopa, alcohols.
    - metabolic disease, e.g. haemochromatosis, Wilson's disease, α_1-antitrypsin deficiency, other inborn errors of metabolism.
    - biliary disease, e.g. primary biliary cirrhosis.
    - vascular lesions, e.g. venous occlusion, chronic cardiac failure.
  - acute disease (fulminant hepatic failure):
    - acute viral hepatitis.
    - drugs, e.g. paracetamol, halothane, chloroform, chlorpromazine, monoamine oxidase inhibitors, phenytoin, isoniazid.
    - others: less common, including:
      - poisons, e.g. carbon tetrachloride.
      - portal vein thrombosis.
      - acute fatty liver of pregnancy.
      - shock.
      - Reye's syndrome.
- Features:
  - chronic liver disease:
    - malaise, GIT symptoms.
    - jaundice.
    - skin: spider naevi, palmar erythema, leukonychia, finger clubbing, Dupuytren's contracture, bruising, pigmentation.
    - hepatic fetor.
    - gynaecomastia and testicular atrophy, caused by decreased metabolism of circulating oestrogens.
    - neurological impairment: thought to be caused by reduced metabolism of toxic waste products, e.g. ammonia, methionine and fatty acids. May be provoked by stress, including surgery, trauma and infection. Classified thus:
      - stage 1: impaired personality or thinking. EEG is usually normal.
      - stage 2: confusion, abnormal sleep and drowsiness. Asterixis (flapping tremor especially affecting the

hands/wrists) and increased reflexes, with plantar response up or down. EEG is abnormal.
- stage 3: marked confusion, with inability to perform fine movement. Responds to painful stimuli.
- stage 4: comatose with depressed reflexes.

Treatment includes reduction of nitrogen intake, and oral administration of lactulose (20–50 ml/day) and/or neomycin (1 g 4–6 hourly) to reduce ammonia-producing GIT bacteria and encourage nitrogen-utilising bacteria.
- portal hypertension is caused by vascular occlusion, possibly due to fibrotic changes in cirrhosis. It may cause splenomegaly and enlargement of portal–systemic vascular anastomoses, e.g. oesophagogastric junction, retroperitoneal and umbilical vessels. Oesophageal varices may cause severe haemorrhage; treatment may include injection of varices with sclerosant, iv infusion of vasopressin or analogues, administration of somatostatin, use of a Sengstaken–Blakemore tube, or rarely surgery.
- GIT haemorrhage: apart from oesophageal varices, may also be caused by gastric erosions or peptic ulcer disease. Coagulation factors and platelets may be reduced. Anaemia is common.
- hypoproteinaemia, with reduced plasma oncotic pressure, drug binding, immunoglobulins, cholinesterase and coagulation factors.
- fluid retention: may cause ascites, pleural effusion, peripheral oedema and hyperdynamic circulation. Treatment includes spironolactone, sodium restriction and drainage of ascites/pleural effusion.
- hypoxaemia is common, caused by $\dot{V}/\dot{Q}$ mismatch, atelectasis, diaphragmatic splinting or pleural effusion.
- infection is common, especially bacterial.
- renal impairment may occur.
- metabolic and respiratory alkalosis may occur.

- acute fulminant hepatic failure: defined as hepatic failure occurring within 8 weeks of illness, in a previously normal liver. It presents with rapidly progressing encephalopathy, coma and cerebral oedema, with hypoglycaemia, hyponatraemia, hypokalaemia, alkalosis, hypothermia, respiratory failure, haemorrhage, and renal failure. Renal failure may be due to hepatorenal syndrome or acute tubular necrosis. Jaundice is uncommon initially. DIC and infection may occur.

  Treatment is supportive and includes O_2 therapy, IPPV, vitamin K, blood products, neomycin/lactulose, H_2 receptor antagonists/omeprazole, prophylactic antibiotics and nutritional support with dextrose. ICP monitoring may be useful and measures (e.g. head-up tilt, mannitol) employed to reduce ICP if raised. Liver dialysis techniques have been used and liver transplantation may be required. Experimental therapies include auxiliary liver transplantation, temporising hepatectomy, artificial liver systems (live liver cells within an extracorporeal circuit), intraperitoneal hepatocyte transplantation, use of liver growth factors and xenotransplantation.

- Anaesthetic management of patients with hepatic failure or chronic liver disease:
  - directed towards the above complications, particularly preoperative assessment for, and improvement of:
    - encephalopathy, and haematological and coagulation abnormalities.
    - pulmonary and renal function.
    - fluid, acid–base and electrolyte disturbance.

    Vitamin K may be administered if coagulation is abnormal, fresh frozen plasma if surgery is urgent.
  - anaesthetic technique: increased doses of iv agents and neuromuscular blocking drugs may be required in cirrhosis, due to increased volume of distribution, but elimination may be prolonged. Opioids should be used cautiously. All sedative drugs require careful use if encephalopathy is present. Drug metabolism is reduced; isoflurane/desflurane and atracurium are often preferred as reliance on metabolism is less than with other agents. Hypocapnia exacerbates the reduction in hepatic blood flow during general anaesthesia.
  - screening for infectious hepatitis should be performed.
  - maintenance of good peri- and postoperative renal function is important (*see Jaundice*).

A scoring system has been devised for assessment of risk, depending on preoperative blood tests and clinical assessment (Table 17). Good operative risk is suggested by < 6 points, moderate by 7–9 points, and poor risk by > 10 points.

[Baron Guillaume Dupuytren (1777–1835), French surgeon; Samuel AK Wilson (1878–1937), US-born English neurologist]

Jackson N, Wendon J (2000). Clin Intensive Care; 11: 127–35

Hepatitis. Acute hepatitis may be:
- viral:
  - hepatitis A:
    - RNA enterovirus, spread via the orofaecal route. Incubation period is 3–5 weeks.
    - causes fever, headache, GIT symptoms, impaired liver function tests, jaundice and hepatomegaly.
    - recovery is usually within 6 weeks, although malaise may persist longer.
    - passive immunisation with immunoglobulin is available.
  - hepatitis B:
    - DNA virus, spread mainly via blood/blood products and body secretions, including homosexual contact, tattooing, iv drug abuse and childbirth. Incubation period is 2–6 months.
    - features are as for hepatitis A but more severe. May lead to recovery, death or a chronic infective state. The last includes asymptomatic carriage or chronic hepatitis which may lead to hepatocellular carcinoma or hepatic failure.
    - serological markers include surface (Australia) antigen (HBsAg), e antigen (HBeAg), corresponding antibodies (anti-HBs, anti-HBe) and antibody to core antigen (anti-HBc). Pattern:
      - HBsAg: increases 1 month after exposure, peaks at 2–3 months, and falls at 4–5 months.
      - HBeAg: increases at 1 month, peaks at 2 months, and falls at 3 months.
      - anti-HBc: increases at 2 months, peaks at 4 months, and falls slowly thereafter.

Table 17 Scoring system for anaesthesia in hepatic failure

	Points scored		
	1	2	3
Bilirubin (μmol/l)	<25	25–40	>40
Albumin (g/l)	>35	28–35	<28
Prothrombin time prolongation (s)	<4	4–6	>6
Encephalopathy stage	0	1–2	3–4

- anti-HBe: increases at 2–3 months, remaining elevated.
- anti-HBs: increases at 1–2 months, remaining elevated.

- asymptomatic carrier state is associated with HBsAg, HBeAg and anti-HBc expression. Its incidence is under 0.1% in the West, and up to 20% in South-East Asia. Serum viral DNA levels may also be measured; they may distinguish between chronic hepatitis B ($> 10^5$ copies/ml) and the inactive state ($< 10^5$ copies/ml). Patients with chronic infection may receive interferon-α or lamivudine.
- prevention:
  - active immunisation (against HBsAg) of medical workers and high risk groups, e.g. homosexuals, drug abusers, multiple blood transfusion recipients, renal dialysis patients, babies of infected mothers, and patients in mental institutions. Universal neonatal immunisation occurs in many countries but not the UK currently although there is pressure to review this policy.
  - passive immunisation using immunoglobulin; preferably performed within 24 h of exposure and certainly within 7 days.
  - screening of blood for transfusion, use of disposable needles, etc.; operating theatre precautions as for HIV infection. Pregnant women should be screened for HbsAg to reduce fetal transmission.

- hepatitis C (causes most cases of what was previously called non-A non-B hepatitis):
  - RNA virus, previously diagnosed by exclusion but now identified with a serological marker.
  - thought to be responsible for over 90% of post-transfusion hepatitis in the Western world. Also common in patients receiving renal dialysis.
  - causes a similar spectrum of disease to hepatitis A and B, but with incubation period up to 60 days. Cirrhosis may follow infection 20–30 years later in 10–20% of cases; a few may develop hepatocellular carcinoma. High rates of chronic infection and cirrhosis occur. Patients with chronic infection may receive interferon-α and ribavirin.
  - screening of blood products began in the UK in 1991.
  - in 2002 in the UK, following reports of transmission of hepatitis C from staff to patients, new guidance was issued restricting infected staff from performing invasive procedures, as for HIV infection. It also recommended the testing of healthcare workers about to start careers or training that would rely on the performance of exposure prone procedures.
- hepatitis D (delta): RNA virus, dependent on coexistent hepatitis B infection.
- hepatitis E (enteral non-A non-B infection): RNA virus, recently characterised.
  - other viral infections include cytomegalovirus, herpes simplex, varicella zoster and glandular fever.

- due to other infections, e.g. toxoplasmosis, leptospirosis.
- chemical:
  - idiosyncratic, e.g. phenothiazines, monoamine oxidase inhibitors, tricyclic antidepressants, halothane, chloroform, methyldopa, indometacin, erythromycin, rifampicin, chlorpropamide.
  - dose-related, e.g. paracetamol, carbon tetrachloride, alcohol.
- metabolic, e.g. Wilson's disease, or associated with pregnancy.
- associated with circulatory abnormalities, e.g. right ventricular failure, severe hypotension.

The cause of postoperative hepatitis is difficult to determine because many factors may be involved. 1 in 700 healthy patients may have incidental impaired liver function tests preoperatively. Chronic hepatitis is one cause of chronic liver disease and cirrhosis leading to hepatic failure.
[Samuel AK Wilson (1878–1937), US-born English neurologist]
See also, Environmental safety of anaesthetists

Hepatorenal syndrome. Renal impairment secondary to severe hepatic dysfunction, usually cirrhosis. Caused by intrarenal vasoconstriction despite systemic vasodilatation; the mechanism is unclear but may involve systemic and intrarenal vasoconstrictor substances overwhelming locally produced vasodilators such as prostaglandins and kallikreins. Excess endotoxin reaching the kidneys caused by bile salt deficiency, and excess bilirubin within the renal tubules, may also contribute. May occur perioperatively in patients with hepatic failure and jaundice, especially if dehydration exists.

Causes oliguria, with concentrated urine with a low sodium concentration (< 10 mmol/l) and few granular casts; i.e. resembles prerenal renal failure, but does not improve with fluid replacement. Blood urea may be low because of impaired production by the liver. May be difficult to differentiate from hypovolaemia.

Prognosis is poor, even with renal replacement therapy, unless hepatic function improves; it often requires liver transplantation for the kidneys to function. Maintenance of adequate urine output, e.g. using mannitol, is generally thought to reduce the incidence of renal failure in hepatic disease.

Ginès P, Guevara M, Arroyo V, Rodés J (2003). Lancet; 362: 1819–27

Herbal medicines. Taken by up to 20–30% of patients presenting for surgery and often overlooked by medical staff. May have unpredictable physiological and pharmacological effects relevant to the perioperative period. Common examples include:

- echinacea: activates the immune system with reports of allergy (including anaphylaxis), decreased effectiveness of immunosuppressive drugs with short-term use and immunosuppression with long-term use.
- ephedra (ma huang): contains ephedrine and other sympathomimetic alkaloids. Causes dose-dependent tachycardia and hypertension with subsequent risk of myocardial ischaemia and CVA. Increases risk of arrhythmias when inhalational anaesthetic agents such as halothane are used. Haemodynamic instability may occur with concomitant use of monoamine oxidase inhibitors. Should be discontinued 24 h preoperatively.
- garlic (ajo): inhibits platelet aggregation (sometimes irreversibly), increasing the risk of perioperative bleeding. Should be discontinued 7 days preoperatively.
- ginkgo: inhibits platelet activating factor with potential for increased bleeding. Should be discontinued 36 h preoperatively.
- ginseng: may cause hypoglycaemia and inhibition of platelet aggregation. Should be discontinued 7 days preoperatively.
- kava and valerian: cause sedation and may potentiate the effects of anaesthetic agents. Should be discontinued 24 h preoperatively.

- St John's wort (hypericum): induces cytochrome oxidase system (especially the cytochrome P_{450} family) causing enzyme induction. Should be discontinued at least 5 days preoperatively.

Hodges PJ, Kam PCA (2002). Anaesthesia; 57: 889–900

Hereditary angio-oedema. Congenital deficiency of C1 esterase inhibitor, leading to complement activation with inflammatory swelling affecting the face, mouth, skin and intestine. Of autosomal dominant inheritance. May occur spontaneously or following trauma, possibly via activation of kinins, plasmins or other proteases. An acquired form may occur in lymphomas. May cause upper airway obstruction. Management of an acute episode is as for airway obstruction; iv adrenaline, corticosteroids, antihistamine drugs, aprotinin, antifibrinolytic drugs and danazol have been tried, with varying results. Synthetic, partially purified C1 esterase inhibitor is available for the termination of acute attacks, but is not recommended for long-term use. 2–3 units of fresh frozen plasma (which contains C1 esterase inhibitor) may also be given. 10 days' preoperative treatment with danazol has been suggested, and avoidance of upper airway instrumentation if possible.

Nzeako UC, Frigas E, Tremaine WJ (2001). Arch Intern Med; 161: 2417–29

Hereditary angioneurotic oedema, *see Hereditary angio-oedema*

Hering–Breuer reflex (Inflation reflex). Inhibition of respiratory muscles following lung inflation, leading to curtailment of inspiration. Afferent pathway is thought to be from pulmonary stretch receptors via the vagus. Of minor importance in humans, but active in many other mammals; bilateral vagotomy produces slow deep breathing in the latter but not the former.

[Karl Hering (1834–1918), German physiologist; Josef Breuer (1852–1925), Austrian psychiatrist]

Heroin, *see Diamorphine*

Hertz. SI unit of frequency. 1 Hz = 1 cycle per second.

[Heinrich Hertz (1857–1894), German physicist]

Hetastarch, *see Hydroxyethyl starch*

Hewer, Christopher Langton (1896–1986). English anaesthetist, of major importance in the establishment and evolution of anaesthesia in the UK. Popularised the use of trichloroethylene in 1941. Edited *Anaesthesia* for its first 20 years, also *Recent Advances in Anaesthesia and Analgesia* for 50 years. Received many honours and medals.

Hewitt, Frederick (1857–1916). English anaesthetist, practised at St George's Hospital. Renowned for many contributions to anaesthesia, including the first fixed proportion N_2O/O_2 machine, also inhalers, airways and other equipment. A strong advocate of teaching and high standards in anaesthesia. Knighted in 1911.

Hexafluorenium. Drug formerly used to prolong the action of suxamethonium by up to 10 times, by inhibiting plasma cholinesterase. Injected before suxamethonium; it may reduce muscle fasciculation due to a mild non-depolarising action. Arrhythmias and bronchospasm have occurred.

Hexamethonium. Ganglion blocking drug, formerly used iv for hypotensive anaesthesia.

Hexastarch, *see Hydroxyethyl starch*

HFJV, HFPPV, HFO, HFV, *see High frequency ventilation*

Hiatus hernia. Protrusion of stomach through the diaphragmatic crura into the thorax. May be sliding (type I), when the oesophagocardiac junction and upper stomach move into the thorax, or rolling (type II), when this junction remains intra-abdominal but part of the fundus herniates. The former is more common and more likely to cause gastro-oesophageal valve incompetence; the latter is more likely to strangulate.

More common in the elderly and in obesity.

- Symptoms:
  - epigastric pain, belching, indigestion.
  - regurgitation; may lead to stricture formation.
  - GIT bleeding may occur.
- Anaesthetic problems:
  - aspiration of gastric contents:
    - chronic pulmonary damage due to repeated aspiration.
    - risk of acute aspiration perioperatively.
  - chronic anaemia.
- Management:
  - medical: weight loss, antacids, H_2 receptor antagonists.
  - surgical: repair of the diaphragmatic defect and fundoplasty: the oesophagogastric junction is invaginated into a sleeve of fundus (Nissen's plication). Requires laparotomy and possibly thoracotomy, and may be lengthy.

[Rudolph Nissen (1896–1981), Swiss surgeon]

See also, Diaphragmatic herniae; Gastro-oesophageal reflux; Lower oesphageal sphincter

Hiccups. Intense synchronous contraction of the diaphragm and inspiratory intercostal muscles lasting about 500 ms, followed approximately 30 ms after its onset by glottic closure. May involve phrenic or vagal efferents. Results in a characteristic inspiratory sound associated with discomfort. On average, occur at a rate of less than 30/min. Frequent in the newborn. Frequency is decreased by breath-holding or a raised arterial $P\text{CO}_2$ and increased by a lowered arterial $P\text{CO}_2$. Episodes may be terminated by a sudden shock. May occur recurrently with neurological disease (e.g. brainstem tumours, encephalitis, meningitis), metabolic disease (e.g. uraemia) and many thoracic, abdominal or cardiac conditions. During anaesthesia, hiccups may be provoked by surgical stimulation, especially around the diaphragm, and particularly in the presence of inadequate paralysis and/or light anaesthesia.

- Rarely troublesome, but the following have been suggested as treatment:
  - hyperventilation.
  - metoclopramide, chlorpromazine, haloperidol, baclofen, anticonvulsant drugs.
  - nasopharyngeal stimulation.
  - during anaesthesia, all the above have been used, as has deepening anaesthesia ± increasing analgesia and muscle relaxation.

Hickman, Henry Hill (1800–1830). English surgeon, practising in Ludlow and Shifnall, Shropshire. First described the production of insensibility in animals by exposure to a gas (CO_2) and suggested its use for painless surgery, in 1824. His efforts to publicise his experiments were unsuccessful, both in the UK and abroad.

Hickman line, *see Central venous cannulation, long-term*

High dependency unit (HDU). Area providing a level of care intermediate between that of a general ward and an ICU. Provides greater monitoring and a higher nurse: patient ratio than a general ward; should not provide IPPV. Usually adopts a step-up, step-down function. Recent guidance suggests that HDUs should be for the care of patients with, or those likely to develop, acute (or acute-on-chronic) single organ failure; they should not manage patients who have developed multi-organ failure but ought to provide monitoring and support to patients at risk of so doing. Currently, most admit patients with medical or surgical conditions, and are used for post-operative care of high risk patients including those undergoing major surgery, monitoring of respiration in patients receiving spinal opioids, care of patients discharged from ICU but not yet ready for general ward care, etc. Costs and nursing requirements are less than for an ICU; they usually have a nurse:patient ratio of 1:2, but no resident doctor.
See also, Care of the critically ill surgical patient; Medical emergency team; Postoperative care team; Safe transport and retrieval team; Transportation of critically ill patients

High frequency ventilation (HFV). Mechanism of respiratory support developed in the 1970s. Small breaths are delivered at high frequencies, maintaining gas exchange without barotrauma or other deleterious effects of IPPV. May be superimposed on spontaneous ventilation.

- Three modes are used:
  - high frequency positive-pressure ventilation (HFPPV): 60–150 cycles/min, delivered via an intratracheal insufflation catheter, bronchoscope or tracheal tube. Tidal volumes of 100–400 ml are used. Fluidic valves are often used, without moving parts. Possible using some conventional ventilators, especially paediatric ones.
  - high frequency jet ventilation (HFJV): 60–600 cycles/min, delivered via a cannula inserted through the cricothyroid membrane, placed within a bronchoscope, etc., or incorporated near the tip of a tracheal tube. Expiration is continuous through the open system. Principles of gas entrainment are as for injector techniques. Tidal volume is up to 150 ml. Produces positive airway pressure of about 5 cmH_2O. Most ventilators employ electrical solenoid valves.
  - high frequency oscillation (HFO): 500–3000 cycles/min; the gas column is oscillated with an O_2 input via a side arm, or more recently using a vibrating membrane (similar to a loudspeaker) applied directly to the gas column (thus providing active exhalation unlike the other systems in which exhalation is passive). Mean airway pressure determines oxygenation, whilst oscillatory amplitude determines CO_2 removal.

The mechanism of gas exchange is unclear but is thought to involve continuous mixing of gases. HFJV is most commonly used and has been advocated for ENT and thoracic procedures such as sleeve resection of the trachea/bronchi and tracheobronchial fistula, in which increased airway pressures and excessive movement may be especially detrimental. HFO has been used in combination with low frequency ventilation. HFO has been used in acute lung injury in all ages. It reduces airway pressures and splints the lungs above closing capacity unlike conventional IPPV in which pressure and volume changes exhibit large swings. HFV has also been used in weaning from ventilators and in ARDS. HFJV via cricothyrotomy has been suggested as an alternative to tracheal intubation and IPPV in respiratory failure.

Hirudin. Peptide (65-amino-acid) originally derived from leech saliva, now manufactured using recombinant techniques. Specifically inhibits the actions of thrombin in the coagulation pathway; unlike heparin it does not require antithrombin III as a cofactor and is not inhibited by anti-heparin proteins. It also does not affect platelets directly and may also inhibit thrombin bound to a fibrin clot. Has been studied as a means of preventing primary and recurrent MI and DVT; initial studies have been encouraging although bleeding may be a problem as with heparin. Lepirudin and bivalirudin are recombinant forms available in the UK.

His bundle electrography. Technique for investigating cardiac conduction defects and tachycardias, using transvenous intracardiac bipolar electrodes at various sites. Concurrent recording of a formal ECG is usually undertaken. Information may be obtained about conduction through different parts of the heart conducting system, and the site of delayed conduction identified. May also be used to distinguish supraventricular from ventricular arrhythmias; ventricular complexes in the former are preceded by His bundle activity. The effects of pacing stimuli at different sites may also be observed, e.g. in assessment of refractory tachycardias.
[Wilhelm His (1863–1934), German anatomist]

Histamine and histamine receptors. Histamine, an amine, is present in mast cells, basophils, gastric mucosa and the CNS. It is involved in the inflammatory response and gastric acid secretion, and is thought to be a neurotransmitter, although its role as the latter is unclear. Involved in many other inflammatory mediator pathways, e.g. cytokines, complement, leukotrienes, and with coagulation and other processes. Synthesised by decarboxylation of L-histidine, and broken down by deamination and/or methylation with renal excretion.

- Histamine receptor subsets have been identified:
  - H_1:
    - cause smooth muscle contraction in the GIT and uterus, and bronchoconstriction via cholinergic pathways following stimulation of irritant pulmonary receptors.
    - cause vascular smooth muscle relaxation and dilatation, with increased vascular permeability.
    - cause stimulation and irritation of cutaneous nerve endings.
  - H_2:
    - cause some vasodilatation (but less than H_1 receptors).
    - have direct inotropic and chronotropic effects on isolated hearts, but hypotension usually results from vasodilatation.
    - increase acid, pepsin and intrinsic factor secretion from gastric mucosa.
  - H_3: present in brain, stomach lung; of uncertain clinical significance. Thought to inhibit histamine release.
  - H_4: identified experimentally only.

The histamine receptors are all G protein-coupled receptors; H_2 actions are thought to be mediated via cAMP, and H_1 via cyclic guanosine monophosphate.

Specific receptor antagonists have been developed; they are called antihistamine drugs (H_1) and H_2 receptor antagonists largely for historical reasons (the latter were discovered many years after the former).

Histamine is released from mast cells following iv injection of certain drugs, e.g. tubocurarine and morphine. The amount released depends partly on the rate of injection. Skin wheals, hypotension and bronchospasm may occur.
See also, Anaphylactoid reactions; Carcinoid syndrome

Histamine receptor antagonists, *see Antihistamine drugs; H_2 receptor antagonists*

HIV, *see Human immunodeficiency viral infection*

HME, *see Heat–moisture exchanger*

Hofmann degradation. Spontaneous degradation of amides ($RCONH_2$) to amines (RNH_2), and quaternary ammonium salts to tertiary ones, under certain physical conditions. Atracurium (a quaternary ammonium compound) spontaneously degrades to laudanosine at body temperature and plasma pH.
[August von Hofmann (1818–1892), German chemist]
Alston TA (2003). Anesth Analg; 96: 622–5

Holmes, Oliver Wendell (1809–1894). US physician, poet and author; Professor of Anatomy at Harvard, Boston. Famous for his treatise on puerperal fever and its prevention, and for his non-medical writing. Suggested anaesthesia as a suitable term for ether narcosis in a letter written to Morton in 1846.

Homeostasis. Concept first proposed by Bernard, relating to maintenance of physiological variables within normal limits, allowing optimal functioning of tissues and cells. Includes maintenance of acid–base balance, fluid balance, temperature regulation, arterial BP, hormone secretion, etc. Most mechanisms involve negative feedback; i.e. an increase of a substance or parameter causes direct inhibition of mechanisms which increase it, bringing about its restoration to normal; deficiency results in stimulation of these mechanisms.

Hormone replacement therapy (HRT). Use of oestrogen or oestrogen/progestogens to prevent unpleasant symptoms, e.g. hot flushes, night sweats and vaginal dryness, associated with the menopause. Also protects against cardiovascular disease and osteoporosis but may increase the risk of strokes and certain cancers (e.g. breast) and DVT, e.g. perioperatively. Perioperative precautions similar to those used for oral contraceptives have been suggested for women on HRT although this is controversial since the risk is thought to be less.
Brighouse D (2001). Br J Anaesth; 86: 709–16

Horner's syndrome. Clinical picture results from interruption of sympathetic innervation to the head. Originally described with cervical lesions, it may be due to lesions anywhere along the sympathetic pathway, including epidural anaesthesia. Consists of partial ptosis, meiosis, apparent enophthalmos, lack of sweating and nasal stuffiness on the affected side.
[Johann Horner (1831–1886), Swiss ophthalmologist]

HRT, *see Hormone replacement therapy*

5-HT, *see 5-Hydroxytryptamine*

5-HT_3 receptor antagonists. Group of drugs including ondansetron, granisetron, tropisetron, dolasetron and palonosetron, used in the prevention and treatment of postoperative or cytotoxic-induced nausea and vomiting. 5-HT is thought to be released by the action of anticancer treatment on enterochromaffin cells in the gut mucosa, stimulating gut 5-HT_3 receptors and activating vagal afferents resulting in vomiting. 5-HT_3 receptors are also thought to be involved centrally in the vagal reflex pathways; 5-HT_3 receptor antagonists therefore have both a central and a peripheral action.

Hüfner constant. The volume of O_2 carried by 1 g haemoglobin; e.g. used in the calculation of O_2 delivery and O_2 flux. Figures vary, according to whether it is measured *in vitro* or *in vivo*; 1.39 and 1.34 ml are most commonly quoted respectively. The latter value is the more relevant clinically.
[Carl von Hüfner (1840–1908), German physician]

Human immunodeficiency viral infection (HIV infection). First recognised in 1981 in the US as the acquired immunodeficiency syndrome (AIDS) in otherwise healthy homosexual males. The retrovirus, human immunodeficiency virus (HIV-1), was previously called human T-cell lymphotrophic virus type III (HTLV-III), or lymphadenopathy associated virus (LAV). HIV-2 has been identified, mainly in West Africa, where the disease is thought to have originated, although most HIV disease worldwide is caused by HIV-1. The virus binds to CD4 and other receptors on T-helper lymphocytes and introduces its RNA into the cells, where the viral enzyme reverse transcriptase generates DNA which is incorporated into the human DNA. Viral protease cleaves viral precursor proteins into their active forms; viral particles can then infect other cells and T cells are eventually destroyed in the process leading to increased susceptibility to infection and malignancy.

Infection has been estimated to be present in up to 1 000 000 people in the USA and 50 000 to 150 000 in the UK, with over 40 million people infected worldwide (30% of them in sub-Saharan Africa) and an estimated 25 million deaths since the disease was first recognised.

- Transmitted mainly via semen and blood, i.e. via:
  - homosexual and heterosexual (especially male to female) contact.
  - transfusion of blood products.
  - infected needles, e.g. used by drug addicts.
  - transplacentally, at delivery or via breast milk.
  - spillage of infected blood on to broken skin, or into the eye.

The virus may be isolated from other body fluids, e.g. vaginal secretions, saliva, tears, etc. Transmission by mouth to mouth contact, e.g. during CPR, is not thought to occur.

High risk groups include promiscuous homo- and heterosexuals and their partners, iv drug abusers, haemophiliacs, Haitians and Central/West Africans.

- Features:
  - most infected people are thought to be asymptomatic.
  - an acute flu-like illness may occur 1–3 weeks after infection. The incubation period may be as long as several years.
  - weight loss, diarrhoea, fever and thrush (AIDS-related complex) commonly progress to AIDS itself. Persistent generalised lymphadenopathy is thought to progress less often. Thrombocytopenic purpura and anaemia, dementia, encephalitis and psychosis may occur, related to HIV infection itself or secondary infection by other organisms.
  - AIDS: presence of indicator diseases, e.g. opportunistic infection (e.g. *Pneumocystis jiroveci* (formerly *P. carinii*) chest infection, pneumonia, candidiasis, cytomegalovirus), Kaposi's sarcoma, lymphoma.

More recently classified according to the CD4 count ($\geq$ 500/μl; 200–499/μl; $\leq$ 200/μl) and clinical presentation:
  - asymptomatic or lymphadenopathy.
  - symptomatic conditions indicating reduced cell-mediated immunity associated with HIV infection, e.g. oral/oesophageal fungal infection, chronic diarrhoea.
  - specific complications of HIV infection, e.g. invasive infections, malignancies, encephalopathy.

Diagnosed clinically and by serum antibody detection. The CD4 count may fall gradually or suddenly; a count below 200/μl (normal 600–1500/μl) may indicate increased risk of opportunistic infection. Early in HIV infection, the suppressor/cytotoxic T cell population (defined by the CD8 antigen) may increase, subsequently becoming normal or reduced. The CD4:CD8 ratio has been used to monitor progress of the infection. Plasma viral load (representing degree of viral replication) refers to the amount of viral RNA measurable in the plasma and correlates with speed of disease progression; current practice favours the use of viral load together with CD4 count to guide management.

Seroconversion occurs on average 1 month after infection, with about two-thirds progressing to AIDS within 10 years, although it is thought that 10–20% of patients may survive for 20 years without developing AIDS. Mortality is unknown but is thought to approach 100% for AIDS. Median survival once AIDS is diagnosed is currently about 15–20 months, with 5-year survival about 20%. In Africa, survival is shorter with about 30% HIV positive cases progressing to death without passing through AIDS itself.

- Treatment:
  - supportive, e.g. nutrition, treatment of infection, etc. Co-trimoxazole and pentamidine are usually used for pneumocystis pneumonia; the latter drug may be given iv, im, or by nebuliser to reduce side effects (and as prophylaxis).
  - nucleoside reverse transcriptase inhibitors, e.g. zidovudine, didanosine, abacavir, zalcitabine, stavudine, lamivudine. GIT upset and less commonly neurological or hepatic impairment may occur.
  - protease inhibitors, e.g. indinavir, ritonavir, lopinavir, nelfinavir, amprenavir, saquinavir. Similar side effects may occur. Inhibition of hepatic cytochrome P_{450} may give rise to interactions with other drugs.
  - non-nucleoside reverse transcriptase inhibitors, e.g. efavirenz, nevirapine: used in combination therapy.

Although originally reserved for AIDS or related states, drug therapy is commonly used before immunosuppression occurs, typically with highly active antiretroviral therapy (HAART) consisting of triple therapy (e.g. two nucleoside reverse transcriptase inhibitors and a protease inhibitor). A CD4 count below 300/μl, plasma viral load above 10 000–50 000 HIV RNA copies/ml or clinical symptoms have been taken as indicators that treatment should start, with the aim of reducing the plasma viral load by as much as possible for as long as possible. Drug therapy has also been advocated even before these indicators are reached.

- Anaesthetic/ICU considerations:
  - features of illness and drug therapy as above.
  - patients are at risk from infection as for immunodeficiency.
  - measures to protect staff and other patients from HIV infection:
    - simple hygiene.
    - avoidance of use of needles/parenteral medication.
    - wearing of gowns, goggles, gloves and overshoes.
    - careful disposal of sharps and other equipment. Needles should not be resheathed after use. Special cannulae that protect against needlestick should be used where possible. Hospitals should have policies for management of accidental needlestick injuries, from which the risk of transmission is about 0.3% (*see Environmental safety of anaesthetists*).
    - use of disposable equipment where possible.
    - minimal equipment in operating theatre.
    - induction of anaesthesia and recovery in theatre.
    - filters on breathing tubing if not disposable.
    - all non-disposable equipment is soaked in hypochlorite or glutaraldehyde solution after use; theatre equipment, walls, floors, etc. are washed down.
    - general considerations:
      - blood and its products are used increasingly sparingly; although donor blood is screened for anti-HIV antibodies, virus infection without seroconversion cannot be excluded.
      - iv equipment should not be used for more than one patient.
    - selection of cases requiring high risk procedures:
      (i) performed on every patient as routine.
      (ii) performed only for high risk groups as above.
      (iii) performed only if seropositive.
      The first option is increasingly employed, especially in the USA, although costly and time consuming. Routine testing is controversial, because of the implications of a positive test result on employment, social standing, life assurance, etc. Testing in the USA is more common than in the UK, and requires full consent and appropriate pretest counselling. This may be difficult in the ICU if the patient does not have capacity; the ethics of testing under these circumstances are controversial.
    - in the ICU, protective wear is required less for routine care. Admission of HIV infected patients is controversial; in general, they are admitted only for treatment of acute, curable episodes, e.g. chest infections.
  - staff who have HIV infection should not perform invasive procedures although they may provide other aspects of medical or nursing care, under the supervision of their occupational health department. If it is discovered that such procedures have been performed, all exposed patients should be contacted and offered counselling and testing. Routine testing of healthcare workers has been called for but is not current practice in the UK.

[Moricz K Kaposi (1837–1902), Austrian dermatologist]

Avidan MS, Jones N, Pozniak AL (2000). Anaesthesia; 55: 344–54

Human Rights Act. Introduced in the UK 1998 (coming into force in 2000), the Act incorporates the European Convention on Human Rights, ratified by the UK in 1951. Has 18 Articles, many of which have particular relevance to clinical anaesthesia/critical care:

- 2: right to life. Withdrawal/withholding of treatment is still permissible if it is in the patient's best interests.
- 3: prohibition of torture and inhuman or degrading treatment. This Article is absolute; i.e. there are no exceptions.
- 5: right to liberty and security. Relevant to treatment or restraint of patients against their will.
- 8: right to respect for private and family life. Relevant to disclosure of information. Requires qualification by balancing individuals' and society's interests
- 9: freedom of thought, conscience and religion. Relevant to refusal of treatments for religious reasons.
- 14: prohibition of discrimination. Relevant to rationing of scarce resources on the grounds of age or race, etc.

Other Articles may be relevant to doctors' rights as employees etc. All public authorities (including the NHS and its employees) must comply with the Convention.

White SM, Baldwin TJ (2002). Anaesthesia; 57: 882–8

Humidification. Inspired air is normally maximally humidified in the naso-/oropharynx, becoming saturated by the time it reaches the trachea. Absolute humidity in the upper trachea is 34 g/m^3 (i.e. fully saturated at 34°C); in alveoli it is 43 g/m^3 (i.e. fully saturated at 37°C). Delivery of dry gases to the trachea, e.g. via a tracheal tube or tracheostomy, may cause drying of the respiratory mucosa with reduced ciliary activity, keratinisation and ulceration, and increased tenacity of mucus with plugging of airways, atelectasis and reduced gas exchange. Humidification of inspired gases prevents this and reduces heat loss, partly by warming the gases (under 2% of total basal heat loss) but more importantly by avoiding the requirement for latent heat of vaporisation (10–15% of total basal heat loss) within the trachea.

Humidification is thus required during ventilation on ICUs. It is also particularly important during prolonged anaesthesia, and in the elderly, children, severely ill patients and those with respiratory disease. It has been suggested as being mandatory during all anaesthetics.

- Humidification of the patient's environment may be achieved, e.g. with an O_2 tent, but it is usually restricted to inspired gases only. Methods:
  - passive:
    - tracheal water/saline instillation; inefficient and potentially dangerous if large volumes are used.
    - bubbling inspired gas through cold water; simple but relatively inefficient (up to 10 g/m^3 produced). Vaporisation cools the water, decreasing efficiency further.
    - heat–moisture exchanger (HME): light, simple and highly efficient with a small dead space. Heat is conserved during expiration allowing inspired gas to be heated and humidified. Most HMEs are hygroscopic, consisting of a foam or chemically coated (calcium or lithium chloride) paper membrane. Many HMEs are also filters. Efficiency is up to 90%. Useful for short-term IPPV provided secretions are not tenacious.
  - active, i.e. energy source required; commonly used in ICU because efficiency is high:
    - hot water bath: up to 60°C is employed in some, to reduce bacterial contamination. Inspired gas is passed over or through the water. Efficiency is increased by passing gas through a perforated screen to form tiny bubbles (cascade humidifier), or using absorbent wicks to increase surface area. Humidified gas is unsaturated at the working temperature, but becomes near-saturated as the temperature falls along the tubing to the patient. Condensation of water within the tubing may be reduced by heating wires within the tubing, giving closer control of the temperature drop between machine and patient. Risk of delivering excessively hot gases is reduced by monitoring the temperature within the humidifier and at the patient end of the tubing (usually kept at about 35°C), using thermostat controls and alarms.
    - other heated humidifiers, e.g. dropping water on to a heated element.
    - nebulisers.

Infection risks (typically with pseudomonas) are reduced by addition of antiseptic to the water, maintenance at high temperature where appropriate, and changing tubing and water regularly (e.g. every 24 h). Condensation within tubing may provide foci for infection, obstruct ventilation, or drain water into the patient's airways. The level of the water source should be kept below that of the patient. Overheating and electrocution may also occur.

Ward B, Park GR (2000). Clin Intensive Care; 11: 169–76

See also, Filters, breathing system

Humidity. Absolute humidity is the amount of water vapour per unit volume of gas at given temperature and pressure, in g/m^3 or mg/l.

Relative humidity (%) is the absolute humidity divided by the amount present when the gas is fully saturated at the same temperature and pressure.

Maximal possible water content varies with temperature (Fig. 81). Thus heating a gas does not affect its absolute humidity, since the amount of water contained remains constant, but relative humidity is reduced, because warmer gas can contain more water vapour.

- Normal values of absolute humidity in:
  - upper trachea: 34 g/m^3 (fully saturated at 34°C).
  - alveoli: 43 g/m^3 (fully saturated at 37°C).

Usual value of relative humidity in operating theatres: 50–60%. Higher values are too uncomfortable; lower values increase risk of sparks. Measured using a hygrometer.

See also, Humidification

Hunter's syndrome, *see Inborn errors of metabolism*

Huntington's disease. Rare autosomal dominant inherited disorder, resulting in neurological degeneration in middle life. Ataxia, dementia and choreiform movements occur, with emaciation and death usually within 15 years. Increased sensitivity to barbiturates and prolonged action of suxamethonium have been reported.

[George Huntington (1850–1916), US physician]

Hurler's syndrome, *see Inborn errors of metabolism*

Hyaline membrane disease, *see Respiratory distress syndrome*

Hyaluronidase. Enzyme which reversibly depolymerises hyaluronic acid, a polysaccharide present in connective tissue. Aids dispersal and absorption of drugs, fluids, etc., given sc or im, by intention or accident. Has also been mixed with local anaesthetic agents to aid spread. Administration: 1500 international units (one ampoule) in 1–2 ml water is injected into the absorption site, before, after or together with the drug. May be injected through a sc cannula prior to administration of fluid (hypodermoclysis), allowing up to 1000 ml to be given into the thigh, calf, chest, abdomen or back regions.

Hydatid disease, *see Tropical diseases*

Hydralazine hydrochloride. Vasodilator drug, acting mainly on arterioles. Used to lower BP, e.g. in hypertension, hypotensive anaesthesia and pre-eclampsia. Half-life is

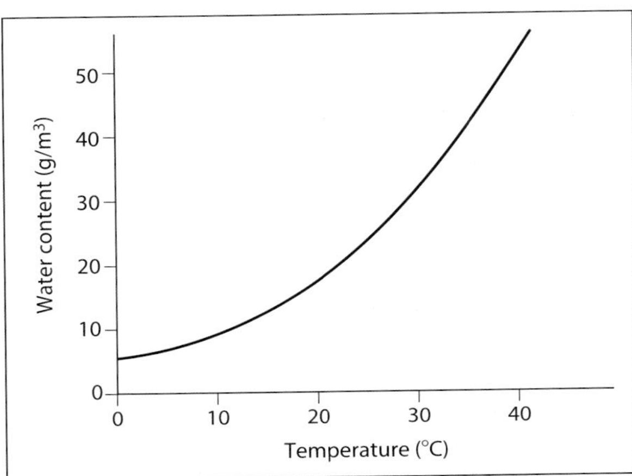

Fig. 81 Water content of saturated air at different temperatures

2–3 h; up to 16 h in renal failure. Certain patients acetylate the drug quickly, reducing half-life to under 1 h. Its onset of action may be up to 15 min after iv bolus, with effects lasting up to 90 min.

- Dosage:
  - 25–50 mg orally 12 hourly.
  - 5–10 mg iv increments.
  - 200–300 μg/min by infusion initially, then 50–150 μg/min.
- Side effects:
  - hypotension, tachycardia, fluid retention, nausea.
  - systemic lupus erythematosus syndrome, especially in slow acetylators and following prolonged oral therapy at a dose greater than 100 mg/day.

Hydrocephalus. Increased CSF volume. May be caused by increased production or decreased drainage, usually the latter:
  - non-communicating: blockage between the lateral ventricles and 4th ventricular outlets.
  - communicating: blockage distal to the 4th ventricular outlets, e.g. at the basal cisterns.
- Causes:
  - congenital, e.g. narrowed aqueduct, obstruction of 4th ventricle outlet by a membrane (Dandy–Walker syndrome), herniation of the cerebellar tonsils through the foramen magnum (Arnold–Chiari syndrome), etc.
  - acquired: meningitis with adhesions, surgery, head injury, subarachnoid haemorrhage, tumour, etc.

Usually accompanied by increased ICP; it may be acute, requiring urgent drainage. Pressure may be normal in some chronic forms, with slow ventricular enlargement. Head size is increased in children, with bulging of fontanelles. Cerebral or cerebellar atrophy may be present.

- Treatment:
  - surgery to the obstructive lesion.
  - shunt insertion: e.g. from the lateral ventricle to the peritoneum or right atrium
- Anaesthetic considerations:
  - as for neonates/paediatric anaesthesia.
  - as for neurosurgery.
  - head enlargement may hinder tracheal intubation.

[Walter E Dandy (1886–1946) and Arthur E Walker (1907–1995), US neurosurgeons; Julius Arnold (1835–1915), German pathologist; Hans von Chiari (1851–1916), Austrian pathologist]

Hydrocodone bitartrate. Opioid analgesic drug, available in the USA together with other ingredients in oral preparations for cough and pain.

Hydrocortisone. Natural corticosteroid, with considerable glucocorticoid activity but little mineralocorticoid activity. Used therapeutically in adrenocortical insufficiency, acute immunological reactions, e.g. anaphylaxis, and various inflammatory/autoimmune conditions.

- Dosage:
  - acutely iv/im as the sodium succinate or sodium phosphate (iv injection of the latter may cause perineal irritation): 100–500 mg 6–8 hourly.
  - orally in replacement therapy: 20–30 mg/day in two doses (most given in the morning to mimic the normal diurnal variation in hydrocortisone levels).
  - other routes: rectally, intra-articularly or topically as the acetate.

Hydrogen ions (H^+). About 12 500–13 000 mmol are produced in the body per day, mainly from the reaction of CO_2 (produced during respiration) with water. Also produced during metabolism of foodstuffs, etc. Acid–base balance requires buffering and excretion to maintain extracellular hydrogen ion concentration at 34–46 nmol/l, equivalent to pH of 7.34–7.46. Hydrogen ion homeostasis is required to maintain proper functioning of proteins (especially enzymes), etc.
See also, Acidosis; Alkalosis; Buffers

Hydromorphone hydrochloride. Opioid analgesic drug, widely used in the USA but less so in the UK. 1.5 mg is equivalent to 10 mg morphine, from which it is derived. Action lasts 3–5 h. Available for rectal, oral and parenteral administration.

Hydrostatic pressure, *see Starling forces*

γ-Hydroxybutyric acid (GHBA). Drug related to GABA and used as an iv anaesthetic agent in the 1960s and 1970s. Present as a neurotransmitter, especially in the hypothalamus and basal ganglia. Causes slow onset of anaesthesia, lasting up to 90 min. Has been used for paediatric anaesthesia (especially cardiac catheterisation) because of its relative lack of cardiorespiratory depression, although bradycardia may occur. No longer available medicinally in the UK, although still used elsewhere in the world, e.g. certain other parts of Europe and Russia.

Has become a drug of abuse for body builders (in an attempt to increase growth hormone production) and as a recreational drug ('liquid ecstasy'). Has also been used by criminals to induce unconsciousness in unwitting victims since the drug is difficult to detect when added to drinks, etc. Overdose has resulted in confusion, ataxia, visual disturbances, hallucinations, coma and convulsions; effects are increased when combined with alcohol. Treatment is largely supportive; gastric lavage and activated charcoal may be of little value because absorption from the GIT is rapid. Classified in the UK as a class C controlled drug from 2003.

Snead OC 3rd, Gibson KM (2005). N Engl J Med; 352: 2721–32

Hydroxydione. Obsolete iv anaesthetic agent, introduced in 1955. A corticosteroid derivative, it produced slow induction of anaesthesia and delayed recovery, with a high incidence of thrombophlebitis.

Hydroxyethyl starch (HES). Synthetic colloid component. Of similar structure to glycogen, consisting of chains of glucose molecules (> 90% amylopectin), etherified with hydroxyethyl groups. Properties of particular colloid products based on HES depend on the degree of hydroxyethyl substitution (n.b. more than one product may exist for each category):
  - hetastarch: 70–75% substitution. Mean mw is 450 000 to 670 000; most molecules are small, but some are very large (mw > 1–2 million). Presented as 6% hetastarch in 0.9% saline (or more recently, in lactated electrolyte solution which results in less hyperchloraemic acidosis although the importance of this is disputed); pH is ~5.5–5.9. Causes sustained increase in plasma volume, by just over the volume infused, for over 24 h. The smallest molecules (mw < 50 000) are excreted rapidly in the urine; the larger ones are broken down slowly, although the glucose-hydroxyethyl bonds remain unbroken. Elimination half-life is approximately 17 days; some remnants have been found in the reticuloendothelial system several years after administration, although the significance of this is unknown.

Slightly prolonged coagulation may occur after large infused volumes. Allergic reactions are very rare and mild. Does not interfere with blood cross-matching after up to 20% of blood volume.
- hexastarch: 60% substitution. Similar to hetastarch but with lower mean mw (200 000). Presented as 6% hexastarch in 0.9% saline; pH is about 5.5.
- pentastarch: 50% substitution. Mean mw is 200 000 to 250 000 depending on the preparation, with median mw about 60 000. Pattern of excretion is as for hetastarch, but 70% is cleared within 24 h and 80% within a week. Presented as a 6% or 10% solution in 0.9% saline; pH is about 5.0 and osmolarity 320 mosmol/l.
- tetrastarch: 40% substitution. mean mw is 130 000. Similar to pentastarch, but with a smaller range of mw in order to have a more predictable action and a lesser effect on coagulation. Degraded to smaller molecules (mw 60 000 to 70 000) at a constant rate, providing a more consistent concentration in the plasma that lasts ~ 4 h, with almost complete renal clearance and low risk of accumulation. Presented as 6% and 10% solutions. Available in saline and also presented in a balanced electrolyte solution (140 mmol/l Na^+; 4 mmol/l K^+; 2.5 mmol/l Ca^{2+}; 1 mmol/l Mg^{2+}; 118 mmol/l Cl^-; 24 mmol/l acetate; 5 mmol/l malate), in order to reduce the risk of hyperchloraemic acidosis.

See also, Intravenous fluids

5-Hydroxytryptamine (5-HT, Serotonin). Substance found throughout the body but especially in GIT enterochromaffin cells (90%), smooth muscle, platelets, mast cells and peripheral and central nervous systems. It acts on at least seven different classes of receptor, several of which have subclasses; all are coupled via G protein-coupled receptor mechanisms except the 5-HT_3 receptor which is a fast ion Na^+/K^+ channel receptor.
- Involved in:
  - inflammatory mechanisms: increases vascular permeability and platelet aggregation, causes bronchoconstriction, and causes vasodilatation and constriction at different vascular beds.
  - GIT function: increases motility, water and electrolyte secretion.
  - arousal, muscle tone, hypothalamic/parasympathetic regulatory mechanisms, mood, memory and spinal modulation of pain sensation. Functions as an inhibitory neurotransmitter in the brainstem, descending spinal pathways, hypothalamic, cortical, limbic and extrapyramidal systems.

Formed by hydroxylation and decarboxylation of tryptophan and stored in cytoplasmic vesicles. Taken up from synaptic clefts via the presynaptic membrane and metabolised mainly by monoamine oxidase to form 5-hydroxyindoleacetic acid (5-HIAA); urinary levels of the latter reflect the rate of metabolism. In the pineal gland and parts of the GIT melatonin is a breakdown product.

Many drugs act by modulating 5-HT activity, including the serotonin reuptake inhibitors (e.g. fluoxetine and related antidepressant drugs); 5-HT_{1D} receptor agonists (e.g. sumatriptan) used in migraine; 5-HT_2 receptor antagonists (e.g. ketanserin) used in various vascular disorders including carcinoid syndrome; and 5-HT_3 receptor antagonists used as antiemetic drugs. Others are currently being developed for possible use in hypertension and psychiatric or GIT disorders. Pizotifen blocks histamine and 5-HT receptors and is used in migraine prophylaxis, as is methysergide. Many other drugs also affect 5-HT as part of a wider spectrum of activity, e.g. octreotide, reserpine, MAO inhibitors, tricyclic antidepressant drugs.

Hygrometer. Device for measuring atmospheric humidity.
- Examples:
  - hair hygrometer: pointer attached to a hair whose length changes with differing humidity. Human hair, animal tissue and paper have been used. Inaccurate but simple.
  - Regnault's hygrometer: silver tube containing ether; cooled by blowing air through it with a rubber bulb. When condensation appears on the outside, the air is saturated with water at that temperature (dew point). From a graph of water content of saturated air against temperature, water content at dew point and that at room temperature may be found. Relative humidity is the latter divided by the former.
  - wet and dry bulb hygrometer: consists of two thermometer bulbs: one dry, the other wrapped in a wet wick. The wet thermometer bulb loses heat due to water evaporation, depending on atmospheric humidity. Humidity is read from tables, according to the temperatures measured by the two thermometers. Accuracy depends on adequate air movement.
  - humidity transducers: electrical properties of certain compounds, e.g. lithium chloride, alter as they absorb water. Electrical resistance or capacitance is usually measured.
  - mass spectrometer.
  - ultraviolet light absorption: depends on water content of air.

[Henri Regnault (1810–1878), French physicist]

Hygroscopic condensers, *see Heat–moisture exchanger*

Hyoscine hydrobromide. Anticholinergic drug, used mainly for premedication. Tertiary ammonium compound, an ester of tropic acid and scopine; found naturally in the henbane plant. Has greater sedative, antiemetic and antisialagogue action than atropine, but with less action on the heart and bronchial muscle. Also used to prevent travel sickness, and (as the quaternary ammonium compound, hyoscine butylbromide) to prevent or reduce gut spasm.
- Effects:
  - sedation, amnesia, mydriasis, antiemetic action via the vomiting centre; may cause the central anticholinergic syndrome.
  - reduced bronchial and GIT secretions; reduced gut motility.
  - tachycardia (bradycardia is possible following a small dose).
- Dosage:
  - 4 µg/kg for im premedication. Confusion is more likely in the elderly.
  - 0.3 mg, repeated twice 6 hourly for travel sickness. Slow-release cutaneous patches are available, and have been used to reduce PONV.
  - 20 mg butylbromide orally/iv/im for GIT spasm.

Hyperaesthesia. Increased sensitivity to a sensory stimulus, excluding the special senses. Includes allodynia and hyperalgesia.

Hyperaldosteronism. Excessive aldosterone secretion. May be:
- primary (Conn's syndrome):
  - causes include adrenal adenoma (most common), hyperplasia and carcinoma. Twice as common in women.

- causes hypertension, hypervolaemia, hypokalaemia and metabolic alkalosis. Plasma sodium level is usually at the upper end of the normal range.
- spironolactone (aldosterone inhibitor) is used to treat hyperplasia. Some forms are corrected by dexamethasone. Adenomas are treated by surgery.
- anaesthetic considerations are related to appropriate preoperative correction of electrolyte, fluid and acid–base imbalances. Spironolactone is useful preoperatively. Cardiovascular instability may occur peri- and postoperatively. Postoperative mineralocorticoid deficiency may be treated with fludrocortisone 50–300 μg/day orally.

▸ secondary: may occur in cardiac and hepatic failure, malignant hypertension and renal artery stenosis.

Measurement of plasma renin activity may aid diagnosis (low in primary disease, increased in secondary forms).

[Jerome Conn (1907–1981), US physician]

Foo R, O'Shaughnessy KM, Brown MJ (2001). Postgrad Med J; 77: 639–44

Hyperalgesia. Increased pain from a normally painful stimulus. The term usually refers to a feature of chronic pain, but is similar to the antanalgesia seen with certain centrally depressant drugs.

Hyperalimentation, *see Nutrition, total parenteral*

Hypercalcaemia. Effects are due to raised ionised calcium levels; symptoms are usually present when total calcium exceeds 3.5 mmol/l.

- Caused by:
  - ▸ hyperparathyroidism.
  - ▸ malignancy, both primary and bony metastases.
  - ▸ less commonly:
    - increased intake, e.g. milk-alkali syndrome.
    - others: hyperthyroidism, sarcoidosis, adrenocortical insufficiency, immobilisation, thiazide diuretics.
- Features:
  - ▸ psychiatric disturbances.
  - ▸ dehydration, polyuria/polydipsia.
  - ▸ nausea/vomiting, constipation.
  - ▸ muscle weakness.
  - ▸ drowsiness, coma.
  - ▸ shortened Q–T interval; prolonged P–R interval on the ECG.
  - ▸ may lead to renal calculi/nephrocalcinosis and renal failure.
- Urgent treatment (before investigation) is required in severe hypercalcaemia:
  - ▸ of underlying cause (if known).
  - ▸ rehydration followed by induced diuresis to increase renal calcium loss, e.g. with furosemide and saline administration (caution with furosemide in renal impairment). Careful fluid balance and CVP monitoring are required.
  - ▸ if severe hypercalcaemia persists, the following may be used:
    - bisphosphonates, e.g.:
      - disodium pamidronate: 15–60 mg, given once or divided over 2–4 days, up to a maximum of 90 mg in total.
      - ibandronic acid: 2–4 mg by a single infusion.
      - sodium clodronate: 300 mg/day for 7–10 days or 1.5 g by a single infusion.
      - zoledronic acid: 4 mg over 15 min by a single infusion.
  - ▸ corticosteroids, e.g. prednisolone up to 120 mg/day.
  - ▸ calcitonin from 5–10 units/kg/day im/sc in 1–2 divided doses up to 400 units 6–8 hourly. Reduces bone resorption.
  - ▸ trisodium edetate up to 70 mg/kg/day iv over 3 h; rapidly acting but may cause renal failure. Chelates circulating calcium.
  - ▸ others include enteral or parenteral phosphate (precipitates calcium phosphate into the tissues including kidneys, thus no longer recommended); and plicamycin (mithramycin; a cytotoxic agent, no longer available in the UK). Dialysis has been used.

Aguilera IM, Vaughan RS (2000). Anaesthesia; 55: 779–90

Hypercapnia. Arterial $P\text{CO}_2$ over 6 kPa (45 mmHg).

- Caused by:
  - ▸ increased production, e.g. MH, TPN using high carbohydrate content. Average normal production is approximately 200 ml/min.
  - ▸ reduced alveolar ventilation.
  - ▸ $\dot{V}/\dot{Q}$ mismatch, e.g. severe COPD.
  - ▸ increased inspired CO_2.
- Effects:
  - ▸ respiratory:
    - arterial O_2 saturation falls below about 90% at an alveolar $P\text{CO}_2$ over about 8 kPa (60 mmHg), breathing air.
    - increased respiratory drive via central/peripheral chemoreceptors. Tidal volume and respiratory rate increase; the extent varies with other factors (*see Carbon dioxide response curve*). Respiration may become depressed at very high levels.
    - response to hypoxaemia is increased.
    - oxyhaemoglobin dissociation curve shifts to the right.
  - ▸ cardiovascular:
    - increased sympathetic activity (causing increases in circulating catecholamine levels, heart rate and arterial BP), overriding CO_2's direct myocardial depressant effect. Arrhythmias may occur.
    - increased cerebral blood flow, ICP and intraocular pressure.
  - ▸ other:
    - dilated pupils, with sluggish response.
    - respiratory acidosis and hyperkalaemia. Initial bicarbonate increase is about 0.76 mmol/l per kPa rise above 5.3 if hypercapnia is acute (1 mmol/l per 10 mmHg above 40). Renal compensation includes bicarbonate retention and excreting hydrogen ions; bicarbonate increase in chronic hypercapnia is about 3 mmol/l per kPa (4 mmol/l per 10 mmHg).
    - confusion, headache and coma may result (CO_2 narcosis).

The CNS may adjust to higher CO_2 levels than normal in chronic hypercapnia.

Treated according to cause. If $P\text{CO}_2$ is reduced too rapidly, alkalosis and potassium shift may occur, causing convulsions, hypotension and arrhythmias. Recent animal data suggest that raised levels of carbon dioxide may be potentially protective in acute organ injury.

See also, Breathing, control of

Hyperglycaemia. Plasma glucose over 6.0 mmol/l (108 mg/dl).

- Caused by:
  - ▸ pancreatic failure, e.g. diabetes mellitus, pancreatitis, sepsis, pancreatectomy.

- stress response, due to actions of catecholamines, growth hormone, glucocorticoids, glucagon. May occur following trauma, surgery, burns, etc. (*see Stress response to surgery*).
- administration of glucose, e.g. TPN.
- drugs, e.g. diethyl ether, thiazide diuretics.

- Effects:
  - osmotic diuresis, causing dehydration, sodium and potassium loss.
  - diabetic coma, e.g. ketoacidosis.
  - increased blood osmolality and viscosity.
  - may impair platelet function, increase susceptibility to infection and exacerbate effects of cerebral ischaemia.
  - chronic effects of diabetes.
- Treatment:
  - of primary cause.
  - hypoglycaemic drugs.

Hyperkalaemia. Plasma potassium over 5.0 mmol/l.

- Caused by:
  - increased intake, e.g. iv administration, rapid blood transfusion.
  - decreased renal output:
    - renal failure:
      - acute: related to intake.
      - chronic: occurs only when GFR falls below 15 ml/min.
    - adrenocortical insufficiency.
    - drugs: ciclosporin, angiotensin converting enzyme inhibitors, potassium-sparing diuretics, e.g. amiloride, spironolactone.
  - movement of potassium out of cells:
    - trauma, crush syndrome, rhabdomyolysis, MH.
    - action of suxamethonium; exaggerated in burns, nerve injury, etc.
    - acidosis.
    - familial periodic paralysis, etc.
  - artefactual, e.g. haemolysed blood sample, very high white cell counts.
- Effects:
  - nausea, vomiting, diarrhoea, muscle weakness.
  - myocardial depression, ECG changes (peaked T waves, absent P waves, widened QRS complexes, and slurring of S–T segments into T waves). Ventricular arrhythmias including VF are common at above 7 mmol/l. Cardiac arrest may occur in diastole.
- Treatment:
  - polystyrene sulphonate resins: 15 g 6–8 hourly orally; 30 g rectally.
  - insulin 5–10 units in 100 ml of 10–20% dextrose iv over 30–60 min (drives potassium into cells).
  - bicarbonate 50 mmol iv may be given (exchanges potassium ions for hydrogen ions across cell membranes). Decreasing the P_aCO_2 by increasing minute ventilation (if artificially ventilated) has the same effect by reducing H^+ concentration.
  - calcium 5–10 mmol iv if severe (acts as a physiological antagonist of potassium).
  - nebulised (5 mg) or iv salbutamol (50 μg bolus/ 5–10 μg/min infusion; increases cellular uptake of potassium).
  - dialysis.

Hyperkalaemia should be corrected before anaesthesia and surgery, although the ratio of intracellular:extracellular potassium is more important than isolated plasma levels.

Evans KJ (2005). J Int Care Med; 20: 272–90

Hypermagnesaemia. Plasma magnesium over 1.05 mmol/l.

- Caused by:
  - renal failure.
  - magnesium administration.
  - laxative/antacid abuse.
  - adrenocortical insufficiency, hypothyroidism.
- Effects:
  - vasodilatation, hypotension, cardiac conduction defects.
  - sedation, coma, weakness, respiratory depression. Potentiation of non-depolarising neuromuscular blockade.
- Treatment:
  - encourage diuresis.
  - iv calcium.

Hypernatraemia. Plasma sodium over 145 mmol/l.

- Caused by:
  - sodium excess (urine sodium > 20 mmol/l):
    - hyperaldosteronism (although it is rare for the sodium concentration to rise above the upper end of normal).
    - Cushing's syndrome.
    - iatrogenic, e.g. sodium bicarbonate, hypertonic saline administration.
  - water depletion (urine sodium variable):
    - renal loss, e.g. diabetes insipidus.
    - other:
      - insensible water loss.
      - insufficient water intake.
  - sodium deficiency, with greater water deficiency:
    - renal loss (urine sodium > 20 mmol/l), e.g. osmotic diuresis caused by mannitol, glucose, urea, etc.
    - other (urine sodium < 10 mmol/l):
      - vomiting, diarrhoea.
      - sweating, weeping wounds.
      - adrenocortical insufficiency.
- Effects:
  - features of dehydration if present.
  - thirst, drowsiness, confusion, coma. Cerebral dehydration, with ruptured vessels and intracranial haemorrhage, may occur.
- Treatment:
  - of underlying cause.
  - oral water is given when possible, and/or diuretics in sodium excess. Normal saline may be given iv, hypotonic saline in severe water and sodium deficiency. Rapid infusion may lead to cerebral oedema and convulsions. Optimal rate of correction is controversial but full correction should take at least 48 h.
  - correction of any accompanying hypovolaemia.

Reynolds RM, Padfield PL, Seckl JR (2006). BMJ; 332: 702–5

Hyperosmolality. Plasma osmolality over 305 mosmol/kg. Features are as for hypernatraemia, which usually accompanies it. May also occur in hyperglycaemia, e.g. due to diabetic coma, TPN, and ingestion/administration of osmotically active substances, e.g. hypertonic mannitol solutions, alcohol poisoning. Detected by hypothalamic osmoreceptors, causing compensatory changes in water ingestion/excretion.

Hyperparathyroidism. Increased parathyroid hormone production:

- primary: usually from a single adenoma; multiple adenomata and carcinoma may also be responsible. May be associated with multiple endocrine adenomatosis.
- secondary: hyperplasia arising from prolonged hypocalcaemia, e.g. in renal failure.

  - tertiary: secondary hyperparathyroidism where autonomous secretion develops, e.g. after renal transplantation.

Hormone secretion may occur in certain tumours, e.g. bronchial carcinoma (pseudohyperparathyroidism). May be asymptomatic.

- Features:
  - those of hypercalcaemia. Renal stones are common.
  - bony erosion and cystic changes may occur.
- Treatment:
  - as for hypercalcaemia.
  - surgery; primary adenomata may be difficult to find.
- Anaesthetic considerations:
  - preoperative hypercalcaemia, dehydration and renal impairment should be corrected before surgery.
  - decalcified bone is easily fractured, e.g. during positioning.
  - practical management of anaesthesia is as for hyperthyroidism.

Marx SJ (2000). N Engl J Med; 343: 1863–75

Hyperpathia. Increased sensation from a sensory stimulus, but with raised threshold of sensation. Pain may increase during stimulation, and linger afterwards.

Hyperphosphataemia. Plasma phosphate above 1.4 mmol/l.

- Caused by:
  - factitious: haemolysis, prolonged contact of plasma with red blood cells.
  - increased intake: diet, iv administration, excess vitamin D.
  - increased release from cells/bone: diabetes mellitus, starvation, rhabdomyolysis, acidaemia, malignancy, renal failure.
  - decreased excretion: renal failure, hypoparathyroidism, excess growth hormone secretion.
- Effects are difficult to distinguish from those of the almost inevitable accompanying calcium abnormality but skin lesions and renal stones have been reported.
- Treatment: reduced protein intake; aluminium hydroxide or calcium carbonate orally (the latter contraindicated in hypercalcaemia); hypertonic dextrose solutions have been used to shift phosphate from the ECF into the cells.

Hyperpyrexia, malignant, *see Malignant hyperthermia*

Hypersensitivity, *see Adverse drug reactions; Atopy*

Hypertension. Raised arterial BP; defined and graded by the British Hypertension Society, European Society of Hypertension and World Health Organization as follows, according to BP measured in the clinic (as opposed to ambulatory):

  - grade 1 (mild): systolic 140–159 mmHg; diastolic 90–99 mmHg.
  - grade 2 (moderate): systolic 160–179 mmHg; diastolic 100–109 mmHg.
  - grade 3 (severe): systolic ≥ 180 mmHg; diastolic ≥ 110 mmHg.
  - isolated systolic hypertension: > 140 mmHg with diastolic < 90 mmHg.

BP increases with age in normal subjects.

- In 5% of cases, hypertension is secondary to:
  - adrenal disorders, e.g. hyperaldosteronism, Cushing's syndrome, phaeochromocytoma.
  - unilateral or bilateral renal disease, e.g. renal artery stenosis, infection, reflux, glomerulonephritis, congenital abnormalities, diabetes mellitus, connective tissue diseases, obstruction, tumour, etc.
  - others: coarctation of the aorta, pre-eclampsia, drugs, e.g. corticosteroids, oral contraceptives.

  In the remaining 95% of cases, hypertension is termed 'essential', i.e. has no apparent cause. Associated with family history and obesity, possibly alcohol and salt intake, diet and stress. Caffeine and smoking increase BP.
- Pathophysiological effects:
  - arteriolar wall thickening, with greater reduction in vessel radius for a given vasoconstrictive stimulus.
  - degenerative changes (e.g. fibrinoid necrosis and atheroma formation) lead to reduced blood flow and propensity to aneurysm formation and rupture.
  - baroreceptor sensitivity is reduced.
  - increased myocardial workload, with left ventricular hypertrophy. Increased end-diastolic pressure and coronary atheromatous plaques reduce coronary blood flow despite increased O_2 demand. Angina and/or cardiac failure may result.
- Features:
  - of ischaemic heart disease.
  - of cardiac failure.
  - CVA, encephalopathy.
  - due to renal impairment.
  - hypertensive crisis may occur.
  - hypertensive retinopathy: arteriovenous nipping, increased light reflex, increased tortuosity, cotton wool exudates, haemorrhages and papilloedema.
  - ECG features include those of ischaemia and left ventricular hypertrophy. Chest X-ray features may include left ventricular dilatation and those of left ventricular failure.
- Treatment:
  - weight loss, cessation of smoking, physical exercise.
  - thiazide diuretics, β-adrenergic receptor antagonists and vasodilator drugs are commonly used first, singly and in combination (*see Antihypertensive drugs*). More recently, the AB/CD algorithm has been suggested: ACE inhibitors or β-antagonists for 'high renin' hypertension, typically younger and non-black patients, and calcium channel blocking drugs and/or diuretics for 'low renin' hypertension, typically older and black patients. NICE guidelines (2006) suggest an ACE inhibitor initially for young patients, and a thiazide or calcium blocker in older or black patients, with combination therapy if required (β- and α-antagonists as fourth line drugs).
  - benefits of treating severe hypertension are undoubted; those of treating milder forms are controversial. The incidence of CVA is thought to be reduced if diastolic pressures above 90 mmHg are treated. Screening is widely practised.
- Anaesthesia for patients with hypertension:
  - preoperatively:
    - assessment for ischaemic heart disease, cardiac failure, cerebrovascular disease and renal impairment.
    - if not on treatment, surgery should be cancelled unless it is an emergency. Patients with diastolic pressure above 110 mmHg should be investigated and hypertension treated before anaesthesia and surgery, since morbidity and mortality are greater if untreated. Antihypertensive drugs are continued up to the morning of surgery.
    - sedative premedication is often advocated to reduce endogenous catecholamine levels.
  - perioperatively:
    - induction and maintenance as for ischaemic heart disease. Large swings in BP are more likely because of

arteriolar hypertrophy; e.g. hypotension due on induction and hypertension on intubation (*see Intubation, complications of*), etc.
- marked cardiovascular instability may accompany spinal/epidural anaesthesia if hypertension is uncontrolled.

- postoperatively:
  - adequate analgesia is particularly important.
  - treatment of persistent hypertension may be required.

- Hypertension during anaesthesia may be due to:
  - inadequate anaesthesia/analgesia.
  - tracheal intubation/extubation.
  - inadequate paralysis.
  - underlying hypertensive disease.
  - aortic clamping.
  - hypercapnia, hypoxaemia.
  - cerebral ischaemia, CVA, etc.; raised ICP.
  - drugs, e.g. ketamine, adrenaline, cocaine.
  - rarely, MH, phaeochromocytoma, thyroid crisis, carcinoid syndrome.

  In the elderly, atherosclerosis is suggested by normal or low diastolic pressure. Altered baroreceptor activity is common.

  Postoperatively, urinary retention, residual neuromuscular blockade, pain and anxiety may cause hypertension, in addition to the above factors. In the ICU, hypertension is often due to inadequate sedation, but many of the factors above should also be considered.

Management is directed towards the underlying cause. Labetalol, hydralazine, nifedipine, sodium nitroprusside and GTN are commonly used to control BP; the first three drugs are usually most convenient. Vasodilator therapy is less likely to be successful in atherosclerosis, since the arterial tree is relatively rigid; labetalol or other β-adrenergic antagonists may be more effective.

Hypertensive crisis. May occur as a feature of hypertensive disease (malignant hypertension), postoperatively after cardiac/vascular surgery, or other conditions including pre-eclampsia and phaeochromocytoma.

- Features:
  - severe progressive hypertension.
  - renal impairment.
  - encephalopathy: confusion, headache, visual disturbances, convulsions, coma.
  - retinal haemorrhage and papilloedema.
  - cardiac failure and CVA may occur.

If associated with hypertensive disease, oral therapy (e.g. atenolol, labetalol or nifedipine) is now preferred, since iv drugs may cause precipitous falls in BP which may result in CVA/blindness, renal impairment or myocardial ischaemia. Thus the previous recommendations for use of rapidly acting iv drugs such as diazoxide, hydralazine, GTN, sodium nitroprusside, labetalol, etc. no longer stand unless in exceptional circumstances. If parenteral treatment is required, sodium nitroprusside is often advised.

Hyperthermia. Raised body temperature, sometimes defined as greater than 41.6°C (107°F). Implies thermoregulatory failure, whereas pyrexia or fever (often defined as body temperature above 38°C (100.4°F) although the cutoff varies between sources) implies intact homeostatic mechanisms. Heatstroke is the clinical syndrome caused by increased temperature itself. May follow several hours' exposure to excessive environmental temperature, especially if unaccustomed, and if temperature regulation is impaired.

- Caused by:
  - hypothalamic lesions, e.g. tumour, surgery, CVA, infection.
  - increased heat production:
    - exertion.
    - drug-induced, e.g. MH, neuroleptic malignant syndrome, salicylate poisoning, cocaine poisoning, methylenedioxymethylamphetamine ingestion.
    - hyperthyroidism.
    - phaeochromocytoma.
    - status epilepticus.
    - tetanus.
  - impaired heat loss:
    - autonomic neuropathy.
    - drug-induced, e.g. anticholinergic drugs, phenothiazines, neuroleptic malignant syndrome.
    - dehydration.
    - excessive warming during anaesthesia.

Features of heatstroke include dry hot skin, confusion, headache, coma and raised temperature. Hyperventilation may be followed by metabolic acidosis, convulsions, and cardiovascular and multisystem failure.

- Treatment:
  - specific, e.g. MH.
  - cooling with tepid water; cold water may induce peripheral vasoconstriction with impairment of further heat exchange. Cold iv fluids and irrigation of body cavities may be used.
  - drugs, e.g. aspirin, paracetamol.

Bouchama A, Knochel JP (2002). N Engl J Med; 346: 1978–88

Hyperthermia, malignant, *see Malignant hyperthermia*

Hyperthyroidism (Thyrotoxicosis). In 99% of cases, hyperthyroidism is caused by primary thyroid overactivity produced by thyroid stimulating autoantibodies (Graves' disease) or hyperactive nodules. It is rarely due to carcinoma, thyroid stimulating hormone secretion, or administration of thyroid hormones. 7–10 times more common in women.

- Features:
  - malaise, anxiety, sweating, heat intolerance, tremor, psychological changes, myopathy (usually proximal).
  - weight loss, increased appetite, diarrhoea.
  - palpitations, tachycardia, AF, cardiac failure.
  - goitre, oligomenorrhoea, gynaecomastia.
  - eye features: usually lid retraction and mild proptosis; occasionally severe with visual disturbances. May be associated with pretibial myxoedema (pink/brown subcutaneous infiltration on the lower leg) and pseudoclubbing.
  - thyroid crisis may occur, triggered by surgery, infection, etc.
- Investigation: measurement of plasma thyroxine and triiodothyronine (either or both of which may be raised), thyroid stimulating hormone, and rarely thyrotrophin releasing hormone. Radioisotope and ultrasound scanning may be performed.
- Treatment:
  - antithyroid drugs:
    - carbimazole (UK) or methimazole (USA); propyluracil: prevent formation of thyroid hormones. Pruritus and rash are common; agranulocytosis may occur. Increase vascularity of the gland, therefore sometimes stopped 2 weeks preoperatively. Usually given for a course of 1–1.5 years. Act within at least 1–2 weeks.

- iodine: temporarily inhibits hormone release; sometimes given for 2 weeks preoperatively to reduce glandular vascularity.
- radioactive iodine: increasingly used as fears of subsequent sterility and tumours diminish.
- β-adrenergic receptor antagonists: reduce the peripheral effects of hyperthyroidism directly and by reducing conversion of thyroxine to triiodothyronine. Act within 12–24 h.
- surgery: requires adequate control of the disease preoperatively, in order to prevent thyroid crisis.

- Anaesthetic management:
  - preoperatively:
    - assessment of thyroid state, especially cardiovascular and neurological aspects. Emergency treatment is as for thyroid crisis. Other autoimmune disease may be present, e.g. myasthenia gravis.
    - assessment for possible upper airway obstruction. Chest X-ray including thoracic inlet views are useful. Elective tracheostomy is sometimes performed if the goitre is very large. Indirect laryngoscopy is performed to assess vocal cord function in case of pre-existing or peroperative damage to the laryngeal nerves.
  - perioperatively:
    - tracheal intubation may be difficult. IPPV is usually used; spontaneous ventilation is preferred by some. Reinforced tracheal tubes are sometimes preferred.
    - because of the risk of damage to the laryngeal nerves, special tracheal tubes have been described through which the vocal cord muscle's electrical potentials may be monitored during surgery. The surgeon stimulates tissues electrically allowing the nerves to be identified and thus avoided. Neuromuscular blocking drugs must be avoided if this technique is used.
    - the eyes should be protected from pressure.
    - operative bleeding may be reduced by infiltration with adrenaline solutions, head-up position, and hypotensive anaesthesia.
    - arrhythmias may result from poor thyroid control or manipulation of the carotid sinus. Risk of air embolism exists in the steep head-up position.
    - pneumothorax and tracheal trauma may occur.
    - regional anaesthesia may also be used in poor risk patients, using 0.5% prilocaine or lidocaine with adrenaline:
      - from the midpoint of the sternomastoid muscle on both sides, 10 ml is injected into the muscle body, 10 ml anteriorly, and 10 ml infiltrated caudally and cranially.
      - 20 ml is injected sc to each side from the midline, below the thyroid gland.
  - postoperatively:
    - assessment of the vocal cords' activity is often requested by the surgeon after extubation, although direct laryngoscopy may be difficult at this stage. Fibreoptic inspection, e.g. through a laryngeal mask airway, has been described.
    - airway obstruction may be caused by:
      - haemorrhage into the tissues of the neck. Skin sutures or clips must be easily removable.
      - floppy collapsible trachea (tracheomalacia) if the goitre is large. Reintubation or tracheostomy may be required.
      - laryngeal nerve damage.
      - hypoparathyroidism causing hypocalcaemia and tetany may occur from several hours to several days later.
  - thyroid crisis or subsequent hypothyroidism may also occur.

[Robert Graves (1796–1853), Irish physician]
Farling PA (2000). Br J Anaesth; 85: 15–28
See also, Neck, cross-sectional anatomy; Thyroid gland

Hypertonic intravenous solutions. Have been used in small volumes (under 500 ml) for initial resuscitation in, e.g. haemorrhage in animals and humans. Thought to draw fluid into the vasculature, possibly to cause vasodilatation and increase myocardial contractility causing increased tissue and organ flow, and possibly to affect central cardiovascular control mechanisms. Have also been used as an alternative to mannitol to reduce ICP after head injury. Various solutions have been used. Combinations of hypertonic 7.5% saline with colloid (usually 6% dextran 70) are thought to maximise the benefits of rapid and sustained plasma expansion by virtue of the saline and colloid components respectively.

Hyperventilation. Commonly performed during IPPV, intentionally or unintentionally. Its main effects are related to resultant hypocapnia, or the adverse cardiovascular effects of IPPV. It may occur in both awake and anaesthetised spontaneously breathing patients, e.g. due to pain, hypoxaemia, hypercapnia, acidosis and pregnancy. Sometimes occurs in midbrain/pontine lesions. Increases the work of breathing, although it aids excretion of the increased CO_2 it produces. Hypocapnia in spontaneously breathing patients caused by anxiety/pain-induced hyperventilation may result in tetany.

Hypnosis. Sleep-like state, with persistence of certain behavioural responses. The subject is susceptible to, and may respond to, the hypnotist's suggestions concerning aspects of behaviour, environment, memory, etc., despite possible contradiction by actual stimuli and character. The effects may persist after return to normal consciousness, but possibly without recall of the hypnotic state.

- Has been used:
  - to help the giving up of smoking, etc.
  - to aid recall of subconscious thoughts, e.g. psychiatric/psychological research and therapy, investigation of awareness under anaesthesia.
  - to modify pain perception, e.g. in obstetrics, perioperatively, and in chronic pain.
  - for entertainment.

Originally expounded as mesmerism in the mid/late 1700s, although evidence of similar techniques dates back thousands of years. The term was coined in the 1840s.

Whether hypnosis represents a separate physiological state, or an interpersonal social interaction (i.e. obeyer/commander) is controversial. Certainly suggestion is widely used, e.g. by doctors and dentists, to reduce fear, anxiety, use of drugs, etc.

Wobst AHK (2007). Anesth Analg; 104: 1199–208
[Hypnos, Greek god of sleep]

Hypoadrenalism, *see Adrenocortical insufficiency*

Hypoaesthesia. Reduced sensitivity to a sensory stimulus, excluding special senses.

Hypoalgesia. Reduced pain from a normally painful stimulus.

Hypocalcaemia. Effects are usually present when total plasma calcium is under 2.0 mmol/l, and are due to decreased plasma ionised calcium. Although total calcium is reduced in hypoproteinaemia, the ionised portion is normal and clinical features are absent.

- Caused by:
  - decreased parathyroid hormone activity, e.g. hypoparathyroidism, hypomagnesaemia.
  - decreased vitamin D activity, e.g. the above, chronic renal failure, intestinal malabsorption, inadequate diet, liver disease.
  - increased calcium loss, e.g. chelating agents, calcification of soft tissues (e.g. rhabdomyolysis, pancreatitis, hyperphosphataemia).
  - decreased ionised calcium, e.g. alkalosis.
- Features (exacerbated by hypomagnesaemia):
  - paraesthesiae.
  - muscle cramps/spasm/tetany. Stridor may occur. Chvostek's sign is facial spasm following tapping over the facial nerve. Trousseau's sign is carpopedal spasm following inflation of a tourniquet around the arm.
  - mental excitability, convulsions.
  - prolonged Q–T interval on the ECG; decreased cardiac output.
- Treatment:
  - of predisposing cause.
  - supportive (airway, etc.).
  - iv calcium if severe, e.g. chloride 5–10 ml or gluconate 10–20 ml slowly, followed by infusion if required.
  - magnesium if deficient.

[Frantisek Chvostek (1835–1884), Austrian physician; Armand Trousseau (1801–1867), French physician]

Aguilera IM, Vaughan RS (2000). Anaesthesia; 55: 779–90

Hypocapnia. Arterial $P\text{CO}_2$ under 4.7 kPa (35 mmHg).

- Caused by:
  - hyperventilation. May be iatrogenic (in ventilated patients), self-induced or a compensatory response to metabolic acidosis.
  - reduced CO_2 production, e.g. in brainstem death.
- Effects:
  - vasoconstriction; reduced cerebral blood flow may cause dizziness, light-headedness and confusion. Risk of convulsions if predisposed, e.g. if enflurane is used. Placental blood flow is reduced. If IPPV is employed, cardiovascular effects are increased.
  - alkalosis, hypokalaemia and hypocalcaemia may occur.
  - reduced respiratory drive; apnoea may occur postoperatively.
  - reduced requirement for anaesthetic agents has been shown in some studies, but not in others.

If iatrogenic, corrected by reducing alveolar ventilation, e.g. by increasing dead space and rebreathing, or reducing minute volume. If compensatory, best not corrected until the underlying cause of acidosis is treated.

Laffey JG, Kavanagh BP (2002). N Engl J Med; 347: 43–53

Hypoglycaemia. Low plasma glucose level; symptoms are uncommon until level falls to 2–3 mmol/l (40–50 mg/dl); the threshold is lower in chronic hypoglycaemia and higher in chronic hyperglycaemia.

- Types:
  - fasting, i.e. only after several hours without food:
    - reduced glucose output from liver:
      - starvation (especially children).
      - alcohol ingestion.
      - hepatic failure.
      - adrenocortical insufficiency.
      - renal failure, growth hormone deficiency, pregnancy.
    - increased insulin activity:
      - insulin/sulphonylurea administration.
      - insulinoma. Over 90% are benign.
      - sarcoma, hepatoma, adrenocortical and other tumours. Thought to be caused by secretion of an insulin-like factor.
      - sepsis, malaria.
  - reactive, i.e. 2–5 h postprandially:
    - idiopathic.
    - gastric surgery; causes rapid glucose absorption and excessive insulin release (cf. dumping syndrome, due to sudden osmotic load and/or other gut hormone release).
    - may occur in diabetes mellitus.
    - inborn errors of metabolism.
  - rebound hypoglycaemia may follow sudden cessation of TPN, due to high levels of circulating insulin.
- Features:
  - secretion of hyperglycaemic hormones, e.g. adrenaline, glucagon, growth hormone and cortisol; the former causes tachycardia, sweating and pallor.
  - confusion, restlessness, dysarthria, diplopia, convulsions, coma. Permanent brain damage may occur with coma of increasing duration, but is rare if under 4 h. May be exacerbated by hypoxaemia and hypotension. Cerebral oedema may contribute.
  - may be masked during anaesthesia, presenting only during recovery.
- Treatment:
  - 25–50 ml 50% glucose iv if unconscious, repeated as necessary. Risk of venous thrombosis is reduced by flushing the cannula with saline after injection. Oral glucose is given if able to drink.
  - glucagon 1 mg has been used im, but is ineffective in hepatic dysfunction and alcohol ingestion, and may exacerbate insulinoma-induced hypoglycaemia.
  - mannitol and dexamethasone have been used if cerebral oedema is suspected and coma persists.

Hypoglycaemic drugs. Strictly, refers to all drugs used to lower plasma glucose concentration although the term is often used to refer to oral drugs only. Used primarily in the treatment of diabetes mellitus, although insulin is also used in the treatment of hyperkalaemia.

Divided into:

- oral:
  - biguanides: decrease gluconeogenesis and increase peripheral glucose uptake.
  - sulphonylureas: increase production of insulin from the pancreas, and possibly increase peripheral glucose uptake.
  - thiazolidinediones: increase peripheral sensitivity to insulin.
  - meglitinides: stimulate release of insulin from the pancreas.
  - acarbose: delays absorption of carbohydrate from the GIT.
- parenteral, i.e. insulin.

Hypokalaemia. Plasma potassium under 3.5 mmol/l. Symptoms usually occur below 2.5 mmol/l. Total deficit may be up to 500 mmol.

- Caused by:
  - reduced intake, e.g. iv fluid therapy without potassium supplementation.

- excessive losses:
  - renal:
    - solute diuresis, e.g. saline, glucose, mannitol, urea.
    - diuretic therapy.
    - hyperaldosteronism and disorders of the renin/angiotensin system.
    - Cushing's syndrome.
    - diuretic phase of acute renal failure.
  - GIT, e.g. diarrhoea, vomiting, fistulae, etc.
- movement of potassium into cells:
  - alkalosis.
  - drugs, e.g. insulin, catecholamines.

- Effects:
  - muscle weakness, ileus.
  - arrhythmias, ECG changes (S–T segment depression, Q–T and P–R interval prolongation, T wave inversion, U wave). Cardiac arrest may occur.
  - impaired renal concentrating ability.
  - increased sensitivity to non-depolarising neuromuscular blocking drugs.
  - increased adverse effects of digoxin.
  - may cause metabolic alkalosis.
- Treatment:
  - oral supplementation: up to 200 mmol (15 g)/day.
  - iv potassium chloride: up to 40 mmol (3 g)/l fluid usually, infused at up to 40 mmol/h. Excessively concentrated solutions may cause vascular necrosis, and too rapid administration may cause VF; in severe cases, the above limits may be exceeded with ECG monitoring.

Hypokalaemia should be corrected before anaesthesia and surgery, although the ratio of intracellular:extracellular potassium is more important than isolated plasma levels.

Hypomagnesaemia. Plasma magnesium under 0.75 mmol/l. Because only 1% of magnesium is present in ECF, plasma levels may not correlate with clinical features.

- Caused by:
  - reduced magnesium intake, e.g. TPN, alcoholism.
  - malabsorption.
  - increased loss, e.g. GIT (prolonged diarrhoea/vomiting), renal (diuretics, diabetes, etc.).
- Features:
  - arrhythmias.
  - neurological: confusion, irritability, tremor, convulsions.
  - exacerbation of the effects of hypocalcaemia.
- Treatment:
  - of primary cause.
  - acutely: 10–20 mmol $MgSO_4$ iv over 1–2 h, repeated as required with plasma monitoring, up to 50 mmol/day.

Hyponatraemia. Plasma sodium under 135 mmol/l. Usually results in hypo-osmolar plasma (not always, e.g. hyperglycaemia or hypertonic mannitol infusion causing hyperosmolar plasma).

- Caused by:
  - water excess:
    - excessive intake (urine sodium < 10 mmol/l):
      - iv administration of sodium-deficient fluids.
      - TURP syndrome.
      - excessive drinking.
    - reduced excretion (urine sodium > 20 mmol/l):
      - syndrome of inappropriate antidiuretic hormone secretion (SIADH).
      - drugs, e.g. chlorpropamide, oxytocin (have antidiuretic effect).
  - water excess with smaller sodium excess (urine sodium < 10 mmol/l):
    - cardiac and hepatic failure.
    - nephrotic syndrome.
  - water deficiency with greater sodium deficiency:
    - renal loss (urine sodium > 20 mmol/l):
      - diuretic therapy.
      - hypoadrenalism.
      - cerebral salt wasting syndrome.
      - salt-losing nephritis.
      - renal tubular acidosis.
      - post-relief of urinary obstruction.
    - other loss (urine sodium < 10 mmol/l):
      - diarrhoea and vomiting.
      - pancreatitis.
  - redistribution of sodium/water:
    - sick cell syndrome in terminally ill patients: thought to be caused by impaired cell membrane sodium/potassium transport, resulting in sodium redistribution to the intracellular compartment.
    - water shift from intracellular to extracellular compartments, e.g. due to hyperglycaemia. Corrected plasma sodium concentration in hyperglycaemia: $[Na^+] + ([\text{glucose}] \div 4)$.
  - pseudohyponatraemia, e.g. in hyperlipidaemia: the sodium-poor lipid portion is analysed together with the aqueous portion. Modern equipment analyses only the aqueous portion.
- Features:
  - of dehydration and hypovolaemia in sodium deficiency.
  - symptoms thought to be caused by water entering cells by osmosis include headache, nausea, confusion, coma and convulsions with possibly permanent neurological defects. Premenopausal women are especially at risk; the threshold for convulsions and/or respiratory arrest in this group may be as high as 130 mmol/l, compared with 115–120 mmol/l in men and postmenopausal women.
- Treatment:
  - of underlying cause.
  - as for SIADH: water restriction, demeclocycline.
  - iv hypertonic saline (1.8%, 4.5% or 5%) has been used in severe cases of sodium and water deficiency (sodium under 115 mmol/l). The optimal rate of plasma sodium increase is controversial, but correction should be slow, since subdural haemorrhage, central pontine myelinosis and cardiac failure may occur if too rapid. 5–10 mmol/l/day has been suggested as the maximal safe rate; up to 2 mmol/l/h until a plasma sodium of 120 mmol/l is reached. Total sodium deficit (mmol) assuming distribution throughout total body water = (125 – measured sodium) × 60% of body weight (kg). Normal saline with furosemide has been used in less severe cases.

Reynolds RM, Padfield PL, Seckl JR (2006). BMJ; 332: 702–5

Hypo-osmolality. Plasma osmolality under 280 mosmol/kg. Features are as for hyponatraemia. Detected by hypothalamic osmoreceptors, causing compensatory changes in water ingestion and excretion.

Hypoparathyroidism. Most commonly occurs postoperatively, e.g. following parathyroid/thyroid/laryngeal surgery; may be acute or occur several years later. May also be idiopathic, sometimes familial.

Pseudohypoparathyroidism: same features, due to peripheral lack of response to parathyroid hormone; may be associated with hypothyroidism.

Pseudopseudohypoparathyroidism: features of pseudohypoparathyroidism but with normal calcium and phosphate levels.
- Features:
  - hypocalcaemia.
  - hyperphosphataemia.
- Treatment: calcium and vitamin D supplements.

Anaesthetic considerations are related to hypocalcaemia.
Marx SJ (2000). N Engl J Med; 343: 1863–75
See also, Thyroid gland

Hypophosphataemia. Plasma phosphate under 0.8 mmol/l.
- Caused by:
  - mild: hyperparathyroidism, osteomalacia, increased carbohydrate metabolism, hypomagnesaemia, haemodialysis, acute alkalosis.
  - severe: ketoacidosis, TPN and refeeding after starvation, chronic alcoholism/withdrawal.
- Effects:
  - muscle weakness, myocardial depression.
  - irritability, dysarthria, encephalopathy, peripheral neuropathy, convulsions, coma.
  - rhabdomyolysis, haemolysis, platelet and leucocyte dysfunction.
- Treatment: sodium or potassium phosphate: 10–20 mmol orally or 5–20 mmol/h iv. Overtreatment and resultant hyperphosphataemia may cause hypocalcaemia and hypomagnesaemia.

Hypopituitarism. Reduced secretion of the anterior pituitary gland (hyposecretion of posterior portion causes diabetes insipidus). Most commonly caused by pituitary tumour; may also follow surgery/radiotherapy, granulomatous disease, cysts and, classically, ischaemic necrosis after haemorrhage during labour (Sheehan's syndrome).
- Features:
  - absent axillary/pubic hair, breast and genital atrophy, pale skin, muscle wasting.
  - of hypothyroidism and adrenocortical insufficiency.

Main anaesthetic considerations are related to the latter two features, and any oversecretion due to tumour, e.g. Cushing's syndrome, acromegaly.
[Harold Sheehan (1900–1988), English pathologist]

Hypoproteinaemia. Plasma proteins under 60 g/l. Most commonly due to low albumin levels (under 35 g/l). May occur in hepatic/renal failure, protein-losing nephropathy or enteropathy, and in severely ill catabolic patients, e.g. on ICU.
- Anaesthetic significance:
  - for drugs which are largely protein-bound, reduced available binding sites increase the proportion of unbound drug after iv injection, increasing the clinical effect; e.g. opioid analgesic drugs, thiopental, antibiotics. Effects are increased further if available binding sites are already occupied by other protein-bound drugs. Albumin is usually involved in protein-binding, but others are also involved, e.g. gammaglobulin and acid α_1-glycoprotein.
  - decreased plasma oncotic pressure may lead to tissue oedema.
  - specific protein deficiencies, e.g. coagulation disorders, plasma cholinesterase deficiency.

Hypotension. Since MAP = cardiac output (CO) × SVR, hypotension may result from reduction of:
- CO:
  - reduced heart rate:
    - vagal reflexes.
    - drugs, e.g. halothane, β-adrenergic receptor antagonists, neostigmine.
    - arrhythmias.
  - reduced stroke volume:
    - reduced venous return, e.g. hypovolaemia, spinal/epidural/caudal anaesthesia, head-up posture, aortocaval compression, IPPV, tension pneumothorax, cardiac tamponade.
    - arrhythmias.
    - increased afterload, e.g. aortic stenosis, PE (including air and amniotic fluid embolism), pneumothorax, tamponade.
    - reduced myocardial contractility, e.g. drugs, hypoxia, hypercapnia, ischaemic heart disease, MI, cardiomyopathy, myocarditis, cardiac failure, acidosis, hypothermia.
- SVR:
  - drugs, e.g. vasodilator drugs, volatile and iv anaesthetic agents.
  - adverse drug reactions.
  - spinal/epidural/caudal anaesthesia.
  - sepsis.

Reduction in blood flow to vital organs may result, with risk of permanent ischaemic damage, e.g. CVA, MI, renal failure. Autoregulation maintains cerebral, coronary and renal blood flows at systolic BP of approximately 70–80 mmHg. Treatment consists of O_2 administration, raising the feet and specific treatment directed towards the cause.

Hypotensive anaesthesia. Usually defined as deliberate lowering of BP during anaesthesia by more than 30% of resting value. Techniques usually involve reduction of systolic BP to about 80 mmHg (MAP 50–60 mmHg), although levels of 60–70 mmHg (MAP 40 mmHg) have been employed. Performed in circumstances where surgery may be hindered by bleeding and to reduce blood loss, e.g. middle ear surgery, neurosurgery, plastic surgery, and extensive major surgery, e.g. cystectomy, pelvic clearance. Its use is controversial, since hypotension may cause organ ischaemia, dysfunction and infarction, particularly of heart, liver, kidneys, brain and spinal cord. Considered by some to be too dangerous for non-life-saving surgery, but by others to be routinely acceptable. Risks are lowest in fit young patients, but consequences of major infarction are more dramatic and tragic in this group.
- Contraindications are also controversial, but include:
  - impaired organ blood flow or function, e.g. ischaemic heart disease, renal disease, cerebrovascular disease, age (implies the foregoing).
  - hypertension.
  - diabetes mellitus: there may be increased sensitivity to hypotensive agents as autonomic function may be impaired already. Increased sensitivity to insulin has followed ganglion blockade.
  - severe respiratory disease. Bronchospasm may follow use of ganglion-blocking drugs or β-adrenergic receptor antagonists in asthmatics.
  - pregnancy, anaemia, hypovolaemia.
  - anaesthetist and surgeon unfamiliar with the technique.
- Originally achieved in the 1940s by deliberate hypovolaemia and/or high spinal anaesthesia. Now achieved by using:
  - anaesthetic drugs/techniques which lower BP:
    - reduced cardiac output, e.g. IPPV, head-up positioning of the patient, halothane.
    - reduced SVR, e.g. tubocurarine, isoflurane, spinal/epidural anaesthesia.
  - specific hypotensive drugs, e.g.:
    - β-receptor antagonists including labetalol.

- vasodilator drugs, e.g. sodium nitroprusside, GTN, hydralazine.
- ganglion-blocking drugs, e.g. trimetaphan.
- Management:
  - preoperative assessment with regard to contraindications.
  - premedication is usually given, to improve smoothness of induction. Atropine is avoided.
  - smooth induction of anaesthesia, with minimal coughing, straining, etc. Attempts may be made to reduce the hypertensive response to intubation (*see Intubation, complications of*). Drugs increasing heart rate or BP are avoided, e.g. atropine, ketamine, pancuronium.
  - tracheal intubation is usually performed. Spontaneous ventilation is preferred by some, since it may indicate adequacy of brainstem blood flow. IPPV is often employed to avoid hypercapnia and vasodilatation associated with spontaneous respiration; it also reduces venous return. PEEP has been used to augment the latter but may increase venous bleeding. Dead space and $\dot{V}/\dot{Q}$ mismatch are increased at low blood pressures, therefore F_IO_2 is usually increased to 0.5.
  - intra-arterial BP measurement is usually employed if profound hypotension or infusions of powerful hypotensive agents are used; otherwise indirect methods of measurement are usually adequate. CVP measurement is useful in major surgery. A large bore iv cannula is required. EEG and its derivatives have been used to monitor cerebral activity.
  - careful positioning of patient, with the site of surgery raised above the heart, and avoidance of venous kinking and obstruction. Head-up tilt is introduced gradually to avoid sudden severe hypotension. 20–30° tilt is usually sufficient; BP at the head is about 15–20 mmHg less than that at the heart.
  - a typical anaesthetic sequence consists of thiopental or propofol, IPPV using, e.g. isoflurane, with increments of labetalol or hydralazine. Infusions of nitroprusside, GTN, or others including trimetaphan may be used. Choice of agent is largely personal. Relative importance of BP over blood flow is controversial, e.g. whether use of vasodilators is better than reduction of cardiac output.
  - careful postoperative observation is important, since cardiovascular instability may persist.

Hypothalamus. Part of the brain forming the floor of the 3rd ventricle. Lies posterior to the optic chiasma and infundibular stalk attached to the posterior lobe of the pituitary gland. Important controlling area for autonomic nervous system activity; sympathetic mainly restricted to the posteromedial part, parasympathetic to the anterolateral part. Involved in temperature regulation and regulation of hormone secretion by the pituitary; also of thirst, hunger, sexual activity, etc.

Hypothermia. Core temperature below 36°C. May result from exposure or immersion (near-drowning), e.g. complicating trauma and coma from any cause, especially involving depressant drug overdose, hypothyroidism and phenothiazine therapy. May also result from excessive heat loss during anaesthesia. Induced for surgery, e.g. cardiac surgery; techniques include surface cooling by sponging or immersion, central cooling with heat exchangers, and irrigation of body cavities with cold solutions. Appears to be beneficial for patients who have suffered prehospital cardiac arrest due to VF. Has been investigated in the treatment of head injury. Permissive hypothermia refers to the technique of allowing body temperature to decrease passively during, e.g. neurosurgery, to afford a degree of cerebral protection.

- Effects:
  - cardiovascular:
    - reduced cardiac output (a 30% reduction at 30°C).
    - J waves (positive deflections at the end of QRS complexes) may appear on the ECG at 30°C (Fig. 82). They are clinically insignificant.
    - ventricular arrhythmias at 30°C, VF at 28°C.
    - vasoconstriction. Vasodilatation occurs below 20°C.
    - increased blood viscosity.
    - increased haematocrit below 30°C. Thrombocytopenia may be caused by sequestration, mainly hepatic but also splenic.
  - respiratory:
    - apnoea at 24°C.
    - reduced tissue O_2 delivery because of reduced cardiac output, vasoconstriction, increased viscosity and shift of the oxyhaemoglobin dissociation curve to the left, despite increased dissolved volume of O_2 in blood.
    - reduced O_2 demand and CO_2 production.
    - arterial blood gas tensions are measured at 37°C; values are traditionally corrected to body temperature but correction is now considered unnecessary.
  - neurological:
    - confusion below 35°C.
    - unconsciousness at 30°C.
    - reduced requirement for volatile agents.
    - cessation of all cerebral electrical activity below 18°C.
  - other:
    - diuresis due to inability to reabsorb sodium and water. GFR is reduced by 50% at 30°C.
    - respiratory and metabolic acidosis. Increased blood glucose and potassium.
    - metabolic rate increases initially, then decreases. Hyperglycaemia and increased fat mobilisation may occur.
- Management:
  - investigation: both routine and as for coma, in particular those causes mentioned above.
  - routine ICU monitoring.
  - treatment of hypoxia/hypoventilation/acidosis as required. Antiarrhythmic treatment may be ineffective at low temperatures.
  - rewarming methods include:
    - heating-blankets and baths.
    - radiant heaters.
    - warmed iv fluids.
    - irrigation of body cavities (e.g. bladder via catheter, peritoneal cavity via dialysis catheter, stomach via nasogastric tube) with warm solution.
    - humidification and warming of inspired gases.
    - extracorporeal circulation using heat exchangers.

    External warming may cause peripheral vasodilatation and hypotension, or subsequent rebound hypothermia if the core is relatively unwarmed. Rapid rewarming is thought to be best in hypothermia of rapid onset; gradual rewarming if of gradual onset (i.e. up to 1°C/h).
  - treatment of the underlying cause.

Complications include chest infection, frostbite and pancreatitis. Residual hypothalamic damage may remain,

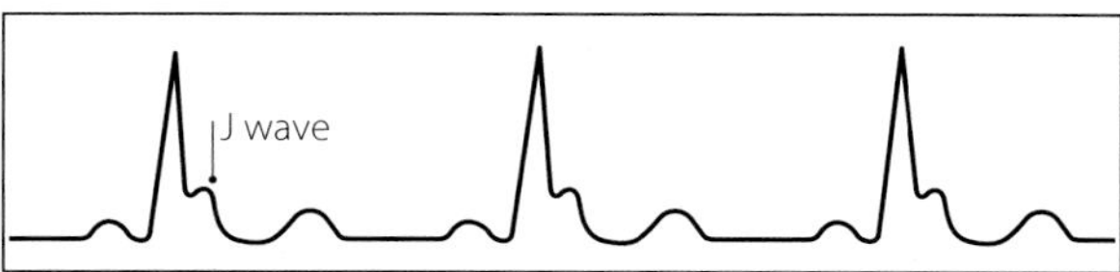

Fig. 82 ECG showing J waves

especially in the elderly, with susceptibility for future episodes of hypothermia.

Epstein E, Anna K (2006). BMJ; 332: 706–9

See also, Temperature regulation

Hypothesis testing, *see Null hypothesis*

Hypothyroidism. Usually follows thyroid disease (e.g. autoimmune) or treatment for hyperthyroidism (including surgery and radiotherapy). May also follow treatment with other drugs, e.g. amiodarone and lithium. Rarely due to pituitary disease. Approximately 10 times more common in women; the incidence increases with age.

- Features:
  - cretinism in children.
  - lethargy, slowed reactions, delayed relaxation of tendon reflexes (classically plantar reflex).
  - coarse skin and hair. Loss of the outer part of the eyebrows is classically described but is uncommon.
  - weight gain, reduced appetite, constipation.
  - hoarse voice, lowered temperature.
  - anaemia: from menorrhagia or associated pernicious anaemia.
  - bradycardia, cardiomegaly and pericardial effusion may occur. Typical ECG findings include low voltage complexes, bradycardia and T wave flattening/inversion. Hyperlipidaemia and ischaemic heart disease are common.
  - nerve entrapment, myopathy, confusion. Coma may occur (see below).
- Investigations: thyroxine (T_4) and triiodothyronine (T_3) are low. Thyroid stimulating hormone is high in primary thyroid failure, and low in pituitary failure.
- Treatment: thyroxine replacement (50–200 μg/day). Initial dosage is reduced in the elderly and those with heart disease, to reduce the risk of myocardial ischaemia.
- Hypothyroid coma (myxoedema coma):
  - particularly common during winter when hypothermia is common, especially in the elderly. May be precipitated by infection, CVA, anaesthesia, etc.
  - mortality may exceed 50%.
  - treatment:
    - T_3 (liothyronine) 5–20 μg slowly iv, repeated 4–12 hourly depending on severity and response. Alternatively, 50 μg iv may be followed by 25 μg 8 hourly, reducing to 25 μg 12 hourly. ECG monitoring is required.
    - hydrocortisone is often given but its place is uncertain if adrenocortical insufficiency is not present.
    - treatment of hypoventilation, hypothermia, hypotension, bradycardia, acidosis, hyponatraemia, hypoglycaemia and convulsions as required. Fluid restriction is usually advocated for treatment of hyponatraemia and prevention of cardiac failure.
- Anaesthetic considerations in hypothyroidism:
  - other autoimmune diseases may be present, e.g. myasthenia gravis.
  - patients show increased sensitivity to depressant drugs, especially opioids.
  - CO_2 and heat production, and drug metabolism/excretion are reduced.
  - hypoventilation and coma may occur.

Farling PA (2000). Br J Anaesth; 85: 15–28

Hypoventilation. Reduced alveolar ventilation; it may result from reduction of respiratory rate and/or tidal volume.

- Caused by:
  - reduced central respiratory drive:
    - drugs, e.g. opioid analgesic drugs, barbiturates, inhalational anaesthetic agents.
    - hypocapnia, e.g. following IPPV. Also may occur in extreme hypercapnia.
    - metabolic disturbances, e.g. primary metabolic alkalosis, hyperglycaemia, etc.
    - administration of high F_IO_2 to patients with COPD who rely on hypoxic respiratory drive.
    - intracranial pathology, e.g. CVA, tumour, infection, head injury, raised ICP, etc.
    - hypothermia.
    - alveolar hypoventilation and sleep apnoea syndromes.
  - impaired peripheral mechanism of breathing:
    - airway obstruction.
    - restriction due to pain, obesity, severe ascites, tight bandages, circumferential chest burns, etc.
    - chest disease, e.g. COPD, pneumothorax, asthma, flail chest, etc.
    - muscular weakness, e.g. electrolyte disturbances, muscular dystrophy, dystrophia myotonica, myopathy associated with critical illness, etc.
    - neuromuscular junction impairment, e.g. non-depolarising and depolarising neuromuscular blockade, myasthenia gravis.
    - nerve lesions, e.g. spinal cord injury, phrenic nerve injury, motor neurone disease, poliomyelitis, Guillain–Barré syndrome, critical illness polyneuropathy, etc.
  - increased dead space, e.g. embolism, anaesthetic apparatus.

Effects are those of hypercapnia, respiratory acidosis and hypoxaemia. During anaesthesia, uptake of inhalational anaesthetic agents, or recovery from them, is slowed.

- Treatment:
  - O_2 therapy. Restores alveolar P_{O_2} as indicated by the alveolar air equation. Assisted or controlled ventilation may be required if arterial P_{CO_2} is high or rising.
  - directed at the cause. Neuromuscular blockade monitoring helps distinguish central from peripheral causes.
  - doxapram has been used perioperatively and in COPD to reduce or treat hypoventilation. Naloxone is used in opioid overdose.

See also, Carbon dioxide response curve

Hypovolaemia. Reduced circulating blood volume. May be caused by deficiency of:

- blood; i.e. haemorrhage.
- plasma; e.g. burns.
- extracellular and/or intracellular fluid; e.g. dehydration, diuretic therapy, haemodialysis/haemofiltration, third space losses (e.g. surgery, sepsis) and evaporative losses (e.g. pyrexia, during surgery).

'Relative hypovolaemia' refers to pooling of blood, e.g. during sepsis, as a result of drugs or following spinal/epidural anaesthesia. Less blood is available for circulation despite an unchanged blood volume.

- Results in increased sympathetic activity, reduced parasympathetic activity and other compensatory mechanisms, as in acute haemorrhage. Important clinically because:
  - many patients presenting with acute illness or for emergency surgery have a degree of hypovolaemia.
  - BP and perfusion of vital organs (e.g. heart, brain) are maintained largely by sympathetically mediated vasoconstriction and tachycardia. Drugs (e.g. sedatives, anaesthetic agents) which cause vasodilatation or reduce

cardiac output may thus cause severe hypotension, as may spinal/epidural anaesthesia.
- vital organs receive a greater proportion of cardiac output than normal, at the expense of other tissues, e.g. skin and GIT. Smaller doses of anaesthetic agents are therefore required to produce clinical effects, including side effects (e.g. myocardial depression).
- renal failure may occur.

Hypovolaemia should therefore be detected and corrected wherever possible before induction of anaesthesia, and treated promptly when it occurs peri- and postoperatively.

- Features:
  - pallor (peripheral vasoconstriction).
  - tachycardia.
  - hypotension with low CVP and pulmonary capillary wedge pressure.
  - oliguria, thirst.
  - reduced O_2 delivery, e.g.:
    - to tissues: lactic acidosis.
    - to brain: confusion, restlessness.
    - to carotid/aortic bodies: breathlessness.
    - to heart: angina if susceptible.
  - haematocrit and urea and electrolyte abnormalities depending on aetiology.
- Treatment:
  - O_2 administration, supine position and raising the feet.
  - fluid replacement.
  - of the cause.

Hypoxaemia. Arterial Po_2 under 12 kPa (90 mmHg).

- Caused by:
  - hypoventilation (*see Alveolar air equation*).
  - diffusion impairment, e.g. due to pulmonary fibrosis, connective tissue diseases; $\dot{V}/\dot{Q}$ mismatch is thought to be more significant.
  - shunt.
  - $\dot{V}/\dot{Q}$ mismatch.
  - reduced F_IO_2, e.g. due to high altitude or inadvertent hypoxic gas delivery during IPPV, resuscitation or anaesthesia.

In acute illness or during anaesthesia, hypoxaemia may occur because of respiratory depression, airway obstruction, atelectasis and $\dot{V}/\dot{Q}$ mismatch, including reduced FRC. It is especially common after upper abdominal surgery, due to the same factors plus hypoventilation caused by pain and depressant drugs and inability to cough. Impaired ciliary activity may also contribute. Hypoxaemia may persist for 2–3 days after upper abdominal surgery. Impaired sleep control may contribute to obstructive apnoea following anaesthesia.

- Effects:
  - direct effects:
    - cyanosis.
    - confusion, drowsiness, excitement, headache, nausea. Unconsciousness, convulsions and death follow unless corrected.
    - myocardial depression, arrhythmias, bradycardia, coronary and cerebral vasodilatation.
    - hypoxic pulmonary vasoconstriction and pulmonary hypertension.
    - renal impairment.
  - effects of carotid and aortic body stimulation:
    - tachycardia, hypertension.
    - hyperventilation.

  Acute hypoxaemia with 85% haemoglobin saturation may cause mental impairment, becoming severe at 75% saturation. Unconsciousness usually occurs at 65% saturation. Chronic hypoxaemia, e.g. at altitude, leads to adaptation.
- Treatment:
  - directed at the cause.
  - O_2 therapy: increases alveolar Po_2, resulting in increased arterial Po_2. The increase will be minimal in shunt.

See also, Breathing, control of; Hypoxia; Respiratory failure

Hypoxia. Reduced O_2 for tissue respiration.

- Classically divided into:
  - hypoxic hypoxia (hypoxaemia).
  - anaemic hypoxia: normal arterial Po_2 but reduced available haemoglobin, e.g. due to anaemia, carbon monoxide poisoning.
  - stagnant (ischaemic) hypoxia: normal arterial Po_2 and haemoglobin availability, but reduced tissue blood flow; may be due to reduced cardiac output or local interruption of blood flow.
  - histotoxic (cytotoxic) hypoxia: normal arterial Po_2, haemoglobin availability and blood flow, but inability of tissues to utilise O_2, e.g. due to cyanide poisoning, carbon monoxide poisoning.
- Effects:
  - aerobic metabolism at the cytochrome oxidase system is replaced by anaerobic metabolism, with increasing lactate production. Membrane pumps cease functioning, with impairment of normal intra/extracellular ion balance; irreversible cell damage may follow. Brain and heart are most susceptible. Other tissues may continue for long periods under hypoxic conditions. The critical value for intracellular O_2 tension is not known, but is thought to be about 0.13 kPa (1 mmHg) at the mitochondrial level (Pasteur point).
  - local stagnant hypoxia effects depending on the tissue involved.
  - general effects of hypoxia are as for hypoxaemia.

Stimulation of the carotid and aortic bodies occurs when arterial Po_2 falls; i.e. it may not occur in anaemic and histotoxic hypoxia.

See also, Oxygen cascade

Hypoxic pulmonary vasoconstriction. Reflex vasoconstriction of pulmonary arterioles in response to low Po_2 (under 11–13 kPa; 80–100 mmHg) in nearby alveoli. Does not rely on innervation of vessel walls, and is less dependent on Po_2 in blood; thus it occurs in isolated lung perfused with blood of high O_2 content and ventilated with gas of low O_2 content. Results in flow of blood away from poorly ventilated areas of lung, helping to reduce $\dot{V}/\dot{Q}$ mismatch.

Before birth, decreased pulmonary blood flow is thought to be caused by pulmonary vasoconstriction, relieved at birth when O_2 enters the lungs at the first breath.

Important in cardiac defects; hypoxaemia may cause a generalised increase in pulmonary vascular resistance, with increased right ventricular work and increased right-to-left shunting, particularly if SVR is lowered. Of major importance in the development of pulmonary hypertension and right heart failure (cor pulmonale) in patients with chronic lung disease.

- Reduced by:
  - hypocapnia.
  - increased distension of arterioles.
  - vasodilator drugs.
  - volatile anaesthetic agents in animal and laboratory experiments; the clinical relevance of this is controversial.

I

Ibandronic acid, *see Bisphosphonates*

Ibopamine. Prodrug, converted to *N*-methyldopamine, a peripheral dopamine receptor agonist (DA_1 and DA_2). Has been studied as a potential oral treatment for severe cardiac failure though associated with an increased incidence of death in early studies. Has been used as a sympathomimetic in ophthalmology.

Ibsen, Bjørn (1915–2007). Danish anaesthetist, considered by many to be the founding father of intensive care. Created a dedicated respiratory care unit to look after patients with poliomyelitis during the Copenhagen outbreak in 1952. Drastically cut mortality by employing positive pressure ventilation, usually via tracheostomy. Opened the first general intensive care unit in 1953, a concept that was rapidly adopted worldwide.
Richmond C (2007). Br Med J; 335: 674
See also, Intensive care, history of

Ibuprofen. NSAID used to treat musculoskeletal pain, headache, etc. Has been used for postoperative analgesia but has weaker anti-inflammatory and analgesic properties than other NSAIDs, although has fewer GIT side effects.

- Dosage: 400–600 mg orally, 3–4 hourly. A modified release preparation (1600 mg once daily or 300–900 mg 12 hourly), a topical gel and a combination preparation with codeine are also available.

ICAM, Intracellular adhesion molecules, *see Adhesion molecules*

Iceberg theory, *see Clathrates*

ICISS, *see International classification injury severity score*

ICNARC, *see Intensive Care National Audit and Research Centre*

ICP, *see Intracranial pressure*

ICU, *see Intensive care unit; Critical care*

ICU psychosis. Loose term denoting abnormal behaviour exhibited by patients in the ICU. Consists of anxiety, confusion, delirium and hallucinosis. Usually occurs 3–5 days after admission; most common post cardiac surgery.
Aetiology is multifactorial:

- patient factors: e.g. premorbid psychological state, age, communication difficulties.
- environmental factors: e.g. unfamiliar surroundings, isolation from friends/family, lack of privacy, disrupted day/night cycle, noise level, monotony.
- staff factors: e.g. insensitivity of staff, inappropriate conversations by the bedside, inadequate explanation.
- physiological factors: e.g. pain, fever, hypoxaemia, drug treatment/withdrawal, metabolic disturbance, immobilisation.

The incidence is thus reduced by consistent and sympathetic staffing, provision of clear explanations to the patient and family, relatively unrestricted visiting hours, providing the patient with familiar objects (e.g. family photographs), frequent reassurance, availability of calendars and clocks and promotion of routine during the day whilst dimming the lights and restricting activity at night. Hypnotic drugs may be required to establish a normal sleep pattern. If delirium persists, sedation with benzodiazepines or major tranquillisers (e.g. haloperidol) may be required.

Psychosis generally resolves within 2–5 days of discharge from the unit.
Pun BT, Ely EW (2007). Chest; 132: 624–36
See also, Confusion in the intensive care unit; Confusion, postoperative

I–D interval. Time between induction of anaesthesia and delivery of the infant in Caesarean section. Infant thiopental levels may be high if the interval is very short. If very long, inhalational anaesthetic agents may accumulate in the infant. An I–D interval of less than 30 min is not thought to influence fetal acidosis if aortocaval compression and hypoxaemia are avoided.

Ideal gas law. For a perfect gas:

$$\frac{\text{pressure, } P \times \text{volume, } V}{\text{temperature, } T} = \text{constant}$$

rearranged as $PV = nRT$,

where n = number of moles of gas
R = universal gas constant

Thus a combination of Boyle's law, Charles' law and Avogadro's hypothesis.

IDICM, *see Intercollegiate Diploma in Intensive Care Medicine*

Idioventricular rhythm, *see Atrioventricular dissociation*

I:E ratio, *see Inspiratory:expiratory ratio*

Ignition temperature. Lowest temperature at which combustible mixtures ignite (energy required = activation energy). Lowest for stoichiometric mixtures.
See also, Explosions and fires

IHD, *see Ischaemic heart disease*

ILCOR, *see International Liaison Committee on Resuscitation*

Ileus. Small bowel atony (although the term is often used to describe gastric and colonic stasis).

- Causes include:
  - GIT pathology, e.g. surgery, haemorrhage, peritonitis.
  - drugs, e.g. anticholinergic drugs, opioid analgesic drugs.
  - severe sepsis.
  - others: spinal cord injury, renal failure, diabetic coma, electrolyte imbalance especially hyperkalaemia.

Clinical features include a distended and silent abdomen, with constant (usually mild) abdominal discomfort. Upright abdominal X-ray may reveal gas-filled loops of small intestine. If prolonged, fluid and electrolyte loss may occur. Distension may impair ventilation if severe. The presence of colicky pain and increased bowel sounds suggest intestinal obstruction, which may follow paralytic ileus. Pseudo-obstruction of the colon occurs in bedridden patients with severe systemic illness and may present in a similar way. Abdominal X-ray however shows greatly dilated colonic loops; urgent decompression (e.g. via a colonoscope) may be required to prevent caecal rupture.

- Management:
  - supportive: restriction of oral intake with free nasogastric drainage. Early oral administration of small amounts of clear fluids is becoming more common in uncomplicated cases. Fluid and electrolyte imbalance should be corrected.
  - metoclopramide and erythromycin have been used to stimulate intestinal activity.
  - methylnaltrexone, a peripherally acting mu opioid receptor antagonist, is currently under investigation as a treatment for postoperative ileus, which is thought to arise from a combination of endogenous endorphins and exogenous opioids given for pain relief.

Iliac crest block. Blocks the ilioinguinal, iliohypogastric and lower 2–3 intercostal nerves, providing anaesthesia of the lower ipsilateral abdomen. An 8 cm needle is introduced 2–3 cm inferior and medial to the superior anterior iliac spine, and directed cranially and laterally to reach the inner ilium. 10 ml local anaesthetic agent is injected whilst the needle is withdrawn. Injection is repeated, directed more deeply.
See also, Inguinal hernia field block

Iliacus compartment block, *see Fascia iliaca compartment block*

Iliohypogastric nerve block/Ilioinguinal nerve block, *see Iliac crest block; Inguinal hernia field block*

ILS, *see Immediate Life Support*

Imaging in intensive care. Many modalities are available; usage depends on the body area involved and whether the patient is stable enough to be transferred to the radiology suite. In general, portable imaging equipment produces less clear images. Close liaison with radiology staff is essential for making the correct choice of imaging.

- Techniques include:
  - conventional radiography:
    - chest X-ray: demonstrates physical (as opposed to functional) abnormalities of the lungs, tracheobronchial tree, pleura, diaphragm, heart and great vessels, chest wall, thoracic spine and soft tissues. May also detect foreign bodies including invasive lines and tubes. Commonly performed every 1–3 days in the ICU (depending on the severity of illness; may require repeating several times per day) to check tubes, etc., monitor progress and check for complications, e.g. pneumothorax, especially after invasive procedures.
    - abdominal X-ray: useful for demonstrating dilated loops of bowel and fluid levels in intestinal obstruction, free abdominal gas, kidney and gallstones, etc.
    - skull X-ray: less useful once admitted to ICU since the main indication is trauma; appropriate X-rays will usually have been taken before admission. May be useful for diagnosing sinusitis.
  - others: include cervical spine and other bony structures, soft tissues for presence of gas in gas gangrene, etc.
  - ultrasound:
    - abdomen:
      - general, e.g. in trauma, intra-abdominal sepsis.
      - kidney in acute renal failure; demonstrates renal size, obstructive nephropathy, vascular occlusion, etc.
      - biliary tract (e.g. in cholecystitis, ascending cholangitis) and pancreas (pancreatitis).
    - chest:
      - echocardiography (including transoesophageal echocardiography).
      - both echocardiography and abdominal ultrasound may provide information about the lungs, diaphragm and pleura.
      - central venous cannulation using hand-held ultrasound devices.
  - CT scanning: remains the most sensitive and appropriate modality for critically ill patients with head injury, cerebral oedema, subdural, subarachnoid and extradural haemorrhage and hydrocephalus. Thoracic CT scanning gives detailed information of all structures including lung pathology in ARDS. Abdominal scanning is especially useful for imaging biliary tract, liver, pancreas and retroperitoneal structures. Portable bedside CT scanners are becoming available.
  - MRI: although more sensitive than CT scanning for imaging cerebral and spinal structures, practical difficulties (including long scan times, problems with monitoring, etc.) preclude it from routine use.
  - positron emission tomography: remains primarily a research tool in critically ill patients although it has provided useful information about cerebral blood flow and metabolism in head injury.
  - radioisotope scanning: used to assess organ blood flow and perfusion, presence of infection and cardiac function.

Imaging techniques, especially ultrasound and CT scanning, may allow percutaneous drainage (e.g. of obstructed ureters, intra-abdominal abscesses, empyema, etc.) to be performed by radiologists and others, thereby reducing the risks of surgery in critically ill patients.
See also, Functional imaging; Radiography in intensive care

Imipenem. Extremely broad spectrum carbapenem and antibacterial drug, active against most pathogenic aerobic and anaerobic Gram-negative and -positive organisms. Broken down in the kidney by the enzyme dehydropeptidase, and thus combined with cilastatin (1:1 ratio by weight) which inhibits the enzyme. Usually reserved for severe or mixed infections (excluding CNS infection).

- Dosage:
  - 250–500 mg iv over 20–30 min, 6–8 hourly, up to 50 mg/kg (≤ 4 g/day) for less sensitive organisms.
  - 500–750 mg im, 12 hourly.
- Side effects: GIT upset, blood dyscrasias, allergic reactions, convulsions, confusion, hepatic/renal impairment, red urine.

Imipramine hydrochloride. Tricyclic antidepressant drug, similar to amitriptyline but with less sedative properties. Used in endogenous depression and panic disorders. Also used in nocturnal enuresis.

- Dosage: 75 mg/day, orally, increased up to 300 mg/day (usually 50–100 mg/day). 25–50 mg is used in pain management.
- Side effects: as for amitriptyline.

Immediate Life Support (ILS). One-day course developed in 2002 by the Resuscitation Council (UK) in order to standardise much of the in-hospital training undertaken already by Resuscitation Officers. Trains healthcare personnel in recognition of sick patients, prevention of cardiac arrest, cardiac arrest rhythms, basic life support (BLS), simple airway management and safe defibrillation (manual and/or automatic). Aims to enable staff to manage patients in cardiac arrest until the arrival of a cardiac arrest team.

Soar J, Perkins GD, Harris S, Nolan JP (2003). Resuscitation; 57: 21–6.

Immune system, anaesthesia and. Normal immune defences are:

- innate (non-specific), e.g. epithelial surface barriers, secreted immunoglobulins, local inflammatory responses including phagocytes and macrophages, complement system, pH of gastric juice, ciliary action, etc.
- adaptive (specific):
  - humoral: B lymphocytes; under the influence of T-cell cytokines, form plasma cells which secrete specific immunoglobulins.
  - cellular: T lymphocytes conditioned in the thymus have killer activity and regulatory effects via helper/suppressor subsets.
  - natural killer cells.
- Main areas of anaesthetic importance:
  - patients with immunodeficiency.
  - adverse drug reactions, blood cross-matching, etc.
  - effects of anaesthesia on immunocompetence, especially against infection and malignancy. Difficult to study clinically, because of other factors, e.g. surgery, drugs, pre-existing disease, stress response to surgery, etc., although phagocyte, monocyte and B lymphocyte activity is reduced during anaesthesia. Ciliary activity may be affected. *In vitro* testing has revealed depression of monocyte and phagocyte activity and migration, e.g. in response to mitogen or antigen provocation. Natural killer cell activity, lymphocyte proliferation and plasma cell formation are also reduced following anaesthesia with most inhalational agents. Lysosomal free radical formation may also be suppressed. Effects on spread and metastasis of malignancy are controversial, although spread in animals may be increased by anaesthesia and blood transfusion may be detrimental in colonic cancer surgery and renal transplantation.

Immunodeficiency. Results in increased susceptibility to infection and malignancy, the former a more common problem acutely. May result from deficient cell-mediated (T cell lymphocyte) or antibody-mediated (B cell lymphocyte) function, phagocytic activity or complement activity. Results in repeated and persistent infection, typically with unusual organisms.

- May be:
  - primary, e.g. B cell or T cell deficiency, often inherited. Specific immunoglobulin types may be deficient. Neutrophil and complement disorders may also be inherited.
  - secondary to:
    - infection, e.g. viral (e.g. HIV infection), sepsis.
    - drugs, e.g. immunosuppressive drugs, gold, penicillamine.
    - connective tissue diseases.
    - severe illness, trauma, burns, etc., i.e. it may occur in any severely ill patient on ICU.
    - malignancy.
    - splenectomy.
- Management:
  - prevention of infection, e.g. meticulous aseptic technique, barrier nursing, prophylactic antibacterial therapy, etc.
  - prompt diagnosis and treatment of infection.
  - treatment of the underlying cause.
  - immunoglobulin administration, (*see Immunoglobulins, intravenous*).
  - immune stimulant therapy is not generally available, although some agents, e.g. interferons, have been used.

Immunoglobulins (Antibodies). Proteins secreted by plasma cells, involved in immunological defence systems. Each molecule consists of two heavy chains (which determine the class of immunoglobulin) and two light chains. The Y-shaped molecule presents two highly specific antigen-binding sites, each made up of portions of heavy and light chains, at one end (the Fab portion). The other end (the Fc portion) is made up of heavy chain only, and may bind to complement, or to the surface of mediator cells, e.g. mast cells, macrophages.

- Types of immunoglobulins:
  - IgG: the most abundant in plasma. Involved in complement fixation.
  - IgA: secreted from epithelial barriers, e.g. GIT.
  - IgM: comprises five joined molecules; involved in complement fixation.
  - IgD: involved in antigen recognition by lymphocytes.
  - IgE: on the surface of mast cells; involved in histamine release and anaphylactic reactions.

Most adverse drug reactions to anaesthetic drugs via immunoglobulins involve IgG and IgM (complement activation) or IgE (anaphylaxis).

- Immunoglobulins may be administered to humans, and are obtained from:
  - pooled human plasma:
    - from blood donated for transfusion (normal immunoglobulin): given im for prophylaxis of certain infections, e.g. measles, hepatitis, rubella in pregnant women. Certain forms may be given iv as replacement therapy in immunodeficiency, and in various other immune related disorders (*see Immunoglobulins, intravenous*).
    - from donors who are convalescing, or whose antibody production has been boosted (specific immunoglobulins): given im and available against hepatitis B, tetanus, rabies, Rhesus D antigen and herpes viruses.

    They are screened for hepatitis and HIV infection.
  - monoclonal cell biology and recombinant genetic engineering: not yet widespread. Infliximab is a monoclonal antibody against tumour necrosis factor, used in rheumatoid arthritis.

Hypersensitivity reactions are more likely with immunoglobulins from pooled plasma. Digoxin specific antibody fragments (Fab) derived from sheep immunoglobulins are available for use in digoxin toxicity.

Immunoglobulins, intravenous (IVIG). Obtained from a plasma pool of 1000–10 000 donors and provide polyclonal immunoglobulins to a wide variety of pathogens. Originally used to treat idiopathic thrombocytopenia and congenital agammaglobulinaemia, have been shown to be effective in

Guillain–Barré syndrome and other peripheral neuropathies, myasthenia gravis and the myasthenic syndrome. Proposed mechanisms of action include an anti-inflammatory and complement effect, reduction in cytokine synthesis and blocking of IgG-binding Fc receptors on macrophages.

Despite pre-donation testing, transmission of hepatitis C has been reported.

- Dosage: 0.4 g/kg iv daily for 5 days.
- Side effects: malaise, fever, acute meningism, acute renal failure, anaphylaxis. Contraindicated in patients with class-specific anti-IgA antibodies.

Kazatchkine MD, Kaveri SV (2001). N Engl J Med; 345: 747–55

Immunosuppressive drugs. Used to treat inflammatory/ autoimmune diseases and connective tissue diseases, and to prevent rejection following transplantation.

- Different types of drug used:
  - cytotoxic drugs, e.g. cyclophosphamide, azathioprine, chlorambucil, mycophenolate. All depress bone marrow haemopoiesis and increase susceptibility to infection.
  - corticosteroids.
  - anti-lymphocyte agents, e.g. ciclosporin, tacrolimus.
  - immunoglobulins or immuno-active receptor agonists/ antagonists, e.g. tumour necrosis factor (TNF) receptor-antibody complexes, anti-TNF antibodies or interleukin-1 receptor antagonist, used to treat rheumatoid arthritis.

Impedance. Resistance to flow of an alternating current in an electrical circuit, dependent on the current's frequency. Represented by the letter Z, although measured in ohms. Different components within circuits, e.g. loudspeakers, monitor screens, etc., should be matched for impedance, to maximise efficiency. Amplifiers in monitoring equipment generally have high input impedance to minimise the effect of poor contact with the patient; any increased impedance because of the latter makes little difference to the overall input impedance.

See also, Impedance plethysmography

Impedance plethysmography. Method of determining changes in intrathoracic gas and fluid volumes by measuring transthoracic impedance, which varies according to the composition of thoracic contents.

- Used for:
  - monitoring respiration, e.g. on ICU: a small high-frequency current is passed between ECG electrodes; the changes in impedance between them represent ventilatory movements. Has been used to detect oesophageal intubation (produces a different impedance pattern to tracheal intubation).
  - cardiac output measurement: two sets of circular wire electrodes are placed around the chest and neck. Current is passed between the outer two, with measurement of potential difference between the inner two. Maximal rate of change of impedance occurs with peak aortic flow, although absolute values do not correlate well.
  - others, e.g. lung water measurement.

May also be applied to other parts of the body, e.g. leg veins to diagnose DVT.

See also, Inductance cardiography

IMV, *see Intermittent mandatory ventilation*

Inborn errors of metabolism. Group of disorders caused by inherited single enzyme defects. Over 200 are known; some are clinically insignificant and others fatal. Most are rare (1:20 000–500 000), are caused by autosomal recessive genes, and are present in infancy/early childhood.

- Include disorders of:
  - porphyrin metabolism (*see Porphyrias*).
  - carbohydrate metabolism, e.g. glycogen storage disorders, galactosaemia and fructose metabolic disorders. Liver, brain, skeletal and cardiac muscle may be affected. Hypoglycaemia is common, also metabolic acidosis and electrolyte imbalance.
  - amino acid metabolism, e.g. phenylketonuria, homocystinuria, alcaptonuria. Mental handicap, neurological abnormalities and metabolic disturbances are common. Skeletal abnormalities may present difficulty with tracheal intubation in the latter two disorders. Hypoglycaemia may occur.
  - lysosomal storage; results in accumulation of macromolecules within lysosomes. Most conditions cause severe mental retardation and neurological abnormalities, with death in childhood. Include:
    - sphingolipidoses, e.g. Gaucher's disease; coagulation abnormalities and hepatosplenomegaly are common.
    - mucopolysaccharidoses, e.g. Hurler's and Hunter's syndromes (the latter is sex-linked recessive). CNS, skeleton and viscera are affected. Characteristic 'gargoyle' facies occur, with possible upper respiratory obstruction, and thoracic spinal deformities. Hurler's syndrome is more severe than Hunter's, with corneal clouding, valvular and ischaemic heart disease.
  - purine metabolism: may lead to gout, with tissue deposition of urate crystals, especially in the joints. This group includes Lesch–Nyhan syndrome, with mental and neurological abnormalities.
  - red blood cell metabolism, e.g. glucose 6-phosphate dehydrogenase deficiency. Haemolysis may also feature in other defects.
  - copper metabolism (Wilson's disease): impaired hepatic and central nervous motor function.
  - iron metabolism (haemochromatosis): hepatic and myocardial impairment are common; diabetes mellitus may occur.

[Philippe Gaucher (1854–1918), French physician; Gertrud Hurler (1889–1965), German paediatrician; Charles Hunter (1872–1955), US physician; Michael Lesch (1939–2008), US cardiologist; William Nyhan, US paediatrician; Samuel Wilson (1878–1937), US-born English neurologist]

Incentive spirometry. Lung expansion technique designed to encourage deep breathing to reduce atelectasis and improve respiratory muscle function, e.g. postoperatively.

- Apart from verbal encouragement and teaching of breathing exercises, the following techniques have been used:
  - inspiration from bellows; when the preset tidal volume has been reached, a light illuminates.
  - inspiration or expiration through flowmeters, e.g. glass cylinders containing coloured balls; the patient attempts to reach preset targets.
  - inflation of a balloon on expiration.
  - expiration through a blow-bottle: the patient breathes out through a tube passing into a sealed jar containing water, which is displaced through a second tube into a second jar.

Recent evidence suggests that the technique is useful in reducing breathlessness in COPD but evidence for its efficacy in preventing postoperative pulmonary complications is lacking.

Overend TJ, Anderson CM, Lucy SD, et al (2001). Chest; 120: 971–8

See also, Physiotherapy

Incident, major. Practical hospital definition: any event involving casualties causing significant disruption of normal running of the hospital. Has also been defined according to the number of casualties. May refer to transport accidents, riots, terrorist activities, natural disasters, etc.

- Main problems:
  - large number of patients to be sorted (triage) for treatment and transfer, with their sudden arrival at hospital. Although there have been arguments over whether pre-hospital treatment is better than a 'scoop and run' policy, it is now generally accepted that certain interventions (e.g. airway management) should ideally be carried out before transfer to hospital if competent staff are available on-site. Adequate record-keeping is difficult, e.g. patient identification, assessment, treatment given, location, etc.
  - coordination of emergency services, with organisation of staff and resources at the scene of the incident and receiving (designated) hospitals.
  - clearing of non-urgent cases from wards, ICU, operating theatre, etc.
  - communication between medical teams, hospitals, police, fire brigade, press and public. Telephone and computer networks may be non-functioning or disabled, and/or the volume of calls from the press, public and staff may be overwhelming.
  - sudden need for specific equipment (e.g. breathing apparatus, protective suits), drugs, blood, blood products, and other support services, e.g. X-ray, etc.
  - dispersal of patients once initially treated; identification and holding of corpses.
- Major Incident plans of most hospitals are similar:
  - affected hospitals are informed, and main receiving hospitals designated. Use is made of nearby specialist centres, e.g. thoracic, neurosurgical, etc.
  - specific duties are assigned to each member of staff on duty, i.e. medical staff (including formation of a mobile team), nursing staff, telephone operators, porters, etc. Assignment of a team leader and establishment of routes of communication in each area is vital.
  - duties of anaesthetists include triage and treatment at the scene of the incident, resuscitation in the receiving area, and anaesthesia for surgery.
  - duties of ICU staff include resuscitation and organising and managing admissions to ICU.
  - previously prepared emergency drug and equipment boxes/bags contain iv fluids, cannulae, self-inflating bag, tracheal intubation equipment, bandages, scissors and drugs. Triservice apparatus has been suggested as suitable for field anaesthesia, but most anaesthetists' experience of this is limited, and anaesthesia is rarely required before transfer to hospital.

Aylwin CJ, König TC, Brennan NW (2006). Lancet; 368: 2219–25

See also, Biological weapons; Chemical weapons; Transportation of critically ill patients; Trauma

Independent lung ventilation, *see Differential lung ventilation*

Indocyanine green. Strongly infra-red absorbing and fluorescent agent, given iv as a marker substance to permit organ blood flow or cardiac output measurement. Has also been used to study cerebral perfusion using near infra-red spectroscopy. Transported on proteins, it is exclusively eliminated by the liver but does not undergo enterohepatic circulation. Elimination is dependent on both liver blood flow and parenchymal cellular function.

Indometacin (Indomethacin). NSAID, available for oral and rectal use. The latter route has been used for postoperative analgesia and to replace oral therapy withdrawn perioperatively. Also used to promote closure of a patent ductus arteriosus (PDA).

- Dosage:
  - 100 mg rectally once/twice daily.
  - 25–50 mg orally, 6–8 hourly.
  - for PDA closure: 200 μg/kg iv initially.
- Side effects: as for NSAIDs; in addition dizziness and headache may occur.

Inductance. Capacity for an electromotive force to be induced in an electrical circuit by a changing current flowing in that circuit, or in a neighbouring one. Flow of current induces a magnetic field, which in turn induces the electromotive force, the magnitude of which depends on the rate of change of current. May give rise to interference in electrical equipment, or occur intentionally in transformers. Has been used as a basis for measuring cardiac output and monitoring respiration, by using two coils placed on the chest, e.g. one anteriorly, one posteriorly.

Inductance cardiography (Thoracocardiography). Used for determining changes in intrathoracic volumes, and thus estimating cardiac output. An insulated electrical conductor placed around the chest, level with the heart, is connected to an alternating current, and changes in cross-sectional area detected via changes in its self-inductance (via changes in the oscillatory frequency of the current induced). Accuracy is generally not as good as other methods of measuring cardiac output; thus absolute values are less useful than trends.

Induction agents, *see Intravenous anaesthetic agents*

Induction of anaesthesia. Transition from the awake to the anaesthetised state, although the end-point is difficult to define.

- Represents a period of great physiological change during which the following may occur:
  - cardiovascular changes, e.g. hypotension, arrhythmias.
  - hypoventilation/apnoea. Particularly dangerous in patients with airway problems.
  - aspiration of gastric contents.
  - laryngospasm, hiccups, vomiting, etc. during the stage of excitement, particularly if disturbed by movement, noise, etc.
  - adverse drug reactions, especially following iv injections.
  - others, e.g. involuntary movement/convulsions, MH/masseter spasm.

Inhalational and iv techniques are most commonly used, although other routes (e.g. im or rectal) of drug administration are possible.

- Inhalational induction:
  - usually reserved for children, patients with airway obstruction, and in difficult intubation. By allowing continuous spontaneous ventilation, the anaesthetist avoids being unable to ventilate an apnoeic patient. May also be used in patients with poor veins or needle phobia.
  - the anaesthetic agent is gradually introduced to the patient in increasing concentrations. The characteristics of induction depend on the inhalational anaesthetic

agent used. More rapid induction has been achieved using maximal breaths of high percentage of volatile agent, e.g. 4–5% halothane or 4–8% sevoflurane ('single breath induction').
- the different stages of anaesthesia may be seen in turn, especially in unpremedicated patients.
- induction is slower than with iv agents. The stage of excitement may be prolonged.

- IV induction:
  - much faster, allowing rapid passage through the stage of excitement. Usually more pleasant for adults than an inhalational technique.
  - an estimated appropriate dose should be given slowly, and the patient observed for its effect before injecting more. Considerable time may be required if the arm–brain circulation time is prolonged, e.g. in the elderly and those with cardiovascular disease.
  - the characteristics of induction depend on the iv anaesthetic agent used.
  - carries risk of extravasation, intra-arterial or painful injection, thrombosis, chemical reaction with other drugs in the cannula, and adverse drug reactions.
  - movement, hiccuping, etc., may occur.
  - overdosage is more likely because induction is faster, especially if injection is rapid and without pausing to observe the effect.

Respiratory and cardiac depression may follow both methods of induction, but are more sudden after iv induction, especially after rapid injection. Use of other depressant drugs, e.g. for premedication, may reduce the amount of induction agent required and allow smoother induction. Respiratory depressants, e.g. opioids, may slow inhalational induction.

Emergency drugs and equipment, a tipping trolley and skilled assistance should always be present before inducing anaesthesia. Equipment should always be checked before use.
See also, Anaesthesia, stages of; Checking of anaesthetic equipment; Induction, rapid sequence

Induction, rapid sequence ('Crash induction'). Induction of anaesthesia in which risks of regurgitation and aspiration of gastric contents are minimised by:
- presence of emergency drugs and equipment, a tipping trolley and skilled assistance (should be present before inducing anaesthesia in any patient, but especially important in rapid sequence induction, as is checking of anaesthetic equipment).
- suction equipment: should be turned on before induction and be within easy reach of the anaesthetist.
- aspiration of gastric tube if in place, prior to induction. Pre-induction passage of a stomach tube is rarely done routinely. A nasogastric tube is usually left in situ during induction.
- use of a rapidly acting iv induction agent and suxamethonium to achieve rapid muscle relaxation. Rocuronium has been suggested as an alternative when suxamethonium is contraindicated, but takes longer for recovery; thus spontaneous ventilation takes at least 30 min to return should intubation fail. Regurgitation and aspiration have been reported during use of the priming principle. Other analgesic or sedative drugs should not precede the iv agent.
- application of cricoid pressure.
- avoidance of manual inflation of the lungs by facepiece to prevent inflation of the stomach and thus increase risk of regurgitation. Preoxygenation is therefore required to prevent hypoxaemia during apnoea until tracheal intubation is achieved.
- tracheal intubation and inflation of the cuff before cricoid pressure is released.

Spare laryngoscopes, tubes, etc. must be prepared in advance, as must a plan in case of unexpectedly difficult or impossible intubation.

Rapid sequence induction should be performed in all cases known to be at risk of regurgitation or aspiration, including all emergency abdominal operations, except in cases where intubation is expected to be particularly difficult.
See also, Intubation, difficult; Intubation, failed; Nasogastric intubation

Inert gas narcosis. Loss of consciousness caused by inhalation of high partial pressures of inert gases, e.g. xenon, neon, argon and nitrogen (nitrogen narcosis). Nitrogen has no anaesthetic properties at sea level pressures, but impairs intellectual and manual functions at partial pressures above 4–5 atmospheres, e.g. diving to depths greater than 30–40 metres whilst breathing air. Use of helium in breathing apparatus allows deeper dives.

Infection. Most common cause of disease worldwide. Anaesthetic and ICU implications may be related to:
- primary cause of illness, e.g. meningitis, chest infection, hepatitis, etc.
- complication of surgery, anaesthesia, intensive care, trauma, etc., e.g. nosocomial infection.
- treatment, e.g. side effects of antibacterial or antiviral drugs, etc.
- risk of transmission to susceptible patients or from infected patients to staff.

Whatever its cause and site, infection may result in SIRS and/or septic shock.
See also, Infection control; individual infections and organisms

Infection control. Important in anaesthetic and ICU practice for prevention of nosocomial infection. Many hospitals have an infection control team (microbiologist, nurse and laboratory staff) with major responsibility for surveillance/investigation of infection, review of antibiotic therapy/resistance and education of staff.
- Achieved by:
  - provision of single bedded rooms in ICUs for patients susceptible to infection or those who pose a cross-infection hazard to other patients. Barrier nursing is often necessary. If possible, patients returning from ICUs to general wards should also be isolated from other patients until they are clear of infections with organisms such as meticillin-resistant *Staphylococcus aureus* (MRSA) and vancomycin-resistant enterococcus.
  - maintaining sufficient nurse:patient ratios to manage fluctuating workload.
  - staff hygiene: though often poor, it is the major controllable factor in cross-infection. Hands should be washed before and after each patient contact, watches/jewellery not worn, and meticulous aseptic technique used during medical and nursing procedures. Gloves (and in ICU, aprons) should be worn during non-sterile procedures.
  - early identification and treatment of infection. Immediate screening, e.g. for MRSA, with decolonisation of high risk patients, is essential when patients are admitted from other ICUs or hospitals, especially from abroad. Regular sampling of sputum, urine, etc. should continue for all patients on ICU.

- identification and avoidance of catheter-related sepsis.
- use of bacterial filters on breathing systems and regular changing of disposable ventilator tubing (e.g. every 48 h).
- use of disposable syringes, pressure transducers, etc. which should not be reused.
- restricting drugs at risk from bacterial infection (e.g. propofol) to single patients only and preparing syringes, etc. immediately before use.
- avoiding contamination of breathing equipment by appropriate cleaning/disposal of equipment after each patient.
- joint daily ward rounds between microbiologists and the ICU team. Antimicrobial therapy should only be used when clinically necessary and the choice of agent dictated by bacterial sensitivity.
- regular cleaning/decontamination of the ICU.
- better ward design to minimise environmental contamination, including air filtration and conditioning.

The routine use of selective decontamination of the digestive tract is controversial.

Scott G (2000). Intensive Care Med; 26: S22–5

See also, Bacterial resistance; Staphylococcal infections

Infiltration anaesthesia. Commonly performed for minor surgery, suturing, etc. Subcutaneous and intradermal infiltration is performed around the lesion, with further injection as required. May also be used for manipulations and more extensive surgery, e.g. Caesarean section, etc., in which the deeper tissues are also infiltrated. The maximal safe dose of local anaesthetic agent should not be exceeded. Dilute solutions are usually adequate. Excessive volumes of injectate containing adrenaline may cause skin necrosis. Adequate time must be allowed before starting surgery.

Inflammatory bowel disease. Chronic inflammatory GIT disease of uncertain aetiology. Comprises:

- Crohn's disease: transmural granulomatous disease; commonly affects the terminal ileum and ascending colon although it may affect the GIT from mouth to anus.
- ulcerative colitis (UC): characterised by inflammation of the colonic and rectal mucosa.

Features include fever, malaise, weight loss, anaemia, vitamin deficiencies, dehydration, abdominal pain and tenderness, diarrhoea (often bloody). Chronic inflammation may lead to intestinal obstruction; Crohn's disease typically is associated with fistula formation. Non-intestinal manifestations include arthritis, sacro-iliitis, ankylosing spondylitis, uveitis, skin involvement and liver/gallbladder disease. Diagnosis is confirmed by intestinal biopsy.

- Management:
  - medical: correction of nutritional deficiencies, anaemia, etc.; sulfasalazine, 5-aminosalicylic acid enemas; corticosteroids.
  - surgical: may be required for Crohn's disease (e.g. for obstruction, fistulae) or UC (e.g. in toxic megacolon when extensive disease is unresponsive to medical therapy, or in total colitis lasting more than 10 years when malignant change becomes more common).

Anaesthetic considerations are related to the above complications and the need for emergency surgery. Severe toxic megacolon may require admission to ICU for resuscitation.

[Burrill B Crohn (1884–1983), US physician]

Inflation pressure, *see Airway pressure*

Inflation reflex, *see Hering–Breuer reflex*

Informed consent, *see Consent*

Infraorbital nerve block, *see Maxillary nerve blocks*

Infratrochlear nerve block, *see Ophthalmic nerve blocks*

Infusion regimens. Used to ease the setting up and administration of potent iv drugs whilst minimising errors. Generally rely on adding a fixed amount of drug to a fixed volume of diluent to produce a set concentration, or varying one component (usually the amount of drug) according to the patient's weight to produce a concentration expressed in terms of amount of drug per kilo. Other considerations relate to the kind of infusion device used and whether the dose is commonly expressed as drug per unit of time (e.g. μg/h), volume per unit of time (e.g. ml/h) or drug per kilo per unit of time (e.g. μg/kg/h). A common and useful method of preparing drugs such as inotropic drugs is to add (body weight × 3) mg of drug to diluent to make 50 ml solution; 1 ml/h is then equivalent to 1 μg/kg/h.

Inguinal hernia field block. May be used as the sole technique for surgery in poor risk patients, or as an adjunct to general anaesthesia to reduce the anaesthetic requirement and to provide postoperative analgesia.

- Anatomy (*see Fig. 66; Femoral triangle*):
  - the inguinal canal represents the path taken by the descending testicle, and contains the spermatic cord in the male (round ligament in the female). It runs downwards and medially, above and parallel to the inguinal ligament, which passes from the superior anterior iliac spine to the pubic tubercle.
  - anterior abdominal wall muscle layers, from within outwards: transversus abdominis, internal oblique, external oblique.
  - the canal emerges through the deep ring of the transversalis fascia and transversus abdominis above the midpoint of the inguinal ligament. The internal oblique lies in front laterally, but its conjoint tendon (formed with transversus abdominis) arches over the canal superiorly to lie behind it medially. The external oblique lies anteriorly along its length. The superficial ring is the defect in the external oblique aponeurosis just lateral and above the pubic tubercle.
  - nerve supply (branches from the lumbar plexus):
    - iliohypogastric (L1): anterior cutaneous branch is given off at the iliac crest; it passes between transversus abdominis and the internal oblique, piercing the latter 2 cm medial to the anterior superior iliac spine. It then runs deep to the aponeurosis of the external oblique, piercing it above the superficial ring to supply the skin above the pubis.
    - ilioinguinal (L1): passes just caudal to the iliohypogastric nerve, passing through the superficial ring to supply the skin of the groin and scrotum/labia majora.
    - genitofemoral (L1, 2): genital branch passes with the spermatic cord through the deep ring, supplying the skin of the scrotum/labia majora.
- Technique of block:
  - iliohypogastric and ilioinguinal nerves: with the patient supine, a short bevelled needle is introduced vertically downwards, 2 cm medial and caudal to the anterior superior iliac spine. A click is felt as the external oblique aponeurosis is penetrated. 10–20 ml local anaesthetic agent is injected, repeated with the needle directed medially and laterally. Subcutaneous infiltration from the pubis, 10 cm cranially, blocks fibres from the other side.

- subcutaneous infiltration along the incision site.
- genitofemoral nerve: injection of 20 ml solution at the deep ring, 1–2 cm above the midpoint of the inguinal ligament, deep to the external oblique aponeurosis as before. This may be left to the surgeon to reduce risk of vascular or peritoneal puncture.
- the neck of the hernia sac may also be infiltrated by the surgeon.

Prilocaine 0.5% with adrenaline is suitable, and allows use of a large volume of solution. The maximal safe dose allowable is calculated and divided between the above injections. For an adjunct to general anaesthesia and postoperative analgesia, smaller volumes of bupivacaine with adrenaline may provide several hours' analgesia. Leg weakness has been reported.

Inhalational anaesthetic agents. Since the discovery of anaesthesia, a variety of gases and volatile agents have been tried and discarded, including: diethyl ether (first used in 1842), N_2O (1844), chloroform (1847), ethyl chloride (1848), ethylene (1923), cyclopropane (1930), divinyl ether (1933), trichloroethylene (1935), xenon (1946), halothane and fluroxene (1956), methoxyflurane (1960), enflurane (1966), isoflurane (1971), desflurane (1994) and sevoflurane (1996). Some properties of inhalational agents are shown in Table 18.

Inhalational agents are popular because alveolar levels (and thus blood levels) are easily controllable by adjusting inspired concentration. However, side effects and pollution fears have led to increased use of iv anaesthetic agents, e.g. TIVA.

Volatile anaesthetic agents are convenient to supply and store, but require special vaporisers. Many are ethers; flammability and risk of explosion and fires are reduced by addition of halogen atoms to the basic molecule.

Gases are supplied in cylinders or via pipelines. Cylinders are bulky to store. Administration of gases is controlled using flowmeters alongside the O_2 flowmeter of an anaesthetic machine.

- Features of the ideal inhalational anaesthetic agent:
  - physical/chemical properties:
    - chemically stable, e.g. in the presence of heat, light, soda lime; long shelf-life. No additive required, e.g. thymol, and non-flammable.
    - non-irritant, with pleasant smell.
    - no corrosion of metal or adsorption on to rubber.
    - SVP should be high enough to enable production of clinically useful concentrations (depends on potency; MAC).
    - low blood/gas partition coefficient.
    - cheap.
  - pharmacology:
    - smooth rapid induction with no breath holding, laryngospasm, coughing, increased secretions, etc.
    - sufficiently potent to allow concurrent high F_IO_2.
    - analgesic, antiemetic and anticonvulsant properties, with skeletal muscle relaxation. No increase in cerebral blood flow or ICP.
    - no respiratory depression. Bronchodilatory action.
    - no cardiovascular depression or sensitisation of myocardium to catecholamines. No decrease in coronary, renal or hepatic blood flow.
    - minimal metabolism, with excretion via the lungs. No fluoride ion production.
    - no adverse renal, hepatic or haematological effects.
    - non-trigger for MH.
    - no effects on the uterus.
    - non-teratogenic/carcinogenic.

No currently available agent fulfils all the above. All of the volatile agents currently used have undesirable effects; in addition to those listed in Table 19, they all depress respiration, reduce uterine tone, and may trigger MH. All increase cerebral blood flow, although isoflurane and sevoflurane less so. N_2O is not potent enough for use as a sole agent and is losing popularity because of its emetic action, effects on methionine metabolism, cardiovascular and cerebral function, expansion of gas-containing cavities (e.g. pneumothorax) and its environmental effects. Trichloroethylene is analgesic and extremely cheap but is no longer produced because of costs associated with renewal of its product licence. Diethyl ether has been available on a named-patient basis. Cyclopropane, previously used mainly in paediatric

Table 18 Properties of inhalational anaesthetic agents

Agent	Structure	Molecular weight	Boiling point (°C)	SVP at 20°C (kPa (mmHg))	MAC (% vol.) (young adults)	Partition coefficients at 37°C: Blood/gas	Oil/gas
Chloroform	$CHCl_3$	119	61	21 (160)	0.5	10	260
Cyclopropane	$(CH_2)_3$	42	−33	—	9.2	0.45	11.5
Desflurane	CF_3–CHF–O–CF_2H	168	23	88 (673)	5–10	0.42	19
Diethyl ether	CH_3–CH_2–O–CH_2–CH_3	74	35	59 (425)	1.9	12	65
Divinyl ether	CH_2=CH–O–CH=CH_2	70	28	74 (553)	3	2.8	60
Enflurane	CHFCl–CF_2–O–CF_2H	184.5	56	24 (175)	1.68	1.9	98
Ethyl chloride	CH_3–CH_2Cl	64.5	13	131 (988)	2	3	—
Ethylene	CH_2=CH_2	28	−104	—	65	0.4	1.3
Fluroxene	CF_3–CH_2–O–CH=CH_2	126	43	38 (286)	3.4	1.4	48
Halothane	CF_3–CHClBr	197.4	50	32 (243)	0.76	2.4	225
Isoflurane	CF_3–CHCl–O–CF_2H	184.5	49	33 (250)	1.28	1.4	97
Methoxyflurane	CF–CHCl–O–CH_3	165	105	3 (23)	0.2	13	970
Nitrous oxide	N_2O	44	−88	—	105	0.47	1.4
Sevoflurane	$(CF_3)_2$CH–O–CH_2F	200	58	21 (160)	2.5	0.69	53
Trichloroethylene	CCl_2=CHCl	131	87	8 (60)	0.17	9	960
Xenon	Xe	131	−108	—	71	0.14	1.9

Table 19 Undesirable features of commonly used volatile anaesthetic agents

Feature	*Halothane*	*Isoflurane*	*Enflurane*	*Desflurane*	*Sevoflurane*
Thymol required	+	–	–	–	–
Decomposed by light	+	–	–	–	–
Approximate cost/100 ml (£)	4–5	15–20	10–13	15–20	45–50
Irritant to breathe	–	+	+/–	++	–
Cardiac output	↓↓	↓	↓↓↓	↓	↓
SVR	(↓)	↓↓	↓	↓↓	↓↓
Heart rate	↓	↑	↑↑	↑	↑↓
Sensitivity to catecholamines	+++	+	++	–	–
Metabolised (%)	20	0.2	2	0.02	3–5
Others	Halothane hepatitis	Coronary steal	Epileptiform EEG	Direct metering vaporiser required	Decomposed by soda lime/baralyme

anaesthesia, is now no longer available. Sevoflurane and desflurane are increasingly being used for day-case surgery since their low blood-gas solubility promotes rapid recovery.

- The potency of anaesthetic agents depends on their solubility in the CNS, estimated by the oil/gas partition coefficient. Brain concentration is related to arterial concentration which approximates to alveolar concentration. Thus steady-state brain concentration requires steady-state alveolar concentration. Drug is distributed from alveoli via bloodstream to:
  - vessel-rich tissues (e.g. brain, heart, kidney, liver; receive 70–80% of cardiac output) until equilibrium is reached, then:
  - vessel-intermediate tissues (muscle, skin; 18% of cardiac output).
  - fat (6% of cardiac output) and other vessel-poor tissues, e.g. bone, ligaments, etc.

In prolonged anaesthesia, the agent accumulates in fat, especially if it is very fat soluble (i.e. potent). Thus it takes 80 min for the partial pressure of N_2O in fat to equal half that in arterial blood; halothane requires 32 h.

- Factors affecting uptake:
  - delivery to alveoli:
    - vaporisation: SVP, gas flow, temperature, vaporiser design, pumping effect.
    - anaesthetic breathing system: gas flow, volume of system and dilution of agent, adsorption on to rubber, etc.
    - alveolar ventilation: agent in each breath is diluted by alveolar gas; the effect is most marked at induction, when uptake of agent is greatest, especially when the blood/gas partition coefficient is high (i.e. blood solubility is high). Hyperventilation thus increases uptake.
    - concentration effect and second gas effect.
  - uptake from alveoli:
    - blood/gas partition coefficient (solubility): if high, uptake into blood is rapid, thus alveolar concentration falls rapidly until the next breath. Build-up of stable alveolar concentration and thus arterial concentration is therefore slow. If solubility is low, only a small proportion of agent passes into blood, leaving a large reserve in the lungs. Thus alveolar and arterial concentrations build up rapidly, with rapid clinical effects. Changes in vaporiser settings are more rapidly reflected in arterial concentrations with insoluble agents than with soluble ones.
    - cardiac output and pulmonary blood flow: uptake is more rapid if cardiac output is high, leading to slow build-up of alveolar concentration. If cardiac output is low, alveolar concentration builds up more quickly; in addition, a greater proportion of cardiac output goes to vital organs, e.g. brain and heart, increasing clinical effects. Thus overdose is more likely if cardiac output is low. The effect is more marked with soluble agents.
    - concentration of agent in the pulmonary artery (i.e. mixed venous). As it approaches pulmonary venous concentration, alveolar and arterial levels approach equilibrium. Occurs as body tissues become saturated, or in severe low output states when tissue perfusion is reduced.
    - $\dot{V}/\dot{Q}$ mismatch: rarely significant unless large, e.g. accidental endobronchial intubation. Effects are greater for insoluble agents.
    - impaired diffusion across alveolar wall is rarely significant.

Factors affecting recovery are similar to those above. If body tissues are unsaturated, recovery is more rapid because the agent moves from arterial blood to both tissues and alveoli. If tissues are saturated after prolonged anaesthesia, recovery is slower, but is hastened by hyperventilation. However, drug movement from tissues into blood may cause reaccumulation of anaesthetic alveolar concentrations after initial wakening.

See also, Anaesthesia, mechanisms of; Coronary steal; Halothane hepatitis; Meyer–Overton rule

Injector techniques. Use of intermittent jets of driving gas, usually O_2, for IPPV by entraining room air. The jet is delivered to the proximal end of a bronchoscope, etc., by a metal cannula (Sanders injector), and entrains stationary gas within the 'scope by jet mixing. Room air is drawn in from the open end to replace the air delivered to the lungs. Expiration occurs by passive recoil of the lungs. A 14–16 G cannula is suitable for adults (delivers up to 30–50 cmH_2O pressure); 17–18 G for adolescents and small adults (up to 25 cmH_2O); 19 G for children (up to 15 cmH_2O). The Carden jetting device was described for attachment to a bronchoscope side-arm; higher inflation pressures and F_IO_2 are achieved with lower driving pressures.

The system usually consists of tubing and a connector for wall socket or gas cylinder, a pressure reducing valve and gauge, a hand-operated trigger and attachment for the cannula. It may also be attached to commercially available cricothyrotomy devices, or to iv cannulae used for emergency cricothyrotomy. Similar principles are also used in high frequency jet ventilation.

Commonly used for bronchoscopy and laryngoscopy because of its convenience.

- Disadvantages:
  - tidal volume and minute ventilation are difficult to assess.
  - trachea is unprotected during airway surgery.
  - possible interference with surgery from movement of vocal cords during ventilation.
  - barotrauma is possible if expiration is obstructed.
  - volatile anaesthetic agents cannot be delivered.

[Richard D Sanders (1906–1977) and Edward Carden, US anaesthetists]
See also, High frequency ventilation

Injury severity score (ISS). Trauma scale used to grade severity of multiple injuries and based on the abbreviated injury scale (AIS). Mostly used for audit purposes, it takes the square of the AIS scores for the three worst affected anatomical regions, with scores ranging from 0 to 75 (any AIS score of 6 automatically converts the total to 75). A score under 24 indicates probable survival, 25–50 reflects progressive increase in mortality and >50 suggests very high mortality rates. Accounts only for anatomical injury, not other factors, and concentrates on only one injury per anatomical site.

The new injury severity score (NISS) differs by including all the most severe injuries rather than the most severe injury per body area. NISS performs better than ISS and is more accurate in distinguishing between survivors and non-survivors.
Baker SP, O'Neill B (1976). J Trauma; 16: 882–5

Inosine. Metabolite of adenosine, with some similar actions. Causes vasodilatation via a direct action on vascular smooth muscle. Also has a positive inotropic effect, but not via β-adrenergic receptors. Thought to improve cell survival following ischaemia and reperfusion, e.g. in cardiac and renal surgery, possibly by increasing intracellular levels of energy-rich phosphates and reducing ATP depletion. Has been used in high vascular and renal surgery; e.g. 30 mg/kg iv before clamping. Hypotension may occur.

Inotropic drugs. Drugs which increase myocardial contractility, increasing cardiac output; used in low cardiac output states.

- Drugs available include:
  - catecholamines: act via G protein-coupled receptors to increase intracellular cAMP levels via adenylate cyclase stimulation; cAMP increases intracellular calcium ion mobilisation and force of contraction.
    - adrenaline: β-adrenergic receptor agonist mainly at low doses, α-adrenergic receptor agonist mainly at higher doses. Causes peripheral and renal vasoconstriction, especially at higher doses. Tachycardia and arrhythmias may occur, increasing myocardial O_2 demand.
    - noradrenaline: α-receptor agonist mainly, with some β-receptor agonist properties. Causes peripheral and renal vasoconstriction, with raised BP and compensatory bradycardia. Myocardial O_2 demand is increased markedly.
    - isoprenaline: β-receptor agonist only. Increases cardiac output and rate, with peripheral and pulmonary vasodilatation. Arrhythmias are common, and myocardial O_2 demand is increased; ischaemia may occur due to lowered BP.
    - dopamine: causes dopamine receptor-mediated renal and mesenteric vasodilatation, with diuresis, at low doses; β_1-receptor agonist at higher doses, with increased cardiac output and BP. α-Receptor-mediated vasoconstriction occurs at even higher doses. Myocardial O_2 demand is increased, but ischaemia is less likely as BP also increases. Tachycardia is less common.
    - dobutamine: mainly a β_1-receptor agonist, with weak β_2- and weaker α-receptor agonist properties. Causes less tachycardia than other catecholamines for a given inotropic effect, possibly due to a smaller effect on the sino-atrial node, and activation of the baroreceptor reflex by increased BP. Coronary perfusion may increase as left ventricular end-diastolic pressure falls.
    - dopexamine. Derived from dopamine; more active at β_2-receptors and less active at dopaminergic receptors. Causes peripheral and renal vasodilatation, with little tachycardia.
    - pirbuterol: mainly a β_1-receptor agonist. Causes some vasodilatation.
    - salbutamol: not a direct inotrope but sometimes used in circulatory failure. A β_2-receptor agonist, reducing SVR. Tachycardia is common.
  - phosphodiesterase inhibitors:
    - specific for cardiac phosphodiesterase: amrinone, milrinone, enoximone. Cause vasodilatation and increased cardiac output.
    - non-specific, e.g. aminophylline.
  - others:
    - calcium: effect lasts for about 5 minutes. Used as a temporary measure. Ventricular arrhythmias may occur.
    - cardiac glycosides, e.g. digoxin. Increase cardiac output and reduce heart rate; possibly also cause vasoconstriction. Thought to increase intracellular calcium ion activity via other ionic effects. Their use in circulatory failure is controversial.
    - glucagon: mechanism is unclear; adrenergic receptors are thought not to be involved. Thought to increase calcium flux into myocardial muscle by stimulating adenylate cyclase.

Choice of drug depends on clinical circumstances. Dopamine is often used in low dosage for its renal effect; dobutamine is commonly used for cardiac support. Adrenaline and noradrenaline are also used, the latter for example when vasodilatation is a particular problem, e.g. septic shock. Enoximone is often used e.g. after cardiac surgery, where tachycardia is particularly undesirable. Isoprenaline is indicated in bradycardia, and raised pulmonary vascular resistance.

Combinations are often used, e.g. with vasodilator drugs, to reduce filling pressures whilst providing inotropic support. Enoximone and dopexamine especially fulfil both functions.

INPB, Intermittent negative pressure breathing, *see Intermittent negative pressure ventilation*

INPV, *see Intermittent negative pressure ventilation*

INR, International normalised ratio, *see Coagulation studies*

Insensible water loss. Unmeasurable volume of pure water lost per day (i.e. without solutes as in sweat), mainly through skin and lungs. Normally up to 1200 ml at rest, increasing with body temperature (by up to 20% per °C above normal) and metabolic rate, and also in tachypnoea. Reduced as ambient humidity increases. During IPPV, exhaled losses may be reduced by humidification of inspired gases.
See also, Fluid balance

Inspiratory capacity. Maximal possible volume of air inspired from FRC. Composed of tidal volume and inspiratory reserve volume. Normally 4.0–5.0 litres.
See also, Lung volumes

Inspiratory:expiratory ratio (I:E ratio). Ratio of inspiratory time to expiratory time. Usually 1:2, allowing recovery from the cardiovascular effects of IPPV during expiration. Adjustable on most ventilators between 1:1 and 1:4. If expiration is too short, air trapping may occur, with increasing intrathoracic volume and pressure, increasing adverse effects of IPPV. However, a reversed I:E ratio of up to 4:1 (inverse ratio ventilation) has been used to improve oxygenation in respiratory failure, especially combined with PEEP.

If expiration is too long, dead space is thought to increase.

Inspiratory pressure support. Augmentation of spontaneous inspiration with supplementary gas flow. A more refined form of assisted ventilation, provided by sophisticated ventilators. Inspiratory flow rate is adjusted to produce a preset inspiratory airway pressure; when flow rate falls to a certain value, inspiration ends. Increases tidal volume, reducing work of breathing and respiratory rate during weaning from ventilators. However, negative pressure must be generated by the patient before augmentation. Tidal volume may vary according to the patient's inspiratory flow pattern. During weaning, the amount of support supplied may be reduced either by lowering the preset airway pressure, or by increasing the negative pressure required to trigger the support.

A combination of pressure support and a decelerating inspiratory flow pattern and a guaranteed tidal volume, 'inspiratory volume support', has recently been developed, in which changes in lung properties during inspiration are continuously monitored.

Inspiratory reserve volume. Inspiratory capacity minus tidal volume. Normally 3.5–4.0 litres.
See also, Lung volumes

Inspiratory volume support. Spontaneous ventilator breathing mode combining the benefits of inspiratory pressure support with a decelerating inspiratory flow pattern and a guaranteed tidal volume. The ventilator automatically monitors the lung properties and modifies the inspiratory pressure support to deliver a predetermined volume. Maximum inspiratory pressure support permitted is just below the preset upper pressure limit and if the tidal volume cannot be delivered with this degree of pressure support, the ventilator alarms indicating that the breath has been pressure limited. Useful mode where lung/chest compliance alters during inspiration, e.g. atelectasis, bronchospasm. As the patient increases spontaneous ventilation, the inspiratory support from the ventilator decreases. If apnoea occurs, volume support also ensures a back-up of pressure regulated volume control ventilation. The maximum pressure change between two breaths is preset by the ventilator (approximately 3 cmH_2O).

Insufflation techniques. Passage of 4–6 l/min fresh gas through a fine bore catheter, passed through the larynx into the trachea; the tip usually lies near the carina (tracheal insufflation). With spontaneous ventilation, fresh gas and room air are inhaled into the lungs, with exhaled gas passing out around the catheter. May also be used to maintain oxygenation in apnoeic patients, although with build-up of CO_2 (apnoeic oxygenation).

First used in the early 1900s. Magill and Rowbotham later provided a separate tube for expired gases, both tubes subsequently replaced by a single wide bore tracheal tube. Still used by some anaesthetists for bronchoscopy, laryngoscopy, etc., especially in children. Fresh gas may also be delivered via the rigid endoscope.

Pharyngeal insufflation is also possible, using a pharyngeal catheter, or by attaching the fresh gas source to a gag or airway.

Barotrauma may occur if escape of gas is obstructed.

Insulin. Hormone secreted by B (β) cells of the pancreatic islets of Langerhans (A (α) cells secrete glucagon, and D (δ) cells somatostatin). Composed of two polypeptide chains specific to species, linked by disulphide bridges. Synthesised as a precursor molecule, subsequently split before secretion.

- Secretion is increased by:
  - glucose, mannose, fructose.
  - amino acids.
  - glucagon and other gut hormones.
  - β-adrenergic receptor stimulation.
  - vagal stimulation.
  - phosphodiesterase inhibition, e.g. due to drugs.
  - sulphonylureas.
  - stress.
- Secretion is decreased by:
  - hypoglycaemia.
  - somatostatin.
  - α-receptor stimulation.
  - insulin itself.
  - drugs:
    - diazoxide.
    - thiazide diuretics.
    - β-adrenergic receptor antagonists.
- Actions:
  - increases:
    - glucose uptake by muscle and fat.
    - glycogen synthesis.
    - fat synthesis and deposition.
    - protein synthesis.
    - potassium uptake by cells.
  - decreases:
    - glycogen breakdown and gluconeogenesis.
    - fat breakdown.
    - protein breakdown.
    - ketone body synthesis in the liver.

  Thus lowers blood glucose levels and increases glucose utilisation. Acts via transmembrane insulin receptors (tyrosine kinase family), via phosphorylation of intracellular enzymes.

Insulins for therapeutic administration, e.g. in diabetes mellitus, have traditionally been derived from beef or pork pancreatic extract, the latter nearer in structure to human insulin than is beef. Human insulin analogues have been obtained using enzymatic modification of pork insulin but are nowadays more commonly produced by recombinant genetic engineering. Substitution/deletion of amino acids at specific sites of the insulin molecule confers different properties with regards to onset and duration of action, mostly via altered absorption from the injection site. Changing from one type to another, especially from beef to human, may result in hypoglycaemia.

Usually administered sc; may also be injected iv, im and intraperitoneally. Recently an inhaled form has been developed.

- Generally classified according to their onset and duration of action:
  - short acting:
    - insulin lispro: recombinant human insulin analogue with a lesser tendency to form hexamers in solution (responsible for slowing uptake). Acts within 15–30 min of sc injection with duration of action 1–3 h.

- insulin aspart: recombinant human insulin analogue; rapidly dissociates into monomers and dimers after injection resulting in rapid absorption. Acts within 10–20 min of sc injection with duration of action 3–5 h.
- insulin glulisine: similar properties to insulin aspart.
- soluble insulin. Acts within 30–60 min of sc injection, with effects lasting up to 8 h (half-life is 5 min after iv injection, with effects lasting 30 min). Used for emergency treatment of hyperglycaemia and perioperatively; also to lower plasma potassium in hyperkalaemia. When added to iv infusions, adequate mixing is essential to prevent uneven administration. May be adsorbed on to the infusion set plastic.

- intermediate and long acting:
  - isophane insulin (suspension with protamine) and amorphous insulin zinc suspension. Acts within 1–2 h, lasting up to 20 h.
  - insulin detemir and insulin glargine: recombinant human insulin analogues: exhibit slower absorption from injection sites via protein-binding and precipitation respectively. Act within 1–2 h with duration of action up to 24 h.
  - crystalline insulin zinc suspension. Acts within 1–2 h, lasting up to 36 h.

The last group is mainly used for maintenance sc administration. Several insulin mixtures (biphasic) are also available. Available as 100 units/ml in the UK; dosage is adjusted for each patient.
[Paul Langerhans (1847–1888), German pathologist]
See also, Glycolysis

Intensive care, costs of, *see Costs of intensive care*

Intensive care follow-up. Programme including ward visits, outpatient clinics and support groups for patients discharged from ICUs. Results in improved communication between ICU and ward staff, and may prevent readmission of patients from wards to ICU by early detection of complications. Clinic appointments allow better identification of the patient's post-ICU quality of life and the identification of late psychological (e.g. anxiety, depression, memory loss) and physical complications (compression neuropathies, impotence, poor balance, voice changes and skin, hair and nail disorders) of intensive care treatment not usually detected during the ICU stay. Specific problems include the undesirable effects of sedation withdrawal (e.g. exaggerated sympathomimetic effects, phobias, perceptual disorders) and post-traumatic stress disorder. Physical status can be measured using pulmonary function testing. Physical and psychological progress can be charted over serial appointments.
Dowdy DW, Eid MP, Sedrakyan A, et al (2005). Intensive Care Med; 31: 611–20

Intensive care, history of. Inseparable from the history of anaesthesia, CPR, pain relief and monitoring. Modern techniques originate from respiratory care units in 1940–1950 along with developments in IPPV and CPR. Coronary care units were the first specialised units, set up in the 1960s. Major developments relating to ICUs include:
- various tank ventilators described and used: 1800s.
- iv salt solutions first used to treat cholera: 1830s.
- concept of keeping all patients requiring 'special' attention and nursing in one place pioneered by Florence Nightingale: 1852.
- curare used in the treatment of tetanus: 1872.
- blood gas analysis performed: 1872.
- venous pressures measured in man: 1902.
- pulse oximetry described: 1913.
- modern oxygen therapy introduced by Haldane: 1917.
- haemodialysis described: 1940s.
- world-wide poliomyelitis epidemic in the 1950s. Early tracheostomy, chest physiotherapy and manual IPPV by medical students used in Copenhagen in 1952 resulted in the establishment of the first ICU by Ibsen: 1953.
- first clinical description of brainstem death: 1959.
- modern CPR developed: 1960s.
- ARDS described: 1967. High frequency ventilation described and developed in the 1970s.
- Intensive Care Society formed in the UK; Society of Critical Care Medicine formed in the USA: 1970.
- critical care training programmes commenced in Canada and the USA: 1970s.
- intermittent mandatory ventilation introduced: 1971.
- bedside pulmonary artery catheterisation described; journal *Critical Care Medicine* first published: 1972.
- *Intensive Care Medicine* first published: 1975.
- first conference of UK Royal Colleges on diagnosis of brainstem death: 1976.
- haemofiltration introduced: 1977.
- APACHE, SAPS and MPM severity of illness scoring systems described: 1980s.
- European Society of Intensive Care Medicine formed: 1982.
- etomidate found to cause adrenal suppression in intensive care patients if used as an infusion: 1983.
- Resuscitation Council (UK) formed: 1982.
- British Association of Critical Care Nurses formed: 1984.
- first CEPOD report: 1987 (*see National Confidential Enquiry into Patient Outcome and Death*).
- European Resuscitation Council formed; European Diploma in Intensive Care Medicine held: 1989.
- International Liaison Committee on Resuscitation formed: 1992.
- Intensive Care National Audit and Research Centre established: 1994.
- Intercollegiate Board for Training in Intensive Care Medicine formed; first running of UK Intensive Care Diploma examination: 1998.
- intensive care medicine granted specialty status by Specialist Training Authority: 1999.
- creation of 'care bundles' summarising best practice: early 2000s.
- first programmes towards Certificate of Completion of Specialist Training in Intensive Care Medicine commenced: 2002.

[Florence Nightingale (1820–1910), English nurse]
See also, Anaesthesia, history of; individual topics

Intensive Care Medicine. Official journal of the European Society of Intensive Care Medicine and European Society of Paediatric Intensive Care, originally published in 1975 as the *European Journal of Intensive Care*.

Intensive Care National Audit and Research Centre (ICNARC). Charitable company established in the UK in 1994 with funding from the Department of Health to develop and undertake comparative audit and evaluative research in intensive care. Its development results directly from the Intensive Care Society's study of the APACHE II severity of illness system. Now a self-financing and non-profit making organisation, with income primarily from subscription of

ICUs to ICNARC's Case Mix Programme; has also received several research grants. Has recently developed an ICU coding method which contains over 700 conditions accessed through a hierarchical selection of type of code, body system, anatomical site, physiological/pathological process and condition, generated from data on over 10 000 patients admitted to 26 UK ICUs.

Intensive care, outcome of. Survival from ICU admission is influenced by:

- patient factors: age, pre-existing morbidity, physiological reserve.
- disease factors: type, site, severity.
- treatment factors: available therapies, appropriate usage, response to therapy.
- organisational factors: early referral/admission, resources, quality of ICU care.

Scoring systems (APACHE, etc.) are used to estimate the risk of hospital mortality for a group of patients. Mortality in ICU varies between ICUs and is dependent upon patient population and case mix factors. In the UK, unadjusted ICU mortality varies between about 11% and 30%; after ICU discharge there is a significant 'step-up' in mortality such that hospital mortality for patients treated in ICUs varies between about 20% and 45%.

There is an increasing awareness that other outcome measures, such as post-ICU morbidity and quality of life, are also important to study.

See also, Intensive care follow-up; Mortality/survival prediction on intensive care unit

Intensive Care Society. British society founded in 1970, for the furtherment of intensive care medicine. Aims include the promotion of education and research, defining standards of intensive care and providing information on the availability, coding and costing of care to its members, the Department of Health and NHS Executive. Currently has over 2400 members, the majority of whom are anaesthetists.

Intensive care, training in. Traditionally obtained in the UK during anaesthetic posts or by ad-hoc arrangements by individual medical/surgical trainees; now coordinated by the Intercollegiate Board for Training in Intensive Care Medicine (formerly the Intercollegiate Committee for Training in Intensive Care Medicine), comprising representatives of the Royal Colleges of Medicine, Surgery and Anaesthesia, and the Intensive Care Society. Recommendations include:

- training undertaken only in ICUs accredited by the Board.
- Educational Adviser for Intensive Care Medicine (ICM) in each area of the UK.
- local Educational Supervisor in each ICU.
- structured training in ICM during undergraduate medical training.
- set periods of training for doctors:
  - junior doctors intending careers in acute hospital specialties: 3 months' training.
  - doctors intending careers in intensive care: minimum of 6-month modules in each of medicine, anaesthesia and intensive care ('Step I' training).
  - prospective ICU Directors: 2 year 'Step II' programme.

The Board oversees dual accreditation on completion of training programmes (i.e. Certificate of Completion of Specialist Training (CCST) in Medicine/ICM, Anaesthesia/ICM or Surgery/ICM) and the Intercollegiate Diploma in Intensive Care Medicine.

Intensive care unit (ICU). Modern techniques originate from postoperative recovery units and respiratory care units in 1940s–50s along with developments in IPPV and CPR. Coronary care units were the first specialised units, set up in the 1960s. An ICU usually provides 1–2% of total hospital beds, although factors affecting this proportion include the number of operating theatres, the type of surgery (e.g. specialised surgery such as cardiac surgery and neurosurgery has greater requirements), location of the hospital (e.g. near major motorways), the overall provision of ICUs within the region and the presence of an accident and emergency department. In general, the unit should have the capacity to accept around 95% of all appropriately referred cases and bed occupancy should be 60–70%. Units larger than 10 beds should be subdivided into specialised units; those smaller than four beds are felt to be uneconomic. Distinction is no longer made between ICU and HDU beds (most units now have a mix of beds), with defined levels of critical care provided according to the type of support required.

- Design considerations:
  - size of unit/bed space (approximately 20 m^2 suggested per patient). Adequate bed separation is important for infection control. Provision of cubicles (e.g. one per six open beds) is necessary for isolation of infected/immunocompromised patients.
  - proximity to theatres, accident and emergency department, X-ray and laboratory facilities.
  - equipment: ventilators, monitoring, infusion pumps, cardiac arrest trolley, etc. Adequate electrical points, gas pipelines, suction, etc.
  - lighting, basins, etc.
  - staff facilities, e.g. on-call room, kitchen, etc.
  - security measures, e.g. single entrance, closed circuit television surveillance.
- Staffing requirements:
  - designated consultant with administrative responsibility for the unit. 85% of ICUs are run by anaesthetists in the UK, although intensive care medicine is rapidly becoming an independent specialty (*see Intensive care, training in*).
  - adequate consultant sessions (15 per week for a unit larger than four beds has been suggested, with more for larger units).
  - resident trainee medical staff with responsibility solely to the unit.
  - nursing staff (one nurse per patient required for 24 h/day).
- Patient selection criteria:
  - according to the requirements in the defined levels of critical care.
  - reasons for admission: the disease state should be potentially reversible.
  - premorbid general health, age and mortality/survival prediction scores (although severity of illness scoring systems cannot be used to predict outcome of intensive care in individual patients).
  - response to treatment so far.
  - anticipated quality of life and the wishes of the patient and relatives.
  - availability of beds.
- Admission to ICU should be:
  - before the patient's condition reaches a point from which recovery is impossible.
  - according to clear criteria to identify at-risk patients.
  - undertaken at senior level using appropriate transfer equipment. Unless the referral area is close to the ICU, full stabilisation (e.g. intubation, IPPV and inotropic therapy) should be undertaken prior to transfer.

- Problems may be related to:
  - original condition.
  - multiple organ failure; may follow many disease processes (e.g. renal failure and ARDS are common in critical illness of any cause). Prognosis worsens as more organ systems are involved.
  - infection, e.g. sepsis.
  - adequate nutrition, and fluid and electrolyte balance.
  - gastric ulceration (stress ulcers). Prophylaxis is as for peptic ulcer disease; H_2 receptor antagonists are most commonly used, sucralfate increasingly so.
  - immobility: DVT and decubitus ulcers may occur. Prophylactic sc heparin is usually administered, and careful skin care, regular turning and physiotherapy instituted.
  - sedation.

Other considerations relate to the cost of intensive care, consent, and the ethics and audit of ICU practice.

See also, Care of the critically ill surgical patient; Intensive care follow-up; Intensive care, history of; Medical emergency team; Postoperative care team; Safe transport and retrieval team; Selective decontamination of the digestive tract; Transportation of critically ill patients

Intensive care unit, transport to, *see Transportation of critically ill patients*

Intercollegiate Diploma in Intensive Care Medicine (IDICM). Instituted in 1997/8 to permit identification of doctors trained to an adequate standard to undertake a career with a large commitment to intensive care medicine in the UK. Aims to test knowledge and its application, and to determine the ability to assess, monitor, investigate and manage critically ill patients. The ability to communicate with medical and nursing staff, patients and their relatives is also examined. Candidates for the Diploma must possess a postgraduate qualification in their primary specialty (e.g. FRCA, MRCP, FRCS), should have completed the stipulated periods of training (*see Intensive care, training in*), and must submit a dissertation.

Intercostal nerve block. Used for peri- and postoperative analgesia, and for analgesia in patients with fractured ribs.

- Technique:
  - may be performed with the patient sitting, with shoulders flexed to pull the scapulae forwards (e.g. with the forearms resting on pillows), or in the lateral position, with the side to be blocked uppermost.
  - identification of selected ribs: by counting down from the spinous process of T1 (the most prominent palpable at the base of the neck) or up from L4–5 (level with the iliac crests). The rib is palpated laterally to the angle, about 6–10 cm from the midline. Injection at the angle blocks the lateral cutaneous branch of the intercostal nerve, which is missed if injection is performed in the mid- or posterior axillary line.
  - a needle (mounted on a syringe to prevent air entry if pleura is pierced) is introduced at the lower edge of the rib, directed cranially. It contacts bone, and is 'walked' inferiorly until it slips off the rib's inferior surface. It is then advanced 2–3 mm. The patient is asked to breath-hold to reduce lung movement and risk of pneumothorax.
  - stretching of the overlying skin cranially before needle insertion has been suggested: release of stretch following insertion aids angling of the needle tip into the subcostal groove.
  - following aspiration for blood, 3–5 ml of local anaesthetic agent is injected whilst moving the needle inwards and outwards 1–2 mm. Bupivacaine 0.25–0.5% with adrenaline may provide analgesia lasting up to 12 h; lidocaine 1% with adrenaline up to 2–4 h. Catheters have been inserted for repeated injections.
  - studies with dyes have shown extensive overlap of injected solution to adjacent spaces (and even to the other side). Systemic absorption of solution is significant; maximal 'safe' doses should not be exceeded.
  - pneumothorax and puncture of intercostal blood vessels may occur. Intra- or epidural spread via a dural cuff surrounding the proximal nerve is also possible.

See also, Intercostal spaces; Interpleural analgesia

Intercostal spaces. Contain the intercostal nerves and blood vessels as they run around the width of the body (Fig. 83).

- Muscle layers between ribs:
  - external intercostal muscle, passing down and forwards.

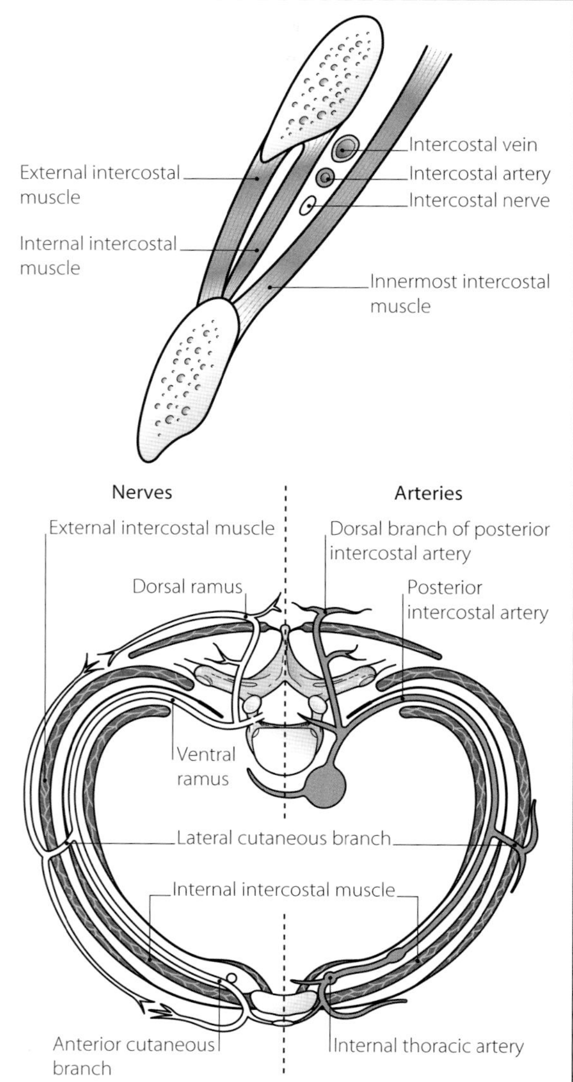

Fig. 83 Anatomy of intercostal spaces

- internal intercostal muscle, passing down and backwards. Becomes the internal intercostal membrane posterior to the rib angles.
- innermost intercostal muscle, attached to the ribs' inner surfaces.

- Intercostal nerves:
  - ventral rami of spinal nerves T1–11. Each spinal nerve has dorsal and ventral roots, which join and then divide into dorsal and ventral rami. The dorsal rami supply the extensor muscles and skin of the back.
  - lie below the blood vessels in the intercostal space.
  - each (except the 1st) gives off a lateral cutaneous branch anterior to the rib angles, and ends as the anterior cutaneous branch.
  - collateral branch arises at the angle, passing forward with main nerve.
- Intercostal arteries:
  - two anterior and one posterior supply each space except the lower two (posterior only).
  - anterior arteries arise from the internal thoracic artery or its terminal branch. They anastomose with the posterior artery and its collateral.
  - posterior arteries arise from the superior intercostal artery (1st and 2nd) or descending aorta. They each give off a collateral branch.

Venous drainage is via two anterior and one posterior intercostal veins, to internal thoracic and azygos veins.

Interferometer, *see Gas analysis*

Interferons, *see Cytokines*

Interleukins, *see Cytokines*

Intermittent flow anaesthetic machines. To be distinguished from apparatus used for draw-over techniques, in which the patient's own inspiratory effort causes gas flow. Intermittent flow machines provide gas flow usually on demand, i.e. when triggered by the patient's inspiration, but are more sophisticated than simple demand valves. Allow mixing of gases, usually O_2 and N_2O, and addition of volatile agents using conventional vaporisers. Minnitt's machine (described in 1933) using a N_2O cylinder with indrawn air was used for analgesia in labour. Inspiration reduces pressure within the apparatus, moving a valve and allowing gas flow. In the McKesson machine, the force opposing fresh gas flow may be adjusted, so that continuous low flow may be provided if required, between breaths. Further adjustment provides continuous high flow, as with conventional anaesthetic machines.

Some machines feature O_2 warning devices, O_2 flushes and valves to cut off N_2O in case of potentially hypoxic gas mixtures.

Traditionally used for dental surgery, but less commonly used now because of unfamiliarity, inaccuracy of flow rates and gas composition, and relative lack of safety features.

[Robert J Minnitt (1889–1974), Liverpool anaesthetist]

Intermittent mandatory ventilation (IMV). Ventilatory mode used to assist weaning from ventilators. A mandatory minute volume is preset and delivered by the ventilator, but the patient is allowed to breathe spontaneously from a gas source between ventilator breaths. As the patient weans, the proportion of minute volume delivered by the ventilator may be reduced, usually by reducing the ventilator rate.

IMV reduces average intrathoracic pressures and risk of barotrauma. The patient's progress may be monitored by counting the spontaneous respiratory rate.

Some sophisticated ventilators will not deliver positive pressure breaths within a certain period of spontaneous breaths, to prevent overdistension of the patient's lungs and barotrauma (synchronised intermittent mandatory ventilation). Others simply incorporate a pressure-relief valve.

Although the weaning process is not shortened, IMV allows it to start earlier and be monitored more easily whilst requiring less sedation, and reducing risks of IPPV.

Intermittent negative pressure ventilation (INPV). Advocated in the 1800s as a means of controlled ventilation without the adverse effects of IPPV, although the latter were then overestimated. Tank ventilators were described first, then cuirass types; motor driven devices were used in the 1930s.

Avoids the risk of barotrauma and other dangers of IPPV, whilst allowing the respiratory muscles to rest. Does not require tracheal intubation, although the risks of regurgitation and aspiration are still present. Indrawing of the soft tissues of the neck may result in upper airway obstruction. Sedation is not required. Continuous end-expiratory negative extrathoracic pressure has similar beneficial effects to PEEP, but without its adverse effects.

Largely superseded by IPPV, but still used for chronic ventilation, e.g. domiciliary night-time ventilation for neuromuscular disease; it has been used to aid weaning from prolonged IPPV.

The Hayek oscillator, first described in the late 1980s, consists of a clear plastic cuirass which fits over the chest and abdomen, connected to a power unit with wide bore tubing. A wide range of frequencies (usually 30–300 Hz) and negative pressures may be generated. It has been used in respiratory failure, for weaning, to allow laryngeal surgery, and perioperatively in cases of failed intubation.

[Zamir Hayek, Israeli-born English neonatologist]

Intermittent positive pressure ventilation (IPPV). Form of controlled ventilation. Performed by Vesalius in 1543 (via a tracheotomy in a pig) and Hooke in 1667 (used bellows via a tracheotomy in a dog). Used initially for CPR; later employed in animal experiments with curare by Waterton in the 1820s. Used in the late 1800s/early 1900s during anaesthesia, but wider acceptance accompanied the introduction of neuromuscular blocking drugs in the 1940s. Use in respiratory failure developed largely following the 1952 Danish poliomyelitis epidemic.

Modified forms, e.g. IMV, pressure control ventilation, pressure regulated volume control ventilation, etc., are mainly used in ICU during weaning from ventilators. High frequency ventilation was developed from the early 1970s. Non-invasive positive pressure ventilation has recently been introduced for patients with neuromuscular respiratory failure and COPD.

- Indications:
  - ICU:
    - respiratory failure.
    - head injury.
    - others, e.g. coma, post-CPR.
  - anaesthesia:
    - when neuromuscular blockade is required; often performed when tracheal intubation is indicated.
    - thoracic surgery.
    - when ventilation is inadequate.
    - to control arterial P_{CO_2}.
    - to reduce requirement for inhalational agents, e.g. in cardiovascular disease.
    - to ensure adequate air entry, e.g. in respiratory disease.

- Technique:
  - tracheal intubation is usually employed, but it may be performed via laryngeal mask airway or even facepiece.
  - manual ventilation was formerly used extensively; ventilators are now widespread. Injector techniques may also be used.
  - a tidal volume of 10–15 ml/kg, at a rate of 10–12 breaths/min, is commonly used, ideally adjusted to arterial (or end-tidal) $P\text{CO}_2$. Intermittent 'sighs' of larger tidal volume were formerly used to reduce atelectasis, but are no longer considered effective. Negative end-expiratory pressure is no longer recommended.

    Mean intrathoracic pressure is lowest with accelerating gas flow, but ventilation is uneven. Ventilation is more uniform with decelerating flow, but mean pressure is highest. Inspiratory:expiratory ratio of 1:2 is usually employed but may be varied according to clinical requirements.
  - neuromuscular blockade is usually employed; deep anaesthesia using volatile agents may also be used, combined with opioid analgesic drugs and hypocapnia to suppress respiratory drive. Sedative/opioid infusions are commonly used in ICU (*see Sedation*).
  - monitoring is important to ensure adequate ventilation and gas exchange, and to detect disconnection.
- Physiological effects/hazards:
  - cardiovascular effects, due to increased intrathoracic pressure:
    - reduced venous return and cardiac output; may reduce BP, especially in autonomic neuropathy or hypovolaemia.
    - increased pulmonary vascular resistance, reducing right ventricular output.
    - reduced left ventricular compliance and filling, especially with PEEP. Bulging of the right ventricle and direct effects of lung expansion are thought to be responsible.
    - measured CVP is raised, and venous drainage from head and neck is reduced. ICP may increase.
  - respiratory effects:
    - intrapleural pressure is about -5 cmH_2O during expiration and up to $+5$ cmH_2O during inspiration, in contrast to spontaneous ventilation.
    - lung compliance and FRC fall. Atelectasis occurs in dependent lung tissue, increasing alveolar–arterial O_2 difference and dead space. Adding PEEP and increasing tidal volume may reduce these effects.
  - others:
    - renal: reduced arterial BP and increased venous pressure lower renal perfusion. Glomerular filtration is reduced, and the renin/angiotensin system stimulated. Atrial natriuretic peptide secretion is lowered and vasopressin secretion may be increased. The overall effect is reduced urine output (by up to 40%) and sodium retention.
    - ileus is common with prolonged IPPV; the cause is unclear but may involve changes in GIT neural activity and pressures. It may also be related to concurrent illness or drug therapy.
    - risks of tracheal intubation.
    - barotrauma, undetected disconnection.

[Andreas Vesalius (1514–1564), German anatomist; Robert Hooke (1635–1703), Curator of the Royal Society, England]

See also, Intermittent negative pressure ventilation; Intubation, tracheal; Ventilator-associated lung injury

Internal jugular venous cannulation. The internal jugular vein lies deep to the sternomastoid muscle, and follows a course from just anterior to the mastoid process to behind the sternoclavicular joint (Fig. 84). Cannulation may be performed at a number of sites; the most common are outlined below.

- Technique:
  - head-down position distends the vein and reduces the risk of air embolism. The head is turned to the contralateral side. Aseptic techniques are used.
  - the distended vein may be palpable (or even visible) in thin subjects, lateral to the carotid pulsation.
  - a right side approach is usually employed, since the right internal jugular vein, superior vena cava and right atrium are more directly aligned than on the left.
  - local anaesthetic is used if the patient is awake.
  - high approach:
    - the carotid pulsation is located level with the cricoid cartilage (C6). With the fingers of one hand guarding the artery, the needle is introduced just laterally, angled at 30° to the skin and directed towards the ipsilateral nipple. When blood is aspirated, the needle is lowered to align it more with the vein, and the cannula advanced or wire inserted (Seldinger technique). If no blood is aspirated, the needle may be redirected slightly medially. Some prefer to locate the vein with a small needle first before using the larger introducer needle.
    - alternatively, a slightly lower approach involves needle insertion at the apex of the triangle formed by the two heads of sternomastoid, a more reliable landmark when the carotid pulsation is weak or absent (e.g. cardiac arrest).
  - low approach: the needle is introduced just above the sternoclavicular joint and directed caudally. A higher incidence of pneumothorax may result from this approach.

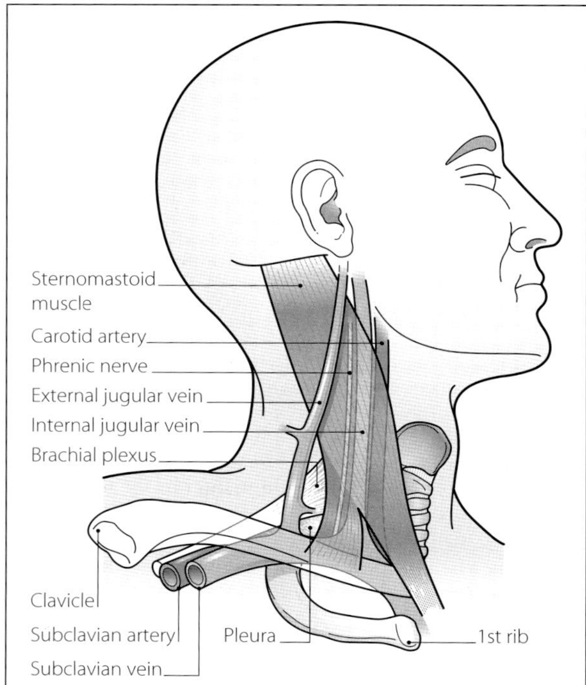

Fig. 84 Anatomy of right internal jugular vein

The routine use of ultrasound probes for location of the vein is now recommended by NICE.
See also, Central venous cannulation, for complications and comparisons with other techniques

International classification injury severity score (ICISS). Trauma scale based on the International Classification of Diseases 9th edition (ICD-9). Has the advantage that most hospitals use the ICD for routine admission and discharge coding. Has been used for predicting survival, costing treatment and assessing outcome. Initial trials suggest it is superior in this respect to the injury severity score and trauma revised injury severity score.
Rutledge R, Osler T, Emery S, Kromhout-Schiro S (1998). J Trauma; 44: 41–9

International Liaison Committee on Resuscitation (ILCOR). Formed in 1992 to provide a forum for liaison between principal resuscitation organisations worldwide. Currently comprises the American Heart Association, the European Resuscitation Council, the Heart and Stroke Foundation of Canada, the Australian and New Zealand Resuscitation Council, the Resuscitation Councils of Southern Africa, the Inter American Heart Foundation and the Resuscitation Council of Asia. It aims to provide consensus opinions on all aspects of resuscitation by considering international research and knowledge relevant to emergency cardiac care, thereby producing consistent international guidelines. ILCOR produced its first advisory statements in 1997.

International normalised ratio, *see Coagulation studies*

Internet. Worldwide network with an estimated 1.4 billion users in 2008. Medical uses include communication (including patient–doctor communication) via email, discussion groups/fora, fax and transmission of files, and remote access to expert systems, databases (e.g. scientific literature, medical registers), documents (e.g. guidelines, official reports), educational resources and patients' records. Strictly, 'intranet' refers to a network within an organisation, while 'internet' refers to links between remote locations and 'Internet' refers to the global network that uses standard communication protocols (IP protocols). The distinction is often blurred and the latter two terms are often used interchangeably. In the UK, 'NHS Connecting for Health', an agency of the Department of Health, was formed in 2005 with the aim of establishing an NHS-wide infrastructure for sharing patients' records, enabling GPs to book hospital appointments directly, and developing electronic prescribing. The project has excited considerable controversy, especially over security of data and spiralling costs.

Interonium distance. Distance between quaternary ammonium groups in molecules of non-depolarising neuromuscular blocking drugs. Thought to relate to drug activity in blocking acetylcholine receptor sites, thought originally to be placed 1.2–1.4 nm apart. Drugs with interonium distances of 0.6–0.7 nm are also active, suggesting cross-linkage between drugs or receptors.

Interpleural analgesia. Injection of local anaesthetic agent into the pleural cavity, performed for analgesia after thoracic and upper abdominal surgery and in rib fractures. Unilateral pain is the most suitable indication. An epidural catheter may be placed either under direct vision during thoracotomy, or via an epidural needle; the midaxillary line or ~10 cm from the dorsal midline, in the 4th–8th interspace is usually employed. The pleural space is identified using a loss of resistance syringe, allowing the syringe plunger to be drawn in by the negative interpleural pressure, or a catheter is pushed through the needle as the latter is advanced; unobstructed passage of the catheter occurs when the parietal pleura is punctured. Alternatively, to avoid entrainment of air when the syringe is removed from the needle, a continuous infusion of saline attached via a three-way tap to the epidural needle allows demonstration of the negative pressure by free flow of saline; the catheter may be threaded though the needle without detaching the saline infusion. Advancement of the needle is during the expiratory phase. Alternatively, straw-coloured pleural fluid may be aspirated. 8–30 ml of 0.25–0.5% bupivacaine with adrenaline has been used, producing up to 24 hours' analgesia. 0.1–0.5 ml/kg/h infusion has also been used. Gravity and positioning may be used to extend the block if inadequate. Solution may also be instilled through a pleural drain. Mechanism of analgesia is unclear, but is thought to involve blockade of intercostal nerves.

Complications are uncommon, and include pneumothorax, local anaesthetic toxicity (maximal levels occur within 20 min of bolus injection), phrenic, recurrent laryngeal or sympathetic nerve blockade and haemorrhage.
Dravid RM, Paul RE (2007). Anaesthesia; 62: 1039–49 and 1143–53

Interstitial fibrosis, *see Pulmonary fibrosis*

Interstitial fluid. Fluid compartment comprising most of the ECF. Volume is approximately 9.5 litres, about 14% of body weight of an average man; it is determined by subtracting plasma volume from ECF volume.
See also, Fluids, body, for composition, etc.

Intestinal obstruction. Physical impairment of transit of GIT contents, to be distinguished from ileus. May be caused by impaction within the lumen (e.g. faeces, foreign object), narrowing arising within the GIT wall (e.g. tumours, strictures) or compression from outside the GIT wall (e.g. strangulation, adhesions). In acute obstruction, gas and intestinal secretions accumulate causing distension of the GIT proximal to the obstruction, resulting in pain, increased bowel activity and vomiting (especially in high obstruction). Dehydration and electrolyte disturbances may rapidly develop. If severe and unrelieved, obstruction may lead to bowel ischaemia, necrosis and perforation. Abdominal X-rays may reveal dilated loops of bowel with fluid levels.

Treatment includes nasogastric intubation and iv fluid replacement; surgery is often required. Anaesthetic and ICU considerations are those of emergency surgery in general, especially relating to dehydration, the risk of aspiration of gastric contents and sepsis if perforation occurs.

Chronic obstruction presents with distension and constipation; emergency surgery is less often indicated although acute-on-chronic obstruction may occur. Malnutrition is more likely to be present than in acute obstruction.

Intra-abdominal pressure (IAP). Usually measured using a closed urinary drainage system, with the bladder acting as a transducer. Has also been measured using nasogastric or gastrostomy tubes. IAP is normally subatmospheric to zero relative to the symphysis pubis. In animals, IAP > 10 mmHg has potentially deleterious effects on hepatic arterial flow, and > 20 mmHg on mesenteric and bowel mucosal blood flow, portal venous flow and intestinal barrier function. In humans, there seems to be a strong relationship between IAP > 20 mmHg and subsequent development of renal failure.

There is consensus that abdominal decompression should occur at levels of IAP > 20–25 mmHg.

Malbrain ML, Cheatham ML, Kirkpatrick A, et al (2006). Intensive Care Med; 32: 1722–32 and Cheatham ML, Malbrain ML, Kirkpatrick A (2007). Intensive Care Med; 33: 951–62

See also, Abdominal compartment syndrome

Intra-abdominal sepsis. The leading cause of death in general surgical practice. May involve a wide variety of anaerobic and aerobic organisms; bacterial translocation has been implicated in many cases.

- Caused by:
  - spontaneous intra-abdominal disease (60%), e.g. perforated appendix, diverticulitis, primary liver abscess, perforated colonic cancer, pancreatitis, etc.
  - trauma (10%).
  - complications of abdominal surgery (30%), especially colonic and biliary.
- Diagnosis:
  - clinical: fever, leucocytosis, localised tenderness.
  - ultrasound: fluid collection may be demonstrated.
  - radiological:
    - plain abdominal X-ray may reveal abnormal fluid and/or gas collections.
    - contrast studies may reveal filling defects suggesting abscess.
    - radiolabelled leucocyte scan or gallium 67 imaging: may reveal collections.
    - abdominal/pelvic CT scan: in general, more sensitive than the above.

If sepsis is strongly suspected, exploratory laparotomy should be performed even in the absence of positive imaging tests.

- Management:
  - prevention: maintenance of careful asepsis during surgery; preoperative bowel preparation; prophylactic antibiotics.
  - treatment: general resuscitation; antibiotic therapy; drainage by either an open surgical procedure or using CT or ultrasound guidance of catheters.

See also, Peritonitis

Intra-aortic counter-pulsation balloon pump. Device used to support cardiac output by inflating a balloon within the descending aorta at the beginning of diastole, with deflation immediately before systole. Introduced percutaneously, e.g. via the femoral artery, and inflated with helium or CO_2. Triggered and timed according to the ECG and arterial waveform. Increases coronary and tissue blood flow, with reduced afterload and left ventricular work; i.e. increases myocardial O_2 supply whilst decreasing demand.

Used as a temporary measure, e.g. in left ventricular failure and cardiogenic shock pre/post cardiac surgery or after MI. Complications include trauma, haemorrhage, etc. during insertion, aortic dissection and rupture, distal thrombus, embolism and ischaemia, and damage to platelets and red cells.

Intra-arterial regional anaesthesia. Injection of local anaesthetic agent, e.g. 10–20 ml 0.5% lidocaine, into the brachial artery, a tourniquet having been inflated proximally to above systolic BP. Produces anaesthesia of the arm using smaller amounts of drug than for IVRA, but now rarely performed. Described in 1908 by Goyanes.

[J Goyanes (1876–1964), Spanish surgeon]

Intracellular fluid. Similar in composition between different cells; thus considered a single fluid compartment comprising about 28 litres (40% of body weight) in an average man. Determined by subtracting ECF from total body water (measured using a dilution technique with deuterium oxide).

See also, Fluids, body, for composition, etc.

Intracranial haemorrhage, *see Cerebrovascular accident; Extradural haemorrhage; Head injury; Subarachnoid haemorrhage; Subdural haemorrhage*

Intracranial pressure (ICP). Pressure exerted by the CSF in the frontal horns of the lateral ventricles of the brain. Normally 7–17 mmHg (1–2 kPa) supine; fluctuations may be revealed by ICP monitoring. Because the skull is a rigid box, and its contents incompressible, ICP depends on the volume of intracranial contents: normally 50–70 ml blood (5–7%), 50–120 ml CSF (5–12%), and 1.4 kg brain tissue (80–85%) (*see Monro–Kellie doctrine*).

- Effects of increased intracranial volume:
  - movement of CSF into the spinal canal, increased absorption of CSF into the venous circulation, and venous sinus compression. Thus ICP is maintained at near normal levels initially.
  - eventually, compensatory mechanisms are overwhelmed; small changes in volume are now accompanied by large increases in ICP (Fig. 85).
  - as ICP rises, cerebral perfusion pressure and cerebral blood flow are decreased. When venous blood vessels are obstructed, massive swelling occurs. Regional ischaemia, structural distortion and coning may follow. During surgery, raised ICP is prevented by the open skull, but the brain may bulge and hinder surgery or closure.
  - clinical features:
    - headache, nausea/vomiting, confusion. Headache is classically worse in the early morning and exacerbated by stooping or straining.
    - papilloedema (may take 24 h of raised ICP for it to occur), impaired consciousness, hypertension and bradycardia (Cushing's reflex) as ICP continues to rise.
    - hypotension, coma, irregular respiration or apnoea, fixed and dilated pupils.
- Raised ICP is caused by increased volume of the following compartments:
  - blood:
    - increased cerebral blood flow due to cerebral vasodilatation, e.g. with use of volatile anaesthetic agents.
    - impaired venous drainage, e.g. coughing, straining, kinked jugular veins, head-down position.
  - brain:
    - tumour, abscess, haematoma.
    - cerebral oedema.
  - CSF: as for hydrocephalus.

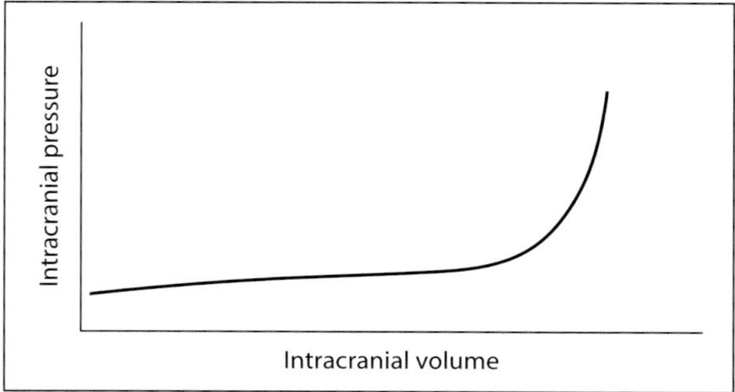

Fig. 85 Effects of increasing intracranial volume on intracranial pressure

Rarely, 'benign' (idiopathic) intracranial hypertension is associated with none of the above, especially in young women. It may cause permanent visual impairment due to optic nerve damage. Its management includes repeated lumbar CSF drainage, corticosteroids, acetazolamide and shunt insertion.

- Treatment of raised ICP involves reduction in volume of:
  - blood:
    - IPPV with hyperventilation to arterial $P\text{CO}_2$ 3.5–4 kPa (27–30 mmHg), to produce cerebral vasoconstriction. Effectiveness may be limited to 24–48 h.
    - encouragement of venous drainage: head-up posture, adequate sedation/relaxation, avoiding jugular compression/kinking.
  - brain:
    - surgical decompression.
    - diuretics and corticosteroids in certain circumstances (*see Cerebral oedema*).
    - fluid restriction to 1.5–2 l/day is often instituted.
  - CSF: drainage, e.g. via the lateral ventricle. Long-term shunts as for hydrocephalus.
- Effects of anaesthetic agents on ICP:
  - iv agents: barbiturates, etomidate, propofol, benzodiazepines: reduce ICP. Opioids: no change or reduction, if normocapnia is maintained. Ketamine increases ICP.
  - inhalational agents: halothane, enflurane, isoflurane, sevoflurane and desflurane: cause a dose-dependent increase in ICP via increasing cerebral blood flow. The effect is counteracted by hyperventilation and hypocapnia; this must be achieved before introduction of halothane or enflurane to prevent the rise in ICP but this is not necessary for isoflurane. N_2O may increase ICP via increased blood flow, or if air is contained in cavities within the skull, e.g. following surgery, head injury, etc.
  - others: non-depolarising neuromuscular blocking drugs cause no change in ICP since they do not cross the blood–brain barrier. Suxamethonium may cause a transient increase during fasciculation, due to an increase in intrathoracic pressure. ICP is increased by laryngoscopy and tracheal intubation.
  - hypotensive drugs: ICP may increase following sodium nitroprusside and nitrates, probably via increased intracranial blood volume due to vasodilatation. No rise is associated with trimetaphan.

Anaesthesia for patients with raised ICP: as for neurosurgery.

Smith M (2008). Anesth Analg; 106: 240–8

See also, Cerebral protection/resuscitation

Intracranial pressure monitoring. Indications vary between units but may include any cause of coma and raised ICP, most commonly head injury, intracranial haemorrhage, postoperatively, encephalopathies, etc. Associated with significant risk of infection, especially with over 3 days' use.

- Types of monitoring:
  - extradural fibreoptic probe, laid between the dura and skull via a burr hole. Easy to position, with low infection rates. CSF drainage is impossible, and accuracy is less reliable. Fully implantable devices have been described.
  - subarachnoid screw, applied via a burr hole. Easy to position, but infection rate is higher. More accurate unless oedema is present. CSF drainage is sometimes possible. Subdural catheters have also been described.
  - ventricular drain, placed during craniotomy, although the ventricle may be difficult to cannulate in the presence of brain swelling. Once placed, therapeutic drainage of CSF is easy. Infection risk is the highest (3–5%), especially if in situ for over 3 days. Fibreoptic devices may also be used, or a catheter attached to a subcutaneous device for percutaneous puncture, for chronic use.
  - intracerebral transducer, placed within brain tissue itself.

Devices are flushed infrequently using small volumes (under 0.2 ml). Continuous flow apparatus is not used. Output is best displayed as a continuous recording, ideally with simultaneous calculation of cerebral perfusion pressure, e.g. using a computer. Injecting small volumes into the ventricular system has been used to calculate ventricular compliance or pressure/volume index (volume required to raise CSF pressure by a factor of 10); these indices of distensibility are not routinely performed. The waveform obtained resembles the arterial waveform, corresponding to the pulsation of large vessels within the brain. The waveform also varies with respiration, reflecting changes in CVP. Mean ICP is calculated in a similar way to MAP and is normally 7–15 mmHg (1–2 kPa) in the supine position.

- Three variations in ICP waveform have been described:
  - A (plateau) waves: amplitude 50–100 mmHg, they last 5–20 min. Associated with cerebral vasodilatation. Most common in patients with intracranial tumours and often represent severely reduced intracranial compliance.
  - B waves: amplitude < 50 mmHg; occur at about 1/min. Associated with changes in respiratory pattern. Less useful clinically. Variations of B waves ('ramp waves') are seen in hydrocephalus.
  - C waves: amplitude < 20 mmHg; occur at 4–8/min. Related to systemic vasomotor tone and BP. Not useful clinically.

Active management is usually advocated at pressures exceeding 15–30 mmHg (2–3 kPa), depending on the underlying condition, speed of deterioration and clinical situation.

Steiner LA, Andrews PJD (2006). Br J Anaes; 97: 26–38

Intractable pain, *see Pain; Pain management*

Intradural . . ., *see Spinal . . .*

Intramucosal pH, *see Gastric tonometry*

Intraocular pressure (IOP). Normally 1.3–2 kPa (10–15 mmHg), increased in glaucoma. Important during open ophthalmic surgery because of the risk of expulsion of intraocular contents and haemorrhage, with subsequent distortion of anatomy, scarring and loss of vision.

- Related to:
  - external pressure on the eye:
    - from facepiece, leaning on the eye, etc.
    - retrobulbar haematoma.
    - extrinsic muscles.
    - venous congestion of orbit.
  - scleral rigidity: increased in severe myopia and in the elderly.
  - intraocular contents:
    - choroidal blood volume:
      - increases with arterial $P\text{CO}_2$ and hypoxaemia, and vasodilatation.
      - increases transiently with acute rises in systolic BP; falls at systolic pressure of under 80–90 mmHg.
      - increases with CVP, e.g. due to straining, coughing, vomiting, head-down or prone position, etc.
    - aqueous humour:
      - formed by the choroidal plexus of the posterior chamber, at about 0.08 ml/h. A small amount is formed in the anterior chamber.

- passes through the pupil to the anterior chamber; drains from the angle between the iris and cornea via the canal of Schlemm into the venous circulation.
- reduced by acetazolamide, although it also increases choroidal blood volume. Also reduced by oral glycerol and meiosis. Control is important in glaucoma, but less so during surgery.

- vitreous humour: may be reduced by administration of mannitol 0.5–1.5 g/kg iv, 45 min preoperatively. Urinary catheterisation is usually required. Sucrose 50% 1 g/kg is shorter acting.
- other structures, e.g. lens.
- sulphur hexafluoride (SF_6) is sometimes injected into the vitreous in retinal surgery to splint the retina; N_2O markedly expands the SF_6 volume and increases IOP by diffusing into the bubble faster than SF_6 diffuses out (blood/gas solubility of N_2O is over 100 times that of SF_6). When N_2O is stopped at the end of surgery, IOP may decrease markedly. N_2O is therefore usually discontinued before SF_6 injection, to reduce large swings in IOP. Atmospheric nitrogen diffuses into the bubble postoperatively, but its effect is smaller and slower because its blood/gas solubility is only 2–3 times that of SF_6.

- Effects of anaesthetic agents on IOP:
  - little effect, if any, of premedicant drugs.
  - no effect of atropine, unless administered topically to glaucomatous eyes (IOP may rise).
  - reduced by all iv induction agents except ketamine; propofol and etomidate cause a greater reduction than thiopental.
  - reduced slightly by benzodiazepines and neuroleptanaesthesia.
  - reduced by all volatile agents; the mechanism is unclear. Unaffected by N_2O.
  - increased by suxamethonium, possibly via choroidal vasodilatation and extrinsic eye muscle contraction, although the increase in IOP still occurs when the muscles are cut. The increase lasts only a few minutes. The use of suxamethonium in the presence of penetrating eye injury is controversial (*see Eye, penetrating injury*).
  - non-depolarising neuromuscular blocking drugs may lower IOP slightly.

Anaesthesia for open eye operations thus involves avoidance of factors increasing IOP, e.g. straining, vomiting, etc. and use of techniques and drugs which lower IOP, e.g. head-up tilt, hypocapnia, smooth anaesthesia, etc.

IOP is estimated by measuring corneal indentation by a weighted plunger, or by measuring the force required to flatten an area of cornea.

[Friedrich Schlemm (1795–1858), German anatomist]

Intraosseous fluid administration. Technique of infusing fluids though a metal cannula into the bone marrow and thence, via a system of non-collapsible veins, into the general circulation. Used for the resuscitation of infants and children under 6 years when conventional venous access is not available (the technique becomes more difficult in older children and adults). The upper tibia (anteromedial surface 1–3 cm below the tibial tuberosity) is the most common site chosen; the iliac crest may be used in older children. A dedicated needle and trocar kit is used to pierce the thin bony cortex, advancement continuing until a loss of resistance is felt. A firm hold of the needle by the bone and easy injection of saline without obvious subcutaneous infiltration suggest correct placement. Aspiration of marrow is not always possible, but if successful, samples can be used for cross-matching. All standard drugs may be given by this route; they should be flushed through with 5–10 ml saline to ensure they reach the circulation. Fluids should be given under pressure to overcome venous resistance. Osteomyelitis is the major complication and can be minimised by sterile technique and by reverting to conventional venous cannulation following resuscitation. Compartment syndrome has been reported.

Intrapleural pressure. Pressure within the pleural cavity, perhaps better termed interpleural pressure. Measured indirectly using a balloon catheter placed within the lower third of the oesophagus (i.e. within the thorax but outside the lungs). Normally negative, due to the thoracic cage's tendency to spring outwards, and the lungs' tendency to collapse inwards. In the erect posture at normal resting lung volume, intrapleural pressure equals approximately −10 cm H_2O at the lung apex, −2.5 cm H_2O at the base.

Increases in magnitude as lung volume (and thus elastic recoil) increases. During spontaneous ventilation, it thus becomes more negative during inspiration. Normally changes by 3–4 cm H_2O, more if airway resistance is increased or breathing forceful. During expiration, it returns to its original value unless expiration is forced or resistance increased; it may then exceed zero.

During IPPV, pressure increases from the resting value, depending on the inflating pressure (usually by 10–20 cm H_2O). Thus it usually exceeds zero during inspiration. Increased by CPAP and PEEP (i.e. towards or beyond zero).

Intrathecal . . ., *see Spinal* . . .

Intravenous anaesthetic agents. Development of drugs and iv techniques occurred later than for inhalational anaesthetic agents, but iv induction of anaesthesia is usually preferred now because it is faster with less risk of excitement, laryngospasm, etc. Popularised in the 1930s by Weese, Lundy and Waters, although Oré had used iv chloral hydrate in 1872. Subsequent agents include hedonal (1905), phenobarbital (1912), paraldehyde (1913), bromethol (1927), hexobarbital (1932; the first widely used iv barbiturate), thiopental (1932), hydroxydione (1955), methohexital (1957), propanidid (1956), γ-hydroxybutyric acid (1962), ketamine (1965), Althesin (1971), etomidate (1973) and propofol (1986). Diethyl ether has been injected iv.

Used for induction and maintenance of anaesthesia, including TIVA, and for sedation. Many iv agents have also been given im or rectally. Benzodiazepines, e.g. midazolam, have been used for induction, as have high doses of opioid analgesic drugs.

- Have been classified thus:
  - rapid onset:
    - barbiturates: thiopental, methohexital.
    - imidazole compounds: etomidate.
    - alkyl phenol: propofol.
    - corticosteroids: Althesin, minaxolone, hydroxydione.
    - eugenols: propanidid.
  - slow onset:
    - ketamine.
    - benzodiazepines.
    - opioids.
- Features of the ideal iv anaesthetic agent:
  - physical/chemical properties:
    - chemically stable; i.e. not requiring storage in a fridge or away from light. Long shelf-life.
    - water-soluble, not requiring reconstitution before use, nor any additives.
    - compatible with iv fluids, other drugs, etc.

- pharmacology:
  - painless on injection, with low incidence of thrombophlebitis. Harmless on extravasation or intra-arterial injection.
  - low incidence of adverse drug reactions.
  - smooth onset of anaesthesia within one arm–brain circulation time, without unwanted movement, coughing, hiccup, etc.
  - anticonvulsant, antiemetic and analgesic properties. No increase in cerebral blood flow, ICP or intraocular pressure. Reduces $CMRO_2$.
  - no respiratory depression. Bronchodilator.
  - no cardiovascular depression or stimulation, or arrhythmias.
  - predictable recovery, related to the dose injected.
  - rapid metabolism to non-active metabolites; i.e. non-cumulative.
  - no impairment of renal or hepatic function or corticosteroid synthesis.
  - no emergence phenomena.
  - no teratogenicity.

No currently available agent fulfils all of the above (Table 20).

Agents should be injected slowly, titrating against effect, especially if the patient has reduced cardiac output. Overdose is easily produced by rapid injection of a large dose.

- Following iv injection, brain levels depend on the amount of drug crossing the blood–brain barrier, related to:
  - protein-binding.
  - ionisation; e.g. at pH of 7.4, 61% of thiopental and over 90% of propofol is unionised.
  - cerebral blood flow: increased as a proportion of cardiac output in hypovolaemia, etc.
  - fat solubility: high for most anaesthetic agents; propofol and ketamine are particularly fat soluble.
  - distribution, metabolism and excretion.

Recovery from, e.g. thiopental occurs by redistribution from vessel-rich tissues (brain, heart, liver, kidney; 70–80% of cardiac output) to vessel-intermediate tissues (muscle, skin; 18% of cardiac output), thence to fat (6%) and vessel-poor tissues such as ligaments, etc. (Fig. 86). Thus significant amounts of thiopental remain in the body after recovery, compared with more rapidly metabolised agents, e.g. propofol.

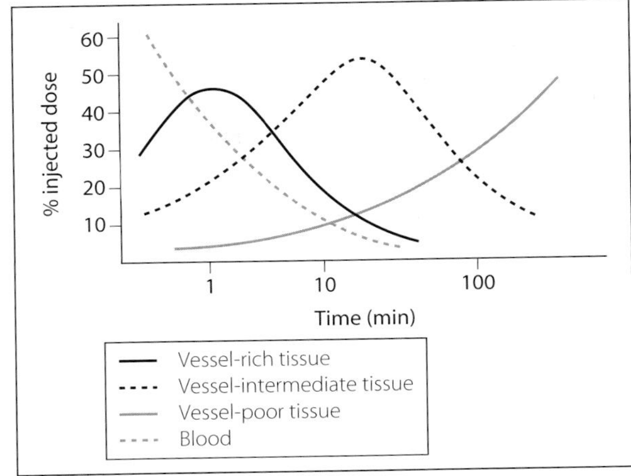

Fig. 86 Fate of thiopental after iv injection

See also, Pharmacokinetics

Intravenous fluid administration. Described in the 1600s. Saline solutions were used sporadically in dehydration due to cholera, diabetes mellitus and diarrhoea in the 1800s. Infusions were widely used in World War I, including acacia as a colloid. Bacterial and chemical contamination and allergic reactions were common. Sterile fluids and administration sets became available in World War II; increasing investigation into fluid balance since then was prompted by subsequent wars, e.g. Korea, Vietnam. Balanced fluid therapy was developed in the 1950s–1960s.

- Practical considerations:
  - site of administration: usually forearm, since it is the least awkward for the patient. The arm or hand is preferred to the legs, since venous stasis is commoner in the latter. Placement near joints or known arteries is avoided when possible. Central venous cannulation is used for irritant or vasoactive drugs, if peripheral cannulation is unsuccessful or if long-term administration or CVP measurement is required.
  - cannulation: venous filling is increased by gentle slapping, squeezing of the hand, or immersion of the limb in

Table 20 Properties of iv anaesthetic agents

Agent	*Thiopentone*	*Methohexital*	*Ketamine*	*Etomidate*	*Propofol*	*Midazolam*
Additives	Sodium carbonate	Sodium carbonate	Benzethonium chloride	Propylene glycol	Soya-bean oil emulsion	–
Aqueous solution	+	+	+	–	–	+
Approximate cost/induction dose in UK (£)	3	unavailable	2–4	1–2	2–4	2–4
Painful injection	–	+	–	+	+	–
Rapid onset	+	+	–	+	+	–
Unwanted movement	–	+	±	+	–	–
Respiratory/cardiovascular depression	+	+	–	±	+	±
Analgesic	–	–	+	–	–	–
Vomiting	–	–	+	+	–	–
Steroid inhibition	–	–	–	+	–	–
Rapid recovery	+	+	–	+	+	–
Emergence phenomena	–	–	+	–	–	–
pK_a	7.6	7.9	7.5	4.2	11	6.2
Protein-binding (%)	85	85	12	75	98	98
Volume of distribution (l/kg)	1.5–2.5	1–2	2–3	2–5	3–5	1–2
Distribution half-life (min)	2–6	5–6	10–15	1–4	1–2	7–15
Elimination half-life (h)	5–10	2–4	2–3	1–5	1–5	2–5
Clearance (ml/kg/min)	2–4	10–12	18–20	18–25	25–30	6–11

warm water for 10 min. Intradermal injection of local anaesthetic or use of EMLA reduces the pain of insertion of large cannulae. Attempts are made to cannulate distal veins first, moving proximally if unsuccessful. Rarely, cut-down may be required:
- an anatomically constant venous site is chosen, e.g. long saphenous vein (above and anterior to the medial malleolus).
- the vein is exposed and two ties placed around it; only the distal one is tightened.
- the cannula is introduced and secured with the proximal tie.

- cannulae: plastic cannulae were developed in the 1970s. Their general design is similar but flow characteristics differ widely between different makes. More recent designs incorporate protective mechanisms to prevent needlestick injury, e.g. a metal clip or plastic cover that automatically shields the sharp point when the needle is withdrawn from the cannula. British Standard for determining flow rate: a constant pressure of 10 kPa is maintained using a constant level tank of distilled water at 22°C. It is connected via 110 cm tubing (inside diameter 4 mm) to the cannula, with the distal 4 cm and the cannula horizontal. The volume of water is collected over at least 30 s; an average of three readings is taken. Thus the flows are different from those achieved clinically, but the values are useful for comparison between differently sized cannulae:
  - 10 G: 550–600 ml/min.
  - 12 G: 400–500 ml/min.
  - 14 G: 250–360 ml/min.
  - 16 G: 130–220 ml/min.
  - 18 G: 75–120 ml/min.
  - 20 G: 40–80 ml/min.

  Gauge ('G') numbers are equivalent to those used for needles. Recently introduced colour-coding standard for iv cannulae:
  - 14 G: orange
  - 16 G: grey
  - 18 G: green
  - 20 G: pink
  - 22 G: blue
  - 24 G: yellow
  - 26 G: black
- giving sets: internal diameter is 4 mm, but extra turbulence and resistance arise from extra length, drip chambers and filter (170 μm pore size). Non-blood giving sets have no filter or float, and are narrower and cheaper.
- syringe pumps, volumetric pumps, drip counters, etc.; high pressures may occur with the former two if obstruction to flow occurs. Some syringe pumps may empty rapidly if placed above the patient.
- microfiltration: not routinely used, but 0.2 μm filters are claimed to reduce phlebitis, especially when repeated drug injections are given. They may also retain endotoxin and prevent air embolism. The routine use of blood filters is controversial.

● Hazards:
- during cannulation: haemorrhage, haematoma, trauma.
- extravasation: especially harmful if the fluid is irritant, e.g. potassium or bicarbonate solutions, thiopental, antimitotic drugs, etc. Flushing with saline, hyaluronidase or corticosteroids has been suggested as treatment.
- thrombophlebitis: venous thrombosis accompanied by venous wall inflammation. Superficial thrombophlebitis does not lead to DVT. More common with small veins and highly concentrated or irritant infusates. Reduced if infusion sites are changed regularly, e.g. 24–48 hourly. Features include pain, redness of the overlying skin and hardening of the vein; there may be swelling and systemic features (e.g. pyrexia) if infection is involved. Infusion life may be prolonged with a GTN patch applied topically. Addition of heparin or hydrocortisone to the fluid bag has also been used. Heparinoid cream is often applied to existing phlebitis.
- interactions between infused drugs or fluids, especially if multiple infusions are used through a single cannula.
- air embolism.
- related to the iv fluid infused, e.g. hyponatraemia, pulmonary oedema, etc.
- when one cannula is used for more than one infusion, temporary blockage of the cannula may lead to one infusion (e.g. of a drug) retrogradely filling the tubing of the second infusion (e.g. a saline infusion), especially if the former is driven by a pump. When the obstruction is relieved, a bolus of drug may be delivered instead of a saline flush; therefore a non-return valve/connector should be used.

Fluids may also be delivered into the circulation by intraosseous fluid administration; other routes, e.g. rectal, im or sc administration (the latter two aided by hyaluronidase), are rarely used now.

See also, Venous drainage of arm

Intravenous fluids. May be divided into colloids and crystalloids (Table 21).

● Simplistic effects of infused fluid on body fluid compartments:
- initial expansion of the vascular compartment. Extent and duration depend on whether it can freely cross the vascular endothelium; i.e. crystalloids do, colloids do so only slowly, e.g. gelatin solutions after a few hours. Colloids may draw water into the vascular space by osmosis in addition to the volume infused (hence 'plasma expanders').
- expansion of the interstitial fluid compartment as fluids pass into it from the vascular compartment. Fluids distribute within the ECF thus: ¾ in interstitial fluid, ¼ in plasma.
- expansion of the intracellular space. Water moves across cell membranes by osmosis only if osmolality on one side of the membrane changes. Thus, if saline 0.9% is added to ECF, osmolality is unchanged, and thus no movement of water occurs; i.e. saline is confined to ECF. With dextrose solutions, the dextrose is rapidly metabolised by erythrocytes, leaving water. The water enters the ECF causing dilution; thus water moves into the cells by osmosis.

● Summary:
- colloids cause greater expansion of the vascular compartment for the volume infused, and are ideally suited to replace plasma/blood losses.
- saline 0.9% and Hartmann's solution expand ECF (¾ interstitial, ¼ plasma), and are ideally suited to replace ECF losses.
- dextrose 5% expands total body water (⅓ ECF, ⅔ interstitial). Thus only 1/12 infused volume of dextrose 5% remains in the vascular compartment. The main use of dextrose is to replenish a water deficit; infusing pure water would cause haemolysis.

See also, Bicarbonate; Colloid/crystalloid controversy; Dextrans; Haemorrhage; Hypertonic intravenous solutions; Intravenous fluid administration

Table 21 Compositions of commonly used iv fluids (in mmol/l unless otherwise stated)

Fluid	*Na^+*	*K^+*	*Ca^{2+}*	*Cl^-*	*Other*	*pH*
*Crystalloids**						
Saline 0.9% ('normal')	154	–	–	154	–	5.0
Dextrose 4%–saline 0.18%	30	–	–	30	Dextrose 40 g	4–5
Dextrose 5%	–	–	–	–	Dextrose 50 g	4.0
Hartmann's solution	131	5	2	111	Lactate 29	6.5
Bicarbonate						
8.4%	1000	–	–	–	HCO_3^- 1000	8.0
1.26%	150	–	–	–	HCO_3^- 150	7.0
Colloids†						
Haemaccel	145	5.1	6.25	145	Gelatin 35 g	7.4
Gelofusine	154	<0.4	<0.4	125	Gelatin 40 g Mg^{2+} <0.4	7.4
Hetastarch	154	–	–	154	Starch 60 g	5.5
Pentastarch	154	–	–	154	Starch 100 g	5.0
Albumin 4.5%	<160	<2	–	136	Albumin 40–50 g Citrate <15	7.4
Dextran						
In saline 0.9%: as above)	60 g dextran 70 or					4.5–5
In dextrose 5%: as above)	100 g dextran 40					5–6

*All have an osmolality of 280–300 mosmol/kg, except for bicarbonate 8.4% (200 mosmol/kg)
†Osmolality ranges between approximately 280 and 320 mosmol/kg

Intravenous oxygenator (IVOX). Intravascular gas exchange device, consisting of a 30–40 cm long bundle of hollow gas-permeable polypropylene fibres (internal diameter 200 μm), which may be introduced into the superior and inferior venae cavae via the right internal jugular or femoral veins. O_2 is passed under low pressure through the lumina of the fibres, whilst blood returning to the heart via normal channels flows over the fibres' external surfaces. O_2 passes into the blood from the fibres, and CO_2 passes in the opposite direction. Was used in the 1990s for acute respiratory failure but its use was hampered by technical and mechanical problems, e.g. obstruction of venous return, bleeding, etc. No longer available.

Intravenous regional anaesthesia (IVRA; Bier block). First described in 1908 by Bier, who injected procaine iv into an exsanguinated portion of the arm between two inflated tourniquets, to provide distal analgesia.

- Modern technique (described in the 1960s):
  - an iv cannula is placed in each hand.
  - the limb is exsanguinated by raising it with the brachial artery compressed, or by using a rubber bandage.
  - a tourniquet is inflated around the upper arm to a value higher than systolic BP (twice systolic BP is usually quoted).
  - local anaesthetic agent is injected slowly.
  - a more distal tourniquet may be inflated after 5–10 min and the original deflated, to reduce discomfort.
  - motor and sensory block occurs within 5–10 min.
  - for prolonged surgery, the cannula is left in situ. The cuff may be deflated after 60–90 min for 5 min, the arm re-emptied of blood and the tourniquet re-inflated. Half the initial dose is then injected. Thus safe tourniquet time is not exceeded.
- Solutions:
  - prilocaine is safest but lidocaine may also used; 3 mg/kg (0.6 ml/kg) 0.5% solution is suitable, without adrenaline. Preservative-free prilocaine is no longer available for IVRA, but solution containing preservative has been safely used for many years.
  - bupivacaine was previously used but is now contraindicated because of its cardiotoxicity.
- Mechanism of action is unclear, but may include:
  - compression by the tourniquet.
  - ischaemia.
  - drug action on nerve trunks.
  - drug action on nerve endings.
- IVRA is a potentially dangerous technique, involving direct iv injection of local anaesthetic; therefore the following must apply:
  - all equipment is checked for leaks, etc.
  - the patient is prepared and starved as for any local anaesthetic procedure, with resuscitative drugs and equipment available.
  - full monitoring is applied throughout.
  - rapid injection is avoided (may force solution past the tourniquet).
  - injection near the antecubital fossa is avoided (solution may be forced into the systemic circulation).
  - the technique is used with caution in patients with severe arteriosclerosis and hypertension, since the tourniquet may not completely compress their arteries. Similar caution has been suggested in obesity.
  - avoidance has been suggested in prepubertal children, since intraosseous vessels may allow local anaesthetic to bypass the tourniquet.
  - the tourniquet is deflated after at least 20 min. Intermittent deflation/reinflation has been suggested to reduce blood drug levels, e.g. deflation for 5–10 s, inflation for 1 s, etc.
  - not to be used in patients with sickle cell anaemia or trait.

May be used for the leg, although larger volumes are required, e.g. 1.0 ml/kg. The block may be less effective than in the arm.

Has also been used for sympathetic nerve block, e.g. using guanethidine 10–25 mg in 20 ml saline for the arm (30–40 mg in 40 ml for the leg); lidocaine or prilocaine is often added. The tourniquet is deflated after 10–20 min. Hypotension may occur up to several hours later. It may be repeated for several weeks, e.g. on alternate days.

Intrinsic activity. Ability of a substance, e.g. drug, to produce a response by interacting with a surface receptor. Refers to the amount of response produced, i.e. efficacy.
See also, Affinity

Intrinsic sympathomimetic activity (ISA). Ability of β-adrenergic receptor antagonists to stimulate β-adrenergic receptors as well as block them. Oxprenolol, labetalol, pindolol, celiprolol and acebutolol have ISA and are therefore partial agonists; they may cause less bradycardia than other β-receptor antagonists, although the importance of this is unclear.

Intubation aids. Used in difficult tracheal intubation.

- Designed for:
  - avoiding obstruction of the laryngoscope handle on the chest during insertion of the blade into the mouth:
    - laryngoscopes with adjustable handles or an increased angle between the blade and handle (e.g. polio laryngoscope blade).
    - adaptor to swing the handle to one side during insertion (Yentis adaptor).
    - short-handled laryngoscope.
  - improving the view of the glottis:
    - specialised laryngoscope blades.
    - fibreoptic instruments: may be flexible, rigid or malleable; extendable forceps, stylets, etc. may be attached.
    - optical devices and mirrors attached to or incorporated in the laryngoscope. The Huffman prism clips to a standard laryngoscope blade, allowing a view of the larynx by refracting light 30° from its original path. It must be warmed before use to prevent misting.
  - enabling intubation despite poor view:
    - long flexible introducer (often called a 'bougie' although this term refers to devices used for serial dilatation of strictures. Traditionally these were made of gum elastic). Usually bears an angled tip which assists placement through the larynx; may be inserted through the tracheal tube before intubation or may be placed first and the tracheal tube passed over it, with gentle rotation if required. It may be placed blindly; correct placement is suggested by feeling the tracheal rings during insertion, and feeling the distal end reach the carina. Directional bougies, controllable from their proximal end, are also available. Airway exchange catheters allow insufflation of O_2 during attempted intubation.
    - malleable stylet, inserted through the tube before intubation. Plastic-coated ones are less traumatic than those of bare metal; trauma is reduced by avoiding protrusion of the stylet from the distal end of the tube.
    - forceps to guide the tube.
    - some tracheal tubes are able to be flexed by pulling a cord within their walls, aiding direction during placement.
    - laryngoscope blades have been described which incorporate forceps, allowing manipulation of the tracheal tube.
    - hooks introduced orally for pulling the tube anteriorly.
  - allowing intubation without laryngoscopy:
    - malleable stylet with a bulb at its distal end (lightwand): passed through the tube and introduced through the mouth, with observation of the anterior neck. The light may be followed down the anterior larynx into the trachea; it disappears if intra-oesophageal.
    - intubating laryngeal mask airway: either blind technique or using a fibreoptic 'scope (the latter may also be passed through a standard laryngeal mask airway or other 'airway support' device).
    - retrograde epidural catheter technique: the catheter is introduced through the cricothyroid membrane via an epidural needle and passed upwards through the larynx and out of the mouth. The tracheal tube is advanced over it from the mouth into the trachea as the catheter is held from above. For nasal intubation, the catheter is tied with thread to a suction catheter passed through the nose and out through the mouth, then both are pulled out of the nose. Central venous cannulae, threads, etc., have also been used.
  - detecting oesophageal intubation.

[John P Huffman, US nurse-anaesthetist; SM Yentis, London anaesthetist]
See also, Intubation, difficult; Intubation, fibreoptic; Intubation, oesophageal; Intubation, tracheal

Intubation, awake. Indications:

  - known or suspected difficult airway or intubation, including an unstable cervical spine.
  - to isolate a leak and/or protect lung segments before applying IPPV, e.g. bronchopleural fistula, tracheo-oesophageal fistula.
  - in neonates: controversial, it is felt to be safer by many but with the possibility of causing undue stress, raised ICP, etc.
- Requires anaesthesia of the pharynx, larynx and trachea, and tongue or nasal passages:
  - nose: cocaine spray 4–10% to provide anaesthesia and vasoconstriction (3 mg/kg maximum). Alternatively, xylometazoline 0.1% and lidocaine 1–4% may be used.
  - tongue and oropharynx: benzocaine lozenge 100 mg, sucked 30 min beforehand.
  - pharynx and larynx above the vocal cords: lidocaine or prilocaine 1–4% via metered spray or swabs at increasing depths into the mouth, using a spatula or laryngoscope. Excessive dosage should not be administered. Glossopharyngeal nerve block has been used, but topical anaesthesia is easier to perform. Superior laryngeal nerve block provides anaesthesia of the epiglottis, base of tongue and mucosa down to the cords, and is performed either by holding a lidocaine-soaked pledget for 2–3 min in the piriform fossa on each side, e.g. using Krause's forceps, or by injecting 2–3 ml 1% lidocaine from the front of the neck just below the greater cornu of the hyoid bone on each side, with the bone displaced towards the side to be blocked with the operator's other hand. A click may be felt as the thyrohyoid membrane is pierced.
  - trachea and larynx below the cords: rapid transtracheal injection of 3–5 ml 1% lidocaine through the cricothyroid membrane, following aspiration of air to confirm correct placement. The patient is asked to breathe out fully before injection; the resultant inspiration and coughing aids spread of solution within the upper tracheobronchial tree. The 21–23 G needle is withdrawn immediately following injection to reduce the risk of breakage during coughing. Use of an iv cannula has been suggested to reduce the risk of this and trauma; the needle is removed leaving the plastic cannula before injection.

- nebulised 4% lidocaine may be used as the sole local anaesthetic.

Tracheal intubation then proceeds as usual, using laryngoscopy or a blind nasal technique.

The upper airways are rendered insensitive to aspirated material, and the patient should be kept nil by mouth for 4 h. Patients already at risk of regurgitation and aspiration are placed further at risk.

A similar technique may be used for awake fibreoptic bronchoscopy. Fibreoptic instruments for bronchoscopy/intubation have injection ports through which local anaesthetic may be sprayed as the 'scope is advanced.

See also, Intubation, blind nasal; Intubation, fibreoptic; Intubation, tracheal

Intubation, blind nasal. Technique of tracheal intubation without using laryngoscopes or other instruments; developed by Magill and Rowbotham as their first method of tracheal intubation (without use of neuromuscular blocking drugs). Of particular use in difficult intubation, since visualisation of the larynx is not required. Also used in awake intubation.

Originally described in spontaneously breathing patients, with use of 5–10% inspired CO_2 to increase ventilation. May also be performed in paralysed patients, although induction of muscle paralysis may be hazardous in difficult intubation. Use of CO_2 is now generally considered dangerous.

- Technique:
  - the patient's head is positioned in the 'sniffing position'.
  - a lubricated tracheal tube is inserted into a nostril (usually the right, since most bevels face left). Uncuffed rubber tubes were originally used; cuffed tubes are also suitable. Epistaxis may occur; it is reduced if a soft tube, little force and cocaine paste or spray are used. Trauma to the nasopharynx may also occur, and the incidence of bacteraemia is higher than with oral intubation.
  - the tube is passed into the pharynx, keeping the head extended and mandible elevated. The head is rotated slightly towards the side of the nostril used.
  - in spontaneous ventilation, the opposite nostril is occluded. Audible breath sounds from the tube are used as a guide to the position of the tube's tip; i.e. if they disappear, the tube is withdrawn slightly and redirected.
  - the tube is gently inserted further; it may:
    - enter the trachea in approximately a third of cases.
    - enter the oesophagus; the tube is partially withdrawn and reinserted with the head extended further. Posterior external pressure on the larynx may help.
    - meet obstruction level with the larynx; the tube's tip may be:
      - lateral to the glottis, e.g. in a piriform fossa, or against a false cord or arytenoid cartilage. A bulge may be visible at one side of the larynx at the front of the neck. The tube is partially withdrawn, rotated and reinserted. Head rotation or lateral external pressure on the larynx may help.
      - against the anterior part of the cricoid or in the vallecula; tube rotation or head flexion may help.

Practice is required to achieve proficiency. Differently curved tubes may be required. Inflation of the tracheal tube cuff when the tube's tip is in the oropharynx may help to centre it and aid insertion into the larynx.

See also, Intubation, awake; Intubation, difficult; Intubation, oesophageal; Intubation, tracheal

Intubation, complications of. Complications may occur at the time of tracheal intubation or afterwards.

- During intubation:
  - trauma:
    - caused by leaning on the eyes.
    - to the neck or jaw.
    - to the teeth, lips, nasal mucosa, mouth, tongue, pharynx, larynx, laryngeal nerves and trachea. Infection, surgical emphysema and bleeding may result. Rigid introducers and bougies are particularly traumatic. Nasal polyps, etc. may be carried into the trachea during nasal intubation.
  - hypertensive response:
    - associated with sympathetic activity and tachycardia.
    - may increase ICP and intraocular pressure.
    - particularly undesirable in patients with hypertension, ischaemic heart disease, etc.
    - caused by laryngoscopy alone; thus not obtunded by lidocaine spray.
    - methods to reduce the response:
      - antihypertensive drugs, e.g. β-adrenergic receptor antagonists, hydralazine, nitroglycerine, sodium nitroprusside. Some may be effective given orally, preoperatively, e.g. β-receptor antagonists, but bradycardia may occur.
      - benzodiazepines.
      - deep inhalational anaesthesia.
      - iv lidocaine 1–2 mg/kg.
      - fentanyl 6–8 μg/kg, alfentanil 30–50 μg/kg or sufentanil 0.5–1.0 μg/kg obtund the response if given 1–2 min before intubation.
  - arrhythmias, particularly if hypoxaemia and hypercapnia are present.
  - laryngospasm, bronchospasm, breath-holding, etc., if intubation is attempted too early.
  - aspiration of gastric contents.
  - misplaced tube, e.g. oesophageal or endobronchial. Auscultation over both lungs and axillae and the stomach should be performed following intubation and positioning.
  - difficult/failed intubation: risk of misplacement of the tube. Hypoxaemia, hypercapnia, awareness, trauma and aspiration may occur during repeated attempts at intubation.
  - bacteraemia has been reported but the clinical significance is unclear. More likely with nasal intubation.
- Once the trachea is intubated:
  - displacement of the tube:
    - extubation.
    - endobronchial intubation. Suggested by:
      - lightening anaesthesia.
      - increased airway pressures.
      - hypoxaemia.
      - unequal lung expansion.

      Usually occurs on the right side. It may cause collapse of the unventilated lung (± right upper lobe) and postoperative infection. On the chest X-ray, the tube's tip should be at T1–3 (carina lies at T4–5). The tube may move up to 2 cm with neck movement (caudad with flexion, cephalad with extension).
    - disconnection from the fresh gas supply.
    - airway obstruction:
      - blockage by sputum, blood, foreign object, etc.
      - compression by mouth gag, surgeon, kinking, etc.
    - related to the cuff.
    - tube ignition by laser.
    - complications of extubation.
- Late complications:
  - cord ulceration and granuloma: uncommon; typically occur at the junction of the posterior and middle thirds of the cord.

- damage to the recurrent/superior laryngeal nerves. Stretching and compression are thought to be the most likely causes. Slow recovery usually occurs.
- tracheal stenosis following prolonged intubation.
- nasal/oral ulceration.
- sinusitis may occur in prolonged nasotracheal intubation.

Tracheostomy is performed to avoid late complications.
See also, Anaesthetic morbidity and mortality; Intubation, difficult; Intubation, failed; Intubation, oesophageal; Intubation, tracheal

Intubation, difficult. Incidence is thought to be about 1% in the general population, although definitions vary.

- Widely accepted classification (of Cormack and Lehane) according to the best view possible at laryngoscopy (Fig. 87a):
  - grade 1: complete glottis visible.
  - grade 2: anterior glottis not seen.
  - grade 3: epiglottis seen but not glottis.
  - grade 4: epiglottis not seen.

Grades 3 and 4 together are often termed 'difficult'. The grading system has been criticised for being too insensitive, especially for laryngoscopies between grades 2 and 3 (grades 2a (cords visible) and 2b (only arytenoids/posterior glottis visible) have been suggested).

- Caused by:
  - inexperienced practitioner.
  - difficulty inserting the laryngoscope into the mouth, e.g. because its handle is obstructed by the patient's chest or by the hand applying cricoid pressure (e.g. obesity, Caesarean section, barrel-chest). This may also occur with reduced mouth opening and neck mobility.
  - reduced neck mobility, e.g. caused by osteoarthrosis, rheumatoid arthritis, ankylosing spondylitis, surgical fixation/traction, etc.
  - reduced mouth opening, e.g. reduced temporomandibular joint (TMJ) mobility, trismus, scarring, fibrosis, local lesions/swelling.
  - lesions/swelling/fibrosis of larynx, pharynx, tongue, etc.
  - congenital conditions, often associated with the above, e.g. facial deformities, achondroplasia, Marfan's syndrome, cystic hygroma, etc.

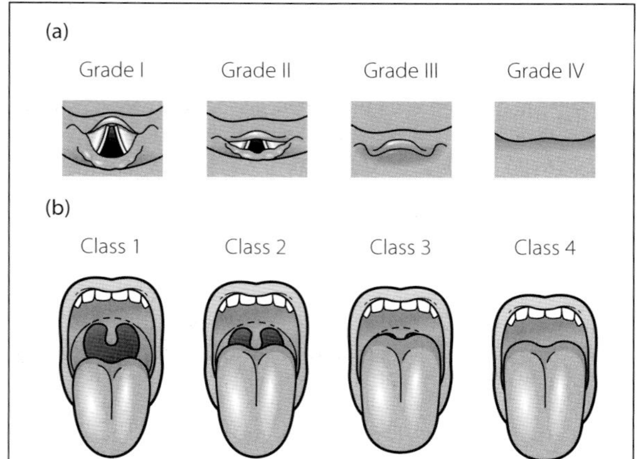

Fig. 87 (a) Cormack and Lehane classification of laryngoscopic views. (b) Modified Mallampati classification of pharyngeal appearance

  - anatomical variants of normal; they may be associated with the above but difficult intubation may occur in otherwise unremarkable patients.

Studies analysing cases of difficult intubation have described many features associated with difficulty; the large number of factors involved may make preoperative anticipation of problems difficult. Although many difficult cases may have common features, many patients with these features present no difficulty; i.e. the specificity of most tests is poor.

- Difficulty may be suggested by:
  - previous difficulty recorded in the medical notes.
  - obesity, with short neck and reduced movement at the cervical spine, especially the atlanto-occipito-axial complex. The latter is tested by asking for full neck flexion, then asking the patient to look up with the examiner's hand at the back of the neck, holding it flexed. Normal movement exceeds 15°.
  - reduced TMJ movement: anterior/posterior sliding of lower jaw (inability to protrude the lower teeth beyond the upper) or mouth opening (less than two fingers' width).
  - protruding teeth, small mouth, high, narrow arched palate, receding mandible.
  - poor view of the pharyngeal structures with open mouth and tongue protruded maximally, with the observer level with the seated patient. The modified Mallampati classification is commonly used (Fig. 87b): soft palate, uvula, fauces and pillars visible (class 1); soft palate, fauces and uvula visible (class 2); only soft palate visible (class 3); and soft palate not visible (class 4). A 'class 0' has been suggested in which the tip of the epiglottis itself is visible. The test is also valid if performed with the patient supine but there may be significant interobserver differences in any position. Phonation during testing misleadingly improves the rating.
  - thyromental distance, with neck extended, of less than three fingers (< 6.5 cm).
  - X-ray assessment: as above plus:

    $$\frac{\text{distance from TMJ to lower incisors}}{\text{distance between top of 3rd molar and}}$$

    Difficulty is suggested if this ratio is under 3.6. Rarely performed.
    - neck in extension/flexion. Middle/upper vertebral movement is particularly important. There should be a gap between the occiput and posterior arch of the atlas. The gap should increase on neck flexion. An absent gap or little change on flexion suggests limited movement at the top of the spine. Rarely performed as routine, unless neck disease is suspected.

Grouping of several tests in various combinations has been proposed to improve the predictive power, although since the incidence of difficulty (and especially failure) is low, even the best tests have poor positive predictive value.

- Management:
  - known case:
    - consideration of alternatives to intubation:
      - regional anaesthesia.
      - facepiece ± airway.
      - laryngeal mask airway.
      - tracheostomy/cricothyrotomy.
    - if oro/nasal intubation is deemed necessary, it may be performed with the patient awake or anaesthetised. In the latter case, inhalational induction is usually employed, with intubation whilst breathing spontaneously. Halothane has traditionally been considered

the agent of choice, but sevoflurane is now preferred by many.

IV induction should be avoided, since ability to maintain the airway or ventilate by facepiece is uncertain, should apnoea occur. If the patient is not at risk of regurgitation, small incremental doses of iv agent may be slowly given, maintaining spontaneous ventilation, and simultaneously deepening inhalational anaesthesia.

- techniques of intubation:
  - the position of the head should be optimised. Cricoid pressure (especially backward, upward and to the patient's right (BURP)) may help if the larynx is anteriorly placed.
  - blind nasal intubation.
  - use of intubation aids, e.g. bougies, forceps, fibreoptic instruments, specialised laryngoscopes and tracheal tubes, retrograde catheter technique, etc.

Preoxygenation must precede all attempts at intubation. Muscle relaxation is avoided until the airway is secure. Experienced help and facilities for tracheostomy or cricothyrotomy should be available. Special considerations apply if airway obstruction is present.

In patients at risk of regurgitation, risk of aspiration is increased if laryngeal protective reflexes are obtunded by local anaesthetic during awake intubation. If inhalational induction is chosen, the left lateral head-down position is considered safest, but intubation may be more awkward.

- unsuspected case:
  - maintenance of oxygenation.
  - consideration of alternative strategies:
    - allowing the patient to wake, with subsequent management as above.
    - continuing inhalational anaesthesia without intubation.
    - persisting in intubation attempts as above. Increases the risk of trauma, awareness, oesophageal intubation, etc.
    - a failed intubation drill should be instituted early, especially if at risk of regurgitation.
- airway obstruction may follow tracheal extubation unless measures are taken to protect the airway; options include tracheostomy/cricothyrotomy, use of an airway exchange catheter, or delaying extubation until further equipment and/or personnel are available or until airway oedema has subsided.
- anaesthetic records and notes should be clearly marked to warn other anaesthetists. The patient should be visited postoperatively, to discuss the events and implications.

The use of a difficult intubation box, containing all the equipment required, and available for emergency use, has been suggested.

[Ronald S Cormack, London anaesthetist; John R Lehane, Oxford anaesthetist; S Rao Mallampati, Indian-born Boston anaesthetist]

See also, Intubation, awake; Intubation, blind nasal; Intubation, complications of; Intubation, failed; Intubation, fibreoptic; Intubation, oesophageal; Intubation, tracheal

Intubation, endobronchial, *see Differential lung ventilation; Endobronchial tubes and blockers; Intubation, complications of*

Intubation, failed. Incidence is approximately 1:2500–3000 in general patients, and 1:300–500 in obstetrics. If it occurs, management is directed towards maintaining oxygenation and preventing aspiration of gastric contents.

- A failed intubation drill is widely practised for Caesarean section, but is applicable to all patients:
  - early recognition of failure is important; i.e. not persisting with attempts at intubation if the patient is becoming hypoxaemic.
  - help should be summoned.
  - cricoid pressure should be maintained, although it may be worth releasing it gradually and momentarily during attempted laryngoscopy to see if the view improves.
  - traditional advice to place the patient in the left lateral head-down position has been criticised as this is an unfamiliar position in which to continue attempts to improve the airway. However, it should be considered if the patient is breathing spontaneously as the airway may improve in the lateral position.
  - oxygenation should proceed via a facepiece, using 100% O_2. Difficult ventilation may be associated with obesity, copious facial hair and poor neck movement. Oxygenation may be aided by:
    - an assistant squeezing the reservoir bag if both hands are needed to support the airway.
    - fully closing the expiratory valve, and turning on and locking the O_2 flush. By applying the facepiece intermittently, IPPV may be performed.
    - laryngeal mask airway: although it does not protect the airway from aspiration of gastric contents, the laryngeal mask airway has proved life-saving in many different situations. Insertion during application of cricoid pressure may be unsuccessful; use of bimanual cricoid pressure or even temporary release may facilitate insertion.
    - an oesphageal obturator/airway if available. Deliberate oesophageal intubation using an ordinary tracheal tube may improve the airway. Oesophageal obturation has been suggested early if the patient cannot be turned into the lateral position.
  - if surgery is not required as an emergency, e.g. elective Caesarean section, the patient should be kept oxygenated and allowed to wake up. Alternative techniques, e.g. regional techniques, awake intubation, etc., should be considered.
  - in emergency surgery, proceeding with inhalational anaesthesia may be considered, but only if the airway is clear. Cricoid pressure should remain applied if the airway is unprotected. The stomach should be emptied only in the head-down, left lateral position, using a wide bore tube. Local anaesthetic infiltration of the surgical field may reduce requirements for volatile agents.
  - if oxygenation is impossible by facemask, laryngeal mask airway or other device, cricothyrotomy should be performed. Difficulty may be encountered, especially if the patient has a fat neck.

See also, Intubation, awake; Intubation, difficult

Intubation, fibreoptic. Usually refers to use of flexible fibreoptic instruments although there are also rigid fibreoptic laryngoscopes available. May be used for awake intubation or as an alternative to direct laryngoscopy in the anaesthetised patient, in both routine and difficult cases. Oral intubation may be assisted by passage of the 'scope via a specialised oral airway (*see Airways*), laryngeal mask airway or other device. Causes less trauma and cardiovascular response than direct laryngoscopy and intubation.

See also, Intubation, awake; Intubation, tracheal

Intubation, oesophageal. A potential complication of attempted tracheal intubation. If undetected, it may lead to severe hypoxaemia resulting in death or brain injury. Particularly likely if intubation is difficult or the intubator unskilled. Detection is often difficult, since observation of chest movement and auscultation over the chest and stomach may wrongly suggest successful tracheal intubation. The belching noise on manual inflation that usually accompanies oesophageal intubation may be absent. The reservoir bag may move convincingly during spontaneous ventilation. Condensation of water vapour within the tube may occur in both oesophageal and tracheal intubation. Preoxygenation may delay subsequent hypoxaemia and cyanosis.

- Methods of detection:
  - tactile test for tracheal tube placement: the index finger is passed along the tube into the pharynx, and attempts made to palpate the interarytenoid groove at the back of the larynx, posterior to the tube. The larynx is moved cranially from the front of the neck, using the other hand.
  - sudden overdistension of the tracheal tube cuff has been suggested, with palpation over the front of the trachea at the sternal notch. Tracheal trauma may occur.
  - injection and withdrawal of air through the tube, using a large syringe or rubber bulb (oesophageal intubation detector device; Wee detector). Oesophageal intubation is suggested by a belch on inflation, followed by absent or obstructed withdrawal of air. Both components are silent and unobstructed if intubation is tracheal.
  - passage of an illuminated stylet down the tube; tracheal placement is suggested by visible light at the front of the neck.
  - use of sound: a simple stethoscope attachment at the proximal end of the tracheal tube has been used to distinguish tracheal and oesophageal tube placement. A hand-held device (SCOTI: Sonomatic Confirmation of Tracheal Intubation) which emits sound waves along the tracheal tube and analyses the reflected waves has also been used but is no longer manufactured because of poor performance.
  - capnography; although CO_2 may be present in the stomach, sustained levels in repeated expirations indicate tracheal intubation. Disposable detectors may be attached to the tube, giving breath-by-breath colour changes in response to exhaled CO_2.
  - fibreoptic endoscopy through the tube.

Removal of the tube has been advocated if there is any doubt as to its position. Alternatively, disconnecting the tube but leaving it in place may allow manual ventilation using a facepiece placed over it.
[Michael Wee, UK anaesthetist]

Intubation, tracheal. Oro/nasal intubation was initially described for resuscitation, e.g. by Kite in 1788, and for laryngeal obstruction, although tracheal insufflation in animals had been described earlier. Macewen was the first to advocate tracheal intubation instead of tracheostomy for anaesthesia for head and neck surgery, in 1880. An intubating tube was described by O'Dwyer in 1885. Laryngoscopy was pioneered by Kirstein, Killian and Jackson between 1895 and 1915. Modern endotracheal anaesthesia and blind nasal intubation were developed by Magill and Rowbotham after World War I. Tracheal tubes and laryngoscopes are continually being developed and adapted.

- Indications for intubation:
  - anaesthetic:
    - restricted access to the patient, e.g. head and neck surgery, prone position.
    - to protect against tracheal soiling by gastric contents, blood, etc., e.g. dental, ENT and emergency surgery.
    - to secure the airway, e.g. in airway obstruction.
    - when muscle relaxation is required, e.g. abdominal surgery.
    - when IPPV is required, e.g. respiratory disease, thoracic or cardiac surgery, neurosurgery, prolonged surgery.
  - non-anaesthetic:
    - CPR.
    - when IPPV is required, e.g. respiratory failure.
    - to secure/protect the airway, e.g. in airway obstruction, unconscious patients, impaired protective laryngeal reflexes, etc.
    - to allow aspiration of sputum/secretions.
- Technique:
  - at least two laryngoscopes, a selection of tubes, syringe for cuff inflation, suction apparatus, intubation aids, emergency equipment and drugs should always be available and checked before use.
  - oral:
    - the patient is positioned with the neck flexed about 35° and head extended about 15° ('sniffing the morning air'). A pillow is required.
    - with the lungs oxygenated and the patient either paralysed or adequately anaesthetised if breathing spontaneously, the mouth is opened with the right hand and the laryngoscope introduced at the right side, using the left hand. The blade's tip is passed back along the upper surface of the tongue until the epiglottis is visible.
    - if a curved blade (e.g. Macintosh's) is used, the tip is placed between the epiglottis and the base of the tongue, and the laryngoscope lifted in the direction of the handle, avoiding pivoting or pressure on the upper teeth. The glottis is visible under the epiglottis as the latter is lifted forward (Fig. 88a). This method is thought to be less stimulating than with a straight blade, because the dorsal surface of the epiglottis (innervated by the superior laryngeal branch of the vagus) is not touched.
    - if a straight blade (e.g. Magill's) is used, the tip is placed posterior to the epiglottis and lifted as above. The glottis is visible beyond the tip (Fig. 88b). Alternatively, the tip is passed into the oesophagus and slowly withdrawn until the glottis appears. Epiglottic bruising is more likely with this technique. In the paraglossal technique, the straight blade is introduced to the (right) side of the tongue and angled so that the blade's tip lifts the epiglottis in the midline (a similar technique is also possible using a curved blade).
    - lidocaine spray 4% is sometimes applied to the larynx, to reduce stimulation by the tube once placed. Lidocaine gel is also available.
    - size 8–9 mm tubes are often used for men, 7–8 mm for women (smaller tubes are associated with a lower incidence of sore throat and hoarseness); average suitable length is 22–25 cm. The tube is inserted under direct vision if possible, from the right side of the mouth with conventional laryngoscopes. The view may be improved by backward, upward and rightward pressure on the larynx (BURP) from the front of the neck. If the view is incomplete or insertion difficult, intubation aids, e.g. stylet, bougie, etc. may help. If the glottis is not seen, the bougie or tube may be placed blindly, by careful advancement posterior to the epiglottis or laryngoscope tip. Tracheal rings may be felt if placement is successful; oesophageal intubation must be excluded.

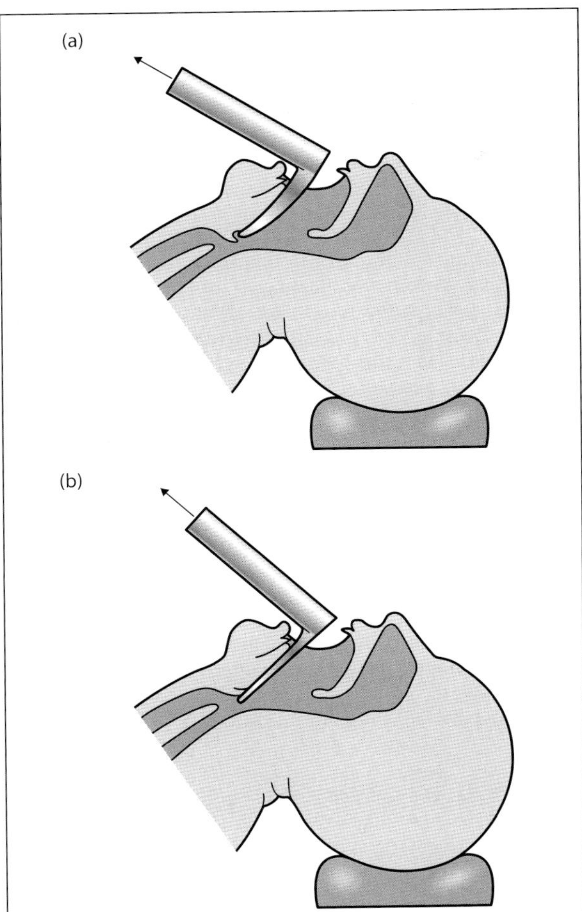

Fig. 88 Tracheal intubation using (a) curved, and (b) straight laryngoscope blades

- the tube cuff is inflated slowly until the audible leak vanishes. Low-pressure inflators are available.
- observation of the chest and auscultation of both lungs, e.g. high in the axilla, are required to exclude accidental intubation of the right main bronchus. Auscultation over the stomach and in the suprasternal notch has also been suggested to help indicate gastric inflation and tracheal leak, respectively.
- the tube is tied or taped in position.
- other techniques include awake intubation, fibreoptic intubation and use of the intubating laryngeal mask airway, retrograde catheters, etc. Intubation may also be performed without instruments, by hooking the fingers or thumb of one hand over the back of the tongue, and guiding the tube by touch.

▸ nasal:
- cocaine paste/spray 10%, or xylometazoline 0.1% is used to reduce epistaxis, which may be severe.
- tubes of diameter 1 mm less than for oral intubation are usually employed; average suitable length is 25–28 cm. The lubricated tube is gently inserted directly backwards, twisting to ease its passage. Intubation is achieved blindly, with fibreoptic instruments or with laryngoscopy as above, using forceps to position the tube if required.
- checking/securing as above.

Special considerations apply for paediatric anaesthesia, or when risk of aspiration is present (*see Induction, rapid sequence*).

In ICU, nasal intubation was previously preferred because of increased patient comfort, easier securing of tube and easier nursing care of the mouth. However, smaller longer tubes are required, and thus suction is more difficult and occlusion more likely. The incidence of nasal sinusitis is also increased. Tracheostomy is an alternative to prolonged oral or nasal tracheal intubation.

See also, Intubation, awake; Intubation, blind nasal; Intubation, complications of; Intubation, difficult; Intubation, oesophageal

Inverse ratio ventilation (IRV). Ventilatory mode used in neonatal IPPV and ARDS. Consists of a prolonged inspiratory phase of up to four times the duration of the expiratory phase. Increases mean airway pressure and is thought to improve oxygenation by keeping collapsible alveoli open for longer periods and by keeping alveoli distended through 'intrinsic PEEP' associated with prolonged expiratory time. May require a few hours for alveolar recruitment to become apparent. Risk of barotrauma may be increased, and air trapping may occur if the expiratory phase is too short. It is therefore contraindicated in obstructive lung disease when hyperventilation may occur. Spontaneous ventilation is prevented by most ventilators during the long inspiratory phase; thus it is unsuitable for weaning from ventilators. Usually requires neuromuscular blockade and sedation.

Investigations, preoperative. Aid clinical preoperative assessment of patients' fitness for surgery and whether improvement is possible, and provide a baseline for subsequent testing. Indications and requirements vary and are sometimes controversial; history and examination are generally considered more useful in routine preoperative screening for disease. Unnecessary testing is expensive, time consuming and may be worrying for the patient; it may be performed because of ignorance, supposed medicolegal security, and to avoid postponement of surgery should a test result be required later. Conversely, anaesthetists are often pressed to proceed with anaesthesia despite inadequate investigation.

- Guidelines for investigation are related to:
  - ▸ cost of testing.
  - ▸ sensitivity and specificity of the test.
  - ▸ incidence of abnormality in the population concerned.
  - ▸ clinical significance of the result if abnormal.
  - ▸ extent of planned surgery.
- Typical guidelines:
  - ▸ chest X-ray:
    - cardiovascular/respiratory disease unless recent (under 6–12 months) films are available.
    - new respiratory symptoms.
    - possible metastases.
    - recent immigrant from an area where TB is endemic, unless recent films are available.
    - as a preoperative baseline in major surgery.
    - age > 60 years.

    The first four indications are recommended by the Royal College of Radiologists.
  - ▸ ECG: age over 40–50 years, earlier in smokers or in patients with cardiovascular disease.
  - ▸ haemoglobin: age > 50–60 years, evidence of anaemia, etc. Routine testing in all women and in all patients has been suggested.
  - ▸ biochemistry: age > 40–50, metabolic diseases, dehydration, etc., drug therapy known to alter biochemistry,

e.g. diuretics, or whose actions are affected by abnormalities, e.g. digoxin. Creatinine has been suggested as a better routine test than urea. Urine testing for glucose has been suggested if blood is not tested.
- other investigations if suggested by history/examination include testing for sickle cell anaemia, liver function tests, lung function tests, coagulation studies, arterial blood gas tensions, cervical spine X-rays, etc.

In 2004 NICE issued guidelines with more detailed recommendations for preoperative testing related to the patient's condition, age and proposed surgery.

Ionisation of drugs. Important determinant of a drug's passage through membranes, since charged (ionised) particles are relatively lipid-insoluble and therefore do not cross easily. Once a drug has dissociated, passage across the membrane depends on the concentration of the unionised form. Weak acids dissociate in alkaline environments; thus passage across membranes is favoured by acid environments. The opposite applies for weak bases.

Degree of ionisation is derived from the Henderson–Hasselbalch equation:

$$\text{acidic drug: pH} - \text{p}K_a = \log\frac{[\text{ionised drug}]}{[\text{unionised drug}]}$$

$$\text{basic drug: pH} - \text{p}K_a = \log\frac{[\text{unionised drug}]}{[\text{ionised drug}]}$$

At 50% ionisation, pH = pK_a.

- Examples of acidic drugs:
  - phenytoin.
  - barbiturates, e.g. thiopental (pK_a 7.6).
  - salicylates.
  - penicillins.
- Examples of basic drugs:
  - diazepam (pK_a 3.3).
  - local anaesthetic agents, e.g. lidocaine (pK_a 7.9), bupivacaine (pK_a 8.1).
  - opioid analgesic drugs, e.g. morphine (pK_a 7.9), pethidine (pK_a 8.5).
  - non-depolarising neuromuscular blocking drugs.
- Examples of anaesthetic relevance:
  - in acidosis, dissociation of thiopental is decreased; thus the concentration of unionised portion increases. The amount of drug entering the brain therefore increases; thus the effect per mg increases.
  - fentanyl passes into the stomach from the circulation and is 'trapped' there by dissociation in acidic gastric fluid. This is now thought to be clinically insignificant.
  - 'trapping' of drugs in the ionised form in urine, by manipulating urinary pH to aid excretion (forced diuresis).

See also, Pharmacokinetics

Iontophoresis. Use of electric current to aid penetration of drug into the tissues. Suitable for drugs of low mw and high lipid solubility and potency, e.g. GTN, fentanyl. The drug is applied to the skin in the ionised form using an electrode of the same charge as the drug; current is applied using a nearby reference electrode to complete the circuit. Drug is repelled from the electrode and passes into the skin and subcutaneous tissues.

Ipecacuanha. Emetic drug, a mixture of plant alkaloids, formerly used in the treatment of poisoning and overdoses. Activates peripheral GIT sensory receptors and stimulates the chemoreceptor trigger zone. Produces vomiting within 20–30 min, with effects lasting up to 2 h. Should only be used if the patient is fully conscious and the ingested substance is not corrosive or a petroleum product. Its efficacy is disputed and its use only advocated where other means of reducing absorption of ingested poisons cannot be used.

- Dosage: 30 ml in adults; 10–15 ml in children.
- Side effects: diarrhoea, aspiration of gastric contents, gastric or diaphragmatic rupture, cerebral haemorrhage.

IPPV, *see Intermittent positive pressure ventilation*

Ipratropium bromide. Anticholinergic drug, used to treat asthma and chronic bronchitis. Has a quaternary amine structure. Of slower onset than salbutamol and similar drugs; there may be synergy between them. Oxitropium (taken 8–12 hourly) and tiotropium (taken once daily) are similar drugs; the latter has been associated with fewer exacerbations of COPD (but more dry mouth) than ipratropium.

- Dosage:
  - 1–2 puffs aerosol (20–40 μg) 6–8 hourly.
  - 0.1–0.5 mg nebuliser solution (0.4–2.0 ml 0.025% solution) 6–8 hourly. Paradoxical bronchospasm in earlier preparations is thought to have been caused by preservatives.
- Systemic anticholinergic effects are rare, although glaucoma has occurred in susceptible patients following delivery of nebulised ipratropium through poorly fitting masks.

IPSP, Inhibitory postsynaptic potential, *see Synaptic transmission*

Iron lung, *see Intermittent negative pressure ventilation*

Iron poisoning. Occurs almost exclusively in children who accidentally consume iron tablets. Doses exceeding 40–60 mg/kg of elemental iron, or serum concentrations exceeding 90 μmol/l in children or 140 μmol/l in adults represent severe poisoning. Early symptoms (within an hour) include nausea, vomiting, upper abdominal pain and GIT bleeding (caused by iron's corrosive action on the gastric mucosa); later symptoms include hypotension, hypoglycaemia, convulsions, renal failure and coma. Hepatic failure and pyloric stenosis may occur. With intensive treatment, mortality is about 1%.

- Management:
  - general measures as for poisoning and overdose, e.g. O_2 therapy, iv fluids. In the absence of shock or coma, induced emesis with ipecacuanha is recommended.
  - in severe cases, desferrioxamine iv up to 15 mg/kg/h to a maximum of 80 mg/kg in 24 h. Instillation of 5 g into the stomach has also been suggested to reduce absorption. Gastric lavage with sodium bicarbonate may convert iron to ferrous carbonate which is less well absorbed. Gastrostomy has been suggested to remove residual tablets if abdominal X-ray suggests large quantities remaining despite emesis and lavage.
  - treatment should be monitored by serial serum iron measurements.

IRV, *see Inverse ratio ventilation*

ISA, *see Intrinsic sympathomimetic activity*

Ischaemic heart disease. Most common cause of death in the Western world (20–30%); its incidence is declining in much of the Western world including the UK.

- Precise aetiology is uncertain but risk factors are as follows:
  - increasing age, male gender.

- family history: incidence is increased if a person has a first degree relative with angina or previous MI aged under 55 years.
- smoking.
- diet: associated with high plasma levels of low-density lipoproteins and cholesterol, and low levels of high-density lipoproteins. Sugar intake may be important although its exact role is controversial. Risk of mortality and morbidity may be lowered by treating hypercholesterolaemia if present.
- hypertension, diabetes mellitus.
- obesity, lack of exercise, poverty, stress, water softness and alcohol have been associated in some studies but the relationships are unclear.

- The main pathophysiological feature is reduction in coronary vessel lumen diameter by lipid atheromatous plaques, which may be exacerbated by coronary spasm. This may lead to:
  - myocardial ischaemia when O_2 demand exceeds supply.
  - fissuring of plaques with thrombus formation; may lead to unstable angina, MI or sudden death.
- Clinical features:
  - angina (*see Myocardial ischaemia*).
  - dyspnoea may occur, related to ischaemia, cardiac failure or associated chest disease caused by smoking.
  - palpitations, fainting attacks due to arrhythmias (including heart block).
  - hypertension, cardiomegaly, peripheral or pulmonary oedema.
  - fatty deposits due to hyperlipidaemia, e.g. around the eyes, arcus senilis in the cornea.
  - sudden death.
- Investigation:
  - ECG.
  - exercise testing.
  - echocardiography.
  - nuclear cardiology ± gated scanning.
  - cardiac catheterisation.
  - CT scanning.
  - MRI.
  - digital subtraction angiography: computerised subtraction of background signals in order to enhance vessel images. Allows iv contrast injection instead of cardiac catheterisation.
- Management:
  - general measures: stopping smoking; treatment of hypertension. Statins decrease mortality by lowering plasma cholesterol levels.
  - first-line specific treatment is with nitrates (e.g. GTN, isosorbide), β-adrenergic receptor antagonists and calcium channel blocking drugs. Oral/sublingual therapy is started first.
  - unstable angina: iv nitrates and β-adrenergic antagonists are used, together with prophylactic heparin and oral aspirin 300 mg orally. Oral diltiazem or verapamil may be used if β-antagonists are contraindicated and left ventricular function is good. The patient should be questioned for use of sildenafil before nitrates are used.
  - drugs affecting coagulation, e.g. warfarin, aspirin, have been investigated. Reduced risk of death has been found using the latter.
  - percutaneous transluminal coronary angioplasty is increasingly used to avoid surgery. Laser ablation of atheroma and stenting of the stenosed vessel have also been used.
  - coronary artery bypass graft.
- Anaesthetic management: the main aim is to prevent perioperative myocardial ischaemia and infarction (reinfarction rate is up to 6%, usually on the third day; infarction rate if none previously is about 0.1–0.2%):
  - preoperatively:
    - preoperative assessment of risk factors and severity of disease. Cardiac risk index is sometimes used. Conditions are optimised before surgery if possible; e.g. treatment of cardiac failure, arrhythmias, etc.
    - continuation of antianginal therapy up to and including the morning of surgery.
    - addition of further therapy if required; e.g. GTN skin patch.
    - sedative premedication is usually prescribed, to reduce anxiety and endogenous catecholamine secretion.
  - perioperatively:
    - direct arterial BP monitoring is useful if disease is severe or surgery extensive. Pulmonary artery catheterisation is controversial.
    - preoxygenation.
    - smooth induction of anaesthesia, using a minimal dose of iv anaesthetic agent given slowly, as the arm–brain circulation time may be prolonged. Etomidate causes less myocardial depression than other drugs, but others are often used. Ketamine may increase cardiac work and is usually avoided.
    - maintenance of adequate oxygenation and avoidance of hypercapnia and excessive amounts of volatile agent are achieved by tracheal intubation and muscle relaxation for most procedures. Alternatively, light inhalational anaesthesia combined with local anaesthetic techniques avoids the cardiovascular effects of intubation. Spinal and epidural anaesthesia risk hypotension and worsening of myocardial ischaemia, although they may reduce preload and afterload.
    - hypertensive response to intubation increases myocardial O_2 demand with risk of myocardial ischaemia (*see Intubation, complications of*).
    - perioperative control of excessive changes in heart rate, BP, etc., is especially important. The combination of tachycardia and hypotension is particularly hazardous. In general, drugs with minimal cardiovascular effects are often chosen, e.g. vecuronium, atracurium, fentanyl, although bradycardia has been reported. Pancuronium has traditionally been preferred because hypotension is less likely. Low concentrations of volatile agents are acceptable; large amounts cause myocardial depression. Halothane decreases heart rate and myocardial O_2 consumption, but enflurane and isoflurane cause tachycardia, which may be detrimental. Isoflurane has been implicated as causing coronary steal.
    - recently, administration of 5–10 mg atenolol iv before surgery, followed by 50–100 mg orally during the hospital stay (up to a week), has been used to reduce mortality in at-risk patients, though this is controversial.
    - myocardial ischaemia may be demonstrated by ECG or also assessed by rate–pressure product, etc.
  - postoperatively:
    - admission to HDU/ICU if severe. Routine ICU admission with aggressive maintenance of cardiovascular stability is controversial.
    - postoperative analgesia is particularly important, to reduce sympathetic overactivity.

See also, Atherosclerosis

Ischaemic preconditioning. Protective effect of short ischaemic periods on subsequent infarct size, originally described in animal experiments and relating to myocardial ischaemia (although has also been applied to the brain and other tissue). Thought to be endogenous adaptation of myocytes; the mechanism is unknown but is thought to involve accumulation of adenosine and other metabolites stimulating protein kinase C production. The effect is transient although some protective effect has been described up to 72 h later; improved ventricular function may also follow. Its importance in humans is uncertain but has been suggested by *in vitro* work, by epidemiological surveys and studies in patients undergoing cardiac surgery or angiography.

Isobestic point. Point at which two substances absorb a certain wavelength of light to the same extent. In oximetry, the different absorption profiles of oxyhaemoglobin and deoxyhaemoglobin are utilised to quantify the percentage saturation of haemoglobin. Isobestic points occur at 590 and 805 nm; these may be used as reference points where light absorption is independent of degree of saturation (*see Fig. 121; Oximetry*).

Isoflurane. 1-Chloro-2,2,2-trifluoroethyl difluoromethyl ether (Fig. 89). Inhalational anaesthetic agent, first synthesised in 1965 with its isomer enflurane, but not introduced until 1980 because of earlier (erroneous) reports of hepatic carcinogenicity in mice.

- Properties:
  - colourless liquid; pungent vapour, 7.5 times denser than air.
  - mw 184.5.
  - boiling point 49°C.
  - SVP at 20°C 33 kPa (250 mmHg).
  - partition coefficients:
    - blood/gas 1.4.
    - oil/gas 97.
  - MAC 1.05% (> 60 years) to 1.28% (young adults); 1.6–1.8% in children.
  - non-flammable, non-corrosive. Dissolves certain plastics, e.g. some makes of syringe, etc.
  - supplied in liquid form with no additive.
- Effects:
  - CNS:
    - smooth rapid induction, but speed of uptake is limited by respiratory irritation. Recovery is also rapid.
    - anticonvulsant properties, unlike enflurane. Causes more reduction of EEG activity than other agents, producing an isoelectric EEG at greater than 2 MAC.
    - reduces $CMRO_2$.
    - increases cerebral blood flow and ICP (prevented by hyperventilation and hypocapnia even if achieved after introduction of isoflurane, unlike halothane).
    - decreases intraocular pressure.
    - has poor analgesic properties.
  - RS:
    - irritant; more likely to cause coughing, etc. than halothane and enflurane.
    - respiratory depressant, with increased rate and decreased tidal volume.
    - causes bronchodilatation.
  - CVS:
    - myocardial depression is less than with halothane and enflurane, but vasodilatation and hypotension commonly occur. Compensatory tachycardia is common, especially in young patients.
    - myocardial O_2 demand decreases, but tachycardia and coronary steal may reduce myocardial O_2 supply, although this is controversial.
    - arrhythmias are less common than with other agents. Little myocardial sensitisation to catecholamines.
  - other:
    - dose-dependent uterine relaxation.
    - nausea/vomiting is uncommon.
    - skeletal muscle relaxation; non-depolarising neuromuscular blockade may be potentiated.
    - may precipitate MH.

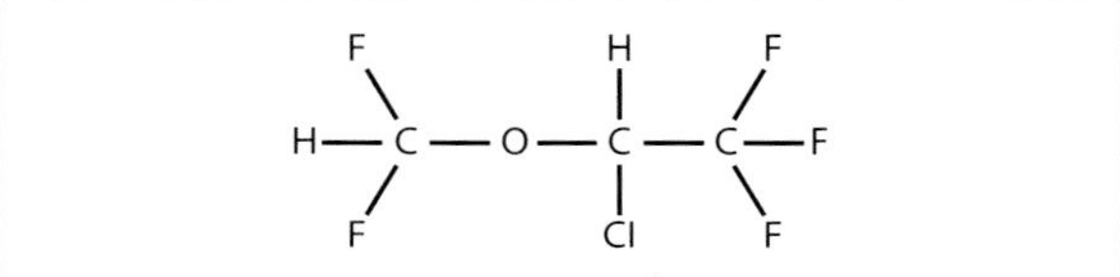

Fig. 89 Structure of isoflurane

Less than 0.2% metabolised, the rest being excreted by the lungs. Widely used in neurosurgery, for the above properties. Fluoride ion production is minimal, even after prolonged surgery; higher levels have been reported after several days' use on ICU.

1–2.5% is usually adequate for maintenance of anaesthesia, with higher concentrations for induction. Tracheal intubation may be performed easily with spontaneous respiration, once the patient is adequately anaesthetised.

See also, Vaporisers

Isolated forearm technique. Method for detecting awareness during anaesthesia. A tourniquet is inflated on the upper arm to above systolic BP, before systemic injection of neuromuscular blocking drug. Arm movement, both spontaneous and in response to verbal command, can be observed during anaesthesia. Patients may respond to command without postoperative recall (wakefulness).

Tunstall ME (1977). BMJ; 1:1321

Isomerism. Existence of two or more ions or compounds that have the same atomic composition but different structural arrangement, often with different properties.

- Two types exist:
  - structural: compounds have the same molecular formula but different chemical structures, that is, their atoms are arranged differently. Structural isomers may have similar actions (e.g. isoflurane ($CF_3CHClOCHF_2$) and enflurane ($CHClFCF_2OCHF_2$)) or different actions (e.g. promazine and promethazine). Tautomerism (or dynamic isomerism) refers to two structural isomers existing in equilibrium. Following iv administration, pH changes convert one isomer into the other, e.g. thiopental, ionised and water soluble in the syringe but rapidly converted to the largely unionised, water insoluble form after injection. Midazolam undergoes similar changes in lipid solubility after injection.
  - stereoisomerism: compounds have the same molecular formulae and chemical structure but have different spatial orientation. Two types exist:
    - enantiomers: (optical isomers; chiral substances): the compounds are mirror images of each other, and have the ability to rotate the plane of polarisation of polarised light to the right (+, dextro, *d* or D) or left (−, laevo/levo, *l* or L). This classification has been largely superseded by the R/S system (standing for rectus and sinister, the Latin for right and left respectively), which describes the configuration of the atoms

around the chiral atom (around which the other components differ between the isomers) according to set rules involving the mw of the other atoms. An R(−) enantiomer thus has its atoms arranged in a clockwise manner; an R(+) enantiomer also rotates light to the right. Each enantiomer typically has very different effects to those of its mirror image. That such closely related isomers may have different effects is one piece of evidence supporting receptor theory. A racemic mixture is one containing equal amounts of the two enantiomers and has no optical activity.
- diastereomers: the compounds are not mirror images but have identical molecular formulae and chemical structure. They generally have more than one chiral centre.

Much attention has been paid to stereoisomers since different spectra of activity of drugs have been identified as resulting from specific isomers, e.g. S(+) ketamine produces more anaesthesia and amnesia than the R(−) isomer, with fewer emergence phenomena and faster recovery. Similarly, levobupivacaine has fewer side effects than the traditional racemic preparation. Future drug development will be directed at production of single stereoisomers. Currently available drugs in single stereoisomer form include *d*-tubocurarine, *l*-hyoscine, etomidate, cisatracurium and ropivacaine. Drugs administered as a mixture of two isomers include ketamine, bupivacaine, atropine, adrenaline, halothane and isoflurane. Mivacurium and atracurium are presented as a mixture of more than two stereoisomers.

Cis-trans isomerism refers to the arrangements of paired atoms or groups around a double bond; *cis* refers to both substituents being on the same side of the double bond, whilst *trans* refers to one on each side.

Nau C, Strichartz GR (2002). Anesthesiology; 97: 497–503

Isoniazid. Antituberculous drug, usually included in all anti-TB regimens.

- Dosage: 300 mg/day iv, im or orally in adults; 10 mg/kg/day up to 300 mg/day in children.
- Side effects: peripheral neuropathy (especially in diabetes, alcoholism, malnutrition or chronic renal failure, when concurrent treatment with pyridoxine 10 mg/day should be given); nausea, hepatitis, agranulocytosis, psychosis, convulsions, lupus-like syndrome and erythema multiforme are rare.

Isoprenaline hydrochloride/sulphate. Catecholamine and inotropic drug. A non-selective β-adrenergic receptor agonist, used for its effects on heart rate, vasomotor tone and bronchial muscle. Only available in the UK on special order.

- Actions:
  - increased heart rate and force of myocardial contraction.
  - peripheral and pulmonary vasodilatation.
  - bronchodilatation.
  - systolic BP may rise or fall; diastolic BP usually falls.
- Dosage:
  - 0.02–0.2 μg/kg/min iv for complete heart block or severe bradycardia. A bolus of 5–20 μg may also be given.
  - may also be given orally, rectally or sublingually: 10–30 mg 8 hourly; absorption may be unreliable.

May cause tachycardia, tremor and ventricular arrhythmias. May worsen coronary perfusion in ischaemic heart disease.

Isoprostanes. Substances related to prostaglandins, formed by peroxidation of arachidonic acid by a reaction catalysed by free radicals and not involving cyclo-oxygenase. Have been studied as markers of oxidative stress, e.g. occurring during reperfusion injury. Isoprostanes themselves have disruptive effects on cell membranes and cause vasoconstriction.

Sakamoto H, Corcoran TB, Laffey JG, Shorten GD (2002). Eur J Anaesthesiol; 19: 550–9

Isoproterenol, *see Isoprenaline*

Isosorbide di- and mononitrate. Vasodilator drugs, with similar actions to GTN but of longer duration (up to 12 h with sustained release preparations). IV infusion of the dinitrate has been suggested in preference to infusion of GTN preparations because the latter contains additives (e.g. propylene glycol). The mononitrate is a metabolite of the dinitrate. Used in ischaemic heart disease, cardiac failure, and as an antihypertensive drug perioperatively.

- Dosage:
  - dinitrate:
    - 5–10 mg sublingually.
    - up to 240 mg/day orally; given 1–4 times daily.
    - 2–10 mg/h iv (0.5–2 μg/kg/min).
  - mononitrate: 20–120 mg/day orally; given 1–3 times daily.
- Side effects: as for GTN.

Isothermal change. Alteration in the state of a gas while temperature remains constant, e.g. by removal of heat produced during compression. Thus Boyle's law applies.
See also, Adiabatic change

Isotherms. Lines on a chart or graph denoting changes in volume or pressure with temperature remaining constant. The graph for an ideal gas would consist of rectangular hyperbolas according to the gas laws. In fact, for N_2O (Fig. 90), the isotherms approach those of an ideal gas at temperatures above its critical temperature (36.5°C). Compression of the N_2O below its critical temperature causes liquefaction, thus resisting an increase in pressure. Once all the N_2O is liquid, further compression causes a large increase in pressure, since liquids are less compressible than gases.

Isoxane. Trade name for premixed Entonox with 0.25% isoflurane. Has been used to provide analgesia during labour and minor surgery, etc. in a similar way to Entonox.
See also, Obstetric analgesia and anaesthesia

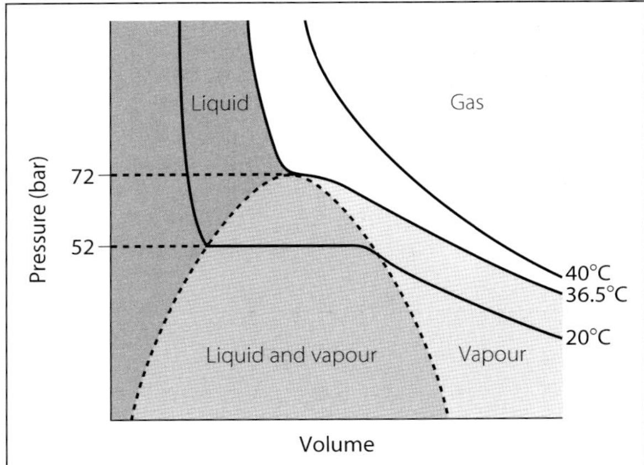

Fig. 90 Isotherms for N_2O

ISS, *see Injury severity score*

Itraconazole. Triazole antifungal drug, related to fluconazole.
- Dosage: 100–400 mg orally/iv daily.
- Side effects: as for fluconazole, though hepatic impairment is more common. Heart failure has been reported.

ITU, Intensive therapy unit, *see Intensive care unit*

Ivabridine hydrochloride. Antianginal drug, licensed for patients in normal sinus rhythm in whom β-adrenergic receptor antagonists are contraindicated or not tolerated. Acts purely on the sinoatrial node, selectively inhibiting the cardiac pacemaker I_f ('funny') current, a mixed sodium/potassium inward current, that controls diastolic depolarisation, and lowering heart rate.
- Dosage: 2.5–7.5 mg orally, twice daily.
- Side effects: bradycardia, first-degree heart block, ventricular ectopics, headache, dizziness, visual disturbances; less commonly GIT upset, supraventricular ectopics.

IVOX, *see Intravenous oxygenator*

IVRA, *see Intravenous regional anaesthesia*

J

J receptors, *see Juxtapulmonary capillary receptors*

J wave, *see Hypothermia*

Jackson, Charles T (1805–1880). US chemist, present at Wells' unsuccessful demonstration of N_2O in 1846; suggested diethyl ether to Morton for dental topical anaesthesia instead. Applied for the patent rights to ether jointly with Morton, the latter subsequently taking over 90% of Jackson's share. Jackson later claimed sole credit for the discovery of anaesthesia.

Jackson, Chevalier (1865–1958). Renowned US laryngologist. Perfected a direct vision laryngoscope in the early 1900s, and wrote extensively on laryngoscopy and tracheal insufflation.

Jaundice. Clinically detectable when plasma total bilirubin exceeds 50 μmol/l (normally under 17 μmol/l).

- Normal formation and metabolism of bilirubin:
  - haemoglobin is broken down to haem in the reticuloendothelial system. Lipid-soluble unconjugated bilirubin is transported to the liver.
  - unconjugated bilirubin is converted to conjugated bilirubin (water soluble) in the liver.
  - conjugated bilirubin is stored in the gallbladder with bile salts and acids, passing into the small bowel.
  - bilirubin is converted to urobilinogen and thence urobilin by gut bacteria. Reabsorbed from the gut, with some urobilinogen passing back to the liver to be re-excreted; a small amount is extracted by the kidneys.
- Causes of jaundice:
  - increased bilirubin production, e.g. haemolysis. Usually mild. Unconjugated and conjugated bilirubin levels are raised, with increased urinary urobilinogen.
  - impaired conjugation of bilirubin, e.g. hepatitis, cirrhosis, drug-induced (e.g. α-methyldopa, paracetamol), hepatic failure. Unconjugated bilirubin is raised; urinary urobilinogen may be raised because the liver is unable to re-excrete it.
  - congenital abnormalities of bilirubin transport are rare, except for Gilbert's syndrome (mild unconjugated bilirubinaemia with otherwise normal liver function tests, and no urinary bilirubin).
  - obstruction of bile drainage, e.g. gallstones, pancreatic carcinoma, cholangitis, cholecystitis (extrahepatic), primary biliary cirrhosis, drug-induced, e.g. contraceptives. Conjugated bilirubin is raised, often markedly, spilling over into the urine, which is dark (but with urobilinogen reduced). Faeces are pale. Itching is common.

The latter two types are frequently mixed and difficult to distinguish.

Assessment should include questioning for a history of tattoos, drug abuse, sexual contacts, contacts with jaundiced people, travel abroad, drugs, blood transfusions, alcohol, acupuncture, abdominal symptoms and recent anaesthetics.

Jaundice in ICU patients is often part of the presenting problem (e.g. in hepatic failure, biliary obstruction, sepsis) or may result from drug therapy, the development of acalculous cholecystitis, haemolysis of intra-abdominal haematoma, ischaemic hepatitis (in shocked patients) or the administration of TPN. It may also be part of multiorgan failure.

- ICU management:
  - support of other organs, e.g. circulation, respiration, etc.
  - treatment of cause, e.g. endoscopic retrograde cholangiopancreatography/surgery for obstructive causes, cessation of drugs likely to cause jaundice.
  - treatment of associated clotting abnormalities, e.g. with clotting factors, vitamin K.
  - early treatment of infection.
- Anaesthetic management:
  - preoperative assessment as above, and for hepatic failure, depending on severity and cause.
  - risk of perioperative acute renal failure due to acute tubular necrosis or hepatorenal syndrome:
    - especially common with obstructive jaundice, since bilirubin levels are often highest.
    - more likely if dehydration or biliary sepsis is present.
    - plasma urea/creatinine is monitored preoperatively.
    - preoperative iv hydration is instituted to maintain urine flow above 1 ml/kg/h.
    - mannitol is usually infused if bilirubin is very high or urine output inadequate despite hydration. Furosemide has also been used.
  - antibacterial therapy.
  - anaesthetic drugs and techniques as for hepatic failure.
- Postoperative jaundice may be due to:
  - Gilbert's syndrome.
  - underlying medical/surgical conditions.
  - drugs, including halothane.
  - haemolysis, e.g. due to blood transfusion reaction, or following extensive bruising and haematoma.
  - infection, e.g. transmitted via transfused blood, needles, etc., sepsis, pre-existing subclinical hepatitis becoming apparent postoperatively, etc.
  - hepatic damage due to severe hypoxia/hypotension.
  - surgical iatrogenic biliary obstruction.

Jaundice is particularly hazardous in neonates; the immature blood–brain barrier allows penetration of bilirubin into the basal ganglia of the brain, causing kernicterus (convulsions may occur leading to brain damage).

[Nicolas Gilbert (1858–1927), French physician]

See also, Biliary tract; Halothane hepatitis

Jaw, fractured, *see Facial trauma*

Jaw, nerve blocks, *see Gasserian ganglion block; Mandibular nerve blocks; Maxillary nerve blocks*

Jehovah's Witnesses. Religious group founded in the USA in the 1870s. Believe that they alone will survive the imminent destruction of the world, to rule over the resurrected.

Also believe that to receive blood products is against God's will, thus causing potential difficulties perioperatively. Special consent forms are usually employed. For paediatric surgery, a court order is required in order to overrule parents' wishes. Although blood, plasma and autologous pre-donation are unacceptable, cardiopulmonary bypass and recombinant erythropoietin and factor VIIa are usually permitted. Autologous blood transfusion is usually permitted only if contact of blood with the body is not broken. Other factors such as platelets, clotting factors, albumin and intravenous immunoglobulin are 'matters of conscience' for individual Witnesses. Special measures to reduce blood loss may be required, e.g. hypotensive anaesthesia, recombinant factor VIIa.
[Jehovah (Old Testament); divine being]
Remmers PA, Speer AJ (2006). Am J Med; 119: 1013–8
See also, Medicolegal aspects of anaesthesia

Jet mixing. Effect of a jet of gas, e.g. O_2, delivered from a nozzle into ambient gas, e.g. air. Energy is transferred from O_2 molecules to adjacent air molecules; the latter are entrained into the jet due to viscous shearing between the gas layers. Employed in injector techniques for IPPV, and in fixed performance O_2 masks. In the latter, air is entrained to a fixed degree depending on O_2 flow rate and the size of side ports in the entrainment device.
See also, Oxygen therapy; Venturi principle

Jet ventilators, *see High frequency ventilation; Injector techniques; Ventilators*

JG cells, *see Juxtaglomerular cells*

Jorgensen technique. Outmoded form of sedation using pentobarbital (30–300 mg), pethidine (up to 25 mg) and hyoscine (0.3 mg) iv, to allow dental surgery. Although maintaining cardiovascular stability, nausea and delayed recovery may occur. Described in 1953.
[Niels B Jorgensen (1894–1974), Danish-born Californian dentist]

Joule. SI unit of energy. 1 joule = work done when the point of application of a force of 1 newton moves 1 metre in the direction of the force (1 J = 1 N × 1 m).
[James Joule (1818–1889), English physicist]

Joule–Thomson effect (Joule–Kelvin effect). Lowering of temperature when a gas expands, e.g. passing from a cylinder under pressure to a large space. The principle is employed in the cryoprobe. Conversely, temperature rises if gas within a small space is compressed.
See also, Adiabatic change

Jugular bulb catheterisation. Performed to allow access to the blood draining the brain, and thus provide information about cerebral metabolism and blood flow. The jugular bulb is a dilatation of the internal jugular vein just below the base of the skull and may be catheterised using a Seldinger technique with the needle inserted lateral to the carotid pulsation at the level of the thyroid cartilage and directed cranially towards the external auditory meatus. It has been argued that the right internal jugular vein is better than the left since it is thought to drain the cerebral hemispheres in most cases whilst the left drains the posterior fossa; however, the side of injury has also been advocated. The correct side can be identified more accurately by ultrasound examination of the internal jugular veins or by identifying the largest increase in intracranial pressure that occurs during manual compression of each internal jugular vein. Blood may be sampled for Po_2 and O_2 saturation (S_jo_2), giving an indication of cerebral blood flow (lower values reflecting greater uptake by the brain and therefore less blood flow, assuming O_2 consumption remains constant), and concentrations of lactate and other substances. Indwelling fibreoptic sensors may also be placed to give a continuous reading of global cerebral O_2 saturation; this has been used particularly during cardiopulmonary bypass, in neurosurgery and after head injury. Desaturation ($S_jo_2 < 55\%$) indicates impending cerebral ischaemia, e.g. caused by hypotension, hypocapnia, increasing cerebral oedema, etc.

Although supported by many enthusiasts, monitoring of jugular bulb O_2 saturation gives information only about global cerebral function, not regional differences. In addition, if cerebral blood flow and O_2 consumption both decrease, e.g. in severe brain injury, S_jo_2 may be unchanged.
Shaaban-Ali M, Harmer M, Latto IP (2001). Anaesthesia; 56: 24–37

Jugular veins. Include the internal, external and anterior jugular veins (Fig. 91; *see also Fig. 110; Neck, cross-sectional anatomy*).
- Internal jugular vein:
  - passes through the jugular foramen at the base of the skull, draining the intracranial structures via the sigmoid sinus.
  - lies at first posterior, then lateral, to the internal carotid artery. Contained within the carotid sheath with the carotid artery and vagus nerve; the cervical sympathetic chain lies behind the sheath.
  - receives tributaries from the pharynx, face, scalp, tongue and thyroid gland. Receives the thoracic duct on the left and right lymph duct on the right.
  - has a dilatation at each end (jugular bulb), with valves above the lower bulb.
  - terminates behind the sternoclavicular joint by joining with the subclavian vein to form the brachiocephalic vein.
- External jugular vein:
  - drains the lateral parts of the head; passes over the sternomastoid muscle to join the subclavian vein behind the clavicle at its midpoint.

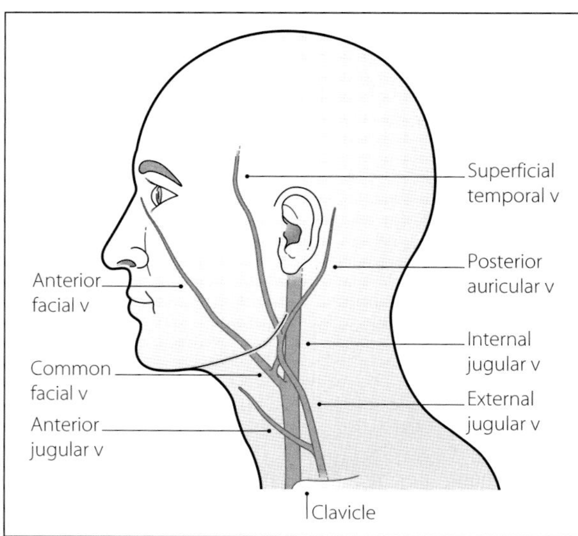

Fig. 91 Venous drainage of head and neck

- receives the anterior jugular vein (passing down from in front of the hyoid bone) behind the clavicle.

See also, Cerebral circulation; External jugular venous cannulation; Internal jugular venous cannulation; Jugular bulb catheterisation

Jugular venous pressure (JVP). Assessed by observing the height (in cm) of visible pulsation in the jugular veins above the sternal angle, with the patient reclining at 45°. The normal value is zero; i.e. the venous pulsations are not normally visible. The JVP falls during inspiration, and rises during expiration and when pressure is applied to the abdomen (Q sign). Pulsations are usually non-palpable. The venous waveform may be apparent. JVP may be difficult to identify in obese patients.

Useful as a clinical guide to right atrial pressure; raised in right-sided cardiac failure, hypervolaemia, and mechanical obstruction, e.g. tricuspid stenosis or superior vena caval obstruction.

See also, Central venous pressure

Junctional arrhythmias (Nodal arrhythmias). Arrhythmias arising from the atrioventricular node. Common during anaesthesia, especially deep inhalational anaesthesia.

- May consist of:
  - ectopic beats.
  - bradycardia.
  - tachycardia.

On the ECG, inverted P waves may precede, follow, or be hidden by, the (normal) QRS complexes. Usually of little clinical significance, although cardiac output may be reduced. Cannon waves may be visible in the jugular venous waveform.

Atropine and ephedrine have been used to restore sinus rhythm in bradycardia; junctional tachycardias may respond to lidocaine and similar drugs.

See also, Heart, conducting system

Juxtaglomerular apparatus. System adjacent to renal glomeruli, composed of:

- juxtaglomerular cells; epithelioid cells within the media of afferent arterioles entering the glomeruli. Contain renin in granules.
- macula densa; specialised tubular epithelial cells, just before the start of the distal convoluted tubule. Thought to be involved in the control of renin secretion.
- granular cells within surrounding connective tissue; contain some renin granules.

Responds to reductions in renal perfusion pressure by secreting renin, although the exact mechanism is unclear. Possibly renal vasodilatation is involved, since β-adrenergic receptor agonists, prostacyclin, bradykinin, dopamine, furosemide and vasodilator drugs all increase renin secretion. Conversely, α-adrenergic receptor agonists, vasopressin, and angiotensin reduce renin secretion.

Richly innervated with adrenergic nerve fibres; β-adrenergic activity increases secretion, and antagonism reduces it, independently of vasodilatation.

See also, Nephron; Renin/angiotensin system

Juxtapulmonary capillary receptors (J receptors). Receptors thought to be present in alveolar walls near the capillaries. Thought to be responsible for the tachypnoea seen in pulmonary oedema and interstitial lung disease, via vagal afferent fibres. Their role in normal lungs is unknown.

Kallikreins. Serine proteolytic enzymes in tissue and plasma, producing kinins from kininogens. May also catalyse formation of renin from prorenin. Plasma kallikrein is produced from prekallikrein by various activating substances, including part of activated coagulation factor XII. Plasmin, a fibrinolytic enzyme, catalyses the reaction, as does kallikrein itself. Inhibited by aprotinin. Prostate-specific antigen (PSA) is a kallikrein used as a biomarker for prostatic cancer.

Kanamycin. Antibacterial drug, now superseded by other aminoglycosides.

Katharometer. Device used for gas analysis, following separation, e.g. by gas chromatography. A heated wire is placed in the gas flow; different gases have different thermal conductive properties and therefore produce different changes in electrical resistance of the wire. Particularly useful in detecting inorganic gases, e.g. helium, CO_2, N_2O and O_2. Used to quantify the amount of a known gas, not to identify unknown ones.

Kawasaki disease (Musculocutaneous lymph node syndrome). Systemic vasculitis of unknown aetiology, usually affecting children under 5 years old. Incidence is 3.4 per 100 000 in the UK; three and 30 times more common in the US and Japan respectively. Important because coronary arteritis may lead to formation of coronary aneurysms in 20–30% of cases if untreated, with mortality of up to 4%. May present with fever (typically for more than 5 days), conjunctivitis, reddened lips, mouth and tongue, desquamating rash, peripheral oedema, and cervical lymphadenopathy. Diagnosis may be difficult because not all these features may be present at once, other non-specific symptoms may be present (e.g. cough, abdominal pain, vomiting, arthralgia) and there is no diagnostic test. Treatment is with iv immunoglobulin 2 g/kg over 10 h and aspirin 30 mg/kg/day in 3–4 divided doses.
[Tomisaku Kawasaki, Japanese paediatrician]
Burns JC, Glode MP (2004). Lancet; 364: 533–44
See also, Vasculitides

KCT, Kaolin cephalin time, *see Coagulation studies*

Kelvin. SI unit of temperature. One kelvin (K) = 1/273.16 of the thermodynamic scale temperature of the triple point of water (point at which solid, liquid and gaseous water are at equilibrium). nK = (n – 273.16)°C.
[William Thomson (1824–1907), Irish-born Scottish physicist; became Lord Kelvin in 1892]

Kerley's lines. Opaque markings seen on the chest X-ray:
- type A: thin unbranched lines, radiating from the hila. Possibly represent interlobular septa.
- type B: transverse lines, under 3 cm long, seen at the lung bases, especially costophrenic angles. Represent thickened interlobular septa, e.g. due to fluid (e.g. pulmonary oedema), fibrosis or tumour.
- type C: spider's web appearance.

[Peter Kerley (1900–1978), Irish radiologist]

Ketamine hydrochloride. IV anaesthetic agent (Fig. 92), first used in 1965. Derivative of phencyclidine ('angel dust'), but less likely to cause hallucinations. An antagonist at NMDA receptors. Presented in 10, 50 and 100 mg/ml solutions, all containing benzethonium chloride (the 10 mg/ml solution since 1997). pH is 3.5–5.5; pK_a 7.5. 12% bound to plasma albumin. Elimination half-life is about 3 h. Metabolised in the liver to weakly active metabolites, excreted in urine. Produces a state of 'dissociative anaesthesia': intense analgesia with light sleep. Increased thalamic and limbic activity occur, with dissociation from higher centres. Commercially available ketamine is a racemic mixture of two isomers with similar pharmacokinetic properties; however the S(+) isomer is 2–4 times as potent as the R(−) isomer and less psychoactive, with more rapid recovery.

Used for induction of anaesthesia, traditionally in shocked patients. May also be used for maintenance as the sole agent, especially in burns, trauma, radiotherapy, radiological investigations, etc., because of its alleged preservation of upper airway reflexes. Has local anaesthetic properties, and has been used for spinal and epidural anaesthesia. Has been given by low dose infusion and orally in some forms of neuropathic pain, although unlicensed.

Has been used increasingly as a recreational drug ('Special K'), leading to its classification as a Class C drug under the Misuse of Drugs Act in 2006.

- Effects:
  - induction: smooth, but slower than thiopental (about 30 s).
  - CVS/RS:
    - BP and heart rate usually increase; cardiac output is maintained. Changes are probably via direct myocardial and central sympathetic stimulation, and blockade of noradrenaline uptake by sympathetic nerve endings. Contraindicated in severe ischaemic heart disease and hypertension.
    - may cause respiratory depression after rapid injection, but less than with other agents.
    - traditionally held to preserve laryngeal and pharyngeal reflexes, with minimal upper airway obstruction.

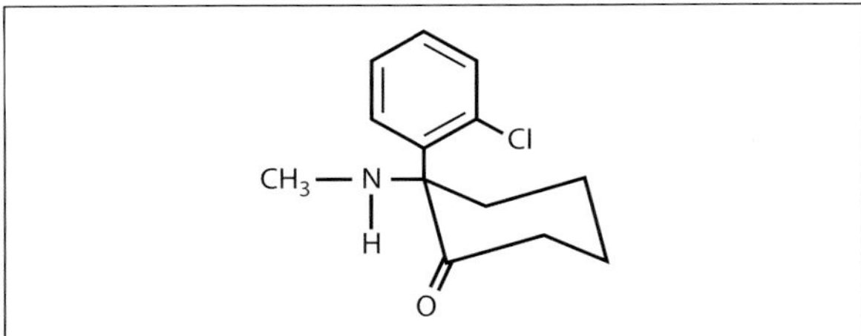

Fig. 92 Structure of ketamine

However, airway obstruction, laryngospasm and aspiration may still occur.
- causes bronchodilatation via a direct action and sympathomimetic effects.
- CNS:
  - causes analgesia, even at subanaesthetic doses.
  - may cause increased muscle tone, twitching, blinking and nystagmus.
  - increases cerebral blood flow and ICP; contraindicated in pre-eclampsia and severe intracranial pathology.
  - may cause anterograde amnesia.
  - may cause vivid dreams and emergence phenomena, e.g. hallucinations which are often frightening. Usually less distressing in patients below 15 years or above 65 years. Dreams are said to be reduced by benzodiazepines, and delirium by butyrophenones. Physostigmine has also been used. Preoperative counselling and opioid/hyoscine premedication may also reduce their incidence. In the past, patients have traditionally recovered in quiet darkened rooms.
- other:
  - may cause nausea and vomiting. Salivation is increased.
  - may increase uterine tone.
  - increases intraocular pressure; contraindicated in open eye operations, although it has been used for anaesthesia for measurement of intraocular pressures in children.
  - does not cause histamine release.
- Dosage:
  - 1–2 mg/kg iv for induction. Effects last for 5–10 min. Supplementary doses 0.5 mg/kg.
  - 10 mg/kg im for induction; acts in 3–5 min, lasting 20–30 min.
  - may be used in smaller doses for sedation, e.g. prior to induction in agitated patients or whilst performing regional techniques, especially when moving painful limbs. Suitable doses: 2 mg/kg im, 10 mg increments iv, or 1–2 mg/kg/h infusion. Has also been used by iv bolus to supplement imperfect regional blocks, e.g. during Caesarean section, and by infusion for sedation in ICU.
  - to treat severe asthma: 0.5–2.5 mg/kg/h infusion.

See also, Isomerism

Ketanserin. 5-HT antagonist, and weak α_1-adrenergic receptor antagonist. Also has Class III antiarrhythmic properties. Has been used to prevent vasoconstriction and bronchospasm in carcinoid syndrome, and also to provide vasodilatation and hypotension in cardiac surgery.

Ketoacidosis. Metabolic acidosis due to accumulation of ketone bodies in plasma. May be associated with hyperglycaemia, especially in diabetic coma. May also occur in chronic alcoholism following a recent binge and starvation; hyperglycaemia is then not a feature.
- Features:
  - of acidosis, including hyperventilation and hyperkalaemia.
  - characteristic sweet smell on the patient's breath due to ketosis (undetectable by a minority of clinicians).
  - nausea and vomiting, dehydration.

Treatment includes rehydration and correction of electrolyte imbalance. Diabetics require insulin; alcoholics require glucose.

Ketobemidone hydrochloride. Opioid analgesic drug, with similar potency and properties to morphine. Mainly used in Scandinavia.

Ketoconazole. Imidazole antifungal drug, active against a wide range of fungi and yeasts. Should not be given for superficial infections because of the risk of fatal hepatotoxicity. Has also been used for treatment of Cushing's disease.
- Dosage: 200–400 mg orally once daily, usually for less than 14 days (3 mg/kg daily in children).
- Side effects include hepatic impairment (liver function must be monitored closely), GIT disturbances, gynaecomastia, rashes.

Ketone bodies. Acetone, acetoacetic acid and hydroxybutyric acid; formed from hepatic metabolism of free fatty acids released from adipose tissue. Normally utilised by brain, heart and other tissues as an energy source, keeping blood levels low. Levels increase when fat metabolism increases, especially when intracellular glucose is deficient, e.g. in diabetes mellitus, starvation, and high fat/low carbohydrate diet. May occur in alcohol abuse, when glucose production is impaired. Increased levels may lead to ketoacidosis. Acetone may be detected on the breath.

Ketoprofen. NSAID, similar to ibuprofen but with greater incidence of GIT side effects.
- Dosage: 50–100 mg 6–12 hourly up to 200 mg/day; may be given orally, pr or by deep gluteal im injection (the latter for up to 3 days). A modified release preparation (100–200 mg orally, once daily) and a topical gel are also available.

Ketorolac trometamol/tromethamide. NSAID, indicated for short-term postoperative analgesia. Has a marked analgesic effect with little anti-inflammatory effect. Maximal plasma levels occur within 60 min of im injection and 5 min of iv injection, with half-life of 5–6 h. Pain relief may not occur until 30 min from injection. Over 99% protein-bound, with hepatic metabolism (reduced in the elderly). Over 95% of metabolites are excreted in urine, with ~6% in the faeces. Recommended parenteral doses have been reduced from those originally proposed, following adverse events including death from GIT perforation/haemorrhage, asthma, anaphylaxis and renal failure. The datasheet specifies intra-operative and prophylactic use before surgery as contraindications because of the increased risk of bleeding.
- Dosage: 10 mg im/iv (the latter over at least 15 s) 4–6 hourly, up to 90 mg/day (60 mg in elderly or patients < 50 kg) for up to 2 days. May also be given orally: 10 mg 4–6 hourly, up to 40 mg/day for up to 7 days.
- Side effects: as for NSAIDs. CNS effects including drowsiness, dizziness, psychological changes and convulsions have been reported. Contraindications include peptic ulcer disease, coagulation abnormalities/anticoagulant drugs (including low dose heparin), asthma, concurrent treatment with or allergy to any other NSAID, renal impairment, hypovolaemia, CVA, pregnancy and lactation.

Kety–Schmidt technique. Method of measuring cerebral blood flow using the Fick principle, using N_2O. 10% N_2O is inhaled for 10–15 min, and the jugular venous concentration is assumed to be equal to the brain concentration. Cerebral N_2O uptake is therefore calculated.

[Seymour S Kety (1915–2000) and Carl F Schmidt (1893–1988), US neuroscientists]

Key filling system. System for filling modern vaporisers with volatile anaesthetic agent, preventing filling with incorrect agent and supposedly reducing spillage and pollution by using closely fitting interlocking components.

- Composed of:
  - filler tube: a base at one end screws on to the bottle; the other end bears a plastic block which only fits into the correct vaporiser filling port.
  - collar round the neck of the bottle of volatile agent; protruding pegs slot into corresponding slots in the filler tube base. Position of pegs and slots are specific for each agent.

Collar, filler tube base and block are colour-coded for the particular agent (halothane – red; enflurane – orange; isoflurane – purple; trichloroethylene – blue; methoxyflurane – green). The name of the correct agent is written on the filler tube base.

Vaporisers for desflurane and sevoflurane do not utilise the key filling system, their bottles fitting to the vaporiser by an agent-specific attachment already on the bottle (desflurane) or fitted to it (sevoflurane).

See also, COSHH regulations; Environmental safety of anaesthetists

Kidney. Situated on the posterior abdominal wall, with the diaphragm and 11th and 12th ribs posteriorly. The renal hila are approximately level with the pylorus. Each kidney is about 10 cm long, 5 cm wide and 3 cm thick. Nerve supply is via the coeliac ganglion from T12 and L1. Blood supply is from the renal arteries which arise from the descending aorta, and venous drainage is via the renal veins into the inferior vena cava. Renal blood flow is 1200 ml/min (22% of cardiac output), about 400 ml/100 g/min. O_2 consumption is 20 ml/min, or 6 ml/100 g/min.

Composed of outer cortex and inner medulla forming pyramids. Functional unit is the nephron, with accompanying arterioles and capillaries.

- Functions:
  - filtration of plasma and excretion of waste products of metabolism, whilst maintaining water, osmolality, electrolyte and acid–base homeostasis.
  - secretion of renin.
  - secretion of erythropoietin.
  - formation of 1,25-dihydroxycolecalciferol (important in calcium homeostasis).
  - metabolism and excretion of drugs.
- May be affected by anaesthesia/surgery:
  - drug effects, e.g. methoxyflurane, diuretics.
  - alteration of renal blood flow, e.g. hypotension, aortic aneurysm repair.
  - renal impairment following incompatible blood transfusion, severe jaundice, sepsis, obstetric emergencies, crush syndrome, etc.

See also, Acid–base balance; Fluid balance; Renal failure; Renal transplantation; Renin/angiotensin system

Killian, Gustav (1860–1921). German laryngologist; published extensively on the structure and function of the larynx. A former student of Kirstein, he helped popularise direct laryngoscopy. Also performed the first translaryngeal removal of a foreign body from the right main bronchus in 1897, using a rigid oesophagoscope and cocaine local anaesthesia, thus pioneering bronchoscopy.

Kilogram. SI unit of mass. The standard kilogram is the mass of a cylindrical piece of platinum–iridium alloy kept at Sèvres, France.

Kilogram weight. Weight of a mass of 1 kilogram. Also called kilogram force.

$$\begin{aligned} 1 \text{ kg wt (or kgf) due to gravity} &= 1 \text{ kg} \times 9.81 \text{ m/s} \\ &= 9.81 \text{ Newton.} \end{aligned}$$

Kinins. Vasodilator peptides derived from precursor molecules (kininogens) by the action of kallikreins. Involved in many inflammatory and immune reactions, and possibly in shock. Also thought to be involved in the carcinoid syndrome. Bradykinin is the main plasma kinin, causing vasodilatation and increased vascular permeability. Glucocorticoids inhibit their release. Broken down by angiotensin converting enzyme, mainly in the lung. Elimination half-life is less than 15 s.

Kirstein, Alfred (1863–1922). German laryngologist; described the first direct laryngoscopy in 1895. His laryngoscopes could be placed anterior or posterior to the epiglottis. Stressed the importance of the 'sniffing the morning air position' for laryngoscopy. Also suggested translaryngeal removal of bronchial foreign bodies as being easier than via tracheostomy.

Hirsch NP, Smith GB, Hirsch PO (1986). Anaesthesia; 41: 42–5

Kite, Charles (1768–1811). English doctor, practising in Gravesend, Kent. Awarded the silver medal by the Humane Society (now Royal Humane Society) in 1787 for his *Essay on the Recovery of the Apparently Dead*, later published as a book. Described oro- and nasotracheal catheterisation for lung inflation, and suggested laryngospasm as a cause for hypoxia in drowning.

Klippel–Feil syndrome. Inherited condition characterised by congenitally fused cervical vertebrae; subdivided according to the extent of vertebral involvement:

- type I: several vertebrae (cervical and upper thoracic) form a single unit.
- type II: one or two cervical vertebrae affected only.
- type III: types I or II with thoracic or lumbar abnormalities too.

Most commonly restricted to C2–3 and C5–6. Scoliosis, other skeletal malformations, and cardiovascular and genitourinary abnormalities may also occur. Typically, the patient has a short neck with limited movement and a low posterior hairline. Both autosomal dominant and recessive inheritance has been suggested for different subtypes.

- Anaesthetic considerations:
  - cervical instability.
  - difficult intubation.
  - epidural and spinal anaesthesia may be technically difficult.
  - related to abnormalities of other systems.

[Maurice Klippel (1858–1942) and Andre Feil (1884–1955), French neurologists]

Naguib M, Farag H, Ibrahim AEW (1986). Can Anesth Soc J; 33: 66–70

Knee, nerve blocks. Performed for surgery to the lower leg and foot.

- Nerves which may be blocked (*see Fig. 65; Femoral nerve block*):
  - tibial nerve (L4–S3): terminal branch of the sciatic nerve; supplies the anteromedial part of the sole of the foot via plantar branches. In the popliteal fossa, the nerve lies superficial and lateral to the popliteal vessels, with vein medially and artery most medial.

With patient prone and knee extended, a needle is inserted in the midline of the popliteal fossa, level with the femoral condyles. 5–10 ml local anaesthetic agent is injected at a depth of 2–3 cm.
- common peroneal (L4–S2): terminal branch of the sciatic nerve; supplies the dorsum of the foot via its superficial peroneal branch, and the area between the first and second toes via the deep peroneal branch. The region posterior to the head of the fibula is infiltrated with 5 ml solution. Some workers claim that neuritis is common, but this has been disputed.
- sciatic (L4–S3): may be blocked before it divides into tibial and common peroneal nerves above the popliteal fossa, at a point 7 cm cranial to the skin crease behind the knee, and 1 cm lateral to the midline. 5–10 ml solution is injected at a depth of 3–5 cm.
- saphenous (L4–5): a continuation of the femoral nerve; supplies the medial part of the lower leg, ankle and foot. May be blocked by infiltration from the medial border of the tibial tuberosity to the posterior edge of the tibia (taking care to avoid the saphenous vein).

Koller, Carl (1857–1944). Austrian ophthalmologist; first described the use of local anaesthetic agent (cocaine) for a surgical operation (for glaucoma) in Vienna in 1884, having previously investigated the drug with Freud. This was reported by a colleague at an ophthalmological congress in Heidelberg on the following day. Disappointed with his career's subsequent progress, he emigrated to New York in 1888.

Korotkoff sounds. Sounds heard during auscultation over the brachial artery, whilst a proximal cuff is slowly deflated from above systolic pressure. Thought to result from turbulent flow within the artery causing vessel wall vibration and resonance. Used in arterial BP measurement. Three phases were originally described by Korotkoff; these were subsequently increased to five:
- phase I: intermittent tapping sound, corresponding to the heartbeat. Represents systolic pressure.
- phase II: sounds quieten or even disappear (auscultatory gap).
- phase III: sounds become louder again.
- phase IV: sounds suddenly become muffled.
- phase V: sounds disappear.

Argument over whether diastolic pressure is best recorded at phase IV or V continues; traditionally phase IV is used in the UK, phase V in the USA. Recording of both has been suggested, e.g. 120/80/75 .
[Nicolai Korotkoff (1874–1920), Russian physician]

Krebs cycle, *see Tricarboxylic acid cycle*

Kuhn, Franz (1866–1929). German physician; wrote extensively on tracheal intubation for anaesthesia. Described tracheal insufflation in 1900 and nasotracheal intubation in 1902.
Sweeney B (1985). Anaesthesia; 40: 1000–5

Kussmaul breathing (Air hunger). Hyperventilation originally described in diabetic hyperglycaemic ketoacidosis. Caused by stimulation of central chemoreceptors by hydrogen ions. Occurs in severe metabolic acidosis of any cause.
[Adolf Kussmaul (1822–1909), German physician]

Kussmaul's sign, *see Cardiac tamponade*

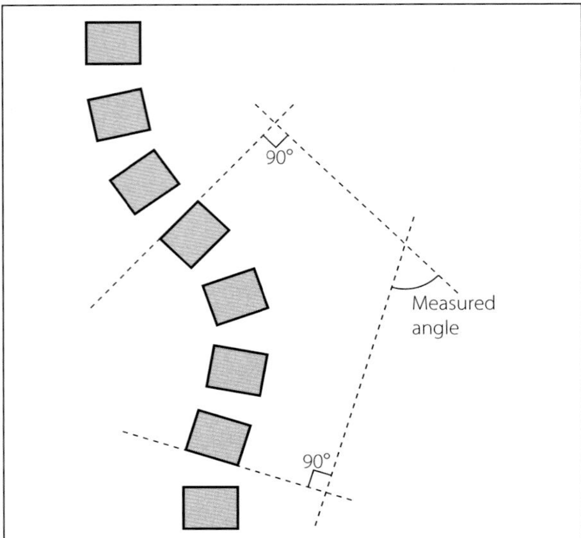

Fig. 93 Measurement of the angle of curvature in scoliosis

Kyphoscoliosis. Definitions:
- kyphosis: posterior curvature of spine.
- scoliosis: lateral curvature.

There may also be rotational deformity.

May be associated with congenital skeletal, muscular or neurological abnormalities and diseases. Idiopathic scoliosis develops in childhood and is the most common form. The angle of curvature is measured from X-rays of the spine (Fig. 93) and an angle $> 10°$ is abnormal. There may be rotation of the vertebrae, with the spinous processes turned inward towards the concavity of the curve. Thoracic, rib and chest wall deformity may cause restriction of ventilation, especially if the curve exceeds 65°. Surgical fixation is usually performed before puberty. This may be performed using metal Harrington rods, allowing distraction of the vertebrae using a ratchet.

- Anaesthetic management:
  - preoperatively:
    - assessment for associated disease.
    - MH is commoner in this group.
    - assessment of RS: lung volumes and compliance are reduced; the main defect is restrictive. $\dot{V}/\dot{Q}$ mismatch may be present. Repeated aspiration may occur in neuromuscular disease. Chest X-ray is mandatory; lung function tests and arterial blood gas analysis are useful.
    - chronic hypoxaemia may lead to pulmonary hypertension and cor pulmonale.
    - preoperative physiotherapy, antibiotics, etc. may be required.
  - perioperatively:
    - tracheal intubation may be difficult, especially if the patient is unable to lie flat.
    - surgery may be prolonged, with risk of major blood loss, hypothermia, etc.
    - transthoracic surgery may involve anterior or posterior approaches.
    - hypotensive anaesthesia is advocated by some, to reduce blood loss and ease surgery. Others argue that possible ischaemia of the spinal cord precludes this. Careful positioning of the patient is required to prevent pressure on the abdominal inferior vena cava.
    - risk of cord damage during distraction of vertebrae may be assessed by the wake-up test or monitoring of evoked potentials.

- access to the patient may be restricted.
- postoperatively: ventilatory failure is possible; close monitoring is required. Chest X-ray is usual to exclude pneumothorax. An epidural catheter may be placed by the surgeon for postoperative analgesia.

Central neural blockade (e.g. for labour) may be difficult in scoliotic patients. The incidence of accidental dural puncture during epidural anaesthesia may be increased, and its efficacy may be reduced following prior surgery.

[Paul R Harrington, Texas surgeon]

L

Labat, Gaston (1877–1934). Anaesthetist, born in the Seychelles; worked in Paris and at the Mayo Clinic and New York University, USA. Pioneer of regional anaesthesia, writing a classic text on the subject in 1922. Founded the American Society of Regional Anaesthesia in 1923.
Brown DL, Winnie AP (1992). Reg Anesth; 17: 249–62

Labetalol hydrochloride. Combined β- and α-adrenergic receptor antagonist, with ratio of activities usually quoted between 2:1 and 5:1 respectively. Selective for α_1-receptors, but non-selective at β-receptors, with some intrinsic sympathomimetic activity. Used to treat severe hypertension and pre-eclampsia, and in hypotensive anaesthesia. 90% protein-bound. Half-life is 4 h. Metabolised in the liver and excreted in urine and faeces. Undergoes extensive first-pass metabolism when given orally.

- Dosage:
  - 5–50 mg iv by slow injection, up to 200 mg. Effects occur usually within 5 min, lasting 6 h but possibly up to 18 h.
  - 10–200 mg/h infusion.
  - 50–100 mg orally 12 hourly; increased up to a maximum 2.4 g/24 h.
- Side effects:
  - as for β-adrenergic receptor antagonists. Synergistic with halothane; marked hypotension may result.
  - jaundice has occurred rarely.

Labour, active management of. Term referring to a collection of medical interventions and management including strict diagnostic criteria for the onset and course of labour, artificial rupture of membranes, early use of oxytocic drugs and continuous obstetric input so that the duration of labour is limited. Despite claims of improved outcome, evidence is at best controversial, apart from the benefit of continued support throughout labour.

Medical intervention depends on the plot of cervical dilatation and descent of the fetal head against time, usually starting from presentation in labour. The curve obtained is compared with curves derived from studies of normal labours, primiparous or multiparous as appropriate (partograms). The normal curve is comprised of latent (up to 3–4 cm cervical dilatation) and active (until 10 cm dilatation) phases. Delay in progress is represented by a lag of more than 2 h to the right of the expected curve.

- Different patterns of delay may occur:
  - prolonged latent phase: its existence is disputed by some obstetricians, since the definition of onset of labour is difficult and variable. Others claim up to 30% instrumental rate and up to 15% Caesarean section (CS) rate. More common in primiparous women.
  - primary delay: i.e. slow progress of the active phase, e.g. due to inefficient uterine contraction. Instrumental rate is 7–8%, CS rate 4–5%. More common in primiparous women.
  - secondary arrest: normal progress to 7–8 cm, then delay. Commonly due to malposition. Instrumental rate is 2–3%, CS rate 1–2%.

Cephalopelvic disproportion may cause delay at any stage, but especially secondary arrest. Most other causes are treated successfully with oxytocic drugs, ensuring fetal monitoring.

Epidural blockade is often instituted to provide analgesia for augmented contractions, possibly to restore coordinated uterine activity, and in case of operative delivery.

Lack breathing system, *see Coaxial anaesthetic breathing systems*

β-Lactams. Group of substances containing the 4-atom β-lactam ring (Fig. 94). Include the penicillins, cephalosporins, the monobactam aztreonam and the carbapenems. The β-lactam ring is a site of breakdown by bacterial β-lactamase, leading to bacterial resistance.

Lactate. Byproduct of anaerobic glycolysis. Hypoxia prevents aerobic metabolism of pyruvate to CO_2 and water; instead lactate is formed, with consequent increases in plasma lactate/pyruvate ratio (normally 10) and plasma lactate (normally 0.3–1.3 mmol/l). The liver removes 70% of lactate and the rest is converted to pyruvate by mitochondria-rich skeletal and cardiac muscle.

- Causes of increased levels:
  - Type A: tissue hypoxia results in faster production than normal: hypoxaemia, anaemia, tissue hypoperfusion, shock, CO poisoning, severe exercise, impaired hepatic flow.
  - Type B: hypoxia is not a feature: increased catecholamine levels, thiamine deficiency, decreased gluconeogenesis (e.g. biguanide therapy).

Lactic acidosis. Metabolic acidosis accompanied by raised plasma lactate levels.

- Causes are divided into:
  - those with overt tissue hypoxia (type A):
    - severe hypoxaemia.
    - severe anaemia.
    - shock/haemorrhage/hypotension.
    - cardiac failure.
    - severe exercise.
    - carbon monoxide poisoning.

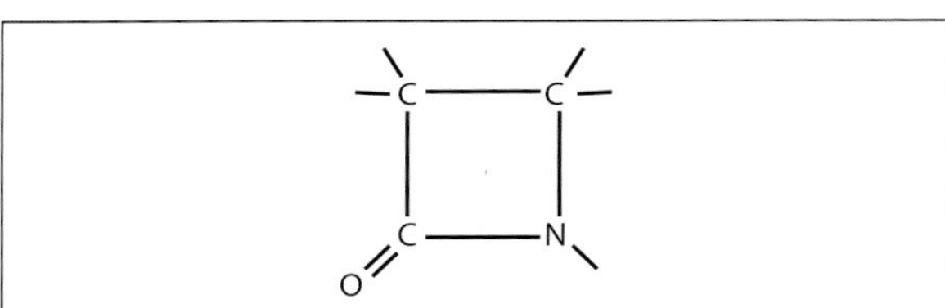

Fig. 94 Structure of β-lactam ring

- mesenteric ischaemia.
  - those without apparent initial tissue hypoxia (type B):
    - hepatic failure/renal failure (cause delayed clearance of lactate).
    - severe infection, thiamine deficiency, alcoholic and diabetic ketoacidosis (cause pyruvate dehydrogenase dysfunction).
    - cyanide poisoning, biguanides, salicylates, sodium valproate (cause uncoupling of oxidative phosphorylation).
    - exercise, severe infection, seizures, xylitol, fructose and sorbitol in TPN, malignancies (cause increase in aerobic glycolysis)
    - glycogen storage disorders, inborn errors of metabolism.
- Treatment:
  - directed at the underlying cause.
  - cautious use of bicarbonate (increased lactate levels have followed its use).
  - amine buffers, insulin and glucose infusions, and stimulation of pyruvate dehydrogenase with sodium dichloroacetate have also been tried.

Laevobupivacaine, *see Bupivacaine*

Lambert–Beer law, *see Beer–Lambert law*

Lamotrigine. Anticonvulsant drug, thought to block voltage gated sodium channels and thus inhibit the pre-synaptic release of glutamate and other excitatory neurotransmitters. Used for partial or secondary generalised seizures, either alone or in combination with other anticonvulsants. Has also been used for the treatment of bipolar disorders and in chronic pain management. Rapidly absorbed after oral administration with peak plasma concentrations at 2.5 h; half-life is 24–36 h. Plasma concentration is increased by sodium valproate but decreased by drugs causing enzyme induction (e.g. other anticonvulsants). It also induces its own metabolism.
- Dosage: depends on the drug combination used; generally starts at 25 mg/day increased up to 500 mg/day, orally.
- Side effects: rash and serious skin reactions, fever, malaise, blood dyscrasias, hepatic impairment, visual disturbances, GIT upset.

Lanreotide. Long-acting somatostatin analogue; actions and effects are similar to those of octreotide. Used mainly in long-term management of acromegaly, either by deep sc or im injection.

Lansoprazole. Proton-pump inhibitor; actions and effects are similar to those of omeprazole.
- Dosage: 15–30 mg orally/day.
- Side effects: as for omeprazole.

LAP, *see Left atrial pressure*

Laparoscopy. Originally used mainly for diagnostic gynaecological procedures, now commonly performed for more extensive procedures (e.g. hysterectomy) and other types of surgery, e.g. cholecystectomy, gastric banding. Requires induction of a pneumoperitoneum, usually with CO_2. N_2O has also been used. In general, whilst postoperative pain and morbidity (and thus stay in hospital) are often reduced compared with conventional surgery, patients may be exposed to prolonged operating times and specific complications, which may be related to:
  - gas insufflation:
    - risk of trauma to intra-abdominal viscera (including stomach if previously distended with air during IPPV via facepiece) and great vessels when the trocar is introduced or gas insufflated.
    - risk of gas embolus if gas is inadvertently insufflated into blood vessels. CO_2 is rapidly absorbed from the blood, reducing the size of embolus, whereas N_2O is not.
    - subcutaneous/mediastinal emphysema and pneumothorax may occur.
    - caval compression reducing venous return if intraperitoneal pressure exceeds 3–4 kPa. Higher pressures may compress the aorta.
    - gas may splint the diaphragm and reduce lung expansion.
    - raised intra-abdominal pressure may increase risk of regurgitation and aspiration of gastric contents.
    - CO_2 may be extensively absorbed across the peritoneum, requiring increased alveolar ventilation to maintain normocapnia. If N_2O is used, absorption provides some analgesia.
    - risk of explosion if laparoscopic diathermy is used with N_2O, but not with CO_2 (though ignition of intestinal methane causing explosion has been reported).
    - presence of peritoneal gas postoperatively may cause pain or discomfort, typically referred to the shoulder tip.
  - patient's position: for upper GIT procedures patients are positioned head-up, which may encourage venous pooling in the legs and further hinder venous return. For gynaecological procedures the semilithotomy position is used, which may be associated with:
    - reduced FRC and diaphragmatic splinting, with risk of hypoxaemia and hypoventilation.
    - exacerbated risks of regurgitation.
    - increased venous return when the legs are raised. Pooling of blood in the legs may occur when they are lowered afterwards, with resultant hypotension.
    - high incidence of severe arrhythmias and hypoventilation occurred in earlier studies involving deep halothane anaesthesia with spontaneous ventilation, thought to be related to the above. Bradycardia may occur even in patients receiving IPPV.
  - surgical procedure:
    - bleeding may be unnoticed if not in the immediate area currently being worked on, unless the surgeon regularly inspects the abdomen.
    - large amounts of irrigating fluid may be used, with the risk of hypothermia if not warmed.
    - sudden coughing during upper GIT surgery may risk damage to vital structures (e.g. bile ducts, vessels) if they are being worked on at the time.
    - may involve laser surgery.

Other considerations include any underlying condition of the patient; e.g. most patients for gynaecological laparoscopy are young fit women, whereas those for gastric banding have severe obesity. The above complications have made many anaesthetists choose tracheal intubation and IPPV as the technique of choice, although the laryngeal mask airway is also commonly used for short gynaecological procedures in suitable patients.
- Recommended maximal safe limits for insufflation:
  - 4 l/min.
  - 3–5 litres total gas volume.
  - 3 kPa maximal intraperitoneal pressure.
  - 30–40 min total duration.

Gynaecological laparoscopy may also be performed using local anaesthesia, with infiltration of the abdominal puncture site. Discomfort may result from peritoneal stretching and pneumoperitoneum. Use of epidural/spinal anaesthesia has been described but is rarely attempted because of the above considerations.
Gerges FJ, Kanazi GE, Jabbour-Khoury SI (2006). J Clin Anesth; 18: 67–78

Laplace's law. For a hollow distensible structure:

$$P = \frac{T}{R_1} + \frac{T}{R_2}$$

where P = transmural pressure
T = tension in the wall
R_1 = radius of curvature in one direction
R_2 = radius of curvature in the other direction

For a cylinder, one radius = infinity, therefore $P = \frac{T}{R}$

For a sphere, both radii are equal, therefore $P = \frac{2T}{R}$

- Physiological/clinical importance:
  - cylinders:
    - arteriolar smooth muscle response to fluctuating intraluminal pressure: wall tension varies in order to maintain constant radius and blood flow (one theory of the mechanism of autoregulation).
    - as intraluminal pressure in arterioles or airways falls, or external pressure rises, there is a critical closing pressure across the wall at which collapse may occur. In the lungs, this may occur during forced expiration, limiting expiratory air flow.
  - spheres:
    - ventricular cardiac muscle must generate greater tension when the heart is dilated than when of normal size, in order to produce the same intraventricular pressure. Thus an enlarged failing heart must contract more forcibly to sustain BP, hence the benefit of reducing preload.
    - in the lungs, alveoli would tend to collapse as they became smaller, were it not for surfactant, which reduces surface tension.
    - if the outlet of an anaesthetic breathing system is obstructed, the reservoir bag distends, thus limiting the dangerous build-up of pressure that would occur within a non-distensible bag.

[Pierre-Simon Laplace (1749–1827), French scientist]

Larrey, Baron Dominique Jean (1766–1842). French surgeon-in-chief to Napoleon. Employed refrigeration anaesthesia in 1807, and again in the Russian campaign to allow painless amputations in half-frozen soldiers. Also employed triage. Supported Hickman when the latter presented his experiments on 'suspended animation' to the French Academy in 1828.
Baker D, Cazalaà J-B, Carli P (2005). Resuscitation; 66: 259–62
[Napoleon Bonaparte (1769–1821), French Emperor]

Laryngeal mask airway (LMA). Device for supporting and maintaining the airway without tracheal intubation. Consists of an oval head attached to a connecting tube (Fig. 95a). The head is inserted blindly into the pharynx to lie against the back of the larynx, and the circumferential cuff inflated to form a seal. Pressing the junction of the head and tube backward and upward against the palate during insertion has been recommended by the inventor; alternative methods include insertion with the bowl facing upwards and rotating it 180° once inserted. Tolerated at lighter levels of anaesthesia than a tracheal tube. Insertion is easier following propofol induction of anaesthesia than thiopental induction, because of the former's greater suppression of laryngeal reflexes.

Has been used for spontaneous or controlled ventilation, the latter using inflation pressures of up to 10–25 cmH_2O. Does not protect against aspiration of gastric contents. May be removed before the patient wakes, or left in position. A bite block is required to prevent obstruction or damage by the teeth.

Available in several sizes from 1 (neonates < 5 kg) to 6 (adults > 100 kg), each with its own recommended volume of air for inflation of the cuff although a maximum of 60 cmH_2O has been suggested as more logical than maximal volumes.

- Used for:
  - routine inhalational anaesthesia.
  - inhalational anaesthesia where holding a facepiece may be difficult, e.g. due to the patient's positioning or site of surgery.

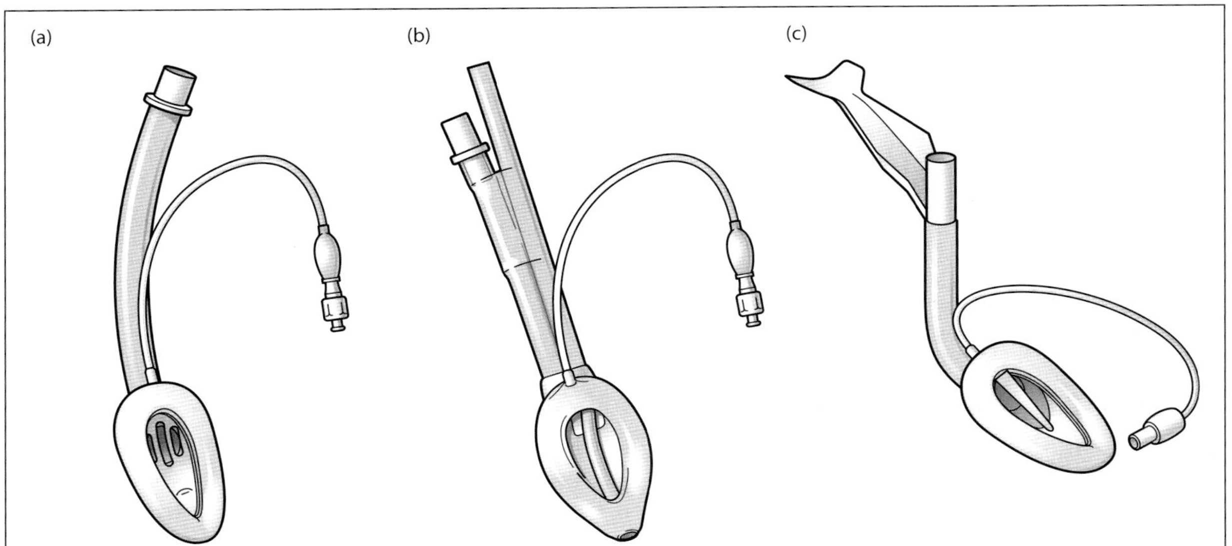

Fig. 95 Laryngeal mask airways: (a) standard; (b) ProSeal; (c) intubating

- airway maintenance in difficult intubation, in both previously unsuspected and known cases.
- emergency management of failed intubation.
- CPR.

Also available with reinforced tubes to prevent kinking. More recent developments include the ProSeal, in which a second tube opens at the tip of the cuff, and through which gastric contents may pass or be aspirated (Fig. 95b); and the intubating laryngeal mask airway, in which the tube is shorter and rigid with a sharp angle. In the latter, the bars covering the laryngeal aperture are replaced by a single flap which lifts the epiglottis when a tracheal tube (a soft silicone one specifically provided for the purpose) is passed blindly through it (Fig. 95c). The intubating and standard laryngeal mask airways have been used (with or without a fibreoptic 'scope) in known and unsuspected cases of difficult intubation. A version of the intubating laryngeal mask airway has also been introduced which incorporates a small display screen mounted at the proximal end of the airway so that intubation can be observed in real time.

Washed and autoclaved between uses; a maximum of 40 uses is recommended by the manufacturer. The standard laryngeal mask airway and the intubating and ProSeal versions are also available in disposable single-use versions, as are many other similar-looking devices based on the same concept but produced by other manufacturers.

Laryngeal nerve blocks, *see Intubation, awake*

Laryngeal nerves. Derived from the vagus nerves:
- superior laryngeal nerve:
  - arises at the base of the skull and passes deep to the carotid arteries.

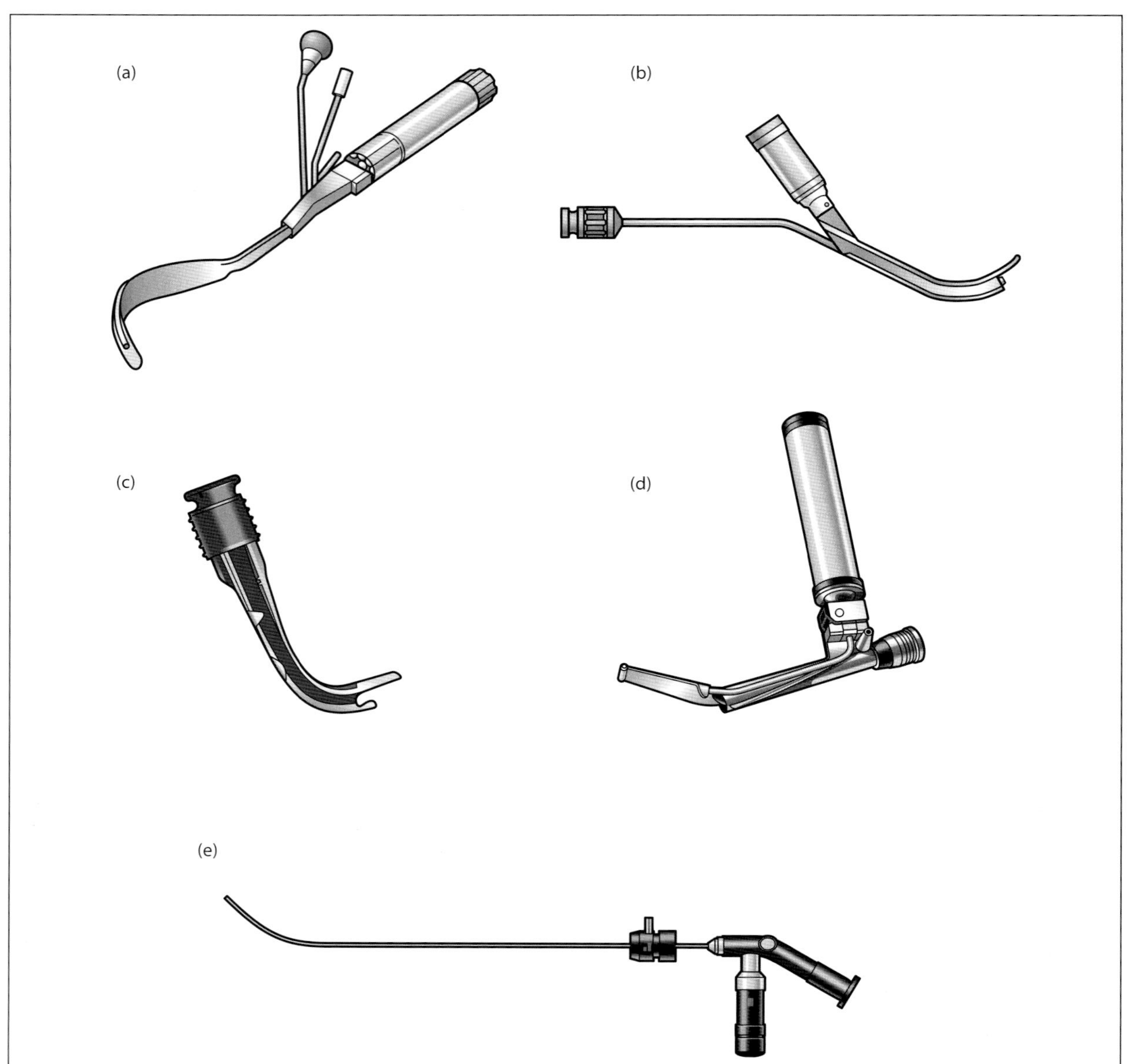

Fig. 96 Rigid laryngoscopes that convey the distal image via viewing channels to an eyepiece: (a) Bullard; (b) Upsher; (c) Airtraq; (d) TruView; (e) Bonfils; or via a screen:

(Continued)

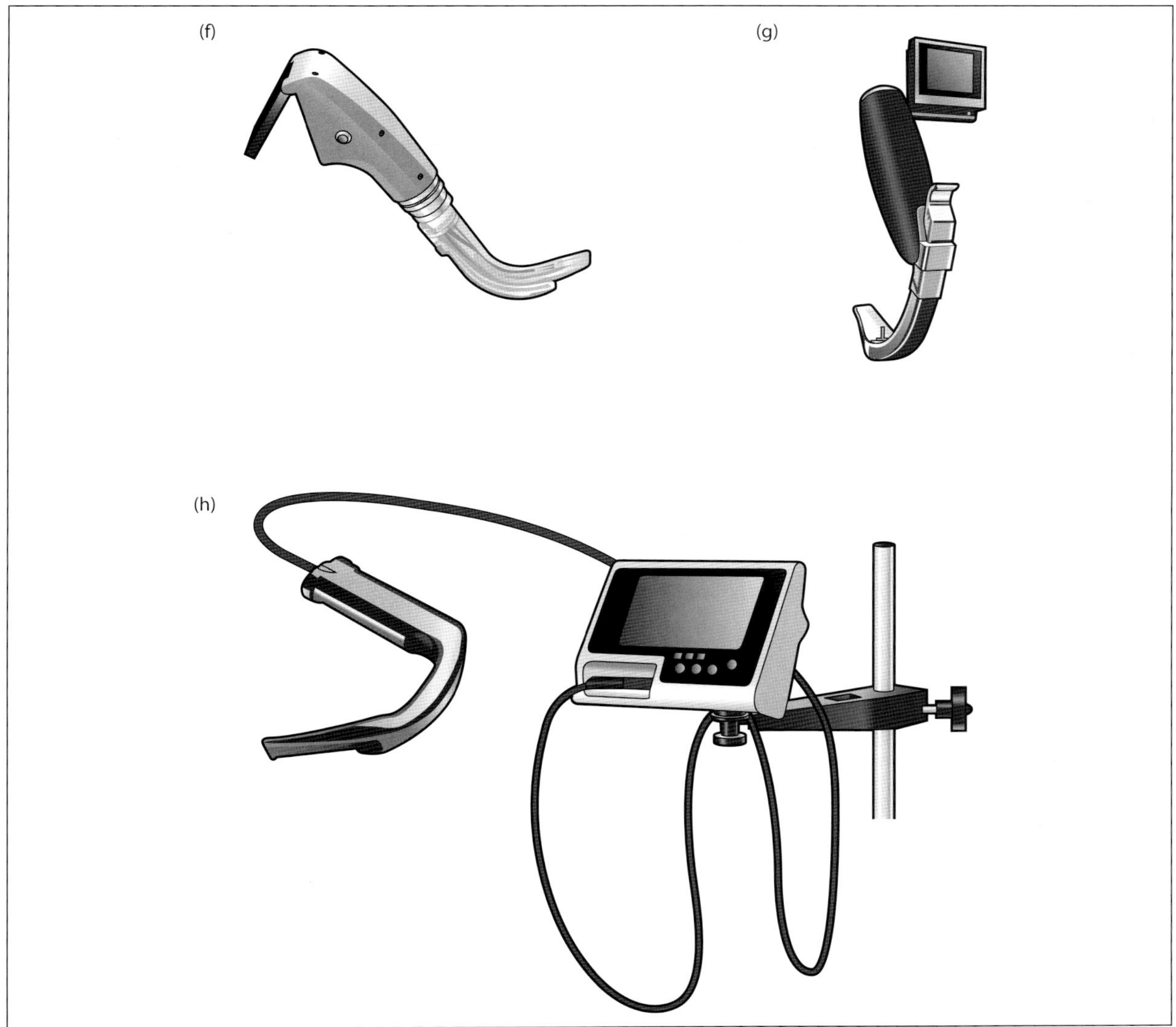

Fig. 96 Cont'd. (f) Airway Scope; (g) McGrath; (h) GlideScope (n.b. various similar devices and versions exist)

- divides into internal and external branches below and anterior to the greater cornua of the hyoid bone.
- the internal laryngeal nerve pierces the thyrohyoid membrane with the superior laryngeal vessels, supplying the mucous membrane of the larynx down to the vocal cords.
- the external laryngeal nerve passes deep to the superior thyroid artery, supplying cricothyroid muscle and the inferior constrictor muscle of the pharynx.

▸ recurrent laryngeal nerve:
- on the left, arises anterior to the ligamentum arteriosus, passes below and behind it and the aorta and ascends in the neck (*see Fig. 110; Neck, cross-sectional anatomy*).
- on the right, given off at the right subclavian artery, passing below and behind it and ascending in the neck.
- in the neck, ascends in the groove between the oesophagus posteriorly and trachea anteriorly.
- enters the larynx posterior to the thyrocricoid joints, deep to the inferior constrictor. Supplies all the intrinsic laryngeal muscles except cricothyroid, and the mucous membrane of the larynx below the vocal cords.

▸ afferent pathways also pass within the above nerves. Sympathetic branches pass with the arterial supply.

- Effects of nerve damage:
  - ▸ superior laryngeal: slack cord and weak voice.
  - ▸ recurrent laryngeal (partial): cord held in the midline because the abductors are affected more than the adductors (Semon's law). The voice is hoarse. If bilateral, severe airway obstruction may occur.
  - ▸ recurrent laryngeal (complete): cord held midway between the midline and abducted position. If bilateral, the cords may be snapped shut during inspiration, causing stridor. The voice is lost.
  - ▸ if one side only is affected, the contralateral cord may move across and restore the voice.

Branches may be damaged during surgery (e.g. thyroidectomy) and also by tracheal intubation, especially if undue force is used or the cuff is inflated within the larynx. The recurrent laryngeal nerve may be involved by lesions in the neck, or thorax or mediastinum (on the left).

The superior laryngeal nerve may be blocked to allow awake tracheal intubation.
[Sir Felix Semon (1849–1921), German-born English laryngologist]
See also, Intubation, awake

Laryngeal reflex. Laryngospasm in response to touching of the laryngeal/hypopharyngeal mucosa. Afferent pathway is via the laryngeal nerves, vagus and brainstem.

Laryngeal tube, *see Airways*

Laryngoscope. Instrument used to perform laryngoscopy. The first direct-vision laryngoscope was invented by Kirstein and later developed by Jackson; the principle was later modified by Magill, Macintosh and others.

- Most consist of:
  - handle:
    - contains a battery power source (originally connected to mains electricity).
    - fibreoptic laryngoscopes have batteries and bulb in the handle, with transmission of light along a fibreoptic bundle set in the blade.
    - short or adjustable handles are available; smaller lighter handles are usually used for paediatric anaesthesia. The Anderson laryngoscope handle bears a hook for the left index finger, allowing laryngoscopy using only the thumb and index finger whilst the other fingers of the left hand are free to apply pressure over the front of the infant's larynx. The hook and blade should be on the same side of the laryngoscope when correctly assembled.
  - blade:
    - usually set at right angles to the handle.
    - many different laryngoscope blades have been described, most of them interchangeable when standard attachments are used.
    - older type of attachment: secured by screwing a pin through the handle and blade seatings (Longworth fitting). Newer forms employ a 'hook on' attachment at the base of the blade, locked on to the handle by a spring-loaded ball-bearing.

Devices incorporating viewing channels or with video chips at the distal end allow either placement of the device in the trachea under visual control, with advancement of the tracheal tube over it, or identification of the glottis and observation of the tube's passage through the vocal cords. The image may be viewed by looking through an eyepiece, attachment to a camera/video system, or via a screen incorporated into the device itself (Fig. 96). Flexible fibreoptic instruments are also available.

Surgical (suspension) laryngoscopes resemble Jackson's more closely; they are comprised of a viewing tube with a right-angled handle, the two components together forming three sides of a rectangle. They are illuminated by an external light source attached to the proximal end of the tube.

Concerns over cross-infection, especially transmission of variant Creutzfeldt-Jakob disease, have led to development of disposable laryngoscope blades, laryngoscopes or blade covers/sheaths.

[Sheila M Anderson (?–1986), London anaesthetist; Longworth Scientific Instrument Co. Ltd, original name for Penlon Ltd; Roger Bullard, Australian anaesthetist; Michael Upsher, US anaesthetist; Matt McGrath, Scottish designer; Pierre Bonfils, Swiss anaesthetist].

Laryngoscope blades. Parts of laryngoscopes inserted into the mouth.

- Consist of:
  - base for attachment to handle.
  - tongue: straight or curved; the former is designed for placement posterior to the epiglottis, the latter for anterior placement. The tip is usually blunt and thickened to reduce trauma.
  - web: forms a shelf along one edge of the tongue, connecting the latter to the flange. Incorporates electric connections and bulb (or fibreoptic bundle). Connection channels are completely removable in older models, and fixed to the web in newer ones.
  - flange: parallel to the tongue; usually only present for the proximal one- to two-thirds of the blade.

  Most are designed for use with the laryngoscope handle held in the left hand; i.e. the tongue is pushed to the left side of the patient's mouth by the flange and web.
- Common varieties (Fig. 97a):
  - Macintosh (1943): tongue, web and flange form a reverse Z shape in cross-section. The most commonly used blade in the UK; also popular in the USA. Available in large adult, adult, child and baby sizes; the latter size was not designed by Macintosh and was criticised by him as being anatomically incorrect. A 'left-handed' version is available, for use when anatomical features of the airway require insertion of the tracheal tube from the left side of the mouth instead of the right. The McCoy blade (1993) is hinged at the tip, and is controlled by a lever on the laryngoscope handle. It allows elevation of the epiglottis whilst reducing the amount of force required during laryngoscopy. Although it may make a difficult laryngoscopy easier, it may also make an easy one more difficult. Another blade with a similar function to the McCoy is actually flexible throughout its length; its curvature is increased by a lever on the handle.
  - polio Macintosh (1950s): mounted at 135° to the handle, to allow intubation in patients confined to iron lung ventilators (e.g. in the Scandinavian polio epidemics of the 1950s). Useful when insertion of the blade into the mouth is hindered, e.g. by barrel chest, enlarged breasts, etc., especially in obstetrics.
  - Magill (1926): U-shaped in cross-section.
  - Miller (1941): similar to Magill's, but with a curved tip and flatter flange and web, requiring less mouth opening for insertion. Available in 4–5 sizes from premature baby to large adult. Popular in the USA.
  - Wisconsin (1941): bigger than Magill's, with the bulb nearer the tip. Available in similar sizes to Miller's blade. Popular in the USA.
  - Soper (1947): straight version of the Macintosh blade. The small transverse slot near the tip was designed to prevent the epiglottis slipping off the blade. Available in adult, child and baby sizes.
  - Bellhouse (1988): angled along its length to give the advantage of a straight blade, whilst the end nearest the anaesthetist is brought anteriorly to avoid obstruction of the anaesthetist's view. May be fitted with an optical prism to enable an indirect view of the glottis when a direct view is impossible.
- Specific paediatric blades (Fig. 97b):
  - Robertshaw (1962): straight tongue with gently curving tip; the flange is folded inwards over the tongue. Available in infant and neonatal sizes.
  - Seward (1957): similar to Robertshaw's but with the flange folded outwards. Available in child and baby sizes.

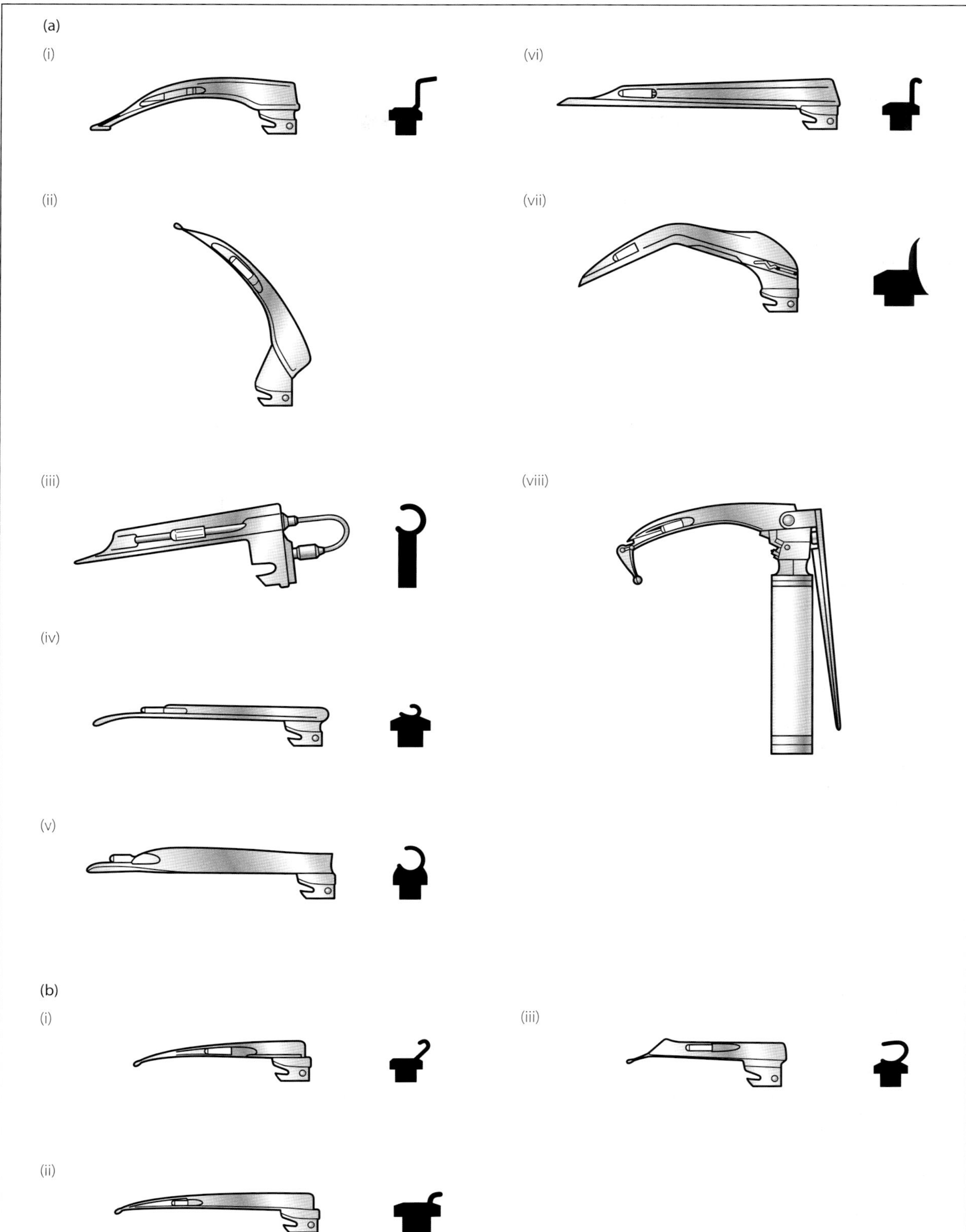

Fig. 97 Laryngoscope blades (not to scale). (a) Adult/paediatric: (i) Macintosh; (ii) polio Macintosh; (iii) Magill; (iv) Miller; (v) Wisconsin; (vi) Soper; (vii) Bellhouse; (viii) McCoy. (b) Paediatric only: (i) Robertshaw; (ii) Seward; (iii) Oxford infant

- Oxford infant (1952): straight tongue with slightly curved tip. Available in one size. Useful for intubation in children with cleft palate.
- Others:
  - Guedel and Flagg (1928): similar to Magill's, but with the bulb at the tip. Guedel's is set at an acute angle to the handle.
  - Bowen–Jackson (1952): similar to Macintosh's but with a cleft tip, designed to straddle the glossoepiglottic fold.
  - Siker (1956): angled blade incorporating a mirror at the angle.
  - Bizzarri–Giuffrida (1958): similar to Macintosh's but with virtually no web and a very small flange; designed for patients with little mouth opening.

Disposable blades (both plastic and metal) and blade covers are available but concern has been raised that although they may reduce the risk of cross-contamination, they may make laryngoscopy more difficult.

[Robert L Soper (1908–1973), RAF anaesthetist; Eamon P McCoy, Belfast anaesthetist; Paul Bellhouse, Australian anaesthetist; Frank L Robertshaw (1918–1991), Manchester anaesthetist; Edgar H Seward (1917–1995), Oxford anaesthetist; Ronald A Bowen (1913–1999) and Ian Jackson, London anaesthetists; Paluel Flagg (1886–1970), Robert A Miller (1906–1976), Ephraim S Siker, Dante V Bizzarri (1914–1994) and Joseph G Giuffrida (?–1993), US anaesthetists]

See also, Intubation aids; Intubation, tracheal

Laryngoscopy. Act of viewing the larynx. Indirect laryngoscopy was first described in 1855 in London by Garcia using a mirror. Direct laryngoscopy was pioneered by Kirstein, Killian and Jackson in the late 1800s/early 1900s, and is now the technique most commonly used for tracheal intubation. The view of the larynx during direct laryngoscopy is shown in Figure 98.

Anaesthesia for diagnostic or therapeutic laryngoscopy must provide relaxation of the jaw and vocal cords, with rapid recovery of laryngeal reflexes without laryngospasm. Problems include sharing of the airway, the hypertensive response to laryngoscopy, contamination of the airway with blood, etc. Usually performed under general anaesthesia, with IPPV through a special 5–6 mm 'microlaryngoscopy' cuffed tracheal tube (resistance is too high for spontaneous ventilation). Other methods include injector and insufflation techniques as for bronchoscopy. Spraying the cords with lidocaine reduces postoperative laryngospasm but at the expense of diminished laryngeal reflexes.

[Manuel Garcia (1805–1906), Spanish singing teacher]

See also, Intubation, complications of; Intubation, difficult; Intubation, tracheal

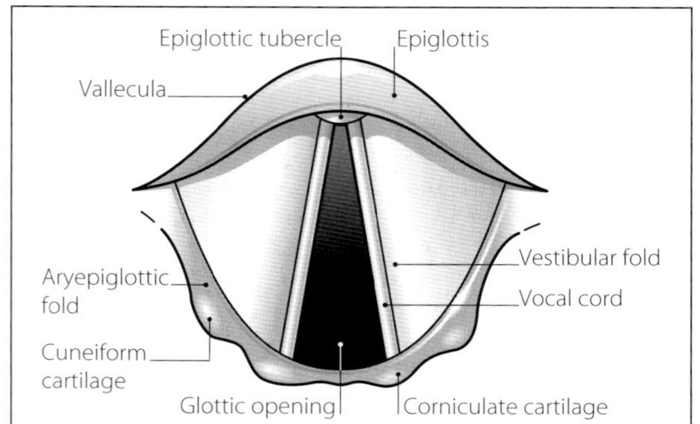

Fig. 98 View obtained during direct laryngoscopy

Laryngospasm. Reflex closure of the glottis by adduction of the true and/or false cords. May persist after cessation of its stimulus. The precise mechanism is controversial; the lateral cricoarytenoid muscles are thought to be most important in adducting the cords whilst cricothyroid tenses them. The extrinsic muscles of the larynx may also have a role.

- Caused by:
  - local stimulation of the larynx by saliva, blood, vomitus, foreign body (including laryngoscope, airway or tracheal tube), etc.
  - response to other stimulation, e.g. surgery, movement, stimulation of anus, cervix, etc. (Brewer–Luckhardt reflex).

The reflex is abolished in planes 2–4 of anaesthesia; thus its occurrence may indicate insufficient depth of anaesthesia. Occurs in about 1% of the general population during general anaesthesia, up to 3% in infants and up to 10% in patients with recent upper respiratory tract infections or smokers.

May cause complete or partial airway obstruction, the latter often presenting as inspiratory stridor. Causes hypoxaemia and hypoventilation; pulmonary oedema has been reported.

- Management:
  - cessation of stimulus.
  - administration of 100% O_2. Positive airway pressure may be applied by tightening the expiratory valve of the breathing system, thus increasing the intake of O_2 with each breath.
  - when laryngospasm has subsided, depth of anaesthesia may be deepened.
  - laryngeal muscle relaxation may be achieved with suxamethonium (as little as 8–10 mg may suffice) or propofol, followed by ventilation with O_2 and tracheal intubation if necessary.
- Prevented by:
  - achieving adequate depth of anaesthesia before attempting laryngoscopy, insertion of airway, surgery, etc.
  - local anaesthetic spray to the larynx and laryngeal nerve blocks.
  - use of neuromuscular blocking drugs and tracheal intubation.

Larynx.

- Functions:
  - protects the tracheobronchial tree and lungs, e.g. during swallowing.
  - allows coughing.
  - allows speech.
  - allows straining, e.g. during defaecation.

Extends from the root of the tongue to the cricoid cartilage, i.e. level with C3–6 (at higher level in children).

- Dimensions:
  - length: 45 mm (men); 35 mm (women).
  - anteroposterior: 35 mm (men); 25 mm (women).
  - transverse: 45 mm (men); 40 mm (women).
- Composed of hyoid bone, and epiglottic, thyroid, cricoid, arytenoid, corniculate and cuneiform cartilages, joined by several muscles and ligaments (Fig. 99):
  - hyoid bone:
    - level with C3.
    - U-shaped, with horizontal body and bilateral greater and lesser horns, which pass backwards and upwards respectively.
    - attached superiorly to the mandible and tongue (by hyoglossus, mylohyoid, geniohyoid and digastric muscles), and styloid process (by stylohyoid ligament and muscle).

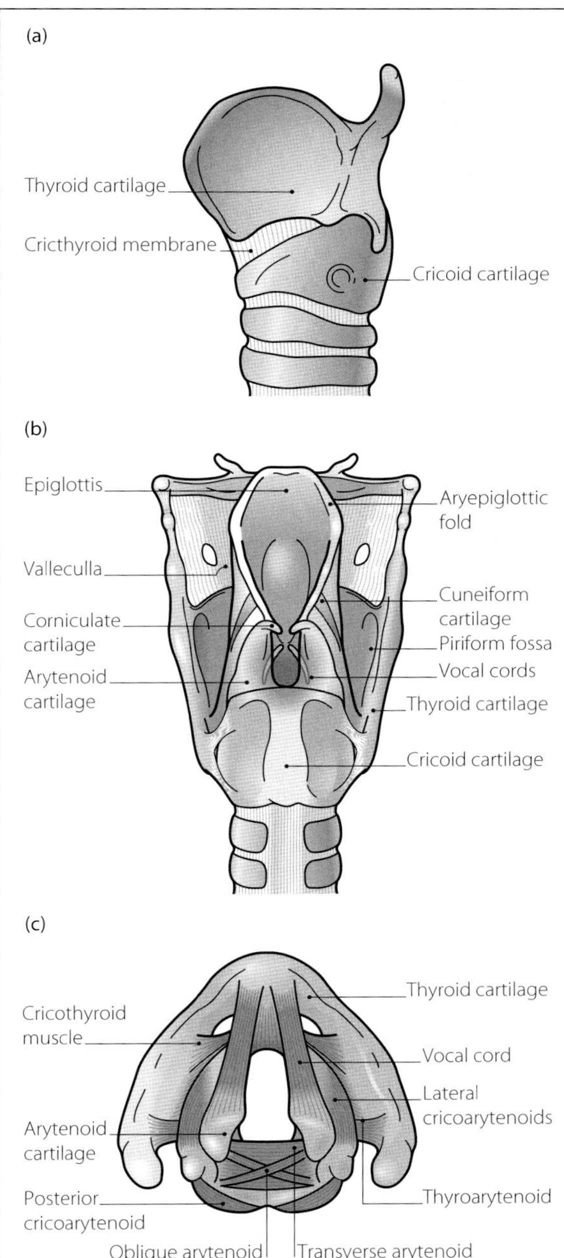

Fig. 99 Anatomy of the larynx: (a) lateral view; (b) posterior view; (c) superior view with intrinsic muscles

- attached inferiorly to the thyroid cartilage (by thyrohyoid membrane and muscle), sternum (by sternohyoid muscle) and clavicle (by omohyoid muscle).
- attached posteriorly to the pharynx by the middle constrictor muscle.

- epiglottis:
  - leaf-shaped, attached anteriorly to the base of the tongue, body of the hyoid and back of the thyroid cartilage above the vocal cords. The depression on either side of the midline glossoepiglottic fold is the vallecula, with the pharyngoepiglottic folds laterally.
  - attached to the arytenoid laterally by the aryepiglottic membrane.
- thyroid cartilage:
  - formed from two quadrilateral halves, meeting anteriorly to form the thyroid notch level with C4. The posterior edge forms superior and inferior horns on each side, the latter articulating with the cricoid cartilage.
  - attached superiorly to the hyoid bone by the thyrohyoid membrane and muscle.
  - attached posteriorly to the pharynx (by inferior constrictor muscle, palatopharyngeus and salpingopharyngeus muscles) and styloid process (by stylothyroid muscle).
  - attached inferiorly to the cricoid (by cricothyroid membrane and muscle) and sternum (by sternothyroid muscle).
  - attached inferomedially to the arytenoids by thyroarytenoid muscle; part of it attaches to the free border of cricothyroid forming vocalis muscle and part attaches to the lateral epiglottis forming thyroepiglottic muscle.
- cricoid cartilage:
  - signet-ring shaped, broadest posteriorly. Level with C6. The lateral surface articulates with the inferior horn of the thyroid cartilage; its upper surface posteriorly articulates with the arytenoids.
  - attached via the superior surface to the thyroid cartilage by the cricothyroid membrane.
  - attached via the lateral surface to the thyroid cartilage (by cricothyroid muscle) and arytenoids (by lateral cricoarytenoid muscles).
  - attached via the posterior surface to the arytenoids by the posterior cricoarytenoid muscles.
  - attached inferiorly to the trachea by the cricotracheal membrane.
- arytenoid cartilages:
  - pyramid shaped, the bases articulating with the back of the cricoid.
  - also attached to the cricoid by posterior and lateral cricoarytenoid muscles.
  - the vocal cords pass from the vocal processes anteriorly to the back of the thyroid cartilage.
  - attached to the epiglottis superomedially via the aryepiglottic folds and muscles.
  - attached anterolaterally to the back of the thyroid cartilages by the thyroarytenoid muscles.
  - attached to each other by the transverse arytenoid muscle.
- corniculate cartilages: form tubercles in the posterior aryepiglottic folds, at the apex of the arytenoids.
- cuneiform cartilages: lie anterior to the corniculate cartilages, in the aryepiglottic folds.

- Membranes and areas of the larynx:
  - aryepiglottic membrane:
    - passes from the anterior arytenoid to lateral epiglottis.
    - forms the vestibular fold at the lower border. The area between vestibular folds is termed the rima vestibuli; that between the aryepiglottic fold and vestibular fold is the vestibule; the recess between the vocal and vestibular cords is the laryngeal sinus (saccule).
  - cricothyroid membrane: free upper border forms the vocal cord (level with C5) between the back of the thyroid cartilage and vocal process of the arytenoid; it contains the vocal ligament beneath its mucosa. The area between vocal cords is the rima glottidis (glottis).
  - thyrohyoid membrane: lateral borders are thickened to form the lateral thyrohyoid ligaments.

The entrance to the larynx slopes downwards and backwards, bounded anteriorly by the epiglottis, laterally by the aryepiglottic folds and posteriorly by the arytenoid cartilages. The piriform fossa is the recess on each side, between the aryepiglottic folds medially and thyroid cartilage and thyrohyoid membrane laterally. The rima glottidis is the narrowest part of the airway in adults; the cricoid is the narrowest in children.

- Epithelium: squamous above the cords, columnar below. Mucosa of the cords is closely adherent.
- Muscle actions (Fig. 99c):
  - the cords are tensed by cricothyroid and relaxed by thyroarytenoid and vocalis muscles.
  - the cords are abducted by the posterior cricoarytenoids, causing outward rotation and movement of the arytenoids.
  - the cords are adducted by the lateral cricoarytenoids (causing inward rotation of the arytenoids) and transverse arytenoid muscle (causing the arytenoids to move together).
  - the inlet is opened by the thyroepiglottic muscle and closed by the aryepiglottic muscle.
  - the larynx is elevated by muscles from the pharynx and those above the hyoid, and depressed by sternothyroid.
- Nerve supply:
  - recurrent **laryngeal nerve**: all muscles except cricothyroid, and sensation below vocal cords.
  - superior laryngeal nerve: cricothyroid muscle, and sensation above vocal cords.
- Blood supply: branches of superior and inferior thyroid arteries and accompanying veins.
- Lymphatic drainage:
  - above cords: to upper deep cervical nodes.
  - below cords: to lower deep cervical nodes.

See also, Laryngoscopy

Laser surgery. Use of laser (Light Amplification by Stimulated Emission of Radiation) radiation to cause tissue destruction by producing intense local heat. Involves stimulation of atoms, ions or molecules within a tube using high voltage. Energy is absorbed and emitted by the particles; the emitted energy is amplified and allowed to escape as a parallel beam of coherent light, of precise wavelength and in phase.

- Effects of the laser beam on tissues depend on its wavelength:
  - CO_2 laser (wavelength 10 600 nm): used for precise surgical cutting and coagulation, e.g. in **ENT surgery**, **neurosurgery**, general and gynaecological surgery and dermatology.
  - neodymium yttrium–aluminium–garnet (NdYAG) laser (1060 nm): used for photocoagulation and debulking of tumours, e.g. bronchial carcinoma.
  - argon or krypton (400–700 nm): used for photocoagulation in ophthalmology and dermatology.
- Risks to patient and operating staff:
  - ocular (corneal and retinal) damage: prevented by containment of the laser beam, and by wearing protective glasses. Most glasses will absorb energy from the CO_2 laser; specifically tinted goggles are required for the other types.
  - skin damage: prevented by appropriate towelling of the patient.
  - **explosions and fires**: particularly problematic during upper airway surgery, when the high energy beams may cause ignition of anaesthetic vapours, rubber, PVC or silicone tracheal tubes, drapes, etc. The following precautions have been suggested:
    - flexible metal tracheal tubes without cuffs.
    - metallic-coated tubes: expensive, and may still be susceptible to damage. Cuff inflation is with saline instead of air.
    - protection of the tube by wrapping in metallic tape: risks detachment of the tape within the airway, or damage to tissues by the tape's sharp edges; no longer recommended now that coated or metal tubes are available.
    - avoidance of tracheal intubation, e.g. use of **insufflation** or **injector techniques**, including **high frequency ventilation**.
    - use of non-explosive mixtures of gases, e.g. under 30% O_2 in nitrogen or helium. Intermittent flushing with 100% nitrogen or helium has been used.
    - limitation of laser power and duration of bursts.

    Vigilance should be high. If ignition occurs, the O_2 source should be disconnected and the operative site doused with water.
  - gas embolism if the probe's tip is gas-cooled.
  - production of noxious/potentially infective fumes: adequate suction is required.

Latent heat. Energy required solely to change the state of a substance, without changing its temperature, e.g.:

- liquid to gas or vice versa (latent heat of vaporisation).
- solid to liquid or vice versa (latent heat of fusion).

Heat is required to change liquid to a gas, in order to overcome the attraction between molecules and expand the substance; heat is given out when the reverse occurs, e.g. when steam condenses.

Specific latent heat is the energy required to alter the state of unit mass of substance at specified temperature; e.g. specific latent heat of vaporisation of water = 2.26 MJ/kg at 100°C. It is greater at lower temperatures, and falls at higher temperatures until it reaches zero at the **critical temperature**.

Lateral cutaneous nerve of the forearm, block, *see Elbow, nerve blocks*

Lateral cutaneous nerve of the thigh, block. Provides analgesia of the lateral thigh, e.g. following skin harvesting, and to reduce leg tourniquet pain. Has also been used in pain states and to diagnose entrapment neuropathy of the nerve caused by the latter's piercing the inguinal ligament instead of passing under it (meralgia paraesthetica), prior to surgical treatment.

The nerve (L2–3) arises from the **lumbar plexus** (may arise from the femoral nerve), passing under the inguinal ligament just medial to the anterior superior iliac spine to supply the skin of the lateral side of the thigh (*see Fig. 66; Femoral triangle*). A needle is inserted 2 cm medial and inferior to the iliac spine, at right angles to the skin. A click is felt as the fascia lata is pierced. 10–15 ml **local anaesthetic agent** is injected fanwise, mediolaterally.

May also be blocked via **femoral nerve block** (three-in-one block).

Latex allergy. Typically occurs in individuals repeatedly exposed to latex, e.g. healthcare workers and patients undergoing repeated urinary catheterisation (e.g. those with spina bifida) or surgery. Thought to be true **anaphylaxis** to various soluble proteins in latex.

May present as cardiovascular collapse during surgery, when the cause may not be easily apparent. A history of allergy to rubber (e.g. rubber gloves, condoms, etc.) may be obtained. Typically associated with allergy to bananas, avocados and chestnuts.

Evaluation includes skin-testing, *in vitro* leucocyte studies and testing for anti-latex IgE. Perioperative management includes avoidance of all latex-containing equipment including

facemasks, gloves, airways/tubes, rebreathing bags/bellows, bungs, drains and catheters. Drugs vials with rubber tops and iv tubing with rubber injection ports should be avoided. Protection of the arm with gauze before application of a rubber BP cuff has been suggested, although cuffs and other equipment are increasingly manufactured without latex. Pretreatment with antihistamine drugs, H_2 antagonist drugs and corticosteroids has been used but may not be necessary if proper precautions have been carried out. Since airborne latex particles have triggered allergic reactions, no latex-containing equipment should be used in the operating room before a known case; scheduling surgery for the beginning of the operating list has been advocated. A high index of suspicion and availability of resuscitative drugs are important; management of a reaction should follow standard lines as for adverse drug reactions.
Hepner DL, Castells MC (2003). Anes Analg; 96: 1219–29

Laudanosine. Tertiary amine, a product of atracurium metabolism via Hofmann degradation. Half-life is about 2–3 h, i.e. considerably longer than for atracurium; approximately doubled in renal failure. In anaesthetised dogs, causes epileptiform EEG changes at blood levels over 17 µg/ml. Blood levels in humans, even after several days' infusion of atracurium in patients with renal and hepatic failure, rarely rise above 5 µg/ml, although fears have been expressed about central stimulation in patients at risk, e.g. those with an impaired blood–brain barrier. Cisatracurium at equipotent doses produces one-fifth of the level of laudanosine. Has recently been found to have analgesic effects in animals, and to interact with central GABA, opioid and acetylcholine receptors.
Fodale V, Santamaria LB (2002). Eur J Anaesthesiol; 19: 466–73

Lavoisier, Antoine Laurent (1742–1794). French chemist. Disproved the phlogiston theory, showing that the gain in weight of sulphur or phosphorus on combustion was due to combination with air. Concluded that air consists of two elastic fluids: one necessary for combustion and respiration, and one that would support neither. Renamed the former (previously called dephlogisticated air) 'oxygene', estimating its concentration in air to be about 25%.

Lawen, Arthur (1876–1958). German surgeon, the first to perform caudal analgesia for abdominal surgery, using large volumes of procaine. Also described paravertebral block, and helped popularise regional anaesthesia. Described the use of curare to produce relaxation during surgery in 1912.

Laxatives. Perioperative/ICU usage:
- to prepare the lower GIT before surgery.
- to reduce pain following rectal or anal surgery.
- to treat constipation, e.g. on ICU or postoperatively.
- to treat poisoning and overdoses, e.g. whole bowel irrigation, especially in children.

- Divided into:
  - bulk-forming laxatives: increase faecal mass and stimulate peristalsis. Useful in patients with enterostomies and colonic disease. Include bran, methylcellulose, ispaghula and sterculia.
  - stimulants: increase GIT motility. Include senna, bisacodyl, dantron, docusate sodium, glycerol (also acts as an osmotic laxative and faecal softener) and sodium picosulfate.
  - faecal softeners: liquid paraffin is rarely used since if aspirated may cause severe pneumonitis. Arachis oil enemas may be useful for impacted faeces.
  - osmotic laxatives: cause retention of water within the bowel. Include lactulose (broken down by gut bacteria to osmotically active compounds; also reduces ammonia production hence its use in hepatic failure), polyethylene glycols and rectal citrate or phosphates (caution in renal impairment since hyperphosphataemia may result). Magnesium salts act within just 2–4 h but should not be used in renal impairment because of systemic absorption.
  - bowel cleansers: usually mixtures of agents; should not be used in constipation. In frail patients, preoperative use may result in significant dehydration. Used in whole bowel irrigation.

Dosage depends on the particular preparation used. Complications include dehydration and electrolyte disturbances. Stimulants may cause abdominal cramps; osmotic laxatives may cause bloating. Laxatives (especially stimulants) are contraindicated in intestinal obstruction.

Lazaroids. Group of 21-aminosteroid analogues which have membrane stabilising properties without the mineralo- or glucocorticoid properties of conventional corticosteroids. Tirilazad is under investigation for its cerebral protection properties in cerebral ischaemia following head injury and subarachnoid haemorrhage and in spinal cord injury. Thought to act by inhibiting membrane lipid peroxidation, thus reducing damage caused by oxygen free radicals.
Kavanagh RJ, Kam PCA (2001). Br J Anaesth; 86: 110–19

LBBB, Left bundle branch block, *see Bundle branch block*

LD_{50}, *see Therapeutic index/ratio*

Le Fort classification, *see Facial trauma*

Left atrial pressure (LAP). Mean pressure approximates to left ventricular end-diastolic pressure, unless the mitral valve is abnormal. Pressure wave abnormalities are similar to the venous waveform, but with reference to mitral and aortic valves and systemic circulation, instead of tricuspid and pulmonary valves and pulmonary circulation.

May be measured via a catheter inserted directly into the left atrium, or indirectly via pulmonary artery catheterisation, which measures pulmonary capillary wedge pressure. Usually measured from mid-axilla or sternal angle. Normal value is 2–10 mmHg.

Left ventricular ejection time, *see Systolic time intervals*

Left ventricular end-diastolic pressure (LVEDP). Reflects the preload of the left ventricle. Provided ventricular compliance is constant, a constant relationship (exponential rather than linear) holds between LVEDP and left ventricular end-diastolic volume. Normal LVEDP does not ensure normal ventricular function, and abnormal LVEDP may not indicate degree of dysfunction. Elevations of LVEDP (normally under 12 mmHg) may reflect increased blood volume, reduced myocardial contractility, reduced ventricular compliance and increased venous return. May be measured directly via a ventricular cannula or arterial cannulation, or inferred via pulmonary artery catheterisation.

Left ventricular end-diastolic volume. Nearest physiological variable to left ventricular preload as described by Starling's law. May be assessed using echocardiography or radiology, but indicators of left ventricular end-diastolic pressure are easier to measure. Normally 70–95 ml/m^2.

Left ventricular failure, *see Cardiac failure*

Left ventricular fractional shortening. Indicator of left ventricular function derived from M-mode echocardiography.

Equals:

$$\frac{\text{(end-diastolic internal dimension)} - \text{(end-systolic internal dimension)}}{\text{end-diastolic internal dimension}}$$

Normally 34–44%; often easier to estimate during echocardiography than doing a formal evaluation of ejection fraction.

Left ventricular stroke work, *see Stroke work*

Legionnaires' disease. Caused by species of legionella, Gram-negative aerobic bacteria. First came to prominence when it killed 29 delegates at an American Legion convention in 1976. More likely to affect elderly patients. Acquired by inhaling contaminated water particles, especially derived from cooling towers; typically occurs in epidemics involving a single building. Presents as an acute febrile chest infection, typically with myalgia, fatigue and GIT upset before respiratory symptoms develop. Pleuritic chest pain and confusion may occur. Widespread infiltrates may be present on chest X-ray. Diagnosis is via sputum culture ± serological testing. Treatment is with erythromycin; 4-quinolones have also been used. The disease lasts for 7–10 days. Mortality rates of 10–30% have been reported.

Lenograstim, *see Granulocyte colony-stimulating factor*

Lepirudin. Recombinant hirudin, used as an alternative to heparin if the latter induces immune thrombocytopenia.

- Dosage: 400 μg/kg slowly iv followed by 150 μg/kg/h up to 16.5 mg/h, adjusted according to coagulation studies.
- Side effects: bleeding; hypersensitivity.

Leptospirosis (Weil's disease). Caused by species of leptospira, Gram-negative aerobic bacteria. Passed from asymptomatic animals (dogs, rodents, livestock and wild animals) via their urine to water, where it may survive for many months. Typically affects sewage workers. Acquired via mucous membranes and broken skin; it causes widespread vasculitis affecting the kidney, liver, lungs and heart. Clinical features include fever, myalgia, headache/neck stiffness, cough, chest pain, confusion, rash and occasionally renal and hepatic failure. Diagnosed retrospectively by increases in antibody titre. Treatment is with benzylpenicillin, erythromycin or tetracyclines. Normal organ function returns usually within 1–2 months. Mortality is up to 11% if hepatic failure occurs.

[H Adolph Weil (1848–1916), German physician]

LES, *see Lower oesophageal sphincter*

Letheon. Name given to diethyl ether by Morton when he patented his discovery. Despite this patent, ether was widely used without acknowledgement of Morton's claim. His attempts to enforce the patent and payments of royalties included approaching the governments of the USA and France, but were unsuccessful.

[Lethe (Greek mythology), river in Hades whose waters induced forgetfulness in those who drank them]

Leucocytes. White blood cells; total count in peripheral blood is 4–10 × 10^9/l.

- Exist as three morphologically different types:
  - granulocytes: derived from common bone marrow precursor stem cells:
    - neutrophils (60–70%; 2.5–7 × 10^9/l): phagocytic with high enzyme content.
    - eosinophils (1–4%; 0.01–0.4 × 10^9/l): contain histamine and are involved in cell-mediated allergic reactions.
    - basophils (0–1%; 0–0.2 × 10^9/l): contain histamine and heparin; non-phagocytic.
  - lymphocytes (23–35%: 1–3.5 × 10^9/l): derived from lymphoid stem cells throughout the body including bone marrow. Mainly concerned with immune mechanisms: B (bursa) cells with immunoglobulin production and T (thymus) cells with immune system regulation and killing of infected cells.
  - monocytes (4–8%; 0.2–0.8 × 10^9/l): formed in spleen, lymphoid tissue and marrow. Differentiate into phagocytic tissue macrophages.

Leucocytosis may be caused by almost any acute illness as part of the inflammatory response. Leucopenia may be caused by reduced production (e.g. drugs, radiation, inflammation, infection, infiltration of bone marrow by malignancy, fibrosis) or increased utilisation (e.g. sequestration into the tissues). Thus in severe illness, white cell count may be increased or decreased. A low count appears to be prognostic of increased mortality in ICU patients.

Bellingan G (2000). Intensive Care Med; 26: S111–18

See also, Erythrocytes; Platelets

Leukotriene pathway inhibitors. Group of drugs which block the synthesis of all leukotrienes; have been used in asthma along with the leukotriene receptor antagonists. Zileuton is an example.

Leukotriene receptor antagonists. Group of drugs which block the action of cysteinyl leukotrienes at their receptors, especially on bronchial smooth muscle. Have been used orally in mild/moderate asthma but not indicated for treatment of acute attacks. Churg–Strauss syndrome (eosinophilia, systemic vasculitis and worsening pulmonary symptoms) has been reported following their use. Examples include montelukast, zafirlukast and pranlukast.

[Jacob Churg (1910–2005; Polish-born) and Lotte Strauss (1913–1985; German born), US pathologists]

Leukotrienes. Series of compounds derived from arachidonic acid by the action of lipoxygenases. Act as mediators of inflammation, and released from mast cells, platelets and some leucocytes following mechanical, thermal, chemical, infective and immunological stimuli. Most leukotrienes cause bronchoconstriction, vasoconstriction and increased vascular permeability; the cysteinyl leukotrienes LTC_4, LTD_4 and LTE_4 account for the activity originally known as slow-reacting substance of anaphylaxis (SRS-A). LTB_4 is a potent chemotactic agent for other inflammatory cells. They have been implicated in the pathophysiology of sepsis and ARDS. The cysteinyl leukotrienes are extremely potent bronchoconstrictors and have been implicated in asthma, especially LTE_4; given experimentally they induce changes which persist for several days. Leukotriene pathway inhibitors and leukotriene receptor antagonists have recently been developed for use in asthma.

Peters-Golden M, Henderson WR (2007). N Engl J Med; 357: 1841–54

Levallorphan tartrate. Opioid receptor antagonist with partial agonist properties, the *n*-allyl derivative of levorphanol.

Synthesised in 1950. 1.25 mg levallorphan has been combined with 100 mg pethidine as Pethilorphan, but hopes of analgesia without respiratory depression were not realised. Its use has been superseded by naloxone.

Levetiracetam. Anticonvulsant drug used as monotherapy or as an adjunct in the treatment of partial or generalised epilepsy and for myoclonic seizures. Mechanism of action is unknown.

- Dosage: 250 mg–1.5 g 12 hourly, orally or iv.
- Side effects: GIT upset, cough, ataxia, visual disturbance, thrombocytopenia.

Levobupivacaine, *see Bupivacaine*

Levofloxacin. Antibacterial drug, one of the 4-quinolones related to ciprofloxacin but more active against pneumococci.

- Dosage: 250–500 mg orally or iv over 60 min, once/twice daily.
- Side effects: as for ciprofloxacin. Hypotension and thrombophlebitis may occur on iv administration.

Levorphanol tartrate. Synthetic opioid analgesic drug, synthesised in 1949. Similar to morphine but less sedating. Onset of action is under 30 min, lasting for up to 8 h. No longer available in the UK.

Levosimendan, *see Calcium sensitisers*

Lidocaine hydrochloride (Lignocaine). Amide local anaesthetic agent, introduced in 1947 (revolutionising regional anaesthesia because of its superior safety to previous agents). The standard drug against which other local anaesthetics are compared. pK_a is 7.9. 65% protein-bound; 95% of an injected dose undergoes hepatic metabolism and is excreted renally. Onset is rapid by all routes; usual duration of action for 1% solution is about 1 h, increased to 1.5–2 h if adrenaline is added.

- Uses:
  - local anaesthesia. Often combined with adrenaline, since lidocaine tends to produce local vasodilatation; 1:200 000 and 1:80 000 solutions are commonly available, the latter usually restricted to dental use.
  - iv administration:
    - depression of laryngeal and tracheal reflexes (e.g. during tracheal intubation/extubation). Commonly used to reduce the increase in ICP caused by laryngoscopy. Possibly reduces muscle pains and potassium increase after suxamethonium. It has been used to produce analgesia and general anaesthesia (although its therapeutic ratio is low). 4–10% lidocaine has been used instead of air to inflate the tracheal tube cuff, thereby reducing postoperative sore throat and hoarseness.
    - class I antiarrhythmic drug in ventricular tachyarrhythmias.
- Many preparations are available, including:
  - 0.25–0.5% solutions for infiltration anaesthesia and IVRA.
  - 1–2% solutions for nerve blocks and epidural anaesthesia.
  - 4% solution for topical anaesthesia of the mucous membranes of the mouth, pharynx and respiratory tract.
  - 10% spray for topical anaesthesia as above. Available in metered dose delivery systems (10 mg/spray).
  - also available in 1–2% gel for urethral instillation, and 5% ointment for skin, rectum and other mucous membranes. A constituent of EMLA cream. In other countries (especially the USA). 5% hyperbaric solution has been used in spinal anaesthesia (but see below).
- Dosage:
  - depends on the block.
  - 1–2 mg/kg iv 2–5 min before intubation/extubation.
  - for ventricular arrhythmias: 1 mg/kg iv initially, then 4 mg/kg/min for 30 min, 2 mg/kg/min for 2 h, and 1 mg/kg/min thereafter.

  May be given via the tracheal tube in emergency at twice the iv dose.

Adverse effects are as for local anaesthetic agents. Lidocaine is thought to be more toxic to nerve tissue when directly applied than other local anaesthetics, hence the increased incidence of transient radicular irritation syndrome following its use for spinal anaesthesia than with other drugs (hyperbaricity of the solution and use of very thin needles/catheters are also thought to contribute by encouraging pooling of drug around spinal nerves). This has led to revision of the drug's data sheet to specify dilution to 2.5% before administration (even this concentration has been implicated in causing transient symptoms). Maximal recommended dose: 3 mg/kg without adrenaline, 7 mg/kg with adrenaline. Toxic plasma levels: above about 10 μg/ml.

Life support, *see Cardiopulmonary resuscitation*

Lightwand. Device used to place a tracheal tube without requiring laryngoscopy. Consists of a flexible malleable stylet incorporating a light bulb at the distal end, with the battery and handle at the proximal end. Placed inside a tracheal tube with the bulb at the tube's tip, the tube/lightwand combination is bent into a J shape and manoeuvred into the larynx, with successful placement indicated by a glow at the anterior neck below the thyroid prominence. The tracheal tube is then passed into the trachea and the lightwand removed. Oesophageal placement is suggested by a more diffuse glow above the prominence.

Several different types exist. The technique has been used for both routine and difficult intubations.

Agro F, Hung OR, Cataldo R, et al (2001). Can J Anesth; 48: 592–9

Lignocaine, *see Lidocaine*

Likelihood ratio. Method of quantifying the probability of two hypotheses. For a predictive test, it equals the probability that a person with the condition has a positive test, over the probability that a person without the condition has a positive test. Also equals sensitivity divided by (one minus specificity).

Limbic system. Part of the brain, formerly termed the rhinencephalon. Composed of left and right lobes, each consisting of:

- rim of cortical tissue around the hilum of the cerebral hemisphere.
- associated deep structures: hippocampus and gyrus, uncus, amygdala, cingulate gyrus, part of insula, septal area, isthmus, Broca's olfactory area and orbital surface of the frontal lobe. Also includes the hippocampal formation and thus associated with memory.

Responsible for olfaction, feeding behaviour, motivation, sexual behaviour and generation of emotions. Damage to the amygdala is associated with rage reactions, hyperphagia and increased sexual activity; lesions in the uncus with olfactory and gustatory hallucinations.

Thought to be one site of action of benzodiazepines and possibly other anaesthetic drugs.
[Pierre P Broca (1824–1880), French surgeon]

LiMON. Commercial non-invasive monitor of liver function and blood volume. Requires peripheral or central venous access and uses a 4-wavelength near infra-red finger sensor. Measures the plasma disappearance rate and the 15-min retention rate of an intravenous marker, indocyanine green. Knowledge of the cardiac output permits estimation of circulating blood volume and indocyanine green clearance within minutes. As the elimination of indocyanine green is dependent on both liver blood flow and parenchymal cellular function, the system cannot differentiate the cause of a reduced clearance of indocyanine green. However, any sudden reduction in clearance will reflect a fall in liver blood flow. Up to 10 measurements are possible in any 24-h period.
See also, Liver function tests

Linear analogue scale (Visual analogue scale). Method of evaluating pain, nausea, anxiety and other symptoms, e.g. for statistical analysis. For example, for pain evaluation, a horizontal 10 cm line is drawn on plain paper, with 'no pain' written at the left-hand end, and 'worst possible pain' at the right-hand end. The patient marks his or her position on the line. Thought to be more reliable than assessments where patients choose the most appropriate number or word from a list, which may be influenced by personal preference for certain words or numbers and limited by the number of choices offered. Thought to be consistent for any individual; however, because patients may interpret the analogue scale differently, comparison between patients may be unreliable. Also, patients tend to avoid the extremes of the scale, clustering their scores around the middle; the scale is thus not truly linear.

Linezolid. Oxazolidinine antibacterial drug active against Gram-positive bacteria including multiresistant staphylococci and enterococci, but poorly active against Gram-negative organisms.
- Dosage: 600 mg orally or iv over 30–120 min, 12 hourly.
- Side effects: GIT disturbance, headache, dry mouth, blood dyscrasias (full blood count must be monitored weekly). Has weak MAOI properties. Has been associated with increased mortality from Gram-negative bacteria when used in critically ill patients with Gram-positive intravascular infections.

Lingual nerve block, *see Mandibular nerve blocks*

Lipopolysaccharide, *see Endotoxins*

Liquid ventilation. Technique of partially or totally filling the lungs with perfluorocarbons (especially perfluorooctylbromide) and ventilating with this liquid instead of O_2 enriched air. First done experimentally in animals in the early 1960s, using pressurised crystalloid solutions. Has been used in neonatal respiratory distress syndrome and ARDS, mostly in animal models but human studies have been and are currently being performed.

In total liquid ventilation, the entire lung volume and ventilator circuit are filled, requiring a specialised ventilator. The liquid is oxygenated to a PO_2 of 50–90 kPa (350–675 mmHg) by either bubbling O_2 through it or by using a standard extracorporeal device. Tidal volumes of 15–20 ml/kg are given at a rate of about 5 breaths/min. In partial liquid ventilation (perfluorocarbon associated gas exchange; PAGE) a volume approximating to FRC is instilled and standard IPPV continued. Results in improved oxygenation and increased compliance, thought to be via increased recruitment of non-aerated alveoli and redistribution of perfusion. A protective effect against further lung injury has been suggested.
Kaisers U, Kelly KP, Busch T (2003). Br J Anaesth; 91: 143–51

Lissive anaesthesia. Technique of anaesthesia, now considered unsafe, in which non-depolarising neuromuscular blocking drugs (originally tubocurarine) were used to produce muscle relaxation without causing complete paralysis. Thus spontaneous respiration was allowed following small doses of tubocurarine, due to presumed 'diaphragmatic sparing'.

Liston, Robert (1794–1847). Scottish-born surgeon; moved to London after quarrelling with his colleagues. Performed the first operation under diethyl ether anaesthesia in England on 21st December 1846, at University College Hospital, London, having been told about ether by Boott. William Squire administered the anaesthetic from a glass inhaler made by his uncle, Peter, whilst Frederick Churchill had an above-knee amputation. The operation allegedly lasted 25 s.
[William Squire (1825–1899), London medical student, later physician; Peter Squire (1798–1884), London chemist; Frederick Churchill (1810–?), English butler]

Lithium carbonate/citrate. Salts used for manic-depressive disease. Lithium mimics sodium in the body, entering excitable cells during depolarisation. It decreases release of central and peripheral neurotransmitters and may prolong depolarising neuromuscular blockade and decrease requirements for anaesthetic agents. Termination 24 h before anaesthesia has been suggested but this is disputed. Has low therapeutic ratio, with optimal plasma concentration of 0.4–1.0 mmol/l. Distributed slowly within the tissues (24–36 h with slow-release preparations). Almost entirely excreted by the kidneys, with half-life 6–12 h initially but over 24 h if the tissue compartment contains significant amounts of drug. Lithium poisoning may occur acutely and deliberately, or insidiously during chronic treatment as a result of dehydration, impaired renal function, infection and use of drugs, e.g. NSAIDs, diuretics.
- Dosage: 200 mg–2.0 g/day according to the preparation used and the indication/individual response.
- Side effects: as for lithium poisoning.

Lithium poisoning. Toxic effects of lithium may be seen at plasma concentrations of < 1.0 mmol/l but are common at > 1.5 mmol/l; severe toxicity is usual at levels > 2.0 mmol/l although acute poisoning may produce high concentrations before the onset of symptoms. Features include lethargy or restlessness initially; then tremor, ataxia, GIT upset, weakness and muscle twitching; finally, hypokalaemia, arrhythmias, renal failure, convulsions and coma.

Management consists of increasing urine output if symptoms have not yet developed; general treatment is supportive with control of electrolyte imbalance and convulsions, and haemodialysis (which may need repeating as tissue lithium enters the circulation) if renal failure is present. The possibility of prolonged absorption of lithium from slow-release preparations should be remembered. Activated charcoal is relatively ineffective at preventing further absorption; whole bowel irrigation has been used but is not standard therapy.

Litre. SI unit of volume. Originally defined as the volume of 1 kg pure water at 4°C, but redefined as equal to 1000 cm^3 in 1964, because of an error in the standard kilogram constructed in 1889.

Liver. Largest body organ, weighing about 1200–1500 g, lying in the right upper abdominal quadrant. Two major lobes, right and left, are divided into lobules based on a central vein connected by a network of sinusoids to peripheral portal tracts. Central veins are tributaries of hepatic veins; portal tracts contain branches of the hepatic artery, portal vein, lymphatics and bile ducts. Blood from the hepatic arterial and portal venous systems is conveyed to the central veins via the sinusoids, lined with endothelial and phagocytic (Kupffer) cells and separated by hepatocytes. Bile canniculi form networks between the hepatocytes, conveying bile towards the biliary tract.

Blood flow is about 20–30% of cardiac output (70% via the portal vein).

- Functions:
  - carbohydrate metabolism: glycogen storage and breakdown.
  - protein metabolism: synthesises many, including albumin, globulins, coagulation factors, complement system components, transferrin, haptoglobulins, caeruloplasmin, plasma cholinesterase and α_1-antitrypsin. Important site of amino acid deamination prior to interconversion and oxidation. Ammonia produced by deamination is converted to urea.
  - fat metabolism: breakdown of dietary triglycerides and fatty acids, and synthesis of triglycerides, phospholipid and cholesterol, released into the bloodstream as lipoproteins. Cholesterol is also used to make bile acids.
  - bilirubin metabolism: unconjugated fat-soluble bilirubin is transported to the liver bound to albumin; it is conjugated with glucuronide to the water-soluble form (*see Jaundice*).
  - formation of bile acids: cholic and chenodeoxycholic acids are produced from cholesterol and secreted in the bile. Reabsorbed via enterohepatic circulation.
  - vitamin storage: A, D, K, B_{12} and folate.
  - hormone metabolism and inactivation: includes cortisol, oestrogens, aldosterone, vasopressin and thyroxine.
  - haematological role: site of haemopoiesis during fetal and early neonatal life. Also acts as a reservoir for blood which can be redistributed to the body by stimulation of the liver's autonomic innervation. Kupffer cells phagocytose antigens and bacteria absorbed from the GIT, and destroy old red cells.
  - drug metabolism: achieved by transforming lipid-soluble compounds into water-soluble ones via enzymes located in the hepatocyte microsomes. Several processes are involved, including oxidation, conjugation, reduction, hydrolysis, methylation and acetylation. Most drugs are metabolised by a combination of oxidation by cytochromes and conjugation (*see Pharmacokinetics*).
- Effects of anaesthetic agents:
  - both hepatic artery and portal vein blood flow are reduced by most agents, probably as a consequence of reduced cardiac output. The effect is opposed by hypercapnia and exacerbated by hypocapnia and IPPV, although this is thought to be rarely significant.
  - drug metabolism may be reduced in the presence of volatile agents, although whether due to alterations in hepatic blood flow or a direct inhibitory effect is unclear.
  - enzyme induction by volatile agents has been reported but is controversial.
  - toxic effects: e.g. halothane hepatitis.

[Karl W von Kupffer (1829–1902), German anatomist]

Liver dialysis. Term used to describe various techniques for extracorporeal detoxification of blood in hepatic failure. Includes the molecular adsorbents recirculation system (MARS) in which a dialysis circuit containing albumin is separated from the patient's blood by a semipermeable membrane, the albumin filtered in a second circuit before being reused. Single pass albumin dialysis (SPAD) uses a single circuit containing albumin, the latter being discarded instead of cleaned and reused. Continuous venovenous haemodiafiltration and other variants of haemoperfusion and haemodialysis have also been investigated. Few are in routine use although MARS was approved in the USA in 2005.

Liver failure, *see Hepatic failure*

Liver function tests. Most commonly measured:
- bilirubin (*see Jaundice*).
- liver enzymes:
  - aspartate aminotransferase (AST) and alanine aminotransferase (ALT): released by damaged hepatocytes. Highly raised values suggest hepatitis. Normally 5–40 iu/l.
  - alkaline phosphatase: highly raised in cholestasis, both intra- and extrahepatic. Isoenzyme analysis differentiates between hepatic and other sources, e.g. bone. Normally 40–110 iu/l.
  - γ-glutamyl transferase (γGT): non-specific, but often raised following drug ingestion, e.g. alcohol. Normally 10–50 iu/l.
- plasma proteins:
  - albumin: reduced in chronic liver disease after a few weeks. Normally 35–55 g/l.
  - globulins: increased to varying extents, depending on the underlying cause. Normally 25–35 g/l.
- coagulation studies.
- others, including:
  - bromosulfothalein excretion: rate of excretion depends on hepatic function.
  - α_1-fetoprotein, increased in hepatoma.
  - cholinesterase.
  - 5′ nucleotidase, increased in biliary obstruction.

Limdi JK, Hyde GM (2003). Postgrad Med J; 79: 307–12

Liver transplantation. First performed in 1963. There are now seven units for liver transplantation in the UK; 1-year survival is > 80%. Indicated for end-stage hepatic failure, e.g. due to inherited disease, chronic hepatitis, acute toxic hepatitis, primary biliary cirrhosis and some cases of liver tumour. Scoring systems are commonly used to prioritise potential recipients, based on the likelihood of death whilst waiting for transplantation. Surgery involves vascular and biliary isolation of the diseased organ (pre-anhepatic and anhepatic phases) with re-anastomosis of a donor cadaveric organ (reperfusion phase); partial donation by live donors has also been used. The recipient's liver is dissected to its vascular pedicle, the portal vein, hepatic artery and inferior vena cava above and below the liver are clamped, and the diseased organ is removed. Venovenous bypass is often employed from the portal and femoral veins to the axillary or internal jugular veins, although different centres vary in its usage. Donor liver viability is up to 8 h from harvesting. It is flushed with crystalloid solution via the portal vein to remove the transport infusate and air bubbles. Anastomosis of the portal vein and hepatic artery is followed by release of vascular clamps, incorporating the donor liver into the recipient's circulation.

- Anaesthesia:
  - as for hepatic failure. Preoperative assessment is directed at establishing cardiovascular status and evaluating concurrent disease. Opioid, volatile agent, neuromuscular blockade and IPPV are usual; N_2O is often avoided to reduce bowel distension and risk of air embolism during re-anastomosis. Aseptic techniques are used to reduce infection. Ciclosporin and corticosteroids are given.
  - monitoring and vascular lines include direct BP and CVP measurement, pulmonary artery catheterisation, several large iv cannulae (e.g. 8 G), temperature probes and urinary catheter.
  - frequent estimation of plasma electrolytes, glucose, haemoglobin, platelets, arterial blood gases and coagulation studies is required. Thromboelastography is useful for coagulation studies.
  - blood loss is usually 8–10 units but may be up to 200 units. Autologous blood transfusion is often used. Rapid transfusion devices are required to keep up with losses; they include a reservoir of several units of blood, driven by a pump. Venous return may also be reduced by surgical manipulation.
  - SVR and cardiac rhythm may change frequently. Myocardial depression may be caused by hypocalcaemia, hypothermia and acidosis. Acidosis is common but treated cautiously, as postoperative metabolic alkalosis is also common, due to metabolism of lactate and citrate. Inotropic drugs are often required.
  - hypoglycaemia and hyperglycaemia may occur, especially during the anhepatic phase.
  - potassium levels fluctuate due to acid–base changes, flushing out of liver perfusate and uptake by the transplanted liver.
  - surgery usually lasts 8–10 h but may be up to 24 h, with major biochemical, haematological and temperature disturbances which may persist postoperatively. IPPV is usually maintained for 24–48 h. Postoperative problems include infection, atelectasis and pleural effusion, graft failure, hepatic artery thrombosis, biliary leaks or obstruction, neurological impairment, renal failure.

Lentschener C, Ozier Y (2002). Eur J Anaesthesiol; 19: 780–8

See also, Organ donation; Transplantation

Living will, *see Advance decision*

Local anaesthesia, *see Infiltration anaesthesia; Local anaesthetic agents; Regional anaesthesia; Topical anaesthesia; specific blocks*

Local anaesthetic agents. Cocaine was introduced in 1884 by Freud and Koller; less toxic agents subsequently introduced include procaine and stovaine (1904), cinchocaine (1925), tetracaine (amethocaine) (1931) and lidocaine (lignocaine) (1947). Lidocaine was particularly non-toxic. Later drugs include chloroprocaine (1952), mepivacaine (1956), prilocaine (1959), bupivacaine (1963), etidocaine (1972), articaine (1974), ropivacaine and levobupivacaine (both 1997). Others are used only for topical anaesthesia, e.g. benzocaine.

- General properties (Table 22):
  - poorly water soluble weak bases with $pK_a > 7.4$.
  - comprised of hydrophilic and hydrophobic portions separated by an alkyl chain. The hydrophilic part is usually a tertiary amine; the lipophilic part (essential for local anaesthetic action) is usually an unsaturated aromatic ring, e.g. *para*-aminobenzoic acid.
  - modification of chemical structure (lengthening the alkyl chain or increasing the number of carbon atoms in the aromatic ring or tertiary amine) may alter lipid solubility, potency, rate of metabolism and duration of action.
  - classified according to the nature of linkage between the amine and aromatic parts into ester or amide drugs:
    - esters:
      - allergic reactions are common.
      - rapidly metabolised by plasma and liver cholinesterase. One metabolite, *para*-aminobenzoic acid, is thought to be responsible for allergic reactions. Metabolism may be prolonged when plasma cholinesterase level is low, e.g. liver disease, pregnancy or atypical enzymes.
    - amides:
      - allergic reactions are rare; they may be associated with the preservative vehicle.
      - metabolised by liver microsomal enzymes, initially to aminocarboxylic acid and a cyclic aniline derivative, subsequently via *N*-dealkylation and hydroxylation respectively. Dependent on liver blood flow and function.
  - presented in solution as acidic hydrochloride salts.
- Mechanism of action:
  - produce reversible blockade of neural transmission in autonomic, sensory and motor nerve fibres, depending on the concentration of drug applied. Active peripherally and at the CNS.
  - bind to fast sodium channels in the axon membrane from within, preventing sodium entry during depolarisation. The threshold potential is thus not reached and the action potential of the nerve not propagated (membrane stabilising effect).
  - fate of injected drug:
    - diffuses to axons; thus more effective the nearer the nerve it is deposited (*see Minimal blocking concentration*).
    - crosses the membrane in the unionised form; thus activity depends on extracellular pH, since the degree of ionisation and thus lipid insolubility is increased by acidosis. The pH of infected tissue is lower than

Table 22 Properties of local anaesthetic agents

Agent	pK_a	*% Protein binding*	*Equivalent concentration (%)*	*Recommended maximal safe dose (mg/kg)*
Esters				
Amethocaine	8.5	76	0.25	1.5
Chloroprocaine	8.7	–	1	15
Cocaine	8.7	–	1	3
Procaine	8.9	6	2	12
Amides				
Bupivacaine	8.1	96	0.25	2
Cinchocaine	7.9	—	0.25	2
Etidocaine	7.7	94	0.5	2
Lidocaine	7.9	64	1	3–7
Mepivacaine	7.6	78	1	5
Prilocaine	7.9	55	1	5–8
Ropivacaine	8.1	94	1	3.5

normal, hence the effects of local anaesthetics are reduced.
- dissociates within the axon to the ionised form; thus dependent on intracellular pH.
- binds to sodium channels in their open state.
- smallest nerve fibres are blocked first.
- Features of block are affected by:
  - patient variables, e.g. age, fitness, pregnancy, etc.
  - individual drug characteristics.
  - concentration and dose used: e.g. higher concentrations and doses reduce onset time, and increase density and duration of block.
  - site of injection, e.g. rapid onset of spinal anaesthesia but slow onset of brachial plexus block.
  - additives:
    - vasoconstrictors, e.g. adrenaline, felypressin, phenylephrine: reduce absorption and prolong the block. Intensity and onset may be improved. Effects are greatest with local anaesthetics that cause vasodilatation, e.g. lidocaine, and less with prilocaine and bupivacaine. Cocaine itself causes vasoconstriction. Noradrenaline is less effective than adrenaline.
    - CO_2 dissolved under pressure (carbonated solutions): passes into axons, lowering pH; intracellular dissociation is thus favoured, with faster block.
    - sodium hydroxide: remains extracellular, raising pH and increasing the unionised fraction of drug; uptake into the axon is thus favoured.
    - potassium: has been shown to increase duration of block.
    - dextrans: used to prolong blocks, perhaps by combining with local anaesthetic and trapping it within the tissues. Results are inconsistent.
    - hyaluronidase: formerly used to increase spread by breaking down tissue stroma. Benefits are doubtful; thus rarely used now except in eye blocks.
    - dextrose to increase baricity for spinal anaesthesia: affects spread.
- Toxicity:
  - due to membrane stabilising effects on other cells, especially heart and CNS. Features:
    - tingling, typically around the mouth and tongue.
    - lightheadedness, agitation and tremor.
    - unconsciousness and/or convulsions.
    - hypotension may be caused by hypoxaemia following central apnoea, direct myocardial depression or vasodilatation. Arrhythmias may occur; resistant ventricular arrhythmias are particularly likely with bupivacaine.
  - may follow accidental iv injection, or systemic absorption, the latter affected by:
    - total dose administered. Recommended maximal 'safe' doses are rough estimations only, since other factors are involved, but are useful as a guide (*see Table 22*).
    - site of injection: e.g. absorption is large after topical anaesthesia and intercostal block and slow after brachial plexus block and infiltration anaesthesia. Affected by blood flow and tissue vascularity.
    - vasoconstrictor additives.
    - individual drug: e.g. lidocaine causes vasodilatation; bupivacaine binds extensively to tissues. Ropivacaine and levobupivacaine are less toxic than bupivacaine.
  - effects are related to age and fitness of the patient, other drugs (e.g. anticonvulsants), etc. Uptake by the lungs reduces blood levels following iv injection, shielding the heart and brain from higher levels.
  - treatment: supportive, with oxygenation/cardiovascular support as for CPR. Thiopental or diazepam/midazolam may be used for convulsions, although hypotension may be exacerbated. Recovery of consciousness is usually within a few minutes. Intralipid 20% (1–2 ml/kg over 1 min, repeated up to twice, followed by 0.25 ml/kg/min increased to 0.5 ml/kg/min if the CVS is stable) has been suggested as a treatment, possibly by binding free drug or replenishing myocardial energy substrates. The intralipid contained within propofol is not recommended as an alternative because of the drug's cardiodepressant actions.
  - other complications may be related to:
    - vasoconstrictors, e.g. tachycardia, arrhythmias, pallor, agitation, etc. caused by adrenaline.
    - regional technique, e.g. intraneural injection, hypotension following spinal anaesthesia, etc.
    - preservatives, e.g. allergic reactions (e.g. to methylparaben), neurological damage and arachnoiditis.

See also, Regional anaesthesia; specific blocks

LODS, *see Logistic organ dysfunction system*

Lofentanil *cis*-oxalate. Opioid analgesic drug derived from fentanyl; developed in 1975. 20 times as potent as fentanyl and 6000 times as potent as morphine in animal studies. Of similar pK_a to fentanyl, highly lipophilic and with a particularly long duration of action due to persistent binding to opioid receptors (about 10 h). Has been used via the epidural route to provide long-lasting analgesia, but not generally available.

Logistic organ dysfunction system (LODS). Scoring system developed to predict hospital mortality from 11 variables measured on the first day of admission to ICU (Glasgow coma scale, heart rate, systolic BP, urea, creatinine, urine output, P_aO_2/F_IO_2 ratio, white cell count, platelets, bilirubin and international normalised ratio). The total score ranges from zero (normal) to 22.

Has been modified by adding infection as a 12th item (organ dysfunction and/or infection; ODIN).

Le Gall JR, Klar J, Lemeshow S, et al (1996). JAMA; 276: 802–10

See also, Mortality/survival prediction on intensive care unit

Long, Crawford Williamson (1815–1878). US general practitioner; administered diethyl ether several times for minor surgery from 1842 in Georgia, but did not report it until after Morton's demonstration.

Hammonds WD, Steinhaus JE (1993). J Clin Anesth; 5: 163–7

Lorazepam. Benzodiazepine, used for insomnia, epilepsy, sedation and premedication. Now the initial drug of choice in status epilepticus. Half-life is approximately 12 h with prolonged duration of action. Said to produce more amnesia than other benzodiazepines. Similar rates of absorption follow im and oral administration.

Metabolised to a non-active metabolite.

- Dosage:
  - 1–4 mg orally. If given the night before surgery, a further 1–2 mg may be given 1–2 h preoperatively.
  - 25–30 μg/kg iv (50–75 μg/kg in status epilepticus).

LOS, *see Lower oesophageal sphincter*

Lower oesophageal sphincter. 2–5 cm portion of oesophagus of increased intraluminal pressure, extending

above and below the diaphragm. Opens reflexly during swallowing, and helps to prevent retrograde passage of gastric contents into the oesophagus via:
- increased muscle tone: muscle of the sphincter zone, especially the inner circular layer, has higher resting tone than other oesophageal muscle, possibly via increased calcium ion uptake and utilisation.
- neural input:
  - vagal: muscle tone reflexly increases as intragastric pressure increases, thus maintaining barrier pressure (normally about 20 cmH_2O). The reflex is abolished by atropine.
  - sympathetic: tone is increased by α-stimulation and β-blockade, and decreased by β-stimulation and α-blockade.
- mechanical factors:
  - oesophageal compression by the diaphragm.
  - acute angle of entry of the oesophagus into the stomach.
  - mucosal flap or rosette at the oesophageal opening.

- Muscle tone is decreased by:
  - anticholinergic drugs given iv; possibly less with glycopyrronium. Atropine im does not affect sphincter pressure, but prevents the action of metoclopramide.
  - gut hormones, e.g. vasoactive intestinal hormone, glucagon and gastric inhibitory peptide. Gastrin may increase tone at very high levels.
  - progesterone.
  - opioid analgesic drugs, volatile anaesthetic agents and most iv anaesthetic agents.
  - ganglion blocking drugs.
- Tone is increased by:
  - metoclopramide, domperidone and prochlorperazine.
  - neostigmine.
  - pancuronium.

No change is found with H_2 receptor antagonists. Although suxamethonium may increase intragastric pressure, the corresponding increase in lower oesophageal sphincter tone maintains barrier pressure.

Sphincter incompetence may result in gastro-oesophageal reflux. It becomes less competent in hiatus hernia, particularly if intra-abdominal pressure increases, e.g. by raising the legs.

Lown–Ganong–Levine syndrome. Tendency to SVT caused by an accessory conducting pathway bypassing the atrioventricular node. Impulses may pass directly from the atria to the distal heart conducting system, without the usual delay at the node.

Characterised by a normal P wave, short P–R interval and normal QRS complex on the ECG. Anaesthetic management is as for Wolff–Parkinson–White syndrome.

[Samuel A Levine (1891–1966) and Bernard Lown, US cardiologists; William F Ganong (1924–2007), US physiologist]

LPS, Lipopolysaccharide, *see Endotoxins*

Lucid interval. Period of apparently normal function and behaviour following an often relatively trivial head injury, but during which blood is accumulating inside the skull from a slowly bleeding vessel. Classically occurring with extradural haematomas, features only become apparent when the collection causes compression of intracranial structures; because this may occur up to several hours after injury, diagnosis may be delayed and significant impairment may result.

Ludwig's angina. Cellulitis of the floor of the mouth and submandibular region, with massive swelling. Often due to anaerobic infection. May progress to laryngeal obstruction and death unless treated with antibiotics initially, or by deep incision of the tissues under the mandible.

Anaesthetic management is as for airway obstruction; antibiotic therapy may reduce the swelling and improve obstruction preoperatively. Local anaesthesia may be preferable in extreme cases.

[Wilhelm von Ludwig (1790–1865), German surgeon]

Lumbar epidural anaesthesia, *see Epidural anaesthesia*

Lumbar plexus. Formed in front of the transverse processes of the lumbar vertebrae from the anterior primary rami of the first four lumbar nerves, occasionally with a contribution from T12 (Fig. 100).

May be blocked via paravertebral, psoas compartment, fascia iliaca compartment and 'three-in-one' femoral nerve blocks. Individual nerves may also be blocked. Block is useful for surgery on the inner and outer aspects of the thigh and anterior gluteal region together with adjacent perineal and suprapubic areas.

See also, Inguinal hernia field block

Lumbar puncture. Procedure for removing CSF either for diagnostic purposes (e.g. meningitis) or treatment (e.g. benign intracranial hypertension, intrathecal injection of chemotherapy, CSF filtration). First performed by Quincke for the treatment of hydrocephalus. Forms part of the procedure of spinal anaesthesia. May be required in the ICU for diagnosis of neurological conditions. Technique, contraindications and complications are as for spinal anaesthesia but without the drug effects. Neurologists, general physicians and radiologists are more likely to use larger needles with cutting points than anaesthetists; whether subsequent post-dural puncture headache (PDPH) is masked by the presenting symptoms is uncertain. The incidence of PDPH may be decreased if the stylet is reinserted after aspiration before removal of the needle, presumably by preventing avulsion of dural strands sucked into the needle's shaft during removal of CSF.

Lumbar sympathetic block. Performed for peripheral vascular disease including incipient gangrene, and in chronic pain management (e.g. post-traumatic dystrophies).

The lumbar sympathetic chain lies on the anterolateral aspect of the lumbar vertebral bodies within a fascial

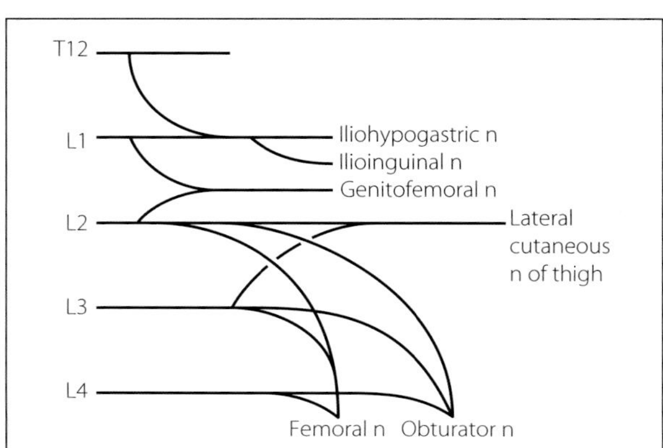

Fig. 100 Plan of the lumbar plexus

compartment formed by the vertebral column, psoas sheath and posterior peritoneum.

With the patient in the lateral position and with a soft pillow between the iliac crest and costal margin to curve the spine laterally, skin wheals are raised 5–8 cm lateral to the upper borders of the spinous processes of L2–4. A 12–18 cm long needle is directed medially, to strike the transverse process at about 3–5 cm. The lateral aspect of the vertebral body is contacted usually 4–6 cm deeper, and the needle advanced a further 1–2 cm. Correct positioning is confirmed by negative aspiration for CSF or blood, and radiographic imaging: the needles should barely reach the anterior borders of the vertebral bodies in the lateral view, and should overlie their lateral edge in the anteroposterior view. Further confirmation of positioning is made by injecting contrast medium. 25–30 ml local anaesthetic solution, e.g. 0.5% lidocaine or prilocaine, is injected at L2, or 15 ml at L2 and L4. Catheters have been inserted for repeated injection. Phenol or absolute alcohol is used for chemical sympatholysis, 3 ml at each of L1, L2 and L3. The block may also be performed with patient prone.

Complications include hypotension, genitofemoral neuritis, bleeding into psoas, and epidural, subarachnoid or iv injection.

Similar blocks have been performed in the thoracic region but with risk of pneumothorax.

Lundy, John Silus (1894–1973). US anaesthetist; he became head of department at the Mayo Clinic in 1924. Co-founder of the American Board of Anesthesiology. An advocate and developer of regional techniques, balanced anaesthesia, thiopental and post-anaesthetic recovery rooms.

Lung. Organ of respiration. Continues to develop after birth, with alveolar proliferation complete at about 8 years.

- Anatomy:
  - cone-shaped, with bases applied to the diaphragm.
  - enveloped in pleura, attached to the mediastinum at the hila.
  - the right lung is larger than the left and divided into three lobes separated by the oblique and transverse fissures.
  - the left lung is divided into two lobes by the oblique fissure. The lingula is the anteroinferior portion of the upper lobe.
  - lobes are divided into segments (*see Tracheobronchial tree*).
  - surface anatomy:
    - as for pleura, except for the lower border, which lies two ribs cranial to the caudal pleural limit.
    - on the left side, the medial anterior border lies 2–3 cm lateral to the sternum at the 5th and 6th costal cartilages (cardiac notch).
    - the oblique fissure follows a line from the spine of T4 downwards and outwards to the 6th costal cartilage.
    - the transverse fissure follows a horizontal line from the 4th costal cartilage until it hits the previous line.
- Blood supply: via bronchial and pulmonary arteries (*see Pulmonary circulation*).
- Nerve supply: sympathetic and vagal plexuses; sensory pathways are mainly via the latter.
- Lymph drainage: via bronchopulmonary, tracheobronchial and paratracheal nodes to mediastinal lymph trunks and thence brachiocephalic veins.
- Functions:
  - gas exchange.
  - synthesis of associated phospholipids, e.g. surfactant, carbohydrates (e.g. mucopolysaccharides) and proteins (e.g. collagen).
  - metabolism and deactivation of certain compounds, e.g. angiotensin, bradykinin and 5-HT. Takes up amide local anaesthetic agents.
  - synthesis and release of compounds, e.g. prostaglandins and histamine.
  - involvement in the immune system and possibly coagulation.
  - acts as a reservoir for blood; the pulmonary circulation contains 500–900 ml blood.

See also, Alveolus; Lung . . . ; Pulmonary . . .

Lung function tests. Used to determine the nature and extent of pulmonary disorders. Clinical assessment, e.g. ability to walk up stairs, breath-hold for >30 s, or blow out a lighted match held 6 inches (15 cm) away, are imprecise and non-specific indicators.

- Include tests of:
  - ventilation mechanics:
    - measurement of static lung volumes: cumbersome apparatus is required. Dead space and closing capacity may be measured.
    - assessment of forced expiration and derived variables (e.g. FEV_1, FVC, forced expiratory flow rate, etc.), e.g. using a spirometer. The FEV_1/FVC ratio typically is reduced in obstructive lung disease, and is normal or high in restrictive disease. Peak expiratory flow rate is another simple bedside test for obstructive disease. Airway reactivity is assessed by challenging with histamine or methacholine whilst measuring FEV_1.
    - flow–volume loops require more sophisticated apparatus, with instantaneous flow rate measurement.
    - airway resistance itself may be measured, and lung compliance.
    - maximal voluntary ventilation is non-specific and related to effort as well as pulmonary function.
    - respiratory muscle function may be assessed, e.g. maximal mouth pressures when breathing against a closed valve. Work of breathing and O_2 consumption may also be measured.
  - gas exchange:
    - analysis of blood gas tensions and pulse oximetry.
    - diffusing capacity for carbon monoxide (transfer factor); now thought to be related more to $\dot{V}/\dot{Q}$ mismatch than to diffusion impairment.
    - distribution of ventilation and perfusion as for $\dot{V}/\dot{Q}$ mismatch.
  - pulmonary circulation: assessment is difficult. Radioisotope scanning may be used as for $\dot{V}/\dot{Q}$ mismatch.
  - control of breathing: CO_2 response curve or response to hypoxia may be used.
  - response to exercise, using the above tests.

See also, Body plethysmograph; Nitrogen washout

Lung protection strategies. Introduced in the 1990s for the management of acute lung injury. Components include:
  - avoidance of overdistension of alveoli.
  - acceptance of permissive hypercapnia.
  - maintenance of alveolar volume.
  - prevention of radial stress associated with cyclical end-expiratory collapse and re-expansion at low lung volumes.

Inspiratory plateau pressure is usually limited to < 35 cmH_2O. Pressure–volume curves may be used to identify an upper inflection point (UIP), thought to represent the point of alveolar overdistension, and a lower inflection point (LIP), thought to represent the point of alveolar recruitment during inflation. PEEP levels are set at or above LIP; maximum inspiratory plateau pressure is set below UIP. Extracorporeal CO_2

removal has also been used to reduce the minute ventilation requirement.

Lung transplantation. First performed in 1963; includes transplantation of a single lung, both lungs (rarely performed now) or sequential single lungs during the same operation. Most commonly performed for COPD but also idiopathic pulmonary fibrosis, cystic fibrosis and other causes of end-stage lung disease. Survival is approximately 45% at 5 years. Similar considerations apply as to heart–lung transplantation:

- Donor:
  - as for heart–lung transplantation; those with significant respiratory disease are excluded. HLA mismatching is not associated with reduced long-term rejection although matching of size is important.
  - up to 9 h is thought to be acceptable before transplantation although up to 3 h is best. Preservative techniques may include iv heparin and prostacyclin (the latter into the pulmonary artery) before removal from the donor. A left atrial cuff, pulmonary veins, main bronchi and pulmonary artery are taken in addition to the lungs themselves.
- Recipient:
  - immunosuppression and antibiotic therapy as for heart–lung transplantation.
  - a double lumen endobronchial tube or single lumen tube with bronchial blocker have been used. Initial problems are those of thoracic surgery in general, especially one-lung ventilation.
  - monitoring may include pulmonary artery catheterisation (the catheter usually flows to the better perfused lung; it may require withdrawal before the lung is removed).
  - control of pulmonary vascular resistance may be difficult. Cardiopulmonary bypass has been used.
  - postoperative problems include non-cardiogenic pulmonary oedema (pulmonary reimplantation response), hypoxaemia, disrupted anastomosis, infection and rejection. Obliterative bronchiolitis may occur.

Anaesthetic management of patients with transplanted lungs is as standard, remembering the risks of infection, impaired lung function, the possibility of rejection and the drugs the patient may be taking.

Lung volumes. Functional, not anatomical, volumes of the lungs, usually expressed as if both lungs comprise one unit. May be derived from a spirometer tracing of inhaled/exhaled volumes, with maximal inspiration and expiration following normal quiet tidal breathing (Fig. 101).

- Approximate normal values for a 70 kg man:
  - tidal volume: 0.5 litres
  - inspiratory reserve volume: 2.5 litres
  - inspiratory capacity: 3.0 litres
  - vital capacity: 4.5 litres
  - expiratory reserve volume: 1.5 litres
  - residual volume: 1.5 litres
  - FRC: 3.0 litres
  - total lung capacity: 6.0 litres.

Capacities are sums of volumes.

Tidal volume, inspiratory reserve volume, expiratory reserve volume, and capacities derived from them may be measured using a wet spirometer. Residual volume may be measured using helium dilution or the body plethysmograph.

Other lung volumes measured include dead space and closing capacity. Differential spirometry is used to examine function of single lungs.

See also, Lung function tests

LVEDP, *see Left ventricular end-diastolic pressure*

LVEDV, *see Left ventricular end-diastolic volume*

LVET, Left ventricular ejection time, *see Systolic time intervals*

LVF, Left ventricular failure, *see Cardiac failure*

LVH, Left ventricular hypertrophy, *see Cardiac failure*

Lyme disease. Tick-borne disease caused by the spirochaete *Borrelia burgdorferi*. First recognised as a cause of paediatric arthropathy in Lyme, Connecticut, USA, in 1975. Widespread in the US and parts of Europe and Asia, becoming more common in the UK. Causes characteristic expanding skin lesions (erythema migrans) at the site of the

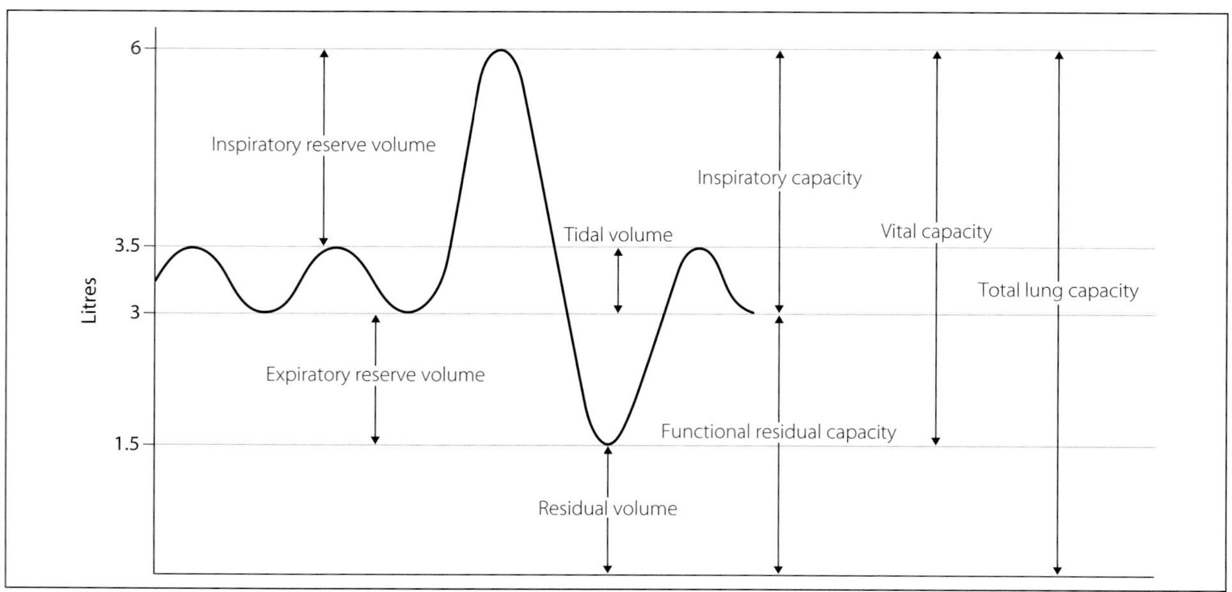

Fig. 101 Lung volumes

tick's bite, associated with systemic flu-like symptoms. Weeks to months later, neurological features (meningitis, encephalitis, cranial neuritis) lasting for months occur in 15% of cases whilst 8% develop cardiac features (heart block, myocarditis) lasting a few days. Arthritis occurs up to 2 years later in 60% of cases. Diagnosis is on clinical grounds aided by serological testing. Treatment is with penicillins, tetracyclines, cephalosporins or macrolides depending on the presentation and stage of illness. Outcome is usually favourable although late neurological complications may persist.
[Willy A Burgdorfer, Swiss-born US entomologist]

Lypressin, *see Vasopressin*

Lytic cocktail. Mixture of chlorpromazine, promethazine and pethidine (e.g. 50–100 mg of each added to an iv infusion), described in the 1940s as a means of sedation, e.g. for unpleasant procedures, premedication and labour. Produced a state of drowsiness and apathy ('artificial hibernation') but effects were long-lasting and accompanied by hypotension. The technique was later refined as neuroleptanaesthesia and analgesia.

Has been used for premedication in children, e.g. a mixture containing chlorpromazine 7 mg, promethazine 7 mg and pethidine 28 mg per ml; 0.05 ml/kg im or 0.1 ml/kg rectally.

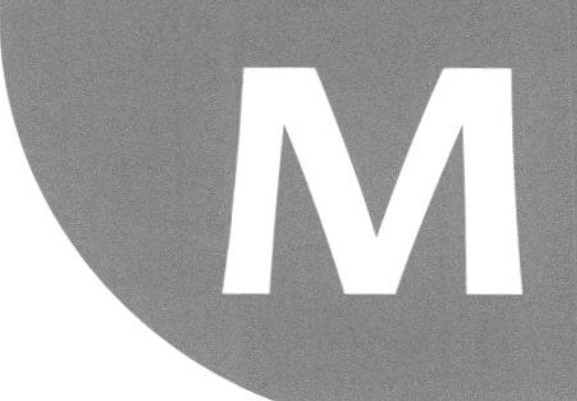

MAC, *see Minimal alveolar concentration*

Macewen, William (1847–1924). Eminent Scottish surgeon; Professor at Glasgow University, knighted in 1902. Advocated and practised tracheal intubation, usually oral, for laryngeal obstruction, e.g. due to diphtheria; he performed this by touch without anaesthetic. Was the first to advocate tracheal intubation instead of tracheotomy for head and neck surgery, in 1880. The tube was inserted prior to introduction of chloroform, and the patient allowed to breathe spontaneously. Packing around the tube achieved a seal.
James CDT (1974). Anaesthesia; 29: 743–53

Macintosh, Robert Reynolds (1897–1989). New Zealand-born anaesthetist, he became the first British Professor of Anaesthetics in Oxford in 1937. Lord Nuffield, a friend of Macintosh, had insisted that such a chair be set up as a precondition for endowing further chairs in Medicine, Surgery and Obstetrics and Gynaecology. Established Oxford as a centre for anaesthesia, and helped to establish anaesthesia as a medical specialty. Wrote books and articles about many aspects of local and general anaesthesia, and designed many pieces of equipment, including his laryngoscope, spray, endobronchial tube, vaporisers and devices for locating the epidural space. Also helped research the hazards of aviation and seafaring. Knighted in 1955, and received many other medals and awards.
[William Morris (1877–1963), English automobile industrialist and philanthropist – became Lord Nuffield in 1934]
Mushin WW (1989). Anaesthesia; 44: 950–2

McKesson, Elmer Isaac (1881–1935). US anaesthetist, practising in Toledo, Ohio. Founder and member of many US and international anaesthetic bodies. Also inventor and manufacturer of expiratory valves, pressure regulators, flowmeters, suction equipment, vaporisers and intermittent flow anaesthetic machines. A major proponent of the use of N_2O in modern anaesthesia.

McMechan, Francis Hoeffer (1879–1939). US anaesthetist, practising in Cincinnati. A pioneer of the development of anaesthesia in the USA. Founded the American Association of Anesthetists in 1912, and instrumental in founding the National Anesthetic Research Society (subsequently the International Anaesthesia Research Society) whose publication (which became *Anesthesia and Analgesia*) he edited.

Macrolides. Group of antibacterial drugs containing a lactam ring but distinct from β-lactams. Interfere with RNA-dependent protein synthesis. Includes erythromycin, azithromycin, clarithromycin and telithromycin. All have similar antibacterial activities (Gram-positive and some Gram-negative bacteria, mycoplasma, rickettsia and toxoplasma) but varying properties otherwise; thus the latter three drugs have longer durations of action than erythromycin and cause less nausea and vomiting.

Macrophage colony-stimulating factor, *see Granulocyte colony-stimulating factor*

Magill breathing system, *see Anaesthetic breathing systems*

Magill, Ivan Whiteside (1888–1986). Irish-born anaesthetist, responsible for much of the innovation in, and development of, modern anaesthesia. With Rowbotham in Sidcup after World War I, he developed endotracheal anaesthesia as an alternative to insufflation techniques, originally for facial plastic surgery. Introduced his own anaesthetic breathing system, forceps, laryngoscope and connectors, and developed blind nasal intubation. A pioneer of anaesthesia for thoracic surgery, he developed one-lung anaesthesia, endobronchial tubes and bronchial blockers. Also introduced bobbin flowmeters, portable anaesthetic apparatus and other equipment.

Helped found the Association of Anaesthetists of Great Britain and Ireland, and was involved in the setting up of the DA examination, the Faculty of Anaesthetists and the FFARCS examination. Worked at the Westminster and Brompton Hospitals, London. Knighted in 1960, and received many other medals and awards.
Edridge AW (1987). Anaesthesia; 42: 231–3

Magnesium. Largely intracellular ion, present mainly in bone (over 50%) and skeletal muscle (20%); the remainder is found in the heart, liver and other organs. 1% is in the ECF. Normal plasma levels: 0.75–1.05 mmol/l (although the value of measurement has been questioned, since most magnesium is intracellular). Required for protein and nucleic acid synthesis, regulation of intracellular calcium and potassium, and many enzymatic reactions including all those involving ATP synthesis/hydrolysis. Its actions are opposed by calcium.
Dubé L, Granry JC (2003). Can J Anaesth; 50: 732–46
See also, Hypermagnesaemia; Hypomagnesaemia.

Magnesium sulphate. Drug used mainly as an anticonvulsant drug in pre-eclampsia and eclampsia. Also causes vasodilatation, helping to lower BP. Traditionally, widely used in the USA and Australia for many years but rarely used in the UK until the late 1990s/early 2000s when evidence strongly supported its improved efficacy over diazepam and phenytoin in reducing the incidence of primary eclampsia by almost 60%, as well as preventing recurrence of seizures. Has also been used as a tocolytic drug, in severe asthma resistant to conventional bronchodilator therapy, and in perioperative management of phaeochromocytoma. Has been shown not to reduce mortality in MI despite initial encouraging studies although useful for treatment of arrhythmias, especially caused by hypokalaemia. Acts peripherally at the neuromuscular junction, decreasing acetylcholine release and reducing end-plate sensitivity to acetylcholine; it may also cause cortical depression.

Magnesium chloride is also used.

- Dosage: 2–4 g (8–16 mmol) initially slowly, followed by 1–2 g/h iv.
- Side effects:
  - cardiac conduction defects, drowsiness, absent reflexes, hypoventilation and cardiac arrest may occur with increasing hypermagnesaemia.
  - may augment non-depolarising and depolarising neuromuscular blockade. Neonatal hypotonia may also occur.

Overdosage may be treated with iv calcium.

- Therapeutic plasma levels: 2.0–3.5 mmol/l; side effects may occur above 4–5 mmol/l, with cardiac arrest above 12 mmol/l. Regular testing for presence of the knee jerk reflex has been found to be a useful way of monitoring magnesium therapy, without the need for blood testing.

Dubé L, Granry JC (2003). Can J Anaesth; 50: 732–46

Magnesium trisilicate. Particulate antacid, used in dyspepsia. Has been used to increase gastric pH preoperatively in patients at risk from aspiration of gastric contents, but may itself cause pneumonitis if inhaled. Has also been used to reduce risk of peptic ulceration on ICU, e.g. by hourly nasogastric administration to keep pH above 3–4.

Magnetic resonance imaging (MRI; Nuclear magnetic resonance, NMR). Imaging technique, particularly useful for investigating CNS and pelvic disease, where tissue movement is minimal. Also used in other parts of the body, including the chest; accurate measurements of the heart's dimensions and movement have been obtained.

Involves placement of the patient within a powerful magnetic field, causing alignment of tissue atoms with an odd number of protons or neutrons, e.g. hydrogen. Radiofrequency pulses are then applied, causing deflection of the atoms with absorption of energy. When each pulse stops, the atoms return to their aligned position, emitting energy as radiofrequency waves. Computer analysis of the emitted waves provides information about the chemical make-up of the tissue studied. MRI can provide graphic tissue slices in any plane, or may be used to analyse metabolic processes, e.g. distribution and alterations of intracellular phosphate (spectroscopy). So-called functional MRI (fMRI) techniques allow examination of regional differences in tissue oxygenation and measurement of cerebral blood flow. Interventional MRI involves surgery within the MRI suite to allow scanning during operative procedures.

- Problems and anaesthetic considerations:
  - magnets used are very powerful but thought not to be directly harmful, although maximal 'safe' levels for exposure to static magnetic fields have been set at 200 mT over a single 8-h period for staff. Indirect problems:
    - metal objects may become dangerous projectiles if they are placed near the magnet. All ferromagnetic metal equipment, including cylinders, needles, laryngoscope batteries, etc., must be kept away from the machine. Intracranial clips, pacemakers, heart valves, etc. may also be affected. Non-ferromagnetic anaesthetic equipment is increasingly available.
    - monitoring may be difficult because of poor access to the patient and the need for special equipment. Remote monitoring from outside the scanning room requires a window and protective brass tubes (waveguides) for cables etc. passing between the scanning and observation rooms, with the ability to communicate with the patient. Audible alarms may not be heard because of the background noise of the scanner and the need for ear protection. Automatic BP devices using plastic connectors, capnography, oesophageal stethoscopes and non-magnetic oximeters using fibreoptic cabling have been used. ECG artefacts (especially in the S–T region) may be caused by currents induced by aortic blood flow within the magnetic field. The length of capnography tubing introduces a long delay before the CO_2 signal is obtained.
    - risk of electric current induction by the magnetic field, e.g. causing VF, is minimised by limiting the allowed induced current density.
    - some magnets may be switched off in emergencies, but may require lengthy and expensive restarting procedures. Rapid sudden shutdown may result in the liquid coolant of the magnet (cryogen; usually helium in modern devices) boiling off and flooding the immediate area if not properly vented (quenching). This may cause a dangerous reduction in available O_2 with the risk of asphyxia; proper procedures and O_2 sensors are therefore required.
  - radiofrequency pulses may cause heating effects, thought to be relatively insignificant. These effects may be increased with metal prostheses.
  - sedation/anaesthesia may be required, especially in children or nervous adults, since the subject has to lie within a very small space and the scans themselves may be accompanied by loud knocking noises. Problems include those of radiology in general, in addition to the above. Scans originally took up to 2–3 h but are quicker with newer machines.

Malaria. Tropical disease caused by the protozoan Plasmodium (*Pl. vivax*, *Pl. ovale* or *Pl. falciparum*), and spread by the Anopheles mosquito which carries infected blood between individuals. Although not endemic in the UK, individual cases occur not uncommonly because of widespread air travel. Usual presentation is within 4 weeks of travel from an infected area, although onset may be delayed by many months. In milder forms, periodic release of the organism from the liver and reticuloendothelial system into the bloodstream causes relapsing fever, rigors and malaise (typically cycles of pyrexia lasting 3 days (tertian) or 4 days (quartan), or having no pattern (subtertain), depending on the infecting organism).

Severe illness and death are more likely with *Pl. falciparum*, particularly common in tropical Africa and South-East Asia. Incubation period is 7–14 days. Many features are thought to result from sludging of damaged infected red blood cells within capillaries, with resultant ischaemia of organs.

- Features include:
  - rigors, fever, vomiting, headache.
  - confusion, convulsions, coma. 80% of deaths result from cerebral malaria.
  - renal failure.
  - hypoglycaemia; thought to be caused by increased insulin secretion; it may also result from quinine therapy.
  - bronchopneumonia, ARDS, pulmonary oedema.
  - diarrhoea, endotoxaemia from bowel bacteria.
  - anaemia, thrombocytopenia, intravascular haemolysis, DIC.

Diagnosis is made by examining blood films, or rarely bone marrow, for parasites.

- Treatment:
  - chloroquine and primaquine for mild infections.
  - quinine; usually reserved for resistant organisms or severe falciparum infection.
  - severe infection: quinine salt 20 mg/kg iv over 4 h, then 10 mg/kg over 4 h repeated 8–12 hourly until able to

swallow (reduced by a third after 72 h if unable to swallow). Oral therapy (10 mg/kg) is continued until 7 days' treatment is completed. It is then followed by a course of either pyrimethamine/sulfadoxime combination or doxycycline.

Malaria may be transmitted by blood transfusion; those with infection are therefore excluded from being donors.

Greenwood BM, Bojang K, Whitty CJM, Targett GAT (2005). Lancet; 365: 1487–98

Malignancy. Second commonest cause of death in the UK after cardiovascular disease. Patients may present to anaesthetists for investigative, therapeutic or unrelated procedures. ICU management may be required after major surgery related to the malignancy or for incidental conditions. Considerable ethical issues surround ICU provision for patients with terminal disease.

- General considerations:
  - effects of malignancy itself:
    - primary:
      - local, e.g. pressure effects, ulceration, haemorrhage, etc.
      - systemic, e.g. anaemia, cachexia, susceptibility to infection, electrolyte disturbances (e.g. hypercalcaemia), endocrine effects (e.g. Cushing's syndrome caused by bronchial carcinoma, carcinoid syndrome, myasthenic syndrome, etc.).
    - metastatic, e.g. lung, liver, bone.
  - effects of previous treatment:
    - surgery/radiotherapy, e.g. scarring, deformities.
    - cytotoxic drugs, corticosteroids, opioid analgesic drugs, antidepressant drugs, etc.
  - possible effects of anaesthesia on the immune system and cancer, e.g. administration of blood during bowel cancer resection may decrease survival.
  - anxiety, depression.
  - pain management.

Malignant hyperthermia (MH). Condition first recognised in 1960 in Australia, consisting of increased temperature and rigidity during anaesthesia. Incidence is reported between 1:5000 and 1:200 000. Results from abnormal skeletal muscle contraction and increased metabolism affecting muscle and other tissues. Susceptibility shows autosomal dominant inheritance; in 50–70% of affected families the predisposing gene is thought to be on chromosome 19, at or near the gene for the ryanodine/dihydropyridine receptor complex at the T-tubule/sarcoplasmic reticulum complex of striated muscle. This receptor is involved in the control of calcium flux in and out of the sarcoplasmic reticulum; this control is lost in MH. The genes for muscular dystrophy and certain metabolic disorders are nearby. Several other genes on different chromosomes have also been implicated, thus reducing the sensitivity of genetic analysis as a test for MH.

MH follows exposure to triggering agents, particularly the volatile anaesthetic agents and suxamethonium, although it is thought that a single dose of the latter by itself will not cause the syndrome. It may occur in patients who have experienced previous anaesthetics without problem. In certain animals, e.g. Landrace pigs, a similar response may be provoked by stress. This has also been reported in a susceptible patient. Thus patients may show different sensitivity to triggering agents at different times. Reactions have been reported up to 11 h postoperatively after triggering anaesthetics.

Most common in young patients undergoing musculoskeletal surgery, including trauma surgery. Whether this reflects an underlying abnormality of muscle predisposing to trauma is unknown. Operations in the young are commonly for squints and orthopaedic problems, and increased incidence in this group may simply represent the first exposure to anaesthesia in susceptible patients. MH is also thought to be more common in patients with certain muscular dystrophies (e.g. central core disease) and related disorders.

- Features are related to muscle abnormality and hypermetabolism, but not all may be present:
  - sustained muscle contraction; results from breakage of the normal impulse/contraction sequence (excitation/contraction uncoupling) relating to abnormal calcium ion mobilisation, and is unrelieved by neuromuscular blocking drugs. Masseter spasm may be an early sign.
  - muscle breakdown with release of potassium, myoglobin and muscle enzymes, e.g. creatine kinase. Hyperkalaemia may cause cardiac arrhythmias.
  - increased O_2 consumption leading to cyanosis.
  - increased CO_2 production and hypercapnia. Hyperventilation may occur in the spontaneously breathing patient.
  - rapidly increasing body temperature (e.g. $> 0.5°C$ every 10 mins) and sweating.
  - tachycardia and unstable BP.
  - metabolic acidosis.
- Management:
  - discontinuation of the triggering agent, and abandonment of surgery if feasible. Changing the anaesthetic machine, tubing and soda lime has been suggested if possible. More recently, since the modern volatile agents are hardly adsorbed on to modern plastic breathing tubing, simply removing the vaporisers and emptying the reservoir bag (or flushing the ventilator bellows) is thought to be sufficient – the bulk of the volatile agent in the breathing system then arising from the patient rather than the anaesthetic apparatus.
  - dantrolene is the only available specific treatment. 1 mg/kg is given iv, repeated as required up to 10 mg/kg.
  - supportive treatment:
    - hyperventilation with 100% O_2. Boluses of, e.g., thiopental iv will maintain anaesthesia.
    - correction of acidosis with bicarbonate, according to the results of blood gas analysis.
    - cooling with cold iv fluids, fans, sponging, irrigation of body cavities, etc. Other causes of hyperthermia should be considered.
    - treatment of hyperkalaemia if severe.
    - diuretic therapy and urinary alkalinisation to reduce renal damage caused by myoglobin. Mannitol or furosemide has been recommended.
    - treatment of any arrhythmias as they occur.
    - corticosteroids, e.g. dexamethasone 4 mg, have been advocated.
    - close monitoring in an ICU for 36–48 h postoperatively, including of temperature. Blood should be taken 12 hourly for 36–48 h, for measurement of creatinine kinase, and the first urine voided should be analysed for myoglobin.
    - renal failure and DIC are treated as necessary.

Treatment should be instituted as soon as the diagnosis is suspected. Arterial blood gas analysis and measurement of plasma potassium should be performed early to detect acidosis and hyperkalaemia.

Prognosis is good if treated appropriately and early; mortality was 80% before dantrolene became available but it is $< 5\%$ today.

- Investigation:
  - serum creatine kinase elevation and myoglobinuria are suggestive but not diagnostic. The former is not reliable

as a screening test. Creatine kinase and myoglobin may both increase after suxamethonium administration in normal patients.
- muscle biopsy may appear normal histologically.
- caffeine and halothane contracture tests are now accepted as investigations of choice. Biopsied muscle is exposed to caffeine and halothane, and tension in the muscle measured. Contractures are induced in susceptible muscle. Results are divided into positive, negative or equivocal. False positive results may occur. All suspected cases and immediate relatives should be tested for susceptibility.

- Management of known cases:
  - pretreatment with oral dantrolene 5 mg/kg over 24 h preoperatively, or 1–2 mg/kg iv before induction has been used, but this is rarely considered necessary now.
  - sedative premedication is sometimes given to reduce 'stress', but this is controversial.
  - avoidance of known triggering agents: volatile agents and suxamethonium. N_2O is considered safe. Many other drugs have been implicated at some time, but the above are the only definite triggers. TIVA has been suggested as a useful technique. Local anaesthetic techniques may be used, but MH may still occur. All local anaesthetic agents are now considered as safe as each other. Some would avoid phenothiazines and butyrophenones because of the neuroleptic malignant syndrome, but there is no evidence that the two conditions are related.
  - formerly, use of an anaesthetic machine not previously exposed to volatile agents was considered mandatory, but a new breathing system, flushed with fresh gas for 10–20 min, has been suggested as being adequate.
  - monitoring should include temperature (rectal and axillary), expired CO_2 and oximetry. Some would consider arterial cannulation mandatory. Close monitoring should continue postoperatively.
  - dantrolene and supportive treatments should be readily available.
  - reactions have been reported following apparently 'trigger-free' anaesthetics, but these have not been severe.

All patients should be questioned for family history of anaesthetic problems, since many susceptible patients give a positive family history. Susceptible patients should wear 'Medic Alert' bracelets.

Wappler F (2001). Eur J Anaesthesiol; 18: 632–52

Mallampati score, *see Intubation, difficult*

Malnutrition. Nutrient deficiency, usually of several dietary components. Protein depletion with near normal energy supply may lead to kwashiorkor, with hypoproteinaemia and oedema. Protein and energy depletion may lead to marasmus, with normal plasma protein concentration.

- Body reserves during total starvation under basal conditions:
  - carbohydrate: about 0.5 kg mainly as liver and muscle glycogen; lasts under 1 day.
  - protein: 4–6 kg mainly as muscle; lasts 10–12 days.
  - fat: 12–15 kg as adipose tissue; lasts 20–25 days.

Protein breakdown is reduced by even small amounts of glucose, possibly by the effects of resultant insulin secretion, which prevents protein catabolism.

- Malnutrition is common to some degree in hospital patients. It may be associated with:
  - decreased intake, e.g. vomiting, malabsorption, anorexia, poor diet, nil-by-mouth orders.
  - decreased utilisation, e.g. renal failure.
  - increased basal metabolic rate, e.g. trauma, burns, severe illness, pyrexia.

Thus common perioperatively, especially in severe chronic illness, GIT disease/surgery, alcoholics, the elderly, immigrants and the mentally ill. May result in impaired healing, bedsores, increased susceptibility to infection, weakness, anaemia, hypoproteinaemia, electrolyte disturbances and dehydration, vitamin deficiency disorders, and predisposition to hypothermia. Respiratory muscle weakness may predispose to respiratory complications.

Long-term nutrition, via enteral or parenteral routes, is thought to be beneficial preoperatively (at least 14 days). The place of short-term feeding is less certain. Progress may be monitored by weight or skin thickness measurements.

Managing Obstetric Emergencies and Trauma course (MOET course). Training programme, devised in 1998, designed for medical staff working within obstetrics, obstetric anaesthesia, and accident and emergency medicine. Similar to other acute life support courses in its systematic approach and structure.

Mandatory minute ventilation (MMV). Ventilatory mode used to assist weaning from ventilators. The required mandatory minute ventilation is preset, and the patient allowed to breathe spontaneously, with the ventilator making up any shortfall in minute volume. Thus with the patient breathing adequately, the ventilator is not required. However, a minute ventilation made up of rapid shallow breaths will also 'satisfy' the ventilator, despite alveolar ventilation being inadequate. In addition, not all ventilators allow spontaneous minute ventilation to exceed the preset one (extended mandatory minute ventilation; EMMV). Thus MMV is less popular than IMV.

Mandibular nerve blocks. Performed for facial and intraoral procedures.

- Anatomy: the mandibular division (V_3) of the trigeminal nerve passes from the Gasserian ganglion through the foramen ovale.
- Divisions:
  - motor nerves to the muscles of mastication and tensor muscles of the palate and eardrum.
  - sensory nerves (*see Fig. 75; Gasserian ganglion block*):
    - meningeal branch: passes through the foramen spinosum and supplies the adjacent dura.
    - buccal nerve: supplies the skin and mucosa of the cheek.
    - auriculotemporal nerve; supplies the anterior eardrum, ear canal, temporomandibular joint, cheek, temple, temporal scalp and parotid gland.
    - inferior alveolar nerve: enters the mandible at its ramus, supplying the lower teeth and gums; the central incisors are innervated bilaterally. Emerges through the mental foramen to supply the mucosa and skin of the lower lip, chin and gum.
    - lingual nerve: passes alongside the tongue to supply its anterior two-thirds, the floor of the mouth and lingual gum.

The supraorbital foramen, pupil, infraorbital notch, infraorbital foramen, buccal surface of the second premolar and mental foramen all lie along a straight line.

- Blocks:
  - mandibular: a needle is inserted at right angles to the skin between the coronoid and condylar processes, just above the bone. After contacting the pterygoid plate, it is

redirected posteriorly until paraesthesiae are obtained, and 5 ml local anaesthetic agent injected (n.b. the pharynx lies 5 mm internally).

- inferior alveolar/lingual: with the mouth wide open, a needle is inserted parallel to the teeth and 1 cm above their occlusal surface, medial to the oblique line of the mandibular ramus. It is advanced 1.5–2.0 cm and the syringe barrel swung across to the opposite side. 1–1.5 ml solution is injected with a further 0.5 ml on withdrawal (to block the lingual nerve).

  May also be performed extraorally, by injecting 1.5–2.0 ml between the mandibular ramus and maxilla, level with the upper teeth gingival margins; the needle is inserted from the front with the mouth shut.

  Buccal infiltration is required for surgery to the molar teeth; 0.5–1.0 ml is injected into the cheek mucosa opposite the third molar. The incisors receive bilateral innervation.
- mental/incisive branches of the inferior alveolar nerve (supplying from the incisors to the first premolar): 0.5–1.0 ml is injected at the mental foramen from behind the second molar intraorally, or extraorally.
- buccal nerve: 0.5–1.0 ml is injected lateral and posterior to the last molar, by the anterior border of the mandibular ramus.
- submucous infiltration on both sides of individual teeth, directed along its long axis, may also be used.
- auriculotemporal nerve: 1.5–2.0 ml is injected in the anterior wall of the ear canal, at the junction of its bony and cartilaginous parts. Allows myringotomy to be performed.

1–2% lidocaine or prilocaine with adrenaline are most commonly used. Systemic absorption of adrenaline may cause symptoms, especially if high concentrations are used, e.g. 1:80 000. Immediate collapse following dental nerve blocks is thought to result from retrograde flow of solution via branches of the external carotid artery, reaching the internal carotid; perineural spread to the medulla has also been suggested.
See also, Gasserian ganglion block; Maxillary nerve blocks; Nose; Ophthalmic nerve blocks

Mandragora (Mandrake). Plant, supposedly human-shaped, thought to hold magic powers including the ability to induce sleep and relieve pain. Contains hyoscine and similar alkaloids. According to legend, its scream on uprooting killed all who heard it, hence the supposedly 'safe' method of collection: a dog is tied to the plant at midnight, whilst its owner retreats to a safe distance with ears stopped with wax. The dog is enticed to run after food, pulling out the mandrake and dying in the process.

Mannitol. Plant-derived alcohol. An osmotic diuretic; it draws water from the extracellular and intracellular spaces into the vascular compartment, expanding the latter transiently. Not reabsorbed once filtered in the kidneys, it continues to be osmotically active in the urine, causing diuresis. Used mainly to reduce the risk of perioperative renal failure (e.g. during vascular surgery, surgery in obstructive jaundice, etc.), and to treat cerebral oedema. Efficacy in the latter depends on integrity of the blood–brain barrier which may be altered in neurological disease, although some benefit is derived from the systemic dehydration produced. Has also been used to lower intraocular pressure. It may also act as a free radical scavenger. Oral mannitol has been used (together with activated charcoal) as an osmotic agent to increase intestinal removal of poisons.

Temporarily increases cerebral blood flow; ICP may rise slightly before falling, especially after rapid injection. Excessive brain shrinkage in the elderly may rupture fragile subdural veins. A rebound increase in ICP may occur if treatment is prolonged, due to eventual passage of mannitol into the brain; the effect is small after a single dose. A transient increase in vascular volume and CVP may cause cardiac failure in susceptible patients.

- Dosage: 0.5–1 g/kg by iv infusion of 10–20% solution over 20–30 min. Effects occur within 30 min, lasting 6 h. 0.25–0.5 g/kg may follow 6 hourly for 24 h, unless diuresis has not occurred, cardiovascular instability ensues or plasma osmolality exceeds 315 mosmol/kg.

Available as 10% and 20% solutions with osmolality 550 and 1100 mosmol/kg respectively.

Mann–Whitney rank sum test, *see Statistical tests*

Manslaughter. Unlawful killing of another person; a criminal charge (as opposed to the civil charge of negligence) that has been applied to anaesthetists in cases where the care provided was so poor as to constitute a reckless or grossly negligent act or omission. Examples have included fatal cardiac arrest following disconnection of the breathing system and inadequate immediate postoperative care.

The charge of corporate manslaughter exists in common law but actions against large organisations have often been unsuccessful because of difficulties identifying the person(s) responsible for the decisions that led to death. The Corporate Manslaughter and Corporate Homicide Act 2007 raises the possibility of senior managers including clinicians (i.e. not just directors and executives) facing charges if they are implicated in playing 'a significant role' that leads to a 'breach in decision making related to operational processes within the organisation that subsequently results in the death of a person'.

Ferner RE (2000). BMJ; 321: 1212–16
See also, Medicolegal aspects of anaesthesia

MAO, *see Monoamine oxidase*

MAOI, *see Monoamine oxidase inhibitors*

MAP, *see Mean arterial pressure*

Mapleson classification of breathing systems, *see Anaesthetic breathing systems*

Marey's law. Increased pressure in the aortic arch and carotid sinus causes bradycardia; decreased pressure causes tachycardia.
[Etienne Jules Marey (1830–1904), French physiologist]
See also, Baroreceptor reflex

Marfan's syndrome. Connective tissue disease, inherited as an autosomal dominant gene. Prevalence is 1:20 000.

- Features:
  - tall stature, with long thin extremities. Joint dislocations, kyphoscoliosis, pes excavatum, inguinal and diaphragmatic herniae are common.
  - subluxation of the ocular lens (50%).
  - cardiovascular:
    - aortic regurgitation (< 90%).
    - ascending aortic aneurysm.
    - mitral valve prolapse.
    - conduction defects.
  - respiratory:
    - kyphoscoliosis.
    - emphysema.
    - pneumothorax.
    - tracheal intubation may be difficult (high arched palate).

Death usually results from aortic dilatation and its complications. Careful preoperative assessment and antibiotic prophylaxis are required as for congenital heart disease.
[Bernard J Marfan (1858–1942), French paediatrician]
Judge DP, Dietz HC (2005). Lancet; 366: 1965–76

MARS, Molecular adsorbents recirculation system, *see Liver dialysis*

Masks, *see Facepieces; Oxygen therapy*

Mass. Amount of matter contained in a body. Under conditions of differing gravity, mass remains constant, whereas weight varies. SI unit is the kilogram.

Mass spectrometer. Device used to analyse mixtures of substances according to mw. The sample passes through an ionising chamber, and becomes charged by electrons arising from a cathode. The charged sample particles are then accelerated by an electric field which imparts a certain velocity. When they subsequently pass through a strong magnetic field, the particles are deflected to varying degrees depending on their mass and momentum. The electrical charge arriving at certain distances from the accelerating chamber is measured, and corresponds to the amount of differently sized particles present in the original sample. Different ranges of particle size may be analysed by altering accelerator characteristics. Compounds of identical mw may be distinguished by identifying breakdown products.

Alternatively, in the quadrupole mass spectrometer, the accelerated beam passes longitudinally between four rods, of variable potential. Particles are removed from the beam unless of a certain mass, depending on the rods' potential.

Mass spectrometers may be used for on-line gas analysis during anaesthesia.

Masseter spasm. Increase in jaw tone occurring after suxamethonium. More common in children and after halothane induction, although the incidence is hard to determine because of difficulty in definition. 1:100–1:3000 incidence has been reported, but amidst controversy. A protective effect of thiopental has been suggested. Spasm may represent a normal dose-related response to suxamethonium, but has been associated with MH susceptibility, especially if spasm is severe and prolonged, and associated with markedly raised serum creatine kinase and myoglobinuria. May also be seen in dystrophia myotonica following suxamethonium and acetylcholinesterase inhibitors.

Management of spasm is controversial: termination of anaesthesia, treatment with dantrolene, proceeding with caution or referral for muscle biopsy have all been recommended.

MAST, Military antishock trousers, *see Antigravity suit*

Mast cells. Basophilic cells in connective and subcutaneous tissues, involved in inflammatory reactions and immune responses. Storage granules contain lytic enzymes (e.g. tryptase) and inflammatory mediators, e.g. histamine, kinins, heparin, 5-HT, hyaluronidase, leukotrienes, platelet aggregating and leucocyte chemotactic factors. Release is caused by injury to tissues, complement activation, drugs, e.g. tubocurarine, and cross-linkage of surface IgE molecules (e.g. in anaphylactic reactions) by antigen. Also involved in presentation of antigen to lymphocytes. Occur in excess (either in the circulation or as tissue infiltrates) in mastocytosis.

Maternal mortality, *see Confidential Enquiries into Maternal Deaths*

Maxillary nerve blocks. Performed for facial and intraoral procedures.

- Anatomy: the maxillary division (V_2) of the trigeminal nerve passes from the Gasserian ganglion through the foramen rotundum into the pterygopalatine fossa, dividing into sensory branches and continuing as the infraorbital nerve (*see Fig. 75; Gasserian ganglion block*). Branches:
  - via the pterygopalatine ganglion to the nose, nasopharynx and palate via nasal, nasopalatine, greater and lesser palatine and pharyngeal nerves.
  - nasopalatine nerve: supplies the anterior third of the hard palate and palatal gingiva of the upper incisors.
  - greater palatine: supplies the posterior hard palate and palatal gingiva of adjacent teeth.
  - zygomatic nerve: supplies the temple, cheek and lateral eye.
  - posterior superior alveolar nerve: supplies the molar/premolar teeth.
  - infraorbital nerve: supplies the lower eyelid, conjunctiva, side of the nose, upper lip, cheek, and via its anterior superior alveolar branch, the upper canines and incisors, maxillary sinus and cheek mucosa.

  The supraorbital foramen, pupil, infraorbital notch, infraorbital foramen, buccal surface of the second premolar and mental foramen all lie along a straight line.
- Blocks:
  - maxillary nerve: a needle is inserted extraorally 0.5 cm below the midpoint of the zygoma and directed medially until bone is contacted. It is redirected anteriorly and advanced a further 1 cm, anterior to the lateral pterygoid plate. 3–4 ml local anaesthetic agent is injected. May also be blocked via the intraoral route: the needle is inserted behind the posterior border of the zygoma and directed upwards, medially and posteriorly 3 cm. Up to 5 ml solution is injected within the pterygopalatine fossa.
  - nasopalatine nerve: 0.5–1.0 ml is injected at the incisive foramen, 0.5–1.0 cm posterior to the upper incisors in the midline.
  - greater palatine nerve: 0.5–1.0 ml is injected at the greater palatine foramen, marked by a depression in the palate opposite the second/third molar 1 cm above the gingival margin.
  - infraorbital nerve: 1–2 ml is injected at the infraorbital foramen, 0.5–1.0 cm below the infraorbital notch. Injection may be performed intraorally or extraorally.
  - superior alveolar nerve branches to individual teeth may be blocked by submucous infiltration above each tooth.
  - for the Cadwell–Luc approach, the mucosa and periosteum above the upper premolars may be infiltrated with 5–10 ml solution, to block branches of the anterior superior alveolar nerve. Topical application of, e.g., lidocaine may assist the block. Further solution may be injected into the mucosa of the maxillary sinus once opened. Alternatively, maxillary or infraorbital nerve blocks may be performed.

1–2% lidocaine or prilocaine with adrenaline are most commonly used. Systemic absorption of adrenaline may cause symptoms, especially if high concentrations are used, e.g. 1:80 000.

Immediate collapse following dental nerve blocks is thought to result from retrograde flow of solution via branches of the external carotid artery, reaching the internal carotid; perineural spread to the medulla has also been suggested.

[George Caldwell (1834–1918), US ENT surgeon; Henri Luc (1855–1925), French ENT surgeon]
See also, Mandibular nerve blocks; Ophthalmic nerve blocks

Maximal breathing capacity, *see Maximal voluntary ventilation*

Maximal voluntary ventilation (Maximal breathing capacity). Maximal minute volume of air able to be breathed, measured over 15 s. Normally about 120–150 l/min. Equals approximately 35 × FEV_1. Rarely used, since very tiring to perform.
See also, Lung function tests

MCH/MCHC/MCV, Mean cell haemoglobin/Mean cell haemoglobin concentration/Mean cell volume, *see Erythrocytes*

MDEA, Methylenedioxyethylamfetamine, *see Methylenedioxymethylamfetamine*

MDMA, *see Methylenedioxymethylamfetamine*

MEA syndrome, *see Multiple endocrine adenomatosis*

Mean (Average). Expression of the central tendency of a set of observations or measurements. Equals the sum of all the observations divided by the number of observations (n), i.e.

$$\bar{x} = \frac{\Sigma x}{n}$$

Population mean is denoted by μ; sample mean by $\bar{x}$.

Means of more than one sample group may be compared using statistical tests.
See also, Median; Mode; Standard error of mean; Statistical frequency distributions; Statistics

Mean arterial pressure (MAP). Average arterial BP throughout the cardiac cycle. The area contained within the arterial waveform pressure trace above MAP equals the area below it.

$$\text{Equals approximately } \frac{(2 \times \text{diastolic}) + \text{systolic}}{3}$$

$$\text{or diastolic} + \frac{(\text{systolic} - \text{diastolic})}{3}$$

Preferred by some clinicians to measures of systolic or diastolic pressures, since it is less liable to errors or differences due to measuring techniques. Also represents the mean pressure available for perfusion of tissues.

Mechanocardiography. Recording of the mechanical pulsations of the CVS; includes tracings of the JVP and venous waveform, arterial waveform and recordings at the apex using an externally applied transducer. Has been used to investigate cardiovascular disease, especially valvular disease, and to determine systolic time intervals.

Median. Expression of the central tendency of a set of measurements or observations.

$$\text{Equals the } \frac{(n+1)\text{th}}{2} \text{ measurement.}$$

Half the population lies above it, half below. Equals the mean for a normal distribution.
See also, Statistical frequency distributions; Statistics

Median nerve (C6–T1). Arises from the medial and lateral cords of the brachial plexus in the lower axilla, lateral to the axillary artery. Passes down the front of the arm to the antecubital fossa, first lateral to the brachial artery, then crossing it anteriorly at mid/upper arm to lie medially. Entering the forearm, it crosses the ulnar artery anteriorly, separated from it by pronator teres's deep head. Passes between flexor digitorum superficialis and profundus; at the wrist it lies between the tendons of palmaris longus (medially) and flexor carpi radialis (laterally).

- Apart from branches to the joints of the wrist and hand, it supplies:
  - superficial flexor muscles (except flexor carpi ulnaris), abductor pollicis brevis, flexor pollicis brevis and opponens pollicis.
  - radial side of the palm and the palmar surface of the radial 3½ digits, extending to their dorsal surface at their tips.
  - via the anterior interosseus branch arising at the distal antecubital fossa: flexor pollicis longus, radial part of flexor digitorum profundus, and pronator quadratus.

May be blocked at the brachial plexus, elbow and wrist.
See also, Brachial plexus block; Elbow, nerve blocks; Wrist, nerve blocks.

Mediastinum. Region of the thorax between the two pleural sacs. It is in contact with the diaphragm inferiorly, and continuous with the tissues of the neck superiorly. Lies between the vertebral column posteriorly and sternum anteriorly. Contains the heart, great vessels, trachea, oesophagus, thoracic duct, vagi, phrenic and recurrent laryngeal nerves, sympathetic trunk, thymus and lymph nodes (Fig. 102).

- Divided into:
  - superior mediastinum: above a horizontal line level with T4/5 and the angle of Louis.
  - inferior mediastinum: below this line. Composed of anterior (between heart and sternum), middle (containing pericardium and contents) and posterior (between heart and vertebrae) portions.

  Thus mediastinal enlargement may be caused by:
  - enlargement of any of the above constituent structures (central).
  - spinal and vertebral masses (posterior).
  - thymic, thyroid, teratoma and dermoid tumours (anterior).

  Tumours, e.g. bronchial carcinoma, may involve local structures within the mediastinum, e.g. recurrent laryngeal or phrenic nerves, pericardium, etc. Bleeding from the aorta following chest trauma or dissection may cause widening of the superior mediastinum.

Patients with mediastinal enlargement may present for biopsy, e.g. via mediastinoscopy through a suprasternal incision, or resection.

- Main anaesthetic considerations:
  - preoperative state, e.g. related to the primary malignancy. Tracheal compression and airway obstruction, superior vena caval obstruction, phrenic and recurrent laryngeal nerve involvement and drug and radiotherapy effects may be present.
  - classically, induction of anaesthesia is inhalational, but some advocate iv induction. Reinforced tracheal/bronchial tubes are often preferable.
  - severe haemorrhage may occur. Fluid replacement via the femoral vein may be required if the superior vena cava and its tributaries are involved.
  - one-lung anaesthesia and even extracorporeal circulation may be required during resection.

[Antoine Louis (1723–1792), French surgeon]
See also, Chest X-ray

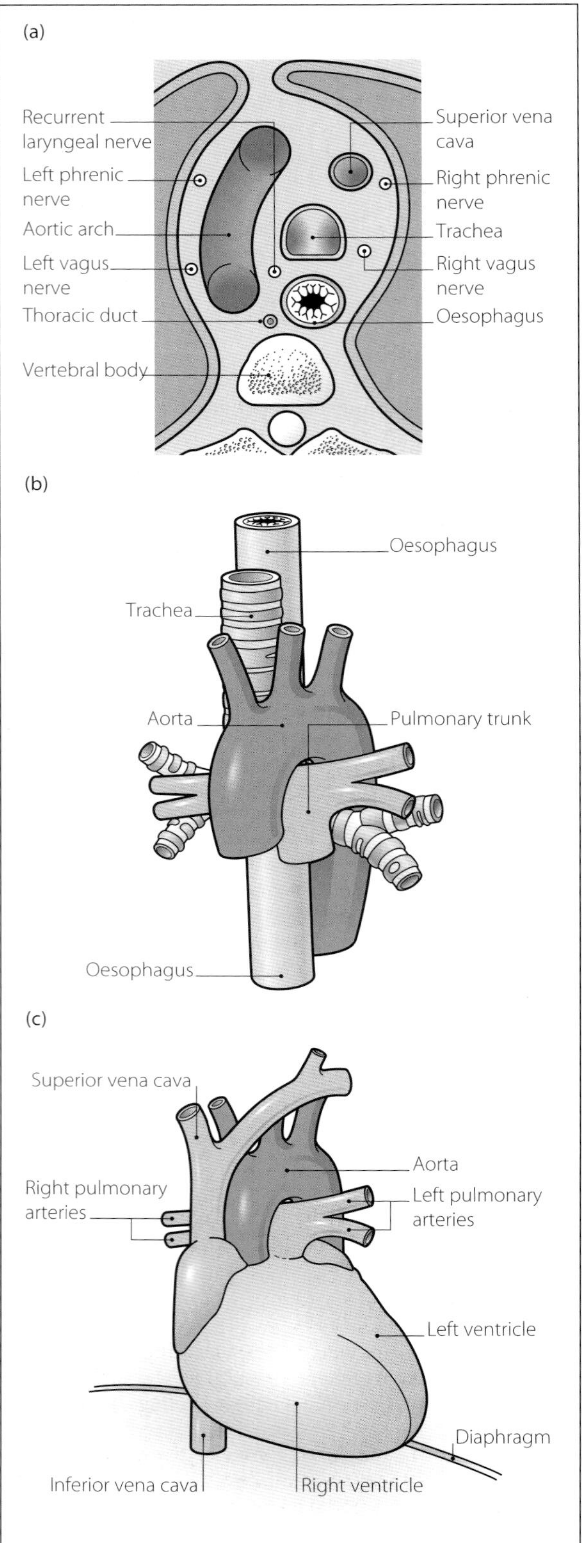

Fig. 102 Anatomy of the mediastinum: (a) transverse section through T4; (b) trachea and relations; (c) heart and great vessels

Medical emergency team (MET). Team consisting of medical and nursing staff skilled in resuscitation (in its broadest sense) responding to standardised calling criteria including abnormal physiological variables (e.g. systolic BP < 90 mmHg), specific conditions or 'any time urgent medical assistance is required'. Originally devised at Liverpool Hospital, Australia, in 1990, but becoming increasingly accepted internationally. Replaces existing cardiac arrest teams on the basis that prevention of cardiac arrest or severe physiological deterioration is likely to have a better outcome than treatment applied after cardiac arrest. Its effect on preventing cardiac arrest, decreasing ICU admission and improving mortality has not been proved.

Lee A, Bishop G, Hillman KM, Daffurn K (1995). Anaesth Intens Care; 23: 183–6

See also, Acute life-threatening events – recognition and treatment; Postoperative care team

Medicines and Healthcare products Regulatory Agency (MHRA). UK government agency formed in 2003 from the Medicines Control Agency and Medical Devices Agency. Responsible for regulating medicines and medical devices and ensuring their safety, via approval/regulation/monitoring of clinical trials, reporting/investigating adverse drug reactions, and licensing/testing medicinal products.

Medicolegal aspects of anaesthesia. In the UK, these usually concern matters of civil law, e.g. negligence, breach of contract or battery; proof must be according to 'balance of probabilities'. Criminal law is involved less commonly (e.g. involving murder or manslaughter), e.g. due to criminal neglect or reckless disregard of clinical duties; proof must be 'beyond reasonable doubt'. Leaving anaesthetised patients unattended has led to criminal prosecution.

- Usually related to:
  - consent for surgery, procedures, etc.
  - negligence: harm resulting from a failure in the duty of care. Expert opinion is obtained and clinical notes scrutinised.

    Individual doctors are responsible privately; in the National Health Service (NHS) responsibilty is shared by the employing Trust. Defence organisations provide advice and indemnity; the latter has been provided by the employer for NHS work from 1990.

    Claims commonly involve:
    - faulty equipment, incorrect drugs or blood, etc.
    - consent.
    - wrong operation, etc.
    - poor preoperative assessment and preparation.
    - absence of the anaesthetist.
    - nerve damage, broken teeth, etc.
    - awareness.
    - hypoxia, cardiac arrest, etc.

    Anaesthesia is considered a high risk specialty because of common minor claims and very expensive major claims.

    Risks are reduced by:
    - checking of anaesthetic equipment, drugs, drips, allergies, patients' names and operation sites.
    - adequate preoperative assessment and preparation, including warning patients of risks, e.g. to teeth, of dural tap, etc.
    - consultation with senior colleagues when appropriate.
    - adherence to generally accepted techniques, including adequate monitoring.
    - careful writing of clinical notes and anaesthetic record-keeping, with copies kept for later use.

Informing defence bodies early is encouraged, should mishaps occur.
- full and honest explanation with patients and/or relatives when anything goes wrong.
- perioperative deaths: those occurring within 24 h of anaesthesia are reported to the coroner, who may order an inquiry or inquest, although the time interval is not specified by law. Once reported, organs may not be harvested for transplantation without the coroner's permission.
- Misuse of Drugs Act.
- fitness to practise: investigated by a committee of the General Medical Council which regulates licensing to practise medicine in the UK; although not a civil court the process may be broadly similar. Recent debate has focused around a proposed change in fitness to practise hearings from the traditional criminal 'standard' – i.e. beyond reasonable doubt – to the civil standard of balance of probabilities.

Similar considerations apply to ICU although claims arising from ICU itself are less common; however ICU may be required for critical illness arising from negligent practice. ICU issues with medicolegal implications include competence (whether the patients are able to make their own decisions), non-provision of life-sustaining treatment or withdrawal of treatment (justified if it is in the patient's best interests to be allowed to die) and brainstem death. The need for attention to detail and proper record-keeping is just as important as in general anaesthetic practice.

See also, Abuse of anaesthetic agents; Anaesthetic morbidity and mortality; Ethics; Sick doctor scheme

Meglitinides. Oral hypoglycaemic drugs used in the management of diabetes mellitus. Stimulate insulin release from the pancreas. Two available agents are nateglinide and repaglinide; the former is only licensed for use in combination with metformin.

Membrane potential. Results from the differential distribution of charged particles across cell membranes. The distribution of each particle is related to its permeability across the membrane, the distribution of other particles (e.g. Donnan effect), and to active transport systems, e.g. sodium/potassium pump. Membranes are impermeable to protein (negatively charged) which thus remains intracellular; membranes are poorly permeable to sodium ions and moderately permeable to chloride and potassium ions.

Concentration and electric gradients exist across membranes for each ion; the membrane potential at equilibrium for each is calculated by the Nernst equation. Membrane potentials at given intracellular/extracellular concentrations of sodium, chloride and potassium ions together are calculated by the Goldman constant-field equation.

Potential is conventionally written as negative; i.e. the inside is negative relative to the outside. The potential's magnitude varies between tissues, e.g. −70 mV for nerves and −90 mV for muscle.

Changes in membrane permeability may alter, or be altered by, membrane potential, e.g. during action potentials.

Membranes. Biological membranes share certain features:
- phospholipid bilayer; the hydrophilic end of each phospholipid molecule faces the membrane surface and the hydrophobic end lies within the membrane substance.
- protein molecules at intervals within the membrane; they may traverse it or project on one side only, according to the water/lipid solubility of the protein subunits. Proteins are able to 'float' within the lipid molecules.
- proteins may function as enzymes, receptors, pumps or channels for ions. They also have antigenic properties.
- resting membrane potential is created by differential permeability for certain ions, together with active transport pumps. Most membranes are relatively permeable to chloride and potassium ions, less so to sodium ions, and relatively impermeable to proteins and anions. Noncharged substances, e.g. CO_2 and non-ionised drugs, are able to cross freely, as is water.
- function of cells is dependent on the features of their membrane proteins, which may be altered by electrical signals or chemicals, e.g. drugs, hormones, neurotransmitters. The action of anaesthetic agents is thought to involve alteration of membrane configuration within the nervous system.

See also, Action potential; Anaesthesia, mechanisms of

Memory. Classically divided into short- and long-term memory; the latter is subdivided into procedural (not requiring conscious retrieval, e.g. driving a car) and declarative (either requiring conscious retrieval of specific events (episodic) or related to information about the world and language (semantic)). The hippocampus, amygdala, frontal lobes, and thalamic and hypothalamic nuclei are thought to be concerned with memory storage and retrieval.

Anaesthetic agents are thought mainly to impair acquisition of short-term memory, although transfer into long-term memory may also be affected.

Warltier DC, Ghoneim MM (2004). Anesthesiology; 100: 987–1002 and Ghoneim MM (2004). Anesthesiology; 100: 1277–97

See also, Amnesia

Mendelson's syndrome, *see Aspiration pneumonitis*

Meninges. Tissue layers surrounding the brain and spinal cord, comprised of:
- pia mater: delicate vascular layer, closely adherent to the brain and cord, following their surfaces into clefts, sulci, etc. Surrounded by CSF within the arachnoid. Thin projections of the latter cross the subarachnoid space to the pia. Blood vessels lie within the space.

  Within the vertebral canal, the denticulate ligament passes laterally from the pia along its length and attaches at intervals to the dura. The subarachnoid septum lies posteriorly, attaching to the arachnoid intermittently. The pia terminates as the filum terminale which passes through the caudal end of the dural sac and attaches to the coccyx.
- arachnoid mater: delicate membrane, containing CSF internally. Does not project into clefts and sulci, apart from the longitudinal fissure. Applied to the dura externally; the potential subdural space lies between them, containing vessels. Fuses with the dura at S2. Arachnoid granulations project into the venous sinuses, for drainage of CSF.
- dura mater: comprised of two fibrous layers: the outer is adherent to the periosteal lining of the skull; the inner attaches to the outer but is separated by venous sinuses. The inner layer forms sheets within the skull:
  - vertical: falx cerebri and falx cerebelli between the cerebral and cerebellar hemispheres respectively.
  - horizontal: tentorium cerebelli above the cerebellum and the diaphragma sellae above the pituitary gland.

  The dura also forms two layers within the vertebral canal: the external adherent to the inner periostium of the vertebrae and the internal lying against the outer surface of the arachnoid. The space between the two dura layers is the epidural space. Projections and fibrous bands have been demonstrated from the dura within the epidural space, especially in the midline. Dura projects intermittently to the posterior longitudinal ligament of the vertebrae, especially lumbar. Dura ends at about S2.

All layers donate a thin covering 'sleeve' to **cranial nerves** and **spinal nerves** as they leave the CNS. These dural cuffs, which contain CSF, may accompany spinal nerves through the intravertebral foramina.

- Blood supply:
  - intracranial:
    - from ascending pharyngeal, occipital and maxillary branches of the external **carotid artery**. The maxillary artery gives rise to the middle meningeal artery (the largest artery), which enters the skull through the foramen spinosum.
    - from branches of the internal carotid and vertebral arteries.
  - spinal: as for the spinal cord.

See also, Meningitis; Vertebral ligaments

Meningitis. Inflammation of the **meninges**. Usually infective:
- viral: usually coxsackie, echo and mumps viruses. Usually has good prognosis, unless associated with generalised **encephalitis**.
- bacterial: *Neisseria meningitidis, Streptococcus pneumoniae* and *Haemophilus influenzae* are the most common organisms. Mortalilty is high unless treated; adhesions, **hydrocephalus** and **cranial nerve** damage are still possible after treatment.
- others, e.g. **TB**, fungi.

Aseptic meningitis may also occur; it may be caused by malignant infiltration, chemical irritation (e.g. alcoholic solutions used to clean the skin before lumbar puncture) and occasionally drugs (e.g. **NSAIDs**, **H_2 receptor antagonists**).

- Features:
  - fever, nausea, vomiting, headache, photophobia, convulsions, coma.
  - neck stiffness, with muscle resistance to passive knee extension from the flexed position with the thigh flexed (caused by stretching of inflamed sciatic nerve roots (Kernig's sign)).
  - cranial nerve lesions or signs of **cerebral oedema** may be present.
  - may be associated with systemic involvement, e.g. effects of severe **sepsis** in **meningococcal disease**.
  - CT scan is usually required to exclude space-occupying lesions and raised **ICP** prior to **lumbar puncture**.
  - **CSF**: Typical findings include:
    - viral: increased lymphocytes, slightly raised protein and normal glucose.
    - bacterial: increased polymorphs and protein, and reduced glucose. Bacteria may be visible on staining.
    - aseptic: increased polymorphs and protein, and normal glucose. The CSF may appear cloudy but no organisms are seen or grown.

Recovery may be complete or there may be neurological deficit, especially in bacterial meningitis and especially if treatment is delayed. Aseptic chemical meningitis is characterised by its short and benign course.

Treatment is directed at the underlying organism. Recent UK guidelines suggest **cefotaxime** or **ceftriaxone** (both 2 g iv) as soon as possible and before definitive microbiological diagnosis is obtained. **Ampicillin** 2 g is added if > 55 years, to cover Listeria or **vancomycin** $\pm$ **rifampicin** if penicillin-resistant pneumococcus is suspected. **Dexamethasone** (e.g. 0.15 mg/kg iv, 6 hourly for 4 days) reduces mortality and neurological morbidity .

[Vladimir M Kernig (1840–1917), Russian neurologist]

Meningococcal disease. Strictly, refers to any illness caused by *Neisseria meningitidis* although the term is often used to describe the severe systemic illness which often results in admission to an ICU. Most infections in the UK are caused by the B serotype, although the C serotype more frequently causes outbreaks. The A serotype may also cause clinical infection. Important because of its innocuous early course, rapid progression and potentially disastrous outcome which is thought to be related to the extremely toxic **endotoxin** (especially the lipid A component) present in the outer wall of the organism. An important cause of morbidity and mortality in children and young adults; epidemics, e.g. in schools/colleges, occur periodically. Asplenia and **complement** deficiency are particular risk factors. Shows seasonal variation (approximately 40% of cases occurring between January and March). The organism is present in the nasopharynx of about 5% of otherwise healthy subjects, increasing to about 30% during epidemics. Mortality is up to 10–12%.

- Features:
  - non-specific (especially initially), e.g. cough, sore throat, fever, vomiting, headache.
  - signs and symptoms of **meningitis**: may develop in about 85% of cases but bacteraemia and severe **SIRS** may occur without overt meningitis being present, and has a higher mortality.
  - petechial rash: present in up to 80% of patients although sometimes limited to the mucous membranes. May become maculopapular. **DIC** is common. Vasculitic lesions or extensive skin digit or limb necrosis (purpura fulminans) may also occur.
  - **MODS** and **septic shock** may occur.
  - **adrenocortical insufficiency** due to sepsis or adrenal haemorrhage.

Diagnosis is often suggested by the history and clinical examination, although similar rashes can occur with staphylococcal, streptococcal or *Haemophilus influenzae* infections. **Blood cultures** reveal the meningococcus in up to 80% of untreated cases. The organism may also be isolated from the skin lesions or CSF although lumbar puncture should be performed with care if at all. Molecular techniques, e.g. polymerase chain reaction (PCR), may also be used to identify the organism.

- Treatment:
  - iv antibiotic therapy as for meningitis.
  - supportive: includes management of meningitis (depressed consciousness, etc.), coagulopathy, cardiovascular impairment, etc. as for septic shock.
  - limb fasciotomies or amputation may be necessary.
  - others: specific **anti-endotoxin antibodies** and anti-**cytokine** therapies, **corticosteroids** and other treatments of severe sepsis have been studied but their place is uncertain.

Close contacts (including ICU staff) should be treated with antibiotics, e.g. **rifampicin**, **ciprofloxacin**. At-risk subjects may be protected by immunisation with a polysaccharide vaccine against types A and C meningococci; the B serogroup has a number of subtypes and an effective vaccine against it has not yet been developed. Public health officials should be contacted (it is a **notifiable disease**) to organise contact tracing and prophylaxis.

Other forms of meningococcal disease are often trivial (e.g. conjunctivitis, pharyngitis, otitis media) but some may be severe (e.g. pericarditis, endocarditis, myocarditis, septic arthritis).

Stephens DS, Greenwood B, Brandtzaeg P (2007). Lancet; 369: 2196–210

Mental Capacity Act 2005. Act providing a framework for decision making on behalf of adults without capacity; came into force in England and Wales in April 2007. Largely building on pre-existing common law, the Act confers formal statutory status on advance directives (termed 'advance decisions') and creates new 'Lasting Powers of Attorney' and 'court-appointed deputies' with the ability to make medical decisions on behalf of incapacitous adults > 16 years.

Based on the following principles:
- capacity must be presumed unless proven otherwise.
- everything practicable must be done to support individuals to make their own decisions, before deciding they lack capacity.
- individuals may make unwise or irrational decisions and doing so is not evidence of incapacity.
- any decision made on behalf of another person must be in their best interests (not necessarily their best *medical* interests).
- if a decision is made on another's behalf, it should be the least restrictive option; i.e. the one that interferes least with his/her freedoms in order to achieve the required aim.

Requires providers of health care to consider advance decisions and to assess capacity before initiating, withholding or withdrawing treatment. The new Court of Protection, created by the Act, has ultimate responsibility for the Act's proper functioning including deciding on individual cases.
White SM, Baldwin TJ (2006). Anaesthesia; 61: 381–9

Meperidine, *see Pethidine*

Mephentermine sulphate. Vasopressor drug, no longer available. Related to amfetamine; causes cerebral stimulation in addition to a rather variable increase in BP.

Mepivacaine hydrochloride. Amide local anaesthetic agent, first used in 1956. Similar to lidocaine, but more protein-bound. Does not cause vasodilatation. Not available in the UK. Used in 1–2% solutions for epidural anaesthesia and 4% solution for spinal anaesthesia, in the same doses as lidocaine. Maximal safe dose is 5 mg/kg; toxic plasma level is about 6 μg/ml. Rarely used in obstetrics because of greater fetal protein-binding and longer fetal half-life than alternative drugs.

MEPP, Miniature end-plate potential, *see End-plate potentials*

Meptazinol hydrochloride. Synthetic opioid analgesic drug, first investigated in 1971. Has partial agonist properties, and therefore antagonises respiratory depression caused by morphine. Causes less respiratory depression or sedation than morphine. Analgesic effects are almost completely reversed by naloxone. 100 mg is equivalent to 10 mg morphine or 100 mg pethidine.
- Dosage: 1–2 mg/kg 2–4 hourly as required, iv/im.; 200 mg 3–6 hourly, orally

Meropenem. Broad-spectrum carbapenem and antibacterial drug, similar to imipenem but not broken down by renal enzymatic action. Less likely to cause convulsions than imipenem, thus more useful in CNS infections.
- Dosage: 500 mg–1 g iv over 5 min, 8 hourly (2 g in meningitis or infection in cystic fibrosis).
- Side effects: as for imipenem.

Mesmerism. Treatment of various maladies by 'animal magnetism', the transmission between individuals of healing force derived from the ubiquitous magnetic fluid that pervaded the universe. Named after Mesmer, who originally passed magnets over his patients' bodies to treat them. He later used only his touch, and then speech, to achieve the same effects. Investigated in Paris by a French Royal Commission in 1784, which included Benjamin Franklin and Lavoisier; mesmerism was declared to have no scientific foundation, relying on suggestion alone. It continued to be popular until the 1840s, when the importance of psychological suggestion by the therapist was emphasised, leading to the concept of hypnotism.
[Franz A Mesmer (1734–1815), Swiss-born French physician; Benjamin Franklin (1706–1790), US statesman and scientist]
See also, Hypnosis

MET, *see Medical emergency team*

Meta-analysis (Systematic review). Technique for determining the efficacy of a treatment by combining trials which may individually have been too small to show a statistically significant difference. Requires careful inclusion of all randomised controlled trials (RCTs) of the particular treatment, some of which may not have been published. The RCTs are then scored according to their methodology, excluding any that are inadequately randomised, blinded, etc. The results of the remaining RCTs are then pooled to increase the overall number of subjects and power; the outcome of each RCT is expressed in a standard format (e.g. odds ratio, number needed to treat, absolute or relative risk reduction) and the value for the combined data given. Typically, each separate RCT's result is shown on a graph, with horizontal lines representing confidence intervals; the size of the central mark represents the sample size (forest plot; Fig. 103). The combined result therefore has smaller confidence intervals and larger central mark than the constituent RCTs, representing the greater certainty of the combined result and the larger number of subjects. Those trials whose confidence intervals cross the line of equivalence (for odds ratio, a value of one) are statistically 'non-significant' whilst those that do not are 'significant'. In the example given, the overall conclusion is that there is a statistically significant difference, as demonstrated by the combined confidence intervals' not crossing the line.

Although meta-analysis has the ability to demonstrate true treatment effects and thus represents the best evidence on which to base clinical practice, the technique may not always be valid because of:

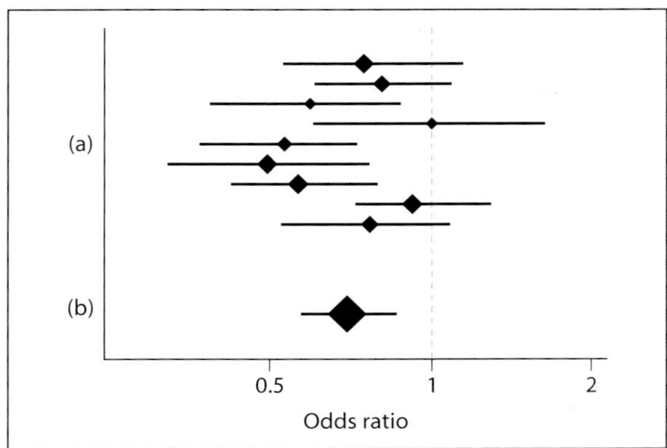

Fig. 103 Meta-analysis (forest plot): 9 small trials (a) are pooled to give a combined result (b)

- bias in the identification of RCTs included (e.g. 'positive' studies are more likely to be published than 'negative' ones).
- differing definitions of selection criteria for RCTs.
- use of different outcomes in the component studies.
- the ability for single RCTs to influence unduly the overall result in certain circumstances.
- uncertainty in applying the result to a particular patient (e.g. man aged 45 years) when the RCTs included all refer to a specific patient population (e.g. men aged 60–70 years).

Thus there have been some famous examples of treatment effects apparently demonstrated by meta-analysis which have not been supported by subsequent huge RCTs, e.g. the 'beneficial' effect of magnesium sulphate following MI. However, meta-analysis has had notable successes too, e.g. by demonstrating clearly the reduction in mortality when β-adrenergic receptor antagonists are given following MI despite conflicting results of the many small RCTs that previously existed.
Akobeng AK (2005). Arch Dis Child; 90: 845–8

Metabolism. Physical and chemical changes occurring in an organism, including alteration in molecules and energy transformation. Involves anabolism (building up; i.e. incorporation of substrate into living cells) and catabolism (breaking down; usually concerned with energy production). Metabolic pathways and steps are controlled by enzymes, subject to hormonal and other control. Basic pathways are related to intake of foodstuffs:

- carbohydrates: digested to monosaccharides, absorbed and passed to liver and muscle. Glucose is converted to glycogen for storage or broken down via glycolysis, tricarboxylic acid cycle and cytochrome oxidase system to CO_2 and water with production of energy, stored by ATP and other compounds.
- fats: digested to fatty acids and glycerol, which pass to the liver. Stored as adipose tissue or oxidised to CO_2, water and energy.
- proteins: digested to amino acids; form new proteins, e.g. enzymes, secretions, cellular components such as muscle. Subsequently broken down to urea.

Carbohydrate, fat and protein subunits are interchangeable via many pathways, and are interlinked with other substances, e.g. purines, nucleic acids, etc.
See also, Basal metabolic rate; Inborn errors of metabolism

Metaraminol tartrate/bitartrate. Vasopressor drug, acting directly via α-adrenergic receptors, and indirectly via adrenaline and noradrenaline release. Increases cardiac output and SVR, and thus arterial BP. Used to raise BP following epidural/spinal anaesthesia and cardiogenic shock. May cause excessive hypertension in hyperthyroidism and monoamine oxidase inhibitor therapy, and myocardial ischaemia in ischaemic heart disease.

- Dosage:
  - 2–10 mg sc or im; acts within 10 min and lasts 1–1.5 h.
  - 1–5 mg iv; acts within 1–2 min, lasting for 20–30 min.

Methadone hydrochloride. Synthetic opioid analgesic drug, prepared in 1947. Used mainly for chronic pain management because of its prolonged duration of action (up to 24 h). Also used as maintenance in opioid addicts, and to relieve cough in terminal care. Has been administered epidurally with good effect but its duration of action is shorter than that of morphine. Has similar actions and side effects to morphine, but is generally milder with less sedation. Elimination half-life exceeds 18 h. Cumulation may be problematic.

- Dosage: 5–10 mg orally, im or sc, 6–8 hourly (12 hourly in chronic use).

See also, Spinal opioids

Methaemoglobinaemia. Increased circulating haemoglobin in which the iron atom of haem is in the ferric (Fe^{3+}) state (normally < 1%).

- May be:
  - congenital:
    - deficiency of reducing enzymes (especially cytochrome b5 oxidase), which normally convert naturally formed methaemoglobin to haemoglobin. Usually autosomal recessive inheritance; heterozygotes may be at risk of acute acquired methaemoglobinaemia.
    - abnormal haemoglobin chains, with fixation of iron in Fe^{3+} state; autosomal dominant inheritance.
  - acquired: drugs and chemicals, e.g. prilocaine, chlorate, quinones, nitrites, phenacetin, sulphonamides, aniline dyes.
- Effects:
  - because methaemoglobin is dark (brownish), patients appear to have cyanosis when levels exceed 10–12% (at normal haemoglobin concentrations). Inaccurate readings of haemoglobin saturation may occur with pulse oximetry (as the level of methaemoglobin increases, measured arterial O_2 saturation tends towards 85% since both oxygenated and deoxygenated forms absorb light equally at 660 nm and 940 nm).
  - the oxyhaemoglobin dissociation curve of the unaffected haem is shifted to the left, reducing O_2 delivery to tissues. Patients already anaemic are more at risk. Dyspnoea and headache are common at above 20% methaemoglobin, although rate of formation is also important.
- Treatment: reducing agents, e.g. methylthioninium chloride (methylene blue) iv, if acute and severe: 1–2 mg/kg over 5 min, repeated as necessary. Oral therapy with methylthioninium chloride or ascorbic acid may suffice in chronic methaemoglobinaemia. In acute severe cases, blood or exchange transfusion may be required.

Johnson D (2005). Can J Anesth; 52: 665–8
See also, Sulphaemoglobinaemia

Methanol poisoning, *see Alcohol poisoning*

Methionine and methionine synthase. Methionine (an amino acid) is the main source of methyl groups in the body, and is involved in many biochemical reactions including myelination. It is also the precursor of glutathione, depleted in the liver by toxins, e.g. paracetamol poisoning, hence its use in the latter. Formation from homocysteine by methionine synthase is involved in folate metabolism, and thymidine and DNA synthesis.

Methionine synthase containing vitamin B_{12} as a cofactor is inhibited by N_2O, which interacts directly with the vitamin. Prolonged exposure to N_2O may result in features of folate/vitamin B_{12} deficiency, e.g. subacute combined degeneration of the cord and megaloblastic anaemia. Myelination may also be affected. Significant effects are thought to be minimal up to 8 h normal anaesthetic use, but biochemical changes have been found after a few hours. Megaloblastic changes have been found in dentists who use N_2O. Effects on DNA synthesis are thought to be involved in teratogenesis following prolonged exposure of experimental animals to N_2O, but risk during anaesthesia in early pregnancy is generally considered negligible.

Methohexital sodium (Methohexitone). IV anaesthetic drug, first used in 1957 and discontinued in the UK in 2000. A methyl barbiturate, presented as a white powder with 6% anhydrous sodium carbonate. pH of 1% solution: 10–11. pK_a is 7.9; thus a greater proportion remains unionised in plasma than with thiopental. Used mainly for day-case surgery and short procedures including electroconvulsive therapy (because of its proconvulsant properties).

Properties are similar to those of thiopental but pain, involuntary movement, hiccup, laryngospasm, etc. are more likely. Adverse effects of intra-arterial injection are less than with thiopental, due to the more dilute solution. Recovery is within 3–4 min of a single dose of 1.0–1.5 mg/kg, with half-life 2–4 h.

Methotrexate. Antimetabolite cytotoxic drug; inhibits dihydrofolate reductase, thus blocking purine and pyrimidine synthesis and preventing cell division. Used in the treatment of various malignancies including acute lymphoblastic leukaemia; also used in severe psoriasis and rheumatoid arthritis. May accumulate in pleural or ascitic fluid, producing systemic toxicity subsequently. Excreted renally; thus NSAIDs are contraindicated since reduced renal function may also increase toxicity.

- Dosage varies widely according to the condition and route; usual range is 7.5–100 mg every 2–7 days. May be given orally, iv, im or intrathecally.
- Side effects: myelosuppression, mucositis, pneumonitis (may be especially likely in rheumatoid arthritis), GIT disturbance, hepatic impairment.

Methoxamine hydrochloride. Vasopressor drug, acting via selective α_1-adrenergic receptor stimulation. Slows the heart rate by reflex baroreceptor-mediated inhibition secondary to raised BP, and possibly via a direct effect on the heart. Used (1–2 mg iv) to raise BP, e.g. during epidural or spinal anaesthesia, and to treat SVT. Discontinued in 2001 because of falling global demand.

Methoxyflurane. $CHCl_3CF_2OCH_3$. Inhalational anaesthetic drug, first used in 1960. Withdrawn because of high output renal failure caused by fluoride ion production following its administration. Has high boiling point (105°C) and therefore difficult to vaporise; the Pentec vaporiser required the double-release of its safety catch to enable higher concentrations to be delivered, following which the whole of the fresh gas flow passed through the vaporising chamber. Very soluble in blood (blood/gas partition coefficient of 13); induction and recovery are therefore slow. Extremely potent (MAC 0.2) and a powerful analgesic. Formerly used for general anaesthesia and draw-over analgesia, e.g. during labour, using the Cardiff fixed output (0.35%) inhaler. Cheap and non-explosive.

***N*-Methyl-D-aspartate receptors** (NMDA receptors). Receptors in the CNS activated by glutamate (but requiring glycine as a co-agonist) and to a lesser extent aspartate; involved in the plasticity of the CNS to afferent impulses, especially pain. Activation by sustained or repeated C fibre stimulation leads to intracellular phosphorylation of proteins and causes opening of specific membrane ion channels (opposed by magnesium). This leads to an increase in intracellular calcium concentration and increased response to glutamate by a positive feedback mechanism. Thus input via NMDA receptors is thought to lead to a hyperexcitable state ('wind-up') whereby repeated stimuli cause increasing degrees of pain sensation and expansion of the receptive field of individual sensory neurones involved in pain pathways. NMDA receptor antagonists are thought to prevent these phenomena and may thus have a role in pre-emptive analgesia. Also has a major role in long-term neuronal potentiation and depression involved in memory and learning. The only NMDA antagonist available for use in the UK is ketamine, which has been used in low doses (e.g. 0.1–0.2 mg/kg) before skin incision to reduce postoperative pain.

NMDA receptor-mediated calcium influx is also thought to contribute to neuronal cell death following cerebral ischaemia and in neurodegenerative disorders.

Petrenko AB, Yamakura T, Baba H, Shimoji K (2003). Anesth Analg; 97: 1108–16

α-Methyldopa. Antihypertensive drug, originally thought to act via uptake into catecholamine synthetic pathways and formation of a 'false transmitter', α-methylnoradrenaline. The latter is now thought to have a direct antihypertensive action of its own, possibly via stimulation of central inhibitory α-adrenergic receptors, or reduction of plasma renin activity. Use has been supplanted by more modern drugs, but it is still occasionally used, e.g. in pre-eclampsia (shown to be non-teratogenic).

- Dosage:
  - 250 mg orally, 8–12 hourly, adjusted according to response (maximum 3 g/day).
  - 250–500 mg iv over 30–60 min (as methyldopate hydrochloride). Onset of action is 4–6 h, lasting up to 16 h.
- Side effects:
  - leucopenia, hepatitis, haemolytic anaemia. 10–20% of patients have a positive direct Coombs' test which may interfere with blood cross-matching (*see Haemolysis*). A systemic lupus erythematosus-like syndrome has been reported.
  - sedation, confusion.
  - bradycardia, hypotension, oedema.
  - GIT disturbances.
  - paradoxical hypertension has occurred after iv use.

[Robin RA Coombs (1921–2006), Cambridge immunologist]

Methylenedioxyethylamfetamine, *see Methylenedioxymethylamfetamine*

Methylenedioxymethylamfetamine (MDMA; 'Ecstasy'). Synthetic amfetamine-related stimulant drug, used as a recreational drug as part of modern youth culture, especially in association with prolonged dancing. Results in a wide variety of acute psychological effects, and has been associated with collapse and sudden death, particularly when associated with extreme physical exertion and dehydration. Has been associated with hyperthermia (thought to involve central 5-HT pathways and not peripheral mechanisms as in MH), arrhythmias and hepatic failure after acute dosage. With increasing awareness that dehydration may increase morbidity and mortality, cases of hyponatraemia have been reported, caused by excessive ingestion of water. Degeneration of central neurones has also been reported after prolonged exposure. Most reported cases of acute critical illness have involved hyperthermia, which may be associated with severe acidosis, DIC and rhabdomyolysis.

Management of acute toxicity is mainly supportive. Hyperthermia is treated with physical methods; dantrolene has been used.

Similar concerns exist for the related drug methylenedioxyethylamfetamine ('Eve'), which is less commonly used.

Hall AP, Henry JA (2006). Br J Anaesth; 96: 678–85

Methylmethacrylate. Acrylic cement used in orthopaedic surgery for fixation of prostheses. Thought to be the cause of hypotension, hypoxaemia or cardiovascular collapse upon prosthesis insertion, although the mechanism is unclear.
- Possible mechanisms:
  - direct cardiotoxicity of the monomer.
  - allergic reaction.
  - peripheral vasodilatation.
  - activation of the coagulation cascade within the pulmonary vasculature.
  - fat or air embolism resulting from insertion of lipid-soluble cement into the bone cavity under pressure.
  - combination of the above, exacerbated by the high temperatures generated (over 90°C) as the cement hardens.

Risks are reduced by washing out the bone cavity with saline before cement insertion, and retrograde insertion avoiding air trapping within the cavity.
Byrick RJ (1997). Can J Anesth; 44: 107–11

Methylnaltrexone. Peripherally acting mu opioid receptor antagonist currently under investigation as a treatment for opioid-induced constipation and postoperative ileus. Does not cross the blood–brain barrier, thus devoid of central effects.

Methylprednisolone, *see Corticosteroids*

α-Methyl-*p*-tyrosine (Metirosine). Antihypertensive drug; inhibits conversion of tyrosine to dopa and thus blocks catecholamine synthesis. Available on a named patient basis in the UK. Has been used to reduce the incidence and severity of hypertensive episodes in phaeochromocytoma, e.g. before or instead of surgery. Should not be used in essential hypertension.
- Dosage: 2–4 g/day orally.
- Side effects include sedation, extrapyramidal movements, renal stones and diarrhoea.

Meticillin-resistant *Staphylococcus aureus*, *see Infection control; Staphylococcal infections*

Metoclopramide hydrochloride. Antiemetic drug, acting via dopamine receptor antagonism at the chemoreceptor trigger zone. Also a prokinetic drug, increasing gastric emptying and lower oesophageal sphincter pressure via a peripheral cholinergic action, but will not reverse the effects of opioid analgesic drugs in this respect unless given iv. It also decreases the sensitivity of visceral afferent nerves to local emetics and irritants. Has been shown to have little effect on PONV if 10 mg is given iv on induction of anaesthesia, but significantly reduces PONV if 25–50 mg is given towards the end of surgery. Half-life is about 4–6 h.
- Dosage:
  - 10 mg iv, im or orally, repeated 8 hourly. Total daily dose: 0.5 mg/kg.
  - has been used in very high doses (up to 5 mg/kg iv) to treat vomiting caused by cytotoxic therapy; thought to antagonise central 5-HT_3 receptors.
- Side effects: Extrapyramidal effects and dystonic reactions (particularly affecting the face), especially following iv administration and in children or young adults. Hypotension and tachy- or bradycardia may occur after rapid injection. Has been associated with sulphaemoglobinaemia if taken chronically or in high dosage.

Metocurine, *see Dimethyl tubocurarine chloride/bromide*

Metoprolol tartrate. β-Adrenergic receptor antagonist, available for oral and iv administration. Relatively selective for β_1-receptors. Uses and side effects are as for β-adrenergic receptor antagonists in general.
- Dosage:
  - hypertension, migraine: 100–200 mg orally once/twice daily; arrhythmias, angina: 50–100 mg 8–12 hourly; thyrotoxicosis: 50 mg 6 hourly.
  - acute administration: 2–4 mg slowly iv, repeated up to 10 mg.
  - acute MI: 5 mg iv over 2 min, then 15 min later 50 mg orally 6 hourly for 48 h, then 200 mg/day thereafter in divided doses.

Metre. SI unit of length. Originally defined according to the length of a platinum–iridium bar kept at Sèvres, France, but redefined in 1960 according to the speed of light in a vacuum, following doubts as to the bar's constant length over time: 1 metre = the distance occupied by 1 650 763.73 wavelengths of a specified orange-red light from gaseous krypton-86.

Metronidazole. Antibacterial drug, active against a wide range of anaerobic bacteria and protozoa. Used in many infections, especially gastrointestinal and gynaecological. Undergoes hepatic metabolism and excreted renally, with a half-life of 8.5 h. Tinidazole has similar actions but a longer duration of action and is given once daily.
- Dosage:
  - 200–500 mg orally/iv, 8 hourly.
  - 1 g pr, 8 hourly for 3 days, then 12 hourly.
- Side effects: disulfiram-like reaction, nausea, vomiting, urticaria; rarely drowsiness, ataxia; on prolonged dosage peripheral neuropathy, convulsions, leucopenia, urine discolouration.

MEWS, *see Modified early warning score*

Mexiletine hydrochloride. Class Ib antiarrhythmic drug; reduces fast sodium entry and shortens the refractory period. Chemically related to lidocaine, but active orally. Half-life is about 10 h. Used to treat ventricular arrhythmias.
- Dosage:
  - 400 mg orally, followed by 200–250 mg 6–8 hourly.
  - 100–250 mg iv over 10 min, followed by 250 mg over 1 h, then 250 mg over 2 h, then 30 mg/h thereafter.
- Side effects:
  - hypotension, bradycardia.
  - confusion, ataxia, nystagmus, tremor, convulsions.
  - hepatitis, jaundice, GIT disturbances.

Meyer–Overton rule. States that inhalational anaesthetic agents act via the lipid-rich cells of the CNS; thus anaesthetic potency increases with lipid solubility. Can be seen if MAC is plotted against oil/gas partition coefficients at 37°C for various agents, using logarithmic scales (Fig. 104).
[Hans Meyer (1853–1939), German pharmacologist; Charles Ernest Overton (1865–1933), English-born German pharmacologist]
See also, Anaesthesia, mechanism of

MH, *see Malignant hyperthermia*

MHRA, *see Medicines and Healthcare products Regulatory Agency*

MI, *see Myocardial infarction*

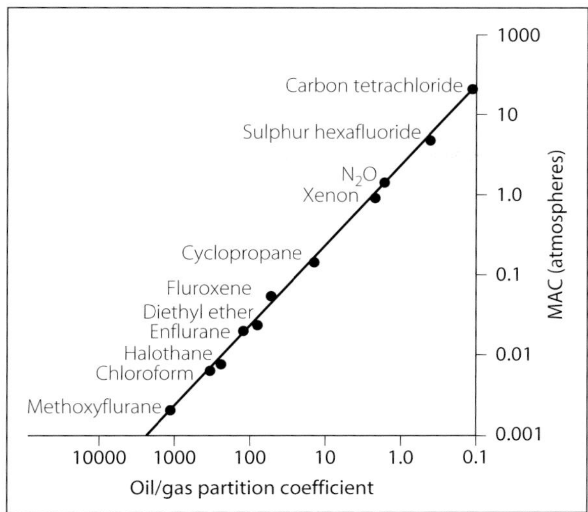

Fig. 104 Meyer–Overton rule

Michaelis–Menten kinetics. Refers to the reaction between a single substrate S and an enzyme E, via an intermediate complex ES to give a single product P:

$$S + E \rightleftharpoons ES \rightleftharpoons P$$

As the concentration of S ([S]) increases from zero, rate of reaction increases, until the enzyme binding sites become saturated, and maximal rate of reaction is reached. Thus initially, velocity of reaction (V) is proportional to [S]; i.e. first order kinetics apply. Eventually, V does not increase as [S] increases; i.e. zero order kinetics apply (Fig. 105).

$$\text{Michaelis–Menten equation: } V = \frac{V_{max}[S]}{K_m + [S]}$$

where V_{max} = maximal reaction velocity
K_m = Michaelis constant, the concentration of S at which $V = ½\, V_{max}$.

V_{max} and K_m are found by plotting $1/V$ against $1/[S]$ to obtain a straight line; the x-intercept is $-1/K_m$, the y-intercept is $1/V_{max}$, and the slope is K_m/V_{max}.

May also be applied to pharmacology, to describe absorption, distribution, elimination, etc. of drugs.

[Leonor Michaelis (1875–1945), German-born US chemist; Maud Menten (1879–1960), US physician]

See also, Pharmacokinetics

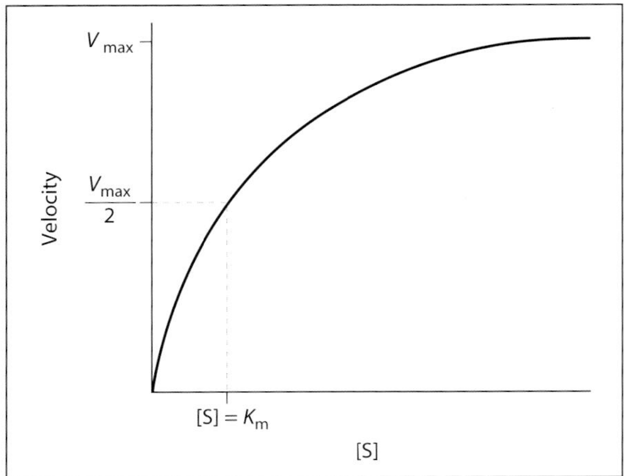

Fig. 105 Michaelis–Menten kinetics

Miconazole. Imidazole antifungal drug, active against a wide range of fungi and yeasts. Used for local treatment, or by mouth (as tablets or oral gel) for intestinal infection.

- Dosage: tablets: 250 mg 6 hourly for 10 days; gel: 5–10 ml 6 hourly.
- Side effects include GIT disturbances and rash. Should be avoided in porphyria.

Microshock, *see Electrocution and electrical burns*

Midazolam hydrochloride. Benzodiazepine, used mainly for sedation; has also been used for premedication and induction of anaesthesia. Water-soluble at pH < 4 because of its open imidazole ring (five-membered ring containing carbon and nitrogen atoms); it becomes highly lipid-soluble at body pH due to ring closure, resulting in rapid onset of action following iv administration (usually under 90 s). Also rapidly absorbed after im injection. Half-life is about 2 h. Metabolised to inactive compounds. Anterograde amnesia is marked.

Has slow onset when used for induction, with prolonged recovery. Effects may be antagonised by flumazenil.

- Dosage:
  - premedication: 0.07–0.1 mg/kg im, 30–60 min preoperatively. Has been administered orally to children: 0.5–0.75 mg/kg 30 min preoperatively.
  - sedation: 0.5–2 mg increments iv. By infusion: 0.05–0.2 mg/kg/h.
  - induction: up to 0.3 mg/kg.

Respiratory and cardiovascular depression may occur, especially in elderly and sick patients, in whom reduced dosage is required.

See also, Intravenous anaesthetic agents; Isomerism

MID-CM, *see Minimally invasive direct cardiac massage*

Midwives, prescription of drugs by. Approved hospital midwives in the UK are usually permitted to administer certain drugs on the labour ward without individual prescription by doctors, according to agreement with the local health authority and obstetricians. Specified drugs thus vary between hospitals, but usually include:

- opioid analgesic drugs, usually pethidine 100–150 mg im, repeated once.
- Entonox and O_2.
- oxytocics, e.g. oxytocin and ergometrine separately or combined.
- antiemetic drugs/H_2 receptor antagonists, e.g. metoclopramide/ranitidine.
- lidocaine 0.5% 10–20 ml for local perineal infiltration.
- vitamin K and naloxone for the neonate.

Others include hypnotics, traditionally chloral hydrate or trichlofos. Temazepam and alternative opioids, e.g. pentazocine, are sometimes given. Community midwives usually have freedom to prescribe iron, antacids, etc., in addition.

Midwives may give epidural solutions (but not the first injection) according to written instructions; responsibility for administration lies with the prescribing doctor. They may also administer TENS.

See also, Nurses, prescription of drugs by

Migraine. Episodic form of headache; classified into migraine without aura (75% of cases; headache is typically unilateral and throbbing; there may be nausea and photophobia) and migraine with aura (25% of cases; headache is preceded by visual disturbances, numbness, etc.). May be difficult to distinguish from tension headaches (caused by muscular contraction), headache caused by cervical spondylosis, temporal arteritis, trigeminal neuralgia/other facial pain syndromes and headache caused by drugs. Subarachnoid haemorrhage, meningitis and post-dural puncture headache may also pose diagnostic difficulties. Neurological features may occasionally be severe and mimic CVA. Typically provoked by triggers such as stress, alcohol and certain foods. The pathophysiology is uncertain but increased cerebral blood flow, cerebral vasoconstriction/dilatation, cortical hyperexcitability and nitric oxide pathways have all been implicated.

- Management is divided into:
  - prophylactic: includes β-adrenergic receptor antagonists, 5-HT receptor antagonists (e.g. pizotifen, methysergide), amitriptyline.
  - therapeutic: includes simple analgesic/antiemetic combinations, 5-HT_{1D} receptor agonists, ergotamine.

Anaesthetic management of a migraine sufferer is along standard lines. Management in the presence of an actual migraine attack is uncertain; if severe it may be wiser to postpone surgery although there is no evidence to support this.

Silberstein SD (2004). Lancet; 363: 381–91

Military antishock trousers, *see Antigravity suit*

Milrinone lactate. Phosphodiesterase inhibitor, used as an inotropic drug. Increases cardiac output and reduces SVR without increasing heart rate or myocardial O_2 demand, although rate of atrioventricular conduction may increase slightly. Elimination half-life is about 2–2.5 h. Excreted mainly via urine.

- Dosage: 50 µg/kg over 10 min iv, followed by 0.3–0.75 µg/kg/min up to 1.1 mg/kg/day; doses should be reduced in renal impairment.
- Side effects: hypotension, ventricular and supraventricular arrhythmias, angina, headache.

Minaxolone. Water-soluble corticosteroid iv anaesthetic agent derived from Althesin, investigated in the late 1970s/early 1980s. Causes rapid induction with involuntary muscle movement, anaesthesia lasting up to 20 min. Development was terminated because of reported toxicity in rats.

Mineralocorticoids. Group of corticosteroids; typically comprise aldosterone physiologically and fludrocortisone therapeutically. Chief function is to regulate the transport of sodium and potassium ions in the kidney and other organs; hence they cause sodium reabsorption and loss of potassium in the kidney tubules. Hydrocortisone and other corticosteroids have some mineralocorticoid effects but these are generally too weak to make hydrocortisone a useful therapeutic mineralocorticoid (although they may limit its usefulness as a long-term glucocorticoid when used for disease suppression).

Miniature end-plate potential, *see End-plate potentials*

Minimal alveolar concentration (MAC). Minimal alveolar concentration of inhalational anaesthetic agent that prevents movement in response to a standard skin incision in 50% of subjects studied, when breathed in oxygen in the absence of any other analgesic or anaesthetic/depressant drugs. Thus inversely related to anaesthetic potency. Useful as a means of comparing different agents, and may be used to guide clinical dosage if end-tidal concentration of agent is monitored. Defined in terms of percentage of one atmosphere; therefore not influenced by altitude.

- MAC is reduced by:
  - other depressant drugs (e.g. opioids, sedatives, other inhalational agents, etc.).
  - CNS depletion of catecholamines, e.g. by α-methyldopa, reserpine.
  - hypothermia.
  - hypoxaemia/hypotension.
  - pregnancy possibly due to increased progesterone levels.
  - extremes of age.
- MAC is increased in:
  - children.
  - hyperthermia.
  - hyperthyroidism.
  - chronic alcoholism.

It is unaffected by duration of anaesthesia, sex, acidaemia/alkalaemia, hypercapnia or hypocapnia.

The term 'MAC-BAR' (blocks adrenergic response) has also been studied; it refers to the minimum alveolar concentration of agent at which the increase in heart rate or BP (or both) provoked by skin incision is prevented in 50% of subjects.

The term 'MAC awake' has been used to describe the alveolar concentration of agent at which 50% of subjects no longer respond appropriately to command, when increasing concentrations are breathed from the awake state. The term has also been applied to the alveolar concentration at which 50% of subjects respond appropriately when recovering from anaesthesia, in the absence of other depressant drugs. It is often presented as the ratio of MAC awake/MAC; in general this ratio is in the order of 0.3–0.5 for the commonly used volatile agents. It has been suggested that MAC awake is the minimum alveolar concentration required to prevent awareness during anaesthesia although this is disputed.

For values of MAC, see Table 18; Inhalational anaesthetic agents

Minimal blocking concentration (C_m). Lowest concentration of local anaesthetic agent that will block a nerve *in vitro* within (usually) 10 min. Temperature, pH, electrolyte composition, etc., are specified. Higher concentrations are required clinically, in order to achieve C_m at the axons. Dependent on the size of axon, not the site (although important clinically because of diffusion across membranes, drug absorption, etc.).

Minimal infusion rate (MIR). Application of the MAC concept to infusions of iv anaesthetic agents, e.g. in TIVA. Equals the minimal infusion rate of agent that prevents movement in response to skin incision in 50% of subjects studied. More complex than MAC of inhalational agents, because of the influence of pharmacokinetic factors associated with the use of iv infusions.

Minimal local anaesthetic concentration/dose/volume (MLAC/MLAD/MLAV). Measurement used to compare the effects of different local anaesthetic solutions and/or dosing regimens, typically for epidural or spinal anaesthesia. For example, for MLAD, it requires a series of patients to receive a standard concentration of local anaesthetic, the response of each patient according to a defined outcome (e.g. for labour analgesia, whether pain scores reach a 'target' reduction within a set time) affecting the dose that the subsequent patient receives (e.g. 'failed' analgesia results in the next patient receiving a 20% higher dose; 'successful' analgesia results in a 20% lower dose). Analysis of the fluctuating dosage requirements over a set number of patients allows calculation of the ED_{50} for that concentration and outcome. Thus akin to MAC for inhalational anaesthetic agents. Criticisms include the lack of usefulness of knowing the ED_{50} (ED_{90} or ED_{95} being more useful), and the arbitrariness of the defined outcomes. However, it has been useful for examining the effects of local anaesthetic dosage, concentration and volume independently, and of the addition of adjuncts, e.g. opioids.

Minimally invasive direct cardiac massage (MID-CM). Variant of open chest cardiac massage that does not require thoracotomy. Uses a hand-held device introduced via a small thoracostomy. The device consists of a 40 FG introducer and a flat umbrella-shaped 'plunger' that is collapsed and retracted during insertion. Once in the chest, the umbrella is opened, expanding to a diameter of 7.5 cm, and used to 'pump' the heart rhythmically from outside the pericardium.

Rozenberg A, Incagnoli P, Delpech P, et al (2001). Resuscitation; 50: 257–62

See also, Cardiac arrest; Cardiopulmonary resuscitation

Minitracheotomy. Commercially available device, enabling cricothyrotomy in emergencies. Also useful as a route for tracheobronchial suction when sputum retention is a problem, e.g. respiratory infection, impaired coughing, or postoperatively. May thus avoid tracheal intubation or formal tracheostomy, e.g. in ICU.

The pack originally included a blade, 4 mm internal diameter tube and introducer, standard 15 mm connector, suction catheter and securing tapes. Because of difficulties inserting the device without a guidewire, one was subsequently introduced into the pack along with a syringe, short 16 G needle and dilator. The needle and syringe are used to locate the trachea through a small vertical incision in the cricothyroid membrane and the guidewire inserted into the trachea. The rest of the insertion proceeds using the Seldinger technique. Complications include haemorrhage, subcutaneous emphysema and misplacement.

Minivent, *see Ventilators*

Minoxidil. Antihypertensive drug causing peripheral vasodilatation. Reserved as third-line treatment after diuretics and β-adrenergic receptor antagonists, because of tachycardia and water and salt retention. Also causes increased hair growth. Taken orally, 2.5–25 mg once/twice daily.

Minute ventilation (Minute volume). Volume of air breathed per minute. Equals tidal volume × respiratory rate; i.e. includes alveolar ventilation and dead space ventilation. Normally 5–7 litres.

Minute volume dividers, *see Ventilators*

MIR, *see Minimal infusion rate*

Misoprostol. Analogue of naturally occurring prostaglandin E_1, licensed for gastric protection and healing of ulcers in patients taking NSAIDs. Has been used to increase uterine contractions, e.g. in medical abortion, and to prevent and treat postpartum haemorrhage, for which doses of 200–800 μg have been given orally, vaginally and rectally. Serious side effects are rare although shivering is common.

Misuse of Drugs Act 1971. Introduced in the UK as a replacement for the obsolete Dangerous Drugs Act. Defined three classes of drugs, according to the penalties for offences:
- class A:
  - opioid analgesic drugs, e.g. morphine, pethidine, fentanyl, alfentanil, diamorphine, methadone.
  - cocaine, methylenedioxymethamfetamine, methylamfetamine, lysergide (LSD), phencyclidine.
  - parenteral forms of class B drugs.
- class B:
  - opioids, e.g. codeine, pentazocine.
  - amfetamines, barbiturates.
  - others, e.g. glutethimide (sedative/hypnotic), phenmetrazine (appetite suppressant).
- class C: includes benzodiazepines, anabolic steroids and certain amfetamine-related drugs. Cannabis was reclassified as a Class C drug in 2004 (previously Class B) but this was reversed in 2008. Ketamine (previously unclassified) was classified as a Class C drug in 2006.

- Misuse of Drugs Regulations 2001: specifies the requirements for handling, storage, record-keeping, etc.:
  - Schedule 1: drugs not used therapeutically, e.g. cannabis, lysergide.
  - Schedule 2: opioids including codeine, pentazocine, morphine, etc. and cocaine (controlled drugs). To be kept in locked cupboards (but not necessarily double-locked); details of patients are recorded in registers with practitioners' signatures and kept for 2 years.
  - Schedule 3: barbiturates, buprenorphine, pentazocine, temazepam (from 1996). Registers and locked cupboards are not required but special prescription requirements are (except for buprenorphine and temazepam).
  - Schedule 4: benzodiazepines, ketamine, anabolic steroids.
  - Schedule 5: products containing low concentrations of substances otherwise in Schedule 2. Exempt from virtually all controlled drug requirements.

Mitral regurgitation. Usually due to mitral valve prolase (45%); previously, most cases were due to rheumatic fever when mitral stenosis usually coexisted. May also be due to papillary muscle dysfunction secondary to MI or degeneration; rare causes include left ventricular dilatation in cardiac failure, cardiomyopathy, bacterial endocarditis, and ruptured chordae tendinae.
- Effects:
  - left atrial dilatation; pulmonary oedema especially if acute. Regurgitant fraction increases if SVR rises.
  - left ventricular hypertrophy and increased stroke volume.
  - AF if severe. Ventricular filling is less reliant on atrial contraction than in mitral stenosis; thus cardiac output is usually maintained.
- Features:
  - left ventricular hypertrophy, with pansystolic murmur usually at the apex, loudest on expiration and sitting forward, and radiating to the axilla. A thrill, third heart sound and diastolic flow murmur may be present. AF, left and later right ventricular failure may be present.
  - systemic embolism.
  - endocarditis.
  - ECG may reveal P mitrale, ventricular hypertrophy, and ventricular ectopics. Chest X-ray features may include cardiac enlargement, particularly of the left atrium, and pulmonary oedema. Echocardiography and cardiac catheterisation are useful.
- Anaesthetic management:
  - prophylactic antibiotics as for congenital heart disease.
  - main principles are as for congenital and ischaemic heart disease. Drugs taken may include diuretics, digoxin and anticoagulant drugs. The following should be avoided: myocardial depression, hypovolaemia, bradycardia

(which increases regurgitation; mild tachycardia is preferable), vasoconstriction, e.g. due to sympathetic hyperactivity (pain, light anaesthesia), cold, etc. If pulmonary artery catheterisation is done, large V waves are typically seen in the pulmonary venous waveform.

See also, Heart murmurs; Valvular heart disease

Mitral stenosis. Rheumatic fever is by far the most common cause; others include congenital, infective and inflammatory causes. Symptoms are usually present if the valve area is reduced from the normal 4–5 cm^2 to about 1–3 cm^2.

- Effects:
  - reduced left ventricular filling, with left atrial hypertrophy and dilatation.
  - increased pulmonary vascular pressures, with pulmonary congestion and reduced pulmonary compliance. Work of breathing is increased.
  - if prolonged, it may cause pulmonary hypertension, with right ventricular overload and/or tricuspid or pulmonary regurgitation. Progression may be rapid in 25–30%; the reason is unknown.
  - AF occurs in up to 50%; ventricular filling is reliant on atrial contraction, thus AF may lead to pulmonary oedema.
- Features:
  - cardiac failure and dyspnoea. Haemoptysis may be caused by recurrent chest infection, pulmonary oedema or infarction, or blood vessel rupture.
  - AF and systemic embolism.
  - malar flush (mitral facies), parasternal heave and features of tricuspid valve regurgitation may be present.
  - 'tapping apex' (palpable first heart sound). The first sound is loud, with opening snap following the second sound. A low-pitched rumbling diastolic murmur follows, heard best at the apex on expiration with the stethoscope bell, leaning forward and to the left. Presystolic accentuation is heard before the first heart sound, due to atrial contraction; it disappears in AF. The opening snap may disappear if the valve is calcified.
  - ECG may reveal P mitrale, AF, and right ventricular hypertrophy. Chest X-ray features may include cardiac enlargement, particularly of the left atrium, and pulmonary oedema. Mitral calcification and features of pulmonary hypertension may be present. Echocardiography and cardiac catheterisation are especially useful. In moderate and severe stenosis the area is reduced to < 2 and < 1 cm^2 respectively.
- Anaesthetic management:
  - prophylactic antibiotics as for congenital heart disease.
  - main principles are as for congenital and ischaemic heart disease. Drugs taken may include diuretics, digoxin, anticoagulant drugs. The following should be avoided: myocardial depression, tachycardia (which reduces left ventricular filling time), hypovolaemia and vasodilatation (reduce atrial and thus ventricular filling), and increased pulmonary vascular resistance, e.g. due to hypoxaemia. In pulmonary artery catheterisation, left ventricular end-diastolic pressure estimation is inaccurate due to stenosis. Percutaneous catheter balloon valvuloplasty is sometimes performed in poor-risk patients.
  - postoperative IPPV may be required.

Carabello BA (2005). Circulation; 112: 432–7

See also, Heart murmurs; Tricuspid valve lesions; Valvular heart disease

Mitral valve prolapse. Thought to occur in up to 15% of the population, sometimes associated with autosomal dominant inheritance. Also associated with Marfan's syndrome and possibly other disorders of collagen formation. Often asymptomatic, but may lead to mitral regurgitation, cardiac failure, bacterial endocarditis and systemic emboli.

- Signs:
  - mid-systolic click, occurring at the onset of the carotid pulsation.
  - late systolic heart murmur, not always present.

Diagnosis is usually aided by echocardiography or angiography.

Prophylactic antibiotics as for congenital heart disease are usually advised preoperatively. Complications are unlikely unless mitral regurgitation is severe or left ventricular dysfunction is present.

Hayek E, Gring CN, Griffin BP (2005). Lancet; 365: 507–18

See also, Heart sounds

Mivacurium chloride. Non-depolarising neuromuscular blocking drug, introduced in the UK in 1993. Tracheal intubation is possible approximately 2 min after a dose of 0.07–0.25 mg/kg (doses above 0.15 mg/kg should be given over 30 s – more slowly in patients with asthma or CVS disease). Effects last 10–20 min. Supplementary dose: 0.1 mg/kg. May be given by iv infusion at 0.2–0.5 mg/kg/h. Causes little or no cardiovascular instability, although histamine release (with bronchospasm, urticaria and hypotension) may accompany high doses, especially if given rapidly. Metabolised by plasma cholinesterase (thus its action may be markedly prolonged in cholinesterase deficiency) to highly water-soluble metabolites, excreted rapidly via the urine; half-life is 2–5 min. Also undergoes some hepatic metabolism. More easily reversed than atracurium or vecuronium. Has been suggested as an alternative to suxamethonium, especially in children, in whom onset and recovery are faster than in adults.

Mixed venous blood. Truly mixed venous blood is obtained from the right ventricle or pulmonary artery, since superior and inferior vena caval blood is different in composition, and mixes during passage through the heart.

Mixed venous O_2 saturation ($S_{\bar{v}}O_2$) is related to arterial O_2 content, O_2 consumption and cardiac output; it may be monitored continuously via a fibreoptic bundle on a pulmonary artery catheter. $S_{\bar{v}}O_2$ has been used as an indicator of O_2 supply/demand in critically ill patients, and as an early indicator of imminent haemodynamic failure; tissue O_2 delivery is considered critical at $S_{\bar{v}}O_2$ of under 50% (normally 75%). The measurement is non-specific, however, and is increased by peripheral shunting, e.g. in septic shock.

See also, Arteriovenous oxygen difference

MLAC/MLAD/MLAV, *see Minimal local anaesthetic concentration/dose/volume*

MMV, *see Mandatory minute ventilation*

Mode. Expression of the central tendency of a set of observations or measurements. Equals that observation, or group of observations, which occurs the most often. Equals the mean for a normal distribution.

See also, Median; Statistical frequency distributions; Statistics

Modified early warning score (MEWS). Scoring system used to aid identification of critically ill patients or those at risk of further clinical deterioration. Uses six parameters

(systolic BP, heart rate, respiratory rate, temperature, neurological status and urine output) to score the degree of abnormality of a patient's physiology, with a possible composite score of 0 (normal) to 17. Used to 'trigger' calls for assistance from the patient's primary team, a medical emergency team, an outreach team or others.
Goldhill DR (2001). Q J Med; 94: 507–10
See also, Acute life-threatening events – recognition and treatment; Early warning scores

MODS, *see Multiple organ dysfunction syndrome*

MOET, *see Managing Obstetric Emergencies and Trauma course*

Moffet's solution, *see Nose*

Molality. Number of moles of solute per kilogram of solvent. A molal solution contains 1 mole/kg.

Molarity. Number of moles of solute per litre of solution. A molar solution contains 1 mole/l.

Mole. SI unit of amount of substance. Defined as that quantity containing the same number of particles as there are atoms in 12 g of carbon-12. This number (Avogadro's number) equals 6.022×10^{23}.

Molecular adsorbents recirculation system, *see Liver dialysis*

Molecular weight (mw). Mass of a molecule, equal to the sum of atomic weights of its constituent atoms.

Molgramostim, *see Granulocyte colony-stimulating factor*

Monitoring. Adequate monitoring during anaesthesia and recovery is now generally accepted as improving patient safety and helping to reduce anaesthetic morbidity and mortality. Standards of minimal monitoring have been published in many countries, e.g. in the USA since 1986 and the UK since 1988. Failure to employ appropriate monitoring equipment is increasingly considered negligent. Devices should warn of adverse changes in the state of the patient, and of altered functioning of anaesthetic equipment.

- Most monitors involve electrical equipment. Technical considerations:
  - signal from patients may be:
    - primary electrical signals, e.g. ECG, EEG.
    - electrical signals derived from other energy forms, e.g. via pressure transducers.
    - evoked signals, e.g. neuromuscular blockade monitoring, evoked potentials.
  - skin electrodes are usually made of silver/silver chloride to reduce alterations in impedance, and to reduce the creation of interfering potentials within the electrode.
  - amplification/processing of the signal via intermediate components. Accuracy of reproduction is related to:
    - signal:noise ratio: improved by filtering, and averaging the signal so that background noise is cancelled out. Recording between two recording leads (differential input) also cancels out background noise, since the noise is in phase in both the leads.
    - baseline drift: may be random or due to the effect of temperature on semiconductors.
    - sensitivity of the amplifier: related to the voltage of the original signal (i.e. appropriate gain).
    - linearity of the response: distortion causes non-linear response characteristics.
    - damping.
    - frequency range: related to the harmonics of the measured signal.
    - matched output/input voltage, current, etc. of components.
    - interference; may be caused by:
      - capacitance between the patient and electrical equipment.
      - inductance of current in the patient, monitor wires, etc. by electrical equipment.
      - other electrical equipment, e.g. diathermy, other monitors, etc.
    - display of the signal, as, e.g. a waveform on oscilloscopes, numerical display, galvanometer and/or paper strip, etc.
    - alarms are usually incorporated into monitors; limits are set to minimise inappropriate warnings without compromising sensitivity. Alarms of different devices are often of random pitch and frequency; standardisation of alarms has been suggested.
    - risk of electrocution and electrical burns from electrical equipment.
- UK recommendations (Association of Anaesthetists):
  - presence of the anaesthetist is mandatory during the whole procedure, with adequate record-keeping and hand-over.
  - monitoring is instituted before induction and continued until recovery.
  - equipment monitoring: O_2 failure warning device, output and delivery O_2 analyser, and disconnection detection by expired tidal volume measurement, capnography and airway pressure measurement. Monitoring of volatile agent whenever one is used. All alarms set at appropriate values and enabled. Infusion devices checked and alarms set.
  - patient monitoring: continuous clinical observation of colour, pupils, respiration, pulse and response to surgery, chest auscultation, urine output and blood loss when appropriate, plus:
    - for induction (and very short procedures, e.g. ECT): ECG, arterial BP measurement, pulse oximetry, capnography, plus a nerve stimulator whenever neuromuscular blocking drugs are used and a means of temperature measurement available.
    - for maintenance (including prolonged 'induction' time, e.g. for insertion of invasive lines/regional blockade): as for induction plus volatile agent analyser.
    - for recovery: oximetry and BP measurement (ECG, nerve stimulator, temperature measurement and capnography immediately available).
    - heart rate and BP recorded at regular intervals as appropriate. Waveforms are preferable to numeric displays. Trend displays/printouts recommended.
    - direct BP measurement, CVP measurement, pulmonary artery pressures, arterial blood gas analysis and blood tests as appropriate.
    - for sedation, regional anaesthesia: at least ECG, oximetry and BP measurement.
    - adequate monitoring (including easily accessible and visible displays) required for transfer of patients.

Buhre W, Rossaint R (2003). Lancet; 362: 1839–46
See also, Anaesthesia, depth of; Blood flow; Carbon dioxide measurement; Cardiac output measurement; Echocardiography; Gas analysis; Oxygen measurement; Pulmonary artery catheterisation; Pulmonary wedge pressure; Respirometer

Monoamine oxidase (MAO). Enzyme present in mitochondria of most tissues, especially liver, intestinal mucosa, lung, kidney and central and peripheral catecholamine secreting nerve endings. Catalyses oxidative deamination of amines to aldehyde derivatives, e.g. R-CH_2–NH_2 → R-CHO. Inactivates active amines including catecholamines, whether circulating, absorbed from the gut, or at adrenergic/5-HT nerve endings. Many products are subsequently metabolised by catechol-*O*-methyl transferase (COMT), and many products of COMT metabolism are subsequently metabolised by MAO.

Two distinct types have been identified: type A, mainly inactivating noradrenaline and 5-HT, and type B, mainly inactivating tryptamine and phenylethylamine. Dopamine and tyramine are inactivated by both. Both are present in liver and brain; type B is thought to be predominant in certain CNS regions, e.g. basal ganglia.

Non-specific and type A-specific MAO inhibitors are used to treat depression; MAO type B inhibitors are used as antiparkinsonian drugs.

Monoamine oxidase inhibitors (MAOIs). The term usually refers to non-specific inhibitors of monoamine oxidase, used as antidepressant drugs and developed in the 1950s from anti-TB drugs. Recently increasing in use following a period of unpopularity. Interact with monamine oxidase irreversibly, resynthesis of the enzyme taking at least 3 weeks.

- Anaesthetic importance:
  - interaction with opioid analgesic drugs: may be:
    - excitatory: may cause agitation, hypertension, tachycardia, hyperreflexia, hypertonus, pyrexia, convulsions, coma. Thought to be caused by excessive central 5-HT activity, and only reported with pethidine, which reduces 5-HT uptake from nerve endings. Treatment includes α-adrenergic receptor antagonists, vasodilator drugs and chlorpromazine. Steroids have been used.
    - depressive: may cause hypoventilation, hypotension, coma. Thought to be caused by impaired hepatic metabolism of opioid. Naloxone and directly acting vasopressors, e.g. noradrenaline, have been used for treatment.

    Morphine has been suggested as the opioid of choice, titrated carefully against effect. Although fentanyl is related to pethidine, it has been safely used; however experience is limited. Pentazocine has also been used safely.
  - sympathomimetic drugs may produce exaggerated hypertensive responses, especially those acting indirectly via catecholamine release, e.g. ephedrine, metaraminol. Directly acting drugs, e.g. noradrenaline, adrenaline and isoprenaline should be used in small amounts, if required. Catecholamines and drugs increasing catecholamine levels should be avoided, e.g. pancuronium, ketamine, cocaine, and adrenaline in local anaesthesic solutions (the last is controversial).
  - other iv and inhalational agents, benzodiazepines and non-depolarising neuromuscular blocking drugs are considered safe; doxapram is considered unsafe.
  - phenelzine may decrease plasma cholinesterase levels.

Crises may also follow oral ingestion of active amines or precursors, e.g. in tyramine-rich food such as cheese and red wine, because of inhibition of the enzyme in the gut wall.

Traditional advice, to stop taking MAOIs 2–3 weeks preoperatively, is rarely given now, because of risks of worsening depression, and possible inadequacy of this interval. Moclobemide is a reversible inhibitor of MAO type A (thus described as a RIMA), and said to be less likely to interact with amines and drugs. No treatment-free period is required after stopping therapy. Selegiline is a MAO type B inhibitor used in Parkinson's disease; it increases central dopamine levels without exhibiting an exaggerated response to dietary amines.

Monro–Kellie doctrine. The cranial cavity is a rigid closed container; thus any change in intracranial blood volume is accompanied by the opposite change in CSF volume, if ICP is maintained.

[Alexander Monro (1733–1817) and George Kellie (1758–1829), Scottish anatomists]

Moracizine hydrochloride. Class I antiarrhythmic drug, structurally related to phenothiazines. Available on a named patient basis in the UK. Used to treat ventricular arrhythmias. Half-life is 3–6 h.

- Dosage: 200–300 mg orally, 8 hourly, or 400–500 mg followed by 200 mg 8 hourly for rapid control.
- Side effects: GIT disturbances, dizziness, arrhythmias, jaundice, thrombocytopenia.

Morbidity and mortality, *see Anaesthetic morbidity and mortality; Mortality/survival prediction on intensive care unit*

Morphine hydrochloride/sulphate/tartrate. Opioid analgesic drug, in use for thousands of years as opium derived from poppy seeds. Isolated in 1803, and synthesised in 1952, although still obtained from poppies. The standard drug against which other opioids are compared.

Used for premedication and as an analgesic drug. Also useful in pulmonary oedema. Peak effect occurs 15–20 min after iv, and 60–90 min after im injection; action lasts 4–5 h. Undergoes significant first-pass metabolism if given orally. Undergoes hepatic dealkylation, oxidation and conjugation to morphine 3- and 6-glucuronide, excreted in urine. The latter compound has analgesic properties, and may be responsible for prolonged action, e.g. in renal impairment or chronic administration.

- Actions:
  - CNS:
    - depression of:
      - respiratory centre; rate is reduced more than tidal volume. Neonates and the elderly are particularly susceptible.
      - cough reflex.
      - pain sensation, especially dull continuous pain. Most effective if given before the painful stimulus. Perception of painful stimuli is altered as well as pain sensation itself.
      - anxiety; morphine causes sedation and euphoria.
      - ACTH and prolactin secretion.
      - metabolic rate.
      - vasomotor centre; depression is now thought to be minimal, if it occurs at all.
    - stimulation of:
      - chemoreceptor trigger zone.
      - parasympathetic nucleus of the 3rd cranial nerve, causing miosis.
      - vasopressin release.
      - vagus nerve; thought to result in occasional bradycardia.
      - higher centres; may cause dysphoria.
    - muscle rigidity following high doses; thought to be caused by central interference with motor function, although the mechanism is unclear.
    - may cause addiction.

- peripheral:
  - histamine release; may cause vasodilatation, bronchoconstriction, itching (typically of the nose), flushing. Hypotension may occur (partly a central effect).
  - constipation, delayed gastric emptying and reduced lower oesophageal sphincter tone. Increases the tone of biliary and genitourinary smooth muscle, including sphincters.
  - increases catecholamine release from the adrenal medulla.
- Dosage:
  - standard im, iv or sc dose: 0.1–0.15 mg/kg.
  - orally: 10 mg increased slowly up to 200 mg, 4 hourly. Sustained release preparation: from 10 mg 12 hourly.
  - has been given via buccal and rectal routes.

  Doses should be reduced in renal or hepatic failure.

[Morpheus, Greek God of Dreams]

See also, Opioid receptors; Spinal opioids

Mortality and morbidity, *see Anaesthetic morbidity and mortality; Mortality/survival prediction on intensive care unit*

Mortality probability models (MPM). Scoring systems, similar to APACHE and simplified acute physiology score, for estimating outcome of ICU patients. The latest version (MPM III) is based on multiple regression analysis applied to data from 125 000 patients at the time of admission to ICU and reflects changes in clinical management since the MPM II system was introduced. Scores are derived from weighting of variables related to physiology, acute and chronic disease, reason for admission, age and therapeutic interventions. A probability of hospital mortality can be calculated at 0, 24, 48 and 72 h after ICU admission. Individual versions of the MPM system are termed MPM_0 (calculation of risk of hospital death on entry to ICU), MPM_{24}, MPM_{48} and MPM_{72} (calculated after 24, 48 and 72 h of ICU care respectively).

Higgins TL, Teres D, Copes WS, et al (2007). Crit Care Med; 35: 827–35

See also Intensive care, outcome of; Mortality/survival prediction on intensive care unit

Mortality/survival prediction on intensive care unit. Many attempts have been made to develop methods of predicting outcomes in critically ill patients, to allow:
- estimation of prognoses for individual patients.
- comparison between different treatments, e.g. in clinical studies.
- comparison between different units (e.g. using the standardised mortality ratio: observed mortality divided by predicted mortality).
- allocation of resources.

Scoring systems may be based on a single set of data (static) or on repeated collections over time (dynamic). Many different systems exist, including:
- simple five-point scale according to clinical judgement, e.g. certain to die; likely to die, etc.
- therapeutic intervention scoring system (TISS): based primarily on treatment interventions.
- acute physiology score (APS), simplified acute physiology score (SAPS), APACHE scoring systems, mortality probability models (MPM), logistic organ dysfunction system (LODS): based mainly on the patient's physiological state ± therapeutic interventions.
- specific systems for certain conditions, e.g. coma scales such as the Glasgow coma scale (GCS), trauma scales, scoring systems for sepsis, burns, subarachnoid haemorrhage, hepatic failure, etc.

None of the general systems has been shown to be superior to the others, although updated systems generally perform better than the original ones.

Strand K, Flaattten H (2008). Acta Anaesthesiol Scand; 52: 467–78

See also, Intensive care, outcome of

Morton, William Thomas Green (1819–1868). US dentist, considered the founder of anaesthesia despite being predated by Clarke, Long and Wells. Briefly practised with Wells in Boston in 1842–3, before entering Harvard Medical School in 1844, although he never completed his medical studies. Present at Wells' unsuccessful demonstration of N_2O at Harvard in 1844. Morton approached Jackson for advice on supplies of N_2O for further experiments. Jackson's suggestion of diethyl ether as a topical analgesic led to Morton's use of ether for inhalational anaesthesia for dental extraction on September 30th 1846. At the Massachusetts General Hospital on October 16th, he successfully anaesthetised Edward Gilbert Abbott, whilst Warren excised a mass from the latter's jaw. Became demoralised by subsequent battles against Jackson's claim to the discovery, and against widespread infringement of his patent. His contribution was recognised only posthumously.

[Edward Gilbert Abbott (1825–1855), US printer]

See also, Letheon

Motor neurone disease. Progressive degenerative disorder characterised by degeneration of motor neurones in the cerebral cortex, brainstem nuclei of the cranial nerves and anterior horn cells of the spinal cord. Prevalence is 5 per 100 000; mainly affects men aged 50–70. Death usually occurs within 3–5 years.
- Types:
  - amyotrophic lateral sclerosis: upper motor neurone lesion with spastic limb weakness.
  - progressive bulbar palsy: lower motor neurone lesions of the brainstem nuclei, causing dysarthria and dysphagia.
  - progressive muscular atrophy: lower motor neurone lesions of the anterior horn cells.
- Anaesthetic problems are related to:
  - possible laryngeal incompetence leading to aspiration of gastric contents.
  - respiratory muscle weakness, with greater sensitivity to respiratory depressant drugs.
  - increased sensitivity to neuromuscular blocking drugs. An exaggerated hyperkalaemic response to suxamethonium is theoretically possible but has not been reported.

ICU concerns include the above and also the ethical issues surrounding respiratory support should respiratory failure occur.

Motor neurone, lower. Term used to describe motor neurones that directly innervate muscle, i.e. without other neurones interposed. Lesions of these neurones (lower motor neurone lesions) therefore result in complete cessation of neural input to the muscle, resulting in characteristic clinical features:
- flaccid paralysis.
- visible fasciculations, thought to be caused by spontaneous firing of neighbouring motor units that have taken over the affected muscle.
- absent reflexes.

- muscular atrophy.
- denervation hypersensitivity. Thought to be the cause of invisible fibrillation of muscle fibres. An increased hyperkalaemic response to suxamethonium may occur from 4 days to 7 months after injury.

See also, Motor neurone, upper

Motor neurone, upper. Term used to decribe neurones of the motor pathways excluding lower motor neurones. Thus include neurones of the motor cortex, cerebellar and extrapyramidal pathways, although the term commonly refers to the former only. Upper motor neurone lesions may thus occur at any level above the lower neurone cell bodies, producing characteristic features, after initial flaccid paralysis:

- increased tone and spastic paralysis. Typically, muscle exhibits 'clasp-knife' rigidity, possibly due to activity of muscle spindles without inhibitory higher input.
- increased reflexes and upwards plantar responses (Babinski reflex).
- no fasciculation.
- no atrophy.
- an increased hyperkalaemic response to suxamethonium may occur from 10 days to 7 months after injury, although the mechanism is unclear.

[Joseph Babinski (1857–1932), French neurologist]

See also, Motor neurone, lower

Motor pathways. Consist of the following systems:

- pyramidal pathways (Fig. 106): fibres arise from pyramidal cells of the motor cortex of the precentral gyrus and premotor area. Legs are represented uppermost, with the head at the lower part of the gyrus. Regions of greatest importance (e.g. face, hands) have a disproportionately greater representation. Fibres then pass via the internal capsule (legs represented behind, face anteriorly), and via the cerebral peduncle and pons to the medulla, forming the pyramids. Most of the fibres decussate in the lower medulla and pass within the lateral corticospinal tract of the spinal cord. Some pass within the anterior corticospinal tract without decussating; these cross within the spinal cord at their spinal levels. Some fibres pass to cranial nerve motor nuclei. Most of the fibres synapse with intermediate neurones.
- extrapyramidal pathways: less well-defined than the above system. Fibres arise from the premotor area and corpus striatum, and pass via the basal ganglia, substantia nigra and nuclear masses of the midbrain and hindbrain. They descend within the rubroreticulospinal and vestibulospinal tracts. Other pathways pass from the tectum of the midbrain and olives of the medulla. Concerned with control of movement.
- cerebellar pathways: involve the thalamus, red nucleus, pons, medulla and cerebral cortex.
- pathways of the autonomic nervous system.

See also, Motor neurone, lower; Motor neurone, upper; Spinal cord lesions

Motor unit. One lower motor neurone and the muscle fibres it innervates. In muscles for fine movement, e.g. of the eye and hand, motor units are small, i.e. under 10 fibres per neurone. Muscles involved in posture may have up to 1000 fibres per neurone. All fibres of a motor unit are of the same type, i.e. fast or slow; the type is thought to be determined by characteristics of the nerve itself.

Mountain sickness, *see Altitude, high*

Mouth, *see Larynx; Pharynx; Teeth; Tongue*

Mouth care. Important aspect of care of the unconscious patient. Involves regular inspection of the oral mucosa, tongue, gums and teeth and their thorough cleansing. The teeth, tongue and palate are cleansed with toothpaste using a toothbrush or sponge-tipped swab. The mouth should be thoroughly rinsed with clean water or a mouthwash solution. The use of a syringe for irrigation is useful. Regular suction of the mouth is important to improve comfort and reduce the risk of aspiration. Immunocompromised patients or those receiving broad-spectrum antibiotics may develop oral candida.

Tracheal or gastric tubes, etc. may exert pressure which may lead to ulceration unless they are adequately supported and gently moved to different parts of the mouth at regular intervals.

Mouth gags. Devices used to hold open the patient's mouth, e.g. during dental surgery (Fig. 107). Held by the anaesthetist from behind the patient's head, they are grasped at the blades' pivot to ensure control of the blades during insertion. The blades' tips are usually covered with plastic or rubber to prevent dental damage, and are placed at the molars.

[Eugene L Doyen (1859–1916), French surgeon; Sir William Fergusson (1808–1877), Scottish-born London surgeon; Francis Mason (1837–1886), London surgeon]

Moxonidine. The first selective imidazoline receptor agonist, introduced as a centrally acting antihypertensive drug. Acts by stimulating imidazoline type 1 (I_1) receptors in the medulla, thereby reducing central and peripheral sympathetic activity. May also stimulate renal I_1 receptors causing increased sodium and water excretion. Has minimal affinity for α_2-adrenergic receptors and thus causes fewer side effects than other centrally acting drugs. Peak plasma levels occur within 1 h of oral administration, with half-life of about 2 h. 90% is excreted unchanged in the urine.

- Dosage: 200 μg orally once daily, increased to 300 μg 12 hourly if required.
- Side effects: sedation, dry mouth, headache, dizziness, sleep disturbances.

MPM, *see Mortality probability models*

MRI, *see Magnetic resonance imaging*

MRSA, Meticillin-resistant *Staphylococcus aureus*, *see Infection control; Staphylococcal infections*

Mucolytic drugs. Used to reduce sputum viscosity (e.g. in COPD, asthma) via cleaving of disulphide bonds in mucus glycoprotein. Their use is controversial since no clear benefit has been shown when administered orally. Include carbocisteine, erdosteine and mecysteine. Inhaled dornase alfa, a genetically engineered DNA-ase (DNase), is indicated in cystic fibrosis but has been used in other lung conditions. *N*-Acetylcysteine has been used orally and by aerosol in ICU, but severe bronchospasm has occurred after the latter. Other strategies to reduce sputum viscosity include use of saline or bicarbonate solutions by instillation.

MUGA, *see Multigated acquisition imaging*

Multigated acquisition imaging (MUGA imaging). Technique of nuclear cardiology in which information from each of many cardiac cycles is combined to allow studies of

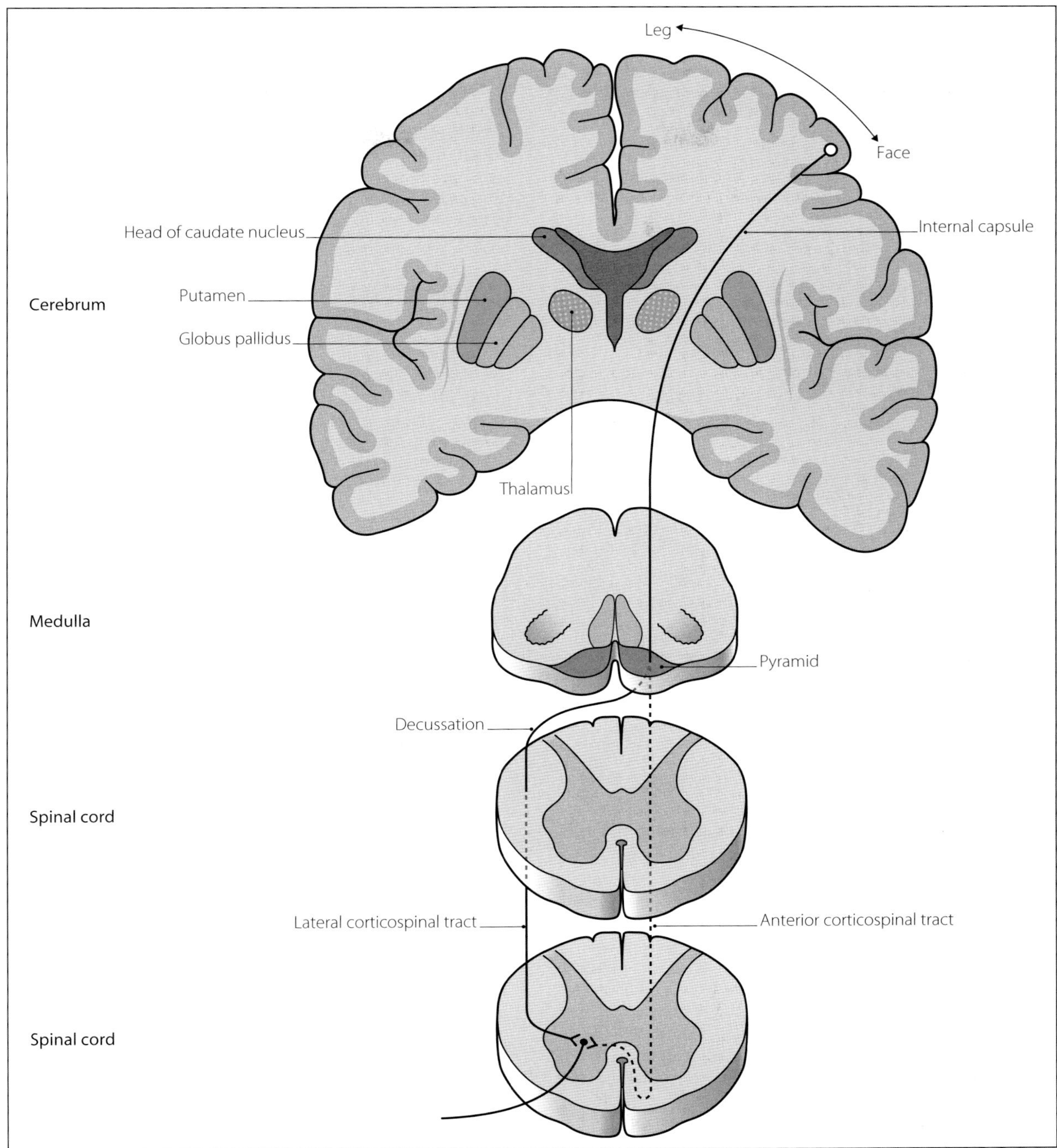

Fig. 106 Pyramidal (corticospinal) motor system

regional ventricular wall function and determination of ejection fraction. The subject's red blood cells are labelled with Technetium-99 m *in vivo* and time allowed for complete mixing of the marker throughout the circulating volume. Scanning then takes place over several cycles. Advantages over single-pass cardiographic techniques include less reliability on the injection technique (crucial in the single-pass method) and the ability to scan before and after exercise or drug administration. Disadvantages include the overlap of the heart chambers on the image and the inability to follow a tracer bolus through the chambers of the heart.

Multiple endocrine adenomatosis (MEA; Multiple endocrine neoplasia, MEN). Syndrome of multiple endocrine tumours; may occur in three groups:

- type I: parathyroid adenoma, pancreatic adenoma or carcinoma, and anterior pituitary adenoma.
- type II: medullary thyroid carcinoma, phaeochromocytoma, and parathyroid adenoma.
- type III: medullary thyroid carcinoma, phaeochromocytoma, and mucosal neuromas.

Patients presenting for endocrine surgery may thus have other tumours and associated syndromes.

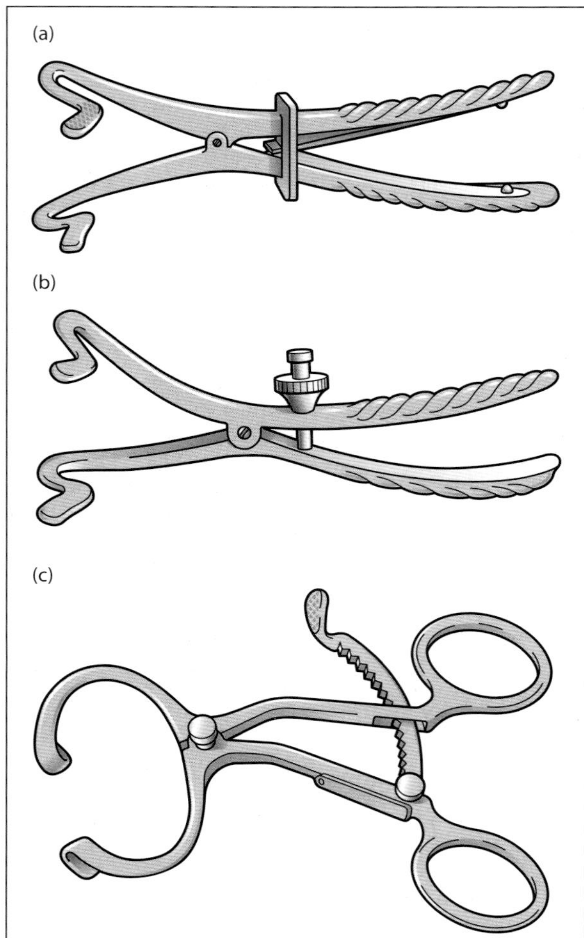

Fig. 107 Examples of mouth gags: (a) Fergusson; (b) Mason; (c) Doyen

All are inherited by autosomal dominant transmission.
See also, Apudomas; Hyperparathyroidism

Multiple organ dysfunction score. Scoring system for evaluating dysfunction of six organ systems: respiratory, renal, hepatic, cardiovascular, central nervous and haematological. Weighted scores (0–4 points) are given for increasing degrees of abnormality of six parameters (arterial $P\text{O}_2$:$F_I\text{O}_2$ ratio, serum creatinine, serum bilirubin, platelet count, pressure-adjusted heart rate (heart rate × CVP:mean arterial BP ratio) and Glasgow coma score). Raw data are collected daily; the value recorded is a representative value for the day (i.e. at a particular time and not necessarily the worst value).
Marshall JC, Cook DJ, Christou NV, et al (1995). Crit Care Med; 23: 1638–52

Multiple organ dysfunction syndrome (MODS). Syndrome of organ dysfunction affecting two or more organs, occurring remote from the site of primary tissue injury or infection. Thought to be caused by dysregulation of the host inflammatory response with consequent release of inflammatory mediators and tissue injury, associated with hypoperfusion. May progress to multiple organ failure (MOF) although the definitions of what constitutes organ dysfunction and failure are controversial. Predominantly affects the respiratory, renal, hepatic, neurological, gastrointestinal, haematological and cardiovascular systems. A major cause of death in ICU; attention is focused on preventing the transition from MODS to MOF which has a mortality of over 50% (higher the more organs are involved). Can be classified into primary and secondary forms: primary MODS is the result of a well-defined insult with early organ dysfunction attributable to an identifiable disease process (e.g. acute renal failure secondary to rhabdomyolysis), whilst secondary MODS occurs days after admission as a result of sepsis or SIRS. The degree of organ dysfunction may be described by the multiple organ dysfunction score.
Johnson D, Mayers I (2001). Can J Anesth; 48: 502–9

Multiple sclerosis, *see Demyelinating diseases*

Murphy eye, *see Tracheal tubes*

Muscarine and muscarinic receptors. Muscarine, an alkaloid extracted from certain mushrooms, mimics certain actions of acetylcholine (hence it is a parasympathomimetic drug) and was used to investigate the physiology of the autonomic nervous system. It stimulates postganglionic acetylcholine receptors (muscarinic receptors) at effector organs of the parasympathetic nervous system, and at sweat glands of the sympathetic nervous system. It also causes Parkinsonian tremor, ataxia and rigidity; thus muscarinic receptors are thought to exist in the CNS. Other receptors may be involved in an inhibitory role at adrenergic nerve endings, e.g. in the heart, and at autonomic ganglia.

Division of receptors into subtypes is suggested by experimental work: M_1 (stimulation of gastric acid secretion; may be present at sympathetic ganglia), M_2 (heart), M_3 (causes smooth muscle contraction, and lacrimal and salivary gland secretion), M_4 (brain and adrenal medulla) and M_5 (brain). Pirenzepine is thought to antagonise M_1 receptors. All subtypes are G protein-coupled receptors.

Muscle. Contractile tissue; may be:
- skeletal (striated; voluntary):
  - the most abundant form.
  - normally contracts only when stimulated.
  - no connections between individual fibres.
  - comprised of elongated cylindrical fibres, each surrounded by its sarcolemma (muscle cell membrane). Each fibre contains myofibrils, containing actin and myosin filaments and surrounded by sarcoplasmic reticulum and mitochondria. The T-tubule system invaginates from the sarcolemma to connect all myofibrils with the extracellular space.
  - microscopically visible striations are due to myosin and actin arrangements, labelled for historical reasons (Fig. 108). The sarcomere (portion between adjacent Z lines) shortens during muscle contraction.

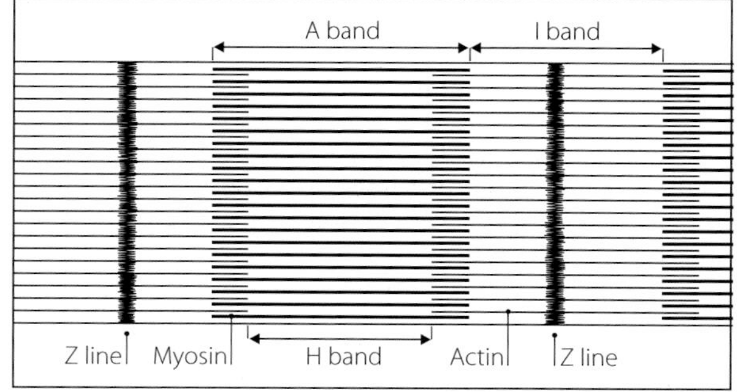

Fig. 108 Microscopic appearance of myofibril

- different types of fibre:
  - type I: red muscle; responds slowly with slow metabolism and high oxidative capacity (high myoglobin, mitochondria and capillary content). Suitable for prolonged contraction, e.g. postural muscles.
  - type IIB: white muscle, short contracting with low oxidative capacity. Suitable for rapid skilled movement, e.g. eye and hand muscles.
  - type IIA: as for IIB but with high oxidative capacity, i.e. red. Uncommon in humans.
- cardiac:
  - similar to slow striated muscle, but fibres are branched, and joined end-to-end by intercalated discs; also connected to adjacent fibres by gap junctions (i.e. forms a functional syncytium). Requires continuous O_2 supply.
  - has spontaneous pacemaker activity, due to slow depolarisation between action potentials.
  - cannot exhibit tetanic contraction, due to a prolonged refractory period.
- smooth:
  - no striations; actin and myosin filaments arranged randomly.
  - occurs in sheets of interconnecting cells (e.g. visceral) or multiunits (e.g. iris).
  - exhibits slow spontaneous activity; also responsive to stimulation of the autonomic nervous system. Visceral muscle contracts if stretched.

See also, Motor unit; Muscle spindles; Neuromuscular junction

Muscle contraction. Involves the following steps:
- depolarisation of the postsynaptic membrane at the neuromuscular junction.
- area of depolarisation spreads across the muscle membrane and into the muscle bulk via the T-tubule system.
- depolarisation causes release and mobilisation of intracellular calcium ions from sarcoplasmic reticulum.
- calcium ions bind to the troponin component of the actin complex, causing displacement of the tropomyosin component from myosin binding sites.
- myosin can now bind to actin, with hydrolysis of ATP, structural alteration of myosin and shortening of muscle fibres. ATPase is present on myosin molecule heads. The process repeats with further muscle shortening. Histologically, contraction leads to shortening of the I band and H band (*see Fig. 108*).
- further hydrolysis of ATP allows uptake of calcium, and muscle relaxation.

A single twitch caused by an action potential of 1 ms lasts up to 200 ms. Contraction may be isometric (force increases but muscle length remains constant) or isotonic (force is constant and muscle shortens). Repeated fast stimulation results in summation of contraction, since there is inadequate time for relaxation between stimuli. Above a certain frequency, tetanic contraction occurs.

ATP is derived from glycolysis and from dephosphorylation of phosphorylcreatine, stored during rest. Anaerobic glycolysis and metabolism of free fatty acids are also used. During severe exercise, anaerobic glycolysis predominates, incurring an O_2 debt which is paid back during recovery.

Muscle relaxants, *see Neuromuscular blocking drugs*

Muscle spindles. Encapsulated structures present in and parallel to skeletal muscle. Contain up to 10 specialised muscle (intrafusal) fibres, attached to the ordinary muscle (extrafusal) fibres or to their tendons. Muscle contraction thus results in shortening of the spindles. Sensory nerve fibres from the spindles end on the motor neurones supplying the extrafusal muscle fibres of that muscle. They transmit impulses when stretched; thus passive muscle stretching causes reflex contraction, e.g. knee jerk reflex arc. Discharge in some afferent fibres is proportional to degree of stretch; discharge in others is also proportional to speed of stretch. Muscle contraction reduces tension within the spindle, reducing the afferent discharge. Activation of the reflex also inhibits contraction of opposing muscle groups (reciprocal innervation) via an inhibitory spinal interneurone.

Small γ-motor fibres innervate the ends of the intrafusal fibres, causing them to contract. This stretches the central portions, with reflex extrafusal fibre contraction as before, and increases the sensitivity of the spindles to passive stretching. γ-Motor activity is controlled by descending pathways in the spinal cord; thus muscle tone and posture are controlled at both spinal and supraspinal levels. Increased muscle tone and clonus seen in upper motor neurone lesions may result from overactive γ-activity due to interruption of inhibitory descending pathways. γ-Activity is also increased in anxiety, resulting in exaggerated tremor.

Increased passive stretching of a muscle eventually causes sudden relaxation, due to stimulation of Golgi tendon organs within the muscle tendons. This inverse stretch reflex is exaggerated in upper motor neurone lesions (clasp-knife effect).
[Camillo Golgi (1843–1926), Italian physician]

Muscular dystrophies. Rare (up to 30:100 000 live births) hereditary disorders of muscle, involving progressive destruction of mainly skeletal, but also cardiac muscle. Result from mutation of the gene for dystrophin, a cytoskeletal protein involved in cell structure and in the interaction between the sarcomeres and the extracellular matrix (via dystrophin-associated protein, DAP). Deficiency of dystrophin (and DAP) results in weakening of the muscle membrane with calcium influx and necrosis of muscle fibres; in Duchenne's dystrophy deficiency is severe whilst in Becker's a reduced amount of abnormal dystrophin still results in some activity. Plasma creatine kinase levels may be markedly increased. Classified according to inheritance: may be sex-linked (e.g. Duchenne's, Becker's), autosomal dominant (e.g. facioscapulohumeral, oculopharyngeal) or recessive (e.g. limb girdle):
- Duchenne's: most common and severe. Affects boys usually from 3 to 5 years old; usually fatal by the early twenties. A similar autosomal recessive form may occur in girls.
- Becker's, facioscapulohumeral, limb girdle: less severe, with later onset and death. Cardiac involvement is less common.

- Orthopaedic surgery is common for limb contractures, etc. Severe forms may present significant anaesthetic risk:
  - weak respiratory muscles and kyphoscoliosis: impaired ventilation, sputum clearance, etc. Pre-existing and postoperative chest infection is more likely. Patients may be more sensitive to respiratory depressant drugs and neuromuscular blocking drugs.
  - rhabdomyolysis may follow suxamethonium or volatile anaesthetic agents, typically following prolonged exposure to the latter. Severe hyperkalaemia and myoglobinuria may result. An MH-like picture may develop as muscle metabolism increases (in the absence of true inherited MH); thus whilst some authorities would use volatile agents for short cases most would avoid prolonged exposure.

- cardiac involvement is common in Duchenne's; characteristically the ECG shows tachycardia, short P–R interval, deep Q waves laterally and tall R waves in V_1. Cardiomyopathy may be more common in Becker's but both may lead to arrhythmias (VF has occurred on induction of anaesthesia). Bradycardia is common in facioscapulohumeral dystrophy.
- delayed gastric emptying and poor bulbar function predispose to aspiration of gastric contents.

Plans for anaesthesia must take account of the above consideration. Regional techniques are popular when feasible. ICU concerns include the above and also the ethical issues surrounding respiratory support should respiratory failure occur.

[Guillaume Duchenne (1806–1875), French neurologist; Peter Becker (1908–2000), German geneticist]

MVV, Maximal voluntary ventilation, *see Lung function tests*

Myasthenia gravis. Autoimmune disease characterised by weakness and increased fatiguability of skeletal muscle. Prevalence is 50–100 per million. More common in young women and older men. May also occur transiently in neonates born to affected mothers, and may be caused by drugs, e.g. penicillamine.

Caused by an immune response in which IgG autoantibodies are produced against the acetylcholine receptors of the neuromuscular junction postsynaptic membrane. The autoantibodies (detectable in 90% of patients) occupy receptors leading to their destruction and reduction in receptor density. The thymus gland is abnormal (either hyperplasia or thymoma) in 75% of cases and is thought to be the site of production of the autoantibodies. Often associated with other autoimmune conditions, e.g. thyroid disease.

- Characterised by muscle weakness (typically worse on exertion and improving with rest); may affect:
  - ocular muscles causing ptosis and diplopia.
  - bulbar muscles causing dysarthria and predisposing to aspiration of gastric contents.
  - respiratory muscles.
  - limb muscles.

Myasthenic crises (suddenly worsening and spreading weakness requiring IPPV) may be provoked by drug omission, infection, stress, pregnancy, drugs (e.g. aminoglycosides), etc.

- Classified according to severity:
  - grade I: confined to eye muscles only (15% of cases).
  - grade IIa: generalised mild muscle weakness.
  - grade IIb: generalised moderate weakness and/or bulbar weakness.
  - grade III: acute fulminating: rapid and progressive and/or respiratory involvement.
  - grade IV: myasthenic crisis requiring IPPV.
- Diagnosis:
  - marked improvement following iv edrophonium 2 + 8 mg (Tensilon test).
  - EMG shows reduced response to single twitch, fade on tetanic stimulation and post-tetanic potentiation.
  - detection of anti-acetylcholine receptor antibodies.
- Treatment:
  - emergency intubation and IPPV for impending/actual respiratory failure or bulbar dysfunction. Blood gas analysis is rarely useful in myasthenia for determining the need for IPPV; clinical indicators are best.
  - acetylcholinesterase inhibitors, e.g. pyridostigmine 30–90 mg 6 hourly, neostigmine 15–30 mg 4 hourly. Muscarinic side effects include miosis, colic, lacrimation, diarrhoea, salivation; atropine may be given to reduce these. May cause cholinergic crisis in overdosage; distinguished from myasthenic crises by injection of edrophonium 2 mg. Myasthenic crises improve transiently, cholinergic crises do not.
  - immunosuppressive therapy includes corticosteroids (e.g. prednisolone 1 mg/kg on alternate days; usually started in hospital because of possible deterioration), azathioprine, cyclophosphamide, ciclosporin, mycophenolate.
  - treatment of any coexistent electrolyte abnormalities, especially hypokalaemia, hypocalcaemia, hypermagnesaemia.
  - plasmapheresis, especially combined with immunosuppressive therapy. Used in severe cases.
  - iv immunoglobulin therapy has been used in severe cases.
  - thymectomy: indications are controversial but most myasthenic patients between 16 and 60 years old benefit with either full remission or reduction in immunosuppressive therapy. Anaesthetic management:
    - preoperatively: assessment of respiratory function is important. Pyridostigmine is usually withheld on the morning of surgery. Preoperative plasmapheresis and corticosteroids have been used. Potassium abnormalities increase muscle weakness and should be corrected.
    - perioperatively: there is increased sensitivity to non-depolarising neuromuscular blocking drugs and relative resistance to suxamethonium with increased tendency to develop dual block. Tracheal intubation and IPPV are usually performed without neuromuscular blocking drugs, using e.g. propofol and/or a volatile agent. Atracurium in reduced doses (50–60% of usual) has been suggested over other drugs. Surgery is performed via a suprasternal or trans-sternal route. Haemorrhage and pneumothorax may occur. The tracheal tube may be left in situ and ventilation monitored on ICU or HDU; tracheal extubation is usually possible within a few hours postoperatively, although 24–48 h intubation is preferred in some centres. Extubation may be possible immediately postoperatively.
    - postoperatively: pyridostigmine may be restarted, usually in reduced dosage. Close monitoring of respiration and physiotherapy are required. Postoperative atelectasis and infection are common.

Anaesthetic management of patients with myasthenia gravis for other surgery should follow the above guidelines. Regional techniques, where feasible, have been suggested as being safer.

Hirsch NP (2007). Br J Anaesth; 99: 132–8

See also, Myasthenic syndrome

Myasthenic syndrome (Eaton–Lambert syndrome). Acquired disorder of the neuromuscular junction in which there is decreased quantal release of acetylcholine from the presynaptic nerve terminal. Caused by IgG autoantibodies interfering with the voltage dependent calcium channels necessary for acetylcholine release. May be associated with small cell bronchial carcinoma or rarely autoimmune disease (e.g. polyarteritis nodosa).

- Distinguished from myasthenia gravis thus:
  - classically improves on exercise (EMG shows an increase in power on tetanic stimulation).
  - usually affects proximal limb muscles.
  - autonomic nervous system involvement is common.
  - tendon reflexes are depressed or absent.

- power is only slightly improved by neostigmine, despite possible improvement following edrophonium.
- caused by defective release of acetylcholine from presynaptic nerve endings, with normal postsynaptic receptors.

May improve with oral guanidine hydrochloride 30–50 mg/kg thrice daily or aminopyridine; corticosteroids, iv immunoglobulins and plasmapheresis have been tried.

General anaesthetic considerations are as for myasthenia gravis. There is increased sensitivity to non-depolarising and depolarising neuromuscular blocking drugs. Atracurium has been suggested as the drug of choice. Postoperative respiratory complications are more likely with severe weakness.

[LM Eaton (1905–1958), US neurologist; Edward H Lambert (1915–2003), US neurophysiologist]

Hirsch NP (2007). Br J Anaesth; 99: 132–8

Mycophenolate mofetil. Cytotoxic immunosuppressive drug used in organ transplantation especially in combination with ciclosporin and corticosteroids. Has also been used in myasthenia gravis. Metabolised to mycophenolic acid.

- Dosage: 1–5 mg/kg orally or iv, daily.
- Side effects: hypersensitivity reactions, myelosuppression, liver toxicity.

Mycoplasma infections. Caused by various species of mycoplasma, the smallest free-living micro-organisms; similar to bacteria but lack cell walls. The most important infection is mycoplasma pneumonia, caused by *M. pneumoniae*:

- typically associated with initial headache, sore throat, fever, malaise and cough; the cough becomes productive and patchy chest signs may develop although classic signs of consolidation are rare. Usually affects a single lower lobe only, although the clinical course is variable. Chest X-ray signs (patchy shadowing) often precede clinical features and persist after clinical recovery.
- extrapulmonary features include haemolytic anaemia, GIT upset including hepatic and pancreatic involvement, rash, arthritis, CNS (meningitis, encephalitis, ascending paralysis, transverse myelitis, cranial nerve palsy) and cardiac (myocarditis, pericarditis) involvement.
- diagnosed by demonstration of a rising antibody titre, since culture of organisms is slow and difficult. Cold agglutinins may also be identified in blood.
- treatment with erythromycin or tetracycline. Death is rare.

Other infections include GIT and genitourinary ones such as non-specific urethritis, pelvic inflammatory disease, vaginitis, pyelonephritis, etc. Most are caused by *M. hominis* or *urealyticum*.

Myelin. Lipoprotein derived from multiple layers of cell membranes, encasing the axons of myelinated neurones. Arises from Schwann cells in the peripheral nervous system (one cell to one axon portion), and from oligodendrocytes in the CNS (one cell to up to 40 axon portions). Deficient at 1 mm intervals (nodes of Ranvier). Unmyelinated peripheral nerves are merely encased in Schwann cell cytoplasm. Acts as an insulating sheath, increasing speed of nerve conduction in myelinated nerves by restricting membrane depolarisation to the nodes of Ranvier; depolarisation 'jumps' from node to node (saltatory conduction) instead of slower, smooth progression along unmyelinated nerves.

[Theodor Schwann (1810–1882), German physiologist; Louis Ranvier (1835–1922), French physician and pathologist]

Myocardial contractility. Ability of the myocardial muscle to contract at a particular length of fibre, thus a major determinant of stroke volume and cardiac output, and myocardial O_2 demand.

- Increased by:
  - intrinsic mechanisms:
    - Anrep effect.
    - Bowditch effect.
  - extrinsic factors:
    - sympathetic nervous system activity.
    - catecholamines via β_1-adrenergic receptors.
    - inotropic drugs.
- Decreased by:
  - parasympathetic nervous system (slight effect).
  - hypoxaemia and hypercapnia (via direct effects; also cause increased sympathetic activity).
  - acidosis and alkalosis.
  - cardiac disease, e.g. ischaemic heart disease, cardiomyopathy, myocarditis, etc.
  - electrolyte disturbances, e.g. hyperkalaemia, hypocalcaemia.
  - drugs, e.g. most iv and inhalational anaesthetic agents, antiarrhythmic drugs.
- Assessment is difficult; indirect methods include measurement of:
  - stroke volume and stroke work.
  - speed of contraction.
  - cardiac output.
  - ratio of left ventricular end-diastolic pressure to left ventricular end-diastolic volume.
  - peak left ventricular pressure.
  - ejection fraction.

See also, Starling's law

Myocardial infarction (MI). Consequence of unrelieved myocardial ischaemia. Usually starts at the endothelium, spreading outwards. The left ventricle is usually affected, but it may involve the right ventricle or atria. Most acute MIs are associated with coronary vessel thrombosis.

- Features:
  - pain as for ischaemia, but more severe and persistent (MI may be silent, especially in the elderly and possibly perioperatively).
  - arrhythmias. Cardiac arrest may occur.
  - sweating, pallor, dyspnoea.
  - hypertension or hypotension.
  - cardiac failure and cardiogenic shock.
  - may lead to:
    - ventricular rupture, usually 5–8 days later.
    - ventricular aneurysm.
    - interventricular septum rupture, usually 4–6 days later.
    - papillary muscle damage and mitral regurgitation.
    - mural thrombus formation and systemic embolism.
    - PE.
    - Dressler's syndrome: pericarditis, pleurisy and pneumonitis, typically 4–6 weeks later.
- Investigations:
  - ECG changes: typically T wave changes and S–T segment elevation with Q waves in leads overlying the infarct. S–T elevation usually lasts for under 2 weeks, T wave inversion for several months, and Q waves for at least several years (Fig. 109). Persistent S–T elevation may indicate ventricular aneurysm or an area of dyskinetic myocardium. Q waves may be absent in

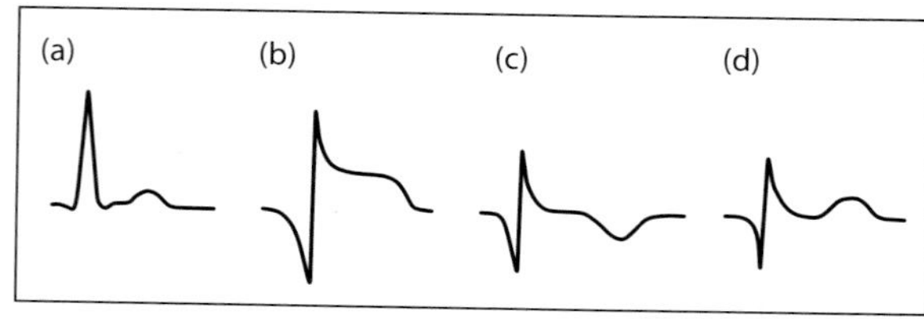

Fig. 109 Typical changes in ECG following MI: (a) normal; (b) immediate: (c) few weeks; (d) few months

subendocardial infarction. Other changes include abnormalities of the P wave and P–R interval in atrial infarction, conduction defects, e.g. bundle branch block and heart block, and arrhythmias.
- cardiac enzymes may show characteristic changes.
- nuclear cardiology may reveal areas of infarcted muscle. Echocardiography and other imaging techniques may reveal areas of reduced or absent contraction.

- Differential diagnosis: pain and ECG changes may occur with lesions of:
  - heart/great vessels, e.g. aortic dissection, pericarditis.
  - lung, e.g. PE, chest infection.
  - oesophagus, e.g. spasm, inflammation, rupture.
  - abdominal organs, e.g. peptic ulcer disease, pancreatitis, cholecystitis.
- Medical management:
  - analgesia, e.g. iv opioid analgesic drugs, Entonox prehospital.
  - systemic fibrinolytic drugs within 24 h. Oral aspirin or clopidogrel is usually commenced but use of heparin is associated with increased risk of bleeding. There is no benefit to adding warfarin to aspirin. For patients with 1 mm or more ST elevation in 2 contiguous limb leads or 2 mm or more in 2 contiguous precordial leads, thrombolysis therapy is indicated (contraindications include active bleeding, recent surgery, trauma or stroke, active peptic ulcer disease and evidence of aortic dissection).
  - monitoring, bed rest and O_2 therapy, usually within a coronary care unit. Management of the above complications. Pulmonary artery catheterisation and use of inotropic and vasodilator drugs may be required.
  - long-term treatment with β-adrenergic receptor antagonists (in patients without cardiac failure) and angiotensin converting enzyme inhibitors (in patients with cardiac failure) has been shown to reduce mortality. Recent studies suggest that magnesium sulphate, nitrates and calcium channel blocking drugs do not reduce mortality.
  - consideration for cardiac surgery if angina or surgical complications develop post infarct.
- Perioperative MI has been investigated by several studies. Summary of findings:
  - with previous MI, overall reinfarction rate is 6–7% (if no previous MI, infarction rate is 0.1–0.2%).
  - reinfarction rate is related to the time since the MI:
    - within 3 months of surgery: 20–30%.
    - within 4–6 months: 10–20%.
    - greater than 6 months: 4–5%.
  - aggressive management, e.g. pulmonary artery catheterisation, use of inotropic and vasodilator drugs, admission to ICU, etc., has been reported to lower the overall infarction rate to 2%, and the reinfarction rates as follows:
    - MI within 3 months: under 6%.
    - within 4–6 months: 2–3%.
    - greater than 6 months: 1–2%.

  However, the statistical analysis used has been criticised, and the value of routine intensive monitoring and treatment remains controversial, especially when the increased cost is considered.
  - perioperative reinfarction carries increased mortality (up to 70%), and is commonest on the 3rd postoperative day.
  - incidence of silent MI may be higher.
  - unstable angina, perioperative hypotension, prolonged surgery, and upper abdominal/thoracic or vascular surgery have been identified as risk factors.
  - risk is not increased by previous cardiac surgery.
  - risk is not associated with the type of anaesthetic or drugs used.
  - cardiac risk index has been developed for assessment of risk of death or severe perioperative cardiovascular complications. Presence of cardiac failure is the most important risk factor. Other factors are related to arrhythmias, age and general condition of the patient.
  - reinfarction is often associated with perioperative myocardial ischaemia detected by S–T depression. It is not always associated with hypertension or hypotension.
- Risk of perioperative MI is thus reduced by:
  - postponement of elective surgery until at least 6 months after MI.
  - treatment of preoperative risk factors where possible.
  - avoidance of myocardial ischaemia as for ischaemic heart disease.

[William Dressler (1890–1969), US cardiologist]

Myocardial ischaemia. Inadequate blood supply to the myocardium. Effects are related to myocardial O_2 supply/demand balance; largely dependent on:
- supply:
  - coronary blood flow:
    - aortic end-distolic pressure minus left ventricular end-diastolic pressure.
    - duration of diastole.
    - coronary vessels: calibre is usually maintained by autoregulation. Stenosis may be caused by atheroma, thrombosis and spasm. Collateral vessels are important (e.g. coronary steal). The subendocardial region is most at risk of ischaemia.
    - blood viscosity.
  - O_2 content.
- demand:
  - myocardial contractility and wall tension.
  - heart rate.

- Effects:
  - reversible increases in hydrogen ion, potassium, phosphate, lactate, adenosine, etc. Unless ischaemia is corrected within about 30 min, permanent damage ensues, with release of cardiac enzymes and myoglobin, i.e. MI occurs.
  - ECG changes: thought to be caused by ion leakage across the ischaemic myocardial membrane, altering membrane potentials and causing current flow between normal and ischaemic areas. S–T segment changes are most common; depression is due to subendocardial ischaemia, elevation due to transmural ischaemia. Arrhythmias may occur.
  - impaired myocardial contraction: first depressed, then absent, then myocardial lengthening with worsening ischaemia.
  - pain (angina): possibly due to increased potassium or substance P. Pain is typically steady, crushing and midsternal, radiating across the chest, to the neck or arms.

Related to exertion, cold or emotion and relieved by rest, it may be absent (silent ischaemia). Dyspnoea and sweating may occur. Crescendo angina is characterised by increasing frequency of attacks with diminishing levels of exertion; unstable angina occurs at rest (diagnosed when MI has been excluded). Repeated small thromboses may be responsible; both types may herald imminent MI.

- Detection:
  - symptoms and signs as above.
  - detection of reduced supply/increased demand. Indices of supply include diastolic pressure time index. Indices of demand include rate–pressure product and tension time index. Endocardial viability ratio has been used to indicate the ratio between supply and demand.
  - ECG. Preoperative 'silent' ischaemia (i.e. without symptoms) has been found in up to 15% of patients over 40 years old; the significance of this in terms of outcome is unknown. The figure is higher for patients presenting for vascular surgery. Similar episodes of silent ischaemia have been found postoperatively, especially in those with risk factors. It has been suggested that patients who exhibit this are more likely to suffer postoperative MI.
  - pulmonary capillary wedge pressure monitoring.
  - echocardiography.
  - nuclear cardiography.
  - coronary sinus catheterisation.
- Management: as for ischaemic heart disease.

See also, Monitoring; Myocardial metabolism

Myocardial metabolism. Myocardial O_2 consumption is normally about 30 ml/min (10 ml/100 g/min). Coronary blood flow is directly proportional; the mechanism is unclear but may involve adenosine, CO_2, potassium ions, prostaglandins, hydrogen ions and lactate. O_2 extraction from blood is about 70%; thus increased demands are met mainly by increasing blood flow. The main energy substrate is free fatty acids; other substrates include glucose, pyruvate and lactate. Utilisation of the latter compounds increases in ischaemia.

O_2 requirements are reduced by volatile anaesthetic agents and other negative inotropes, e.g. β-adrenergic receptor antagonists. Effects on other factors determining myocardial O_2 supply/demand may be important, e.g. possibility of coronary steal and tachycardia with isoflurane. Etomidate and propofol may decrease demand; other iv agents may increase it if tachycardia occurs.

Myocardial preconditioning, *see Ischaemic preconditioning*

Myocarditis. Inflammation of the cardiac muscle; the definition is difficult because clinical diagnosis (acute cardiac failure, arrhythmias or ECG changes in a cardiologically previously healthy person) is often not supported by the results of biopsy or post-mortem histology (i.e. with lymphocytic infiltration).

- Caused by:
  - infective invasion of cardiac muscle, e.g. viruses (especially coxsackie B and echovirus), many bacteria, rickettsia, fungi, trypanosomiasis. Myocarditis is thought to be a common feature of apparently mild viral upper respiratory tract infections. Features may be prompted by vigorous exercise or anaesthesia and especially if the diagnosis is unsuspected.
  - post-infective inflammation: thought to represent a different mechanism to the above and includes post-viral, HIV infection, rheumatic fever, diphtheria. In the last, bacterial toxins are thought to be responsible.
  - primary autoimmune processes: rheumatic fever, connective tissue diseases, sarcoidosis, thyroid disorders, diabetes mellitus (microangiopathy may also be involved), amyloidosis.
  - other allergic processes, e.g. drug-induced (e.g. penicillin, sulphonamides), rejection of cardiac transplants, serum sickness.
  - direct drug toxicity, e.g. lithium, cyclophosphamide, alcoholism.
  - physical trauma, e.g. radiation.
  - other infiltration or inflammation, e.g. diabetic, myxoedema, haemochromatosis, connective tissue disease, drug-induced (e.g. cytotoxic drugs).

Treatment includes corticosteroids, antiviral drugs and supportive therapy.

Medical and anaesthetic management is as for cardiac disease in general; in acute disease surgery should be deferred if feasible, and as cardiostable an anaesthetic provided as possible. General treatment is supportive according to the presenting features.

Feldman AM, McNamara D (2000). N Engl J Med; 343: 1388–98

Myofascial pain syndromes. Dysfunction and usually pain in one or more muscles/muscle groups, associated with trigger point activity. May follow acute strain or repeated use. Typically associated with patterns of referred pain, e.g. trigger points in the neck with facial pain, trigger points in the shoulder with arm pain, etc. Identified trigger points may be injected with local anaesthetic, treated with acupuncture, ultrasound, pressure, etc., or the muscles passively stretched using a cold spray to allow adequate relaxation.

Myoglobin. Iron-containing molecule with mw 17 000. Similar to haemoglobin, but binds only one molecule of O_2 per molecule. Its O_2 dissociation curve is to the left of that of haemoglobin, being a rectangular hyperbola with a steep rise to a plateau. The Bohr effect does not occur. 95% saturated at P_{O_2} of 5.3 kPa (40 mmHg), falling below 65% saturation only at P_{O_2} below 1 kPa (7.5 mmHg). Found in skeletal and heart muscle, where it binds O_2 from arterial haemoglobin, releasing it at O_2 tensions close to zero. Thus it acts as an O_2 transporter and reservoir for contracting muscle.

See also, Oxyhaemoglobin dissociation curve

Myoglobinuria. Presence of myoglobin in the urine, colouring it red. Results from skeletal muscle breakdown (rhabdomyolysis) due to:

- crush injury (crush syndrome).
- prolonged immobility/hypothermia from any cause, especially poisoning and overdoses (and particularly opioid, alcohol and cocaine overdose).
- extreme exertion.
- polymyositis, myopathies, e.g. alcoholic, deficiency states, congenital conditions, or associated with viral infections.
- toxins, e.g. of sea snakes, multiple wasp stings.
- MH.
- neuroleptic malignant syndrome
- carbon monoxide poisoning
- heatstroke.
- paroxysmal myoglobinuria: rare disorder of muscle pain, weakness, paralysis and myoglobinuria. Most common in young men/children.

Affected muscles are classically painful and oedematous. Creatine kinase levels may be markedly raised. Myoglobin is readily filtered by the kidneys because of its small size. May be associated with renal failure, thought to be caused by ferrihemate, a nephrotoxic breakdown product of myoglobin in acid conditions (myoglobin itself is not thought to be directly nephrotoxic). Tubular obstruction may also be involved. Maintenance of good hydration and urine output is thought to prevent renal impairment. Administration of bicarbonate helps to increase urinary pH and reduce formation of ferrihemate.

Myosin. Muscle protein (mw 460 000), consisting of two heavy and four light chains. Globular portions of the molecules contain ATPase and actin binding sites, and project sideways from myosin filaments.
See also, Muscle contraction

Myotomes. Inner parts of embryonic somites, differentiating into skeletal muscle and related to their corresponding dermatomes. Although the origins of certain skeletal muscle groups are controversial, they tend to retain their original somatic nerve supply; thus particular spinal nerves may be assessed clinically by testing specific muscles or groups (Table 23). Used to assess neurological lesions and the extent of spinal/epidural anaesthesia, etc.

Table 23 Segmental innervation of limb muscles

Movement	*Muscle(s)*	*Level*
Shoulder		
Abduction	Supraspinatus	C4–5
External rotation	Infraspinatus	C4–5
Adduction	Pectoralis	C6–8
Elbow		
Flexion/supination	Biceps	C5–6
Pronation	Pronators	C6–7
Extension	Triceps	C7–8
Wrist		
Extension/radial flexion		C6–7
Ulnar flexion		C7–8
Fingers		
Extension	Long extensors	C7
Flexion	Long flexors	C8
Spreading and closing	All short muscles of the hand	T1
Hip		
Flexion	Iliopsoas	L1–3
Extension	Gluteal	L5–S2
Knee		
Extension	Quadriceps	L3–4
Flexion	Hamstrings	L5–S2
Ankle		
Extension	Anterior tibial	L4–5
Flexion	Calf muscles	S1–2

Myotonia congenita. Autosomal dominant disorder of skeletal muscle. No systemic symptoms occur other than myotonia (involuntarily sustained muscle contraction following stimulation) exacerbated by cold and rest, and relieved by exercise. A more common, milder form is inherited as autosomal recessive. Anaesthetic management is as for dystrophia myotonica. Hypothermia should be avoided. An association with MH has been suggested although there are difficulties in interpreting the caffeine–halothane contracture test in myotonic patients.

Myotonic syndromes. Group of inherited muscle diseases including dystrophia myotonica and myotonia congenita characterised by an increase in muscle tone (myotonia) following muscular contraction. Myotonia may also be present in hyperkalaemic periodic paralysis. Anaesthetic considerations are related to systemic manifestations of the disease and the effects of certain anaesthetic drugs worsening myotonia, e.g. suxamethonium.

Myxoedema, *see Hypothyroidism*

N

Nabilone. Cannabinoid antiemetic drug, acting on CB_1 and CB_2 cannabis receptors, used in chemotherapy-induced nausea and vomiting. Has also been used in terminal care.
- Dosage: 1–2 mg orally 8–12 hourly.
- Side effects: drowsiness, ataxia, visual disturbances, sleep disturbances, hypotension, tachycardia.

Nalbuphine hydrochloride. Opioid analgesic drug and opioid receptor antagonist, synthesised in 1968. Partial agonist at kappa and sigma opioid receptors, and antagonist at mu receptors. Used for premedication, anaesthesia and treatment of pain. Active within 2–3 min of iv, or 15 min of im, injection. Half-life is about 5 h. Undergoes hepatic metabolism and excreted renally. Side effects such as vomiting are thought to be less than with morphine, although maximal analgesia attainable is also less. Psychomimetic effects are less problematic than with pentazocine.
- Dosage: 0.1–0.3 mg/kg iv/im/sc. Up to 1.0 mg/kg iv has been used during anaesthesia.

Nalmefene hydrochloride. Opioid receptor antagonist, introduced in the USA in 1995. Longer half-life (10.8 h) than naloxone, thus less likely for opioid effects to recur following reversal.

Nalorphine hydrochloride/hydrobromide. Opioid analgesic drug and opioid receptor antagonist, synthesised in 1941. Partial agonist at kappa and sigma opioid receptors, and antagonist at mu receptors. Psychomimetic effects are common at analgesic doses (5–10 mg). No longer available.

Naloxone hydrochloride. Opioid receptor antagonist, synthesised in 1961. *N*-Allyl derivative of oxymorphone. Although it has a high affinity for the mu receptor, it has no intrinsic activity. Used to reverse unwanted effects of opioid analgesic drugs, e.g. sedation, respiratory depression, spasm of the biliary sphincter. Also reverses opioid-mediated analgesia. Reverses the effects of pentazocine but not buprenorphine. Has been used to reverse ventilatory depression and pruritus following spinal opioids, without reversing analgesia. Has also been used in poisoning and overdoses due to other depressant drugs, e.g. alcohols, benzodiazepines, barbiturates, although its efficacy is disputed. Reportedly useful in septic shock, increasing BP and cardiac output; the mechanism is unclear but may involve increase of endogenous catecholamine release or antagonism of increased levels of endorphins that occur in sepsis. Effective within 1–2 min of iv injection, with a half-life of 1–2 h; thus depressant effects of opioid analgesic drugs may recur after a few hours. Metabolised in the liver and excreted mainly renally.
- Dosage:
  - opioid poisoning: 0.4–2.0 mg iv/im/sc, repeated after 2–3 min to a total of 10 mg. Administration by infusion (3–10 μg/kg/h) may be required.
  - postoperatively: 1.5–3 μg/kg iv, followed by 1.5 μg/kg repeated every 2 min as required. Infusion or im injection may be used to prevent later resedation.
  - neonatal resuscitation: 10 μg/kg im, iv or sc repeated every 2–3 min or 60 μg/kg im as a single injection.
- Side effects: hypertension, arrhythmias, pulmonary oedema and cardiac arrest have followed sudden iv injection, possibly due to sudden catecholamine release secondary to reversal of sedation and analgesia.

  Acute withdrawal may be precipitated in patients addicted to opioids.

NALS, Neonatal Advanced Life Support, *see Neonatal Resuscitation Program*

Naltrexone hydrochloride. Opioid receptor antagonist, synthesised in 1965. Derived from naloxone, with similar actions but longer duration (24 h after a single dose). Used in the treatment of opioid and alcohol dependence.
- Dosage: 25–50 mg/day orally. Has also been given via subcutaneous implants.

Naproxen. NSAID derived from propionic acid. Has a favourable side effect profile among NSAIDs, and can be given just twice daily.
- Dosage:
  - 250–500 mg orally, 12 hourly.
  - 500 mg pr, 12–24 hourly.
- Side effects: as for NSAIDs.

Narcotic drugs. Strictly, drugs which induce sleep, but the term usually refers to morphine-like drugs. Preferred terms include opiates, opioids and opioid analgesic drugs.

Nasal inhalers. Used instead of facepieces for dental anaesthesia. Designed to fit over the nose, leaving the mouth free. During induction of anaesthesia, the patient is instructed not to 'mouth breathe'. During anaesthesia, a mouth pack prevents mouth breathing.
- Different types:
  - Goldman's: black rubber, with an inflatable rim as for facepieces. Incorporates an adjustable pressure-limiting valve, and attaches to the breathing system over the patient's forehead. It should be held from behind the patient's head using both thumbs whilst the other fingers support the jaw. May also be held with a head harness using two studs incorporated into the sides.
  - McKesson's: made of malleable black rubber, thus adjustable. Connected to the breathing system via two tubes which pass around the sides of the head to meet behind, helping to hold the inhaler in place. Incorporates an expiratory valve.
  - newer types are made of plastic, and may incorporate unidirectional gas flow, e.g. through inspiratory and expiratory tubes passing around the head. Scavenging of exhaled gases is thus aided.

[Victor Goldman (1903–1993), London anaesthetist]

Nasal positive pressure ventilation, *see Non-invasive positive pressure ventilation*

Nasogastric intubation. Performed for enteral nutrition, or gastric drainage. Fine bore tubes are used for the former, usually inserted using a wire stilette, which is removed after placement. Larger tubes (e.g. 10–16 Ch) are used for gastric drainage, e.g. following abdominal surgery or in intestinal obstruction. They may be placed in the awake patient (who aids placement by swallowing or sipping water) or unconscious patient (e.g. after induction of anaesthesia, either before or after tracheal intubation). Placement can often be performed blindly, and may be aided by passage through a plain nasal tracheal tube placed into the pharynx or by prior transient inflation of the upper oesophagus via a tightly fitting facepiece. Placement may require direct vision using a laryngoscope and forceps (the oesophagus lies posterior to the larynx and to the left of the midline). Correct placement is confirmed by aspiration of gastric contents (may be tested for acidity), auscultation over the left hypochondrium during injection of air, palpation by the surgeon during surgery or abdominal X-ray. If already in place, withdrawal of the tube prior to induction of anaesthesia has been suggested, to avoid increasing gastro-oesophageal reflux or rendering cricoid pressure inefficient. However, this is rarely done.

National Confidential Enquiry into Patient Outcome and Death (NCEPOD). Ongoing study originally commissioned by the Association of Anaesthetists of Great Britain and Ireland, together with the Association of Surgeons of Great Britain and Ireland, and published in 1987 as the Confidential Enquiry into Perioperative Deaths (CEPOD). The first UK study to involve both anaesthetists and surgeons, it analysed all 4000 NHS deaths in three regions, occurring within 30 days of surgery during 1986, excluding obstetric and cardiac surgery. Individual consultants involved with deaths were invited to fill out forms for further assessment. The first national Report (NCEPOD; 1989) focused on children under 10 years; subsequent Reports have focussed on particular aspects, e.g. deaths following specific surgical or interventional procedures or in specific age groups, out-of-hours operating, etc.

The scheme now includes independent hospitals and also involves the Royal Colleges of Anaesthetists, Obstetricians and Gynaecologists, Ophthalmologists, Pathologists, Physicians, Radiologists and Surgeons, and the Faculties of Dental Surgery and Public Health Medicine of the Royal Colleges of Surgeons and Physicians respectively. The name changed in 2002 to the National Confidential Enquiry into Patient Outcome and Death, reflecting extension of NCEPOD's remit to include physicians and primary care and to review near-misses as well as deaths. NCEPOD is funded mainly by the Department of Health via the National Patient Safety Agency though is an independent body.

- General findings and recommendations:
  - most deaths occur in elderly and/or the sickest patients.
  - overall care is good but there are identifiable deficiencies:
    - inadequate consultation between trainees and their seniors and between anaesthetists and surgeons.
    - inadequate supervision and training of locum and trainee (and in later reports, of non-consultant career grade) anaesthetists and surgeons. Also, inappropriate vetting of locum staff.
    - inappropriate decisions to operate in hopeless cases.
    - operating outside the surgeon's subspecialty.
    - inadequate prophylaxis against DVT.
    - insufficient appreciation of the importance of preoperative resuscitation, especially in the elderly and non-elective surgery.
    - inappropriate operating at night.
    - insufficient emergency operating theatre, ICU and HDU facilities.
    - lack of involvement of senior staff in emergency lists and paediatric cases.
    - non-availability of fibreoptic intubating equipment.
    - sending inappropriate staff with critically ill patients during transfer.
    - poor quality and unavailability of medical records.
  - the need for post-mortem examination, audit and morbidity/mortality assessments has been repeatedly stressed.

National Halothane Study, *see Halothane hepatitis*

National Institute for Clinical Excellence (NICE). NHS Special Health Authority for England and Wales, established in 1999 to provide authoritative, robust and reliable guidance on current 'best practice'. Its guidance covers both individual health technologies (including medicines, medical devices, diagnostic techniques and procedures) and the clinical management of specific conditions. In 2005, NICE took on the functions of the Health Development Agency to become the National Institute for Health and Clinical Excellence (though still known as NICE). Is thus responsible for providing national guidance on the promotion of good health and the prevention and treatment of ill health.

National Patient Safety Agency (NPSA). NHS Special Health Authority formed in 2001 to coordinate reports of adverse events or 'near misses' and their analysis. Now incorporates three main services:

- Patient Safety Division: collection and analysis of information on patient safety incidents in the NHS, producing reports and recommendations to reduce future risk. Recent reports or campaigns of anaesthetic interest/relevance include hand hygiene/infection control, accidental iv administration of local anaesthetics and other drug errors, and management of throat packs. Also commissions the national confidential enquiries (into maternal and child health, patient outcome and death, and suicide and homicide).
- National Clinical Assessment Service (NCAS): provision of advice and support to the NHS regarding concerns about doctors' and dentists' performance.
- National Research Ethics Service (formerly the Central Office of Research Ethics Committees; COREC): administration of a structure for ethical review of research across the UK.

See also, Confidential Enquiry into Maternal Deaths; National Confidential Enquiry into Patient Outcome and Death

Natriuretic hormone, *see Atrial natriuretic peptide*

Nausea, *see Postoperative nausea and vomiting; Vomiting*

NCEPOD, *see National Confidential Enquiry into Patient Outcome and Death*

Near-drowning. Defined as initial survival following immersion in liquid, usually water; death at the time of immersion may be due to anoxia (drowning), or cardiac arrest caused by sudden extreme lowering of temperature (immersion syndrome). Secondary drowning refers to death following near-drowning after a period of relative wellbeing and is usually due to ARDS/acute lung injury.

Autopsy following drowning reveals little or no lung water in 15% of cases (dry drowning); laryngospasm following initial laryngeal contamination has been suggested. In 85% of cases, pulmonary aspiration of water occurs (wet drowning); this may involve:

- fresh water: systemic absorption may cause haemolysis, haemodilution and electrolyte disturbances.
- salt water: draws water into the lungs.

Both types cause pulmonary oedema and hypoxaemia. Haemodynamic changes due to fluid shifts are rare; thus in practice the type of water may have little clinical significance.

Other adverse factors include hypothermia, aspiration of gastric contents, and predisposing conditions, e.g. alcoholism or drug abuse, trauma, epilepsy, MI, CVA, etc.

Complications include ARDS, cerebral oedema, renal failure, pneumonia, pancreatitis, acidosis and shock. Sepsis is especially likely if the water is contaminated.

- Management:
  - CPR.
  - treatment of complications as appropriate.
  - rewarming.
  - antibiotics as appropriate. Use of corticosteroids is controversial and declining.
  - nasogastric aspiration to remove gastric water.

Recovery has been reported after up to 60 minutes' immersion followed by prolonged CPR, especially in children and if hypothermic. Cerebral damage may occur.

Harries M (2003) BMJ; 327: 1336–8

Near infra-red oximetry/spectroscopy (NIRS). Monitoring technique based on the principle that light with wavelengths in the near infra-red region (650–900 mm) transmits through biological tissues. Increasingly used to image biological events in the cerebral cortex. Photons produced by a laser photodiode are directed into the skull; whilst many are reflected and dispersed, a proportion are transmitted. Coloured compounds within the tissues (chromophores), especially oxyhaemoglobin, deoxyhaemoglobin and oxidised cytochrome oxidase, have characteristic absorption spectra. The emergent light intensity is detected and a computer converts the changes in light intensity into changes in chromophore concentration. Clinical applications include monitoring of cerebral oxygenation and cerebral blood flow and volume, e.g. in neurosurgery, cardiac surgery and head injury.

Owen-Reece H, Smith M, Elwell CE, Goldstone JC (1999). Br J Anaesth; 82: 418–26

See also, Functional imaging

Nebulisers. Devices used to provide a suspension of droplets in a gas, for administration of inhaled drugs or humidification. Droplets of 5 μm are deposited in the trachea and bronchi; those of 1 μm pass to alveoli and may impair gas exchange. Thus the ideal droplet size is between 1 and 5 μm.

- Nebulisers may be:
  - gas-driven: water is entrained by the gas flow (Venturi principle) and broken into a spray; this may be directed against an anvil which breaks up the drops into smaller droplets. May be combined with a heater.
  - ultrasonic: droplets are formed from water lying on a vibrating plate, or from water dropped on to the plate. Water overload may occur, since the droplets are very small and the water content of the gas is high.
  - mechanical: water is dispersed into a mist by a spinning disc.

  Gas-driven devices are used for drug delivery; all types may be used for humidification.

Neck, cross-sectional anatomy. At the level of C6, major anatomical structures within the layer of skin, fat and subcutaneous tissue are related to fascial layers (Fig. 110):

- superficial fascia: encloses platysma muscle and deep fascial layers.
- deep fascia: comprised of three layers:
  - investing fascia: lies posterior to the anterior and external jugular veins. Splits to enclose sternohyoid, sternothyroid, omohyoid, sternomastoid and trapezius muscles.
  - prevertebral fascia: extends laterally on scalenus anterior and medius to form the floor of the posterior triangle of the neck, and passes downwards to form the axillary sheath. Separated from the oesophageal/pharyngeal junction in the midline by the retropharyngeal space.

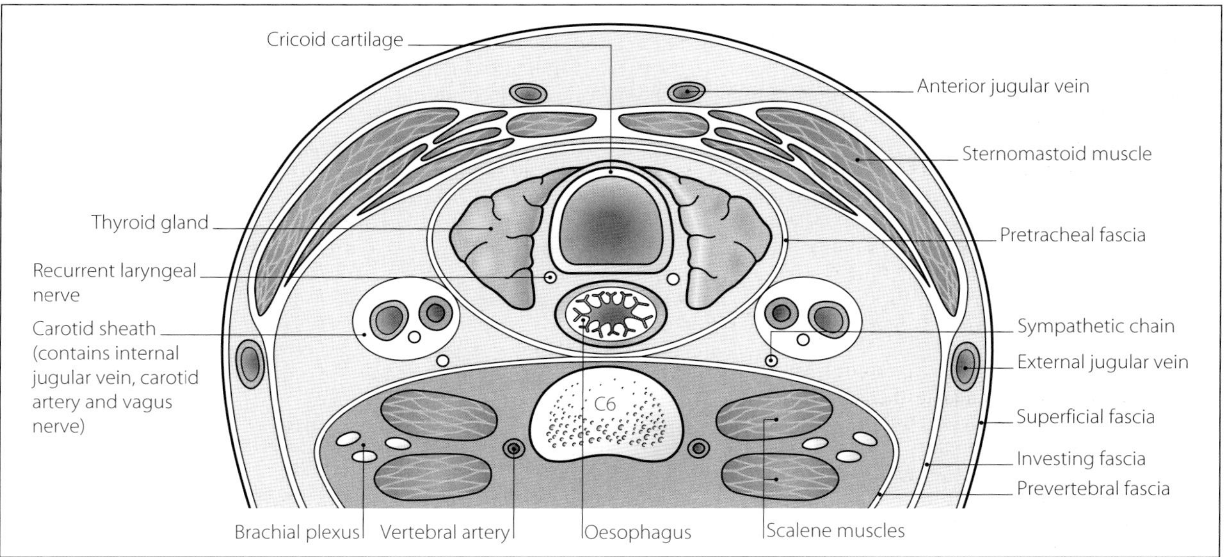

Fig. 110 Cross-section of neck at C6

- pretracheal fascia: contains the trachea, oesophagus and thyroid gland.

See also, Carotid arteries; Tracheobronchial tree

Necrotising enterocolitis (NEC). Necrosis of GIT mucosa (especially terminal ileum, caecum and ascending colon) seen in neonates, usually within the first week of life. Prevalence is up to 8% in premature and low birth weight babies; predisposing factors include asphyxia, hypotension and umbilical catheterisation. Mucosal damage follows hypoperfusion and ischaemia, leading to abdominal distension, vomiting and faecal blood and mucus, although the onset may be insidious. Pallor, bradycardia, jaundice, intestinal perforation and DIC may occur. Plain abdominal X-ray shows dilated loops of bowel and intramural gas bubbles.

Management is largely supportive, with iv fluids, IPPV, correction of anaemia, antibacterial drugs (including anaerobic cover), probiotic agents and TPN. Surgery may be required if perforation occurs or there is no improvement despite medical therapy. Mortality remains 5–10%.

Lin PW, Stoll BJ (2006). Lancet; 368: 1271–83

Necrotising fasciitis. Uncommon deep-seated infection of subcutaneous tissue resulting in destruction of fat and fascia. Predisposing factors include immunosuppression, alcoholism, diabetes, peripheral vascular disease, surgery, penetrating injuries (which may be minor) and varicella infection, although it may affect young healthy individuals. Systemic upset is thought to result from bacterial toxins and endogenous cytokines and other inflammatory mediators. May be rapidly fatal unless aggressively treated. May be caused by:

- Gram-negative bacilli, enterococci and mixed anaerobes. Infection involves fat and fascia although the skin is usually spared. Includes Fournier's gangrene of the perineum.
- group A streptococci. Features include systemic toxicity, pain, necrosis of subcutaneous tissue and skin, gangrene, shock and MODS.

- Management:
    - prompt diagnosis; made on clinical grounds although MRI and biopsy may help distinguish it from acute cellulitis.
    - early surgical debridement (the diagnosis is usually confirmed at surgery), with fasciotomy to prevent compartment syndrome.
    - antibacterial drug therapy and general supportive care; hyperbaric oxygen has been suggested.

[Jean A Fournier (1832–1914), Paris dermatologist]

Hasham S, Matteucci P, Stanley PRW, Hart NB (2005). BMJ; 330: 830–3

Needles. Christopher Wren described injection via a quill and bladder in 1659. Metal tubes and stylets were subsequently used, but the hypodermic cannula and trocar were first described by Rynd in 1845. Different sizes and types are available for different uses, e.g. for iv/hypodermic use, epidural and spinal anaesthesia. Short-bevelled needles are traditionally preferred for regional anaesthesia. Internal lumina are not required for needles used for acupuncture or electrical stimulation/recording.

Needle size is described by a wire gauge classification (G; Stubs Gauge; Birmingham Gauge) which originally referred to the number of times the wire was drawn through the draw plate (Table 24). It differs slightly from the American and Standard Wire Gauges. Inside diameter varies according to different materials and needle strengths. The system is also used for iv cannulae. For hypodermic needles, colour-coding is mandatory in the UK for certain sizes: 26 G brown; 25 G orange; 23 G blue; 22 G black; 21 G green; 20 G yellow; 19 G cream.

[Sir Christopher Wren (1633–1723), English scientist and architect; Francis Rynd (1801–1861), Irish surgeon; Peter Stubs (1756–1806), English toolmaker and innkeeper]

Table 24 Diameter of needles of different gauge number

Gauge number (G)	Outside diameter (mm)
36	0.10
30	0.30
29	0.33
28	0.36
27	0.41
26	0.46
25	0.51
24	0.56
23	0.64
22	0.71
21	0.81
20	0.90
19	1.08
18	1.27
17	1.50
16	1.65
15	1.83
14	2.11
13	2.41
12	2.77
11	3.05
10	3.40
9	3.76
8	4.19
7	4.57
6	5.16
1	7.62

Needlestick injury, *see Environmental safety of anaesthetists*

NEEP, *see Negative end-expiratory pressure*

Nefopam hydrochloride. Analgesic drug, unrelated to opioid analgesic drugs and NSAIDs. Peak action occurs 1–2 h after im injection. Drowsiness and respiratory depression may occur, but less than with opioids.

- Dosage:
    - 30–90 mg orally, 8 hourly.
    - 20 mg im, 6 hourly.
- Side effects: nausea, headache, confusion, anticholinergic effects. Should be avoided in patients with epilepsy and those taking monoamine oxidase inhibitors.

Negative end-expiratory pressure (NEEP). Adjunct to IPPV, popular in the 1960s–1970s as a method of reducing the adverse cardiovascular effects of IPPV by maintaining a subatmospheric airway pressure at end-expiration. However, NEEP increases airway collapse, alveolar–arterial O_2 difference and dead space, whilst reducing FRC. Thus no longer used.

Negligence. Civil charge in which the following must be established:

- duty of care owed to the patient by the doctor, other professional or institution.

- failure in that duty.
- harm suffered as a result of that failure.

Although the duty of care and failure in that duty may be easy to demonstrate, establishing according to the 'balance of probabilities' that harm is a direct result of that failure is usually more difficult. A doctor's action (or lack thereof) is judged against that of a 'reasonable' body of medical opinion – even if that body is a minority (Bolam test); traditionally the fact that such a body of opinion exists has usually been enough for a successful defence against a charge of negligence in the UK. More recently the courts have scrutinised the reasoning and evidence behind such opinion before accepting that it is 'reasonable'. In the UK, since negligence must be proved in order for compensation to be paid, inability to establish this link will result in no compensation. Thus there have been calls for no-fault compensation schemes similar to that in New Zealand, in which the fact that harm has occurred is enough to result in compensation without having to prove negligence.

[John Bolam, UK psychiatric patient; suffered fractures in 1954 during electroconvulsive therapy administered without anaesthetic or restraint, then claimed negligence by the hospital. The claim was dismissed because withholding of anaesthesia was accepted medical practice at the time.]

Neisserial infections. Mostly caused by two species of the Gram-positive cocci genus:

- *N. gonorrhoeae*: may cause acute endocarditis, urethritis, pelvic inflammatory disease and pelvic abscesses.
- *N. meningitidis* (meningococcus): causes meningococcal disease including meningitis. The organism may be carried in the nasopharynx of about 5% of otherwise healthy subjects, increasing to about 30% during epidemics.

Neisserial infection is common in complement deficiency.
[Albert Neisser (1855–1916), German physician]

Neomycin sulphate. Aminoglycoside and antibacterial drug, used topically for skin or mucous membrane infections and orally in hepatic failure, prior to bowel surgery, and in selective decontamination of the digestive tract.

- Dosage: 1 g orally, 4 hourly.
- Side effects: as for aminoglycosides. May be absorbed systemically in hepatic failure resulting in toxicity.

Neonatal resuscitation, *see Cardiopulmonary resuscitation, neonatal*

Neonatal Resuscitation Program (NRP). Programme of training in neonatal CPR, established in 1988 in the US and administered by the American Heart Association and American Academy of Pediatrics. Similar in concept to the ATLS and related courses. Has been referred to as 'NALS' (Neonatal Advanced Life Support) but the term is not an official one.

Neonate. Child within 28 days of birth. Usually weighs 3–4 kg, with body surface area approximately 0.19 m^2.

- Major changes at birth include the following:
  - change from fetal circulation to adult circulation via transitional circulation. The fibrous left ventricle, which is of similar size to the right ventricle at birth, gradually increases in compliance and contractility.
  - expansion of fluid-filled alveoli; requires negative intrapleural pressures exceeding 70 cmH_2O. Increasing numbers of alveoli are expanded in successive breaths. Most fluid is rapidly expelled via the upper airway, with the remainder drained via capillary and lymphatic vessels over 1–3 days.

Anatomical and physiological features, and principles of anaesthesia are as for paediatric anaesthesia. Perioperative risks are higher than for older children, especially in premature neonates; surgery is usually deferred if possible.

See also, Cardiopulmonary resuscitation, neonatal; Fetal haemoglobin; Fetal monitoring; Neurobehavioural testing of neonates; Obstetric analgesia and anaesthesia; Paediatric advanced life support; Paediatric intensive care; Surfactant

Neostigmine methylsulphate/bromide. Acetylcholinesterase inhibitor, synthesised in 1931. Used to increase acetylcholine concentrations at the neuromuscular junction, e.g. reversal of non-depolarising neuromuscular blockade and myasthenia gravis. Also has a direct stimulatory effect on skeletal muscle acetylcholine receptors; in addition, it is thought to have significant presynaptic action, increasing the amount of acetylcholine released. May cause depolarising neuromuscular blockade in overdosage. Other effects are those of muscarinic stimulation, e.g. bradycardia, increased GIT motility and bladder contractility, sweating, salivation, miosis, bronchospasm. Has been used to treat urinary retention and ileus, e.g. postoperatively. Effects on autonomic ganglia are small, consisting of stimulation at low doses and depression at high doses. A quaternary ammonium compound, it crosses the blood–brain barrier poorly and has few CNS effects. Routinely given with atropine or glycopyrronium when administered iv to prevent muscarinic effects. Active within 1 min of iv injection, with action lasting 20–30 min. Active for up to 4 h after oral administration. Excreted mainly renally, mostly unchanged. Elimination half-life is 50–90 min. May be administered parenterally (as methylsulphate) or orally (as bromide). Has also been given intrathecally; produces analgesia but with increased nausea and vomiting.

- Dosage:
  - reversal of non-depolarising blockade: 0.04–0.08 mg/kg iv with 0.02–0.04 mg/kg atropine or 10–20 μg/kg glycopyrronium.
  - myasthenia gravis: 15–30 mg orally or 1.0–2.5 mg sc/im, 2–4 hourly.
  - other uses: as for myasthenia gravis.
- Side effects: as above. Cholinergic crisis may occur in overdosage.

Neosynephrine, *see Phenylephrine*

Nephritic syndrome. Acute glomerular disease characterised by reduction of glomerular filtration rate, haematuria, salt and water retention, increased intravascular volume and hypertension. Usually mild; severe cases may result in acute renal failure. Distinction between it and nephrotic syndrome has been overplayed in the past and both share common aetiologies.

Nephron. Basic renal unit; each kidney contains about 1.3 million.

- Structure (Fig. 111a):
  - glomerulus: formed by a 200 μm diameter invagination of capillaries into the blind end of the nephron (Bowman's capsule). Water is filtered from the blood across the glomerular membrane, together with substances under 4–8 nm in diameter. GFR equals about 120 ml/min (180 l/day).

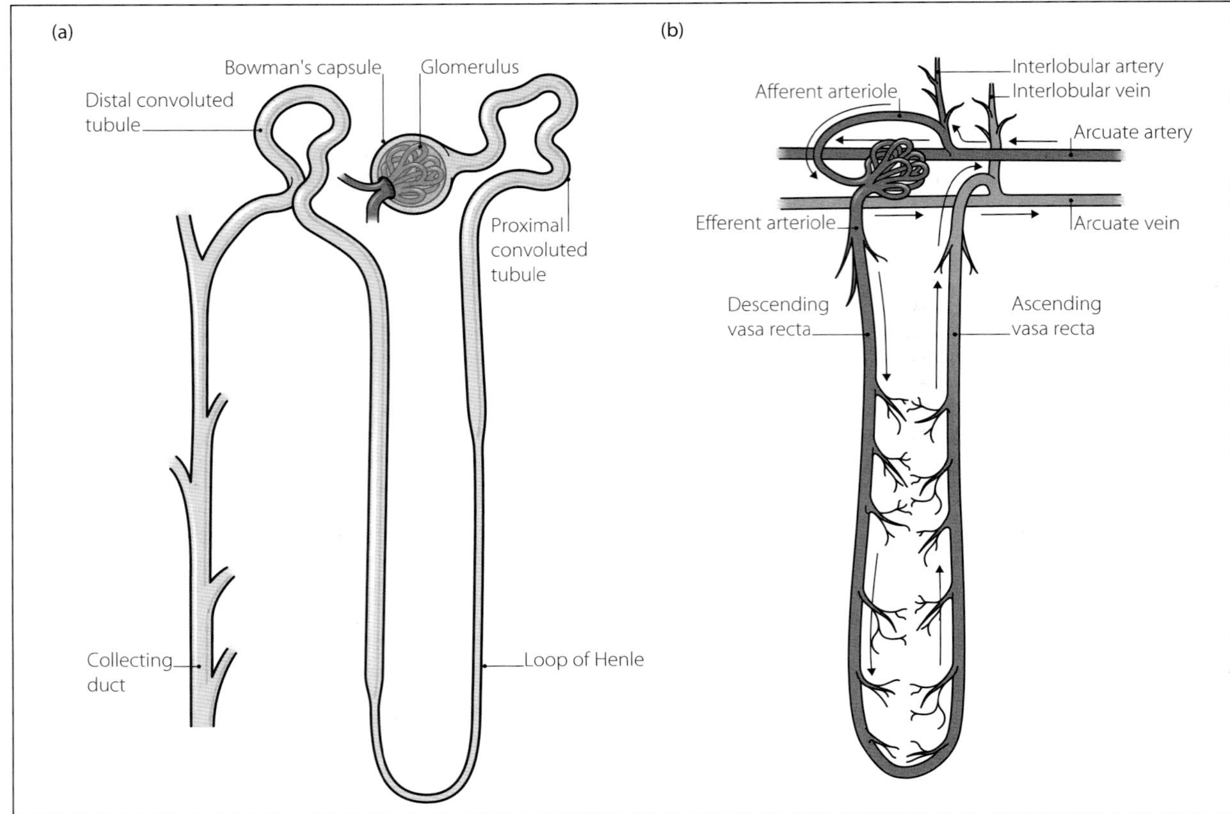

Fig. 111 Structure of nephron: (a) glomerulotubular system; (b) vascular system

- tubule: 45–65 mm long. The site of reabsorption/secretion of substances from/into the filtrate, giving rise to the eventual composition of urine. Consists of:
  - proximal convoluted tubule: 15 mm long. Lies within the renal cortex. Lined by a brush border. Site of active reabsorption of sodium and potassium ions, bicarbonate, phosphate, glucose, uric acid and amino acids. Water moves passively from the tubule by osmosis. Up to 80% of filtered water and solutes are reabsorbed.
  - loop of Henle: about 15–25 cm long; length depends on whether the glomerulus lies within the outer or inner renal cortex (short in the former, long in the latter). A further 15% of filtered water is reabsorbed. 15% of loops extend into the medulla, where interstitial osmolality is very high (up to 1200 mosmol/l). Water moves out of the descending limb, followed by sodium ions along a concentration gradient as the tubular fluid becomes more concentrated. In the ascending limb, which is impermeable to both water and sodium ions, sodium and chloride ions are actively co-transported from the tubule. The fluid thus becomes more dilute as it ascends. Urea is relatively free to pass across the tubular membranes. The solutes remain in the region of the medulla because of the countercurrent multiplier mechanism whereby the blood vessels supplying the loop pass close to those draining it. Solutes pass down concentration gradients from ascending vessels to descending vessels, and thus recirculate at the tip of the loop. Water passes from the descending vessels to the ascending vessels, and is thus removed from the area. This maintains the high osmolality in the medullary region. The thick ascending segment forms part of the juxtaglomerular apparatus where it passes near the glomerulus.
  - distal convoluted tubule: 5 mm long. A further 5% of filtered water is reabsorbed. Sodium ions are reabsorbed in exchange for potassium or hydrogen ions, under the influence of aldosterone.
- collecting ducts: 20 mm long. Each receives several tubules. Pass through the cortex and medulla, opening into the renal pelvis at the medullary pyramids. Some sodium/potassium/hydrogen ion exchange occurs at the cortical part. Water is reabsorbed depending on the amount of vasopressin present, which increases tubular permeability to water and thus increases urine concentration.

- Blood supply (Fig. 111b):
  - afferent and efferent arterioles supply and drain the capillaries to the glomerulus respectively.
  - efferent arterioles subsequently divide to form peritubular capillaries or vasa recta (long loops which accompany the loop of Henle).
  - peritubular capillaries and ascending vasa recta drain into interlobular veins.

[Sir William P Bowman (1816–1892), English surgeon; Friedrich GJ Henle (1809–1885), German anatomist]

See also, Acid–base balance; Clearance; Diuretics; Renin/angiotensin system

Nephrotic syndrome. Defined by daily urinary protein excretion exceeding 3.5 g/1.73 m^2 body surface area. May be caused by primary or secondary (e.g. to diabetes mellitus, pre-eclampsia, connective tissue disease, post-viral hepatitis or streptococcal infection, drugs such as NSAIDs or captopril) glomerular disease. Features include generalised oedema, susceptibility to infection and thromboembolism (especially renal vein thrombosis and DVT), and hyperlipidaemia. Hypoalbuminaemia may lead to altered drug binding.

Treatment includes a low sodium diet and diuretic therapy to reduce oedema, and a low protein diet and angiotensin converting enzyme inhibitors to reduce proteinuria. Other treatment is directed against the cause, e.g. corticosteroids in glomerulonephritis.

See also, Renal failure

Nernst equation. Equation for calculating the membrane potential at which individual ions are at equilibrium across the membrane. For ion X:

$$E = \frac{RT}{FZ} \ln \frac{[X]_o}{[X]_i}$$

where E = equilibrium potential
R = universal gas constant
T = absolute temperature
F = Faraday constant (coulombs per mole of charge)
Z = valence of the ion
$[X]_o$ = extracellular concentration of X
$[X]_i$ = intracellular concentration of X.

For chloride, potassium and sodium, $E = -70$ mV, -94 mV and $+60$ mV respectively. Since the normal resting membrane potential is about -70 mV, other factors must affect potassium and especially sodium distribution (i.e. the sodium/potassium pump).

[Hermann W Nernst (1864–1941), German physicist; Michael Faraday (1791–1867), English scientist]

Nerve. Excitable tissue whose function is the transmission of nerve impulses. Typical peripheral nerves consist of several groups of fascicles. Each fascicle is surrounded by the perineurium and contains a group of neurones, the axons of which are encased in the endoneurium (Fig. 112).

Peripheral nerves originate in the spinal cord, and may be sensory, motor or mixed. Some also carry autonomic nervous system fibres.

See also, Motor pathways; Sensory pathways

Nerve conduction. Passage of an action potential along neurones; involves waves of depolarisation and repolarisation that move longitudinally across the nerve membrane.

In unmyelinated nerves, impulses spread at up to 2 m/s. Positive charge flows into the depolarised area from the membrane just distally, altering the distal permeability to ions (especially sodium and potassium) as for action potential generation. When the threshold potential is reached, depolarisation occurs. Retrograde conduction is prevented by the refractory period of the membrane proximally.

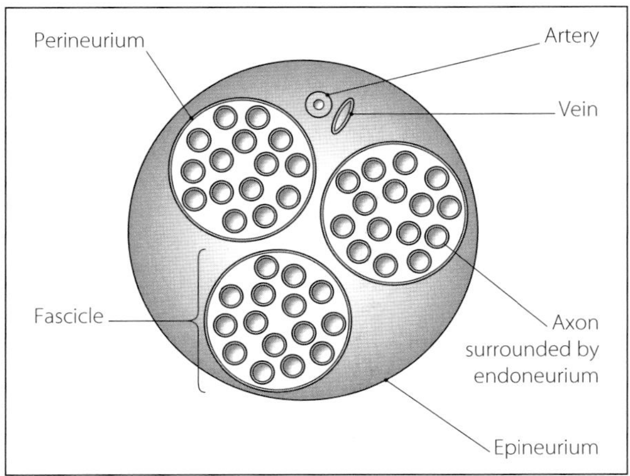

Fig. 112 Cross-section of a typical nerve

The myelin sheath of myelinated nerves acts as an insulator that prevents the flow of ions across the nerve membrane. Breaks in the myelin (nodes of Ranvier), approximately 1 mm apart, allow ions to flow freely between the neurone and the ECF at these points. Depolarisation 'jumps' from node to node (saltatory conduction), a process that increases conduction velocity (up to 120 m/s) and conserves energy.

[Louis A Ranvier (1835–1922), French pathologist and physician]

Nerve growth factor (NGF). Protein produced by many cell types; taken up by small sensory and sympathetic nerve fibres via specific receptors and retrogradely transported to the cell body. Required for growth and survival of neurones in the fetus and neonate; released from connective tissue and inflammatory cells following tissue injury in adults in response to cytokine stimulation. Causes hyperalgesia via both central and peripheral effects and thus thought to be important in acute pain and possibly chronic pain states, perhaps by involvement in adaptation to painful stimuli.

Sofroniew MV, Howe CL, Mobley WC (2001). Ann Rev Neuroscience; 24: 1217–81

Nerve injury during anaesthesia. May occur during general, local or regional anaesthesia.

- Causes of neuronal injury include:
  - general anaesthesia:
    - poor positioning of the patient; thought to cause local nerve ischaemia.
    - ischaemia caused by hypotension or use of tourniquets.
    - hypothermia.
    - extravasation of drugs into perineural tissue.
    - toxicity of degradation products of anaesthetic agents, classically trichloroethylene with soda lime.
  - local/regional anaesthesia: positioning/ischaemia/hypothermia as above plus:
    - direct trauma from a needle or catheter.
    - intraneural injection of local anaesthetic agent.
    - cauda equina syndrome following use of microspinal catheters for continuous spinal anaesthesia.
    - infection.
    - haematoma formation.
    - chemical contamination of local anaesthetic, or injection of the wrong solution.
    - poor positioning of the part rendered anaesthetic with ischaemia as above.
  - other:
    - central venous cannulation.
    - tracheal intubation.
- Classic division of nerve injuries:
  - neurapraxia: caused by compression. Typically incomplete, affecting motor more than sensory components (when present, touch and proprioception predominate). Usually recovers within 6 weeks. Damage during general anaesthesia is usually of this nature, and associated with positioning.
  - axonotmesis: axonal and myelin loss within the intact connective tissue sheath. Typically there is complete motor and sensory loss, with slow recovery due to nerve regeneration from proximal to distal nerve.
  - neurotmesis: partial or complete severance. Recovery is rare.

Electromyographic and conduction studies may aid differentiation between types of injury, and are most useful 1–3 weeks after injury.

- Many specific neuropathies have been described, including lesions of the following:
  - brachial plexus: usually stretched, typically by shoulder abduction and extension, with supination. Stretch is exacerbated by bilateral abduction. Upper roots are usually affected; weakness lasts up to several months, although recovery usually occurs within 2–3 months. Lower roots may be damaged during sternal retraction in cardiac surgery. Compression may be caused by shoulder rests in the steep head-down position, resulting in temporary palsy.
  - ulnar nerve (most common nerve injury reported): may be compressed between the humeral epicondyle and the operating table, or injured by the stretcher poles during transfer of the patient.
  - radial nerve: caused by the patient's arm hanging over the side of the operating table.
  - median nerve: may be damaged by direct needle trauma, or drug extravasation in the antecubital fossa.
  - facial nerve: compressed between the anaesthetist's fingers and the patient's mandible during mask anaesthesia.
  - abducens nerve: temporary lesions may follow spinal or epidural anaesthesia.
  - trigeminal nerve: typically damaged by the trichlorοethylene/soda lime interaction.
  - supraorbital nerve: compressed by the tracheal tube connector, catheter mount, head harness or ventilator tubing.
  - common peroneal nerve: compressed between lithotomy pole and fibular head.
  - saphenous nerve: compressed between lithotomy pole and medial tibial condyle.
  - sciatic nerve: damaged by im injections or compressed against the operating table in emaciated patients.
  - pudendal nerve: compressed between a poorly padded perineal post and the ischial tuberosity.

Nerve injury may also be caused by surgical trauma/compression.

Similar concerns exist for patients undergoing prolonged treatment on ICU.

Sawyer RJ, Richmond MN, Hickey JD, Jarrett JA (2000). Anaesthesia; 55: 980–91

See also, Cranial nerves; Critical illness polyneuropathy

Nerve stimulator, *see Neuromuscular blockade monitoring; Regional anaesthesia; Transcutaneous electrical nerve stimulation*

Netilmicin. Aminoglycoside and antibacterial drug with similar activity to gentamicin but less active against pseudomonas. Less ototoxic than gentamicin.

- Dosage: 4–6 mg/kg im/slowly iv, daily or up to 2.5 mg/kg im/slowly iv, 8–12 hourly. Blood concentrations: 1 h post-dose < 12 mg/l; pre-dose < 2 mg/l.
- Side effects: as for aminoglycosides.

Neuralgia. Pain in distribution of nerve(s).

Neuritis. Inflammation of nerve(s).

Neurobehavioural testing of neonates. Investigation of the effects of obstetric analgesia and anaesthesia on the neonate is difficult because of many variables, e.g. obstetric details, fetal distress, method of delivery, type and route of drugs administered, methods of analysis of data, etc. In many early studies, aortocaval compression was not avoided.

- Tests used:
  - neonatal behavioural assessment scale (NBAS): very detailed, taking up to 1 h to perform. More sensitive than the others.
  - early neonatal neurobehavioural scale (ENNS): directed more towards disorders of tone. Quicker and easier to perform.
  - neurological and adaptive capacity score (NACS): even more directed towards tone. Takes a few minutes to perform. The least sensitive test of subtle effects.
- Summary of results:
  - pethidine: reduces alertness and responsiveness before respiratory depression is evident. Greatest effect is at 2 days. Rapid placental transfer follows maternal iv injection.
  - anaesthetic agents: thiopental causes more neonatal depression than ketamine (but tone is increased by ketamine, giving higher scores). Low concentrations of volatile inhalational anaesthetic agents produce little, if any, effects. Regional techniques consistently produce higher scores.
  - local anaesthetic agents: initial fears of hypotonia following lidocaine have now been dispelled. All local anaesthetic drugs have similar effects, lowering scores only when very sensitive testing is employed. The significance of this is unknown.

Neurofibromatosis. Group of neurocutaneous diseases characterised by multiple tumours derived from the neurilemma sheath of cranial and peripheral nerves/nerve roots.

- Classified into:
  - neurofibromatosis 1 (NF-1; von Recklinghausen's disease). Autosomal dominant disease with gene locus at chromosome 17, with an incidence of 1:3000. Flat, brown 'café au lait' spots occur in all sufferers, six or more spots larger than 1.5 cm being diagnostic. Neurofibromata may be subcutaneous/cutaneous, or may occur in deeper peripheral nerves or autonomic nerves supplying viscera. They may also occur at the foramen magnum or within the theca, causing nerve root or spinal cord compression. Pulmonary fibrosis occurs in 20% of cases; hypertension is present in 6% of patients and may be associated with phaeochromocytoma (in 1%) or renal artery stenosis. Intracranial tumours occur in 5–10% of cases, and skeletal abnormalities (including kyphoscoliosis) in 10%. Potential anaesthetic problems result from the distribution of neurofibromata and may include difficulty with tracheal intubation or regional blocks. Despite earlier reports, patients exhibit normal sensitivity to neuromuscular blocking drugs.
  - neurofibromatosis 2 (NF-2): very rare condition in which bilateral acoustic neuromas are present. Gene has been mapped to chromosome 22.

[Friedrich D von Recklinghausen (1833–1910), German pathologist]

Hirsch NP, Murphy A, Radcliffe JJ (2001). Br J Anaesth; 86: 555–64

Neurokinin-1 receptor antagonists. Antiemetic drugs, acting via inhibition at neurokinin-1 (NK1) receptors present in the GIT and CNS. Aprepitant is currently licensed for nausea and vomiting induced by cancer chemotherapy. Have also been studied in PONV.

See also, Tachykinins

Neurolepsis, *see Neuroleptanaesthesia and analgesia*

Neuroleptanaesthesia and analgesia. Use of very potent opioid analgesic drugs (e.g. fentanyl and phenoperidine) combined with butyrophenones (e.g. droperidol and haloperidol) to produce a state of reduced motor activity and passivity (neurolepsis). Introduced in 1959. The term neuroleptanaesthesia is usually restricted to the combination of opioid, butyrophenone and N_2O. Characterised by profound analgesia, sedation and antiemesis, with cardiovascular stability (although mild hypotension may occur). Has been used for premedication, sedation and as the sole anaesthetic technique, with/without neuromuscular blocking drugs, for surgical procedures (rarely employed for the latter use now because of prolonged recovery).
See also, Lytic cocktail

Neuroleptic malignant syndrome (NMS). Rare condition first described in 1960, characterised by altered consciousness, hyperthermia, autonomic dysfunction and muscle rigidity. Usually follows medication with butyrophenones and phenothiazines although it has been reported during withdrawal of L-dopa in patients with Parkinson's disease and in patients treated with metoclopramide, lithium and reserpine. Thought to be related to the antidopaminergic activity of the drugs, caused by receptor blockade in the basal ganglia and hypothalamus. Occurs in under 1% of patients, mostly young males. Increased by dehydration, CNS disease and exhaustion.

- Features develop over 1–3 days:
  - hyperthermia and tachycardia (thought to be caused mostly by increased muscle metabolism, although a central component may be present).
  - extrapyramidal dysfunction: rigidity, dystonia, tremor.
  - autonomic dysfunction: labile BP, sweating, salivation, urinary incontinence.
  - increased creatine kinase (> 1000 units/l) and white cell count.

Differential diagnosis is as for hyperthermia (in particular MH), Parkinson's disease, catatonia, central cholinergic syndrome, monoamine oxidase inhibitor reaction, and infection including tetanus. Although similar to MH, NMS is generally considered an entirely separate entity.

- Management:
  - supportive: O_2, cooling, hydration, DVT prophylaxis.
  - increased central dopaminergic activity, e.g. with bromocriptine (dopamine agonist) 2.5–20 mg 8 hourly (orally only). Amantidine and L-dopa have also been used.
  - dantrolene and non-depolarising neuromuscular blocking drugs have been used to treat the peripheral muscle effects, reducing fever, rigidity and tachycardia. The latter drugs are effective in NMS, in contrast to MH.
  - anticholinergic drugs have also been used.

Mortality is 20–30%, from renal failure, arrhythmias, PE or aspiration pneumonitis.

Adnet P, Lestovel P, Krivosic-Horber R (2000). Br J Anaesth; 85: 129–35

Neuromuscular blockade monitoring. Ideally, this should be undertaken whenever non-depolarising neuromuscular blocking drugs are used since residual block is common in the recovery room even after the use of intermediate acting drugs such as atracurium and vecuronium. Performed using a nerve stimulator, with assessment of the appropriate muscle response to stimulation of a peripheral nerve via surface or needle electrodes.

- Assessment may be:
  - visual.
  - tactile.
  - mechanical: reflects both neuromuscular transmission and muscle contractility. Assessed by:
    - measurement of tension developed in a muscle with a strain gauge or pressure transducer.
    - accelerometry: the transducer consists of a piezoelectric ceramic wafer with electrodes on both sides. Following changes in velocity, an electrical voltage proportional to the acceleration is generated between the electrodes. Force = mass × acceleration; thus the muscle tension response may be evaluated.
  - electrical: registers the EMG response via two surface/needle electrodes. Only monitors transmission across the neuromuscular junction, and thus is more specific than mechanical assessment.
- Stimulation:
  - unipolar square waveform lasting 0.2–0.3 ms (ensures constant current during stimulation).
  - in order to eliminate variation in muscle response caused by partial depolarisation of the nerve, supramaximal stimulation is required, which results in simultaneous depolarisation of all nerve fibres within the nerve. Required current may vary between 20 and 60 mA, and is minimised by placing the positive electrode proximally.
  - direct stimulation of the muscle should be avoided, since any response will be independent of neuromuscular blockade.
  - commonly used sites:
    - ulnar nerve: electrodes are placed along the ulnar border of the forearm, with assessment of thumb adduction. More sensitive than the diaphragm and vocal cords to neuromuscular blocking drugs.
    - facial nerve: electrodes are placed anterior to the tragus of the ear, with assessment of facial muscle contraction. Underestimation of the degree of blockade is common, because of direct muscle stimulation and relative insensitivity of the facial muscles to neuromuscular blocking drugs.
    - accessory nerve: one electrode is placed behind the mastoid process and the other at the posterior border of sternomastoid. Stimulation causes contraction of sternomastoid and trapezius muscles and is easier to see than following stimulation of the facial nerve. Asystole has followed tetanic stimulation when the upper electrode was placed anterior to the ear, attributed to stimulation of the vagus via the cranial root of the accessory nerve.
    - tibial nerve: electrodes are placed behind the medial malleolus, with assessment of big toe plantar flexion.
    - common peroneal nerve: electrodes are placed lateral to the neck of the fibula, with assessment of foot dorsiflexion.
  - patterns of stimulation:
    - single pulses (0.1–1.0 Hz).
    - tetanic stimulation (50–100 Hz) for 3–5 s. Painful in the awake patient. May be repeated every 5–10 min.
    - post-tetanic stimulation using single pulses.
    - train-of-four (TOF; four pulses at 2 Hz). TOF count is the number of palpable muscle twitches; TOF ratio is force of the fourth twitch divided by force of the first. May be repeated every 10–15 s.
    - post-tetanic count: used to assess intense blockade. Following 5 seconds' tetanus at 50 Hz, the number of twitches produced by single pulses at 1 Hz is counted. Should not be performed more than once in 5 min.

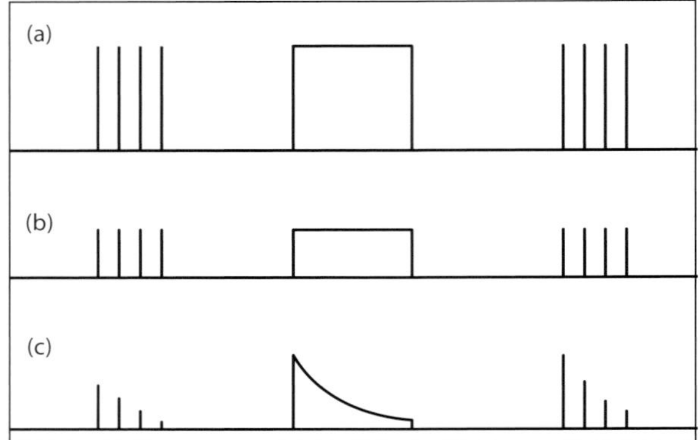

Fig. 113 EMG response to peripheral nerve stimulation in a train-of-four, tetanus, train-of-four pattern: (a) normal; (b) partial depolarising block; (c) partial non-depolarising block

- double-burst stimulation: used to assess recovery from non-depolarising blockade. Two short tetanic stimulations, e.g. 50 Hz for 60 ms, are applied 750 ms apart. The second response is weaker than the first in non-depolarising blockade. More sensitive at detecting fade than TOF.

- Observed responses:
  - normal neuromuscular function:
    - equal twitches in response to single pulses (Fig. 113a).
    - sustained tetanic contraction, with post-tetanic potentiation (PTP) revealed by mechanical assessment only.
  - depolarising neuromuscular blockade:
    - equal but reduced twitches in response to single pulses and TOF (Fig. 113b). TOF ratio thus equals unity.
    - sustained but reduced tetanic contraction, with neither fade nor PTP.
    - dual block may supervene if large amounts of suxamethonium are administered.
  - non-depolarising neuromuscular blockade.
    - progressively decreasing twitches in response to single pulses (Fig. 113c), with eventual disappearance.
    - tetanic contraction exhibits fade and PTP.
    - TOF: successive decrease in the four responses, with eventual disappearance of the 4th, 3rd, 2nd and 1st twitches at 75%, 80%, 90% and 100% blockade respectively. During recovery, the twitches reappear in the reverse order. Suggested suitable values during anaesthesia:
      - TOF count of 1 for tracheal intubation.
      - TOF count of 1–2 for maintenance; deeper levels may be required for complete diaphragmatic paralysis.
      - TOF count of 3–4 before attempting reversal of blockade, especially with long-acting drugs.
      - TOF ratio (at the thumb) of 0.9 for adequate maintenance of spontaneous ventilation.
    - post-tetanic count and double-burst stimulation as above.
    - sustained head-lift for 5 s is the most useful clinical indicator of adequate neuromuscular function (under 30% blockade). Other suggested indicators include the ability to open the mouth, protrude the tongue, cough, maintain sustained hand-grip, and achieve adequate tidal volume, vital capacity (15 ml/kg) and inspiratory pressure (−20 cmH_2O). However, these may all be possible at 50–80% blockade.

Hemmerling TM, Le N (2007). Can J Anesth; 54: 58–72

Neuromuscular blocking drugs. Drugs used to impair neuromuscular transmission and provide skeletal muscle relaxation during anaesthesia or critical care.

- May be one of two types:
  - non-depolarising: include tubocurarine (first used as curare in 1912), gallamine (1948), dimethyl tubocurarine (1948), alcuronium (1961), pancuronium (1967), fazadinium (1972), atracurium (1980), vecuronium (1983), pipecuronium (1990), doxacurium (1991), mivacurium (1993), rocuronium (1994), cisatracurium (1995), and rapacuronium (1999). Non-depolarising agents are competitive antagonists at postsynaptic acetylcholine (ACh) receptors of the neuromuscular junction. They are highly ionised at body pH, containing two quaternary ammonium groups (tubocurarine and vecuronium contain one each, but acquire a second following injection). Poorly lipid-soluble and poorly protein-bound. Following injection, the drugs are rapidly redistributed from blood to the ECF and other tissues, e.g. kidney, liver. The clinical effect depends on individual drug characteristics and drug concentration at the neuromuscular junction which depends on the drug's pharmacokinetics.
  - depolarising: cause depolarisation by mimicking the action of ACh at ACh receptors, but without rapid hydrolysis by acetylcholinesterase. An area of depolarisation around the ACh receptor–drug complex results in local currents which open sodium channels before the continuing current flow inactivates them. Propagation of an action potential is prevented by the area of inexcitability that develops around the ACh receptors. Thus fasciculations occur before paralysis. Examples are suxamethonium (1951) and decamethonium (1948); only the former is available for clinical use in the UK.

Apart from the presence or absence of fasciculation, non-depolarising and depolarising neuromuscular blockade may be distinguished by neuromuscular blockade monitoring.

In general, suxamethonium is used for paralysis of rapid onset and short duration, e.g. to allow rapid tracheal intubation. The non-depolarising drugs are traditionally used for prolonged paralysis when rapid intubation is not required, although atracurium and vecuronium (and more recently, mivacurium and rocuronium) have bridged the gap between these drugs and suxamethonium (Table 25).

See also, Interonium distance; Nicotine and nicotinic receptors

Neuromuscular junction. Synapse between the presynaptic motor neurone and the postsynaptic muscle membrane. On approaching the junction, the axon divides into terminal buttons that invaginate into the muscle fibre. The synaptic cleft is 50–70 nm wide and filled with ECF. The muscle membrane is folded into longitudinal gutters, whose ridges conceal orifices to secondary clefts. The orifices lie opposite the release points for acetylcholine (ACh) and contain high concentrations of acetylcholinesterase (Fig. 114).

- Three types of acetylcholine receptor have been identified at the neuromuscular junction:
  - postjunctional: involved in traditional neuromuscular transmission. Following activation of both α subunits, sodium and calcium move into the muscle and potassium exits, along specialised ion channels (*see Fig. 2b; Acetylcholine receptors*).
  - prejunctional: control an ion channel specific for sodium and respond to released ACh by mobilising further ACh storage vesicles to the active zone of the junction, ready

Table 25 Properties of neuromuscular blocking drugs

Drug	Onset time (min)	Half-life (min)	Vol. of distribution (l/kg)	Clearance (ml/kg/min)	Clinical duration of action (min)	Route of elimination	Histamine release	Autonomic effects
Alcuronium	3–5	180–200	0.1–0.3	1.5	20–40	Renal	±	–
Atracurium	1.5–2	20	0.16–0.18	5.5–6.0	20–30	Hofmann degradation + plasma hydrolysis	+	–
Cisatracurium	1–1.5	100	0.23	3.9	30–40	As for atracurium	–	–
Dimethyl tubocurarine (metocurine)	3–5	345	0.5	1.0	90–120	Renal	+	Weak ganglion blockade
Doxacurium	4–5	85–100	0.2	2.2–2.6	100–200	Renal + hepatic	–	–
Fazadinium	0.5–1.5	40–80	0.2	4.0	40–60	Renal	–	Muscarinic + ganglion blockade
Gallamine	1–2	160	0.25	1.2	20–30	Renal	–	Muscarinic blockade
Mivacurium	1.5–2	2–5	–	–	10–15	Plasma cholinesterase + hepatic	±	–
Pancuronium	2–3	120–140	0.25–0.3	1.8	40–60	Renal + hepatic	–	Weak muscarinic blockade + sympathomimetic action
Pipecuronium	2.5–3	140	0.3	2.5	90–120	Renal + hepatic	–	–
Rapacuronium	0.5–3.5	28	0.29	6–11	6–30	Renal + hepatic	++	–
Rocuronium	2	22–29	0.12–0.16	4.7–5.7	30	Hepatic	–	±
Tubocurarine	3–5	150–190	0.5–0.6	2–3	30–50	Renal + hepatic	++	Ganglion blockade
Vecuronium	1.5–2	55–70	0.27	5.2	20–30	Renal + hepatic	–	–
Suxamethonium	0.5–1.5	2.5	–	–	2–5	Plasma cholinesterase	+	Muscarinic + ganglionic stimulation

for release. Thought to be involved in the phenomenon of fade in non-depolarising neuromuscular blockade.
- extrajunctional: normally present in small numbers, but proliferate over the muscle membrane in denervation hypersensitivity, burns and certain muscle diseases.

Hirsch NP (2007). Br J Anaesth; 99: 132–8

See also, Neuromuscular blocking drugs

Neuromuscular transmission. Stages of transmission:
- depolarisation of the motor nerve leading to action potential propagation to the nerve endings at the neuromuscular junction.
- opening of presynaptic voltage-gated calcium channels. Resultant increase in intracellular calcium causes mobilisation of acetylcholine (ACh) vesicles to the active zone and subsequent release into the synapse.
- binding of ACh to postsynaptic nicotinic ACh receptors, causing an end-plate potential. If the latter is large enough, depolarisation of the muscle membrane occurs.

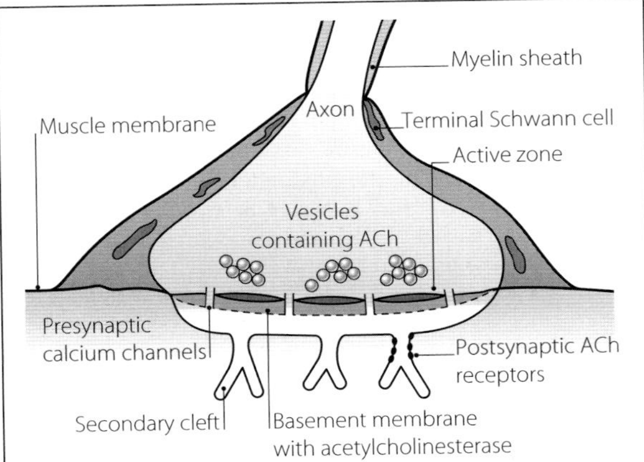

Fig. 114 Structure of neuromuscular junction

- resultant action potential causing muscle contraction.
- hydrolysis of ACh by acetylcholinesterase within 1 ms.

● Transmission may be impaired by:
  - inhibition of ACh synthesis, storage or release, e.g. by hemicholinium, β-bungarotoxin and botulinum toxins respectively. Aminoglycosides are also thought to impair ACh release, as does the myasthenic syndrome.
  - blockade of ACh receptors, e.g. by neuromuscular blocking drugs, α-bungarotoxin, receptor destruction in myasthenia gravis.
  - acetylcholinesterase inhibitors.

Naguib M, Flood P, McArdle JJ, Brenner HR (2002). Anesthesiology; 96: 202–31

See also, Synapse

Neurone. Basic unit of the nervous system. Consists of:
- cell body: contains the nucleus and most of the cytoplasm. Usually at the dendritic end of the neurone. The dendritic zone is the site of integration of incoming impulses via dendrites, and of initiation of the action potential.
- axon: may exceed 1 metre in length. May be myelinated or unmyelinated (*see Myelin; Nerve conduction*). Anterograde and retrograde flow of organelles and proteins occurs along the axon.
- terminal buttons (nerve endings): situated near the cell body or dendrites of other neurones and contain neurotransmitters.

● Divided into classes in 1924 according to the compound action potential obtained when a mixed nerve is stimulated:
  - A: 1–20 μm diameter myelinated fibres. Subdivided into:
    - α: 70–120 m/s conduction; somatic motor and proprioception sensation.
    - β: 50–70 m/s; touch and pressure sensation.
    - γ: 30–50 m/s; motor fibres to muscle spindles.
    - δ: < 30 m/s; pain, cold, touch sensation.

- B: 1–3 μm diameter; < 15 m/s conduction: myelinated preganglionic autonomic fibres.
- C: < 1 μm diameter; < 2 m/s conduction: unmyelinated post-ganglionic autonomic fibres, and pain and temperature sensation.

Local anaesthetic agents block C fibres first, then B then A fibres. Pressure blocks A, B and C fibres in order, and hypoxia B, A and C fibres.

- An alternative classification has been suggested:
  - I:
    - a: muscle spindles.
    - b: Golgi tendon organ.
  - II: muscle spindles, touch, pressure.
  - III: pain, cold, touch.
  - IV: pain, temperature, others.

[Camillo Golgi (1843–1926), Italian physician]
See also, Nociception

Neuropathy of critical illness, *see Critical illness polyneuropathy*

Neuroradiology. Most neuroradiological procedures are painless and do not require anaesthetic intervention; sedation or anaesthesia may be required in children, uncooperative or neurologically impaired patients or for prolonged procedures. Principles are as for radiology and neurosurgery.

- Specific techniques:
  - myelography: injection of contrast into the thecal sac to examine the spinal cord. Usually performed via lumbar puncture but occasionally via a cervical approach. Steep tilting is often required to aid spread of the contrast. Complications include headache, convulsions and arachnoiditis.
  - CT scanning.
  - MRI.
  - positron emission tomography.
  - cerebral angiography: injection of radiological contrast media via femoral or carotid puncture. Hyperventilation improves the arteriogram quality by increasing cerebrovascular resistance. Complications include CVA (1% of patients), haemorrhage, haematoma, thrombosis, arterial spasm and bradycardia (especially during vertebral angiography).
  - ventriculography and pneumoencephalography: injection of gas (usually air) into the ventricular system, with imaging in different positions. N_2O is usually avoided. Bradycardia may occur. Rarely performed now.
  - therapeutic interventions:
    - embolisation: e.g. of cerebral and spinal arteriovenous malformations and cerebral aneurysms. Usually requires anticoagulation. Control of BP is essential to avoid rupture.
    - balloon angioplasty: e.g. of occlusive cerebral disease and vasospasm secondary to subarachnoid haemorrhage. Deliberate hypertension may be required to maintain cerebral perfusion pressure and avoid ischaemia.
    - carotid artery stenting for stenosis.
    - thrombolysis of acute thromboembolic stroke. Cerebral haemorrhage may occur postoperatively.

Varma MK, Price K, Jayakrishnan V, et al (2007). Br J Anaesth; 99: 75–85

Neurosurgery. Encompasses procedures involving the cranium, brain, meninges, cranial nerves, spinal cord and vertebral column, and those performed for pain management. Basic principles for intracranial surgery are related to maintenance of normal cerebral perfusion pressure and cerebral blood flow, with avoidance of cerebral ischaemia, cerebral steal and increased ICP. Cerebral protection has been employed.

- Main considerations:
  - preoperatively:
    - preoperative assessment of neurological status, hydrocephalus, etc. Endocrine abnormalities may be present (e.g. pituitary gland surgery).
    - fluid and electrolyte imbalance may be present, especially if associated with reduced oral intake and vomiting.
    - hypertension may be present, especially in association with subarachnoid haemorrhage.
    - drug therapy may include anticonvulsant drugs and corticosteroids.
    - other injuries may accompany head injury.
    - sedative premedication is usually avoided because of possible pre- or postoperative respiratory depression and decreased conscious level.
  - perioperatively:
    - iv induction of anaesthesia is usual; most iv anaesthetic agents are suitable apart from ketamine. Smooth induction avoiding hypoxaemia, hypercapnia, hypertension and tachycardia is required. Hyperkalaemia has followed suxamethonium in certain upper and lower motor neurone lesions. β-Adrenergic receptor antagonists may be given to reduce the hypertensive response to laryngoscopy, whilst lidocaine 0.5–1.5 mg/kg may be given iv to reduce the increase in ICP. Adequate time should be allowed for full paralysis before tracheal intubation is attempted. Lidocaine spray may be employed during laryngoscopy. Use of a non-kinkable tracheal tube is usual, with thorough fixation. The eyes and face should be protected with padding.
    - a large-bore iv cannula is necessary, since blood loss may be considerable. CVP measurement may be required, especially if the patient is to be positioned sitting. Arterial cannulation is usual. End-tidal CO_2 measurement, pulse oximetry and temperature measurement are considered mandatory in addition to ECG. Neuromuscular blockade monitoring is especially useful, since inadequate paralysis may have disastrous results. ICP monitoring, evoked potentials and EEG derivatives are sometimes employed.
    - permissive hypothermia (to 33°C) is increasingly popular in an attempt to reduce cerebral metabolism.
    - perioperative problems include:
      - those related to positioning of the patient. The supine position is common; others also used include:
        - lateral/prone: vena caval obstruction and damage to the face, eyes, etc. may occur.
        - sitting (for posterior fossa lesions): air embolism, hypotension, and obstruction of neck veins may occur. The first two may be reduced by the anti-gravity suit, PEEP and administration of iv fluids.
      - inaccessibility of the airway.
      - those of prolonged surgery, e.g. heat loss, fluid balance.
      - acute control of ICP.
      - arrhythmias and cardiovascular instability during manipulation of brainstem structures (posterior fossa lesions).
    - maintenance is usually with N_2O/O_2 (although the former is often avoided because of the risk of

expansion of a pneumoencephalocoele), supplemented by a volatile inhalational anaesthetic agent (isoflurane or sevoflurane is usually preferred) with or without a short-acting opioid, e.g. fentanyl, remifentanil. TIVA has been used. Hyperventilation to arterial $P\text{CO}_2$ of 4.0–4.5 (30–38 mmHg) is considered optimal.
- hypotensive anaesthesia is sometimes employed, especially for vascular lesions.
- bradycardia may follow application of suction to intracranial and extracranial drains.
- some procedures involving CT scanning (e.g. stereotactic surgery) require moving the anaesthetised patient between operating and imaging rooms.
- local anaesthetic techniques may also be used (e.g. for awake craniotomy). Once the skull and dura are opened, there is usually little discomfort and the patient's neurological state is easily monitored.

- postoperatively:
  - tracheal extubation is usually possible at the end of surgery; coughing or straining should be avoided. Elective IPPV may be required, e.g. following prolonged operations and when ICP is critically raised. Airway obstruction caused by acute swelling of the tongue has been reported following posterior fossa surgery.
  - close observation is required, in case of bleeding, vasospasm, increased ICP, convulsions, hypotension, hypertension, etc. The Glasgow coma scale is employed for monitoring progress. ICP monitoring may be used.
  - the patient should be rewarmed to prevent postoperative shivering.
  - analgesia was traditionally provided by im codeine although this has been superseded by morphine.
  - diabetes insipidus or the syndrome of inappropriate antidiuretic hormone secretion may occur.
  - increased risk of DVT has been associated with neurosurgery. Mechanical methods of prophylaxis are usually preferred to heparin.

Dinsmore J (2007). Br J Anaesth; 99: 68–74

See also, Spinal surgery

Neurotransmitters. Substances secreted from presynaptic nerve endings, which act at the postsynaptic membrane to cause excitatory or inhibitory effects. Act via specific receptors, binding to which opens or closes membrane channels. The same neurotransmitter may be excitatory at one synapse, and inhibitory at another.

- Examples:
  - amines, e.g. noradrenaline, adrenaline, dopamine, 5-HT, histamine.
  - amino acids, e.g. glycine, glutamate, GABA, aspartate.
  - polypeptides, e.g. substance P, enkephalins. Substances active as circulating hormones may also function as neurotransmitters, e.g. vasopressin, oxytocin, vasoactive intestinal peptide, glucagon, somatostatin.
  - others, e.g. acetylcholine, nitric oxide.

In general, acetylcholine and the amino acids are involved with fast point-to-point signalling whereas the polypeptides, amines and nitric oxide have a slower, more diffuse regulatory function. More than one neurotransmitter may be secreted by one neurone, e.g. vasoactive intestinal peptide is often secreted with acetylcholine, and is thought to potentiate the latter's actions. Amines are often secreted with peptide neurotransmitters.

See also, Neuromuscular junction; Synaptic transmission

Neutral thermal range, *see Thermoneutral range*

New injury severity score, *see Injury severity score*

New York Heart Association classification. Method of assessment of cardiac disease (originally cardiac failure), used, e.g. in preoperative assessment:
- class I: no functional limitation.
- class II: slight functional limitation. Fatigue, palpitations, dyspnoea or angina on ordinary physical activity, but asymptomatic at rest.
- class III: marked functional limitation. Symptoms on less than ordinary activity, but asymptomatic at rest.
- class IV: inability to perform any physical activity, with or without symptoms at rest.

Newton. Unit of force. 1 N is the force required to accelerate a mass of 1 kg by 1 m/s^2.
[Sir Isaac Newton (1643–1727), English physicist]

Newtonian fluids, *see Fluids*

NGF, *see Nerve growth factor*

Nicardipine hydrochloride. Calcium channel blocking drug. Used in the UK for treatment of hypertension and ischaemic heart disease; also available parenterally in the USA for short-term reduction of BP, e.g. perioperatively. Given as a 0.1 mg/ml solution. Incompatible with bicarbonate and Hartmann's solutions.

NICE, *see National Institute for Clinical Excellence*

NiCO. Commercial non-invasive cardiac output measurement system that employs partial CO_2 rebreathing and the Fick principle to estimate cardiac output. A small rebreathing loop is inserted into the patient's breathing circuit and is used to increase intermittently the volume of the circuit. Concentration and flow of CO_2 are measured by a sensor placed between the patient and the rebreathing loop. The change in cardiac output is proportional to the ratio of the change in CO_2 elimination and the resulting change in end-expiratory CO_2.

Nicorandil. Potassium channel activator with a nitrate component, used to prevent and treat angina. Causes arterial and venous vasodilatation. Peak plasma levels occur within 30–60 min of administration. Only slightly protein-bound.
- Dosage: 5–30 mg orally, 12 hourly.
- Side effects: headache, vomiting, dizziness, hypotension.

Nicotine and nicotinic receptors. Nicotine, a toxic alkaloid derived from tobacco, mimics certain actions of acetylcholine, and was used to investigate the physiology of the autonomic nervous system. At low doses, it stimulates postsynaptic nicotinic acetylcholine receptors of the neuromuscular junction, autonomic ganglia and adrenal medulla; at high doses, it blocks them. Also causes CNS stimulation, followed by depression. Neuromuscular and ganglionic nicotinic receptors have different properties, since neuromuscular blocking drugs and ganglion blocking drugs each act at one site predominantly, although some cross-over effect occurs. For example, tubocurarine causes some ganglion blockade.

Nifedipine. Calcium channel blocking drug, affecting coronary and peripheral vascular smooth muscle more than myocardial muscle. Negative inotropic effect is usually insignificant because of baroreceptor-mediated tachycardia.

Has no antiarrhythmic action. Used in hypertension, ischaemic heart disease and Raynaud's phenomenon. Active within 20–30 min of oral administration, but a faster response follows sublingual retention of the capsule's contents (though not licensed for sublingual use). May thus be administered sublingually during anaesthesia. 95% protein-bound. Half-life is 3–5 h. Metabolised in the liver and excreted renally.

- Dosage:
  - 5–20 mg orally, 8–12 hourly. A long-acting formulation is also available: 10–90 mg, once daily.
  - 100–200 µg may be infused into the coronary arteries, e.g. for spasm during coronary angiography.
- Side effects: headache, flushing, dizziness, GIT disturbance, peripheral oedema. Has been implicated in increasing risk of MI in patients with hypertension, although this has been disputed.

[Maurice Raynaud (1834–1881), French physician]

Nikethamide. Analeptic drug, formerly used as a respiratory and cardiovascular stimulant but rarely used now because of its non-specific actions. Dose: 0.25–1.0 g slowly iv. Side effects are common and include restlessness, arrhythmias, tremor and convulsions.

Nimodipine. Calcium channel blocking drug, preferentially affecting cerebral vascular smooth muscle. Increases cerebral blood flow, especially to poorly perfused areas, e.g. those affected by arterial spasm following subarachnoid haemorrhage (SAH).

- Dosage:
  - prophylactically following SAH: 60 mg orally, 4 hourly, for 21 days.
  - in established vasospasm: 15 µg/kg/h iv, doubled after 2 h if BP is stable. Continued for 5–14 days.

Reacts with PVC infusion tubing; polypropylene and polyethylene are suitable. May be degraded by light.

- Side effects: hypotension, flushing. Should be used with care in raised ICP.

NIPPV, *see Non-invasive positive pressure ventilation*

NIRS, *see Near infra-red spectroscopy*

NISS, New injury severity score, *see Injury severity score*

Nitrazepam. Benzodiazepine widely used as a hypnotic drug. Has also been used as an anticonvulsant in childhood myoclonic epilepsy. Onset of sleep occurs within an hour; duration of action is 4–8 h. Extensively protein-bound; elimination half-life is up to 30 h resulting in hangover effects during the day.

- Dosage: 5–10 mg orally at night.
- Side effects: disorientation, confusion, drowsiness. Dependence may occur.

Nitric oxide (NO). Oxide of nitrogen, active as a biological mediator throughout the body but especially in:

  - vascular endothelium: responsible for vascular relaxation. Reduced production has been implicated in vasospasm associated with various disease states, e.g. diabetes mellitus, hypertension and following subarachnoid haemorrhage. NO is thought to be the effector molecule for all nitrate vasodilator drugs.
  - brain tissue: acts as a neurotransmitter.
  - macrophages: involved in the response to infection.
  - platelets: involved in aggregation and adhesion.

Synthesised in endothelial cells during the oxidation of L-arginine to L-citrulline, the reaction being catalysed by NO synthase (NOS). The NO thus produced diffuses into vascular smooth muscle and converts inactive guanylate cyclase into the active form; the latter converts guanosine triphosphate into cyclic guanosine monophosphate which causes vascular relaxation (Fig. 115). Two forms of NOS exist, the constitutive form present in vascular and brain tissue which produces small quantities of NO continuously (eNOS) and the inducible form present in macrophages (iNOS).

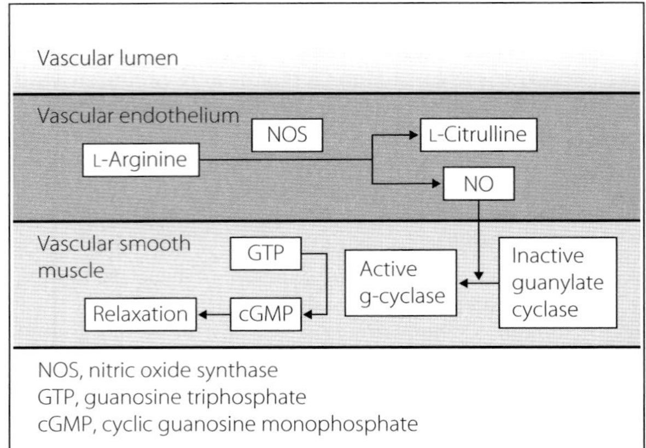

Fig. 115 Synthesis and action of nitric oxide (NO)

In sepsis, NO production is thought to be increased by endotoxin, the action of cytokines e.g. tumour necrosis factor, and certain interleukins. The amount of the inducible form of NOS increases, resulting in overproduction of NO with resultant excessive vasodilatation. NOS inhibitors have been investigated experimentally in the treatment of sepsis.

In neonatal, paediatric or adult pulmonary hypertension, inhaled NO (1–150 ppm) has been used to produce selective pulmonary vasodilatation without systemic effects. A clear effect on outcome in ARDS has not been conclusively demonstrated.

NO has a biological half-life of 4–40 s, its action being terminated by combining with haemoglobin to form methaemoglobin.

Measured in gaseous form using a chemiluminescence reaction ($NO + ozone \rightarrow O_2 + NO_2 + light$) or electroanalysis using a specific electrode. Levels in tissues are measured using electron paramagnetic resonance or fluorescence spectroscopy.

Nitrogen. Non-metallic element existing in the atmosphere as a colourless, odourless 'inert' gas (isolated in 1772). Forms 78.03% of atmospheric air. Atomic weight is 14; boiling point is –195°C. Obtained by fractional distillation of air. Reacts poorly with other substances. Blood/gas solubility coefficient is 0.014. Has anaesthetic properties at hyperbaric pressures (*see Inert gas narcosis*). Converted into organic compounds by nitrifying bacteria and plants, and present throughout the body in amino acids and proteins.

See also, Nitrogen balance; Nitrogen washout

Nitrogen balance. Difference between the amount of nitrogen ingested (as amino acids or proteins) and the amount of nitrogen excreted (mainly urinary). Usually measured within a 24-h period. Negative if losses exceed intake, e.g. catabolism, starvation; positive if intake exceeds losses, e.g. during recovery from severe illness.

- Estimated thus:
  - intake = the nitrogen content of all foods/fluids taken.
  - output = the sum of nitrogen losses calculated from the following three components:

- from urinary urea: nitrogen (g/24 h) = urea (mmol/24 h) × 6/5 because ⅙ is excreted as substances other than urea
  × 1/1000 to convert mmol to mol
  × 60 to convert mol urea to g
  × 28/60 to convert g urea to g nitrogen
  i.e. urea (mmol/24 h) × 0.0336.
- from blood urea: nitrogen (g/24 h) = change in urea (mmol/l/24 h) × 1/1000
  × 60
  × 28/60 as above
  × 60% × body weight (kg) since urea is distributed amongst total body water
  i.e. change in urea (mmol/l/24 h) × 0.0168 × body weight
- from other routes of loss, e.g. proteinuria: nitrogen loss (g/24 h) = protein loss (g/24 h)
  × 1/6.25 since 6.25 g protein contains 1 g nitrogen.

Other losses occur from sweat and stools (e.g. 2–4 g per l GIT fistula fluid lost per 24 h).

Calculation is a useful guide to appropriate nutrition in critical illness. A normal adult requires about 0.15 g N/kg/day; this may double in severe sepsis.

See also, Energy balance

Nitrogen, higher oxides of. Nitric oxide (NO), nitrogen dioxide (NO_2) and nitrogen trioxide (N_2O_3); the latter decomposes to form NO and NO_2. NO reacts with O_2 forming NO_2, which dissolves in water to form nitrous and nitric acids. The gases are produced during some fires, during manufacture of N_2O, and in the metal industry. Irritant if inhaled, they cause mild upper airway symptoms initially but pulmonary oedema several hours after initial recovery. Severe pulmonary fibrotic destruction may follow 2–3 weeks later. Formation of nitrates in the body may result in vasodilatation and hypotension, and cause methaemoglobinaemia. Treatment is supportive. Contamination of some N_2O cylinders in 1967 in the UK led to their widespread recall. May be tested for using moistened starch iodide paper, which turns blue on exposure. NO is involved in intercellular communication and control of vascular tone.

See also, Smoke inhalation

Nitrogen narcosis, *see Inert gas narcosis*

Nitrogen washout. Elimination of nitrogen from the lungs whilst breathing non-nitrogen-containing gas. During successive breaths, the concentration of nitrogen exhaled falls as an exponential process, falling to about 2.5% after 7 min in normal patients. During anaesthesia using circle systems, 7–10 min high fresh gas flow is required to remove most body nitrogen. Elimination is prolonged if ventilation is distributed unevenly (see below).

- Tests employing nitrogen washout:
  - measure of FRC.
  - single-breath nitrogen washout (Fowler's method).
  - multiple-breath nitrogen washout: the patient breathes 100% O_2, with nitrogen measurement at the lips. Log nitrogen concentration is plotted against number of breaths. If lung ventilation is uniform, expired nitrogen concentration decreases by the same fraction with each breath, as demonstrated by a straight line on the graph. A curved line is obtained if ventilation is uneven, as nitrogen is quickly washed out from well-ventilated alveoli but only slowly from poorly ventilated ones (Fig. 116).

Nitroglycerin, *see Glyceryl trinitrate*

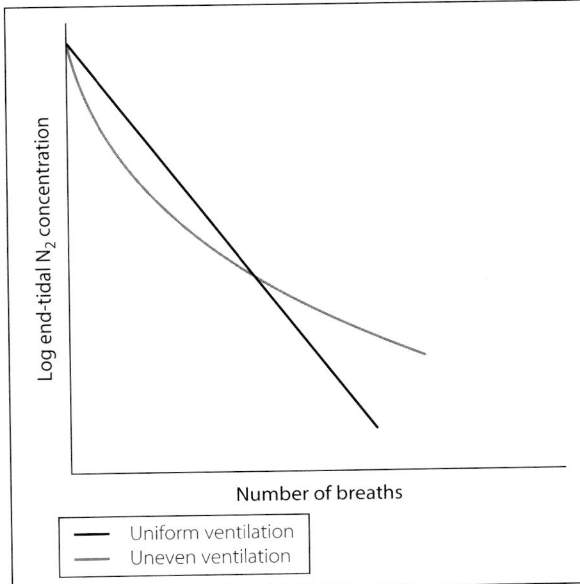

Fig. 116 Multiple-breath nitrogen washout

Nitroprusside, *see Sodium nitroprusside*

Nitrous oxide (N_2O). Inhalational anaesthetic agent, first isolated by Priestley in 1772. Suggested as being potentially useful for analgesia by Davy in 1799; first used for dental extraction by Wells in 1844 but superseded by diethyl ether. Reintroduced by Colton in 1863.

Manufactured by heating ammonium nitrate to 240°C and removing impurities, e.g. higher oxides of nitrogen, ammonia and nitric acid, by passage through scrubbers and washers. Water vapour is also removed.

- Properties:
  - colourless, slightly sweet-smelling gas, 1.53 times denser than air.
  - mw 44.
  - boiling point −88°C.
  - critical temperature 36.5°C.
  - partition coefficients:
    - blood/gas 0.47.
    - oil/gas 1.4.
  - MAC 105%.
  - non-flammable but supports combustion, breaking down to O_2 and nitrogen at high temperatures.
  - supplied as a liquid/gas in French blue cylinders with pin index positions 3 and 5: pressure is 40 bar at 15°C and 54 bar at room temperature. Ice often forms on the cylinder during use because of latent heat of vaporisation. Also supplied as gaseous Entonox.
- Effects:
  - CNS:
    - fast onset and recovery; strongly analgesic but weakly anaesthetic.
    - increases cerebral metabolism, cerebral blood flow and ICP slightly.
    - has inhibitory effects on NMDA receptors; stimulatory on opioid and adrenergic receptors.
  - RS:
    - non-irritant. Depresses respiration slightly.
    - may cause diffusion hypoxia (Fink effect) at the end of surgery.

- CVS: little effect on heart rate and BP usually, although it decreases myocardial contractility, especially when combined with volatile agents or opioids.
- GIT: associated with PONV; expansion of gas-containing bowel or inner ear cavities or a direct central effect (possibly via opioid receptors) have been suggested as possible causes.
- other:
  - does not affect hepatic or renal function, nor uterine or skeletal muscle tone.
  - interacts with methionine synthase; prolonged use may cause bone marrow depression, megaloblastic anaemia and peripheral neuropathy. Implicated in causing fetal abnormalities and spontaneous abortion, but no direct evidence exists. Generally considered as being safe during pregnancy.
  - expands air-filled cavities because it is over 40 times as soluble as nitrogen; thus passes from the blood into the cavity faster than the nitrogen can diffuse out. Can double the size of a pneumothorax in 10 min at 70%. Also expands air embolism and may cause pneumoencephalocoele following neurosurgery.

Excreted unchanged from the lungs; a small amount diffuses through the skin.

Commonly used for analgesia (above 20%) and as a carrier gas for other inhalational agents and O_2, usually in concentrations of 50–66%. Although weakly anaesthetic and rarely adequate alone, it reduces the requirement for other agents. Its adverse effects and concern about its effects on the environment have led to a reduction in its use and replacement by air. Recent evidence suggests an increased incidence of major cardiovascular and respiratory complications after major surgery if N_2O is used, though the findings are controversial and may be related to differences in F_IO_2 rather than to N_2O itself.

Also used in the cryoprobe.

See also, Environmental safety of anaesthetists; Nitrogen, higher oxides of; Pollution; Relative analgesia

Nizatidine. H_2 receptor antagonist used in peptic ulcer disease; similar to cimetidine but does not cause enzyme inhibition. Well absorbed orally, it is 40% protein-bound with 90% excreted by the kidneys.

- Dosage:
  - 150–300 mg orally, 12–24 hourly.
  - 100 mg iv over 15 min, 8 hourly, or 10 mg/h iv up to 480 mg/day.
- Side effects: as for ranitidine.

NMDA receptors, *see N-Methyl-d-aspartate receptors*

NMJ, *see Neuromuscular junction*

NMR, Nuclear magnetic resonance, *see Magnetic resonance imaging*

NO, *see Nitric oxide*

No reflow phenomenon. Reduction in organ blood flow following a period of ischaemia or infarction, without mechanical vessel obstruction. Has been observed affecting the heart and brain, e.g. after MI/myocardial ischaemia and CVA/cerebral ischaemia respectively. The aetiology is unclear but small vessel vasospasm, endothelial oedema or extrinsic compression by tissue oedema, increased blood viscosity, platelet aggregation and venous congestion have all been suggested. Treatment has been aimed at all these factors, with varying degrees of success.

Rezkalla SH, Kloner RA (2002). Circulation; 105: 656–62

Nociceptin, *see Orphanin FQ*

Nociception. Sensation of noxious stimuli, i.e. associated with injury or threatened injury.

- Occurs via specialised nerve endings (nociceptors) of certain neurones:
  - C-fibres: respond to heat, mechanical and chemical stimuli, giving rise to pain. They also respond to endogenous pain-producing substances, e.g. bradykinin, histamine and potassium ions. Because of their responsiveness to many stimuli, they are also known as 'polymodal nociceptors'.
  - Aδ-fibres:
    - type I: respond to heat and mechanical stimuli, with high threshold. Thought to give rise to pain from long-standing stimuli.
    - type II: respond to heat and mechanical stimuli, with fast response and low threshold. Thought to give rise to initial pain sensation.
    - receptors responding to cold and mechanical stimuli, thought to give rise to pain associated with cold.

Other types may also exist. Although initially described and most abundant in skin, they also exist in other tissues, e.g. muscle, joints, teeth. Injury increases their response and sensitivity.

See also, Pain; Pain pathways

Nodal arrhythmias, *see Junctional arrhythmias*

Non-depolarising neuromuscular blockade. Caused by competitive antagonism of acetylcholine (ACh) by non-depolarising neuromuscular blocking drugs at the ACh receptors of the neuromuscular junction. The end-plate potential produced by ACh diminishes as receptor occupancy by the neuromuscular blocking drug increases; when it fails to reach the threshold value neuromuscular transmission fails. This occurs when 80–90% of ACh receptors are blocked, confirming the wide margin of safety of neuromuscular transmission.

- Features:
  - absence of fasciculation following administration of drug.
  - exhibits fade and post-tetanic potentiation.
  - antagonised by acetylcholinesterase inhibitors.
  - potentiated by aminoglycosides, volatile inhalational anaesthetic agents, acidosis, electrolyte disturbances (especially hypokalaemia, hypermagnesaemia, hypocalcaemia), myasthenia gravis, myasthenic syndrome.

  Blockade may also be potentiated by excess drug at the neuromuscular junction, e.g. caused by overdose, or reduced metabolism, excretion or muscle blood flow.

See also, Neuromuscular blockade monitoring; Priming principle

Non-invasive positive pressure ventilation. An alternative to IPPV via tracheostomy in patients who require nocturnal IPPV, e.g. central sleep apnoea, severe respiratory muscle weakness and skeletal deformities. Has been suggested for treatment of exacerbations of COPD or during weaning from IPPV. Has also been used in pulmonary oedema. Applied via a tightly fitting nasal mask, facial mask or nasal 'pillows' which fit into the nostrils. Requires a ventilator capable of delivering twice-normal tidal volumes, since dead space is very high and the facial tissues very compliant. Ventilators may deliver a set volume or more commonly a set pressure. The soft palate moves against the tongue and prevents escape of air through the mouth during inspiration.

BIPAP (bi-level positive airway pressure) is the trade name for a technique in which two levels of positive pressure are provided. During exhalation, pressure is variably positive or near atmospheric; during inspiration pressure is variably positive. Airflow in the patient circuit is sensed by a transducer and augmented to a preset level of ventilation even if leaks occur around the mask. Cycling between inspiratory and expiratory modes may be triggered by the patient's spontaneous breaths, or timed according to preset controls (cycling either fully automatically or only if the patient fails to take a spontaneous breath within a certain time period). CPAP may also be delivered in either mode. BIPAP may also be administered via an oral mask.

Pressure necrosis, e.g. to the bridge of the nose, has occurred following prolonged continuous use. Newer gel masks decrease the problem.

Non-parametric tests, *see Data; Statistical tests*

Non-rebreathing valves. Prevent exhaled gas from passing upstream from the patient in anaesthetic breathing systems, thus almost eliminating rebreathing (but reducing efficiency because dead space gas is wasted). Most commonly used in draw-over techniques and for CPR with self-inflating bags. Also used in demand valves. For use with a fixed fresh gas supply, a reservoir bag is required unless fresh gas flow rate exceeds peak inspiratory flow rate. Should be placed as near to the patient as possible, e.g. attached directly to the facepiece/tracheal tube.

- Valves may be designed for either spontaneous ventilation or IPPV; commonly used ones may be used for both, and include:
  - Ambu-E valve (Fig. 117a): contains silicone rubber flaps (mushroom valves) within a clear plastic housing. Those designed for CPR contain one mushroom valve; those for anaesthetic use contain a second distal one to prevent indrawing of room air.
  - Laerdal valve (Fig. 117b): contains a circular silicone rubber internal valve and a ring-shaped rubber expiratory valve.
  - Ruben valve (Fig. 117c): contains a bobbin which is held against the upstream port by a spring at rest and moved downstream by gas flow during inspiration.

Malfunction, e.g. due to condensation of water vapour, may cause sticking of the valve or rebreathing. Barotrauma may occur if high internal pressure holds the expiratory port closed, e.g. during apnoea with high fresh gas flow.

[Ambu: from ambulant, Danish for movable; Asmund S Laerdal (1913–1981), Norwegian businessman and manufacturer; Henning M Ruben (1914–2004), Danish anaesthetist]

Non-steroidal anti-inflammatory drugs (NSAIDs). Group of chemically dissimilar compounds with anti-inflammatory, antipyretic and analgesic actions. Widely used for mild pain (e.g. musculoskeletal disease, headache, dysmenorrhoea, etc.) and inflammatory disease (especially musculoskeletal). Widely used for postoperative analgesia. Individual responses to NSAIDs are variable and many drugs may have to be tried before achieving optimal benefit.

- Classified into:
  - salicylic acids: e.g. aspirin, benorilate, diflunisal.
  - propionic acids: e.g. fenbufen, ibuprofen, naproxen.
  - acetic acids: e.g. diclofenac, indometacin.
  - fenamates: mefenamic acid, flufenamic acid.
  - pyrazolones: e.g. phenylbutazone, azapropazone.
  - oxicams: e.g. piroxicam, tenoxicam, meloxicam.
  - pyrroles: e.g. ketorolac.

Effects are via inhibition of cyclo-oxygenase resulting in reduced prostaglandin, prostacyclin and thromboxane production (*see Fig. 14; Arachidonic acid*). Inhibitors of cyclo-oxygenase-2 (COX-2) (e.g. parecoxib, celecoxib) have been produced for their potential relative lack of GIT side effects.

- Side effects:
  - GIT disturbance, e.g. nausea, discomfort, diarrhoea, bleeding and ulceration (for the non-selective NSAIDs, the risks are greatest with azapropazone and least with ibuprofen; piroxicam, ketorolac, naproxen, indometacin and diclofenac are intermediate. The selective COX-2 inhibitors are associated with a lower risk than non-selective NSAIDs).
  - renal impairment (may occur with both selective and non-selective NSAIDs); may arise from:
    - renal hypoperfusion: especially common in patients with sodium depletion (e.g. those taking diuretics), hypovolaemia or pre-existing renal disease. Results from inhibition of protective prostaglandin-mediated renal vasodilatation; usually occurs soon after administration of the NSAID, in most cases with recovery following discontinuation. May progress to acute tubular necrosis.
    - acute interstitial nephritis: typically occurs after chronic administration, with slow recovery in most cases after discontinuation. Has also been reported after acute perioperative use. Acute renal failure

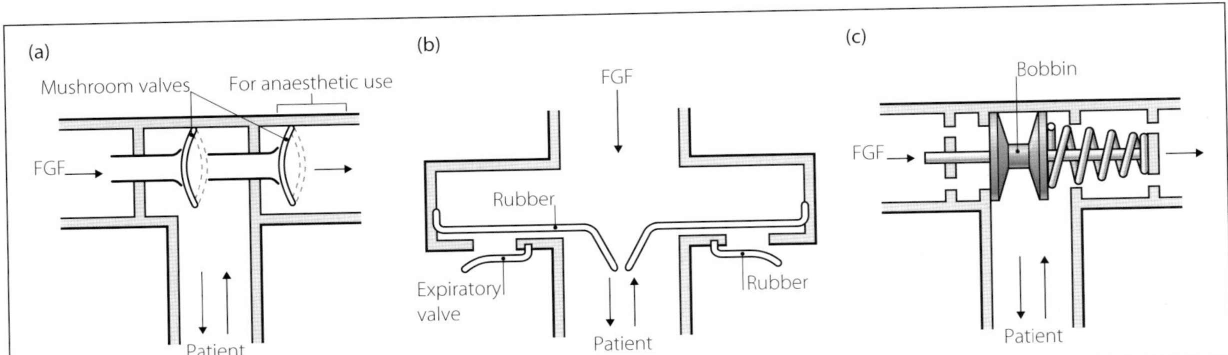

Fig. 117 Examples of non-rebreathing valves: (a) Ambu-E; (b) Laerdal; (c) Ruben. FGF, fresh gas flow

may result, usually associated with severe proteinuria. Corticosteroids have been suggested as being helpful.
- systemic vasculitis (rare) leading to glomerulonephritis and papillary necrosis.
- decreased platelet function and impaired coagulation. Although platelet dysfunction has been shown after perioperative use, bleeding problems are rare, although care is required if other drugs with anticoagulant actions are co-prescribed, e.g. prophylactic heparin. The selective COX-2 inhibitor rofecoxib was withdrawn in 2004 because it was associated with an increased incidence of cardiovascular side effects, particularly MI, that was originally attributed in early studies to a cardioprotective effect of naproxen in the control group. The mechanism is thought to be unequal inhibition of prostacyclin and thromboxane synthesis.
- adverse drug reactions are common (cross-sensitivity may occur between different drugs).
- others, e.g. fluid retention, hyperkalaemia and metabolic acidosis (via inhibition of renin secretion with resultant hypoaldosteronism), rarely hepatotoxicity. NSAIDs have been implicated in reducing bone healing after fractures, leading some orthopaedic surgeons to suggest they should be avoided perioperatively, but the evidence is weak and they continue to be widely used.

Evidence suggests that NSAIDs reduce opioid requirements and enhance opioids' effects when used intra-/postoperatively. Should be used cautiously if there is a risk of increased perioperative bleeding or renal impairment (the latter, for instance, in the elderly, diabetics, and after cardiac, hepatobiliary, renal or major vascular surgery) or sensitivity to aspirin. Postoperative renal dysfunction and GIT ulceration/bleeding should lead to cessation of therapy.

Noradrenaline (Norepinephrine). Catecholamine, the immediate precursor of adrenaline (differing by one methyl group on the terminal amine). A neurotransmitter in the sympathetic nervous system, ascending reticular activating system and hypothalamus. Also a hormone, forming about 20% of the catecholamines released from the adrenal medulla.

Predominately stimulates α-adrenergic receptors (non-selectively), although with some β_1-receptor stimulation. After secretion, 80% is taken up by postganglionic sympathetic nerve endings for reuse (uptake$_1$); the remainder is metabolised by catechol-*O*-methyltransferase and monoamine oxidase or taken up by other cells, e.g. vascular smooth muscle (uptake$_2$).

Used as an inotropic drug when SVR is low, e.g. in sepsis. An extremely potent vasopressor drug, it increases both systolic and diastolic arterial BP via arterial and venous vasoconstriction. There may be compensatory bradycardia caused by baroreceptor reflex activation. Coronary perfusion is increased but with increased myocardial O_2 demand. Cardiac output may increase or decrease depending on clinical circumstances. Cerebral blood flow and O_2 demand may fall. Although hypotension may be corrected, renal and mesenteric vasoconstriction may reduce renal blood flow.

Supplied commercially as noradrenaline tartrate.

- Dosage: 0.03–0.2 μg/kg/min although higher doses may be needed in sepsis.

Tachyphylaxis may occur. Tissue necrosis may follow extravasation.

Norepinephrine, *see Noradrenaline*

Normal solution. One containing one gram equivalent weight of substance per litre. So-called 'normal' saline solution (0.9%) is incorrectly described, being less than ⅙ normal. *See also, Equivalence*

Noscapine, *see Papaveretum*

Nose. Entrance to the pharynx and thence larynx and lungs. Apart from its olfactory role, it filters, humidifies and warms inspired air with its extensive vascular surfaces (turbinates and septum). Filtering relies on the mucous lining which traps particles larger than 4–6 μm, sweeping them back to the pharynx. Sneezing also rids the nose of irritants.

- Divided into:
  - external nose:
    - bones:
      - nasal part of frontal bones.
      - frontal process of maxillae.
      - nasal bones.
    - cartilages (lower part and septum).
    - fibrofatty tissue (ala).
  - nasal cavity: subdivided by the septum into two separate compartments, opening anteriorly by the nares and posteriorly by the choanae. The small dilatation immediately within the nares (vestibule) is lined with stratified squamous epithelium bearing hairs and sebaceous and sweat glands. The remainder is lined with columnar ciliated cells and mucus-secreting goblet cells. Subdivided into:
    - roof: slopes upwards and backwards forming the bridge of the nose; it then has a horizontal part (cribriform plate of the ethmoid bone) and finally a downward sloping part (palatine bone).
    - floor: composed of the palatine process of the maxilla and horizontal plate of the palatine bone. A tissue flap (soft palate) extends into the nasopharynx, closing off the nasal passages during swallowing.
    - medial wall: nasal septum.
    - lateral wall: ethmoidal labyrinth, nasal surface of the maxilla and perpendicular plate of the palatine bone. The three scroll-like conchae hang down over the nasal meatus. The olfactory organ of the first cranial nerve lies above and beside the upper concha. The orifices of the maxillary, sphenoid, frontal and ethmoidal sinuses open on to the lateral nasal wall.
- Blood supply:
  - upper: anterior and posterior ethmoidal branches of the ophthalmic artery.
  - lower: sphenopalatine branch of the maxillary artery.
  - anteroinferior septum: septal branch of the superior labial branch of the facial artery.

Venous drainage is via a submucous plexus which drains into the sphenopalatine, facial and ophthalmic veins.

- Nerve supply is from branches of the ophthalmic (V^1) and maxillary (V^2) divisions of the trigeminal nerve:
  - skin:
    - supratrochlear branch of the frontal nerve (V^1).
    - anterior ethmoidal branch of the nasociliary nerve (V^1).
    - infraorbital branch of V^2.
  - maxillary antrum: V^2 via sphenopalatine ganglion.
  - frontal sinus: frontal nerve (V^1).
  - ethmoid region: anterior and posterior branches of the nasociliary nerve (V^1).
  - nasal cavities:
    - anterior: anterior ethmoidal branch of the nasociliary nerve (V^1).

- posterior: short sphenopalatine and posterior nasal branches of V^2 (septum); long sphenopalatine branch (lateral wall).

Trauma to the nose may result from passage of a tracheal or nasogastric tube, or nasal airway. Resultant epistaxis may be severe, and may be reduced by prior administration of cocaine spray or paste, or other vasopressor solutions, e.g. xylometazoline 0.1%.

- For topical anaesthesia of the nose, many techniques have been described. Moffett's method is one of the best known:
  - solution consists of 2 ml 8% cocaine, 2 ml 1% sodium bicarbonate and 1 ml 1:1000 adrenaline.
  - one-sixth of the solution is instilled into each nostril and retained for 10 min in each of the following positions: right lateral head down, face down, and left lateral head down.

  Other techniques involve application of 8–10% cocaine or other agent plus 1: 200 000 adrenaline swabs to the anterior septum and posterior nasal cavity.

Maxillary and ophthalmic nerve blocks may be used for operations on or around the nose.

[Arthur J Moffett (1904–1995), Birmingham otolaryngologist]

See also, Ear, nose and throat surgery

Nosocomial infection. Infection acquired as a result of a patient's admission to hospital. Occurs in up to 10% of patients, with mortality of up to 5%. More common in the acutely ill (e.g. on ICU).

- Aetiology may be related to:
  - hospital factors: widespread presence of pathogens, poor general hygiene and transfer between staff and patients.
  - patient factors: increasingly elderly population with reduced resistance, immunodeficiency states, diabetes, smoking, malnutrition, alcoholism, trauma, drug therapy, etc.
  - interventions: surgery, tracheal intubation, catheter-related sepsis, bladder catheterisation, use of broad spectrum antibacterial drugs resulting in resistant organisms, blood transfusion, TPN, stress ulcer prophylaxis, etc.

  Sites of infection in order of decreasing frequency: urinary tract infection, surgical wound infection, nosocomial pneumonia and bacteraemia. Organisms most commonly involved in order of decreasing frequency: *S. aureus*, pseudomonas, coagulase negative staphylococci, Candida species and *Escherichia coli*. Fungal infection is especially common in immunosuppressed patients.
- Management:
  - reduce incidence:
    - effective infection control.
    - selective decontamination of the digestive tract may be appropriate in certain circumstances.
  - treat with appropriate anti-infective agents.

Vincent JL (2003). Lancet; 361: 2068–77

See also, Ventilator-associated pneumonia

Nosocomial pneumonia. Hospital-acquired chest infection occurring > 48 h after hospital admission; excludes infections incubating on admission. May occur in up to 25% of ICU patients and increases hospital mortality, length of stay and costs.

- Originates from:
  - environment (air, water, food, etc).
  - equipment (tracheal tubes, suction catheters, bronchoscopes, etc).
  - other patients.
  - hospital staff (inadequate hygiene).
- Other contributing factors include:
  - patient's age and general medical condition.
  - drugs (antacids, corticosteroids, H_2 receptor antagonists, sedatives, broad spectrum antibiotics, etc).
  - supine position.
  - aspiration of gastric contents.
  - reintubation.
- Typical pathogens include:
  - *Streptococcus pneumoniae.*
  - *Haemophilus influenzae.*
  - *Staphylococcus aureus.*
  - Gram-negative bacilli.

  Often more than one organism is involved.

Clinical diagnosis requires new, progressive or persistent chest X-ray abnormalities, with evidence of infection (two of: purulent sputum, hypo- or hyperthermia, and a low (< 5000/mm^3) or raised (> 10 000/mm^3) white cell count). Isolation of the responsible organism(s) is best undertaken using bronchoalveolar lavage, either blind or via fibreoptic bronchoscopy. Therapy should be organism specific when possible, but broad-spectrum antibiotics are frequently necessary until the organism is identified.

- Prevention is assisted by:
  - vaccination, e.g. against *Haemophilus influenzae*, pneumococcus and influenza virus.
  - hygiene, e.g. handwashing policies, removal of wristwatches, use of non-sterile gloves.
  - control of gastric pH (avoidance of alkaline pH reduces bacterial overgrowth).
  - control of gastric volume and motility (distension risks reflux and aspiration).
  - rotational therapy.
  - good airway protocols, e.g. avoiding nasal intubation (risks sinusitis) and the supine position (patients should be nursed 30° head up), regular aspiration of subglottic secretions.
  - selective decontamination of the digestive tract, although this remains controversial except in trauma.

Waldemar G, Johanson JR, Dever LL (2003). Intensive Care Med; 29: 23–9

See also Infection control; Nosocomial infection; Sepsis; Ventilator-associated pneumonia

Notifiable diseases. Diseases that an attending doctor is required by law to report to the Local Authority Proper Officers, usually via the consultant in communicable disease or chief environmental health officer. The scheme allows epidemiological surveillance and early identification of potential epidemics. Failure to send details of the case on a certificate may result in conviction and a fine. Include the following:

Acute encephalitis	Measles	Scarlet fever
Acute poliomyelitis	Meningitis	Smallpox
Anthrax	Meningococcal septicaemia	TB
Cholera	Mumps	Tetanus
Diphtheria	Ophthalmia neonatorum	Typhoid fever
Dysentery	Paratyphoid fever	Typhus
Food poisoning	Plague	Viral haemorrhagic fever
Leprosy	Rabies	Viral hepatitis
Leptospirosis	Relapsing fever	Whooping cough
Malaria	Rubella	Yellow fever

NPSA, *see National Patient Safety Agency*

NRP, *see Neonatal Resuscitation Program*

NSAIDs, *see Non-steroidal anti-inflammatory drugs*

Nuclear cardiology. Assessment of cardiac function using gamma cameras to trace radioisotopes, using data processors. Technetium-99 m labelled blood may be followed through the heart during first pass of a bolus, or over many cardiac cycles linked to the ECG (multigated acquisition imaging; MUGA). Individual chamber movement and valve function may be observed, and ejection fraction calculated by recording the number of counts in systole and diastole. Alternatively, the uptake of thallium-201 by cardiac tissue may be observed (uptake by normal myocardium is proportional to blood flow). Thallium scanning may be enhanced by giving intravenous dipyridamole to precipitate ischaemia by causing coronary steal. Recently infarcted myocardium may be labelled with technetium-99 m pyrophosphate. Other tracers used to identify areas of infarction, necrosis or inflammation include indium-111, gallium-67 citrate, and radiolabelled myosin-specific antibodies.

Nuclear magnetic resonance, *see Magnetic resonance imaging*

Null hypothesis. In statistics, the assumption that the observed frequency of an event equals the expected frequency. It may state that any observations are due to chance alone, or that the groups studied come from the same population, etc.; statistical tests aid the acceptance or rejection of this hypothesis (and whether an alternative hypothesis, e.g. that observed differences are caused by treatment, can be accepted). Results are expressed in terms of the probability that the null hypothesis does not hold for the case concerned.
See also, Confidence intervals; Statistical significance

Number needed to treat (NNT). Indicator of treatment effect in clinical trials. Equals (1 ÷ absolute risk reduction). Gives an indication of the size of treatment effect in a form that is easily understandable by clinicians, e.g. for an antiemetic with NNT for PONV of 5, one needs to treat 5 patients with the drug in order to prevent one patient suffering PONV. Combines both the efficacy of the drug and the incidence of the condition treated; for example, an antiemetic that is effective in 100% of patients will have a NNT of 5 if the incidence of PONV is 1:5, but if it is only 50% effective the NNT will be 10. Number needed to harm (NNH) is a similar concept, indicating the number of patients needed to receive a drug before one suffers a complication.
See also, Meta-analysis; Odds ratio; Relative risk reduction

Nurses, prescription of drugs by. In the UK, specially trained nurses have been able to prescribe from a limited formulary since 1998; from 2006, new regulations allow certain nurses (and pharmacists) to prescribe any licensed drug (including opioids) so long as it is within their specific competence and local clinical governance frameworks. Other nurses and pharmacists are able to prescribe within specific management plans drawn up by a doctor for individual cases. Likely to have most relevance to acute and chronic pain management, premedication and intensive care.
See also, Midwives, prescription of drugs by

Nutrition. An adequately balanced daily supply of carbohydrates, fats, proteins, vitamins, electrolytes, trace elements and water is essential to maintain normal health.

- Average normal adult daily requirements:
  - water: 30–40 ml/kg.
  - nitrogen: 0.2 g/kg.
  - energy : 30–40 Cal/kg.
  - electrolytes:
    - sodium: 1 mmol/kg.
    - potassium: 1 mmol/kg.
    - chloride: 1.5 mmol/kg.
    - phosphate: 0.2–0.5 mmol/kg.
    - calcium: 0.1–0.2 mmol/kg.
    - magnesium: 0.1–0.2 mmol/kg.
  - trace elements:
    - iron: 0.2 mg/kg.
    - zinc: 0.2 mg/kg.
    - selenium: ~1 μg/kg.
  - vitamins: vary from under 0.1 g/kg to 1.0 mg/kg (*see Table 37; Vitamins*).

Energy requirements depend on the particular circumstances for each individual, e.g. they increase after trauma, burns, etc. (*see Catabolism*), and with pyrexia (by about 10% for every °C above normal). Patients should be fed via the oral route if possible, preferably with normal food.

For critically ill patients, more precise estimation of energy balance is necessary, whatever the route of administration. Once energy requirements have been determined, it is divided into carbohydrate (4 Cal/g) and fat (9 Cal/g) components to accompany nitrogen (150–200 Cal per g nitrogen). Carbohydrate should comprise 40–50% of energy requirements. Appropriate enteral or parenteral solutions are then selected from commercially available products (some pharmacies make up their own solutions), satisfying requirements for energy, fluid and electrolytes. Vitamins, etc. may be added as required.

Bistrian BR, McCowen KC (2006). Crit Care Med; 34: 1525–31

See also, Malnutrition; Metabolism; Nitrogen balance; Nutrition, enteral; Nutrition, total parenteral

Nutrition, enteral. Ingestion of foodstuffs via the GIT. Ideal route is by mouth using normal or liquidised food and calorific/protein supplements, if necessary. In patients recovering from critical illness or major surgery, it is preferable to TPN as it is more physiological, provides protection against stress ulcers (thereby decreasing the requirement for H_2 receptor antagonists) and maintains intestinal barrier integrity, thus reducing the occurrence of bacterial translocation. The presence of nutrients within the small intestine also promotes biliary flow and prevents the cholestasis commonly seen with TPN.

Commonly performed via fine-bore nasogastric tubes although this is usually limited to about 6 weeks because of the risk of aspiration, especially in depressed consciousness. Alternatives include a nasoenteric feeding tube (using a weighted tube or passed via endoscopy) into the small intestine, percutaneous endoscopic gastrostomy or a jejunostomy tube placed at the time of surgery. Principles are those of nutrition generally.

Carbohydrate is the usual energy source in most enteral feeds, but high concentrations increase osmolality, causing diarrhoea. The protein source is usually whole protein although preparations containing oligopeptides or amino acids are useful in pancreatic disease and malabsorption syndromes. Medium chain triglycerides are the usual source of fat.

- Complications:
  - mechanical, e.g. tube blockage, passage of the tube into the trachea, regurgitation.

- nausea and vomiting: occurs in 10% of cases; may require antiemetic drugs or prokinetic drugs.
- diarrhoea: occurs in up to 60% of cases; may be caused by intolerance of high osmotic load, underlying bowel disorder, infected feed or concurrent antibacterial drug therapy.
- electrolyte and liver function test disturbances.

Zaloga GP (2006). Lancet; 367: 1101–11

See also, Energy balance; Nutrition, total parenteral

Nutrition, total parenteral (TPN). Administration of total nutritional requirements by iv infusion; it may be required in patients who are hypercatabolic and/or have an abnormal GIT. Commonly required in critically ill patients on ICU with intra-abdominal conditions or multiorgan failure. Only indicated if enteral nutrition fails or is impossible to use. May also be used to support enteral nutrition.

Principles are those of nutrition generally, i.e. calculation of nitrogen balance, energy and fluid requirements. Nitrogen and the energy source should be given together, preferably continuously. 5–6 mmol potassium and 1–2 mmol magnesium are required per gram of nitrogen.

The nitrogen component is given as mixtures of essential and non-essential amino acids (the nitrogen content varies considerably between different solutions). Some amino acid solutions contain electrolytes and most are hypertonic. Some contain energy sources, e.g. glucose and fructose. Carbohydrate is usually given as glucose 10–50%, and requires central venous infusion to avoid venous thrombosis. Other energy sources, e.g. sorbitol, xylitol and ethanol, have also been used. Insulin is usually required to control hyperglycaemia associated with glucose-rich infusions. Fat is usually administered as 10 or 20% soya bean oil emulsions; allergic reactions may occur rarely with the 20% preparation. Trace elements and vitamins must be added.

Most solutions are administered from one large bag via a pump and a single dedicated central venous cannula, although a peripheral line is acceptable for temporary infusion of fat emulsion.

The patient should be encouraged to mobilise to prevent muscle breakdown.

- Complications:
  - those associated with central venous cannulation.
  - sepsis.
  - metabolic disorders:
    - hyperglycaemia.
    - hypophosphataemia.
    - metabolic acidosis.
    - hypernatraemia.
    - lipaemia.
    - trace element or vitamin deficiency.
  - cholestasis resulting in acute cholecystitis.
- Routine monitoring should include:
  - clinical signs, weight and fluid balance daily. Skinfold thickness and arm circumference have been used.
  - plasma urea, creatinine, electrolytes and osmolality daily. Glucose should be measured more frequently, e.g. by stick-testing. Liver function and plasma calcium, phosphate and magnesium should be assessed at least twice a week.
  - urine urea and osmolality daily.
  - full blood count every 1–3 days; prothrombin time once a week. Iron, folate and vitamin B_{12} should be measured at least weekly.

See also, Energy balance; Nutrition, enteral

Nystatin. Polyene antifungal drug, principally used for treatment of *Candida albicans* infections of skin, mucous membranes and GIT. Not absorbed when administered by mouth and too toxic for parenteral use. Available as tablets, oral suspension, cream or pessaries.

- Dosage: 500 000–1 000 000 units orally, 6 hourly (in children 100 000 units 6 hourly); 1 000 000 units/day for prophylaxis or oral infection.
- Side effects: GIT upset, rash.

O

Obesity. Common and increasing problem in the Western world. Body mass index (weight in kg divided by height in m^2) is often used for definition: < 25 kg/m^2 = normal; 25–30 kg/m^2 = overweight; > 30 kg/m^2 = obese. Approximately 20% of UK adults are obese by this definition and this number has trebled in the last 20 years. Morbid obesity is defined as twice ideal body weight; general mortality in this group is twice that of normal. Distribution of fat is thought to be more important than weight per se, with abdominal deposition particularly detrimental. Thus for a BMI ≥ 25 kg/m^2, a waist (just above the navel) circumference of ≥ 94 cm indicates increased risk and ≥ 102 cm substantially increased risk for men; corresponding values for women are 80 cm and 88 cm respectively.

- Effects:
  - RS:
    - increased body O_2 demand and CO_2 production, because of increased tissue mass. Minute ventilation required to maintain normocapnia is thus increased, which further increases O_2 demand.
    - reduced FRC because of the weight of the chest wall. FRC is especially reduced in the supine position, due to the weight of the abdominal wall and contents. Thoracic compliance is thus reduced, increasing work of breathing and O_2 demand. $\dot{V}/\dot{Q}$ mismatch results in hypoxaemia.
    - hypoxic pulmonary vasoconstriction increases work of the right ventricle and may lead to pulmonary hypertension and right-sided cardiac failure.
    - obstructive sleep apnoea and alveolar hypoventilation syndrome may occur.
  - CVS:
    - cardiac output and blood volume increase, to increase O_2 flux.
    - hypertension occurs in 60%; thus left ventricular work is increased. Left ventricular hypertrophy and ischaemia may occur, with resultant left-sided cardiac failure. Arrhythmias are common.
  - other diseases are more likely, e.g. non-insulin dependent diabetes mellitus (caused by insulin resistance and inadequate insulin production, the latter worsening with age), hypercholesterolaemia, gout and arthritis, gallbladder disease, hepatic impairment, CVA, breast and endometrial malignancies.

Patients may require surgery for related or unrelated conditions, or for 'treatment'. The latter procedures are increasingly done laparascopically and include gastric banding, partial gastrectomy and gastric bypass, as single procedures or in combination.

- Anaesthetic considerations:
  - preoperatively:
    - preoperative assessment for the above complications and appropriate management. Patients may be taking amfetamines or related drugs for weight loss.
    - heparin prophylaxis is usual, because patients are less mobile and risk of DVT is increased. The ideal dose of heparin is not certain in morbidly obese patients.
    - im injection may be difficult because of subcutaneous fat, while anti-DVT stockings may not fit properly.
  - perioperatively:
    - veins may be difficult to find and cannulate.
    - hiatus hernia is common, with risk of aspiration of gastric contents. Volume and acidity of gastric contents may be increased. In addition, tracheal intubation may be difficult: insertion of the laryngoscope blade into the mouth may be hindered, the neck may be short and movement reduced.
    - hypoxaemia may occur rapidly during apnoea, since FRC (hence O_2 reserve) is reduced, and O_2 utilisation increased. FRC is increased if the patient is positioned head-up before induction of anaesthesia.
    - airway maintenance is often difficult, because of increased soft tissue mass in the upper airway. Spontaneous ventilation is often inadequate because of respiratory impairment, which worsens in the supine position (especially in the head-down position or with legs in the lithotomy position). Thus IPPV is usually employed; high inflation pressures may be required.
    - lifting and positioning the patient may be difficult. The typical maximum weight limit for manual operating tables is 135 kg, and for electrical operating tables is 250–300 kg. Two operating tables placed side by side may be necessary if the patient is too wide for a single table.
    - monitoring may be difficult, e.g. BP cuff too small, ECG complexes small.
    - surgery is more likely to be difficult and prolonged, with increased blood loss.
    - drug use:
      - appropriate dosage may be difficult; e.g. neuromuscular blocking drugs are given according to lean body weight. Distribution of drugs is affected by the increase in adipose tissue mass.
      - increased metabolism of inhalational anaesthetic agents is thought to occur, e.g. increased fluoride ion concentrations after prolonged use of enflurane.
    - although regional techniques may have potential advantages over general anaesthesia, they are often technically difficult.
  - postoperatively:
    - atelectasis and hypoventilation are common, with increased risk of infection, hypoxaemia and respiratory failure. Patients are often best nursed sitting. Elective IPPV may be required; weaning may be difficult. Difficulty mobilising may also be a problem.
    - postoperative analgesia, O_2 therapy and physiotherapy are especially important. HDU or ICU admission may be required.

Similar considerations apply to admission of obese patients to ICU for non-surgical reasons.
Cheah MH, Kam PCA (2005). Anaesthesia; 60: 1009–21

Obesity hypoventilation syndrome (Pickwickian syndrome, after a character from Dickens' *Pickwick Papers*). Obesity, daytime hypersomnolence, hypoxaemia and hypercapnia often in the presence of right ventricular failure. Pulmonary hypertension is present in 60% of patients. In addition to the alveolar hypoventilation, patients often have $\dot{V}/\dot{Q}$ mismatch. Cyanosis and plethora are common, due to polycythaemia secondary to hypoxia. The syndrome is associated with severe obstructive sleep apnoea and a disordered central control of respiration during sleep. Sudden nocturnal death is common.

General and anaesthetic management is as for obesity and cor pulmonale. The F_IO_2 should be increased cautiously to avoid depression of the hypoxic ventilatory drive. CPAP may be useful. Respiratory depressant drugs should also be used cautiously; postoperative respiratory failure may occur.
[Charles Dickens (1812–1870), English author]
Olson AL, Zwillich C (2005). Am J Med; 118: 948–56

Obstetric analgesia and anaesthesia. Strictly, 'analgesia' refers to removal of pain during labour and 'anaesthesia' is provided for operative delivery and other procedures. Pain during the first stage of labour is thought to be caused by cervical dilatation, and is usually felt in the T11–L1 dermatomes. Back and rectal pain may also occur. Pain often worsens at the end of the first stage. Pain during the second stage is caused by stretching of the birth canal and perineum.

Early attempts at pain relief included the use of abdominal pressure, opium and alcohol. Simpson administered the first obstetric anaesthetic in 1847, using diethyl ether. He used chloroform later that year, subsequently preferring it to ether. Moral and religious objections to anaesthesia in childbirth declined after Snow's administration of chloroform to Queen Victoria in 1853. Regional techniques were introduced from the early 1900s, and have become increasingly popular since the 1960s.

Choice of technique is related to the physiological effects of pregnancy (especially risk of aortocaval compression and aspiration pneumonitis), and effects of drugs and complications on the fetus, neonate and course of labour. Anaesthesia has until the last 20–30 years been a major cause of death during pregnancy as revealed in the Reports on Confidential Enquiries into Maternal Deaths.

- Methods used:
  - non-drug methods, e.g. TENS, acupuncture, hypnosis, psychoprophylaxis, audioanaesthesia, abdominal decompression: generally safe for mother and fetus, but of variable efficacy and thus rarely used except for TENS and psychoprophylaxis.
  - systemic opioid analgesic drugs:
    - morphine was used with hyoscine to provide twilight sleep in the early 1900s. However, it readily crosses the placenta to cause neonatal respiratory depression. Pethidine was first used in 1940 and approved for use by UK midwives in 1950; it is the most commonly used opioid (e.g. 50–150 mg im up to two doses), but 30–75% of women gain no benefit from its use and there is little evidence that opioids actually reduce pain scores. Nausea, vomiting, delayed gastric emptying and sedation may occur, with neonatal respiratory depression especially likely between 2 and 4 h after im injection. Subtle changes may be detected on neurobehavioural testing of the neonate. Neonatal respiratory depression is marked after iv injection.
    - other opioids have been used with similar effects. A lower incidence of neonatal depression has been claimed for partial agonists and agonist/antagonists, e.g. nalbuphine, pentazocine, meptazinol, but they are not commonly used.
    - patient-controlled analgesia has been used, e.g. pethidine 10–20 mg iv or nalbuphine 2–3 mg iv (lockout time 10 min), or fentanyl 10–25 μg following 25–75 μg loading dose (lockout time 3–5 min). More recently, remifentanil has been used (e.g. bolus 40–50 μg with lockout 2 min).
    - opioid receptor antagonists, e.g. naloxone may be given to the neonate if respiratory depression is marked.
  - sedative drugs: rarely used nowadays; promazine, promethazine, benzodiazepines, chloral hydrate, clomethiazole and chlordiazepoxide have been used. All may cause neonatal depression.
  - inhalational anaesthetic agents:
    - ether and chloroform were first used in 1847. Trichloroethylene was used in the 1940s, and methoxyflurane in 1970; formerly approved for midwives' use with draw-over techniques, their use in the UK ceased in 1984.
    - N_2O was first used in 1880. Intermittent flow anaesthetic machines were developed from the 1930s, using N_2O with air or O_2. The Lucy Baldwin apparatus (funded by the Lucy Baldwin fund for supplying labour wards) was developed in the late 1950s, delivering preset N_2O/O_2 mixtures. Entonox was used in 1962 by Tunstall, and approved for use by midwives in 1965. It is usually self-administered using a facepiece or mouthpiece and demand valve, although continuous administration via nasal cannulae has been described. Slow deep inhalation should start as soon as (ideally just before) a contraction begins, in order to achieve adequate blood levels at peak pain. May cause nausea and dizziness; it is otherwise relatively safe with minimal side effects although maternal arterial desaturation has been reported, especially in combination with pethidine. Useful in 50% of women but of no help in 30% and like opioids, there is little evidence that it reduces pain scores. Isoflurane has been added with good effect (Isoxane).
    - enflurane, isoflurane, desflurane and more recently sevoflurane have been used with draw-over inhalation.
  - general anaesthesia: no longer used for normal vaginal delivery. Problems are as for Caesarean section.
  - regional techniques: involve blockade of the nerve supply of:
    - uterus:
      - via sympathetic pathways in paracervical tissues and broad ligament to the spinal cord at T11–12, sometimes T10 and L1 also.
      - the cervix is possibly innervated via separate S2–4 pathways in addition.
    - birth canal and perineum: via pudendal nerves (S2–4), genitofemoral and ilioinguinal nerves and sacral nerves.
- Regional techniques used:
  - epidural anaesthesia/analgesia:
    - caudal analgesia was first used in obstetrics in 1909 by Stoeckel; a continuous technique was introduced in the USA in 1942.
    - continuous lumbar techniques were used in 1946; they have become popular in the UK from the 1960s, with most units now providing a 24-h service. Uptake varies

widely, with up to 70–80% for primiparae in some centres. The overall epidural rate in the UK is around 20–30%.
- advantages:
  - reduces maternal exhaustion, hyperventilation, ketosis, and plasma catecholamine levels.
  - avoids adverse effects of parenteral opioids.
  - reduces fetal acidosis and maintains or increases uteroplacental blood flow if hypotension is avoided.
  - may improve contractions in incoordinate uterine activity.
  - thought to reduce morbidity and mortality in breech delivery, multiple delivery, premature labour, pre-eclampsia, maternal cardiovascular or respiratory disease, diabetes mellitus, forceps delivery and Caesarean section.
- disadvantages:
  - risk of hypotension, extensive blockade, iv injection and other complications. Post-dural puncture headache is more common than in non-pregnant subjects following accidental dural tap (the maximum acceptable incidence of the latter has been set at about 1% in the UK). Shivering and urinary retention may occur.
  - motor block may be distressing, and if extensive may be associated with delayed descent of the fetal head.
  - requires iv cannulation (although the need for routine administration of iv fluids has been questioned if low-dose techniques are used), and 24-h dedicated anaesthetic cover.
  - increased incidence of backache has been reported, but this has been shown to reflect selection of patients prone to backache (e.g. complicated labour, lower pain threshold, etc.), plus the natural tendency of patients to link back pain with any procedure performed on the back, rather than a result of regional analgesia or anaesthesia itself.
  - effect on labour:
    - temporary reduction in uterine activity has been reported following injection of solution, though this may be caused by the bolus of crystalloid traditionally given concurrently.
    - incoordinate uterine activity may improve.
    - ventouse/forceps rate is increased; thought to occur because:
      - patients likely to require forceps delivery are more likely to receive epidural analgesia.
      - muscle tone is reduced as above.

    The relative importance of these two factors is hotly disputed, with non-anaesthetists claiming that epidurals cause an increase in instrumental delivery rates whilst anaesthetists claim that epidural analgesia is merely a marker of abnormal and/or high risk labours. Randomised clinical trials are few and suffer from practical problems such as lack of obstetric blinding and non-compliance with the allocated treatment. The argument is therefore likely to continue, although studies suggest that low dose techniques are more likely to result in spontaneous delivery than the older, higher dose methods (though even with the latter, normal vaginal delivery rates are thought to occur if adequate time is allowed for the second stage). Perineal tears may occur if the second stage is very prolonged.
- technique:
  - standard techniques are used, but low doses of local anaesthetic agent are used to minimise motor block and risk of adverse effects. If higher doses are used, smaller volumes are required because venous engorgement reduces the volume of the epidural space. Hypotension is common with higher doses of local anaesthetic, especially in the presence of hypovolaemia; it is reduced by preloading with iv fluid, usually crystalloid (e.g. 0.9% saline/Hartmann's solution, 500 ml. Ketosis and hyponatraemia may occur with excess administration of dextrose solutions). L2–3 or L3–4 interspaces are usually chosen although because identification of the lumber interspaces by palpation is not reliable (especially in pregnancy when the pelvis tilts), anaesthetists often place the catheter at a higher interspace than that intended.
  - bupivacaine is traditionally preferred, since fetal transfer is least. Others have been used, e.g. lidocaine, chloroprocaine. Prilocaine is rarely used because of the risk of methaemoglobinaemia. Ropivacaine is claimed to cause less motor block than bupivacaine when higher concentrations are used. Levobupivacaine has a better safety profile but with low dose regimens this difference becomes less relevant.
  - use of a test dose is controversial. With low dose regimens, the first dose is also the test dose.
  - suitable dose regimens:
    - bupivacaine 0.1% 10–15 ml with fentanyl 1–2 μg/ml as boluses. More concentrated solutions provide analgesia lasting slightly longer, but with more motor blockade. 0.75% solution is contraindicated in obstetrics. Top-up injections are usually given by midwives. Aspiration through the catheter should precede top-ups, which should be given in divided doses except for low dose solutions. A maximum of 25 mg bupivacaine has been suggested for any single injection. Ropivacaine 0.2% has been used as an alternative.
    - infusions: provide more consistent analgesia, with less motor block and hypotension than high dose top-ups, and reduce the risk from accidental iv or subarachnoid injection. Bupivacaine 10–20 mg/h is usually employed, usually as a 0.1–0.2% solution, and often combined with fentanyl 1–2 μg/ml. Large volumes of more dilute solutions have been used, supporting the concept of an 'extended sleeve' of anaesthetic solution over the appropriate segments. The height of the block must be regularly assessed, and the infusion adjusted accordingly.
    - patient-controlled epidural analgesia is also used, e.g. with 0.1–0.125% bupivacaine with fentanyl 1–3 μg/ml, and boluses of 8–12 ml without a background infusion, or of 3–6 ml with a background infusion of 3–6 ml/min, and a lockout time of 10–20 min.
    - epidural opioids have been used alone, but but rarely in the UK (*see Spinal opioids*). Fentanyl is usually added to weak solutions of bupivacaine as above. In the USA, sufentanil is often used. Epidural pethidine is popular in Australia.
    - inadequate blockade: includes 'missed segment' (commonly in one groin, the cause is unclear), backache (especially with occipitoposterior presentation), rectal or perineal pain, and unilateral blocks. Remedial measures include further injection of solution, with the unblocked part dependent. Use of a stronger solution, a different local anaesthetic,

or fentanyl 50–75 μg, may be helpful. Infiltration of the unblocked dermatome with local anaesthetic has been described but is rarely done. The catheter should be withdrawn 1–2 cm if unilateral block occurs. Resiting of the catheter may be required. Suprapubic pain may result from a full bladder, and may be relieved by urinary catheterisation. Breakthrough pain in the presence of a uterine scar may indicate uterine rupture. Overall about 10% of epidurals require adjustment or extra doses.
- contraindications, complications and management are as for epidural analgesia/anaesthesia. Care should be taken in antepartum haemorrhage (see below). Extensive blockade and accidental iv injection of local anaesthetic are possible following catheter migration. All blocks should be regularly assessed and an anaesthetist should be readily available, with resuscitative drugs and equipment. Maximal doses of local anaesthetic agents should not be exceeded in a 4-h period.

  Backache and neurological damage may be caused by labour itself, although epidural analgesia is often blamed by the patient and non-anaesthetic staff.

- spinal anaesthesia was first used in 1900. Popular in the USA in the 1920s, it only increased in popularity in the UK towards the end of the 1900s. Technique and management are as standard, but with more rapid onset of hypotension and greater incidence of post-dural puncture headache and variable blocks (especially using plain bupivacaine) than in non-pregnant subjects. Dose requirements are reduced, possibly due to altered CSF dynamics, although changes in CSF pH, proteins and volume have been suggested. Effects are as for epidural anaesthesia. Mostly used for Caesarean section, forceps and ventouse delivery, removal of retained placenta, etc. Doses for vaginal procedures: 1.0–1.6 ml heavy bupivacaine 0.5%; lower doses with opioids have also been used.
- CSE has been advocated because of its rapid onset and intense quality of analgesia (from the spinal component), with subsequent management as for epidural analgesia. Its routine place in labour is controversial because of its increased cost, the increased risk of post-dural puncture headache, and (theoretical) fears over a possibly increased risk of infection. There have been reports of damage to the conus medullaris associated with CSE, possibly related to the use of pencil-point needles since they need to be inserted more deeply in order to obtain CSF. In addition, the unreliability of identifying the lumbar interspaces by palpation may result in insertion of the needle at a higher vertebral level than intended. The lowest easily palpable interspace should therefore be chosen, and an epidural-only technique used above L3–4.

  A widely used starting intrathecal dose is 1 ml plain bupivacaine 0.25% mixed with fentanyl 25 μg, made up to 2 ml with saline. 3–5 ml boluses of the low dose epidural mixture above has also been used. Continuous spinal analgesia has been described, using the same low dose solution.
- paravertebral block: bilateral blocks are required at either L2 (for sympathetic block) or T11–12 (somatic block).
- paracervical block: rarely performed because of fetal arrhythmias.
- pudendal nerve block and perineal infiltration/spraying with local anaesthetic: only of use for the second stage. Pudendal block is used for forceps and ventouse delivery.
- local infiltration of the abdomen for Caesarean section.

● Particular problems in obstetric anaesthetic practice:
- obstetric conditions, e.g. pre-eclampsia, placenta praevia, placental abruption, postpartum haemorrhage. Haemorrhage may follow any delivery, and facilities for urgent transfusion should be available, including a cutdown set and O negative uncross-matched blood. DIC may also occur in septic abortion, intrauterine death, hydatidiform mole and severe shock.
- maternal disease, e.g. cardiovascular, respiratory, diabetes, etc. Epidural blockade is usually preferred.
- fluid overload associated with oxytocin administration; pulmonary oedema associated with tocolytic drugs.
- specific procedures/presentations:
  - premature labour: spinal/epidural analgesia/anaesthesia is usually preferred, since it allows smooth controlled delivery with or without forceps. The immature fetus may be especially susceptible to drug-induced depression. Tocolytic drugs may have been used.
  - twin delivery: epidural analgesia is usually employed. The block should be adequate for Caesarean section, in case this is required for delivery of the second twin (this is required in up to 10% of cases). Blood loss at delivery is greater than with a single fetus. The enlarged uterus is more likely to cause aortocaval compression.
  - breech presentation: most deliver by Caesarean section nowadays because of evidence that neonatal outcome is better.
  - manual removal of placenta: spinal/epidural anaesthesia is usually considered preferable to general anaesthesia, since the latter risks aspiration of gastric contents, and inhalational agents cause uterine relaxation.
- collapse on labour ward:
  - causes include: shock associated with abruption and DIC, postpartum haemorrhage, total spinal blockade, overdosage or iv injection of local anaesthetic, amniotic fluid embolism, PE, eclampsia, inversion of the uterus, and pre-existing disease.
  - CPR is hindered by aortocaval compression, relieved by tilting the patient to one side or manually displacing the uterus laterally. Caesarean section may be required.

[Lucy Baldwin (1859–1945), wife of the British Prime Minister; Walter Stoeckel (1871–1961), German obstetrician; Michael E Tunstall, Aberdeen anaesthetist]

See also, Cardiopulmonary resuscitation, neonatal; Ergometrine; Fetal monitoring; Flying squad, obstetric; Labour, active management of; Midwives, prescription of drugs by; Obstetric intensive care

Obstetric intensive care. Required in 0.2–9 cases per 1000 deliveries, depending on the population served and the ICU admission criteria used. Most common reasons for admission are haemorrhage, pre-eclampsia and HELLP syndrome; mortality of 3–4% is reported in UK series but up to 20% has been reported from elsewhere. Main problems are related to the risks to the fetus and the physiological changes of pregnancy: obstetric patients have increased oxygen demands and reduced respiratory reserves, and are more susceptible to aspiration of gastric contents, aortocaval compression, acute lung injury, DVT and DIC.

General management is along standard lines, with attention to the above complications. Excessive fluid administration should be avoided since ARDS is a common feature of obstetric critical illness. Fetal monitoring should be ensured if antepartum, although the needs of the mother outweigh those of the fetus. Uteroplacental blood flow may be impaired by vasopressors and the mother may be too sick to receive tocolytic drugs should premature labour occur. Caesarean section may be required to improve the mother's condition. Breast milk may be unsuitable for use because of maternal drugs; if required lactation can be suppressed with bromocriptine (although hypertension, CVA and MI have followed its use, hence it should be avoided in hypertensive disorders).

Martin SR, Foley MR (2006). Am J Obstet Gynecol; 195: 673–89

See also, Placenta praevia; Placental abruption; Postpartum haemorrhage

Obturator nerve block. Performed to accompany sciatic nerve block or femoral nerve block, or in the diagnosis and treatment of hip pain. The obturator nerve (L2–4), a branch of the lumbar plexus, passes down within the pelvis and through the obturator canal into the thigh, to supply the hip joint, anterior adductor muscles and skin of medial lower thigh/knee.

With the patient supine and the leg slightly abducted, an 8 cm needle is inserted 1–2 cm caudal and lateral to the pubic tubercle, and directed slightly medially to encounter the pubic ramus. It is then withdrawn and redirected laterally to enter the obturator canal, and advanced 2–3 cm. If a nerve stimulator is used, twitches in the adductor muscles are sought. After careful aspiration to exclude intravascular placement, 10–15 ml local anaesthetic agent is injected.

In an alternative approach, the leg is externally rotated and abducted and an 8–10 cm needle inserted behind the adductor longus tendon near its pubic insertion, and directed posteriorly and slightly cranially and laterally. 5–10 ml solution is injected at a depth of 2–3 cm.

Occipital nerve blocks, *see Scalp, nerve blocks*

Octreotide. Long-acting somatostatin analogue, used in carcinoid syndrome and related GIT tumours and acromegaly. Also licensed for use in treating complications of pancreatic surgery. Has also been used in bleeding oesophageal varices, and to reduce vomiting in palliative care. Plasma levels peak within an hour of sc administration, and within a few minutes of iv injection. Half-life is 1–2 h. Lanreotide is a similar agent.

- Dosage:
  - 50 μg once-twice daily sc, increased to 200 μg 8 hourly if required (rarely up to 500 μg 8 hourly in carcinoid syndrome).
  - 50–100 μg iv in carcinoid crisis, diluted to 10–50% in saline.
  - 50 μg iv followed by 50 μg/h in bleeding varices.
- Side effects: GIT upset, glucose intolerance, hepatic impairment.

Oculocardiac reflex. Bradycardia following traction on the extraocular muscles, especially medial rectus. Afferent pathways are via the occipital branch of the trigeminal nerve; efferents are via the vagus. The reflex is particularly active in children. Bradycardia may be severe, and may lead to asystole. Other arrhythmias, e.g. ventricular ectopics or junctional rhythm, may occur. Bradycardia may also follow pressure on or around the eye, fixation of facial fractures, etc. Reduced by anticholinergic drugs administered as premedication or on induction of anaesthesia. If it occurs, surgery should stop, and atropine or glycopyrronium administered. Retrobulbar block does not reliably prevent it; local infiltration of the muscles has been used instead.

See also, Ophthalmic surgery

Oculogyric crises, *see Dystonic reactions*

Oculorespiratory reflex. Hypoventilation following traction on the external ocular muscles. Reduced respiratory rate, reduced tidal volume or irregular ventilation may occur. Thought to involve the same afferent pathways as the oculocardiac reflex, but with efferents via the respiratory centres. Heart rate may be unchanged, and the reflex is unaffected by atropine.

ODAs/ODPs, *see Operating department assistants/practitioners*

Odds ratio. Ratio of the odds of an event's occurrence in one group to its odds in another, used as an indicator of treatment effect in clinical trials. For example, if a disease is suspected to be caused by exposure to a certain factor, a 2 × 2 table may be drawn for proportions of patients in the following groups:

	With disease	*Without disease*
Exposed	*a*	*c*
Not exposed	*b*	*d*

$$\text{Odds ratio} = \text{the ratio of } a/b \text{ to } c/d$$
$$= ad/bc.$$

Harder to understand (but more useful mathematically) than other indices of risk commonly used.

See also, Absolute risk reduction; Meta-analysis; Number needed to treat; Relative risk reduction

ODIN, Organ dysfunction and/or infection, *see Logistic organ dysfunction system*

O'Dwyer, Joseph (1841–1898). US physician; regarded as the introducer of the first practical intubation tube in 1885, although the technique had been described previously by others, e.g. Kite. His short metal tube, used as an alternative to tracheostomy in diphtheria, was inserted blindly into the larynx on an introducer; the flanged upper end rested on the vocal cords. He mounted his tube on a handle for use with Fell's resuscitation bellows in 1888; the Fell–O'Dwyer apparatus could be used for CPR or anaesthesia. Later modifications included addition of a cuff.

[George Fell (1850–1918), US ENT surgeon]

Oedema. Generalised or local excess ECF. Caused by:

- hypoproteinaemia and decreased plasma oncotic pressure.
- increased hydrostatic pressure, e.g. cardiac failure, venous or lymphatic obstruction; salt and water retention (e.g. renal impairment, drugs, e.g. NSAIDs, oestrogens, corticosteroids).
- leaky capillary endothelium, e.g. inflammation, allergic reactions, toxins.
- direct instillation, e.g. extravasated iv fluids, infiltration.

Several causes often coexist, e.g. hypoproteinaemia, portal hypertension and fluid retention in hepatic failure. Characterised by pitting when prolonged digital pressure is applied, although fibrosis reduces this in chronic oedema. Generalised oedema occurs in dependent parts of the body, e.g. ankles if ambulant, sacrum if bed-bound. Treatment is directed at the cause. If localised, the affected part is raised above the heart.

See also, Cerebral oedema; Hereditary angioedema; Pulmonary oedema; Starling's forces

Oesophageal contractility. Used as an indicator of anaesthetic depth and brainstem integrity. Skeletal muscle is present in the upper third of the oesophagus, smooth muscle in the lower third, and both types in the middle third. Afferent and efferent nerve supply is mainly vagal via oesophageal plexuses, but also via sympathetic nerves.

- Normal pattern of contractions:
  - primary: continuation of the swallowing process; propels the food bolus down the oesophagus.
  - secondary (provoked): caused by presence of food, etc. within the oesophageal lumen. Unrelated to swallowing.
  - tertiary (spontaneous): non-peristaltic; function is uncertain.

Measured by passing a double-ballooned probe into the lower oesophagus. The distal balloon is filled with water and connected to a pressure transducer; the other balloon (just proximal) may be inflated intermittently to study provoked contractions.

- Altered by:
  - anaesthesia: provoked contractions diminish in amplitude as depth increases, and spontaneous contractions become less frequent. Oesophageal contractility index ((70 × spontaneous rate) + provoked amplitude) is used as an overall measure of activity. Thought to be analogous to BP, heart rate, lacrimation, sweating, etc., during anaesthesia; i.e. suggestive of anaesthetic depth but not reliable. Activity may be decreased by atropine and smooth muscle relaxants, e.g. sodium nitroprusside, and increased by neostigmine.
  - brainstem death: spontaneous contractions disappear, and provoked contractions show a low amplitude pattern. Has been used to indicate the presence or absence of brainstem activity in ICU, but its role is controversial. Presently not included in UK brainstem death criteria.

See also, Anaesthesia, depth of

Oesophageal obturators and airways. Devices inserted blindly into the oesophagus of unconscious patients to secure the airway and allow IPPV when tracheal intubation is not possible, e.g. by untrained personnel. They have been used in failed intubation. Consist of a cuffed oesophageal tube, often attached to a facepiece for sealing the mouth and nose and preventing air leaks. The cuff reduces gastric insufflation and regurgitation but may not prevent it.

The epiglottis is pushed anteriorly, creating an air passage for ventilation. An ordinary tracheal tube may be used to isolate the stomach and improve the airway in a similar way.

- Two main types are described:
  - blind-ended cuffed tube, perforated level with the hypopharynx for passage of air. Inflation is through the tube and via the perforations to the lungs.
  - open-ended tube, to allow gastric aspiration. Inflation is through a separate port of the facepiece. If accidental tracheal placement occurs, IPPV may be performed through the tube.

  The above features have been combined in a double-lumen device (Combitube), which may be placed in either the oesophagus or trachea (Fig. 118). A distal cuff (15 ml) seals the oesophagus or trachea, whilst a proximal balloon (100 ml) seals the oral and nasal airways. IPPV may be performed through either tube depending on the device's position; it enters the oesophagus in over 95% of cases initially and ventilation via the longer proximal tube (A) will result in pulmonary ventilation via the proximal openings (C). The shorter distal tube (B) may then be used for gastric suction via the distal opening (D). If the device is tracheal, IPPV may be achieved via tube B and opening D. Has been suggested as a suitable device for non-medical personnel, e.g. for CPR, although trauma is more common than with alternative devices such as the laryngeal mask airway.

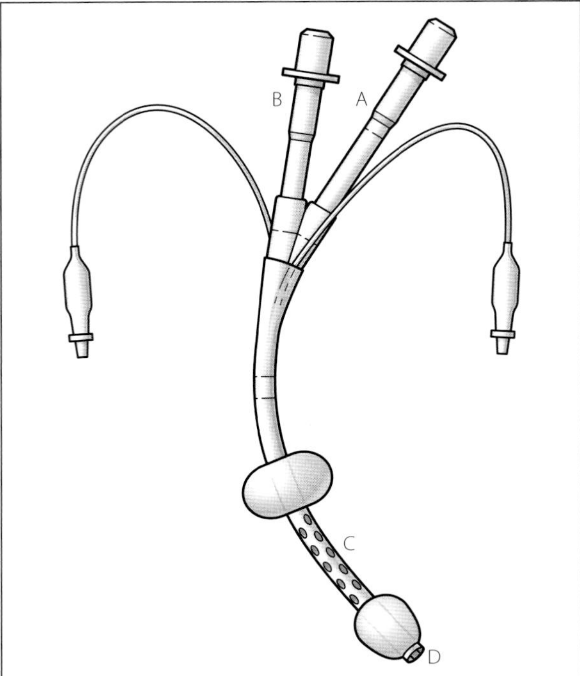

Fig. 118 The Combitube (see text)

Oesophageal stethoscope, *see Stethoscope*

Oesophageal varices. Dilated oesophago-gastric veins occurring in portal hypertension, e.g. in hepatic cirrhosis; the veins represent one of the connections between the systemic and portal circulations. Account for up to a third of cases of massive upper GIT haemorrhage. Mortality is up to 30% if bleeding occurs, partly related to the underlying severity of liver disease.

- Management:
  - prevention of haemorrhage: β-adrenergic receptor antagonists, e.g. propranolol, have been used to reduce portal BP if hepatic function is not too impaired. Endoscopic sclerotherapy (e.g. with ethanolamine oleate or sodium tetradecyl sulphate; causes variceal thrombosis and fibrosis) and ligation (e.g. with rubber bands) have also been used. Portocaval shunt procedures, e.g. distal splenorenal shunts (requiring surgery) or transjugular intrahepatic portasystemic shunts (TIPS; performed under radiological control) decompress the portal circulation but at the expense of hepatic encephalopathy (possibly less common after TIPS). The effect of all these procedures on survival is disputed.
  - if bleeding occurs:
    - resuscitation as for acute hypovolaemia. Airway management is complicated by haematemesis and steps to avoid aspiration of blood and gastric contents must be taken.
    - pharmacological reduction of portal venous pressure:
      - vasopressin 20 U over 15 min iv or its analogue terlipressin 2 mg iv followed by 1–2 mg 4–6 hourly up to 72 h. Controls bleeding in 60–70% of cases.
      - somatostatin 250 μg followed by 250 μg/h or its analogue octreotide 50 μg followed by 50 μg/h.

- endoscopic sclerotherapy or ligation may be performed acutely.
- radiological procedures include embolisation or TIPS.
- acute surgical shunt procedures.
- balloon tamponade using a Sengstaken–Blakemore tube.

Sharara AI, Rockey DC (2001). N Engl J Med; 345: 669–81

'Off-pump' coronary artery bypass graft, *see Coronary artery bypass graft*

Ofloxacin. Antibacterial drug, one of the 4-quinolones related to ciprofloxacin. Used for respiratory and genitourinary tract infections.
- Dosage: 200–400 mg orally or iv over 30 min, once/twice daily.
- Side effects: as for ciprofloxacin. Hypotension and thrombophlebitis may occur on iv administration.

Ohm's law. Current passing through a conductor is proportional to the potential difference across it, at constant temperature. Thus: voltage = current × resistance. (i.e. V = IR). An analogous form exists for flow of a fluid: pressure = flow × resistance.
[Georg S Ohm (1787–1854), German physicist]

Old age, *see Elderly, anaesthesia for*

Oliguria. Reduced urine output; definition is controversial but usually described as under 0.5 ml/kg/h. Common after major surgery or in ICU.
- Caused by:
  - urinary retention, blocked catheter, etc.
  - poor renal perfusion, e.g. hypotension, hypovolaemia, low cardiac output. Urine formation usually requires MAP of 60–70 mmHg in normotensive subjects.
  - effect of drugs, e.g. morphine causes vasopressin secretion.
  - increased intra-abdominal pressure: the mechanism is unknown but ureteric stents do not prevent it, suggesting mechanisms other than ureteric compression.
  - renal failure.
- Management:
  - exclusion of retention or blocked catheter.
  - urinary and plasma chemical analysis, e.g. sodium, osmolality, etc., is useful in distinguishing renal from prerenal causes (*see Renal failure*). Management is according to the underlying cause.

Omeprazole. Proton pump inhibitor used to reduce gastric acidity. A prodrug, its effects last for up to 24 h after single dosage.
- Dosage: 10–40 mg orally once daily. For reduction of risk from aspiration of gastric contents, 40 mg orally the night before, and 40 mg on the morning of surgery. May also be given iv: 40 mg over 5 min.
- Side effects: uncommon and usually mild: diarrhoea, rash, headache, rarely dizziness, hepatic enzyme and haematological changes.

Omphalocele, *see Gastroschisis and exomphalos*

Oncotic pressure (Colloid osmotic pressure). Osmotic pressure exerted by plasma proteins, usually about 3.3 kPa (25 mmHg). Important in the balance of Starling forces, and movement of water across capillary walls, e.g. in oedema. Although related to plasma protein concentration, the relationship is thought to be an upwards curve, not a straight line, because of molecular interactions and effects of charge.
See also, Intravenous fluids

Ondansetron hydrochloride. 5-HT_3 receptor antagonist, introduced in 1990 as an antiemetic drug following anaesthesia and chemotherapy. Although claimed to be superior to alternative antiemetics for PONV, convincing evidence supporting this is lacking. However, it does not affect dopamine receptors and unwanted central effects are rare. Its relatively high cost has led to calls for it to be reserved for severe PONV when cheaper drugs have proved unsuccessful, especially since evidence suggests greater efficacy for treatment of PONV, than for its prophylaxis. Has also been used to treat intractable pruritus following spinal opioids although evidence for its effectiveness is weak. Only 70–75% protein-bound. Undergoes hepatic metabolism and renal excretion. Half-life is 3 h.
- Dosage:
  - PONV:
    - prophylaxis: 4 mg slowly iv/im on induction, or 16 mg orally 1 h preoperatively, or 8 mg orally preoperatively repeated twice 8 hourly postoperatively. In children > 2 years, 0.1 mg/kg slowly iv up to 4 mg.
    - treatment: 1–4 mg slowly iv/im.
  - nausea following radiotherapy or chemotherapy: 8 mg orally/iv or 16 mg pr, followed by further doses to 16 mg/day for up to 5 days. In severe cases, a single loading dose of 32 mg pr or iv over 15 min may be given before treatment. In children, 5 mg/m^2 iv before treatment followed by 4 mg orally 12 hourly.
- Side effects: headache, constipation, flushing sensation, hiccups, occasionally hepatic impairment, visual disturbances, rarely convulsions. Prolongation of ECG intervals including heart block has been reported. Rectal irritation may follow pr use.

Ondine's curse. Hypoventilation caused by reduced ventilatory drive, originally described following CNS surgery (classically to medulla/high cervical spine). Despite being awake, victims may breathe only on command, with apnoea when asleep. The term has also been applied to respiratory depression caused by opioid analgesic drugs, and a congenital form of hypoventilation.
[Ondine, German mythological sea-nymph; the curse of having to remember when to breathe, and thus being unable to sleep for fear of dying, was inflicted on her unfaithful husband by her father, King of the Sea]

One-lung anaesthesia. Deliberate perioperative collapse of one lung to allow or facilitate thoracic surgery, whilst maintaining ventilation and gas exchange on the other side. Requires the use of endobronchial tubes or blockers. Commonly performed for surgery to the lungs, oesophagus, aorta and mediastinum, but most operations are possible without it (sleeve resection of the bronchus being a notable exception). Its main problem is related to hypoxaemia caused by the $\dot{V}/\dot{Q}$ mismatch produced, exacerbated by the lateral position used for most thoracic surgery.
- Effects of lateral positioning on gas exchange:
  - awake:
    - ventilation: FRC of the upper lung exceeds that of the lower lung, because of mediastinal movement to the other side, and pushing up of the lower hemidiaphragm by abdominal viscera. Thus the upper lung lies on a flatter part of the compliance curve, i.e. is less compliant, whilst the lower lung lies on the steep part

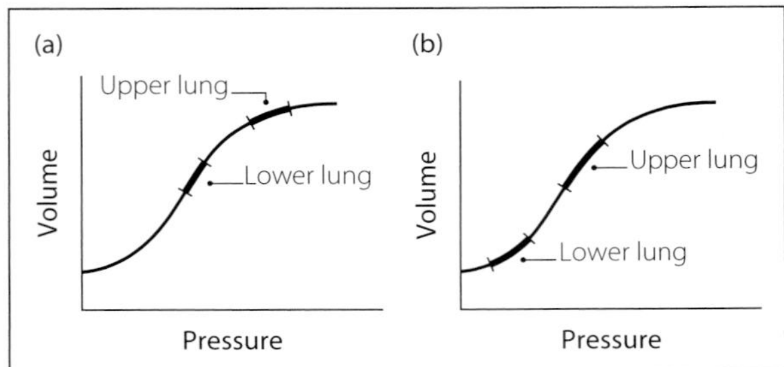

Fig. 119 Compliance curve for upper and lower lungs in the lateral position: (a) awake; (b) anaesthetised

of curve, i.e. is more compliant (Fig. 119a). In addition, the higher hemidiaphragm contracts more effectively. Thus most ventilation is of the lower lung.
- perfusion: mainly of the lower lung because of gravity; i.e. is matched with ventilation.

- anaesthetised:
  - FRC of both lungs is reduced; the upper lung now lies on the steep part of the curve and the lower lung on the flatter part (Fig. 119b). Thus the upper (more compliant) lung is ventilated in preference to the lower (less compliant) lung.
  - perfusion is still mainly of the lower lung, i.e. $\dot{V}/\dot{Q}$ mismatch occurs (usually of minor importance in normal patients, since both blood flow and ventilation usually differ by up to 10% between the two sides).
- one-lung anaesthesia: all ventilation is of the lower lung, whereas considerable perfusion is still of the upper lung. Thus significant shunt occurs in the upper lung, with $\dot{V}/\dot{Q}$ mismatch usual in the lower lung.
  - CO_2 exchange increases via the lower lung; thus CO_2 elimination is thought to be maintained if minute ventilation is unchanged.
  - degree of hypoxaemia is affected by:
    - pre-existing state of the lungs: decrease in oxygenation is greatest in normal lungs, e.g. during non-pulmonary surgery. In abnormal lungs, blood flow is usually already reduced preoperatively, thus the drop in arterial P_{O_2} is smaller.
    - $F_{I}O_2$: increases above 0.5 may not improve oxygenation, since pure shunt is not corrected by raising $F_{I}O_2$.
    - cardiac output: hypoxaemia worsens if cardiac output falls because of a decrease in the P_{O_2} of mixed venous blood passing through the shunt. The situation is complicated by altered distribution of pulmonary blood flow caused by changes in cardiac output.
    - hypoxic pulmonary vasoconstriction: whether it is attenuated by use of anaesthetic agents, or whether it contributes any protection against shunt, is unclear.
    - PEEP to the ventilated lung: may exacerbate hypoxaemia by reducing cardiac output, or by forcing more blood to flow through the uppermost lung.
    - pattern of ventilation: 12 ml/kg tidal volume is thought to be optimal. IPPV with excessive volumes or pressure can result in acute lung injury.
    - content of the collapsed lung: hypoxaemia worsens after about 10 min as contained O_2 is absorbed. Arterial P_{O_2} is increased by application of O_2 at 5–7 cmH_2O positive pressure, or by intermittent inflation, e.g. every 10–15 min.
    - surgery: e.g. leaning on mediastinum, reduction of venous return, etc. Tying the uppermost pulmonary artery stops shunt to the uppermost lung.
- Practical management:
  - preoperative assessment as for thoracic surgery; patients particularly at risk during one-lung anaesthesia may be identified.
  - close monitoring using oximetry and/or arterial blood gas analysis.
  - $F_{I}O_2$ is usually increased to 0.4–0.5; further increases or use of PEEP may improve oxygenation.
  - administration of O_2 to the uppermost lung (especially with positive pressure) or intermittent inflation.
  - surgical ligation of the pulmonary artery is performed early.
  - reinflation and ventilation of both lungs should be performed if hypoxaemia is unacceptable.
  - suction is applied to the collapsed lung before reinflation, to remove accumulated secretions.
  - slow manual inflation is performed at the end of the procedure, to encourage expansion. The surgeon may request sustained pressures (e.g. 30–40 cmH_2O) to test the integrity of the bronchial suturing.

Open-drop techniques. Common and convenient techniques for administering inhalational anaesthetic agents in the 1800s/early 1900s. The volatile anaesthetic agent, e.g. chloroform, diethyl ether, ethyl chloride, was dripped on to a cloth (originally a folded handkerchief) on the patient's face from a dropper bottle. Concentration of agent depended on the rate of drop administration. Specially designed bottles and masks were later developed; the best known mask is that of Schimmelbusch, although this was adapted from Skinner's earlier model. After covering the face with gauze wadding, with a hole for the mouth and nose, the wire mask was placed on the face, and further layers of wadding laid on it. Some masks had retaining clips or wire loops for securing the wadding. The eyes were usually covered to reduce irritation by liquid agent. Poor fitting of the mask allowed inhalation of air around it. Some incorporated channels for O_2 insufflation, or gutters around the edge to catch liquid anaesthetic. Freezing of exhaled water vapour on the wadding was problematic during prolonged procedures.
[Curt Schimmelbusch (1860–1895), German surgeon; Thomas Skinner (1825–1906), Liverpool obstetrician]

Operant conditioning. Manipulation of behaviour by reinforcing wanted or unwanted behaviour with rewards or punishments respectively. Has been used in chronic pain management, with several weeks' admission to hospital, involving reduction in drug therapy and encouragement of activity and independence. Thus concentrates on behaviour secondary to pain instead of pain itself.

Operating department assistants/practitioners (ODAs/ODPs). Non-medical anaesthetic support staff; the role arose from the requirements of military surgeons and anaesthetists for specialist non-nursing assistance during World War II, although 'box carriers' (so-called because they carried the surgeon's instruments in a box) were in use in the UK in the early 1800s. City & Guilds of London Institute training for ODAs was introduced in 1976, offering specific training in the areas of anaesthesia and surgery without passage through the nursing training system, whilst the term ODP was introduced in 1989 to further the concept that adequately trained staff could equally come from nursing or traditional ODA backgrounds. A National Vocational Qualification (NVQ) in

Operating Department Practice was introduced in 1991. Repeated attempts to bring the two ODP career structures (i.e. ODA and non-ODA) closer together was hampered for many years by (i) different pay scales and (ii) lack of central registration of ODAs compared with nurse ODPs' statutory requirement to be registered with the nursing authorities. A voluntary register of ODAs was established in the late 1980s/early 1990s and compulsory registration of all ODPs was established in 2004. The professional body for ODPs is the College (formerly Association) of ODPs, which publishes the monthly *Journal of Operating Department Practice*.

ODPs have an invaluable role in supporting most anaesthetic activity, e.g. preparing and ordering drugs and equipment, setting up the operating theatre for cases, helping to organise operating lists, etc. They may also assist the surgical staff (including 'scrubbing') and the concept of 'multiskilling' supports their activity in various roles within the operating theatre suite and beyond, e.g. ICU. More extended practical roles are supported in some units, e.g. assisting at cardiac arrests, placing iv cannulae, etc., although this is controversial.

Ophthalmic nerve blocks. Performed for procedures around the eye, nose and forehead, and certain intraoral procedures.

- Anatomy (*see Fig. 75; Gasserian ganglion block*):
  - ophthalmic division of the trigeminal nerve (V^1) is entirely sensory and passes from the Gasserian ganglion, where it divides into branches which pass through the superior orbital fissure:
    - lacrimal nerve; supplies the lateral upper eyelid and conjunctiva, lacrimal gland and skin of the lateral angle of the mouth.
    - frontal nerve; supplies the upper eyelid, frontal sinuses and anterior scalp via the supraorbital branch; upper eyelid and medial forehead via the supratrochlear branch.
    - nasociliary nerve; supplies the anterior dura, anterior ethmoidal air cells, upper anterior nasal cavity and skin of the external nose via the anterior ethmoidal branch; posterior ethmoidal and sphenoid sinuses via the posterior ethmoidal branch; medial upper eyelid, conjunctiva and adjacent nose via the infratrochlear branch; eyeball via the long ciliary nerves and branches to the ciliary ganglion.
  - supraorbital foramen, pupil, infraorbital notch, infraorbital foramen, buccal surface of the second premolar and mental foramen all lie along a straight line.
- Blocks:
  - supraorbital nerve: 1–3 ml local anaesthetic agent is injected at the supraorbital notch.
  - supratrochlear nerve: 1–3 ml is injected at the superomedial part of the opening of the orbit.
  - both the above nerves may be blocked by subcutaneous infiltration above the eyebrow.
  - frontal nerve: 1 ml is injected at the central part of the roof of the orbit.
  - anterior ethmoidal nerve: 2 ml is injected at the superomedial side of the orbit, at a depth of 3–4 cm.

See also, Mandibular nerve blocks; Maxillary nerve blocks

Ophthalmic surgery. Historically, first performed without anaesthesia and then under topical anaesthesia, because of the eye's accessibility and the disastrous effects of coughing during general anaesthesia. Subsequently, increasingly performed under general anaesthesia because of patients' expectations and the ability to control intraocular pressure (IOP). More recently local anaesthesia has been favoured again, especially in the elderly. Children (for strabismus repair) and the elderly (for cataract extraction) form the largest groups of patients.

- Local anaesthesia:
  - cornea and conjunctiva: 4% lidocaine (with or without adrenaline) or 2–4% cocaine is instilled into the conjunctival sac. Cocaine is not used in glaucoma, as it dilates the pupil.
  - retrobulbar block, peribulbar block or sub-Tenon's block: retrobulbar block is less commonly performed now because of associated complications.
  - prevention of blepharospasm: infiltration between the muscles and bone parallel to the lower and lateral orbital margins from a point 1 cm behind the orbit's lower lateral corner; alternatively, local anaesthetic may be injected above the condyloid process of the mandible. These injections are rarely required with large-volume modern regional techniques.
  - sedation may be used. Close monitoring is required as the patient's head is covered by drapes. Supplementary O_2 should be delivered.
- General anaesthesia:
  - preoperatively:
    - preoperative assessment of children with strabismus for muscle disorders and MH susceptibility. Cataracts may occur in dystrophia myotonica, inborn errors of metabolism, chromosomal abnormalities, diabetes mellitus, corticosteroids or following trauma. Lens subluxation may occur in Marfan's syndrome and inborn errors, e.g. homocystinuria. The elderly should be assessed for other diseases, e.g. diabetes, hypertension (*see Elderly, anaesthesia for*).
    - drugs used in eye drops may be absorbed and active systemically, e.g. ecothiopate, timolol.
    - opioid premedication is usually avoided because of its emetic properties. Benzodiazepines are popular.
  - perioperatively:
    - procedures include the above operations, repair of retinal detachment, vitrectomy, repair of eye injuries (*see Eye, penetrating injury*) and operations on the lacrimal system.
    - the airway is usually not easily accessible to the anaesthetist.
    - for children, considerations include those for paediatric anaesthesia, the very active oculocardiac and oculorespiratory reflexes, and the increased incidence of PONV after strabismus repair (thought also to be associated with traction on extraocular muscles). Atropine or glycopyrronium should be available; some advocate routine administration to all patients preoperatively or on induction of anaesthesia. Standard techniques are employed, with tracheal intubation or laryngeal mask airway and spontaneous or controlled ventilation.
    - for adults, standard agents and techniques are used. Control of IOP is usually achieved by iv induction, IPPV and hyperventilation, and use of a volatile inhalational anaesthetic agent (*for effects of specific drugs, use of sulphahexafluoride, etc., see Intraocular pressure*). Administration of iv acetazolamide may be required. Spontaneous ventilation may be suitable for extraocular procedures. The laryngeal mask airway is often used, since coughing and straining are less problematic than with tracheal intubation. The oculocardiac reflex may still occur in adults.

- systemic absorption of topical solutions, e.g. adrenaline, cocaine, may occur.
- coughing, straining, vomiting, etc. may increase IOP, especially undesirable if the globe is open.

- postoperatively: avoidance of straining and vomiting is desirable. Postoperative pain tends to be mild.

Opiates. Strictly, substances derived from opium. Formerly used to describe agonist drugs at opioid receptors; the terms opioids and opioid analgesic drugs are now preferred.

Opioid analgesic drugs. Opium and morphine have been used for thousands of years; morphine was isolated in 1803 and codeine in 1832. Diamorphine was introduced in 1898, papaveretum in 1909. Other commonly used drugs include pethidine (1939), phenoperidine (1957), fentanyl (1960), alfentanil (1976), sufentanil (1984) and remifentanil (1997). Drugs with opioid receptor antagonist properties include pentazocine (1962), nalbuphine (1968), meptazinol (1971) and buprenorphine (1968).

May be divided into naturally occurring alkaloids (e.g. morphine, codeine), semisynthetic drugs (slightly modified natural molecules, e.g. diamorphine, dihydrocodeine), and synthetic opioids (e.g. pethidine, fentanyl, alfentanil, remifentanil). May also be classified according to their opioid receptor specificity and actions, or according to their onset and duration of action.

Each drug has slightly different effects on the body's systems, but their general effects are those of morphine. The 'purer' drugs, e.g. fentanyl, alfentanil, sufentanil, do not cause histamine release, and may be used in very high doses with relative cardiostability, e.g. for cardiac surgery. In lower doses, they are used to provide intra- and postoperative analgesia, and to prevent the haemodynamic consequences of tracheal intubation and surgical stimulation. Also used as general analgesic drugs and for premedication, anxiolysis, cough suppression and treatment of chronic diarrhoea.

See also, Opioid . . . ; Spinal opioids

Opioid detoxification, *see Rapid opioid detoxification*

Opioid poisoning. Presents with nausea and vomiting, respiratory depression, hypotension, pinpoint pupils and coma. Depressant effects are exacerbated by alcohol ingestion. Hypothermia, hypoglycaemia and rarely pulmonary oedema and rhabdomyolysis may occur. Convulsions may occur with pethidine, codeine and dextropropoxyphene. Drug combinations containing opioids include atropine–diphenoxylate for diarrhoea and paracetamol–dextropropoxyphene/codeine/dihydrocodeine for pain. The former combination may cause convulsions, tachycardia and restlessness; the latter may cause delayed hepatic failure.

- Management:
  - supportive; includes gastric lavage, iv fluids, O_2 therapy and IPPV.
  - naloxone 0.4–2.0 mg iv repeated after 2–3 min as required to a total of 10 mg; infusion may be necessary as naloxone's duration of action is short. Respiratory depression due to buprenorphine may not be responsive.

Opioid receptor antagonists. Different types:

- pure antagonists, e.g. naloxone, naltrexone: antagonists at all opioid receptor subtypes. Methylnaltrexone is a peripherally acting mu antagonist, currently under investigation as a treatment for postoperative ileus.
- agonist–antagonists: agonists at some receptors but antagonists at others, e.g.:
  - pentazocine: agonist at kappa and sigma, antagonist at mu receptors.
  - nalorphine: partial agonist at kappa and sigma, antagonist at mu receptors.
  - nalbuphine: as for nalorphine, but a less potent sigma agonist.
- partial agonists, e.g. buprenorphine, meptazinol (mu receptors); may antagonise mu effects of other opioids, e.g. morphine, although not themselves antagonists.

Their main clinical use is to reverse effects of opioid analgesic drugs, e.g. in opioid poisoning. Those with agonist properties are also used as analgesic drugs; some have been used to reverse unwanted effects of other opioids, e.g. respiratory depression, whilst still maintaining analgesia. In practice, this is very difficult to achieve. Also used in diagnosis and treatment of opioid addiction. Receptor-specific compounds have been developed for research and identification of receptor subtypes.

Many result from modification or substitution of the side chain on the nitrogen atom of parent analgesic drugs, e.g. *N*-allyl group substitution for the *N*-methyl group (hence the name, nal . . .).

Opioid receptors. Naturally occurring receptors to morphine and related drugs, isolated in the 1970s. All are G protein-coupled receptors and activation is thought to result in increased potassium and/or decreased calcium conductance across the cell membrane. Found mainly in the CNS but also GIT; thought to be involved in central mechanisms involving pain and emotion. Only three types of receptor are considered true opioid receptors now (each subdivided into two or more subtypes), although others have been suggested in the past. The picture is confused by different terminology used (e.g. opioids, opiates, narcotics), the use of different animal experiments (e.g. rat and guinea-pig in particular), and the effects of different drugs at the various receptors.

- Subtypes:
  - mu (MOP):
    - activation causes analgesia, respiratory depression, euphoria, hypothermia, miosis, bradycardia, physical dependence; i.e. the classic effects of morphine.
    - responsible for 'supraspinal analgesia'; i.e. drugs act at brain level.
    - the mu_1 receptor is thought to be responsible for supraspinal analgesia; the mu_2 for most of the other effects.
    - agonists: most opioid analgesic drugs.
    - partial agonists: buprenorphine, meptazinol (thought to be specific at mu_1 receptors).
    - antagonists: nalorphine, nalbuphine, pentazocine.
  - delta (DOP):
    - activation has been experimentally shown to produce analgesia, especially at spinal level, but their precise role is unclear.
    - agonists: enkephalins.
  - kappa (KOP):
    - activation causes analgesia, respiratory depression, miosis, sedation, different sort of dependence.
    - responsible for 'spinal analgesia'; i.e. drugs thought to act at spinal level.
    - agonists: pentazocine, butorphanol, dynorphins, morphine.
    - partial agonists: nalorphine, nalbuphine.

Sigma receptors, previously considered opioid receptors, are not considered so now because the effects of their stimulation are not reversed by naloxone. They bind to phencyclidine and its derivatives, e.g. ketamine. Epsilon receptors have been found only in rat vas deferens and are not considered true opioid receptors. All subtypes are antagonised by naloxone and naltrexone (mu and kappa more than delta).

The 'orphan' opioid receptor is related to the above receptors but less strongly bound by opioids. It is found throughout the brain and spinal cord; a naturally occurring ligand, orphanin FQ, produces antanalgesia supraspinally and analgesia at spinal level.

Opioids. Substances which bind to opioid receptors; include naturally occurring and synthetic drugs, and endogenous compounds.

Opium. Dried juice from the unripe seed capsules of the opium poppy *Papaver somniferum*. Contains many different alkaloids including morphine (9–20%), codeine (up to 4%) and papaverine. Used for thousands of years as a recreational drug and for analgesia, especially in the Far East. Use as a therapeutic drug is rare now, purer drugs and extracts being preferred.

Oral rehydration therapy. Method of treating dehydration when mild or where facilities for iv fluid administration are lacking, e.g. in the community or developing countries. Particularly useful in gastroenteritis and in children; it has also been used in less serious burns. Various commercial mixtures exist; all contain glucose, the presence of which in the intestinal lumen facilitates the reabsorption of sodium ions and thus water. A simple version can be made by adding 20 g glucose (or 40 g sucrose since only half becomes available as glucose after ingestion), 3.5 g sodium chloride, 2.5 g sodium bicarbonate and 1.5 g potassium chloride per litre of water. In the developing countries, suitable solutions have been made by taking three 300 ml soft drink bottles of water and adding a level bottle capful of salt and eight capfuls of sugar.

Orbeli effect. Increase in strength of contraction of fatigued muscle following sympathetic nerve stimulation.
[Leon A Orbeli (1882–1958), Russian physiologist]

Orbital cavity. Cavity containing the eye and extraorbital structures. Roughly pyramidal with the apex posteriorly, its roof is formed by the orbital plate of the frontal bone (and lesser wing of the sphenoid posteriorly); its floor by the maxilla and zygoma; its medial wall by the frontal process of the maxilla and lacrimal bone anteriorly and orbital plate of the ethmoid and body of the sphenoid posteriorly; and its lateral wall by the zygoma and greater wing of the sphenoid (Fig. 120). Has three openings posteriorly:

- superior orbital fissure: transmits the 3rd, 4th and 5th (the three branches of the ophthalmic division) cranial nerves. Also transmits branches of the middle meningeal and lacrimal arteries, ophthalmic veins and sympathetic fibres.
- inferior orbital fissure: transmits the maxillary nerve.
- optic canal: transmits the optic nerve and ophthalmic artery.

The extraocular muscles are supplied by the 3rd, 4th and 6th cranial nerves and have the following actions on the pupil:

- superior rectus: elevates.
- inferior rectus: lowers.
- medial and lateral rectus: moves medially and laterally respectively.
- superior oblique: moves downwards and laterally.
- inferior oblique: moves upwards and laterally.

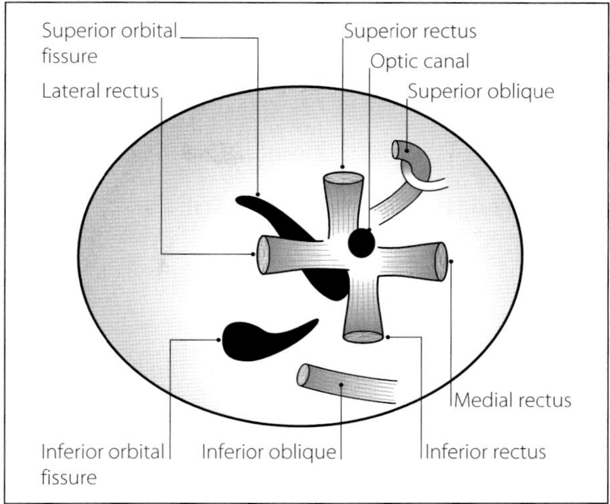

Fig. 120 Frontal view of right orbital cavity

The rectus muscles attach posteriorly to a common tendinous ring surrounding the optic canal and part of the superior orbital fissure; they attach anteriorly to the sclera of the eyeball in front of the equator. The superior oblique muscle attaches posteriorly above the tendinous ring, hooking round the pulley-like trochlea before attaching posterolaterally to the eyeball, behind the equator. The inferior oblique attaches posteriorly to the floor of the orbit and attaches to the posterolateral surface of the eyeball, behind the equator.
See also, Peribulbar block; Retrobulbar block; Skull; Sub-Tenon's block

Oré, Pierre-Cyprien (1828–1889). French physician; Professor of Physiology at Bordeaux. Investigated blood transfusion and the effects of iv injection of drugs. Produced general anaesthesia with iv chloral hydrate, thus becoming the first to employ TIVA.

Orexins. Neuropeptides derived from an amino acid precursor, prepro-orexin. Postulated as playing an important role in arousal, maintenance of the waking state, neural control of food intake and neuroendocrine function, including energy metabolism and reproduction. May be involved in the pathophysiology of neurodegeneration and head injury.

Organ donation. Organs for transplantation may be donated by living subjects, e.g. kidney and bone marrow. The main issue concerns the undertaking of anaesthesia and surgery (with their attendant risks) by a healthy patient for altruistic reasons.

Many organs may be obtained from patients following diagnosis of brainstem death. They include kidney, heart, lung, liver, small bowel, pancreas, skin and cornea. Demand for organs outstrips supply. At present in the UK, members of the public identify themselves as potential donors (e.g. by completing a 'donor card' or joining a national registry); in some countries, an 'opt-in' system operates in which permission is assumed unless specified otherwise, and this has been proposed in the UK though amongst considerable controversy.

Even more controversial is the use of non-heart beating donors, e.g. patients who arrive in hospital dead, patients in whom CPR is unsuccessful, those in whom cardiac arrest occurs after brainstem death and those in whom treatment has been withdrawn but in whom formal brainstem death testing cannot be done because of sedation, metabolic abnormalities, etc. In the latter group, treatment may be withdrawn once the surgical team is ready; death is pronounced 2 min after asystole and surgery to retrieve organs begins 5–10 min after asystole.

- Non-living patients have traditionally been considered unsuitable for donation for a number of reasons:
  - systemic infection or transmissable disease.
  - age: e.g. approximately 40 years for hearts; > 50 years for livers; > 70 years for kidneys.
  - malignancy.
  - disease of the organ or organ system concerned.
  - direct trauma to the organ.
  - poisoning or overdose, until the drug is cleared from the body.

More recently, given the relative shortage of organs, only HIV infection or Creutzfeldt–Jakob disease are considered absolute contraindications.

Maintenance of tissue oxygenation, organ function and metabolic and cardiovascular stability should be pursued as for critically ill patients, until and during organ removal. Endocrine therapy with methylprednisolone, triiodothyronine and control of blood sugar with insulin may improve donor organ function.

Wood KE, Becker BN, McCartney JG, et al (2004). N Engl J Med; 351: 2730–9.

Organe, Geoffrey Stephen William (1908–1989). English anaesthetist, born in India. A major influence on the development of anaesthesia in the UK and abroad, and involved in much research, particularly into the newly introduced neuromuscular blocking drugs. Professor of Anaesthesia at Westminster Hospital, London, and knighted in 1968.

Organophosphorus poisoning. Organophosphorus compounds are acetylcholinesterase inhibitors, commonly used as insecticides but also manufactured as chemical weapons. One, ecothiopate, is used in glaucoma. Those used in insecticides are usually ester, amide or thiol derivatives of phosphoric or phosphonic acids, or their mixtures. They may be absorbed via the GIT, lungs or skin, and are rapidly distributed to all tissues, especially liver and kidney. Half-lives vary from minutes to hours, with metabolism by oxidation, ester hydrolysis and combination with glutathione, and excretion in faeces or urine.

- Toxic effects:
  - peripheral enzyme inhibition:
    - phosphorylation of acetylcholinesterase: may be irreversible depending on the compound involved. Features are those of cholinergic crisis and include muscarinic effects (bronchospasm, sweating, increased secretions, abdominal cramps, bradycardia, miosis) and nicotinic effects (muscle twitching, weakness, hypertension and tachycardia). Spontaneous enzyme 'reactivation' may occur; this process is induced by pralidoxime if administered within 24–36 h.
    - phosphorylation of other enzymes, e.g. lipases, GIT enzymes.
  - myopathic effects: predominantly shown in animals. Weakness may occur within 24 h of poisoning, with recovery taking up to 3 weeks. Muscle paralysis in humans may occur after recovery from the initial cholinergic crisis, 24–96 h after poisoning. Mainly affecting proximal muscles, it is thought to involve postsynaptic dysfunction at the neuromuscular junction.
  - delayed polyneuropathy: usually follows poisoning with non-insecticide compounds. Develops 2–4 weeks after the cholinergic crisis, with weakness and paraesthesiae. Pyramidal signs may be present. Recovery is variable.
  - CNS effects: anxiety, tremor, confusion, coma and convulsions may occur, with EEG abnormalities.

  Respiratory failure may result from peripheral weakness, central depression and increased tracheobronchial secretions.

Diagnosis is based on history, tolerance to atropine therapy, acetylcholine assay and measurement of blood and urine organophosphorus and metabolite levels.

- Treatment:
  - supportive measures as for poisoning and overdoses in general. Care should be taken to avoid self-contamination.
  - drug therapy:
    - atropine 2 mg (20 μg/ml in children) iv each 5–10 min until dry flushed skin, dilated pupils and tachycardia.
    - pralidoxime 30 mg/kg diluted in 10–15 ml water, iv over 5–10 min. May be repeated up to twice if no improvement is seen within 30 min, up to a usual maximum of 12 g/24 h. Rarely, iv infusion of up to 500 mg/h may be required. For children, a bolus dose of 20–60 mg/kg.

Roberts DM, Aaron CK (2007). BMJ 334: 629–34

Orphanin FQ (OFQ; nociceptin). 17 amino acid peptide; activates the orphan opioid receptor producing an antanalgesic effect supraspinally but analgesia at spinal level. Structurally related to dynorphin (and to a lesser degree, other endogenous opioid ligands), its effects are not affected by naloxone. Its role as a neurotransmitter is unclear.

Orthopaedic surgery. Anaesthetic considerations may be related to:

- reasons for surgery:
  - trauma: presence of other injuries, risks of emergency surgery (e.g. aspiration of gastric contents). Adequate resuscitation is important preoperatively, especially in the elderly, e.g. following fractured neck of femur (NOF). Cases with risk of infection, ischaemia or nerve damage are particularly urgent.
  - musculoskeletal disease, e.g. rheumatoid arthritis, connective tissue diseases, muscular abnormalities, etc. There is a higher than normal incidence of MH susceptibility in young patients with musculoskeletal abnormalities.
  - congenital malformations: may be accompanied by other system involvement, e.g. cardiac lesions.
  - risk of massive hyperkalaemia following suxamethonium if neurological or muscle lesions are present.
- surgical procedure:
  - may involve repeated anaesthesia.
  - use of tourniquets.
  - use of methylmethacrylate cement.
  - problems of specific procedures, e.g. kyphoscoliosis.
  - regional techniques are particularly useful, e.g. hip surgery (arthroplasty, fractured NOF). Epidural and spinal anaesthesia are associated with fewer postoperative complications (including DVT) than after general anaesthesia, although mortality after fractured NOF is the same at 1 year.
  - DVT and PE are common, especially after hip surgery; prophylactic measures should be taken. Fat embolism is common after trauma.

Oscilloscope. Device for displaying recorded signals, especially of high frequency and when analysis of their shape is required, e.g. ECG or arterial waveform.

An electron beam is produced by heating a cathode at one end of an evacuated glass tube (cathode ray tube) and accelerated by anodes along the tube's length. It is focused on to one edge of a fluorescent screen at the other end of the tube, and is visible as a bright dot. If a sawtooth patterned potential is applied horizontally (transversely across the beam), the beam is deflected across the screen as the potential increases, flipping back to its original position as the potential returns to zero. The dot appears to sweep across the screen continuously from one side to the other.

The signal potential is applied vertically across the beam, causing vertical deflection; a spatial reconstruction of the signal against time is seen on the screen. The pattern may be made to persist by altering the characteristics of the fluorescent material, or by using a second cathode system. It may also be achieved using rapid computer-controlled repeated movements of the electron beam. Further manipulation allows the frozen pattern to track across the screen, e.g. by storing the signal as a series of digital values, and displaying each in turn for a predetermined period.

May also be used without the time-base to plot two signals applied at right angles to each other, e.g. flow–volume loops.

Oscillotonometer. Device for indirect arterial BP measurement, using one cuff for occluding the brachial artery and a second cuff for detecting pulsations, often incorporated into a double cuff. The cuffs connect via separate tubing to a circular chamber containing aneroid gauges and a lever amplification system, with an indicator dial on its face.

- Principles of use:
  - the upper (occluding) cuff is about 5 cm wide; the lower (sensing) cuff is about 10 cm wide; they overlap by 2–3 cm.
  - with the control lever in its normal (up) position, both cuffs are inflated by hand to above systolic BP; the dial indicates the pressure within both cuffs.
  - moving the lever down connects the sensing cuff to a more sensitive aneroid gauge and connects both cuffs to atmosphere via an adjustable screw-valve. The cuffs are allowed to deflate slowly, whilst observing the pointer needle for changes in sensing cuff pressure.
  - as pressure falls, small oscillations of the needle may occur, representing transmitted pulsations from the occluding cuff. At systolic BP, the oscillations suddenly increase in amplitude, representing pulsations reaching the sensing cuff under the occluding cuff.
  - the lever is released to the up position, and systolic pressure read from the dial.
  - the lever is pressed down and the process continued until the oscillations diminish suddenly, representing diastolic BP, which is read as before. Peak amplitude may occur between systolic and diastolic pressure, and is thought to represent MAP.

Automated devices employ similar principles.

May be used for continuous measurement, by keeping the cuffs inflated at around systolic BP, and the control lever held down: rising BP is indicated by increasing amplitude of oscillations, falling BP by decreasing amplitude. Periodic deflation allows circulation in the arm, e.g. for 1 minute out of every 5. Less accurate at high BP and low pulse pressure. Accuracy is decreased if the cuffs are reversed.

Hutton P, Prys-Roberts C (1982). Br J Anaesth; 54: 581–91

Osmolality and osmolarity. Expressions of concentration of osmotically active particles in solution:

- osmolality = the number of osmoles per kilogram solvent.
- osmolarity = the number of osmoles per litre solution.
- osmoles = the mw of a substance divided by the number of freely moving particles liberated in solution.

Thus 1 mmol of a salt which dissociates completely into two ions provides 2 mosmol. In the body, the solvent is water, with density 1 kg/l; thus osmolality and osmolarity are often used interchangeably, although proteins and fats in plasma give rise to a small difference.

Osmolality of plasma is maintained at 280–305 mosmol/kg. Regulatory mechanisms include stimulation of thirst by osmoreceptors, baroreceptors and the renin/angiotensin system. Osmoreceptors also stimulate vasopressin release. Most contribution to plasma osmolality arises from sodium and its anions, glucose and urea; thus plasma osmolality may be estimated thus:

$$\text{mosmol/kg} = [\text{glucose}] + [\text{urea}] + (2 \times [\text{Na}^+]) \text{ (all in mmol/l).}$$

Alcohols, proteins, triglycerides, mannitol, etc., are not accounted for. Proteins usually contribute little since, despite their high concentration, few particles are liberated in solution because of their high mw.

Osmolality/osmolarity is determined by measuring ionic concentration with a flame photometer, measuring osmotic pressure or by employing the colligative properties of solutions (e.g. depression of freezing point, lowering of vapour pressure).

Urinary and plasma osmolality measurement is useful in investigating oliguria and renal failure.

See also, Fluid balance; Hyperosmolality; Hypo-osmolality; Osmolar gap; Tonicity

Osmolar gap (Osmolality gap). Difference between calculated and measured plasma osmolality. Normally under 10 mosmol/kg; increased by high levels of osmotically active substances, e.g. alcohols, mannitol, glycine (in the TURP syndrome), etc. May also be applied to urine osmolality, e.g. to indicate the presence of osmotically active substances such as ammonium ions.

Osmoreceptors. Cells in the anterior hypothalamus, outside the blood–brain barrier; respond to changes in plasma osmolality. Control thirst and secretion of vasopressin, possibly via separate groups of osmoreceptors.

Osmosis. Movement of solvent molecules across a semipermeable membrane from a dilute solution to a concentrated one, so as to equalise the concentrations on both sides. Thus water moves across cell membranes from the ECF following dextrose infusion, once the dextrose has been metabolised. Similarly, water in very hypotonic iv fluids may move into red blood cells after infusion, causing haemolysis.

Osmotic clearance, *see Clearance, osmotic*

Osmotic diuretics, *see Diuretics*

Osmotic pressure. Pressure required to prevent movement of solvent molecules by osmosis across a semipermeable membrane.

Equals $\frac{nRT}{V}$ as for the **ideal gas law**,

Where n = number of particles,
R = universal gas constant,
T = absolute temperature,
V = volume.

Thus proportional to the number of particles per volume, not mw. Ideal ionic solutions dissociate completely in solution, whereas in the body incomplete dissociation and interactions between ions result in lower osmotic pressure than predicted. Plasma osmotic pressure is approximately 7.3 atmospheres.
See also, Oncotic pressure; Osmolality and osmolarity; Tonicity

Ouabain. Cardiac glycoside, poorly absorbed from the GIT and administered iv. Faster acting than digoxin; thus used when rapid action is required. 5% protein-bound, with half-life about 24 h, and excreted via kidneys and liver.

- Dosage: 100–250 μg by iv infusion.

Not commercially available in the UK.

Outreach team. Concept, similar to the medical emergency team, for improving identification and care of acutely ill patients throughout hospitals but especially on general wards. Usually nurse-led, but may also contain experienced medical and physiotherapy staff, often from ICUs, who may provide the following services: rapid response team to manage acutely ill patients in general ward areas, critical care education for ward clinicians, facilitation of early admission to ICU/HDU, early recognition of patients for whom CPR and/or ICU admission is inappropriate, and early post-ICU follow-up. Calling criteria include specific clinical scenarios or the results of early warning scores.
Goldhill DR (2005). Br J Anaesth; 95: 88–94
See also, Acute life-threatening events – recognition and treatment

Ovarian hyperstimulation syndrome. Condition caused by artificial stimulation of the ovaries by gonadotrophin therapy in order to produce ovulation in assisted conception programmes. Characterised by ovarian enlargement, pleural effusion and ascites; the latter in particular may be massive and unrelenting. Clinical features range from abdominal discomfort and swelling to hypovolaemic shock, hepatic impairment, renal failure and acute lung injury. DVT may also occur. Mild symptoms occur in up to a quarter of cases of induced ovulation, whilst the severe form occurs in 1–2%.

Treatment is mainly supportive, with correction of hypovolaemia, careful attention to fluid balance and correction of metabolic disturbances. Prophylactic therapy against DVT is generally recommended. Abdominal paracentesis and pleural drainage is usually performed in severe cases; ultrafiltration and re-infusion of the ascitic fluid iv has been used to replace the protein-rich fluid otherwise lost.
Budev MM, Arroliga AC, Falcone T (2005). Crit Care Med; 33 Suppl: S301–6

Overdoses, *see Poisoning and overdoses*

Oximetry. Determination of arterial O_2 saturation of haemoglobin (S_aO_2) by measuring absorbance of light by blood. Described in 1934 using open blood vessels, and in 1940 using ear/hand probes, but the technique was cumbersome and difficult to perform. Modern pulse oximeters became widespread from the 1980s following advances in microchip technology, allowing manipulation of the recorded signal.

Relies on the principle that absorbance of light energy by haemoglobin depends upon its level of oxygenation. Oxygenated and deoxygenated haemoglobin (HbO and Hb respectively) have different absorbance spectra (Fig. 121). Isobestic points occur where the lines cross. Thus comparison of absorbances at different wavelengths allows estimation of the relative concentrations of HbO and Hb (i.e. S_aO_2). Earlier machines used two wavelengths including one isobestic point as a reference; modern pulse oximeters may use two or more wavelengths, not necessarily including an isobestic point.

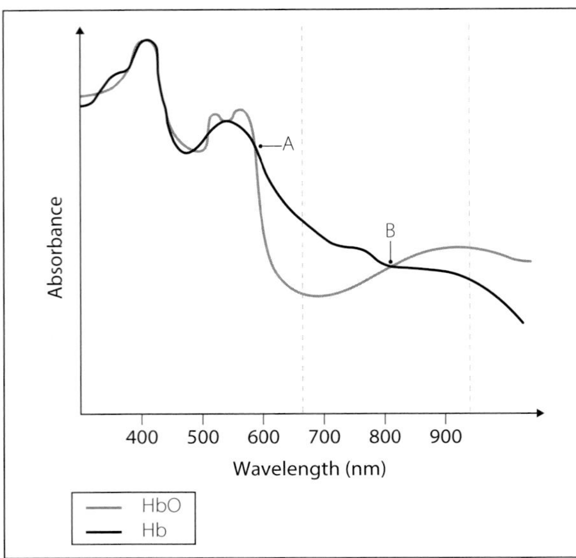

Fig. 121 Absorbance of light by oxygenated (HbO) and deoxygenated (Hb) haemoglobin: A and B are isobestic points. The vertical dashed lines indicate the wavelengths (660 nm and 940 nm) most often used by modern pulse oximeters

Blood gas machines estimate S_aO_2 from arterial samples, whereas pulse oximeters read from ear or finger probes measuring light passing through tissue. Analysis of reflected light has also been used to determine S_aO_2; surface probes have been developed which may be stuck on to skin at any site, e.g. the head of a fetus.
See also, Beer–Lambert law

Oxpentifylline, *see Pentoxifylline*

Oxycodone hydrochloride. Opioid analgesic drug derived from morphine, described in 1916. Action lasts 4–7 h.

- Dosage: 10 mg orally 12 hourly, increased to 200 mg in chronic pain although higher doses may occasionally be required. May also be given sc/slowly iv: 1–10 mg 4 hourly.

Also available as suppositories (as the pectinate) by special order.

Oxygen. Non-metallic element existing as a colourless odourless diatomic gas (O_2) in the lower atmosphere, and as triatomic oxygen (O_3, ozone) and monatomic oxygen (O) in the upper atmosphere. The most plentiful element in the Earth's crust (as opposed to nitrogen, the most plentiful in the atmosphere), it makes up 21% of air by volume. Discovered independently in 1771 by Scheele and Priestley, the latter calling it 'dephlogisticated air'. Recognised as a gas by Lavoisier who named it and explained the process of combustion. Combines with many other elements and molecules, and most abundant as water.

Essential for cellular respiration in animals and lower plants; higher plants take in CO_2 and release O_2 during photosynthesis. Boiling point is −183°C; melting point is −218°C; critical temperature is −118°C. Atomic weight is 16; specific gravity is 1.1 for liquid O_2 and 1.4 for gaseous O_2.

Commercial O_2 is supplied in liquid form, manufactured by the fractional distillation of air. Available in hospitals by piped gas supply, O_2 concentrators or in cylinders at 137 bar.
[Carl W Scheele (1742–1786), Swedish chemist]
See also, Oxygen…; Phlogiston; Vacuum insulated evaporator

Oxygen cascade. Series of steps of Po_2 from atmospheric air to mitochondria in cells:

- dry atmospheric gas: 21 kPa (160 mmHg): influenced by barometric pressure and inspired O_2 concentration
- humidified tracheal gas: 19.8 kPa (150 mmHg)
- alveolar gas: 14 kPa (106 mmHg): influenced by alveolar ventilation and O_2 consumption
- arterial blood: 13.3 kPa (100 mmHg): influenced by $\dot{V}/\dot{Q}$ mismatch
- capillary blood: 6–7 kPa (45–55 mmHg): influenced by blood flow and haemoglobin concentration
- mitochondria: 1–5 kPa (7.5–40 mmHg).

Reduction in Po_2 at any stage, e.g. due to hypoventilation, lung disease, etc., causes reduction in subsequent steps, risking inadequate mitochondrial Po_2 for aerobic metabolism (below the Pasteur point).
See also, Hypoxia; Oxygen, tissue tension; Oxygen transport

Oxygen concentrator. Device for extracting O_2 from atmospheric air. Air is passed under pressure through a column of zeolite which acts as a molecular sieve, trapping nitrogen and water vapour whilst leaving O_2 and trace gases. Nitrogen is removed by depressurising the column. Two columns are used, each alternatively adsorbing or expelling nitrogen. Produces a continuous supply of over 90% O_2, suitable for most medical uses. Range in size from small units for home use to large ones supplying whole hospitals.

Oxygen delivery ($\dot{D}o_2$). Calculated O_2 flux. Used with O_2 consumption ($\dot{V}o_2$) to optimise treatment in critical illness.

$$\dot{D}o_2 = \text{cardiac output (CO)} \times \text{arterial } O_2 \text{ content} = 850\text{–}1200 \text{ ml/min } (500\text{–}700 \text{ ml/min/m}^2)$$

$$\dot{V}o_2 = \text{CO} \times (\text{arterial } O_2 \text{ content} - \text{mixed venous } O_2 \text{ content}) = 240\text{–}270 \text{ ml/min } (120\text{–}160 \text{ ml/min/m}^2)$$

May be used to supplement traditional measurement of cardiovascular variables, e.g. BP, CVP, CO, etc. As $\dot{D}o_2$ falls, a critical point is reached after which $\dot{V}o_2$ also falls, representing tissue anaerobic respiration. Maintenance of $\dot{D}o_2$ above 600 ml/min/m^2, and $\dot{V}o_2$ above 170 ml/min/m^2, has previously been suggested as increasing survival in critical illness, but this is no longer considered to be the case.

O_2 extraction ratio has also been used (normally 22–30%):

$$\frac{\text{arterial} - \text{mixed venous } O_2 \text{ contents}}{\text{arterial } O_2 \text{ content}}$$

Vincent JL (1991). Can J Anaesth; 38: R44–7
See also, Oxygen extraction ratio; Oxygen, tissue tension; Shock

Oxygen extraction ratio. Ratio of oxygen uptake ($\dot{V}o_2$) to oxygen delivery ($\dot{D}o_2$) expressed as a percentage. Normally about 25%, it increases during periods of increased tissue demand e.g. exercise.

Oxygen failure warning device. Device attached to (or incorporated into) the anaesthetic machine; designed to alert anaesthetists to failure of the O_2 supply. Earlier models were often unreliable, e.g. Bosun device (required batteries to power a warning light which could be switched off, and only operated when the N_2O supply was connected).

- Ideal features of mechanical devices:
    - audible warning activated when O_2 pressure falls below a certain value; powered by O_2 itself.
    - warning continues when O_2 is exhausted; powered by N_2O.
    - delivery of N_2O turned off.
    - breathing system opened to atmosphere, allowing inhalation of air.
    - cannot be switched off.

Most consist of a spindle, kept at one end of its casing by the normal working O_2 pressure; a spring moves the spindle towards the other end as O_2 pressure falls, allowing O_2 to pass to a whistle via a port previously blocked by the spindle. Further movement as O_2 pressure continues to fall allows N_2O to flow to a whistle, stops N_2O delivery to the patient, and opens the system to air. Many have a visual indicator too, e.g. producing a colour change.

More recent devices are electronic rather than gas powered.

Oxygen flux. Amount of O_2 delivered to the tissues per unit time.

Equals: CO × arterial O_2 content
= (CO × O_2 bound to haemoglobin + O_2 dissolved in plasma)
= CO × [(10 × Hb × S_ao_2 × 1.34) + (10 × P_ao_2 × 0.0225)]

where CO = cardiac output
Hb = haemoglobin concentration in g/dl
S_ao_2 = arterial O_2 saturation of haemoglobin
1.34 = Hüfner's constant
P_ao_2 = arterial Po_2
0.0225 = ml of O_2 dissolved per 100 ml plasma per kPa (0.003 ml per mmHg).

Normally 850–1200 ml/min, or 500–700 ml/min/m^2 if cardiac index is used.

The tissues cannot utilise all of the transported O_2: the last 20–25% remains bound to haemoglobin. Tissue O_2 supply can increase during times of extra demand, e.g. exercise, via increases in cardiac output. If the O_2 carrying capacity of blood is reduced, e.g. in anaemia, cardiac output must increase at rest in order to maintain O_2 flux, and reserves are less. Cardiac depression during anaesthesia in this situation is thus particularly hazardous.
See also, Oxygen delivery; Oxygen extraction ratio; Oxygen, tissue tension; Oxygen transport

Oxygen, hyperbaric. O_2 therapy at greater than atmospheric pressure, usually 2–3 atmospheres. Increases the amount of dissolved O_2 in blood according to Henry's law. In 100 ml blood, 0.3 ml O_2 dissolves at Po_2 of 13.3 kPa (100 mmHg). Thus for 100% O_2 at 3 atmospheres, dissolved O_2 = 5.7 ml. Since haemoglobin is always saturated, even in venous blood, its binding capacity for CO_2 and buffering capacity are reduced, and pH falls. The resultant hyperventilation may result in hypocapnia.

Used in the treatment of carbon monoxide poisoning, air embolism, gas gangrene, decompression sickness, and has been investigated as an adjunct to radiotherapy and in multiple sclerosis. Single-patient chambers filled with 100% O_2 may be used, or large pressurised chambers containing patient and attendants, with a tightly fitting mask applied to the patient.
Gill AL, Bell CNA (2004). QJM; 97: 385–95
See also, Oxygen transport

Oxygen measurement. Methods include:

- gas analysis:
  - chemical, e.g. conversion to non-gaseous compounds, with reduction in overall volume of gas mixture (Haldane apparatus).
  - physical:
    - O_2 electrode (Clark electrode; polarographic cell): silver/silver chloride anode and platinum cathode in potassium chloride solution inside a cylinder, with a gas-permeable plastic membrane covering its end. 0.6 V potential is applied across the electrodes. O_2 diffuses to the cathode, picking up electrons with water present to become hydroxide ions and causing current flow proportional to the O_2 concentration. May be used with gas or liquid samples. Maintained at 37°C. Falsely high readings caused by halothane are prevented by using a membrane impermeable to halothane.
    - fuel cell: similar to the O_2 electrode but produces its own potential. Consists of lead anode and gold mesh cathode within potassium hydroxide solution. Hydroxide ions are produced at the cathode as above; they combine with lead at the anode to form lead oxide and give up electrons. Thus current flows, proportional to the number of O_2 molecules diffusing through the plastic membrane. No external power source is required, but lifespan is limited. May be affected by N_2O unless special cells are used.
    - paramagnetic cell: most gases are diamagnetic, i.e. repelled by magnetic fields. O_2 and nitric oxide are paramagnetic, i.e. attracted. The cell contains two nitrogen-filled glass spheres joined by a bar which is suspended on a vertical wire within a magnetic field. O_2 introduced into the cell is attracted into the magnetic field, displacing the spheres and rotating the bar against the torque of the wire. Degree of rotation is proportional to the number of O_2 molecules. It may be measured by observing the deflection of a beam of light reflected by a mirror mounted on the wire, or by measuring the current required to prevent rotation when passing through a coil mounted on the bar. A rapid response paramagnetic device employs an alternating magnetic field applied to two streams of gas, one sample and the other reference; the O_2 concentration in the sample gas is represented by a difference in pressure between the two streams. Alternatively, an alternating magnetic field is applied to the gas, producing a sound wave; its amplitude is proportional to the concentration of O_2 (magnetoacoustic technique). Accuracy of these techniques is high.
    - non-specific methods, e.g. mass spectrometer, ultraviolet light absorption.
- measurement of arterial $P\text{O}_2$:
  - O_2 electrode as above. Tiny intravascular probes have been developed for continuous arterial measurement.
  - transcutaneous electrode: similar to the O_2 electrode, but with a heating coil to cause vasodilatation, increase rate of O_2 diffusion, and reduce the difference between arterial and skin $P\text{O}_2$. Inaccurate, especially in adults, and with slow response time; they may also cause burns.
  - fibreoptic sensor placed intravascularly; measures intensity or wavelength of reflected light.
- measurement of arterial O_2 content:, e.g. liberation of gas from blood with chemical analysis (van Slyke apparatus) or use of an O_2 electrode.
- measurement of oxygen saturation of haemoglobin.

[Leland C Clark (1918–2005), US biochemist]

Oxygen radicals, *see Free radicals*

Oxygen saturation. Refers to percentage saturation of haemoglobin with O_2; equals

$$\frac{O_2 \text{ content of haemoglobin}}{O_2 \text{ capacity of haemoglobin}}$$

May be calculated for whole blood, and the dissolved O_2 component subtracted, or measured using oximetry. Normal range in arterial blood at 37°C, pH 7.40 and normal barometric pressure is 97–100%. Reduced in cardiac or respiratory disease.

Oxygen therapy. Used to:

- correct hypoxaemia due to $\dot{V}/\dot{Q}$ mismatch, hypoventilation or impaired alveolar gas diffusion. Only partially corrects hypoxaemia due to shunt.
- increase pulmonary O_2 reserves, e.g. in case of apnoea, hypoventilation, etc.
- increase the amount of dissolved oxygen, e.g. in anaemia, cyanide poisoning and carbon monoxide poisoning (also increases rate of carboxyhaemoglobin dissociation).
- other uses include reduction of pulmonary hypertension, reduction of air-filled cavities (e.g. subcutaneous emphysema, pneumothorax, air embolism, intestinal distension), and special uses of hyperbaric O_2 (*see Oxygen, hyperbaric*).

The effects of breathing 100% O_2 compared with air are shown in Table 26.

- Methods of administration:
  - fixed performance devices; i.e. $F_{\text{I}}\text{O}_2$ is constant despite changes in inspiratory flow rate:
    - O_2 tent.
    - anaesthetic breathing system.
    - high air flow O_2 enrichers (HAFOE): the feed connector to a plastic mask incorporates holes designed to allow entrainment of atmospheric air into the O_2 stream by jet mixing.

      Specific connectors produce set $F_{\text{I}}\text{O}_2$ values at certain O_2 flow rates, assuming the patient's peak inspiratory flow rate does not exceed 30 l/min. For total gas flow of 30 l/min, calculations are as follows:
      - O_2 flow rate $= a$.
      - entrained air flow rate $= b$.
      - $a + b = 30$.
      - volume of O_2 delivered per minute $= (a \times 100\%) + (b \times 21\%)$.
      - but volume of O_2 delivered also $= 30 \times$ required %.

Table 26 Effects of breathing air or 100% O_2

	Air	*100% O_2*
Alveolar $P\text{O}_2$ (kPa (mmHg))	14 (106)	88 (667)
Arterial blood		
$P\text{O}_2$ (kPa (mmHg))	13.3 (100)	84 (638)
O_2 saturation (%)	99	100
O_2 content (ml/100 ml blood):		
bound to haemoglobin	19.7	20.1
dissolved	0.3	1.9
Venous blood		
$P\text{O}_2$ (kPa (mmHg))	5.3 (40)	7 (53.2)
O_2 saturation (%)	75	85
O_2 content (ml/100 ml blood):		
bound to haemoglobin	14.9	17.2
dissolved	0.1	0.2

- therefore $100a + 21b = 30 \times$ required %, and $a + b = 30$.
- thus the values for a and b may be determined.
- variable performance devices; i.e. actual F_IO_2 depends on inspiratory flow rates:
  - nasal cannulae. A nasal catheter, with a foam cuff to aid placement in the nostril, is also available.
  - plastic masks, e.g.:
    - moulded hard plastic.
    - Edinburgh: soft plastic.
    - MC: soft plastic with foam-padded edges.

  All perform similarly, delivering approximately 25–30% O_2 at 2 l/min O_2 flow, and 30–40% at 4 l/min flow.
- other means of administration include IPPV and its variations, CPAP, apnoeic oxygenation and hyperbaric therapy. Transtracheal administration has also been used in chronic lung disease requiring continuous O_2 therapy, via a narrow bore catheter inserted above the sternal notch.

- Problems of O_2 therapy:
  - reduction of hypoxic ventilatory drive in a small group of patients who have chronic CO_2 retention, e.g. COPD. Apnoea may result if chronic hypoxaemia is reversed, thus necessitating controlled O_2 therapy. 24% O_2 is administered initially; if arterial $P\text{CO}_2$ has not risen by more than 1–1.5 kPa (7.5–10 mmHg), and $P\text{O}_2$ has not improved adequately, 28% O_2 is administered, then 30%, etc., until satisfactory $P\text{O}_2$ and $P\text{CO}_2$ have been achieved. It has recently been suggested that this phenomenon is related to an acute decrease in pulmonary vascular resistance following O_2 administration, rather than a reduction in hypoxic ventilatory drive itself.
  - pulmonary and CNS O_2 toxicity.
  - absorption atelectasis.
  - increased risk of explosions and fires.
  - retinopathy of prematurity.

[MC: Mary Catterall, London physician]

Oxygen, tissue tension ($P_T\text{O}_2$). Partial pressure of O_2 in tissues; represents the balance between local supply and consumption of O_2. Most often measured in subcutaneous tissue because of its ease of measurement and relative stability (normally 1 ml/kg/min). Measured using an O_2 electrode mounted on a microcatheter or a fibreoptic probe placed under the skin. Has been used to indicate tissue perfusion; thought to be important in wound healing and susceptibility to infection.

Ragheb J, Buggy DJ (2004). Br J Anaesth; 92: 464–8

Oxygen toxicity. May be:
- respiratory: pulmonary toxicity is related to actual $P\text{O}_2$, not concentration. Tracheobronchial irritation and substernal discomfort is noticed by healthy volunteers after 12–24 h breathing 100% O_2. Reduced vital capacity, compliance and diffusing capacity, and increased arteriovenous shunt and dead space may occur after 24–36 h. Changes include endothelial damage, with reduced mucus clearance and infiltration by inflammatory cells including macrophages and neutrophils. Surfactant may decrease and capillary permeability increase. Eventually fibrosis may occur, although maximal safe concentrations and duration of O_2 therapy are unclear. Up to 48 h breathing 100% O_2 is thought not to be associated with permanent damage; up to 50% is thought to be safe for any period. Certain cytotoxic drugs increase the incidence and severity of fibrosis, e.g. bleomycin. Mechanisms are uncertain, but free radical formation is thought to be most likely. Neutrophil involvement is controversial. Arachidonic acid metabolites may also be involved. Free radical scavengers, surfactant and leukotriene blocking drugs have been studied as possible protective or therapeutic treatments, but prevention is considered more important at present. The lowest F_IO_2 that produces an acceptable arterial $P\text{O}_2$ should be used whenever O_2 is administered.
- neurological: at above 2–3 atmospheres, convulsions may occur (Bert effect).
- ocular: exposure to high arterial $P\text{O}_2$ for long periods may lead to retinopathy of prematurity.

Oxygen transport. In a normal person with a haemoglobin concentration of 15 g/dl breathing air, arterial blood carries approximately 20 ml O_2 per 100 ml:
- 19.7 ml combined with haemoglobin.
- 0.3 ml dissolved in plasma.

In venous blood, 15 ml is carried per 100 ml blood:
- 14.9 ml combined with haemoglobin.
- 0.1 ml dissolved.

Normally, the amount carried by haemoglobin is only slightly increased with O_2 therapy, since haemoglobin is already over 97% saturated; the dissolved O_2 is increased in proportion to the arterial $P\text{O}_2$: 0.0226 ml per kPa per 100 ml blood (0.3 ml per 100 mmHg).

See also, Oxygen flux

Oxygenation index. Indicator of the degree of impairment of oxygenation, often used in studies of neonatal respiratory support as a means of assessing severity of respiratory failure when comparing different respiratory therapies.

$$\text{Equals } \frac{F_I\text{O}_2(\%) \times \text{mean airway pressure (cmH}_2\text{O)}}{P\text{O}_2\text{(mmHg)}}$$

Values above 40 are associated with about 80% mortality with conventional treatment.

Oxygenators, *see Cardiopulmonary bypass*

Oxyhaemoglobin dissociation curve. Plot of oxygen saturation of haemoglobin against $P\text{O}_2$, for normal haemoglobin and $P\text{CO}_2$ at 37°C (Fig. 122a). The curve is sigmoid-shaped because of the increasing affinity of haemoglobin for successive O_2 molecules after the first.
- Important points on the curve:
  - P_{50}: $P\text{O}_2$ at which saturation is 50%; normally about 3.5 kPa (27 mmHg).
  - venous blood: normally corresponds to 75% saturation and $P\text{O}_2$ of 5.3 kPa (40 mmHg).
  - arterial blood: normally corresponds to 97% saturation and $P\text{O}_2$ of 13.3 kPa (100 mmHg).

Thus a small drop in $P\text{O}_2$ from normal levels causes only slight reduction in arterial saturation, because the curve is flat at this point. If $P\text{O}_2$ is already reduced, e.g. in lung disease, the same small drop may cause significant desaturation, corresponding to the steep part of the curve.

The curve is shifted to the right (i.e. $P_{50} > 3.5$ kPa) by acidosis, hyperthermia, hypercapnia (Bohr effect) and increased 2,3-DPG levels (Fig. 122b). Saturation becomes lower for any given $P\text{O}_2$; i.e. O_2 is bound less avidly. Thus O_2 unloading to the tissues is favoured.

The curve is shifted to the left (i.e. $P_{50} < 3.5$ kPa) in the opposite situations, and in fetal haemoglobin, methaemoglobinaemia and carbon monoxide poisoning. Saturation becomes greater for any given $P\text{O}_2$; i.e. O_2 is bound more avidly. Thus fetal haemoglobin can bind O_2 from maternal haemoglobin, but with reduced tissue liberation.

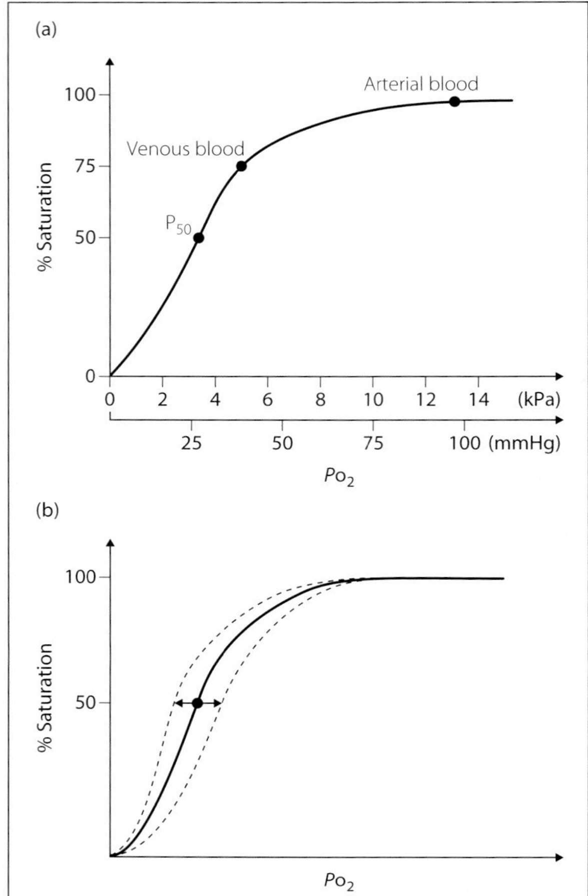

Fig. 122 Oxyhaemoglobin dissociation curve: (a) normal; (b) shift to right or left

Oxymorphone hydrochloride. Opioid analgesic drug, derived from morphine and 6–8 times as potent. Prepared in 1955. Available in the USA for parenteral and rectal use. Action lasts 4–5 h.

Oxytocin. Hormone secreted by the posterior pituitary gland, causing smooth muscle contraction in the uterus and milk ducts. Used to stimulate uterine contraction, e.g. during labour, postpartum or postabortion. Less effective in early pregnancy. Acts within 2–3 min of iv injection. Synthetic preparation (Syntocinon) is free of vasopressin, and thus preferable to pituitary extract.

Causes less nausea/vomiting than ergometrine and does not cause hypertension (but see below). Available as 5 U and 10 U, and as 5 U in combination with ergometrine 500 μg.

- Dosage:
  - to stimulate labour: 1–4 mU/min iv, increased in at least 20-min steps up to 20 mU/min.
  - at Caesarean section or after vaginal delivery: 5 U slowly iv (may also be given im although not licensed by this route).
  - to treat postpartum haemorrhage: 5–10 U slowly iv followed by 5–40 U/500 ml crystalloid, infused as required.
- Side effects:
  - uterine hyperstimulation and fetal distress.
  - reduction in SVR and BP and increased cardiac output results from vasodilatation together with autotransfusion from the uterus to the systemic circulation. Tachycardia may also occur. These changes may be severe, especially when a single bolus of oxytocin is given rapidly, in doses > 5 U and following ephedrine administration. Severe hypotension may occur when oxytocin is given to patients with cardiac disease.
  - severe hyponatraemia has followed prolonged infusion if diluted in dextrose solutions, exacerbated by a direct antidiuretic effect of the hormone itself.
  - rashes, nausea, allergic reactions.

P

P_{50}, *see Oxyhaemoglobin dissociation curve*

P wave. Component of the ECG representing atrial depolarisation. Normally positive (i.e. upwards) in lead I, and best seen in leads II and V_1 (*see Fig. 57b; Electrocardiography*). Maximal amplitude is normally 2.5 mm in lead II, and its duration 0.12 s (three small squares). In right atrial enlargement, the P wave is tall and peaked (P pulmonale); in left atrial enlargement, it is wide and notched (P mitrale).
See also, P–R interval

Pacemaker cells. Cardiac muscle cells which undergo slow spontaneous depolarisation to initiate action potentials. Their activity results from a slow decrease in membrane potassium ion permeability, resulting in gradual increase in intracellular potassium concentration. Rate of discharge depends on the slope of phase 4 depolarisation, resting membrane potential and threshold potential. Pacemaker cells exist in the sinoatrial (SA) node, atrioventricular (AV) node, bundle of His, and ventricular cells. Spontaneous rates of discharge for the different sites: SA node 70–80/min, AV node 60/min, His bundles 50/min and ventricular cells 40/min. Impulses from the faster SA node usually reach and excite the slower pacemaker cells before the latter can discharge spontaneously.
See also, Heart, conducting system

Pacemakers. Usually refers to devices implanted subcutaneously, usually outside the thorax, that provide permanent cardiac pacing (to distinguish them from temporary pacing devices).

Modern devices consist of a titanium casing, containing the pulse generator and lithium iodide battery (the latter nowadays lasting over 10 years). Electrodes are usually unipolar; i.e. one intracardiac electrode, with current returning to the pacemaker via the body. The heart electrode is usually endocardial, passed via a central vein; epicardial electrodes have been used. Leads may be steroid-eluting to reduce inflammation at the site of contact. Modern pacemakers may be checked and adjusted via radiofrequency programming without requiring removal, and recorded data downloaded for analysis of cardiac function.

Indicated if an arrhythmia is associated with syncope, dizziness, cardiac failure, etc., e.g. in sick sinus syndrome, heart block or post-MI. Prophylactic use is controversial.

A generic pacemaker code identifies function (Table 27), the first three positions indicating basic pacing function. Thus VVI denotes ventricular pacing, with inhibition of pacing should any spontaneous ventricular complex occur (e.g. as would apply in temporary transvenous pacing). DDD denotes pacing and sensing of both chambers, with inhibition or triggering to maintain sequential atrial and ventricular contraction, allowing spontaneous activity should it occur. Rate modulation implies the ability to alter the heart rate in response to the patient's level of activity; rate-adaptive devices respond to physiological parameters normally associated with changes in heart rate (e.g. body movement, Q–T interval, respiration, temperature, pH, myocardial contractility, haemoglobin saturation) by increasing the pacing rate. The fifth position is rarely used but has previously been allocated to both multisite pacing, which refers to stimulation of different sites either within one chamber (e.g. right ventricle) or within two chambers of the same type (e.g. both ventricles), and to 'active' anti-tachycardia functions (none/pacing/shock/both). With the development of implantable cardioverter defibrillators, much of the latter functions are covered within the defibrillator codes (*see Defibrillators, implantable cardioverter*).

- Anaesthesia for patients with pacemakers:
  - preoperatively:
    - preoperative assessment is particularly directed towards the CVS.
    - pacemaker type and indication are ascertained. Pacemakers are usually checked regularly.
    - ECG:
      - if pacing spikes occur before all or most beats, heart rate is pacemaker-dependent.
      - although traditional advice was to convert older demand pacemakers to fixed rate by placing a magnet over the pulse generator, this is no longer recommended outside of specialist cardiac pacing units since the effect on the device's programming may be unpredictable.
    - CXR: pulse generator and number of leads may be identified.
  - perioperatively:
    - potential electrical interference or pacemaker damage by diathermy is more likely if the latter is applied near the device. Sensing may be triggered, with resultant

Table 27 North American Society of Pacing and Electrophysiology/British Pacing and Electrophysiology Group generic pacemaker code

Position 1: chamber paced	*Position 2: chamber sensed*	*Position 3: response*	*Position 4: rate modulation*	*Position 5: multisite pacing*
0 = None	0 = None	0 = None	0 = None	0 = None
A = Atrium	A = Atrium	T = Triggered	R = Rate modulation	A = Atrium
V = Dual	V = Ventricle	I = Inhibited		V = Ventricle
D = Dual	D = Dual	D = Dual		D = Dual

chamber inhibition, or arrhythmias induced. Diathermy may also reprogramme the pacemaker to a different mode.
- if avoidance of diathermy is not possible, risks are reduced by using bipolar diathermy, or placing the plate distant from the pacemaker if unipolar diathermy is used. Current should not be applied across the chest, and its strength and duration of use should be minimal.
- care should be taken with CVP/pulmonary artery catheters since they may dislodge the electrodes.
- temporary pacing facilities (or non-invasive transthoracic pacing) and an external defibrillator should be available.
- isoprenaline may be required if pacemaker failure occurs.
- alteration of pacemaker sensitivity by halothane has been described in older pacemaker models.
- avoidance of suxamethonium has been suggested in case fasciculations are sensed as arrhythmias.
- MRI may be hazardous since the pacemaker may be switched to asynchronous mode, may fail altogether or may move within the chest.

- postoperative pacemaker checking may be required.

Allen M (2006). Anaesthesia; 61: 883–90

Packed cell volume, *see Haematocrit*

PADP, Pulmonary artery diastolic pressure, *see Pulmonary artery pressure*

Paediatric Advanced Life Support (PALS). Course set up in the USA by the American Heart Association and the American Academy of Pediatrics. Intended for healthcare professionals caring for acutely ill children (e.g. those working in paediatric, anaesthetic, intensive care and emergency departments). Course objectives include:

- recognition of the infant or child at risk of cardiopulmonary arrest and the development of strategies for its prevention.
- identification of the cognitive and psychomotor skills necessary for resuscitating and stabilising the neonate, infant or child in respiratory failure, shock, or cardiopulmonary arrest (e.g. drug dosages, airway and ventilation techniques, identification of normal and abnormal cardiac rhythms, defibrillation, vascular access).

The course is predominantly practical with an emphasis on 'hands-on' training. Technical skills and cognitive processes are first taught separately in small group sessions. Practical application of these skills and knowledge in critical situations is then emphasised by using case presentations.

American Heart Association (2005). Circulation; 112: iv, 167–87

See also, Advanced Paediatric Life Support

Paediatric anaesthesia. Main considerations are related to the anatomical and physiological differences between adults and children, especially neonates (defined as up to 1 month old; infants are defined as up to 1 year old).

- Thus in children compared with adults:
  - RS:
    - the tongue is large and the larynx is situated more anteriorly and more cephalad (C3–4). The epiglottis is large and U-shaped. Airway management and tracheal intubation may thus be difficult, compounded by the large size of the head compared with the body. A straight laryngoscope blade is often preferred.
    - the cricoid cartilage is the narrowest part of the upper airway up to 8–10 years of age (cf. glottis in adults). A small decrease in diameter (e.g. caused by oedema or stricture formation following prolonged tracheal intubation) may lead to airway obstruction.
    - the left and right main bronchi arise at equal angles from the trachea. At birth, the tracheobronchial tree is developed as far as the terminal bronchioles. Alveoli number 20 million, increasing to 300 million by 6–8 years.
    - respiration is predominantly diaphragmatic, and sinusoidal and continuous instead of periodic. Neonates are obligatory nose breathers. Respiratory rate is increased. Tidal volume is about 7 ml/kg as in adults. The infant lung is more susceptible to atelectasis because the chest wall is more compliant and therefore pulled inwards by the lungs, decreasing FRC. Closing capacity may exceed FRC during normal respiration in neonates and infants. Surfactant may be deficient in premature babies.
    - response to CO_2 is reduced at birth, and irregular breathing may also occur. Premature babies may suffer from apnoeic episodes; they may be at risk from postoperative apnoea up to about 50 weeks postconceptual age. Gasp and Hering–Breuer reflexes are active.
    - basal metabolic rate and O_2 consumption are high (the latter is 5–6 ml/kg/min, compared with about 3–4 ml/kg/min in adults). Hypoxaemia thus occurs more rapidly than in adults.
    - the oxyhaemoglobin dissociation curve of fetal haemoglobin is shifted to the left (P_{50} of 2.4 kPa (18 mmHg)). Haemoglobin concentration falls from 18 g/dl (1–2 weeks of age) to 11 g/dl (6 months–6 years).
  - CVS:
    - cardiac output is 30–50% higher than in adults, largely due to increased heart rate. Arterial BP is lower (Table 28).
    - left and right ventricles are similar at birth, the former fibrous and non-compliant, making stroke volume relatively fixed.
    - blood volume at birth is up to 90 ml/kg (or 50 + haematocrit). It falls to 80 ml/kg for children and 70 ml/kg by 14 years.
    - veins are more difficult to cannulate.
    - reversion to fetal circulation may occur in severe hypoxaemia.
  - CNS:
    - the spinal cord ends at L3 at birth, receding to L1–2 by adolescence.
    - the immature blood–brain barrier results in increased sensitivity to centrally depressant drugs, particularly opioid analgesic drugs. These drugs have traditionally been avoided in children because of the fear of respiratory depression and the theory that neonates do not feel pain because their nervous system is

Table 28 Normal heart rate and BP at different ages

Age	Heart rate (beats/min)	BP (mmHg)
0–6 months	120–180	80/45
3 years	95–120	95/65
5 years	90–110	100/65
10 years	80–100	110/70

insufficiently developed. This theory is now generally disbelieved, and opioids are widely used to provide analgesia for children.
- vagal reflexes are particularly active in children. Bradycardia readily occurs in hypoxaemia.
- subependymal vessels are fragile in premature neonates, with risk of rupture if BP and ICP increase.

- temperature regulation is impaired. Ratio of body surface area to body weight is greater than in adults and there is less body fat. Thus heat loss is rapid, compounded by impaired shivering and increased metabolic rate. Brown fat is metabolised to maintain body temperature. Insensible water loss is increased in premature babies.
- prolonged fasting may cause hypoglycaemia in small children, and oral clear fluids are usually allowed up to 2 h preoperatively (4 h for milk). IV administration of dextrose may be required.
- fluid balance is delicate, since a greater proportion of body water is exchanged each day. Thus dehydration readily occurs in illness. Total body water is normally increased, with a higher ratio of ECF to intracellular fluid (ECF exceeds intracellular fluid in premature babies). The kidneys are less able to handle a water or solute load, or to conserve water or solutes.

  Appropriate maintenance fluid requirements (using dextrose/saline) have traditionally been calculated thus:
  4 ml/kg/h for each of the first 10 kg, plus
  2 ml/kg/h for each of the next 10 kg, plus
  1 ml/kg/h for each kg thereafter.

  More recently, because of the risk of perioperative hyponatraemia (children being at particular risk from resultant encephalopathy), and because perioperative hypoglycaemia is less of a problem than traditionally thought, there has been a move away from hypotonic solutions such as dextrose/saline, with maintenance fluids given as 0.45–0.9% saline or Hartmann's solution, and isotonic fluids avoided if plasma sodium concentration is under 140 mmol/l.

  Other losses, e.g. blood, must be added. Blood is traditionally given above 10% of blood volume loss, but larger blood losses are increasingly allowed if starting haemoglobin concentration is high. In hypovolaemia, 10 ml/kg colloid is a suitable starting regimen.
- actions of drugs may be affected by the above factors, or by lower plasma albumin levels (up to 1 year of age), resulting in greater amounts of free drug. Renal and hepatic immaturity may contribute to delayed excretion. MAC of inhalational anaesthetic agents is increased in neonates, but may be reduced in premature babies. Neonates are more sensitive to non-depolarising neuromuscular blocking drugs, probably due to altered pharmacokinetics. They may be resistant to suxamethonium, requiring up to twice the adult dose.

- Practical conduct of anaesthesia:
  - children are placed first on the operating list, to allow as short a fasting time as possible, etc.
  - most standard drugs are used, administered according to weight. As a rough guide the following scheme may be useful:
    - 14 years: adult dose.
    - 7 years: ½ adult dose.
    - 4 years: ⅓ adult dose.
    - 1 year: ¼ adult dose.
    - newborn: ⅛ adult dose.
    - premature: ⅒ adult dose.
  - premedication is often given orally, to avoid injections, but standard im drugs are also given. Rectal administration has also been used. Atropine is often given to reduce excessive secretions and vagal reflexes.
  - induction of anaesthesia:
    - cyclopropane has been popular but is no longer available in the UK. Halothane has been largely replaced by sevoflurane. Inhalational induction is rapid because of increased alveolar ventilation, a low FRC and a high cerebral blood flow.
    - standard iv anaesthetic agents are suitable. Administration im (e.g. ketamine, methohexital) or rectally (e.g. methohexital) has also been used. EMLA or topical tetracaine (amethocaine) is routinely used before iv induction.

    The presence of parents at induction is usually allowed, depending on the circumstances.
  - awake tracheal intubation has traditionally been used in neonates, but fears have been expressed over adverse effects, e.g. raised ICP. However, ICP has been shown to rise markedly during normal crying, and awake intubation is often felt to be the safest technique, especially in inexperienced hands. Small laryngoscope handles and blades are usually employed. Uncuffed tracheal tubes have traditionally been employed (usually until ~10 years), with a small air leak at 15–25 cmH_2O airway pressure, to avoid subglottic stenosis. The approximate size may be calculated thus:
    - diameter = (age/4) + 4.5 mm.

      For neonates:
      - under 750 g/26 weeks gestation: 2.0–2.5 mm.
      - 750–2000 g/26–34 weeks: 2.5–3.0 mm.
      - over 2000 g/34 weeks: 3.0–3.5 mm.
    - length = (age/12) + 12 cm.

    More recently, cuffed tubes have been used in term neonates and children, on the basis that a smaller tube with a low pressure, high volume cuff is better able to provide an adequate conduit for ventilation whilst minimising pressure on the cricoid cartilage (from the tube itself) and the trachea (from the cuff). A formula for cuffed tubes has been suggested: diameter = (age/4) + 3.0 mm.
  - dead space and resistance should be minimal in anaesthetic breathing systems; adult forms are suitable if the child weighs over 20–25 kg but the Bain system is often avoided because of increased resistance to expiration. Ayre's T-piece is suitable up to 25 kg. Spontaneous ventilation via a facepiece or laryngeal mask airway is usually suitable for short procedures in children older than 3 months. Below this, tracheal intubation and IPPV is traditionally performed although the laryngeal mask airway is preferred by some.
  - for IPPV using a T-piece, the following fresh gas flows have been suggested, producing slight hypocapnia:
    - 10–30 kg: 1000 ml + 100 ml/kg per min.
    - > 30 kg: 2000 ml + 50 ml/kg per min.

    Set minute volume should equal twice fresh gas flow.
  - monitoring: precordial or oesophageal stethoscope and temperature measurement are especially useful.
  - anaesthetic rooms and operating theatres should be warmed. Warming blankets, reflective coverings, etc. should also be used, with humidification of inspired gases.
  - tracheal extubation is usually performed with the child awake, to reduce the risk of aspiration or laryngospasm.
  - regional techniques are popular for peri- and postoperative analgesia, e.g. caudal analgesia, inguinal field block, penile block. Local wound infiltration is also effective. Spinal and epidural anaesthesia have also been used.

- paracetamol and codeine are often used for postoperative analgesia, with pethidine or other opioids for severe pain. Antiemetic drugs are usually avoided, since dystonic reactions are more common in children.
- Other problems are related to the procedure performed, e.g.:
  - repair of congenital defects, e.g. tracheo-oesophageal fistula, pyloric stenosis, gastroschisis, diaphragmatic hernia, congenital heart disease, etc.
  - related to trauma.
  - ENT, dental and ophthalmic surgery, etc.

The National Confidential Enquiry into Patient Outcome and Death (as NCEPOD) focused for its first year on paediatric anaesthesia. It concluded that general care was good, although outcome was related to clinicians' experience.

Paediatric intensive care. Classified into levels 1, 2 and 3, primarily on the basis of interventions undertaken. Level 1 is high dependency care; level 3 is almost always provided in tertiary paediatric centres with specialist medical and nursing staff trained in paediatric intensive care and with specialised equipment necessary for paediatric care. In general, differs from adult intensive care by virtue of anatomical and physiological differences between adults and children (*see Paediatric anaesthesia*) and the range of conditions seen.

- Main clinical problems encountered include:
  - acute respiratory failure:
    - upper airway obstruction:
      - neonates: choanal atresia, congenital facial deformities, laryngeal/tracheal abnormalities.
      - infants/children: inhaled foreign body, tonsillar/adenoidal hypertrophy, croup, epiglottitis, angioedema, etc.
    - lung disorders:
      - neonates: meconium aspiration, respiratory distress syndrome, diaphragmatic hernia, pneumothorax, chest infection, etc.
      - infants/children: pneumonia, asthma, bronchiolitis, cystic fibrosis, congenital heart disease, trauma, near-drowning, burns, etc.

      In neonates, respiratory impairment may result in the development of a persistent fetal circulation.
  - neurological disease:
    - neonates: birth asphyxia, central apnoea, convulsions, etc.
    - infants/children: meningitis, encephalitis, status epilepticus, Guillain–Barré syndrome, etc.
  - trauma: the leading cause of death in children under a year old and the third leading cause in older children (after sudden infant death syndrome and congenital abnormalities). Non-accidental injury must always be considered.
    - head injury occurs in 50% of cases of blunt trauma. A modified Glasgow coma scale is used for assessment; otherwise management is along similar lines to that of adults.
    - spinal cord injury and thoracic/abdominal trauma is usually caused by road traffic accidents.
  - poisoning and overdoses.
- Specific attention must be paid to:
  - smaller equipment, drug doses, fluid volumes, etc.; specialised equipment.
  - nutrition and electrolyte/fluid balance.
  - temperature regulation.
  - sedation and analgesia.
  - educational and psychological needs.
  - the risk of retinopathy of prematurity in neonates.

In 1997, the Department of Health recommended that level 3 paediatric intensive care should be primarily delivered in Lead Centres supported by District General Hospitals (capable of initiating intensive care), Major Acute General Hospitals (large adult ICUs already managing critically ill children at level 2 or 3) and Specialist Hospitals (e.g. those caring for children with burns or requiring cardiac or neurosurgery). Each centre would comply with specific standards relating to training, equipment, the experience of medical and nursing staff, access to specialist services or advice, treatment protocols, facilities for families, and audit. Regional paediatric retrieval teams would also be established.

Overall mortality ranges from 5 to 10% depending on admission criteria. Scoring systems such as the paediatric trauma score, injury severity score and paediatric risk of mortality score attempt to predict outcome and allow audit of care within and between units.

Frey B, Argent A (2004). Intensive Care Med; 30: 1041–6 and 1292–7

See also, Brainstem death; Cardiopulmonary resuscitation, neonatal; Cardiopulmonary resuscitation, paediatric; Necrotising enterocolitis

Paediatric logistic organ dysfunction score (PELOD). Scoring system described as a measure of severity of multiple organ dysfunction in paediatric intensive care. Based on 12 variables relating to six organ systems (neurological, cardiovascular, renal, respiratory, haematological and hepatic). Has been used as daily indicator of organ dysfunction.

Leteurtre S, Martinot A, Duhamel A, et al (2003). Lancet; 362: 192–7

Paediatric risk of mortality score (PRISM). Scoring system used in paediatric intensive care to help predict mortality. Originally used weighted scores for 14 variables related to acute physiological status; the latest version (PRISM III) has 17 and includes additional risk factors including acute and chronic diagnosis. Has been validated for most categories of paediatric ICU.

Pollack MM, Patel KM, Ruttimann UE (1996). Crit Care Med; 24: 743–52

Paediatric trauma score. Trauma scale designed to allow triage of paediatric patients. Six variables (weight, patency of airway, systolic BP, conscious level, presence of skeletal injury and skin injuries) attract scores of 2 (normal), 1 or −1 (severely compromised); scores under 8 indicate increased morbidity and mortality and require referral to a paediatric trauma centre.

Tepas JJ, Ramenofsky ML, Mollitt DL, et al (1988). J Trauma; 28: 425–9

PAF, *see Platelet activating factor*

Pain. Usually defined as an unpleasant sensory and emotional experience resulting from a stimulus causing, or likely to cause, tissue damage (nociception), or expressed in terms of that damage. Thus affected by subjective emotional factors, making pain evaluation difficult. Chronic pain may arise from nervous system dysfunction rather than tissue damage (neurogenic pain, e.g. trigeminal neuralgia, postherpetic neuralgia, complex regional pain syndrome type 2, phantom limb pain, central pain), and may be associated with damage to pain pathways. Substances released from damaged tissues, and/or reorganisation of somatic and sympathetic spinal reflex pathways, are thought to be involved in the aetiology of chronic pain. Chronic pain is usually more

difficult to diagnose and treat than acute pain, and psychological and emotional factors are more important.
See also, Allodynia; Dysaesthesia; Hyperaesthesia; Hyperalgesia; Hyperpathia; Hypoalgesia; Myofascial pain syndromes; Pain clinic; Pain management; Postoperative analgesia

Pain clinic. Outpatient clinic run by consultants (usually anaesthetists) with a special interest in the management of chronic pain. Developed from the 1950s. Its role includes diagnosis of the underlying condition and management directed at reducing subjective pain experiences, reducing drug consumption, increasing levels of normal activity and restoring a normal quality of life. Requires appropriate facilities for consultation, and performance of nerve blocks and surgical procedures. Anaesthetists, physicians, psychologists and neurologists may be involved. Primary referrals to the clinic are usually from general practitioners or hospital consultants.
See also, Pain management

Pain evaluation. Difficult to perform, because pain is a subjective experience.
- Methods used depend on the setting and whether the pain is acute or chronic:
  - experimental methods (e.g. assessing analgesic effects of new drugs):
    - animals: tail-flick response to pinching; pedal withdrawal response to pinching the foot; head shaking response to ear pinching.
    - humans: degree of tolerated digital pressure; tolerated duration of immersion of the forearm into icy water.
  - acute pain, e.g. postoperative: linear analogue scale; using numbers or words to rate the degree of pain (patient and observer assessment may be used); demand for analgesia. Babies have been studied by recording and analysing their cries.
  - chronic pain: the pain is characterised by noting its type, duration, location, quality, intensity, modifying factors (e.g. food, exercise, etc.), time relations, and associated symptoms and mental changes. Full clinical examination is performed, with investigations as appropriate. Linear analogue and rating scales may be used as above. More complicated psychological questionnaires for analysis of personality and pain (e.g. Minnesota multiphasic personality inventory, McGill questionnaire) have been used.

Pain, intractable, *see Pain; Pain clinic; Pain management; individual conditions*

Pain management. Acute pain, e.g. postoperative, is usually treated with systemic analgesics and regional techniques (*see Postoperative analgesia*).
- Chronic pain management may involve the following, after full pain evaluation:
  - simple measures, e.g. rest, exercise, heat and cold treatment, vibration, etc.
  - systemic drug therapy:
    - analgesic drugs: different drugs, dosage regimens and routes of administration may be chosen, depending on the severity and temporal pattern of the pain, and efficacy and side effects of the drugs. Drugs used range from mild NSAIDs to opioid analgesic drugs. The latter are usually reserved for severe pain of short duration, or pain associated with malignancy; they may require concurrent antiemetic and aperient therapy. Implantable devices may be used for intermittent iv, epidural or subarachnoid injection or continuous infusion of opioids.
    - other drugs used include:
      - psychoactive drugs, e.g. antidepressant drugs (especially tricyclics), anticonvulsant drugs (e.g. gabapentin, carbamazepine, phenytoin, clonazepam), phenothiazines, butyrophenones. Thought to have a direct analgesic effect in addition to their other actions.
      - corticosteroids, either by local injection or oral therapy. Particularly useful in neuralgia or pain associated with oedema, e.g. malignancy. Often injected with local anaesthetic agents, e.g. epidurally for back pain.
      - muscle relaxants, e.g. baclofen, dantrolene, benzodiazepines; may be useful if muscle spasm is problematic.
      - others, e.g. antimitotic drugs, calcitonin in bony pain, β-adrenergic receptor antagonists, clonidine.
  - local anaesthetic nerve blocks: may be diagnostic, prognostic (to allow assessment prior to destructive lesions) or therapeutic. Include:
    - injection of trigger points in myofascial pain syndromes.
    - facet joint injection.
    - caudal analgesia, epidural anaesthesia, spinal anaesthesia.
    - paravertebral nerve blocks.
    - sympathetic nerve blocks, e.g. stellate ganglion, coeliac plexus and lumbar sympathetic blocks, iv guanethidine block.
  - destructive procedures: usually reserved for severe pain associated with malignancy, since relief may not be permanent and unacceptable side effects may be produced (e.g. anaesthesia dolorosa). X-ray control is usually employed to aid correct positioning before percutaneous destruction. Methods include:
    - regional techniques as above, using phenol or absolute alcohol. The former is hyperbaric compared with CSF, the latter hypobaric. Thus for intrathecal neurolysis the required posterior sensory roots may be selectively destroyed with appropriate positioning of the patient. Pituitary ablation has also been used.
    - extremes of temperature, e.g. cryoprobe, radiofrequency probe. The latter delivers a high frequency alternating current, producing up to 80°C heat. It is used at peripheral nerves, facet joints, dorsal root ganglia and trigeminal ganglion, and for percutaneous cordotomy.
    - surgery: includes peripheral neurectomy, dorsal rhizotomy or lesions in the dorsal root entry zones (DREZ), commissurotomy (sagittal division of the spinal cord), mesencephalotomy and thalamotomy.
  - electrical stimulation:
    - TENS and electroacupuncture.
    - dorsal column stimulation.
    - stimulation of deep brain structures has also been used, e.g. via electrodes implanted in the periventricular grey matter or thalamus.
  - acupuncture.
  - psychological techniques, e.g. psychotherapy, cognitive behavioural therapy, operant conditioning, hypnosis, biofeedback, relaxation techniques.

The World Health Organization has suggested a 'pain ladder' in which mild pain is treated by a non-opioid ± adjuvant; moderate pain by a mild opioid ± non-opioid ± adjuvant;

and severe pain with a strong opioid ± non-opioid ± adjuvant.

Pain pathways. Most pain arises in pain receptors (nociceptors) widely distributed in the skin and musculoskeletal system. Those responding to pinprick and sudden heat (thermomechanoreceptors) are related to myelinated Aδ fibres, and are responsible for rapid pain sensation and reflex withdrawal. Receptors responding to pressure, heat, chemical substances (e.g. histamine, prostaglandins, acetylcholine, etc.) and tissue damage (polymodal receptors) are associated with unmyelinated C fibre endings, and are responsible for slow pain sensation and immobilisation of the affected part.

- Afferent impulses pass centrally thus:
  - first order neurones have cell bodies within the dorsal root ganglia of the spinal cord. Aδ fibres synapse with cells in laminae I and V of the cord, whilst C fibres synapse with cells in laminae II and III (substantia gelatinosa).
  - most second order neurones synapse with Aδ fibres in the posterior horn, crossing to the opposite side immediately or within a few segments. They ascend within the anterolateral columns (spinothalamic tract) to the ventroposterior nucleus of the thalamus and periaqueductal grey matter.

    The substantia gelatinosa does not project directly to higher levels, but contains many interneurones involved in modification of pain transmission (e.g. described by the gate control theory of pain). Some fibres are projected to deeper layers of the spinal grey matter, from which arises the spinoreticular tract to the ascending reticular activating system (ARAS). Fibres are then relayed to the thalamus and hypothalamus (some fibres reach the thalamus without passing to the ARAS, via the palaeospinothalamic tract).
  - third order neurones transmit from the thalamus to the somatosensory cortex.

Pain sensation may thus be modified by ascending or descending pathways at many levels.

See also, Nerves; Nociception; Sensory pathways

Pain, postoperative, *see Postoperative analgesia*

Palliative care. Overall care of patients whose disease (often malignancy but also neurological, inflammatory, etc.) is not amenable to curative treatment. Includes not only control of pain but also psychological, spiritual and social support. Requires a team approach including the expertise of general physicians, oncologists, surgeons, nursing staff, physiotherapists, religious advisers, etc. Anaesthetists are increasingly involved as they have expertise in controlling symptoms such as pain, anxiety, nausea and vomiting; they also care for patients with terminal disease in the ICU. Since 1987, palliative care has been recognised as a separate specialty in the UK.

See also, Ethics; Euthanasia; Withdrawal of treatment in ICU

Palonosetron. 5-HT_3 receptor antagonist licensed as an antiemetic drug in chemotherapy-induced nausea and vomiting.

- Dosage: 250 μg iv over 30 s. No further dose for 7 days.
- Side effects include GIT upset, arrhythmias, angina and peripheral neuropathy.

PALS, *see Paediatric advanced life support*

Pancreatitis. Acute pancreatitis is an autodigestive process in which pancreatic proteolytic enzymes are activated and cause haemorrhagic necrosis of the pancreatic parenchyma. The gland may be destroyed by haemorrhage, oedema and fat necrosis, releasing serosanguinous exudate into the peritoneal cavity causing peritonitis. There is also local and systemic release of toxins. Mortality may be high because of resulting sepsis, respiratory failure, shock and renal failure.

Commonly associated with biliary tract disease or alcoholism. May occasionally follow upper abdominal surgery, pancreatic ductal obstruction (e.g. by carcinoma), trauma, mumps, cystic fibrosis, hypothermia, hypercalcaemia, hyperlipidaemia, diuretics or corticosteroids.

- Features:
  - severe epigastric pain (typically radiating through to the back), nausea and vomiting, fever, occasionally mild jaundice.
  - epigastric tenderness on palpation, progressing to features of peritonitis.
  - discolouration in flanks caused by tracking of blood from the retroperitoneal space (Grey Turner's sign) or via the falciform ligament to the umbilicus (Cullen's sign).
  - hypotension, oliguria, respiratory failure.

Investigations reveal raised serum and urinary amylase (secondary to leakage from the pancreas), leucocytosis, hyperglycaemia, hypocalcaemia (secondary to calcium sequestration in areas of fat necrosis), hypoproteinaemia and hyperlipidaemia. Since many other disorders also result in increased amylase levels, measurement of the more specific marker serum lipase is increasingly used for diagnosis. Abdominal X-ray may reveal a 'sentinel loop' of small bowel overlying the pancreas. Chest X-ray may show a raised hemidiaphragm, pleural effusion, atelectasis or acute lung injury. Abdominal CT scanning may be helpful in confirming the diagnosis and assessing the severity of pancreatic damage.

Poor prognosis may be indicated by: age >55 years; systolic BP <90 mmHg; white cell count > 15 × 10^9/l; temperature >39°C; blood glucose >10 mmol/l; arterial P_{O_2} <8 kPa (60 mmHg); plasma urea >15 mmol/l; serum calcium <2 mmol/l; haematocrit reduced by over 10%; abnormal liver function tests.

- Management:
  - supportive, e.g. O_2 therapy, iv fluid administration, analgesia, nasogastric drainage, insulin therapy where indicated, TPN. Multiple organ failure is treated along conventional lines. Correction of electrolyte derangement (especially calcium and magnesium) is important.
  - aprotinin, peritoneal lavage, prophylactic antibiotic therapy, glucagon, calcitonin and somatostatin have been used, but with little evidence of efficacy.
  - surgery may be required for drainage of an abscess or pseudocyst or for relief of biliary obstruction. Resection of necrotic pancreas has been performed but mortality from surgery in early disease is high.

Chronic pancreatitis usually occurs in alcoholics, and is characterised by pancreatic calcification and impaired enzyme secretion with malabsorption, and repeated episodes of pain. Surgery may be required; anaesthetic considerations are related to alcohol abuse, and the consequences of malabsorption and malnutrition.

[George Grey Turner (1877–1951), English surgeon; Thomas S Cullen (1868–1953), Canadian-born US gynaecologist]

Swaroop VS, Chari ST, Clain JE (2004). JAMA; 291: 2865–8

Pancuronium bromide. Synthetic non-depolarising neuromuscular blocking drug, first used in 1967. Bisquaternary amino-corticosteroid, but with no corticosteroid activity. Initial dose is 0.05–0.1 mg/kg, with tracheal intubation possible after 2–3 min. Effects last 40–60 min. Supplementary dose: 0.01–0.02 mg/kg. Histamine release is extremely rare. May cause increases in heart rate, BP and cardiac output, caused by vagolytic and sympathomimetic actions. The latter may be due to release of noradrenaline from sympathetic nerve endings or blockade of its uptake. Pancuronium is strongly bound to plasma gammaglobulin after iv injection, and metabolised mainly by the kidney but also by the liver. Elimination is delayed in renal and hepatic impairment.

Traditionally used in shocked patients requiring anaesthesia, because of its cardiovascular effects. Formerly commonly used in ICU, but superseded by atracurium and vecuronium.

Pantoprazole sodium. Proton-pump inhibitor; actions and effects are similar to those of omeprazole.

- Dosage: 40 mg orally or slowly iv, once daily.
- Side effects: as for omeprazole.

Papaveretum. Opioid analgesic drug, first prepared in 1909 and consisting of opium alkaloids: morphine 47.5–52.5%, codeine 2.5–5.0%, noscapine (narcotine) 16–22%, papaverine 2.5–7.0% and others, e.g. thebaine < 1.5%. Said to have greater sedative power than morphine, but generally their effects are similar. Widely popular for many years, especially as premedication; indications and use are as for morphine. The Committee on Safety of Medicines issued a warning in 1991 that noscapine (an alkaloid with similar effects to papaverine) induces polyploidy in mammalian cell lines *in vitro* and may be genotoxic. A new formulation was made available in 1993, consisting of morphine, papaverine and codeine alone in the ratio 253:23:20 at 15.4 mg/ml or 7.7 mg/ml. Confusion over dosage regimens has led to many anaesthetists abandoning papaveretum in favour of morphine.

- Dosage: 7.7–15.4 mg sc, im or iv.

Also available in combination with hyoscine (15.4 mg papaveretum and 0.4 mg hyoscine per ml).

Papaverine. Benzylisoquinoline opium alkaloid, without CNS activity. Used for its non-specific relaxant effect on smooth muscle, especially vascular. May be injected iv or applied directly during surgery. Its use has been advocated following intra-arterial injection of thiopental.

- Dosage: up to 30 mg slowly iv (may cause histamine release). Also used in combination oral preparations to relieve GIT spasm.

Paracelsus (1493–1541). Swiss philosopher and physician; his real name was Theophrastus Bambastus von Hohenheim. Lectured at the University of Basle. Revolutionised the theory of medicine, encouraging the science of research and experimentation. Described the effects of diethyl ether on chickens in 1540. He is also credited with introducing the use of bellows for ventilating the lungs.

Davis A (1993). J Roy Soc Med; 86: 653–6

Paracentesis. Strictly, the term refers to puncture of any hollow organ or cavity for removal or instillation of material; however it usually refers to drainage of ascites from the peritoneum, e.g. in hepatic failure. Removal of large volumes improves cardiac output and respiratory function, decreasing portal venous pressure. It also reduces the patient's weight and makes them more comfortable and mobile. However, rapid aspiration may be followed by cardiovascular collapse and oliguria, thought to be related to sudden release of the splinting effect of the intra-abdominal fluid.

With the patient supine and with the bladder emptied, a needle is inserted through the abdominal wall, usually in the left and right upper and lower quadrants, after infiltration with local anaesthetic. The avascular linea alba below the umbilicus is also commonly used. Insertion of the needle along a Z-shaped path through the layers has been suggested, to reduce subsequent persistent leakage.

See also, Peritoneal lavage

Paracervical block. Used to provide analgesia during the first stage of labour, or for gynaecological procedures, e.g. dilatation and curettage. First performed in 1926.

With the patient's legs apart, a special sheathed needle (with tip protected) is directed into the lateral vaginal fornix by the operator's fingers. The needle tip is advanced 0.5–1 cm to point cranially, laterally and dorsally, and 5–10 ml local anaesthetic agent injected into the parametrial tissue on either side, blocking the uterine nerves which form a plexus at the base of the broad ligament. Vaginal, vulval and perineal sensation is unaffected.

Seldom used in modern obstetrics, because of the high incidence of fetal arrhythmias (especially bradycardia), thought to be caused by alterations in uteroplacental blood flow or absorption of local anaesthetic.

See also, Obstetric analgesia and anaesthesia

Paracetamol (Acetaminophen). Analgesic drug, derived from para-aminophenol; introduced in the 1950s. Inhibits central prostaglandin synthesis and has a central antipyretic action. Traditionally held to have minimal peripheral anti-inflammatory effects, although this has been questioned. Does not cause gastric irritation or alter platelet adhesiveness. Used to treat minor pain.

Rapidly absorbed after oral administration, with peak plasma levels within 60 min. Minimally protein-bound in plasma. Conjugated with glucuronide and sulphate in the liver; under 10% is oxidised by the hepatic P_{450} system to form *N*-acetyl-*p*-benzoquinoneimine, a potential cellular toxin. Normally, this is safely conjugated with glutathione, but it may cause hepatic necrosis in paracetamol poisoning, when the glucuronide and sulphate pathways are saturated and glutathione stores are depleted. Half-life is about 2 h, but its effects last longer.

- Dosage:
  - 0.5–1.0 g orally/rectally 4 hourly, up to 4 g maximum daily.
  - in children, traditionally recommended dosage of 10–15 mg/kg 4 hourly × 4/day has been challenged based on pharmacokinetic data; an initial loading dose of 20 (oral) or 40 (rectal) mg/kg may be followed by doses of 10–15 mg/kg 4–6 hourly up to 40 (premature), 60 (< 3 months old) or 90 (> 3 months) mg/kg/day for up to 48 h (72 h if > 3 months).
  - an iv preparation was introduced in the UK in 2004:
    - adult/child >50 kg: 1 g 4–6 hourly up to 4 g daily.
    - adult/child 10–50 kg: 15 mg/kg 4–6 hourly up to 60 mg/kg daily.
    - adult/child <10 kg: 7.5 mg/kg 4–6 hourly up to 30 mg/kg daily.
- Side effects: nausea, vomiting, rashes.

Available in combination with other analgesics, e.g. dextropropoxyphene, codeine. Over-the-counter sale of 500 mg tablets/capsules in the UK is limited to packs of 32 (packs of 100 tablets/capsules may be purchased from pharmacists in special circumstances).

Paracetamol poisoning. Hepatocellular necrosis may occur if more than about 7.5 g (15 tablets) are taken, due to saturation of the normal metabolic pathways for paracetamol and exhaustion of hepatic glutathione stores. Lower doses may also be toxic, especially in the presence of pre-existing hepatic enzyme induction (e.g. in patients on phenytoin, barbiturates, carbamazepine or rifampicin therapy), or in malnourished, alcoholic or HIV-positive patients. The commonest cause of acute hepatic failure in Europe.

Patients may be asymptomatic for 24 h after ingestion. Early features include nausea and vomiting, anorexia and right upper quadrant pain. Early impaired consciousness suggests concurrent depressive drug ingestion, e.g. alcohol, opioid analgesic drugs. Liver function tests become abnormal after about 18 h, with prolonged prothrombin time and raised bilirubin at 36–48 h. Hepatotoxicity peaks at about 3–4 days, with hepatic failure if severe. Lactic acidosis, hypoglycaemia and renal failure may also occur. Prognostic factors include the presence of acidaemia (mortality ~95% if pH < 7.3), renal impairment, severe hepatic encephalopathy and a Factor V level < 10% (~90% mortality).

- Treatment:
  - as for poisoning and overdoses. Activated charcoal is given if > 150 mg/kg body weight of paracetamol has been ingested or if the patient presents within 1 h of the overdose. Gastric lavage and ipecacuanha are no longer recommended. Ingestion of opioid/paracetamol combinations (e.g. containing codeine, dextropropoxyphene) should be considered if level of consciousness is depressed on presentation to hospital, and naloxone given.
  - replenishment of hepatic glutathione stores with glutathione precursors:
    - methionine: suitable within 10–12 h of ingestion of paracetamol and if vomiting is not excessive. 2.5 g is given orally, followed by 2.5 g 4 hourly for 12 h. Vomiting is common.

    or
    - *N*-acetylcysteine: traditionally thought to be effective only within 16 h of poisoning, but evidence now supports later administration too. 150 mg/kg is given in 200 ml 5% dextrose iv over 15 min, followed by 50 mg/kg in 500 ml dextrose over 4 h, then 100 mg/kg in 1 litre dextrose over 16 h.
  - liver transplantation may be required (*see Hepatic failure*).

A single measurement of plasma paracetamol concentration taken more than 4 h after ingestion (earlier measurements are unreliable) identifies patients at risk of hepatic damage and thus requiring treatment (Fig. 123). Treatment should be started if the concentration lies above the appropriate 'treatment line' depending on whether the patient is at high risk for toxicity as described above.

Brok J, Buckley N, Gluud C (2006). Cochrane Database Syst Rev; 2: CD003328

Paradoxical pain. Type of chronic pain which does not respond to opioid analgesic drugs in the usual way. Usually associated with cancer pain. Increasing the dose may increase side effects without apparent reduction in pain. Altered drug metabolism has been suggested, e.g. for morphine, production of 6-glucuronide (analgesic) reduced in comparison to 3-glucuronide (antanalgesic), but this has been disputed. Management includes giving the drug by an alternative route, using a different opioid or combination with adjunct drugs such as tricyclic antidepressant drugs.

Paraesthesia. Abnormal positive sensation similar to 'pins and needles', occurring when neural tissue is irritated (e.g. peripheral nerve, spinal cord, sensory cerebral cortex). May be produced accidentally or intentionally during regional anaesthesia. Elicitation of paraesthesia may increase the chances of successful nerve block but also of neurological damage.

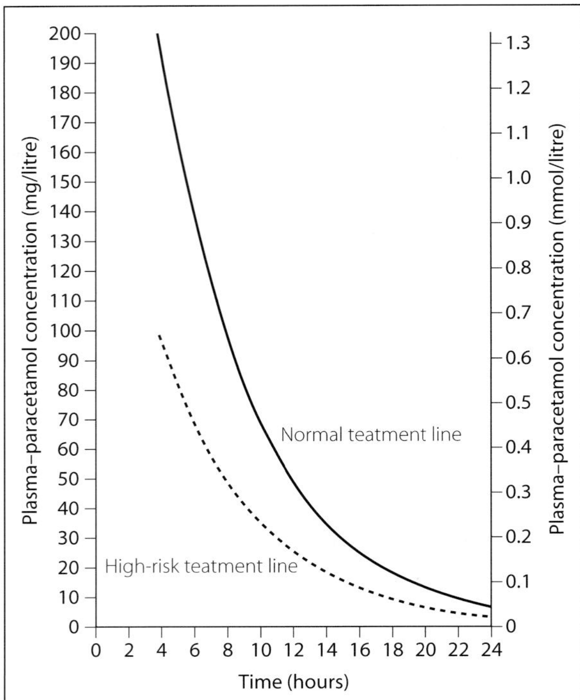

Fig. 123 Treatment lines for normal and high risk patients after paracetamol poisoning

Paraldehyde. Hypnotic and anticonvulsant drug, introduced in 1882. Has an offensive smell, and is irritant and flammable (but not explosive). Decomposes with heat and light to acetic acid, and dissolves plastic. Has been used in the treatment of psychiatric disturbance, status epilepticus and for premedication. Metabolised in the liver; 10–30% is excreted in the breath. Duration of action is about 8 h.

- Dosage: 10–20 ml im or rectally, given with a glass syringe (0.5–6.0 ml in children). Sterile abscesses may occur following im administration. Previously given iv, diluted several times in saline. Cardiovascular depression may occur.

Paralysis, acute. May result in paraplegia (diplegia) with paralysis of the legs and lower part of the trunk or quadriplegia (tetraplegia) with paralysis of all four limbs and trunk. The suffix 'plegia' denotes complete paralysis; 'paresis' denotes partial paralysis. 'Hemiplegia' refers to unilateral paralysis, e.g. associated with CVA and other neurovascular conditions including migraine.

- May be caused by lesions affecting the:
  - cerebrum/brainstem:
    - neoplastic, e.g. frontal lobe or brainstem tumours.
    - vascular, e.g. bilateral carotid or basilar artery thrombosis.
    - demyelinating disease, e.g. multiple sclerosis, central pontine myelinosis.
    - hydrocephalus, cerebral palsy.

- spinal cord:
  - spinal cord injury.
  - neoplastic (primary or metastatic).
  - vascular, e.g. arteriovenous malformations, anterior spinal artery thrombosis, epidural haematoma.
  - inflammatory, e.g. transverse myelitis, multiple sclerosis.
  - infectious, e.g. viral myelitis (e.g. herpes, poliomyelitis, HIV infection), epidural abscess, syphilis, TB.
  - degenerative, e.g. motor neurone disease, bone disease affecting the spinal column.
  - nutritional, e.g. vitamin B_{12} and E deficiency.
  - hereditary, e.g. Friedreich's ataxia.
- peripheral nerve:
  - inflammatory, e.g. Guillain–Barré syndrome, diphtheria.
  - metabolic, e.g. acute intermittent porphyria.
  - poisoning, e.g. heavy metal poisoning.
- neuromuscular junction:
  - poisoning, e.g. botulism, organophosphorus poisoning, aquatic toxins (e.g. tetrodotoxin).
  - bites and stings, e.g. snakes.
  - immunological, e.g. myasthenia gravis, myasthenic syndrome.
- muscle:
  - inflammatory, e.g. polymyositis.
  - congenital, e.g. periodic paralysis.
  - electrolyte imbalance, e.g. hypo/hyperkalaemia, hypercalcaemia, hypermagnesaemia, hypophosphataemia.

Diagnosis is based largely on history and examination. The most common cause of acute paralysis is spinal cord injury caused by fracture dislocation of the cervical spine. Thoracic and lumbar spine damage is less common but may also cause paraplegia. In the absence of trauma, vascular insult to the spinal cord may produce paralysis which may be sudden or may evolve over several hours. This usually follows thrombosis of a spinal segmental artery and results in the anterior spinal artery syndrome. Spinal subarachnoid haemorrhage similarly causes rapid paralysis as will basilar thrombosis causing pontine infarction. Peripheral causes usually produce subacute paralysis with the exception of periodic paralysis (may occur over minutes).

- Anaesthetic/ICU implications:
  - respiratory failure requiring ventilatory support, e.g. IPPV; this may be exacerbated by aspiration of gastric contents if the pharyngeal and laryngeal muscles are affected. Support is likely to be required for a long time since most conditions resolve slowly.
  - control of the airway: suxamethonium may cause severe hyperkalaemia depending on the age of the lesion or whether the process is ongoing. Other alternative methods include use of rapidly acting non-depolarising drugs, e.g. vecuronium, rocuronium; awake intubation, tracheostomy, etc. The latter is often used in the long term.
  - there may also be autonomic disturbance depending on the cause.
  - other features of the primary disease.
  - long-term supportive care includes nutrition and fluid balance, regular turning and prevention of decubitus ulcers, prophylaxis against DVT and nosocomial infection, prompt treatment of infection, and psychological support.

See also, Intubation, awake

Paramagnetic oxygen analysis, *see Oxygen measurement*

Paramedic training. Extended skills training for ambulance personnel in the UK was introduced in certain areas in the early 1970s. In 1984, a national training programme was adopted under the regulation of the NHS Training Directorate. Currently, there are two routes to becoming registered as a paramedic:

- via a Health Professions Council approved Diploma course in Paramedic Science: takes a year of full-time study followed by part-time study for a further 2–3 years while working as an ambulance technician.
- working as an ambulance technician for at least a year then applying for paramedic training (intensive 10–12 week course), leading to an Institute of Health Care Development qualification.

Topics covered include anatomy, physiology, pharmacology, and immediate assessment and management. Trainee paramedics attend local hospitals (including operating departments, coronary care and intensive care units, and emergency departments) and are required to perform a minimum of 25 tracheal intubations and 25 iv cannulations under supervision. Ambulance services underwent major review in 2007–8, with new roles and a preference for the higher education route suggested.

Parametric tests, *see Data; Statistical tests*

Paraplegia, *see Paralysis, acute*

Paraquat poisoning. A common domestic garden weedkiller, paraquat is rapidly absorbed when ingested orally, peak plasma levels occurring in 1–2 h. Can also be absorbed through the skin. Industrial preparations contain 10–20% paraquat; those for home use contain 2.5%. Lethal dose is 3–5 g; mortality is up to 75%.

- Features:
  - corrosive burns to mouth, pharynx and oesophagus.
  - dyspnoea, pulmonary oedema, acute lung injury, rapidly progressive pulmonary fibrosis. Lung damage is exacerbated by high inspired O_2 concentrations.
  - cardiac, hepatic and renal impairment.
- Management:
  - general support as for poisoning and overdoses.
  - oral administration or gastric instillation of an adsorbent such as activated charcoal 100 g followed by 50 g 4 hourly, or fuller's earth 1000 ml 15% aqueous suspension (or 500 ml 30%) 2 hourly, together with 200 ml 20% mannitol or magnesium sulphate as a laxative; administration is repeated until the charcoal or fuller's earth is seen in the stool. Gastric lavage is controversial.
  - haemoperfusion has been advocated but paraquat's large volume of distribution limits its usefulness.

Paraquat concentrations can be measured in the serum or (more easily) in the urine.

Parasympathetic nervous system. Part of the autonomic nervous system. Myelinated preganglionic efferent fibres emerge with cranial nerves III, VII, IX and X, and spinal nerves S2–4. They pass directly to their target organs, where they synapse with short non-myelinated postganglionic fibres (cf. sympathetic nervous system). The vagus nerves carry about 75% of all parasympathetic fibres and innervate the heart, lungs, oesophagus, stomach, other viscera and GIT as far as the splenic flexure. The sacral nerves run directly as the pelvic splanchnic nerves to the pelvic viscera (*see Fig. 20; Autonomic nervous system*). Afferent fibres travel in cranial nerves IX and X and in the sacral nerves.

- Effects of parasympathetic stimulation:
  - pupillary and ciliary muscle contraction, increased lacrimal secretion.
  - bradycardia, reduced velocity of cardiac conduction. Vasodilatation occurs in skeletal muscle, abdominal viscera, and coronary, pulmonary and renal circulations.
  - bronchoconstriction and increased secretions.
  - increased GIT motility, relaxation of sphincters and increased secretions (profuse watery secretion from salivary glands). Increased insulin and glucagon secretion.
  - bladder contraction and relaxation of sphincter.
  - variable effect on the uterus.
  - penile erection.
  - generalised sweating.

Acetylcholine is the neurotransmitter at all synapses. Its actions are divided into nicotinic (at ganglia) and muscarinic (at postganglionic synapses).
See also, Acetylcholine receptors; Muscarine and muscarinic receptors; Nicotine and nicotinic receptors

Parasympathomimetic drugs. Drugs producing the effects of stimulation of the parasympathetic nervous system. Include:
  - drugs which stimulate acetylcholine receptors:
    - acetylcholine: has diffuse actions, therefore not used therapeutically.
    - synthetic choline esters, e.g. carbachol, methacholine: the former has nicotinic and muscarinic actions, the latter mainly muscarinic. Both are resistant to hydrolysis by cholinesterases. Carbachol is used in glaucoma and urinary retention. Bethanechol is a similar drug, and used in urinary retention and as a laxative.
    - cholinomimetic alkaloids, e.g. pilocarpine: used in glaucoma.
  - acetylcholinesterase inhibitors.

Paravertebral nerve block. Used to block the lumbar plexus, e.g. in abdominal or leg surgery. May also be used in the thoracic region. Blocks nerves as they pass through the intervertebral foramina into the paravertebral space; solution may track medially through the foramina into the epidural space, or laterally into the intercostal space.

With the patient in either the lateral or prone position, with a soft pillow between the iliac crest and costal margin, a skin wheal is raised 3–5 cm lateral to the cephalic end of the L1–4 spinous processes. An 8 cm needle is inserted approximately 3–4 cm perpendicular to the skin until the transverse process is encountered, then walked off the cephalad border and advanced a further 1–2 cm. 5 ml local anaesthetic agent is then injected. Must be performed at both sides for bilateral blockade.

A loss-of-resistance technique has been used to confirm correct needle placement, as for epidural anaesthesia. A catheter may be passed into the paravertebral space for prolonged analgesia. Complications include epidural, subarachnoid and iv injection.

Parecoxib. NSAID acting preferentially on cyclo-oxygenase-2, licensed for short-term (< 2 days) treatment of postoperative pain. Onset of action is 7–13 min, with effects lasting up to 12 h. A prodrug of valdecoxib, to which it is rapidly converted (half-life 22 min); valdecoxib itself has a half-life of 8 h.
- Dosage: 40 mg iv/deep im injection followed by 20–40 mg 6–12 hourly up to 80 mg/day.
- Side effects: as for NSAIDs. Hyper- or hypotension, back pain and peripheral oedema may also occur. Valdecoxib has been associated with severe hypersensitivity reactions, especially in patients allergic to sulphonamides.

Parenteral nutrition, *see Nutrition, total parenteral*

Parkinson's disease. Degenerative disorder of the CNS involving the basal ganglia and extrapyramidal motor system, with loss of dopamine in the striatum and substantia nigra. Causes abnormal control of movement, which normally depends on the balance between cholinergic and dopaminergic activity within the basal ganglia. Usually idiopathic, it may follow encephalitis, CVA, heavy metal poisoning, or drugs which antagonise dopamine receptors (e.g. phenothiazines). Affects 3% of the population > 66 years old; the aetiology is in most cases unknown but may include genetic, toxic and environmental factors.
- Features:
  - bradykinesia, rigidity ('lead-pipe' or 'cogwheel'), rest tremor (4–6 Hz). Initiation, speed, strength and precision of movement are impaired. The face is typically expressionless and the gait shuffling.
  - autonomic dysfunction is characterised by salivation, postural hypotension and abnormal control of breathing.
  - a restrictive ventilatory defect may occur.
- Treatment is aimed at restoring the dopaminergic/cholinergic balance, and includes:
  - increasing brain levels of dopamine by administering its precursor levodopa (dopamine itself does not cross the blood–brain barrier). Conversion of levodopa to dopamine outside the CNS with resultant side effects is prevented by concurrent administration of carbidopa or benserazide. These inhibit dopa decarboxylase peripherally, but do not cross into the brain themselves. Bradykinesia and rigidity are improved more than tremor. Side effects include involuntary movements, nausea, vomiting, and psychiatric disturbances. Improvement may be intermittent (on–off effect).
  - anticholinergic drugs: benzatropine, trihexyphenidyl (benzhexol), orphenadrine: improve tremor and rigidity more than bradykinesia.
  - other drugs: bromocriptine, apomorphine and lisuride (dopamine agonists), selegiline (type B monoamine oxidase inhibitor), amantadine, pergolide.
  - stereotactic surgery (especially stimulation of the subthalamic nucleus) may be successful. Fetal tissue implantation has been performed experimentally.
- Anaesthetic considerations:
  - pre-existing restrictive lung disorders and postural hypotension. Excessive salivation and dysphagia may result in tracheal aspiration of secretions.
  - levodopa is continued up to surgery, since its half-life is short. It has been given iv.
  - symptoms may be exacerbated by dopamine antagonists, e.g. phenothiazines and butyrophenones (including antiemetic drugs).
  - the risk of massive hyperkalaemia following suxamethonium is controversial.
  - postoperative sleep apnoea has been reported, especially in the postencephalitic disease.

[James Parkinson (1755–1824), London physician]
Nicholson G, Pereira AC, Hall GM (2002). Br J Anaesth; 89: 904–16

Paroxysmal nocturnal haemoglobinuria. Rare acquired chronic haemolytic anaemia, resulting from blood cell membrane abnormality and increased sensitivity to lysis by complement. Haemoglobinuria is classically noticed on waking.

Platelet destruction may lead to bleeding, or abnormal function may lead to venous thrombosis. Renal impairment is common. Drugs causing complement activation should be avoided, and red blood cells washed before blood transfusion to reduce risk of complement activation. Haemolysis may be precipitated by surgery, infection and cold.

PART team, Patient-at-risk team, *see Outreach team*

Partial liquid ventilation, *see Liquid ventilation*

Partial pressure. Pressure exerted by each component of a gas mixture. For a gas dissolved in a liquid, e.g. blood, the term 'tension' is used, although denoted by the same symbol (P).
See also, Dalton's law; Respiratory symbols

Partial thromboplastin time, *see Coagulation studies*

Partition coefficient. Ratio of the amount of substance in one phase to the amount in another phase at stated temperature, with the two phases being of equal volume and at equilibrium with each other. Depends on the relative solubility of the substance in the two phases. May refer to solids, liquids or gases; when the phases are liquid and gas it equals the Ostwald solubility coefficient. Blood/gas and oil/gas partition coefficients of inhalational anaesthetic agents are related to speed of uptake and potency respectively.

Pascal. SI unit of pressure. 1 pascal (Pa) = 1 N/m^2.
[Blaise Pascal (1623–1662), French physicist]

Pasteur point. Critical mitochondrial Po_2 below which aerobic metabolism cannot occur. Thought to be 0.15–0.3 kPa (1.4–2.3 mmHg).
[Louis Pasteur (1822–1895), French scientist and microbiologist]
See also, Oxygen cascade

Patent ductus arteriosus, *see Ductus arteriosus, patent*

Patient-at-risk team, *see Outreach team*

Patient-controlled analgesia (PCA). Technique whereby small doses of analgesic drugs (usually opioid analgesic drugs) are administered (usually iv but other routes including epidural, sc and intranasal have been used) by patients themselves according to their pain. Widely used for postoperative analgesia. Systems usually consist of sophisticated infusion devices which allow on-demand bolus injections, with or without continuous background infusions. Size and rate of bolus injection may be altered. Inadvertent overdosage is avoided by limiting the size of individual boluses and total dose administered within a set period; the minimal time between boluses can also be preset (lock-out interval). The controls must be inaccessible to the patient (or relatives), and the infusion connected downstream from a non-return valve if attached to another iv infusion (to prevent retrograde flow into the second infusion set with subsequent overdosage when the latter is flushed).

PCA has been shown to provide more consistent plasma drug levels when compared with standard im techniques. The usefulness of background infusions is controversial, the risk of overdosage balanced by possibly improved analgesia. Patients may 'save up' their drug allowance for potentially painful procedures, e.g. physiotherapy. Preoperative explanation of the technique is desirable but not vital.

Drugs with relatively short half-lives are usually employed. Widely varying dosage regimens have been described; individual adjustment is usually required (Table 29). Complications may be related to incorrect programming and setting-up, patients' misunderstanding of the technique, and equipment malfunction. Patients require adequate monitoring, since respiratory depression may still occur. Nausea and vomiting may be a problem if regular antiemetics are not prescribed, firstly because drug levels remain constant, and secondly because the 'as required' antiemetics which would be routinely given along with im opioids tend not to be given if 'as required' opioids themselves are no longer necessary. PCA has also been used (epidural and iv) for analgesia in labour (*see Obstetric analgesia and anaesthesia*).
Grass JA (2005). Anesth Analg; 101 Suppl: S44–61

Table 29 Dosage regimens for different opioids for iv patient-controlled analgesia

Drug	Bolus dose (mg)	Lock-out interval (min)
Diamorphine	0.5–1.5	3–5
Fentanyl	0.02–0.1	3–10
Morphine	0.5–2.0	5–15
Nalbuphine	1–5	5–15
Pethidine	5–20	5–15

PAV, *see Proportional assist ventilation*

PCA, *see Patient-controlled analgesia*

PCV, Packed cell volume, *see Haematocrit*

PCWP, *see Pulmonary capillary wedge pressure*

PDA, Patent ductus arteriosus, *see Ductus arteriosus, patent*

PDPH, *see Post-dural puncture headache*

PE, *see Pulmonary embolism*

PEA, *see Pulseless electrical activity*

Peak expiratory flow rate (PEFR). Maximal rate of air flow during a sudden forced expiration. Most conveniently measured with a peak flowmeter; may also be measured from a flow–volume loop, or with a pneumotachograph. Highly dependent on patient effort. Reduced by obstructive airways disease, e.g. asthma, COPD. Normal values: 450–700 l/min (males), 250–500 l/min (females).

Peak flowmeters. Simple and inexpensive hand-held flowmeters for measuring peak expiratory flow rate (PEFR). The Wright peak flowmeter is a constant pressure, variable orifice device, able to measure peak flow rates of up to 1000 l/min. It has a flat circular body, with a handle and mouthpiece. Exhaled air is directed by a fixed baffle within the body on to a movable vane, which is free to rotate around a central axle against the force of a small spiral spring. There is a circular slot in the base of the chamber, through which expired air escapes to the atmosphere. As the vane moves, the slot is uncovered, thus increasing the effective orifice size. The vane reaches its furthest excursion according to PEFR, and is held there by a ratchet. PEFR is read from a dial on the face of the meter, according to a pointer attached to the vane. It slightly underreads in comparison with a pneumotachograph.

A simpler, cheaper version consists of a cylindrical tube, employing a piston which is blown along its length. As it does so, it uncovers a linear slot along the tube. A ratchet mechanism operates as before. PEFR is read from a scale at the top of the cylinder.
[B Martin Wright (1912–2001), London engineer]

PEEP, *see Positive end-expiratory pressure*

PEFR, *see Peak expiratory flow rate*

PEG, *see Percutaneous endoscopic gastrostomy*

Pelvic trauma. Usually caused by blunt trauma (e.g. road accidents or falls) and often associated with abdominal trauma, chest trauma and head injuries.

- Damage may involve:
  - pelvic ring: disruption causes pain on movement. Diagnosis is confirmed with X-ray or CT scanning.
  - bladder: rupture occurs in 10–15% of pelvic trauma cases. Suggested by lower abdominal peritonism and inability to pass urine. IV urography (or cystography if a urinary catheter is in place) shows extravasation of contrast from the torn bladder wall.
  - urethra: damage is suggested by disruption of the pubis symphysis on X-ray, perineal bruising, blood at the meatus, inability to pass urine and a high-riding prostate on pr examination in males. IV urography should be performed to exclude total disruption.
  - vaginal and bowel perforation from bony fragments.
  - pelvic blood vessels: arteriography may be necessary for diagnosis.
  - pelvic nerves.
- Management:
  - basic resuscitation as for trauma generally.
  - simple pelvic fractures require bed rest only, whereas complicated fractures require early operative fixation. External fixation is now common.
  - intraperitoneal bladder rupture requires laparotomy and drainage of the bladder with both suprapubic and urethral catheters. Extraperitoneal rupture requires drainage via a urethral catheter with subsequent confirmation of healing using cystography. Broad-spectrum antibacterial drugs should be given.
  - urethral injuries generally should be treated by suprapubic catheterisation and drainage; however, if pelvic X-ray shows no disruption of the symphysis and there is no blood at the meatus, a urethral catheter may be passed cautiously.
  - pelvic vessels may require embolisation if haemorrhage is severe.

Pendelluft. Phenomenon originally believed to cause the hypoxaemia occurring in flail chest. The theory suggested that air is drawn from the affected side into the unaffected lung during inspiration, due to the disrupted chest wall integrity on the damaged side. During expiration, air passes from the normal lung back into the affected lung; thus air moves to and fro between the two sides, instead of in and out of the chest via the trachea. Hypoventilation and $\dot{V}/\dot{Q}$ mismatch due to pain, lung contusion and sputum retention are now thought to be more important.
[German: 'oscillating breath']

Penicillamine. Degradation product of penicillin used as a chelating agent especially in copper, lead, gold, mercury and zinc poisoning. Also used in the treatment of rheumatoid arthritis and chronic active hepatitis.

- Dosage: from 125–250 mg/day orally for chronic inflammatory conditions to 1–2 g/day in divided doses for chronic copper overload or lead poisoning.
- Side effects: blood dyscrasias, convulsions, neuropathy, nausea and vomiting, colitis, renal and hepatic impairment, bronchospasm, myasthenia gravis, systemic lupus erythematosus-like syndrome, rashes. Blood counts and urine testing for proteinuria should be performed regularly.

Penicillins. Group of natural and synthetic bactericidal antibacterial drugs with a β-lactam structure. Act by interfering with bacterial cell wall synthesis by binding with various penicillin binding proteins. Penetrate body tissue and fluids well except for the CNS (unless the meninges are inflamed). Excreted renally. Bacterial resistance is caused by production of β-lactamases which hydrolyse the β-lactam ring.

- May be classified into:
  - benzylpenicillin and phenoxymethylpenicillin.
  - penicillinase resistant penicillins: flucloxacillin, temocillin.
  - broad-spectrum penicillins: ampicillin, amoxicillin, co-amoxiclav, co-fluampicil.
  - antipseudomonal penicillins: piperacillin, ticarcillin.

Problems include hypersensitivity (related to the basic penicillin structure – thus all penicillins cross-react; only 7–23% of 'allergic' patients are truly allergic), cerebral irritation (causing encephalopathy) especially in high dosage or renal failure, and excessive administration of sodium or potassium in parenteral preparations.

Penile block. Used to provide peri- and postoperative analgesia for circumcision and other procedures on the penis, especially in children.

The dorsal nerves of the penis (terminal branches of the pudendal nerves, S2–4) travel medial to the ischiopubic rami into the deep perineal pouch, and pierce the perineal membrane to pass to the penis. They may be blocked within a triangular space bounded by the symphysis pubis above, corpora cavernosa below, and superficial fascia anteriorly. The penile vessels lie in the midline. Some innervation of the skin at the base of the penis arises from the genital branch of the genitofemoral nerve.

A needle is introduced at right angles through a skin wheal in front of the symphysis, and passed below its caudal edge. It is inserted up to 3–5 mm deeper than the symphysis (a click may be felt). After careful aspiration, 1–2 ml local anaesthetic agent is injected for children up to 3 years old, 3–5 ml for older children, and 5–10 ml for adults. Adrenaline may cause ischaemia and necrosis and must not be used. Solution diffuses to block both sides following midline injection, but risk of haematoma is greater; therefore the needle may be tilted to each side and solution injected in two halves. 1–5 ml solution is also injected around the base of the penis.
See also, Lumbar plexus; Sacral plexus

Pentamidine isethionate. Antiprotozoal agent used in the treatment and prophylaxis of pneumocystis pneumonia. Because of its side effects, used as a second line drug if infection is resistant to co-trimoxazole. Has also been used to treat leishmaniasis and trypanosomiasis.

- Dosage:
  - pneumocystis treatment: 4 mg/kg/day slowly iv for at least 14 days or 600 mg daily by inhalation of nebulised solution, for 3 weeks.
  - pneumocystis prophylaxis: 300 mg every 4 weeks (or 150 mg every 2 weeks) by nebulised solution.
  - other infections: 3–4 mg/kg iv/im every 1–7 days.

- Side effects: severe, sometimes fatal hypotension, hypoglycaemia and ventricular arrhythmias, pancreatitis, renal failure, blood dyscrasias, bronchospasm, nausea, vomiting.

Pentastarch, *see Hydroxyethyl starch*

Pentazocine hydrochloride/lactate. Agonist–antagonist opioid analgesic drug described in 1962. Benzomorphan derivative, with agonist activity at kappa and sigma opioid receptors, and antagonist activity at mu receptors. Used for moderate to severe pain; has been used to reverse the respiratory depression caused by morphine or fentanyl whilst maintaining analgesia.

Undergoes extensive first-pass metabolism; conjugated with glucuronides and excreted renally. Half-life is about 2–3 h.

- Dosage: 0.5–1.0 mg/kg, iv/im/sc. 50–100 mg orally, 3–4 hourly; up to 50 mg rectally, 6 hourly.
- Side effects:
  - sedation, dizziness.
  - hallucinations and dysphoria, especially in the elderly.
  - sweating, hypertension, tachycardia.
  - precipitation of withdrawal reactions in opioid addicts.

Its side effects have contributed to its unpopularity.
See also, Opioid receptor antagonists

Pentolinium tartrate. Ganglion blocking drug, no longer commercially available. More potent and longer-lasting than hexamethonium. Previously used orally in hypertension, and iv in hypotensive anaesthesia.

Pentoxifylline (Oxpentifylline). Xanthine used in peripheral vascular disease and vascular dementia. Reduces blood viscosity. Also inhibits tumour necrosis factor production by macrophages; has thus been studied as a potential therapeutic agent in sepsis.

- Dosage: peripheral vascular disease: 400 mg orally, 8–12 hourly.
- Side effects: nausea, headache, GIT disturbances, thrombocytopenia.

See also, Cytokines

PEP, Pre-ejection period, *see Systolic time intervals*

Peptic ulcer disease. May occur at any site where peptic acid digestion occurs, e.g. oesophagus, stomach, duodenum. Thought to be due to imbalance between gastric acid digestion and the normal protective mechanisms of the upper GIT mucosa. Abnormal gastric emptying, gastro-oesophageal reflux, drugs (e.g. NSAIDs, corticosteroids), alcohol, psychological and epidemiological factors are thought to contribute. It is now recognised that infection with *Helicobacter pylori* has a fundamental role in the development of chronic gastritis and peptic ulcer disease and the presence and persistence of serum antibodies against the organism reflect the chronicity of the infection. About 70% of patients with gastric ulcers have evidence of *H. pylori* infection which can be detected with the ^{13}C-urea breath test. Infected patients have an increased rate of GIT bleeding in the ICU.

- Treatment:
  - neutralisation of existing acid with antacids.
  - increased surface protection (postulated mechanism):
    - sucralfate.
    - bismuth compounds.
    - carbenoxolone.
  - reduction of acid production:
    - H_2 receptor antagonists.
    - proton pump inhibitors.
    - anticholinergic drugs, e.g. pirenzepine.
    - eradication of *H. pylori* infection. Triple therapy (tetracycline, metronidazole and bismuth subcitrate) is effective in 80% of cases. A 98% cure rate has been claimed if omeprazole is added to the regimen.
  - surgery: indications include failed medical treatment, malignant change, or complications as above. Surgery may involve highly selective vagotomy or vagotomy and drainage procedure (duodenal ulcer), or partial gastrectomy (gastric ulcer).

Anaesthesia in chronic disease requires no special precautions unless gastro-oesophageal reflux or anaemia is present. Acute haemorrhage or perforation may present with vomiting, shock and hypovolaemia.

Percentile. Value which indicates the percent of a distribution equal to or below it; e.g. 97% of measurements are equal or less than the 97th percentile. Often used in charts, e.g. of children's height against age. The 3rd, 50th and 97th percentiles plotted on the chart indicate the heights which include 3%, 50% and 97% of the population respectively, at each age. May thus be used to follow a child's growth, since height would be expected to remain within the same percentile during normal development. The 3rd and 97th percentiles approximate to ± two standard deviations from the mean, for normally distributed data.

Often used to indicate variability (scatter) around the median for ordinal data.

Percutaneous endoscopic gastrostomy (PEG). Technique for establishing enteral nutrition which avoids the discomfort and complications of long-term nasogastric intubation. Useful for patients with neurological dysphagia. After passing a gastroscope into the stomach, the latter is inflated so that its anterior wall makes contact with the anterior abdominal wall. Using the light from the gastroscope, an appropriate site (usually 2 cm below the left costal margin and 2 cm from the midline) is marked on the skin. Under local anaesthesia, a trocar is introduced into the stomach and a thread fed through it into the stomach. This is grasped by the endoscope and pulled out through the mouth; the PEG tube is attached to the thread and pulled through the mouth into the stomach. The PEG is secured to the anterior abdominal wall with a clip.

Percutaneous endoscopic jejunostomy (PEJ). Technique for enteral nutrition, similar to percutaneous endoscopic gastrostomy. Used to administer nutrition and drugs directly to the small bowel.

Percutaneous tracheostomy, *see Tracheostomy, percutaneous*

Percutaneous transluminal coronary angioplasty (PTCA). Non-surgical technique, first described in 1977, for treating ischaemic heart disease by dilating stenosed coronary arteries using a balloon catheter. Most suitable for dilatation of tight proximal stenoses without calcification. Usually performed electively on patients with angina, but it has been performed acutely in unstable angina or following MI if there is a contraindication to fibrinolytic drugs. Patients may be pre-treated with antiplatelet drugs and calcium channel blocking drugs to reduce coronary vasospasm. Considerably cheaper than formal coronary artery bypass graft, with a similar risk of death or MI but with an initial chance of achieving sustained relief from angina of about 60% compared with 90% for surgery. Restenosis may occur in up to 30% of cases within 6 months, and emergency coronary artery surgery may be required if PTCA results in critical ischaemia. PTCA to some vessels has been combined with surgery to others, in an attempt to reduce the risks of surgery in especially high-risk patients.

The basic angioplasty technique has also been used for dilatation of occluded vessels throughout the body. It may be combined with fibrinolytic therapy, microlaser ablation, revolving cutting devices and insertion of rigid stents.

Perfluorocarbons (PFCs). Generally inert organic compounds in which all the hydrogen atoms have been replaced by halogens. Clear liquids, they absorb O_2 and CO_2 to an extent directly proportional to the gas concentration to which they are exposed, and have therefore been investigated as possible artificial blood substitutes. PFCs can dissolve about 20 times as much O_2, and 4 times as much CO_2 as plasma. They have also been investigated as a suitable medium for liquid ventilation, since their high density means they displace exudate from the airways and alveoli whilst their low surface tension is thought to contribute to the increased compliance that results. Also used in eye surgery as a temporary replacement for vitreous humor.

See also, Blood, artificial

Perfusion pressure. Represents the pressure head for blood flow to an organ or tissues. Equals MAP minus mean venous pressure; e.g. cerebral perfusion pressure equals MAP minus ICP.

Peribulbar block. Used in ophthalmic surgery as an alternative to retrobulbar block, since risk of complications (e.g. retrobulbar haemorrhage) is minimal. Facial nerve block is not required. Involves injection of local anaesthetic agent outside the muscle cone.

Several techniques have been described. In one, a needle is inserted through the lid margin between the superior orbital notch and the medial canthus, and directed upwards between the globe and orbital roof. 3–4 ml solution is injected at a depth of 2.0–2.5 cm. The needle is then inserted through the lid margin at the junction of the outer ⅓ and inner ⅔ of the lower orbital rim, and directed downwards between the globe and orbital floor. 4–5 ml solution is injected at a depth of 2.0–2.5 cm. Gentle pressure is applied to the eye for 10 min. Modifications include a more superficial injection (anterior peribulbar block) and the use of a single injection through either the upper or lower lid. A mixture of lidocaine 2% and bupivacaine 0.5–0.75% in equal proportions with or without adrenaline 1: 400 000 is suitable; alternatives include prilocaine 3% or ropivacaine. Hyaluronidase 5 units/ml promotes spread of solution.

See also, Orbital cavity

Pericardiocentesis. Removal of fluid from within the pericardium. Usually performed to relieve acute cardiac tamponade although may also be used for diagnostic purposes. If ultrasonography is available, needle aspiration may be performed from any reasonable area on the chest wall. For blind pericardiocentesis, the subxiphoid approach is most commonly used:

- a long 18–22 G needle attached to a syringe is introduced between the xiphisternum and the left costal margin, and directed towards the left shoulder at 35–40° to the skin. Aspiration is performed as the right ventricle is approached, until pericardial fluid is obtained. A three-way tap is used. Pericardial blood does not clot, whereas intracardiac blood does.
- an ECG chest lead may be attached to the needle; S–T elevation and ventricular ectopics may indicate contact with the ventricle.
- trauma to myocardium and coronary vessels is reduced by inserting a plastic iv cannula over the needle into the pericardial space.

Alternative approaches:

- in the 5th intercostal space just lateral to the left sternal edge (approaches the left ventricle).
- one intercostal space lower, and 1–2 cm lateral to the apex beat, directed towards the right shoulder (approaches the apex).

Pericarditis. Inflammation of the pericardium. May be:

- acute:
  - caused by infections, connective tissue diseases, renal failure, hypothyroidism, MI, trauma, drugs, radiation and tumours. Postviral pericarditis is the most common form.
  - features include sudden central chest pain, worse lying down or on moving, often with fever and tachycardia. Auscultation may reveal a pericardial friction rub. ECG may reveal S–T segment elevation, possibly with T wave inversion later.
  - NSAIDs are often effective in providing analgesia.
  - pericardial fluid may accumulate, with disappearance of the rub. Slow accumulation may cause little cardiovascular disturbance, whereas rapid accumulation may cause cardiac tamponade.
- chronic constrictive:
  - the pericardium becomes fibrous or calcified, and thus rigid.
  - usually follows radiation, chronic renal failure, rheumatoid arthritis, TB, or is idiopathic.
  - resembles cardiac tamponade, with restriction of diastolic cardiac filling. A sharp drop in right atrial pressure ('y' descent) occurs just before right ventricular filling, due to rapid blood flow across the tricuspid valve (cf. tamponade, where atrial pressures remain high throughout diastole). The heart sounds may be quiet, and ECG complexes small. Pericardial calcification may be present on the chest X-ray.
  - management: as for cardiac tamponade. Surgery may be required.

Troughton RW, Asher CR, Klein AL (2004). Lancet; 363: 717–27

Pericardium. Sac enclosing the heart and roots of the great vessels. The outer fibrous pericardium fuses below with the central tendon of the diaphragm, and above and superiorly with the adventitia of the great vessels. The inner serous pericardium has visceral and parietal layers, enclosing the pericardial cavity. The visceral layer covers the heart and is termed the epicardium.

See also, Mediastinum; Pericardiocentesis; Pericarditis

Peridural, *see Epidural.*

Periodic paralysis. Group of diseases, usually inherited as an autosomal dominant trait, characterised by episodic skeletal muscle weakness.

- Classified into different types:
  - hypokalaemic: occurs in young men, often following a large carbohydrate load. May be associated with hyperthyroidism. Thought to be caused by a disorder of ATP

sensitive potassium channels in muscle. May result in respiratory failure. Treatment of acute attacks is with iv or oral potassium; prophylaxis is with acetazolamide.
- hyperkalaemic/normokalaemic: results in mild weakness only, often following exercise. Patients may have an associated myotonic syndrome. Caused by a disorder of sodium channels in skeletal muscle. Acute attacks are treated with iv glucose; prophylaxis is with acetazolamide or thiazide diuretics.

The risk of perioperative muscle weakness and acute changes in plasma potassium levels are the main considerations for anaesthetic management; avoidance of suxamethonium has been suggested but experience is limited. In general, maintenance of normothermia and careful perioperative monitoring have been employed in published cases. No link with MH has been found.

Peripheral neuropathy. Term encompassing any disorder affecting the peripheral nerves (motor and/or sensory).
- Divided into:
  - polyneuropathy: generalised process characterised by widespread and symmetrical degeneration of the:
    - axon, e.g. drugs, metabolic disorders.
    - myelin sheath, e.g. diphtheria, Guillain–Barré syndrome.
    - neurone cell body, e.g. motor neurone disease.
  - focal and multifocal neuropathies: asymmetrical involvement of one or more peripheral nerves, e.g. by ischaemia, trauma (including nerve injury during anaesthesia), vasculitis, infiltration (e.g. by tumour).

Diabetes mellitus is the most common cause of peripheral neuropathy (causing both polyneuropathy and focal neuropathy), followed by carcinoma, vitamin B_1 and B_{12} deficiency (e.g. in alcoholism), and drug therapy (e.g. isoniazid, amiodarone, cimetidine). Other causes include renal failure, hypothyroidism, connective tissue diseases, leprosy, amyloidosis, porphyria and heavy metal poisoning.

Clinical features include weakness and sensory disturbance, usually initially distal in polyneuropathies. Autonomic neuropathy may occur.
- Anaesthetic and ICU considerations:
  - underlying disease.
  - bulbar involvement.
  - autonomic involvement.
  - risk of exaggerated increase in plasma potassium following administration of suxamethonium in motor neuropathy.
  - difficulty weaning from ventilators.

Hughes RAC (2002). Br Med J; 324: 466–9

See also, Critical illness polyneuropathy

Peripheral vascular resistance, *see Systemic vascular resistance*

Peritoneal dialysis (PD). Dialysis technique used primarily in renal failure and less commonly in poisoning and overdose. Following insertion of an intraperitoneal PD catheter through the lower anterior abdominal wall (surgically or percutaneously), prewarmed dialysate fluid is introduced into the peritoneal cavity. The peritoneum acts as a semipermeable membrane between blood and dialysate; the latter is allowed to remain within the cavity for a period ('dwell time') to allow equilibration between the two compartments. The speed and degree of equilibration depends on the frequency and volume of exchanges and dwell time (2 litres dialysate is usually exchanged over 1 h), the permeability and blood supply of the peritoneum and the tonicity of the dialysate (contains sodium, chloride, calcium, magnesium, lactate and a variable amount of glucose and potassium; osmolality is 346–485 mosmol/kg depending on the glucose content, which varies from 1.3 to 4.5%; potassium-free solutions are also available).

Advantages of PD are its simplicity, its non-dependence on vascular access or anticoagulation and lack of haemodynamic instability; disadvantages include its inefficiency and slowness. Complications include pain, bleeding, visceral perforation, peritonitis, hyperglycaemia, hypoproteinaemia and respiratory embarrassment if large volumes of dialysate are used. As with haemodialysis, drugs are removed from the plasma during PD and alterations in dosage may be required. Contraindications include previous abdominal surgery, drains, ileus, adhesions, etc. PD may be performed continuously (e.g. in ICU) to improve its efficacy and reduce respiratory embarrassment.

Peritoneal lavage. Technique for diagnosis of intra-abdominal bleeding following blunt abdominal trauma. Following bladder drainage and decompression of the stomach using a nasogastric tube, a peritoneal lavage catheter is introduced using local anaesthesia into the abdominal cavity, 1–2 cm below the umbilicus in the midline. A Seldinger or cut-down technique may be used. If no fluid is aspirated, 10 ml/kg (up to 1000 ml) of warm saline is introduced into the cavity and then drained by gravity. The resultant aspirate is sent for analysis; the presence of significant numbers of white (> 500/ml) or red cells (> 100 000/ml), or bacteria, indicates the need for diagnostic laparoscopy or laparotomy. Introduction of blood during the procedure itself may lead to a false positive result. Abdominal ultrasound has been used as a less invasive method of diagnosis.

Continuous peritoneal lavage has been used in acute pancreatitis, peritonitis and postoperatively in intra-abdominal sepsis in an attempt to wash away bacteria and toxins.

See also, Paracentesis

Peritonitis. Inflammation or infection of the peritoneum. Infection is usually with bacteria, most commonly involving mixed anaerobic and aerobic organisms although 'spontaneous' (primary) peritonitis is caused by a single species (usually streptococci, pneumococci or haemophilus).
- Caused by:
  - perforation of part of the GIT.
  - penetrating trauma (including postoperative infection from drains, etc.).
  - direct spread from an infected organ, e.g. appendicitis, cholecystitis.
  - haematogenous spread in bacteraemia.

Clinical features include fever (hypothermia in later stages), tachycardia, pain (worse on movement and breathing), guarding and rigidity. Bowel sounds may be sparse or absent, with abdominal distension. Untreated, shock may occur. Diagnosis may be aided by peritoneal aspiration; imaging may reveal an underlying cause. If the diagnosis remains in doubt, exploratory laparotomy may be indicated as for intra-abdominal sepsis.
- Treatment:
  - general resuscitative measures: iv fluids, inotropes, etc., respiratory support.
  - nasogastric tube.
  - broad-spectrum antibacterial drug therapy, e.g. a cephalosporin, metronidazole and aminoglycoside.
  - surgical correction of the underlying cause.
  - peritoneal lavage with or without antibiotics has been used, especially postoperatively.

Complications include MODS, GIT obstruction caused by adhesions, and persistent ileus. TPN may be required. Overall mortality is approximately 10%, although postoperative peritonitis and faecal peritonitis carry mortalities of 50% and 70% respectively.

Permissive hypercapnia. Acceptance of a higher than normal arterial $P\text{CO}_2$ in patients undergoing IPPV, e.g. for respiratory failure especially asthma and acute lung injury. The technique is used when ventilation to a normal $P\text{CO}_2$ might result in detrimental increases in airway pressure and overdistension of alveoli, with consequent adverse effects of barotrauma.
Laffey JG, O'Croinin D, McLoughlin P, Kavanagh BP (2004); Intensive Care Med; 30: 347–56

Peroneal nerve block, *see Ankle, nerve blocks; Knee, nerve blocks*

Perphenazine. Phenothiazine, used as an antiemetic drug and tranquilliser. More potent than chlorpromazine, with fewer side effects. Dystonic reactions are common.

- Dosage: 2–5 mg orally/im, 6–8 hourly (to a maximum of 24 mg).

Persistent vegetative state (PVS). Neurological condition, usually following cerebral trauma or hypoxia, in which the patient appears to be awake with eyes open, but shows no awareness of self or environment. There is an inability to interact with others and there is no evidence of reproducible responses to auditory, tactile or noxious stimuli. The patient is able to breathe spontaneously, and gag, cough and swallowing reflexes are maintained. Sleep–wake cycles are preserved. The vegetative state becomes persistent when it has continued for 1 month; recovery at this stage is possible. If the state continues for 6–12 months the term permanent vegetative state has been applied; recovery at this stage is unlikely. Ethical issues centre around the possible misdiagnosis of the state and whether supportive interventions such as enteral nutrition may be withdrawn if the prognosis is felt to be hopeless. There have been recent reports of temporary 'awakening' of a few patients in PVS following administration of the hypnotic zopiclone.

PET, Pre-eclamptic toxaemia, *see Pre-eclampsia*

PET scanning, *see Positron emission tomography*

Pethick's test, *see Checking of anaesthetic equipment*

Pethidine hydrochloride. Synthetic opioid analgesic drug, developed in Germany in 1939 whilst atropine-like compounds were being investigated. One-tenth as potent as morphine, with duration of action of 2–4 h and half-life of about 3–4 h. Approximately 60% protein-bound in plasma. 5–10% is excreted unchanged in urine, more if the urine is acidic. 90% undergoes hepatic metabolism to norpethidine, an active substance (half-life 20–40 h) which may cause hallucinations and convulsions.

Has similar effects to morphine, but also has local anaesthetic and anticholinergic actions. May cause bronchodilatation, but may also cause histamine release. May relax contracted GIT and urinary smooth muscle. High doses may cause convulsions and myocardial depression.

Indications for use are as for morphine.

- Dosage: 1 mg/kg. Also used in obstetric analgesia and anaesthesia (100–150 mg im, up to 200 mg/patient), and has been given by subarachnoid injection (50–100 mg).

Has been used as a component of the lytic cocktail.

Should be avoided in patients taking monoamine oxidase inhibitors.

PFA-100, *see Coagulation studies*

pH. Negative logarithm to base 10 of hydrogen ion concentration (lower case 'p' being the symbol for $-\log_{10}$); i.e. pH = $-\log\,[\text{H}^+]$. Used as an indication of acidity; the more acid a solution, the lower the pH (Table 30). pH of normal arterial blood is 7.34–7.46, corresponding to $[\text{H}^+]$ of 34–46 nmol/l.
See also, Acid–base balance

pH measurement. Relies on the principle that when different metals are placed in solutions of their own salts, the metallic ions pass into solution to different extents. If two different metal/salt systems are separated by a porous barrier, a potential difference is produced between the two metal electrodes. By using saturated salt solutions, the concentrations of the salts are effectively maintained and the potential difference produced is constant; actual measured potential difference then depends on the presence of other ions, e.g. H^+.

In the pH electrode, a mercury/mercurous chloride/potassium chloride electrode system makes contact with the blood (indirectly via a membrane to avoid contamination with blood) as a reference electrode, with a silver/silver chloride/hydrogen chloride system as the active electrode (via low-conductivity glass, hence 'glass electrode'). In both cases the final chloride solution acts as the bridge or buffer between the electrode itself and the sample. The system is maintained at 37°C; potential output is linear at approximately 60 mV per pH unit.
See also, Blood gas tensions

Phaeochromocytoma. Rare tumour secreting catecholamines developing in chromaffin tissue, usually in the adrenal gland. 6% occur at other sites within the sympathetic nervous system. 10% are bilateral and 10% malignant. May occur as part of multiple endocrine adenomatosis or in association with neurofibromatosis.

Usually presents with headache, psychosis, palpitations, sweating and hypertension (episodic or sustained). Tumours secreting mainly adrenaline cause tachyarrhythmias; those secreting noradrenaline cause vasoconstriction, ischaemia and hypertension. Some tumours secrete both these catecholamines, and also dopamine. Glucose intolerance and cardiomyopathy may occur.

Table 30 Corresponding values for pH and hydrogen ion concentrations

pH units	*[H⁺] (nmol/l)*
6.8	158
6.9	126
7.0	100
7.1	79
7.2	63
7.3	50
7.4	40
7.5	32
7.6	25
7.7	20
7.8	16
7.9	13
8.0	10

- Diagnosis is confirmed by:
  - measuring plasma catecholamines or urinary catecholamine metabolites (e.g. metanephrine, hydroxymethylmandelic acid; HMMA).
  - suppression tests (e.g. using pentolinium, clonidine) with measurement of plasma catecholamines.
  - provocation tests (e.g. using histamine, tyramine or glucagon). Rarely used now, since dangerous hypertension may occur.

Tumours may be located using selective venous catheterisation and catecholamine assays, arteriography (may provoke hypertensive crises), CT scanning, and radioactive *meta*-iodobenzyl guanidine (MIBG) scintigraphy.

- Anaesthetic considerations:
  - preoperatively:
    - preparation includes oral therapy with α-adrenergic receptor antagonists (e.g. traditionally phentolamine or phenoxybenzamine but more recently prazosin up to 12 mg/day or doxazosin 2–8 mg/day). With the older non-selective α-receptor antagonists, β-adrenergic receptor antagonists are administered when α-receptor blockade is complete, but doxazosin has been used without β-receptor antagonists since it does not block presynaptic α_2-receptors and thus is not associated with increased cardiac sympathetic activity unless tumours are predominantly adrenaline secreting. Initiation of β-receptor blockade before α-receptor blockade may exacerbate hypertension because of antagonism of β_2-mediated vasodilatation in muscle. Labetalol and atenolol are often used but others have also been described. α-Methyl-*p*-tyrosine and calcium channel blocking drugs have also been used
    - fluid therapy may be required; this may be aided by central venous cannulation or possibly pulmonary artery catheterisation.
  - perioperatively:
    - drugs causing minimal cardiovascular disturbance are used for anaesthesia.
    - direct arterial BP measurement and CVP with or without pulmonary capillary wedge pressure monitoring are required.
    - catecholamines may be released in response to surgical stress, anaesthetic drugs and handling of the tumour. Sodium nitroprusside, phentolamine, GTN, prazosin, calcium channel blocking drugs and magnesium sulphate have been used to control peroperative hypertension. β-Receptor antagonists or other antiarrhythmic drugs may be used to control tachycardia.
    - following the tumour's removal, iv fluids and occasionally phenylephrine or dopamine may be required to maintain BP.
  - postoperatively:
    - ICU care is required.
    - hypoglycaemia, cardiovascular instability and fluid imbalance may occur.

Rarely, phaeochromocytoma may present for the first time during incidental surgery, pregnancy or labour. Morbidity and mortality are high.

Phantom limb. Sensation of the continued presence of an amputated limb, occurring in up to 80% of patients. More common after arm amputation, and when amputation is delayed after the original injury. May be associated with tingling or usually intermittent pain, which is severe in 15% of cases and usually described as burning or throbbing. The 'limb' may be felt to be in an abnormal position. Thought to be a state of central pain, due to abnormal afferent activity in the interrupted intermediate neurones. Treatment has included phenytoin, carbamazepine, local somatic and sympathetic nerve blocks, injection of trigger points, TENS, dorsal column stimulation and cordotomy. Although spinal anaesthesia has been reported to exacerbate the pain, there have been reports of successful treatment with intrathecal opioids.

Pre-emptive analgesia with epidural anaesthesia has been claimed to prevent the development of phantom limb pain when instituted before surgical amputation but the evidence for this is weak.

Nikolajsen L, Jensen TS (2001). Br J Anaesth; 87: 107–16

Pharmacodynamics. Describes the effects of drugs on the body. Drugs may act by physical interactions (e.g. antacids, general anaesthetics), or by interacting with receptors (receptor theory) or enzymes.

See also, Dose–response curves; Gender differences and anaesthesia; Pharmacogenetics; Pharmacokinetics

Pharmacogenetics. (Pharmacogenomics). Describes the variability of drugs' actions according to the genetic make-up of the individual. Examples include a prolonged action of suxamethonium due to variations of plasma cholinesterase, and variation in metabolism of opioid drugs, benzodiazepines, paracetamol and other NSAIDs due to genetic variation in the cytochrome P_{450} enzyme system. May involve both pharmacodynamic and pharmacokinetic phenomena. Potential applications include the 'tailoring' of drug therapy to individual patients based on their genotype, which could be analysed from a single blood sample. Current obstacles include the incomplete understanding of many drugs' mechanism of action, the involvement of multiple genes in a given response to a drug, and the difficulty in characterising actual patients' responses in terms of their genotypes.

Iohom G, Fitzgerald D, Cunningham AJ (2004). Br J Anaesth; 93: 440–50

See also, Gender differences and anaesthesia; Genetics; Pharmacodynamics; Pharmacokinetics

Pharmacokinetics. Describes the absorption, distribution, metabolism and elimination of drugs, i.e. effects of the body on drugs. These factors determine the concentration of a drug at its effector site, and its temporal effect. Population differences in pharmacokinetic data may arise from general individual variations and genetic factors (*see Pharmacogenetics*).

- Absorption:
  - may be via oral, sublingual, buccal, inhalational, iv, im, sc, rectal or topical routes.
  - rate of absorption determines the intensity and duration of drug action. Most drugs are absorbed by simple diffusion; i.e. rate depends on drug solubility, tissue permeability, surface area of the absorption site, and blood supply to the site of absorption. Permeability depends on the degree of ionisation of the drug, which depends on pH. Some drugs are absorbed by active transport, e.g. L-dopa, α-methyldopa.
  - absorption from the GIT also depends on drug characteristics, gut motility, vomiting, destruction of drug by digestive enzymes, interaction with food or other drugs, GIT disease, and intestinal microflora. First-pass metabolism reduces the bioavailability of many orally administered drugs, e.g. opioid analgesic drugs. Other routes may avoid this.
  - absorption occurs via the lungs for inhalational anaesthetic agents.

- Distribution:
  - related to lipid solubility, pK, body fluid pH, protein binding, regional blood flow, and specific properties of the drug (e.g. iodine taken up by thyroid tissue).
  - protein binding limits both the amount of drug free to cross membranes, and redistribution of drugs from the blood. Volume of distribution and clearance of a drug are inversely proportional to its protein binding.
  - initial redistribution may reduce blood levels of a drug with recovery from its effects, although the total amount in the body has hardly changed, e.g. thiopental and other iv anaesthetic agents.
  - compartment models have been devised to explain the distribution of drugs in the body:
    - one-compartment model: plasma concentration declines as a simple negative exponential process after a bolus injection (first order kinetics; Fig. 124a), i.e.:

$$C_t = C_0 e^{-kt}$$

where C_t = concentration at time t
C_0 = concentration at time zero
k = a constant

A straight line is obtained when the graph is plotted on semilogarithmic paper (Fig. 124b).

$$\text{The slope of the line} = \frac{k}{2.303}$$

$$\text{and half-life} = \frac{0.693}{k}$$

$$\text{Clearance} = k \times \text{volume of distribution}$$

$$= \frac{D}{\text{AUC}}$$

where AUC = area under the plasma concentration/time curve
D = dose of drug at time zero

    - two-compartment model: bi-exponential decline in plasma level; an initial rapid α distribution phase is followed by a slower β elimination phase (Fig. 124c). Each component of the curve may be analysed separately.

      Drug is thought to be distributed from a central compartment (i.e. blood, brain, lungs, etc.) to a peripheral one (e.g. ECF, tissues). The central compartment does not necessarily correspond to an anatomical volume, but is defined in terms of its apparent volume. Elimination occurs from the central compartment.
    - three-compartment distribution: one central and two peripheral compartments are assumed.
- Metabolism:
  - drug activity may be enhanced (e.g. chloral hydrate converted to trichloroethanol), decreased (most drugs) or unaltered (e.g. certain benzodiazepines).
  - usually occurs in two phases in the liver. Phase I involves oxidation, reduction or hydrolysis, often involving the cytochrome P_{450} enzyme system. Phase II reactions involve conjugation with glucuronic acid, glycine, glutamine, sulphate, etc., increasing water solubility. Rate of metabolism may be altered by enzyme induction/inhibition.
  - other sites may be involved, e.g. plasma cholinesterase (suxamethonium), kidney (e.g. dopamine).
- Elimination:
  - may occur via lungs, bile, urine, GIT, saliva or breast milk. Renal excretion depends on GFR, water solubility and extent of active tubular secretion and resorption.
  - most drugs are eliminated by first order kinetics, whereby rate of elimination is proportional to the amount of drug in the body (i.e. simple exponential decay).
  - in zero order kinetics, a constant amount of drug is eliminated per unit time (e.g. alcohol, phenytoin). Zero order kinetics may replace first order kinetics when elimination pathways are saturated, i.e. at high drug concentrations.

These analyses allow prediction of drug kinetics, and calculation of appropriate dosage regimens for achieving desired plasma concentrations. For a continuous drug infusion, 50% of steady-state levels are reached after one half-life, 75% after two half-lives, 87.5% after three, 93.75% after four, 96.875% after five, etc. A loading dose achieves steady-state levels more quickly, but is limited by adverse effects if a large dose is given, depending on the drug's therapeutic ratio/index. In the BET (bolus, elimination, transfer) regimen, a bolus loading dose is followed by an infusion which equals rate of drug elimination, with extra drug infused to allow for transfer between compartments. Alternatively, two or three sequential infusion rates are used. At steady state, the infusion rate equals the rate of elimination of drug for a one-compartment model, or the rate of transfer to a peripheral compartment for a multi-compartment model.

See also, Drug interactions; Gender differences and anaesthesia; Genetics; Michaelis–Menten kinetics

Pharynx. Common upper end of the respiratory and alimentary tracts, extending from the base of the skull to the level of C6.

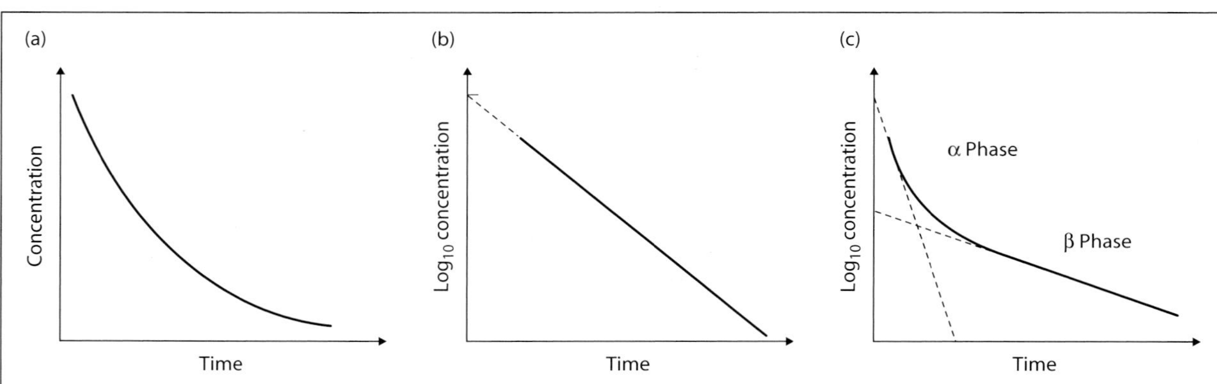

Fig. 124 Drug concentration against time: (a) and (b) one-compartment model; (c) two-compartment model

- Divided into:
  - nasopharynx: lies behind the nasal cavities, above the soft palate. Contains the adenoids, and the Eustachian tube orifice on its side wall.
  - oropharynx: lies behind the mouth and tongue, below the soft palate. Bounded anteriorly by the anterior pillars of the fauces (with buccal cavity anteriorly), superiorly by the palate and inferiorly by the tip of the epiglottis. Contains the tonsils, lying between the anterior and posterior pillars (containing palatoglossus and palatopharyngeus muscles respectively).
  - laryngopharynx: lies behind and around the larynx, extending from the level of the epiglottic tip to the C6 level. The larynx projects into the laryngopharynx, leaving a deep recess (piriform fossa) on each side.

Composed of mucosa (ciliated columnar type in the nasopharynx; stratified or squamous elsewhere), submucosa, muscle layer and loose areolar sheath. The muscles (superior, middle and inferior constrictors) are arranged so that the upper parts of each overlap the lower fibres of the muscle above. They arise thus:
  - superior: from the pterygomandibular raphe, and bony points at either end.
  - middle: from the hyoid bone and stylohyoid ligament.
  - inferior: from the thyroid and cricoid cartilages.

Their anterior borders are open to form the nasal, buccal and laryngeal cavities. Their posterior borders insert into a median raphe along the length of the pharynx.
- Blood supply:
  - arterial: via superior thyroid and ascending pharyngeal branches of the external carotid artery.
  - venous: via pharyngeal plexus to the internal jugular vein.
- Nerve supply: 9th and 10th cranial nerves, with additional nasal innervation via the 5th nerve.

[Bartolomeo Eustachio (1513–1574), Italian physician]
See also, Nose

Phase II block, *see Dual block*

Phase shift. Delay between the arrival of a signal at a monitoring device, e.g. transducer, and the latter's output. Distortion of the signal is minimised by applying the same delay to all components of the waveform, thus maintaining the phase relationship between harmonics. This is achieved by adjusting the damping of the system to about ⅔ critical damping, at which there is a linear relationship between phase lag and the frequency of the wave.

Phenazocine hydrobromide. Synthetic opioid analgesic drug related to morphine, but causing less sedation. Has less effect on sphincter of Oddi tone than other opioids. May be administered sublingually. 5 mg is equivalent to 25 mg morphine.
- Dosage: 5 mg orally, 4–6 hourly; up to 20 mg may be given.

[Ruggero Oddi (1845–1906), Italian physiologist]

Phenobarbital/Phenobarbital sodium (Phenobarbitone). Long-acting barbiturate and anticonvulsant drug, introduced in 1912. Used in all types of epilepsy except absence attacks. Although absorbed slowly after oral administration, it has an has an oral bioavailability of 90% with duration of action up to 16 h. Elimination half-life is about 90 h. 20–45% protein-bound, and 75% metabolised by hepatic microsomal enzymes; 25% is normally excreted unchanged in urine.
- Dosage:
  - 60–180 mg orally once daily (5–8 mg/kg/day in children);
  - 200 mg im 6 hourly.
  - status epilepticus: 15 mg/kg iv at < 50 mg/min
- Side effects include sedation and ataxia. Paradoxical excitement may occur in children.

Hepatic enzyme induction may reduce the effectiveness of other drugs, e.g. warfarin, oral contraceptives, corticosteroids.

Phenol. Neurolytic agent used for nerve blocks in chronic pain management. Thought to spare large myelinated fibres whilst damaging unmyelinated C pain fibres by protein denaturation. Hyperbaric 5% solution in glycerin is used for subarachnoid neurolysis of posterior nerve roots; 0.5–2.0 ml has an effect lasting up to 14 weeks. 6–7% solution in water is used for sympathetic nerve blocks.

Also used for sclerotherapy of haemorrhoids, and as a throat gargle. 1–5% solution (carbolic acid) is also used for disinfection of equipment. Irritant to the skin. Used for antisepsis in surgery by Lister in Glasgow in 1865.
[Joseph Lister (1827–1912), English surgeon]

Phenoperidine hydrochloride. Synthetic opioid analgesic drug related to pethidine, developed in 1957 and discontinued in the UK in 1997. Used during anaesthesia (especially neuroleptanaesthesia and analgesia) and for sedation in ICU. Undesirable features include vasodilatation, hypotension, increased ICP and metabolism to pethidine and norpethidine.

Phenothiazines. Group of drugs used as antipsychotic and sedative drugs. Also have antimuscarinic, antiemetic, antihistamine, antidopaminergic and α-adrenergic receptor antagonist properties. Some may potentiate the effects of opioid analgesic drugs. Different drugs have varying degrees of these properties, depending on the side chains of the molecule. Act mainly on the ascending reticular activating system, limbic system, basal ganglia, hypothalamus and chemoreceptor trigger zone. Cause sedation, with reduced muscular, GIT and cardiovascular activity. Effect on respiration is variable. Central temperature regulatory mechanisms, shivering, and peripheral vasoconstriction are impaired, but metabolic rate is unaffected. Highly lipid soluble and extensively protein-bound. Metabolised in the liver to mostly inactive metabolites.
- Side effects:
  - extrapyramidal symptoms, e.g. tardive dyskinesia, tremor, facial grimacing, etc.
  - drowsiness, insomnia, depression, hypothermia, prevention of shivering.
  - anticholinergic effects, e.g. tachycardia, arrhythmias, dry mouth, urinary retention, blurring of vision.
  - galactorrhoea, menstrual irregularity, gynaecomastia, weight gain.
  - blood dyscrasias, haemolysis.
  - photosensitivity, contact dermatitis, rash.
  - obstructive jaundice.
  - hypotension.
  - neuroleptic malignant syndrome.
  - potentiation of other depressant drugs.

Chlorpromazine is the standard phenothiazine; others include alimemazine (trimeprazine), promethazine, perphenazine, promazine, thioridazine, fluphenazine and trifluoperazine.

Phenoxybenzamine hydrochloride. Irreversible α-adrenergic receptor antagonist, chemically related to the nitrogen mustards; forms covalent bonds with α-adrenergic receptors. Used mainly to control hypertension caused by phaeochromocytoma. More active at α_1-receptors than at α_2-receptors. Onset of action may be up to 1 h after iv injection, due to conversion to an active form. Effects last for several days, although its elimination half-life is about 24 h.

- Dosage:
  - 10 mg orally daily, increased by 10 mg/day as required.
  - 1 mg/kg in 200 ml saline over 2 h, once daily (profound hypotension may occur).
- Side effects: postural hypotension, tachycardia, retrograde ejaculation, nasal congestion, miosis, rarely GIT disturbances.

See also, Vasodilator drugs

Phenoxymethylpenicillin (penicillin V). Natural penicillin used especially in streptococcal infections and in rheumatic fever prophylaxis. Also used for pneumococcal prophylaxis after splenectomy or in sickle cell anaemia. Similar to benzylpenicillin but less active and more acid stable; thus suitable for oral administration following which peak serum levels occur in about 60 min (although somewhat variably, hence the recommendation that it not be used for severe infections). 80% of the drug is protein-bound. Excreted in urine (the dose should be reduced in renal impairment) and faeces. Elimination half-life is 40 min.

- Dosage:
  - 500–1000 mg orally, 6–12 hourly.
  - for prophylaxis, 250 mg (rheumatic fever) or 500 mg (splenectomy, sickle cell) 12 hourly.
- Side effects: as for benzylpenicillin.

Phentolamine mesylate. Non-selective α-adrenergic receptor antagonist, with an additional direct relaxant action on vascular smooth muscle. Used to control hypertensive crises, e.g. caused by phaeochromocytoma, monoamine oxidase inhibitor interactions and clonidine withdrawal, and in hypotensive anaesthesia. An oral preparation is used for the treatment of erectile dysfunction. Previously used for diagnosing phaeochromocytoma and in the assessment of sympathetically mediated pain syndromes. Its place in the management of phaeochromocytoma has now been superseded by prazosin and doxazosin. Acts within 2 min of iv injection, with duration of action 10–15 min.

- Dosage: 2–5 mg iv repeated as required; 0.1–2.0 mg/min by infusion.
- Side effects: postural hypotension, tachycardia, abdominal pain, diarrhoea, nasal congestion.

See also, Vasodilator drugs

Phenylephrine hydrochloride. Directly acting synthetic sympathomimetic drug, used as a vasopressor drug, e.g. in spinal anaesthesia. Has recently become popular in obstetric regional anaesthesia, since it appears more effective than ephedrine, and fetal acid–base profile is better than if large doses of ephedrine are used. Has been administered topically to the nasal mucosa and eye to cause vasoconstriction and mydriasis respectively, and as a vasoconstrictor agent for local anaesthesia. Has also been used to treat SVT. Of similar structure to adrenaline, lacking only the 4-hydroxyl group. Acts at α-adrenergic receptors, causing intense vasoconstriction and compensatory bradycardia.

- Dosage:
  - 2–5 mg im or sc.
  - 100–500 μg iv (5–10 μg/kg in children); 30–180 μg/min by infusion. Boluses of 25–100 μg have been used to treat hypotension in obstetric regional anaesthesia.
  - 2.5–5 mg added to 100 ml local anaesthetic solution.
- Side effects: hypertension, bradycardia, vomiting.

Phenytoin/phenytoin sodium. Hydantoin anticonvulsant drug, introduced in the late 1930s. Used to treat all types of epilepsy except petit mal, in chronic pain management, and previously as a class Ib antiarrhythmic drug (especially for digoxin-induced arrhythmias). Has membrane stabilising effects on all neuronal cells including peripheral nerves and cardiac muscle, thought to involve decreased sodium and calcium flux during depolarisation.

A poorly water-soluble weak acid, with pK_a of about 8.3. Variably absorbed from the GIT, it may cause gastric irritation. Erratically absorbed after im injection, probably due to local precipitation. About 90% protein-bound, and metabolised in the liver to inactive metabolites which are excreted renally. Elimination follows first order kinetics at plasma levels below 10 mg/l; zero order kinetics occur above 10 mg/l, due to saturation of enzyme systems (*see Pharmacokinetics*). Elimination half-life is about 24 h but varies. Susceptible to hepatic enzyme induction, and is itself an enzyme inducer.

- Dosage:
  - 3–4 mg/kg daily as one or two oral doses, increased up to 600 mg/day.
  - for status epilepticus: 15 mg/kg iv slowly, with ECG monitoring, followed by 100 mg 6–8 hourly. Plasma levels should be monitored.
  - for arrhythmias: 3.5–5.0 mg/kg iv slowly, repeated once if required.

  IV administration should be via a large vein at no more than 50 mg/min. Flushing with saline should follow as the solution is strongly alkaline and irritant. Arrhythmias and hypotension may occur.
- Plasma therapeutic range is 10–20 mg/l (40–80 μmol/l).
- Side effects:
  - headache, vomiting, confusion, tremor. Ataxia, nystagmus and blurred vision may indicate overdosage.
  - skin eruptions, lymphadenopathy, hirsutism, fever, hepatitis, gingival hyperplasia. The purple glove syndrome (blue/purple discolouration followed by oedema and necrosis) may occur around the site of iv administration.
  - osteomalacia.
  - rarely, megaloblastic anaemia (due to impaired folate absorption and storage), other blood dyscrasias.
  - fetal abnormalities and neonatal bleeding may follow its use in pregnancy.

  Chronic usage may increase fluoride ion production from enflurane, and cause resistance to non-depolarising neuromuscular blocking drugs.

Available as a prodrug, fosphenytoin.

PHI, *see Prehospital index*

Phlogiston. Imaginary substance proposed in the 1720s, thought to separate from combustible material during burning. Following experiments in the 1770s, Priestley concluded that 'dephlogisticated air' (O_2) and 'dephlogisticated nitrous air' (N_2O) were deficient in phlogiston and could thus support combustion, whereas 'nitrous air' (NO_2) was saturated with it and was unable to do so. The phlogiston theory was subsequently disproved by Lavoisier.

Phonocardiography. Technique employing contact microphones placed on the chest, for amplification and recording of heart sounds. Used to obtain an objective record of heart sounds and heart murmurs. May be performed simultaneously with ECG and arterial waveform recording, allowing

calculation of systolic time intervals. A similar technique is employed in fetal monitoring.
See also, Cardiac cycle

Phosphate. Total body content is about 25 000 mmol, most of which is intracellular. 80% is in bone, 15% is in soft tissues and only 0.1% is in ECF. Most intracellular phosphate is in the organic form. Normal plasma inorganic phosphate levels: 0.8–1.45 mmol/l.

Involved in cell membranes (phospholipids), enzyme regulation, energy storage (ATP), O_2 transport (2,3-DPG) and acid–base buffering.

Levels are controlled by renal excretion; most of the filtered phosphate is reabsorbed in the proximal tubule of the nephron. Excretion is increased by parathyroid hormone, calcitonin, adrenaline and increased phosphate intake. Decreased excretion occurs when intake is low or in response to thyroxine or growth hormone. Hyperphosphataemia causes no specific clinical sequelae but may disturb calcium metabolism. Hypophosphataemia is uncommon but may occur during TPN, ketoacidosis, etc.

Phosphodiesterase inhibitors. Substances which prevent conversion of 3′,5′-adenosine monophosphate (cAMP) to 5′-adenosine monophosphate, or 3′,5′-guanosine monophosphate (cGMP) to 5′-guanosine monophosphate by the enzyme phosphodiesterase (PDE; *see Fig. 5; Adenosine monophosphate, cyclic*). Both cAMP and cGMP are important intracellular messengers. Many isoenzymes of PDE exist:
- PDE I: stimulated by calcium/calmodulin.
- PDE II: stimulated by cGMP.
- PDE III: inhibited by cGMP.
- PDE IV: cAMP specific.
- PDE V: cGMP specific.

PDE inhibitors have antithrombotic, anti-inflammatory, vasodilator, inotropic and bronchodilator properties. Amrinone, milrinone, enoximone, piroximone and pimobendan are examples of PDE III inhibitors. Aminophylline, papaverine and caffeine are non-specific inhibitors and sildenafil and dipyridamole are PDE V inhibitors.

Phrenic nerve pacing. Intermittent electrical stimulation of the phrenic nerves (usually bilaterally), to pace the diaphragm in chronic hypoventilation due to brainstem, medulla or upper cervical cord lesions. Has also been used in COPD. Described in the 1960s, it requires intact phrenic nerves and diaphragm function, thus excluding its use in lower motor neurone lesions and myopathies.

Platinum electrodes are implanted around the nerves in the neck or thorax and connected to a subcutaneous radio receiver, which is triggered by an external power source. Respiratory rate, inspiratory time, sighs, etc., may be adjusted. Neck electrodes risk inadvertent stimulation of the brachial plexus. Nerve trauma at surgery, infection and poor contacts may cause failure. Diaphragmatic fatigue may also occur. Obstructive apnoea may be precipitated in some cases of central alveolar hypoventilation.
Shehu I, Peli E (2008). Eur J Anaesthesiol; 25: 186–91

Phrenic nerves. Originate from the ventral rami of C3–5 on each side, supplying the motor innervation of the diaphragm. Also convey sensory fibres from the diaphragm, hence the shoulder-tip referred pain caused by diaphragmatic irritation. Sensory fibres from the mediastinal pleura, fibrous pericardium and parietal serous pericardium are also conveyed.

Descend vertically on the scalenus anterior muscles, which they cross from lateral to medial sides. Each nerve passes to the root of the neck beneath the sternomastoid muscle, inferior belly of omohyoid, internal jugular vein and (on the left) the thoracic duct. The right phrenic nerve enters the thorax behind the subclavian/internal jugular venous junction, descending subpleurally next to the right brachiocephalic vein, superior and inferior venae cavae and pericardium. Some of its branches pass through the caval foramen of the diaphragm, spreading over its peritoneal surface. The remainder pierce the diaphragm just lateral to the caval orifice. The left nerve enters the thorax between the subclavian artery and vein. It passes superficially to the aortic arch, to pierce the diaphragm anteriorly and to the left of the caval opening. Some of the divisions of each nerve cross to the other side.

Local anaesthetic block has been advocated as a cure for chronic hiccups. 10 ml local anaesthetic agent is injected 1–2 cm deep at a point 2 cm above the sternoclavicular joint and for 5 cm laterally.

Phrenic paralysis may complicate brachial plexus block, trauma, tumour, etc. Paradoxical inward abdominal movement may occur on inspiration, with a raised hemidiaphragm on chest X-ray.
See also, Phrenic nerve pacing

Physician's Assistants (Anaesthesia). Non-medically qualified personnel able to deliver anaesthesia under supervision by a qualified anaesthetist. In the UK, the term is specific to graduates of programmes approved by the Royal College of Anaesthetists, set up as pilots initially in 2003, in response to predicted shortfalls in manpower. The scheme mirrors those introducing other support roles within the NHS, taking on some of the activities and duties traditionally exclusive to qualified doctors. The original term 'Anaesthesia Practitioners' was replaced by the new title in 2008 to bring it into line with Physicians' Assistants in other specialties and to aid understanding of the role.

Physiological and operative severity score for the enumeration of mortality and morbidity (POSSUM). Scoring system described in 1991 as a method of comparing outcome (morbidity and mortality) for operative surgical patients. Patients are scored before operation (using measures of physiological derangement) and at operation (using an operative severity score) to give predictions of morbidity and hospital mortality. Has been shown to be valid for a wide range of surgical procedures.
Prytherch DR, Whiteley MS, Higgins B, et al (1998). Br J Surg; 85: 1217–20

Physiotherapy. Treatment and prevention of disease using passive and active movement, vibration, massage and application of heat. Used for neurological, musculoskeletal and respiratory disorders. Has an important role in the ICU in preventing stiffness of limbs and joints during prolonged immobility, and in helping the patient mobilise during recovery.

Chest physiotherapy aims to maintain clear airways, increase lung expansion and thus reduce atelectasis and sputum retention. It is thought to be most useful when excessive sputum production is present; its place in uncomplicated COPD, chest infection without sputum production, and routine postoperative management has been questioned. It is thought to have little place if disease is mainly peripheral; thus it is most efficient if secretions are within the bronchi. Often beneficial pre- and postoperatively in patients with respiratory disease, helping to optimise respiratory function. It is also valuable in the ICU management of patients with respiratory failure, before, during and after IPPV.

- Techniques include:
  - postural drainage: positioning according to the anatomy of the tracheobronchial tree, with or without breathing exercises, etc.
  - breathing exercises, e.g. incentive spirometry, coughing. Forced expirations may be more effective than cough alone, especially if combined with postural drainage.
  - intermittent lung inflations using ventilators, to increase lung expansion.
  - chest wall percussion and vibration: their efficacy has also been questioned.
  - upper airway suction: usually combined with the above.

Administration of nebulised bronchodilator drugs before physiotherapy may produce a better sputum yield. Nebulised saline, humidified O_2 and mucolytics are also commonly used.

May be painful, especially postoperatively, and may require administration of N_2O/Entonox, ketamine or even opioid analgesic drugs.

Physostigmine salicylate/sulphate. Acetylcholinesterase inhibitor, derived from the West African calibar bean. Causes reversible inhibition of acetylcholinesterase by binding to its esteratic site, lasting 1–2 h. Readily crosses the blood–brain barrier because of its tertiary amine structure. Used to treat the central anticholinergic syndrome, and topically in glaucoma. Formerly used as a general CNS stimulant, e.g. in tricyclic antidepressant drug poisoning and to reverse opioid-induced respiratory depression. No longer available in the UK.

- Dosage: 0.04 mg/kg slowly iv.
- Side effects: nausea, hypertension, tachycardia. Large doses may result in cholinergic crisis.

PiCCO. Commercial non-invasive cardiac output measurement system combining the principles of transpulmonary thermodilution, in which the 'cold' transverses the lungs after injection, and arterial pulse contour analysis. Requires injection of a single bolus injection of cold saline through a central venous catheter and its detection by a specially modified peripheral arterial cannula. Permits rapid estimation of continuous pulse contour cardiac output, intrathoracic blood volume, left ventricular afterload, extravascular lung water and stroke volume variation. Reported to provide cardiac output measurements with an accuracy similar to that obtained from pulmonary artery catheterisation.

Pickwickian syndrome, *see Obesity hypoventilation syndrome*

Pierre Robin syndrome, *see Facial deformities, congenital*

Pin index system. International system introduced in 1952, preventing accidental connection of the wrong gas cylinder to the wrong anaesthetic machine yoke. The cylinder valve block bears holes into which fit pins protruding from the yoke. A flush connection is only achieved if the holes and pins align correctly. The positions of the holes on the valve block (and corresponding pins on the yoke) are specified by an international standard (Fig. 125):

- O_2: positions 2 and 5.
- N_2O: positions 3 and 5.
- air: positions 1 and 5.
- CO_2: positions 1 and 6.
- Entonox: position 7.

The system may be circumvented, e.g. by removing pins, or using several Bodok seals. When piped gas supplies were first introduced, pin-indexed fittings were attached to the pipelines; these could be inserted upside-down into the cylinder yokes, allowing incorrect gas connection. The positions for cyclopropane were 3 and 6.

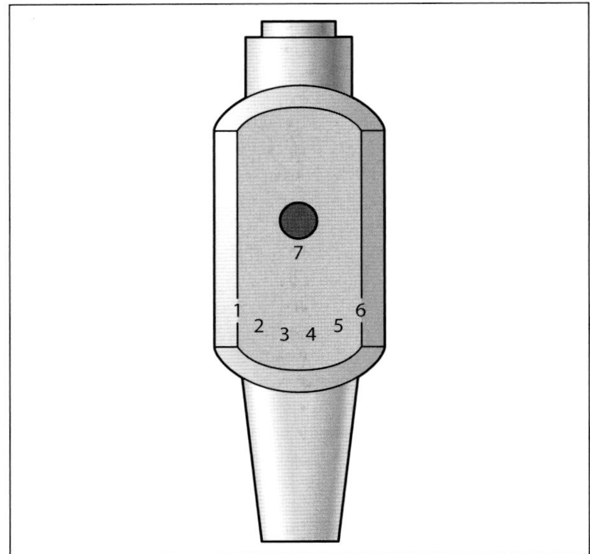

Fig. 125 Position of holes (1–7) in pin index system

Pipecuronium bromide. Non-depolarising neuromuscular blocking drug, synthesised in Hungary in the late 1970s and made available in the USA in 1990. A more potent analogue of pancuronium, which it resembles in its clinical action but with fewer CVS side effects. 40% excreted by the kidneys, it accumulates in renal failure. Reversibly inhibits plasma cholinesterase, and does not release histamine. A 0.07–0.08 mg/kg intubating dose acts within 2.5–3 min, lasting for 1.5–2 h.

Piped gas supply. Networks of pipes and socket outlets that distribute medical gases from a central source to points of use. In the UK, only O_2, N_2O, Entonox, CO_2 (rarely) and compressed air may be distributed by such systems. All are supplied at 4 bar except air which may be required at 7 bar for orthopaedic instruments, etc. Medical vacuum is also supplied by a pipeline system.

- Essential features include:
  - indexing system to prevent cross-connection.
  - prevention of contamination of gases.
  - automatic function, especially when switching over supplies.
  - anticombustion and anti-explosion controls.
- Systems consist of:
  - central gas source: either a large primary source and small reserve supply, or large primary and secondary sources used alternately with a small reserve supply. The primary source may be a manifold of cylinders, vacuum insulated evaporator, air compressor or O_2 concentrator.
  - pipeline distribution network: made of phosphorus deoxidised non-arsenical copper, greased and specially cleaned with steam, shot and medical air. Joints are usually made with a silver alloy although some are threaded. They should be colour-coded and marked with the name of the gas contained. Isolation valves should be supplied.
  - terminal distribution system: includes self-closing sockets, probes, flowmeters, and hoses and their connections with anaesthetic machines. The probes and sockets should be specific for the service supplied, the probe of one gas fitting only the socket for the same gas.

Some probes (e.g. for ward use) may incorporate flowmeters. Connecting hoses to probes should only be possible if specialised equipment is used, reducing the risk of misconnection. Hose connections to anaesthetic machines are made specific for each service by non-interchangeable screw-thread connectors. UK colour coding of hoses:
- N_2O: French blue.
- O_2: white.
- air: black/white.
- Entonox: French blue/white.
- vacuum: yellow.

- system failure alarms: predominantly low pressure alarms, they sound when secondary and reserve systems are in use. Usually situated at hospital telephone switchboards.

Howell RS (1980). Anaesthesia; 35: 676–98

See also, Suction equipment

Piperacillin. Semisynthetic penicillin derivative with broad-spectrum antibacterial activity; especially effective against pseudomonas infections. Often given together with an aminoglycoside in severe pseudomonas infections since the combination results in synergy (but the two drugs should not be mixed in the same syringe). Also available combined with the β-lactamase inhibitor tazobactam. Piperacillin is 20% protein-bound with volume of distribution 15–20 l. Excreted via urine and faeces. Elimination half-life is approximately 1 h.

- Dosage: 100–300 mg/kg iv slowly or by infusion per day, in divided doses (up to 4 g 6 hourly in severe infections).
- Side effects: as for benzylpenicillin. The high sodium content of the preparation (2 mmol/l) may result in hypernatraemia.

Pirbuterol. β-Adrenergic receptor agonist, available for the treatment of asthma but also investigated as an orally active inotropic drug. Active at β_1-adrenergic receptors, with some activity at β_2-receptors. Thus increases cardiac output and causes vasodilatation; BP may fall. Tachycardia is uncommon.

Piritramide. Opioid analgesic drug, developed in 1960 and available in oral and iv forms. 20 mg is equivalent to 15 mg morphine. Of faster onset than morphine, with similar duration of action. Causes less hypotension, nausea and vomiting, but with greater hypnotic effect. Not available in the UK.

Pirogoff, Nicholai Ivanovich (1810–1881). Russian surgeon at St Petersburg, best known for introducing rectal diethyl ether for surgery in 1847. Also studied the effects of ether, designed apparatus for its rectal and inhalational administration, and published a book on the subject in 1847.

Secher O (1986). Anaesthesia; 41: 829–37

Piroxicam. Oxicam NSAID, available for enteral and im use. Rapidly absorbed after oral administration, it is 99% protein-bound and has a long (50 h) half-life; thus can be given once daily. Also available as impregnated wafer-like material which dissolves in the mouth to release the active drug; this method is popular perioperatively because it does not require oral fluids although it is often assumed (erroneously) that the drug is absorbed via the buccal membrane. Since it requires swallowing to make the drug pass into the stomach, the buccal route is not suitable for anaesthetised patients.

- Dosage: 10–20 mg orally, pr or by deep im injection, once/twice daily.
- Side effects: as for NSAIDs, though associated with an increased risk of GIT upset and serious skin reactions compared with most others.

Pituitary gland. Lies in the pituitary fossa of the sphenoid bone, above the sphenoid air sinuses and below the optic chiasma. Composed of anterior and posterior lobes, connected to the hypothalamus by the infundibular stalk which contains nerve fibres and the hyophyseal portal blood system. The infundibulum pierces the diaphragma sellae, a dural sheet, which covers the gland.

- Function:
  - anterior lobe:
    - contains cells formerly classified by their staining properties (chromophobe, eosinophil and acidophil cells); now identified on an immunocytochemical basis into 5 cell types:
      - somatotrophs: secrete growth hormone.
      - lactotrophs: secrete prolactin.
      - corticotrophs: secrete ACTH.
      - thyrotrophs: secrete thyrotrophin.
      - gonadotrophs: secrete luteinising and follicle-stimulating hormones.
    - secretion is controlled by hypothalamic inhibitory or releasing factors, carried to the anterior pituitary by the portal blood system.
  - posterior lobe: secretes vasopressin and oxytocin.

Pituitary gland disease may be associated with over- or under-secretion of hormones (usually the latter). Enlargement may cause visual field defects, optic atrophy and raised ICP.

Smith M, Hirsch NP (2000). Br J Anaesth; 85: 3–14

See also, Acromegaly; Cushing's disease; Diabetes insipidus; Hypopituitarism

p*K*. Negative logarithm (to base 10) of the dissociation constant for a chemical reaction. The law of mass action states that for the reaction $HA \rightleftharpoons H^+ + A^-$:

$$\text{dissociation constant } K_a = \frac{[H^+][A^-]}{[HA]}$$

$$\text{Thus } -\log[H^+] = -\log K_a + \log\frac{[A^-]}{[HA]}$$

Substituting pH for $-\log[H^+]$, and pK_a for $-\log K_a$:

$$pH = pK_a + \log\frac{[A^-]}{[HA]}$$

The p*K* represents the pH value at which the solute is 50% dissociated; i.e. $[A^-] = [HA]$.

Whilst pK_a strictly refers to an acidic substance and pK_b to a basic one, by convention pK_a is used to refer to both acids and bases.

The stronger an acid, the lower its pK_a, and the stronger a base, the higher its pK_a. Thus important when considering ionisation of drugs and passage of drugs or other substances across membranes.

Placenta. Structure dividing the fetal and maternal circulations. Approximately 5–6 days after conception the fertilised egg (now a mass of uniform cells) attaches to the endometrium. The endometrium is invaded by the outer layer of the trophoblast of the egg, the syncytiotrophoblast. Further proliferation of the trophoblast forms finger-shaped masses of tissue, the chorionic villi, between which spaces (lacunae) appear. The tips of the villi erode the walls of the endometrial spiral arteries so that the lacunae expand to form large spaces filled with maternal blood within which float the villi. Primitive blood vessels appear in the villi from about 18 days after fertilisation, eventually joining the fetal umbilical vessels. Densely packed masses of fetal villi (fetal cotyledons) are supplied by branches of the umbilical arteries, distributed radially as end-arteries. Several cotyledons form a single placental lobe. Thus the barrier between fetal and maternal circulations is two cells thick, consisting of the fetal capillary endothelium and its covering of syncytial trophoblast.

- Blood supply:
  - fetal: blood arrives via two umbilical arteries and leaves by a single umbilical vein. Umbilical blood flow is up to 100 ml/min at 22 weeks and 300 ml/min at term, of which about 20% does not participate in exchange with maternal blood.
  - maternal: delivered via the uterine arteries. Uterine blood flow (UBF) at term is 500–700 ml/min, 80% of which passes to the placenta. There is no autoregulation in the placental circulation and therefore flow is directly related to mean uterine perfusion pressure and inversely related to uterine vascular resistance. UBF may be reduced by maternal hypotension, hyperventilation and stress, and by vasopressor drugs.

Placental function is related to its total surface area and UBF. Impaired function causes fetal hypoxaemia and acidosis if acute, and may lead to delayed fetal growth if chronic.

- Functions:
  - gas exchange: O_2 and CO_2 exchange is favoured by fetal haemoglobin and the double Bohr effect respectively.
  - nutrient exchange: all energy substrates, water, minerals, electrolytes, etc. enter the fetus via the placenta by facilitated or active transport.
  - hormonal synthesis and release: hormones include chorionic gonadotrophin, oestrogens, progesterone, prolactin, somatomammotrophin and renin. Several corticosteroid hormones are synthesised by the fetoplacental unit, e.g. placental pregnenolone is metabolised by the fetus before further placental metabolism to form oestrogens.

See also, Fetus, effect of anaesthetic agents on; Obstetric analgesia and anaesthesia; Placenta praevia; Placental abruption

Placenta praevia. Encroachment of the placenta upon the cervical os. Overall risk is about 0.25%, increased if there has been previous Caesarean section (CS), e.g. up to 10% after four previous CS. May coexist with placental abruption in 10% of cases.

- Classified into:
  - grade I: the placenta is low-lying, i.e. within the lower uterine segment; the placenta does not reach the internal os.
  - grade II: the placenta reaches the os.
  - grade III: the placenta covers the whole of the os but most of the placenta is positioned to one side.
  - grade IV: the placenta is placed squarely over the os.
- Problems:
  - may cause antepartum haemorrhage with cardiovascular collapse and fetal distress.
  - requires CS especially in the higher grades since the presenting part will compress the placenta and obstruct blood flow during labour and vaginal delivery. Malpresentation is more common.
  - associated with postpartum haemorrhage since the lower uterine segment is unable to contract as effectively as the upper segment, being less muscular.
  - may be associated with placental invasion (placenta accreta) or even penetration of the uterine wall (placenta percreta); delivery of the placenta may be accompanied by torrential haemorrhage which may require hysterectomy, uterine artery embolisation or iliac artery ligation. Placenta accreta occurs in about 0.04% of all pregnancies, increased to 5–9% in mothers with placenta praevia and up to 40–50% if there have been 2–3 previous CS.
- Anaesthetic management:
  - standard techniques as for obstetric analgesia and anaesthesia.
  - choice of anaesthetic according to standard criteria; in emergency CS general anaesthesia is usually preferred unless the amount of bleeding is small and there is no cardiovascular instability. Traditionally, general anaesthesia has been preferred for elective CS because of the impaired compensatory CVS reflexes during extensive regional block and the difficulty managing an awake patient should severe haemorrhage occur. Recent opinion has shifted to accept regional anaesthesia even in grades III and IV placenta praevia, although many obstetric anaesthetists would prefer general anaesthesia if there has been previous CS.
  - for grades III and IV cases, at least two large bore iv cannulae (plus blood warmer), immediately available cross-matched blood and appropriate senior staff should be ensured. Coagulopathy is uncommon unless massive transfusion is required; thus CS should wait until these facilities and back-up are present.

See also, Placental abruption

Placental abruption. Retroplacental haemorrhage; thought to occur to some degree in up to 4–5% of all pregnancies although only 10–50% of these present clinically. Has been classified into asymptomatic (grade 0); vaginal bleeding without maternal or fetal distress (grade I); fetal distress present (grade II); and fetal and maternal distress (grade III), although this classification is not used as commonly as that for placenta praevia. More common in multiparity; may follow abdominal trauma. May coexist with placenta praevia in 10% of cases.

- Problems:
  - a cause of antepartum haemorrhage; presents with abdominal pain and, usually, fetal distress. The amount of vaginal bleeding (if present) may underestimate the extent of haemorrhage, which may be visible on ultrasound as retroplacental clot.
  - associated with DIC (in up to 10%) and renal cortical necrosis (although renal impairment more often results from acute tubular necrosis caused by hypovolaemia). The extent of DIC may be out of proportion to the amount of bleeding; it may worsen (or develop if not already present) if Caesarean section (CS) is delayed. Thus, urgent CS is required in significant abruption although mild cases may be managed expectantly.
- Anaesthetic management:
  - standard techniques as for obstetric analgesia and anaesthesia.
  - general anaesthesia is usually preferred for CS because of the risk of hypovolaemia and DIC. Coagulation studies are mandatory before regional anaesthesia is performed, if chosen.
  - at least two large bore iv cannulae (plus blood warmer), cross-matched blood and appropriate senior staff should be arranged. Since coagulopathy may worsen unless delivery is achieved, CS should not be delayed.

Plasma. Non-cellular portion of blood; represents the ECF component within the vascular space. A clear, yellowish fluid.

- Normal composition:
  - water.

- proteins:
  - albumin (35–50 g/l).
  - globulins including immunoglobulins (25–35 g/l).
- electrolytes:
  - main cations:
    - sodium (135–145 mmol/l).
    - potassium (3.5–5.5 mmol/l).
    - calcium (2.12–2.65 mmol/l).
    - magnesium (0.75–1.05 mmol/l).
  - main anions:
    - chloride (95–105 mmol/l).
    - bicarbonate (24–33 mmol/l).
    - phosphate (0.8–1.45 mmol/l).
    - lactate (0.6–1.8 mmol/l).
- others, e.g. urea (2.5–7.0 mmol/l), creatinine (60–130 μmol/l), fats, carbohydrates, e.g. glucose (4.0–6.0 mmol/l), amino acids, enzymes, vitamins, hormones, bilirubin.

Osmolality is 280–305 mosmol/kg.

Plasma clots on standing; the supernatant solution is termed serum. Plasma volume is about 3.5 litres in adults (5% of body weight), and measured by dye dilution techniques, using dyes or radioactive markers.

Available for transfusion as fresh frozen plasma.

See also, Blood products; Coagulation

Plasma exchange, *see Plasmapheresis*

Plasma expanders. IV fluids which increase plasma volume by an amount greater than that infused, because of indrawing of water from the extracellular and intracellular spaces by osmosis. The term is usually reserved for colloids, although hypertonic iv solutions act as short-term plasma expanders.

Plasma, fresh frozen, *see Blood products*

Plasma substitutes, *see Colloids*

Plasmapheresis. Selective removal of small volumes (up to 600 ml) of plasma from the body. Replacement with iv fluids is not required. Removal of larger volumes with fluid replacement is termed plasma exchange. Used to remove plasma constituents associated with disease, e.g. antibodies, antigens, immune complexes, drugs, etc. Rate of removal must exceed that of renewal. Not always beneficial, and usually reserved for disease resistant to conventional therapy.

- Often beneficial in:
  - myasthenia gravis and myasthenic syndrome.
  - Guillain–Barré syndrome and other demyelinating neuropathies.
  - multiple myeloma.
  - Goodpasture's syndrome.
  - thrombotic thrombocytopenic purpura.
  - poisoning with mushrooms and digoxin.
- May be beneficial in:
  - bullous pemphigoid.
  - rhesus haemolytic disease.
  - SLE.
  - rheumatoid arthritis.
  - multiple sclerosis

Requires extracorporeal centrifugation or filtration. Removal of over 1000 ml requires replacement with albumin to prevent a fall in plasma oncotic pressure. Partial substitution with colloids or crystalloids is often used. A single volume exchange (40 ml/kg) reduces plasma components by 50–60%, usually lasting 24–48 h. Usually, 1.5 plasma volumes are exchanged during each session, repeated every 1–2 days according to clinical response.

Practical considerations and complications are as for extracorporeal circulation and iv fluid administration.

Plasmin and plasminogen, *see Fibrinolysis*

Plastic surgery. Anaesthetic considerations:
- related to the reason for surgery, e.g. burns, trauma, facial deformities, etc. (*see Ear, nose and throat surgery*).
- possible requirement for hypotensive anaesthesia.
- problems of prolonged surgery, e.g. heat loss, blood loss, positioning of the patient.
- skin grafts may be taken from trunk or limbs, reducing sites of access to the patient.
- regional techniques may be useful for graft donor sites, e.g. femoral nerve block, lateral cutaneous nerve of the thigh block.
- a low haematocrit is thought to improve perfusion and healing of grafts. Dextran solutions may be used to improve perfusion of grafted areas.
- tourniquets may be required.

Platelet activating factor (PAF). Phospholipid autocoid produced by platelets, polymorphonuclear leucocytes and other blood cells. Thought to be a major mediator (along with cytokines) in sepsis. Natural and synthetic PAF antagonists have been investigated as possible treatment for sepsis, with mixed results. PAF has also been shown to modulate CNS activity, e.g. neuronal differentiation, and increased levels are associated with neuronal injury.

Platelet function analysers, *see Coagulation studies*

Platelets. Non-nucleated, smooth, disc-shaped blood cells derived from cytoplasmic fragments of megakaryocytes (bone marrow stem cells). Maturation of megakaryocytes, and thus platelet production, is controlled by a feedback mechanism involving the humoral agent thrombopoietin. Measure 2–4 μm in diameter and 5–8 fl in volume, with a circulatory life span of 8–14 days. Normal adult count is $150–400 \times 10^9$/l blood; 10–20% of the total platelet population lies within the spleen. Platelet deficiency and excess are termed thrombocytopenia and thrombocytosis respectively.

Essential for normal coagulation, spontaneous haemorrhage occurring at counts below $20–30 \times 10^9$/l. Cytoplasmic granules within platelets contain many substances including ATP, ADP, 5-HT, adrenaline, calcium, fibronectin, fibrinogen, β-thromboglobulin and thrombospondin, which contribute to platelet aggregation, blood coagulation, local vasoconstriction, chemotaxis and vessel repair. Also present is an enzyme, thromboxane synthetase, which is activated when platelets contact damaged vascular endothelium. Release of thromboxane stimulates platelet aggregation via increased ADP levels, the ADP binding to specific receptors and activating the glycoprotein IIb/IIIa complex (at which fibrinogen, von Willebrand factor and adhesive proteins bind). Aggregation leads to further ADP release and release of the other substances, eventually resulting in formation of a plug. During this process, the platelets become more spherical and extend pseudopodia. Conversely, prostacyclin, present in the vascular endothelium, stimulates production of platelet cAMP and reduces release of ADP, inhibiting aggregation. Thus a fine balance exists between the two processes.

Apart from coagulation disorders arising from abnormal platelet numbers, prolonged bleeding may arise from abnormal function despite apparently normal counts, e.g. renal failure, hepatic failure, pre-eclampsia, and use of antiplatelet drugs. Platelet function may be assessed using the bleeding time.

George JN (2000). Lancet; 355: 1531–9
See also, Coagulation studies; Platelet activating factor

Plethysmography. Recording of volume changes of an organ, part of the body or the whole body.

- Clinical applications:
  - body plethysmograph.
  - photoelectric plethysmography, used for arterial BP measurement (Finapres device).
  - impedance plethysmography.
  - measuring limb blood flow:
    - recording pressure changes in a circumferential cuff or strain gauges.
    - inflating a proximal cuff to between venous and arterial pressures, and recording volume changes by immersing the limb in water.

Pleura. Double-layered sac enclosing the lungs. The outer parietal layer attaches to the diaphragm, mediastinum and chest wall. The inner visceral layer is closely applied to the lung surface and enters its fissures. The layers meet at the lung hila. They are held together by the negative intrapleural pressure within the pleural cavity which normally contains a small amount of serous fluid.

- Surface markings:
  - apex: 3.5 cm above the clavicular midpoint.
  - medial border: passes behind the sternoclavicular joint, meeting the opposite pleura level with the 2nd costal cartilage. Descends to the costoxiphoid angle on the right; deflects laterally to the lateral sternal edge on the left.
  - inferior border: lies level with the 8th rib in the midclavicular line, 10th rib in the midaxillary line, and passes up to the spine of T12 posteriorly.

Pleural effusion. Serous fluid between the parietal and visceral layers of pleura (interpleural pus and blood are called empyema and haemothorax, respectively). May be unilateral or bilateral. Divided according to the protein content into:

- transudates (< 30 g/l), e.g. cardiac failure, hypoproteinaemia.
- exudates (> 30 g/l), e.g. tumours, inflammatory disease (e.g. connective tissue diseases), infection (e.g. TB), PE, abdominal disease (e.g. subphrenic abscess, pancreatitis, ovarian carcinoma).

Features include dyspnoea, usually related to the size of the effusion. Chest wall movement and breath sounds are reduced over the effusion, with percussion typically 'stony dull'. Large unilateral effusions may displace the mediastinum (and thus the trachea) towards the opposite side. Confirmed by chest X-ray; examination of the fluid aids diagnosis.

Treatment includes chest drainage and is otherwise directed towards the cause.

Large pleural effusions may hinder lung expansion and should be drained preoperatively. Other anaesthetic considerations are related to the underlying cause.

Pneumatics, *see Fluidics*

Pneumocystis pneumonia (PCP). Chest infection caused by the fungus *Pneumocystis jiroveci* (formerly *P. carinii*), particularly common in patients with immunodeficiency associated with HIV infection or organ transplantation. The organism produces an acute interstitial pneumonitis which is rapidly followed by pulmonary fibrosis and impaired pulmonary diffusion and decreased lung compliance. Features include hypoxaemia, dyspnoea and dry cough. Often, patients have an associated picture of systemic sepsis. The chest X-ray typically shows subtle diffuse interstitial shadowing, but may be normal or occasionally grossly abnormal. The diagnosis is confirmed by obtaining specimens, in most cases by using bronchopulmonary lavage. The incidence has decreased recently with more effective prophylaxis and treatment with co-trimoxazole and pentamidine. Corticosteroids have also been used.
Thomas CR Jr, Limper AH (2004). N Engl J Med; 350: 2487–98

Pneumonia, *see Chest infection*

Pneumonitis. Inflammation of the lung caused by physical or chemical agents, e.g. inhalation of toxic or irritant substances and fumes, radiation, etc. Clinical features vary from slight dyspnoea to those of ARDS. Inflammation caused by infection is termed pneumonia; that caused by an allergic reaction is termed alveolitis.
See also, Aspiration pneumonitis

Pneumotachograph. Constant orifice, variable pressure flowmeter, used widely in anaesthetic and respiratory research. Senses the pressure difference across a fixed resistance using pressure transducers; using the Hagen–Poiseuille equation, if flow is laminar, the pressure difference is proportional to flow. In the Fleisch pneumotachograph, the resistance is produced by an array of tubes 1–2 mm in diameter, the number of tubes being matched for the desired flow range. Enclosing the resistor within an electrical coil prevents condensation when moist gases are used. In other devices, the resistance consists of a layer of metal or plastic gauze, the latter less likely to cause condensation.

The instrument head should be appropriately sized to avoid turbulence, and the gas flow spread evenly over the resistance unit. The pressure gradient depends not only on the gas flow but also on its composition, viscosity and temperature; thus difficulties may arise if gas composition varies throughout breaths.
[Alfred Fleisch (1892–1973), Swiss physiologist]

Pneumothorax. Free gas, usually air, within the pleural cavity.

- Has been classified as:
  - simple: the gas is not under tension. May be:
    - open: continuing communication between the source of the gas and the pleural cavity. Intrapleural and atmospheric pressures are equal and lung expansion is poor, causing marked hypoxaemia. Pendelluft may occur. Mediastinal shift may occur in phase with respiration, causing cardiovascular collapse. Gas exchange may improve with IPPV, which increases expansion of the collapsed lung (but tension pneumothorax may develop if gas is forced into the pleural cavity and unable to return).
    - closed: no continuing communication with the gas source; lung collapse is proportional to the volume of gas introduced into the pleural cavity, usually via the bronchi. Gas exchange is unaltered by IPPV, if there is no risk of further gas leakage.
  - tension: gas flow into the pleural cavity is unidirectional and a 'valve' mechanism prevents its escape. The pressure within the pleural cavity increases, with worsening pulmonary collapse, hypoxaemia, hypercapnia, mediastinal shift and obstruction to venous return. Tension is increased by IPPV.

- May occur by three mechanisms:
  - intrapulmonary rupture: retrograde perivascular dissection of gas towards the lung hilum, which may result in mediastinal emphysema. May follow use of high inflation pressures during IPPV, or severe cough or Valsalva manoeuvre. May also occur spontaneously if the alveolar septum is weakened by infection or chronic lung disease.
  - injury to the visceral pleura: air escapes through the hole into the pleural cavity; the lung collapses and the hole may seal or act as a valve. Causes include spontaneous rupture of an emphysematous bulla, fractured ribs, regional anaesthetic techniques or central venous cannulation, tracheostomy and lung biopsy.
  - injury to the parietal pleura: gas enters from the atmosphere (e.g. open chest wound, during central venous cannulation, etc.) or from adjoining structures:
    - peritoneal cavity: gas passes upwards through the retroperitoneal tissue and ruptures through the mediastinal parietal pleura, or passes through defects in the diaphragm.
    - mediastinum: gas ruptures through the pleura as above; it may arise following oesophageal perforation and procedures such as tracheostomy and thyroidectomy.
- Features:
  - range from mild dyspnoea and chest pain to respiratory distress. If the pneumothorax is very large or under tension, severe hypoxaemia and cardiovascular collapse may occur.
  - clinical signs may be absent in small pneumothoraces, but there may be subcutaneous emphysema and ispilateral reduction of chest wall movement and breath sounds, and increased resonance to percussion. There may be audible wheezing, or a 'crunch' caused by air in the mediastinum (Hamman's sign). Inflation pressures may rise during anaesthesia with IPPV.
  - erect chest X-ray in expiration may reveal absent lung markings beyond the edge of the collapsed lung, with the characteristic lung edge usually visible. Diagnosis may be difficult from a supine film. Pleural gas under tension causes marked lung collapse, hyperexpansion of the ipsilateral lung and mediastinal shift.

Treatment depends on the size of the pneumothorax; small ones often resolve spontaneously. If symptomatic, or if IPPV is planned, chest drainage should be performed. A tension pneumothorax may be life-threatening and requires urgent relief, e.g. with a needle or iv cannula. N_2O, being more soluble than atmospheric nitrogen, may rapidly expand a pneumothorax (by 100% in 10 min at inspired concentration of 70%); it should therefore not be used unless a chest drain has been placed.

[Louis Hamman (1877–1946), US physician]

See also, Chest trauma; Flail chest

Poise. Unit of viscosity in the cgs system of units. 1 P = 1 dyne s/cm^2.

[Jean Poiseuille (1797–1869), French physiologist]

Poiseuille's equation, *see Hagen–Poiseuille equation*

Poisoning and overdoses. May be deliberate, or may follow accidental exposure or ingestion. Substances responsible include those found in the home, industrial or agricultural chemicals, plant or animal toxins, and therapeutic drugs.

- Principles of management:
  - removal of the patient from the source of the toxic substance, e.g. from scene of a fire, chemical spillage, etc. Medical staff should be adequately protected, since absorption through skin and lungs may occur.
  - CPR and standard management of the unconscious patient, including monitoring.
  - blood analysis for drug, glucose and electrolyte levels, specific organ function tests, etc.
  - prevention of further absorption of ingested substances, e.g. using activated charcoal, gastric lavage, emetic drugs. Whole bowel irrigation has also been used.
  - specific antidotes and treatments, e.g. naloxone, flumazenil, chelating agents, digoxin antibody fragments, thiosulphate in cyanide poisoning.
  - increasing elimination of ingested substances, e.g. forced diuresis, haemoperfusion, dialysis, activated charcoal.

Common problems include respiratory depression, hypotension, arrhythmias, coma, convulsions and disturbances of temperature regulation. Pulmonary oedema, ARDS, hepatic failure and renal failure may also occur.

Regional or national poisons units provide information and advice.

Zimmerman JL (2003). Crit Care Med; 31: 2794–801

See also, Alcohol poisoning; Barbiturate poisoning; Carbon monoxide poisoning; Chemical weapons; Opioid poisoning; Organophosphorus poisoning; Paracetamol poisoning; Salicylate poisoning; Smoke inhalation; Tricyclic antidepressant drug poisoning

Polarographic oxygen analysis, *see Oxygen measurement*

Poliomyelitis. Disease caused by one of three small RNA enteroviruses transmitted by the respiratory or faeco-oral routes. Now uncommon in the West following successful immunisation programmes. Following 7–14 days incubation period, an acute febrile illness occurs, with upper respiratory or GIT symptoms lasting a few days. Over 90% of cases of infection are subclinical. Pyrexia may recur with features of acute viral meningitis. Asymmetrical lower motor neurone weakness develops in 1% of cases of infection, caused by destruction of the anterior horn cells of the spinal cord and cranial nerve nuclei. Ventilatory support is required during the acute illness in approximately 30% of cases, because of intercostal or diaphragmatic involvement. Bulbar involvement may impair swallowing, cough reflexes and vocal cord function. Rarely, medullary involvement may cause cardiovascular instability or sleep apnoea.

Most patients have residual disability, but improvement may continue for up to 2 years after the acute episode. Progressive weakness may occur 20–30 years later (postpolio syndrome). 10–30% of those requiring ventilatory support acutely require long-term support.

Lambert DA, Giannouli E, Schmidt BJ (2005). Anesthesiology; 103: 638–44

Pollution. Traditionally, most attention has been paid to the effects of inhalational anaesthetic agents on the wellbeing of nearby staff, e.g. in the operating theatre. More recently the contribution of anaesthetic agents to atmospheric ozone depletion and global warming has been a concern. N_2O is degraded in the atmosphere by ultraviolet light to form radicals which damage the ozone layer; it is also a 'greenhouse gas'. Anaesthetic use has been estimated to contribute 10% of all N_2O emissions, in turn accounting for 10% of all atmospheric chemical pollutants – though this figure has been disputed. Volatile agents such as halothane, enflurane and isoflurane also deplete atmospheric ozone. Recent international agreements on reduction of atmospheric pollutants

have included agents such as these, leading to renewed interest in alternative anaesthetic agents such as xenon.
See also, COSHH regulations; Environmental safety of anaesthetists; Scavenging

Polyarteritis nodosa. Connective tissue disease characterised by a necrotising arteritis affecting small and medium sized arteries which causes aneurysm formation, haemorrhage and infarction in major organs. Incidence peaks at 40–50 years, with men affected twice as commonly as women.

- Features:
  - malaise, fever, weight loss, myalgia.
  - arthralgia, rash, peripheral neuropathy. Myasthenic syndrome may occur rarely.
  - GIT involvement including haemorrhage, pancreatitis, intestinal and gallbladder infarction.
  - renal impairment (may be part of a triad of haematuria, haemoptysis and asthma); includes nephritic syndrome or nephrotic syndrome.
  - CVS involvement: hypertension, ischaemic heart disease, cardiac failure, pericarditis.
  - CNS involvement: cerebral ischaemia, blindness, subarachnoid haemorrhage, encephalopathy, seizures.
- Anaesthetic considerations include any pre-existing organ damage as described above, plus possible drug therapy which may include corticosteroids and immunosuppressive drugs.

See also, Vasculitides

Polycythaemia. General term for a haemoglobin concentration above 16–17 g/dl, red cell count above 5.6–6.4 × 10^{12}/l, or haematocrit above 0.47–0.54 (all values female–male respectively).

- May be:
  - relative (reduced plasma volume, e.g. burns, dehydration).
  - absolute (increased red cell volume):
    - primary (polycythaemia rubra vera, PRV): myeloproliferative disorder, occurring mainly in men over 50 years. Features are caused mainly by hypervolaemia and hyperviscosity (headaches, plethora, pruritus, dyspnoea, visual disturbances, reduced cardiac output, thrombotic and haemorrhagic episodes) and a high metabolic rate (night sweats, weight loss). Hepatosplenomegaly may occur. White cell and platelet counts may also be increased; platelet function may be abnormal.

      The main perioperative risks are haemorrhage (caused by abnormal platelets) and thrombosis. Elective surgery should be delayed to allow treatment; emergency surgery should proceed only after venesection and volume replacement. Treatment is directed at keeping the haematocrit below 0.5, usually with repeated venesection, radioactive phosphorus or myelosuppressive drugs (busulfan). PRV progresses to myelosclerosis in 20–30% of cases.
    - secondary to raised erythropoietin levels, e.g. in response to chronic hypoxaemia (e.g. pulmonary disease, cyanotic heart disease, high altitude) or inappropriate secretion (e.g. renal carcinoma, hepatocellular carcinoma, haemangioblastoma). Risks are related to increased blood viscosity and thrombosis as above.

Polymyositis. Group of idiopathic autoimmune inflammatory diseases including dermatomyositis, affecting muscle and skin. May involve multiple systems. Usually presents with myalgia, muscle tenderness and weakness (mainly proximal). Bulbar weakness may lead to dysphagia, dysphonia and regurgitation. Intercostal and diaphragmatic weakness may result in respiratory failure, exacerbated by interstitial pneumonitis which is also a feature of the disease. Cardiac manifestations include arrhythmias, conduction defects, myocarditis and cardiomyopathy. In dermatomyositis, there is a characteristic erythematous rash of the face and neck. Malignancy is common, especially in older men.

Creatine kinase is raised; muscle biopsy is confirmatory. Treatment includes corticosteroids and other immunosuppressive drugs.

An abnormal sensitivity to neuromuscular blocking drugs has been suggested but is unproven.

Polymyxins. Group of antibacterial drugs which include polymyxin E (colistin) which is active against Gram-negative organisms including pseudomonas and polymyxin B which is used in otitis externa. May enhance the action of non-depolarising neuromuscular blocking drugs via their postsynaptic blocking action at the neuromuscular junction.

Polyneuropathy, acute post-infective, *see Guillain–Barré syndrome*

Polyneuropathy of critical illness, *see Critical illness polyneuropathy*

Polystyrene sulphonate resins. Ion exchange resins used to treat mild or moderate hyperkalaemia. Available as calcium (calcium resonium) or sodium (resonium A) preparations. Given orally, they remain in the GIT without renal or hepatic excretion. Decrease in plasma potassium occurs 2–24 h after administration. Electrolytes must be monitored closely during therapy. Contraindicated in hyperparathyroidism, multiple myeloma, sarcoidosis, metastatic bone disease (calcium resins) and cardiac failure (sodium resins).

- Dosage:
  - 15 g 6–8 hourly orally; 30 g rectally retained for 9 h.
  - 0.5–1.0 g/kg/day in children.
- Side effects: cardiac failure, headaches, encephalopathy, metabolic alkalosis, fluid retention, nausea, vomiting, constipation, colonic necrosis, GIT obstruction.

Popliteal fossa. Diamond-shaped space behind the knee joint, bounded inferiorly by the two heads of gastrocnemius muscle and superiorly by biceps femoris (laterally) and semimembranosus/semitendinosus muscles (medially).

- Contents (medially to laterally):
  - popliteal artery: continues from the femoral artery, and divides into anterior and posterior tibial arteries at or below the lower part of the fossa. The popliteal vein lies superficially.
  - tibial nerve: arises from the sciatic nerve, usually at the upper pole of the fossa. Lies superficial to the popliteal vessels. The common peroneal nerve passes laterally around the fibular head, lateral to the fossa.
  - fat pad.

See also, Knee, nerve blocks

Pop-off valve, *see Adjustable pressure-limiting valve*

Populations. In statistics, any group of similar objects, events or observations. Usually contains too many individuals to be studied as a whole, thus samples are studied and any conclusions drawn are applied to the whole population. A population may be described by its:

- shape, i.e. statistical distribution curve, e.g. normal, binomial.
- central tendency, e.g. mean, median, mode.
- scatter, e.g. standard deviation, percentiles.

Porphyria. Group of diseases characterised by overproduction and excretion of porphyrins (intermediate compounds produced during haemoprotein synthesis) and their precursors. Caused by specific enzyme defects within the haem metabolic pathway. Several forms exist, divided into hepatic and erythropoietic varieties. Only three forms, all of them hepatic varieties transmitted by autosomal dominant inheritance, affect the conduct of anaesthesia:

- acute intermittent porphyria (AIP): results in increased amounts of urinary porphobilinogen and δ-aminolaevulinic acid (D-ALA) during attacks. May present with acute abdominal pain, vomiting, acid–base disturbances, motor and sensory peripheral neuropathy, autonomic dysfunction, cranial nerve palsies, mental disturbances, convulsions and coma. Common in Sweden. Diagnosed by urinalysis.
- variegate porphyria: may present with similar features to AIP. Photosensitivity is common. Common in South African Afrikaners. Diagnosed by stool examination for copro- and protoporphyrin.
- hereditary coproporphyria: photosensitivity may occur.

Acute attacks may be precipitated by drugs, stress, infection, alcohol ingestion, menstruation, pregnancy and starvation, although not at every exposure. Information about drugs is obtained from case reports, animal studies and analysis of drug effects on cell cultures.

- Effects of drugs:
  - definite precipitants: include barbiturates, phenytoin and sulphonamides.
  - implicated in laboratory or animal studies but not in humans: etomidate, lidocaine, chlordiazepoxide.
  - considered safe to use: opioid analgesic drugs, N_2O, suxamethonium, tubocurarine, gallamine, atropine, neostigmine, bupivacaine, prilocaine, procaine, propranolol, chlorphenamine, droperidol, chlorpromazine, chloral hydrate, aspirin, paracetamol, insulin.
  - controversial: diazepam, halothane, corticosteroids, ketamine, propofol. All have been used safely despite conflicting evidence.

James MF, Hift RJ (2000). Br J Anaesth; 85: 143–53

See also, Inborn errors of metabolism

Poseiro effect. Decrease in arterial BP during uterine contraction; thought to be caused by exacerbations of aortocaval compression.

[JJ Poseiro (described 1967), Uruguayan obstetrician]

See also, Obstetric analgesia and anaesthesia

Positioning of the patient. Undertaken to:

- facilitate surgery, imaging, etc.
- encourage venous drainage (for surgery) or distension (for central venous cannulation).
- allow the performance of and control the extent of regional anaesthesia.
- protect the airway (e.g. recovery position).
- improve oxygenation (prone ventilation).
- reduce ICP.
- encourage drainage of sputum, e.g. postural drainage.

Often performed when the patient is anaesthetised; damage to limbs, joints, pressure areas and nerves may occur unless care is taken. Tracheal tube, iv lines, etc. may be displaced during movement.

- Specific problems associated with certain positions:
  - supine: $\dot{V}/\dot{Q}$ mismatch may occur, especially if closing capacity exceeds FRC. Regurgitation of gastric contents may occur. The calves should be raised off the bed to reduce risk of DVT. In pregnancy, aortocaval compression may occur.
  - prone: similar considerations to the supine position apply. Chest wall and abdominal movement during respiration may be hindered. Supports should be positioned under the iliac crests and shoulders, leaving the abdomen free. Venous return may be impeded if the abdomen is compressed. Acute hepatic failure has been reported in a small number of patients following prolonged surgery in the prone position; intraoperative hepatic ischaemia related to positioning has been implicated though not proven; nevertheless regular checking of acid–base status and plasma lactate concentration has been advised. The face and eyes should be carefully padded (*see Eye care*). Particular care is required to prevent undue extension or rotation of the neck; the fully neutral position has been suggested since neurological lesions have been reported, especially after long procedures.
  - lateral: $\dot{V}/\dot{Q}$ mismatch occurs (*see One-lung anaesthesia*). The lower arm may be compressed and its venous drainage impaired.
  - Trendelenburg: originally described as supine with steep head-down tilt, with the knees flexed over the 'broken' end of the table. Diaphragmatic movement is limited by the weight of the abdominal viscera, reducing FRC and increasing atelectasis. Risk of regurgitation is increased. Venous engorgement of the head and neck may be accompanied by raised ICP and intraocular pressure. Brachial plexus injury may occur if shoulder supports are used.
  - reversed Trendelenburg: hypotension may occur if the head-up tilt is achieved rapidly.
  - lithotomy position: similar considerations to the Trendelenburg position. Injury to the lower back, hips and knees may occur. Common peroneal or saphenous nerves may be compressed against the lithotomy poles. Sciatic nerve injury has been reported after prolonged procedures. DVT may follow calf compression against the poles.
  - sitting: difficult to position the unconscious patient. Hypotension and air embolus may occur (*see Dental surgery; Neurosurgery*).

Neurological lesions or those relating to tissue ischaemia (e.g. bald areas on the scalp, compartment syndrome) are thought to be more likely if there is prolonged hypotension associated with long procedures.

[Friedrich Trendelenburg (1844–1924), German surgeon]

See also, Nerve injury during anaesthesia

Positive end-expiratory pressure (PEEP). Adjunct to IPPV, introduced in 1967. Produced by maintaining a positive airway pressure during expiration: usually 5–20 cmH_2O, although higher levels have been used ('super-PEEP'). Minimises airway and alveolar collapse and increases compliance, by increasing FRC. Thus improves oxygenation and reduces pulmonary shunt. High levels may increase dead space. Also, the adverse effects of IPPV related to intrathoracic pressure are increased. Thus barotrauma and reduced cardiac output are more likely. Urine output is reduced, and vasopressin secretion and ICP increased.

Has been used to reduce O_2 requirement and improve oxygenation in respiratory failure of any cause, except where its adverse effects are especially dangerous, e.g. asthma. The following terms have been used to describe the adjustment of PEEP:

- best PEEP: produces the least shunting without significant reduction of cardiac output.

- optimum PEEP: produces maximal O_2 delivery with the lowest dead space/tidal volume ratio.
- appropriate PEEP: that with the least dead space.

Auto-PEEP (intrinsic PEEP) is the difference between alveolar pressure and airway pressure at end-expiration, and exists when expiration continues right up to inspiration (i.e. no expiratory pause). It may occur in airway obstruction, asthma, COPD, ARDS, and in forced expiration.

Positron emission tomography (PET). Technique for imaging the distribution of inhaled or injected positron-emitting radioisotopes, e.g. ^{15}O, ^{13}N, ^{11}C and ^{18}F. Tomographic techniques similar to those used for CT scanning are used. Usually restricted to brain imaging, providing information about cerebral blood flow, O_2 and glucose metabolism, etc.

POSSUM, *see Physiological and operative severity score for the enumeration of mortality and morbidity*

Post-dural puncture headache (PDPH). Headache occurring after dural puncture, e.g. spinal anaesthesia or investigative lumbar puncture. First described by Bier in 1899. May rarely develop after epidural anaesthesia without an obvious dural tap. Thought to be due to CSF leaking through the dural hole, with settling of the brain and stretching of intracranial nerves, dura and blood vessels in the upright position. There may be cerebral vasodilatation demonstrable with imaging techniques. The incidence is increased by using large gauge needles, especially if the longitudinal dural fibres are cut transversely by the needle bevel instead of being split longitudinally, e.g. by non-cutting pencil-point spinal needles. More common in obstetrics and in young patients. Reported incidence varies but is under 1% with pencil-point 25–29 G needles in non-pregnant patients, and up to 75% with 16 G epidural needles in obstetric analgesia and anaesthesia.

Headaches usually occur within 1–3 days of dural puncture, normally lasting for 1–2 weeks but occasionally for months. They are classically severe, frontal or occipital, and exacerbated by sudden movement, getting up from the supine position, and coughing and straining. Neck stiffness may occur. Diagnosis is from the history and on clinical grounds. Typically, manual pressure over the right hypogastrium causes lessening of the headache, possibly via epidural venous congestion secondary to hepatic compression. MRI and CT scanning have been used to demonstrate CSF leaks. Rarely, cranial nerve palsies, convulsions and subdural or intracranial haemorrhage have been reported.

Prophylactic bed rest after dural puncture is now thought to be unnecessary.

- Treatment:
  - avoidance of dehydration.
  - simple analgesics, e.g. paracetamol, NSAIDs.
  - specific therapy: caffeine 150–200 mg orally, 6–8 hourly, has been shown to reduce the severity of headache. Sumatriptan 6 mg sc once only; caffeine/ergotamine mixture 100 mg/1 mg; ACTH 1.5 µU/kg iv in 1–2 l saline over 1 h or its synthetic analogue Synacthen 1 mg im have also been used, although evidence is anecdotal and the mechanisms of action unclear.
  - epidural administration of fluids, e.g. saline, dextran, blood: thought to displace CSF cranially and possibly reduce further leakage across the dura. Epidural blood patch is generally reserved for when headache is persistent. The use of prophylactic epidural injection of saline or blood near the time of dural puncture (e.g. after delivery in obstetrics) is controversial.

Turnbull DK, Shepherd DB (2003). Br J Anaesth; 91: 718–29

Posterior tibial artery. Arises (with the anterior artery) from the popliteal artery at the lower border of the popliteal fossa. Runs downwards on the surface of the posterior tibial muscle deep to soleus; lower down it becomes superficial and lies medial to tendo calcaneus. Divides into lateral and medial plantar arteries. The artery can be palpated between the medial malleolus and the prominence of the heel and may be used for arterial cannulation.

Postherpetic neuralgia. Persistent pain in the distribution of one or more peripheral nerves following shingles (herpes zoster). Usually defined as pain lasting for over 1 month. Shingles is caused by reactivation of dormant varicella zoster virus seeded during an earlier episode of primary chickenpox. It usually affects adults and occurs spontaneously although predisposing factors include age > 55 years and immunodeficiency (especially associated with HIV infection and leukaemia). The virus lies dormant in the dorsal root ganglia but may multiply and invade the corresponding sensory nerves. The T_5 and T_6 dermatomes are most commonly affected. Pain usually precedes the appearance of cutaneous vesicles on an inflamed base, which last 2–4 weeks. In 10% of cases, scarring and pain persist; the latter may be severe and intractable, triggered by contact, draughts and stress.

Treatment may be disappointing, but includes tricyclic antidepressant drugs, anticonvulsant drugs, local counter-irritants, TENS, acupuncture, local anaesthetic agent creams, repeated epidural anaesthesia, peripheral or sympathetic nerve block and the dorsal root entry zone procedure. Modification with aciclovir or corticosteroids is unproven. In most cases the pain is self-limiting.

Postoperative analgesia. Increasingly managed by acute pain teams; duties include education of medical and nursing staff, audit, research, and visiting postoperative patients specifically to monitor and adjust analgesia regimens.

Analgesic requirements vary according to the type of surgery, fitness of the patient, psychological factors and inter-patient differences.

- Techniques available:
  - opioid analgesic drugs:
    - im: painful to administer, and result in variable plasma drug levels. The time from the patient's expressing pain to the drug's administration depends on the patient's persistence, the level of nursing staffing and the procedures for obtaining and checking controlled drugs. Commonly used, however, because of its convenience and low cost.
    - iv: more reliable; methods include:
      - incremental small boluses titrated against effect; reduces accidental overdosage but still may allow windows of inadequate analgesia.
      - continuous infusion: may be adjusted to the minimal effective rate with minimal side effects. Steady-state plasma levels may be slow to achieve, and overdosage may still occur.
      - patient-controlled analgesia: less demanding on the nursing staff, and the patient's sense of being in control may be beneficial.
    - spinal opioids: usually administered via epidural catheters which remain in situ for a few days. Although analgesia is usually extremely good, large interpatient variability exists. Side effects include urinary retention, nausea, pruritus and respiratory depression; careful monitoring is required to detect the latter.

- sc: useful if iv access is limited but confers no advantage over iv administration.
- oral: use may be restricted by inability to drink, nausea and vomiting, delayed gastric emptying and first-pass metabolism.
- transdermal: slow-release patches are stuck to the skin; does not require cannulae or catheters, but adjustment of the release rate is impossible. Fentanyl and buprenorphine are available in transdermal preparations.
- sublingual/buccal: avoids injection but suffers the disadvantages of intermittent administration. Buprenorphine is administered in this way.
- rectal: drug absorption may be variable; the technique is less common in the UK.

- NSAIDs: popular as a method of reducing opioid requirements, particularly after day-case surgery, dental surgery and orthopaedic surgery. May be given parenterally, orally or rectally. They may cause GIT upset and impair renal and platelet function. Increased perioperative bleeding has been reported, but this is rarely clinically significant.
- local anaesthetic agents: provide excellent analgesia but with the risk of motor blockade and toxicity of local anaesthetics, and variable duration of action (depending on the technique and drug chosen). Duration may be prolonged by the use of repeated injections or infusions via catheters. Methods:
  - infiltration or nerve block: performed before or after surgery.
  - caudal analgesia, epidural anaesthesia or spinal anaesthesia: limited by hypotension and motor paralysis. May be combined with opioids.
- inhalational anaesthetic agents: some postoperative benefit is derived from the agents used perioperatively. Entonox is the only agent used postoperatively, e.g. for physiotherapy or changes of dressings, and is limited by its adverse effects on the haematological system.
- nerve destruction, e.g. cryoanalgesia has been used in thoracic surgery, but has limited application elsewhere.
- other methods less widely used include TENS, acupuncture and hypnosis.

See also, Analgesic drugs; Pain; Pain evaluation; Pain management; Pre-emptive analgesia

Postoperative care team. Proposed system of comprehensive postoperative care which includes regular rounds and a team of specialist 'postoperative care' nurses who are able to support ward nursing and medical staff by providing additional expertise and equipment. An extension of the concept of acute pain teams. Aims include better maintenance of vital organ function, decreased postoperative complications, reduced postoperative mortality, greater comfort and satisfaction and a shorter hospital stay.

Goldhill DR (1997). BMJ; 314: 389

See also, Care of the critically ill surgical patient; Medical emergency team; Outreach team; Safe transport and retrieval team

Postoperative nausea and vomiting (PONV). Consistently rated by patients as the most feared postoperative symptom. Apart from its unpleasantness, it may also increase pain, disturb dressings/surgical repairs, increase bleeding, and increase the risk of aspiration of gastric contents. May lead to electrolyte imbalance and dehydration if prolonged.

- In the absence of prophylaxis, PONV occurs after up to 90% of surgical procedures, the following increasing the risk:
  - patient factors:
    - young age.
    - female gender. Incidence increases during menstruation and decreases after the menopause, i.e. is presumably hormonally mediated.
    - anxiety, especially in patients who 'always vomit'. Increases in circulating catecholamine levels may be important.
    - previous history of PONV or motion sickness.
    - non-smoking.
    - early postoperative mobilisation, eating and drinking.
  - surgical factors:
    - gynaecological/abdominal/ENT/squint surgery.
    - laparoscopic procedures.
    - severe pain.
  - anaesthetic factors:
    - use of opioid analgesic drugs, including premedication.
    - use of certain anaesthetic drugs e.g. diethyl ether, trichloroethylene, cyclopropane, etomidate, N_2O (the last via a direct central effect, GIT distension and/or expansion of middle ear cavities).
    - possibly prolonged anaesthesia and the use of neostigmine (though these are disputed).
    - physical factors, e.g. gastric insufflation, pharyngeal stimulation.
  - other factors:
    - hypoxaemia/hypotension.
    - dehydration.

Various scores have been devised for predicting the likelihood of PONV in a particular case, based on the presence or absence of the following factors: female gender; history of PONV/travel sickness; non-smoker; postoperative opioids; ± prolonged procedure.

- Reduced by:
  - avoidance of triggers where possible, e.g. anxiety, opioids, N_2O, vigorous pharyngeal suction, and possibly general anaesthesia altogether.
  - use of specific antiemetic drugs and procedures (e.g. acupuncture at the wrist), especially in combination.
  - use of drugs, techniques and procedures associated with low incidence of nausea and vomiting, e.g. propofol.
  - administration of iv fluids.

With prophylaxis the incidence is usually under 30% in high risk cases. The most effective approach for preventing PONV is thought to be the use of multiple strategies and different drugs.

Habib AS, Gan TJ (2004). Can J Anaesth; 51: 326–41

See also, Vomiting

Postpartum haemorrhage (PPH). Defined as more than 500 ml blood loss associated with vaginal delivery and greater than 1000 ml loss with Caesarean section, although accurate measurement is notoriously difficult at this time. A common cause of morbidity and also mortality associated with pregnancy, it is associated with a number of predisposing factors including multiple pregnancy, multiparity, pre-eclampsia, placenta praevia and prolonged augmented labour. Problems include not identifying women at risk (even though risk factors are well known), not recognising significant hypovolaemia when it occurs and a lack of an appropriate sense of urgency when resuscitating the patient. The problems of DIC and dilutional coagulopathy may rapidly be superimposed upon the underlying condition.

- Caused by:
  - obstetric factors, e.g. uterine atony, retained placenta, uterine/vaginal tears, uterine inversion, instrumentation or intrauterine manipulation.

- non-obstetric factors, e.g. coagulation disorders.

Typically, PPH presents with tachycardia and other features of haemorrhage and hypovolaemia, although since most cases are fit young women, cardiovascular compensation is very efficient until severe volume depletion occurs, when sudden collapse may ensue. Uterine inversion may be associated with profound hypotension and bradycardia.

Initial management consists of basic fluid resuscitation. Specific treatment is aimed at the underlying cause, e.g. oxytocin and carboprost for uterine atony, evacuation of the uterus for retained products, surgical repair of tears, reduction of uterine inversion, etc. Anaesthetic management for obstetric intervention depends on the state of the circulation, whether there is an epidural catheter already in situ and the possibility of coagulopathy. The risks of regional anaesthesia must be weighed against the risks of general anaesthesia in each individual case.
See also, Caesarean section; Obstetric analgesia and anaesthesia

Post-tetanic count, *see Neuromuscular blockade monitoring*

Post-tetanic potentiation (PTP; Post-tetanic facilitation). Increased response to a single pulse stimulus following tetanic contraction. Seen during non-depolarising neuromuscular blockade and in myasthenia gravis; thought to be caused by increased presynaptic mobilisation and release of acetylcholine in response to the tetanus. Absent in depolarising neuromuscular blockade. Mechanical PTP occurring in normal subjects without neuromuscular blockade is thought to be caused by calcium ion accumulation resulting in increased muscle strength. EMG recording does not exhibit PTP in unblocked muscle.
See also, Neuromuscular blockade monitoring

Post-traumatic stress disorder. Psychological disorder following a severe physical or mental trauma, e.g. accident or natural disaster; has also been reported after awareness during anaesthesia or after an acute critical illness, e.g. requiring ICU care. In order to make the diagnosis the following must exist:

- the stressor is considered exceptional, e.g. severe trauma or accident.
- onset within 6 months of the event.
- prominent memories: often distressing, intrusive, recurrent and causing the sufferer to relive the experience.
- avoidance behaviour, e.g. refusing to undergo anaesthesia.
- hyperarousal, e.g. irritability or jumpiness.

Management includes psychological support and counselling, with specific psychological treatment according to the individual requirements. Drug therapy may also be required. The advice of a psychologist or psychiatrist with a specific interest is recommended.

Potassium. Principal intracellular cation, present at 135–150 mmol/l. Present in the plasma at 3.5–5.0 mmol/l. Total body content is about 3200 mmol, of which 90% is intracellular, 7.5% within bone and dense connective tissue, and 2.5% in interstitial fluid, transcellular fluid and plasma. About 90% is exchangeable. Essential for maintenance of the cell membrane potential and generation of action potentials.

Filtered potassium is reabsorbed mainly at the proximal convoluted tubule of the nephron. It is secreted at the distal tubule, in effect in exchange for sodium and hydrogen ions under the influence of aldosterone.

- Daily requirement: about 1 mmol/kg/day.

Potassium channel activators. New class of antianginal drugs. Act by opening potassium channels primarily in smooth muscle but also in other excitable tissues, causing arterial and venous dilatation. Result in improved blood flow to poststenotic areas of myocardium. Nicorandil is the first to be developed.

Potency. Ability of a drug to produce a certain effect. Influenced by the drug's absorption, distribution, metabolism, excretion and affinity for its receptor. Very potent drugs are effective in very small doses.
See also, Dose–response curves

Potentiation, post-tetanic, *see Post-tetanic potentiation*

Power. Rate of performing work. SI unit is the watt:

$$1\ \text{W} = 1\ \text{J/s}.$$

Also refers to the ability of statistical tests to reveal a difference of a certain magnitude. Power analysis is performed before a clinical trial to determine the sample size required to show a certain difference, or retrospectively when analysing a statistically insignificant result. Increased if groups are equally sized and large, and if the difference between them is large. Power equals $1 - \beta$, where β = type II error; power of 80–90% ($\beta = 0.1$–0.2) is usually considered acceptable.
Yentis SM (1996). Anaesthesia; 51: 413–14

Power spectral analysis. Fourier analysis of 2–16 second sections (epochs) of the EEG, with graphical representation of the distribution of frequencies within each epoch. The frequency distribution of successive epochs may be plotted consecutively on continuous paper as a series of peaks and troughs (compressed spectral array) representing frequencies of high and low activity respectively. Has been used to monitor depth of anaesthesia. The technique has also been applied to beat-to-beat variability of heart rate and BP to determine the relative influence of sympathetic and parasympathetic activity, e.g. perioperatively.

More recently, the technique has been combined with analysis of the relationship between different frequency components (phase coupling), together with information about other aspects of EEG measurements, e.g. degree of burst suppression. The resultant output, the bispectral index, is a single number between 0 and 100 and has been used to guide anaesthetic dosage and administration, although claims of better 'control' of anaesthesia and shorter recovery following its use have been disputed.
See also, Anaesthesia, depth of

Poynting effect. Dissolution of gaseous O_2 when bubbled through liquid N_2O, with vaporisation of the liquid to form a gaseous O_2/N_2O mixture.
[John H Poynting (1852–1914), English physicist]
See also, Entonox

PPF, Plasma protein fraction, *see Blood products*

PPH, *see Postpartum haemorrhage*

P–R interval. Represents atrial depolarisation. Measured from the beginning of the P wave to the beginning of the QRS complex of the ECG, irrespective of whether the QRS complex starts with a Q wave or an R wave (*see Fig. 57b; Electrocardiography*). Normally 1.2–2.0 ms. Shortened in junctional arrhythmias, Wolff–Parkinson–White syndrome and Lown–Ganong–Levine syndrome. Prolonged in heart block and hypothermia.

Pralidoxime mesylate/chloride. Acetylcholinesterase reactivator, used with atropine to treat organophosphorus poisoning. Has three main actions:
- converts the acetylcholinesterase inhibitor to a harmless compound.
- protects acetylcholinesterase transiently against further inhibition.
- reactivates the inhibited acetylcholinesterase.

Does not reverse the muscarinic effects of organophosphorus compounds, but highly active at nicotinic sites. Must be given within 24–36 h of poisoning to be effective. Its effects usually occur within 10–40 min of administration.
- Dosage: 30 mg/kg diluted in 10–15 ml water, iv over 5–10 min. May be repeated up to twice if no improvement is seen within 30 min, up to a usual maximum of 12 g/24 h. Rarely, iv infusion of up to 500 mg/h may be required. For children, a bolus dose of 20–60 mg/kg.
- Side effects: drowsiness, visual disturbances, nausea, tachycardia, muscle weakness.

Prazosin hydrochloride. α-Adrenergic receptor antagonist, highly selective for α_1-adrenergic receptors. Used as a vasodilator drug, e.g. in hypertension and cardiac failure, and as a bladder smooth muscle relaxant in outflow obstruction. Rarely causes compensatory tachycardia, presumably because of its α_1-receptor specificity. 97% protein-bound, with a half-life of 2–3 h. Excreted mainly via bile and faeces. Doxazosin and terazosin are related drugs.
- Dosage: 0.5–5.0 g orally, 6–12 hourly.
- Side effects: postural hypotension (especially after the first dose), nausea, drowsiness, headache.

Predictive value. In statistics, a test to predict or exclude a condition. May be:
- positive: proportion of patients with positive test results who have the condition.
- negative: proportion of patients with negative test results who do not have the condition.

Altman DG, Bland JM (1994). BMJ; 309: 102
See also, Errors; Sensitivity; Specificity

Prednisolone. Corticosteroid with predominantly glucocorticoid activity, used in the long-term suppression of allergic, autoimmune and inflammatory disease. Four times as potent as hydrocortisone.
- Dosage: initially 10–60 mg orally, once daily, usually reduced after a few days but occasionally longer. Maintenance dose: 2.5–15 mg daily. The acetate preparation may be given im (25–100 mg once or twice weekly) or into inflamed joints (5–25 mg).
- Side effects: as for corticosteroids.

Pre-eclampsia (Pre-eclamptic toxaemia, PET; Pregnancy-induced hypertension, PIH). Defined as the following occurring after the 20th week of pregnancy:
- hypertension: systolic, mean or diastolic BP > 140, 105 or 90 mmHg respectively, or an increase in systolic or diastolic BP greater than 30 and 15 mmHg respectively.
- peripheral oedema.
- proteinuria > 0.3 g/l.

Represents a multisystem disease with many other manifestations. Thus there has been a move in definition away from the classic triad of PET above, towards the definition of PIH with or without other features. PIH occurs in 10–12% of pregnancies whilst PET itself has an incidence of 2–3%. More common in first pregnancies with a particular partner (typically the features are less severe or present later in subsequent pregnancies), diabetes mellitus, polyhydramnios, obesity, black race and multiple pregnancy. Usually improves rapidly following delivery of the fetus, although the clinical picture may first worsen before recovery. Aetiology is unknown but may be related to prostaglandin metabolism, although aspirin has no overall preventative or therapeutic effect despite initial encouraging trials (but may be of value in patients at risk of early PET or premature labour). An increase in the thromboxane/prostacyclin ratio has been suggested, with platelet aggregation within the placental vascular bed causing release of vasoactive substances and intravascular fibrin deposition. Thus increasingly considered a disorder of endothelium, possibly explaining the widespread organ system effects. Apart from maternal effects, placental perfusion is decreased, and secondary trophoblastic invasion of the maternal spiral arteries usually occurring at 16 weeks is absent. Perinatal mortality is increased.
- Maternal features:
  - cardiovascular: thought to involve increased sensitivity to angiotensin II (sensitivity is normally decreased in pregnancy) and catecholamines, with vasoconstriction, reduced plasma volume, oedema and increased arterial BP.
  - renal: renal blood flow, GFR and urine output are decreased, with proteinuria.
  - haematological: fibrinogen, fibrin and platelet turnover is increased. HELLP syndrome (haemolysis, elevated liver enzymes, low platelets) may occur. Platelet function may be impaired.
  - neurological: hyperexcitability and hyperreflexia; visual symptoms and headache may forewarn of impending convulsions (eclampsia).

Severe PET is heralded by BP > 160/110, severe proteinuria or oliguria < 500 ml/24 h, DIC, pulmonary oedema, neurological symptoms and epigastric (hepatic) pain.

Consistently one of the most common causes of maternal mortality, especially in the developing world; death may result from aspiration of gastric contents, CVA, hepatorenal failure or cardiac failure. In the UK, most deaths are now caused by CVA (previously by ARDS).
- Treatment includes bed rest, control of hypertension, prevention of convulsions, and delivery of the fetus if possible:
  - antihypertensive drugs used include α-methyldopa, labetalol, hydralazine and calcium channel blocking drugs orally. Severe hypotension has been reported if the latter (e.g. nifedipine sublingually) is given concurrently with magnesium sulphate, but the risk is smaller than originally feared. Severe hypertension may require iv treatment with:
    - labetalol 5–10 mg increments, or 10–200 mg/h infusion.
    - hydralazine 5–10 mg increments, or 5–50 mg/h infusion.
    - sodium nitroprusside or GTN 0.1–5.0 µg/kg/min.

  Concurrent administration with iv fluids is important since the intravascular compartment is generally depleted; central venous cannulation or pulmonary artery catheterisation may be required (the latter because myocardial dysfunction may be present, although the place of pulmonary artery catheters is controversial). The choice of fluid and degree of volume expansion required is also controversial, but administration of fluids (by consensus, preferably colloids) should begin before iv vasodilators are given to avoid precipitous falls in BP and/or placental perfusion. Since oliguria is common, these patients are often given low dose dopamine or furosemide along with fluid replacement; however, it is relatively easy for inexperienced staff to overload the circulation in an

attempt to improve urine output. As the urine output usually improves spontaneously 1–2 days after delivery, many anaesthetists and obstetricians now feel that allowing the urea and creatinine to increase in the short term is preferable to causing pulmonary oedema and possibly the requirement for ventilatory support.
- anticonvulsant drugs: magnesium sulphate has been shown to reduce the incidence of eclampsia by almost 60%, although the number needed to treat is large (60–90; even higher in developed countries where the disease tends to be less aggressive) and side effects are relatively common, albeit mild. Magnesium has also been shown to reduce the incidence of recurrent convulsions after eclampsia, compared with diazepam and phenytoin. Clomethiazole has traditionally been used in the UK but is rarely used now.

Anaesthetic involvement may be required for analgesia during labour, Caesarean section or assistance with management of fluids, BP, etc.

- Anaesthetic techniques:
  - epidural anaesthesia:
    - prevents the increases in catecholamines associated with pain, thus increasing placental blood flow.
    - avoids the risks of general anaesthesia.
    - contraindicated if there is a coagulopathy or low platelet count (below 50 000 × 10^9/l constitutes an absolute contraindication; 50–100 000 × 10^9/l has been suggested as acceptable if the bleeding time is under 10 min, depending on clinical circumstances. However, bleeding time has been criticised as being unreliable and its performance may vary between investigators.).
    - careful fluid management and local anaesthetic administration is required to avoid cardiovascular instability following blockade. Sensitivity to sympathomimetic drugs is increased.
    - use of relatively large doses of local anaesthetic agents has been questioned in patients with neurological symptoms.
    - avoidance of adrenaline in local anaesthetic solutions has been suggested but this is controversial.
  - spinal anaesthesia has traditionally been avoided because of the fear of sudden severe hypotension, but this may not necessarily occur if there is adequate volume expansion and pretreatment of the condition.
  - general anaesthesia:
    - risks include difficult intubation (because of facial and laryngeal oedema), the hypertensive response to intubation and cardiovascular instability. Administration of antihypertensive drugs or opioid analgesic drugs (e.g. alfentanil 7–10 μg/kg or fentanyl 1–4 μg/kg, especially in combination with magnesium) before intubation has been used.
    - the anticonvulsant effect of thiopental may be beneficial.
    - magnesium sulphate may result in increased sensitivity to neuromuscular blocking drugs.

Careful monitoring should continue after delivery.

Duley L, Meher S, Abalos E (2006). BMJ; 332: 463–8

See also, Obstetric analgesia and anaesthesia

Pre-ejection period, *see Systolic time intervals*

Pre-emptive analgesia. Concept that suppression of dorsal horn neuronal activity involved in pain pathways, before a painful stimulus (e.g. surgery), results in reduced analgesic requirements postoperatively. Techniques of suppression include central neuronal blockade (e.g. epidural/spinal anaesthesia), local anaesthetic infiltration of tissues, use of NSAIDs and opioid analgesic drugs, and antagonism of NMDA receptors, e.g. with ketamine, in order to manipulate CNS plasticity and reduce 'wind-up'. Supported by animal and some human studies, although the clinical relevance is uncertain.

Kissin I (2005). Anesth Analg; 100: 754–6

Pregabalin. Anticonvulsant drug, related to gabapentin. Licensed for adjunctive therapy of partial seizures and also treatment of neuropathic pain.

- Dosage: 150 orally/day in 2–3 doses, increased after 1–2 weeks to 300–600 mg/day.
- Side effects: dry mouth, GIT upset, CNS impairment, weight gain; rarely neutropenia, heart block, pancreatitis.

Gajraj NM (2007). Anesth Analg; 105: 1805–15

Pregnancy. Usually lasts 40 weeks. Most physiological changes occur in response to the increased metabolic demands of the uterus, placenta and fetus, and include alterations in the following systems:

- cardiovascular:
  - increased intravascular volume from the first trimester, returning to normal within 2 weeks of delivery. Plasma expansion (50%) exceeds red cell expansion (20%), resulting in the 'physiological anaemia' of pregnancy. Haemoglobin concentration is usually about 12 g/dl at term. White cell count increases throughout and peaks after delivery.
  - increased heart rate, peaking at 28–36 weeks when it may exceed normal rate by 10–15 beats/min.
  - increased cardiac output from 10 weeks, reaching 140% of normal at term with further increases during labour. Stroke volume increases by 30%. Ejection systolic heart murmurs are common, and 3rd or 4th heart sounds may occur.
  - decreased SVR as a result of the smooth muscle relaxation caused by progesterone. Sites of venous engorgement include cutaneous and epidural vessels, the latter affecting height of block in epidural anaesthesia.
  - reduced MAP, being lowest at the time of maximal cardiac output.
  - aortocaval compression in the supine position.
  - ECG changes caused by cephalad displacement of the diaphragm by the uterus include left axis deviation and inverted T waves in leads V_2 and V_3.
- respiratory:
  - increased minute ventilation (by 50% in the first trimester), mainly caused by increased tidal volume (thought to be a central effect of progesterone).
  - reduced arterial $P\text{CO}_2$ to about 4 kPa (30 mmHg) with resulting respiratory alkalosis by the 12th week of pregnancy; arterial $P\text{O}_2$ increases by about 1.3 kPa (10 mmHg). Arterial pH remains normal due to renal excretion of bicarbonate.
  - reduced FRC (both expiratory reserve volume and residual volume decrease) from the 20th week onwards, caused by the upward displacement of the diaphragm by the uterus.
  - increased O_2 consumption throughout pregnancy, but especially in the third trimester (up to 20%).
  - increased risk of hypoxaemia during anaesthesia results from reduced FRC and increased O_2 demand.
  - venous engorgement of the upper airway, which may lead to spontaneous epistaxis or haemorrhage on instrumentation.
- gastrointestinal: gastric emptying is probably normal apart from during labour, when it may be reduced

(markedly if opioids are given). Gastric acidity is probably normal, despite initial studies suggesting it is increased. Gastro-oesophageal reflux occurs in at least 80% of women, caused by the effects of progesterone on the lower oesophageal sphincter, and the uterus pushing the stomach into a horizontal position. The time after conception at which the GIT effects occur, and the time after delivery at which they revert to normal, are unknown. 16–20 weeks has been suggested as the time of onset; progesterone levels fall to non-pregnant levels by 24 h of delivery, and reflux usually resolves by 36 h.
- coagulation: increased levels of fibrinogen and all clotting factors except XI and XIII, predisposing towards thromboembolism. Platelet count falls slightly. Systemic fibrinolytic activity is depressed, but localised activity (i.e. ability to lyse clots from within) is maintained. Thus the level of fibrin degradation products increases as pregnancy progresses. However, in normal pregnancy neither bleeding nor clotting times are increased.
- renal: dilatation of the renal pelvises and ureters from the end of the first trimester. Renal blood flow and GFR increase by 40%. Increased renin-angiotensin system activity increases sodium and water retention, with falls in serum creatinine and urea; glycosuria may occur.
- endocrine: peripheral insulin resistance due to antagonism by hormones such as human placental lactogen may aggravate or precipitate gestational diabetes.
- hepatic: blood flow is unaltered. Serum albumin and cholinesterase levels fall, whilst hepatic enzyme levels may increase.

Non-urgent surgery is usually delayed until the second trimester, because of the possible risk (although never proven) of teratogenic effects on the fetus. Conditions requiring abdominal surgery are associated with increased risk of miscarriage or premature labour.

See also, Fetus, effect of anaesthetic agents on; Obstetric analgesia and anaesthesia

Pregnanolone, *see Eltanolone*

Prehospital index (PHI). Scoring system used to assess trauma victims according to their BP, pulse rate, respiratory status and conscious level, each of which is scored up to 5. The PHI is the sum of the individual scores, with an extra 4 points given for penetrating abdominal or thoracic injuries. A PHI > 3 has been used to define major trauma.

Koehler JJ, Baer LJ, Malafa SA, et al (1986). Ann Emerg Med; 15: 178–82

Preload. End-diastolic ventricular wall tension. Usually inferred from ventricular end-diastolic pressure, itself approximating to pulmonary capillary wedge pressure (left) or CVP (right). Related to myocardial contractility and cardiac output by Starling's law.

Also refers to prophylactic administration of iv fluids to reduce hypotension, e.g. before spinal or epidural anaesthesia.

Premedication. Administration of medication prior to anaesthesia.

- Aims:
  - allay anxiety.
  - alleviate pain.
  - facilitate smooth induction of anaesthesia and reduce the amount of anaesthetic agents required.
  - reduce secretion formation.
  - reduce awareness.
  - reduce PONV.
  - reduce the risks of specific complications associated with anaesthesia/surgery or the patient's pre-existing condition, e.g.:
    - bradycardia, e.g. in ophthalmic surgery.
    - hypertensive response to tracheal intubation.
    - aspiration pneumonitis.
    - adverse drug reactions.
    - bronchospasm.
    - DVT.
- Drugs suitable for premedication include:
  - opioid analgesic drugs, e.g. morphine, papaveretum, pethidine.
  - benzodiazepines, e.g. diazepam, temazepam, lorazepam.
  - barbiturates, e.g. pentobarbital.
  - butyrophenones, e.g. droperidol.
  - phenothiazines, e.g. alimemazine (trimeprazine), promethazine.
  - anticholinergic drugs, e.g. atropine, hyoscine, glycopyrronium.
  - other antiemetic drugs, e.g. metoclopramide.
  - H_2 receptor antagonists, e.g. ranitidine, cimetidine.
  - antacids, e.g. sodium citrate.

In addition, certain drugs already taken regularly by the patient are usually continued up to and including the day of surgery, e.g. antiarrhythmic drugs, antihypertensive drugs, drugs used in ischaemic heart disease and asthma, anticonvulsant drugs, etc.

Oral premedication (e.g. with benzodiazepines) is often used in place of traditional im injection of opioid and anticholinergic drugs.

- Many anaesthetists do not routinely prescribe premedication because of disadvantages such as:
  - excessive sedation.
  - difficulty with timing of drug administration.
  - pain from im injections.
  - nausea and vomiting (with opioids).
  - dry mouth with anticholinergic drugs.
  - unnecessary drug administration.
  - antanalgesia and restlessness.
  - delayed recovery.

Preoperative assessment. Main objectives include assessment of:
- the risks to the patient of suffering perioperative deterioration in health.
- whether the patient's condition may be improved prior to surgery, e.g. by changing medication, treating pre-existing disease, administering fluids, etc.
- how otherwise to minimise the perioperative risk, e.g. by enlisting more experienced help, rescheduling the time of surgery, using special anaesthetic or analgesic techniques, booking a bed on ICU or HDU, etc.

Preadmission clinics (involving assessment by an anaesthetist, surgeon or nurse) represent an attempt to reduce the rate of delay and cancellation of surgical procedures caused by inadequate preparation of patients. Use of strict protocols may be helpful if non-anaesthetic staff assess the patients.

- Assessment is directed towards the individual patient's circumstances but in general is divided into:
  - history:
    - medical and surgical history, including the nature of the proposed surgery.
    - previous anaesthetic history including adverse reactions, PONV, other problems, etc.

- family history of medical or anaesthetic problems.
- drug history (past and present).
- smoking and alcohol intake.
- known allergies and atopy.
- weight of the patient (especially children).
- presence of capped, crowned, chipped or loose teeth.
- anxiety.
- time of last oral intake.
- systems review, in particular:
  - CVS: hypertension, features of ischaemic heart disease, cardiac failure, arrhythmias.
  - RS: recent chest infection, features of COPD or asthma.
  - GIT: hiatus hernia or other risk factors for aspiration of gastric contents.
  - CNS: epilepsy, pre-existing neurological lesions.
- examination:
  - airway, teeth, cervical spine (including assessment for possible difficult tracheal intubation).
  - CVS: for hypovolaemia, dehydration, cyanosis and anaemia; pulse, BP, JVP, cardiac impulse, heart sounds, lung bases, periphery (for oedema).
  - RS: for clubbing and cyanosis, position of the trachea, chest expansion, air entry, respiratory sounds.
  - CNS: cranial nerves, spinal cord and peripheral nerves including dermatomes and myotomes.
  - suitable veins for cannulation.
  - suitability for regional techniques where intended.
- preoperative investigations.

Scoring systems may be used for classifying patients according to preoperative status, e.g. ASA physical status, cardiac risk index, New York Heart Association classification, Glasgow coma scale, subarachnoid haemorrhage and hepatic failure scoring systems.

More recently cardiopulmonary exercise testing has been used as a means of predicting outcome in high risk surgical cases.

The need for blood cross-matching and premedication is also assessed. The forthcoming anaesthesia is explained and the patient's consent confirmed.

García-Miguel FJ, Serrano-Aguilar PG, López-Bastida J (2003). Lancet; 362: 1749–57

See also, individual diseases and drugs; Emergency surgery

Preoperative fasting, *see Gastric emptying*

Preoperative optimisation. Technique of preoperatively increasing cardiovascular variables with iv fluids, inotropic and vasodilator drugs to produce supranormal levels of oxygen delivery in patients undergoing major surgery. Has been claimed to reduce morbidity and mortality in certain groups of patients, e.g. those undergoing major vascular surgery. Since it requires preoperative admission to the ICU and invasive monitoring, the process has huge implications in terms of costs and utilisation of ICU beds.

Tote SP, Grounds RM (2006). Br J Anaes; 97: 4–11

Preoxygenation. Administration of 100% O_2 prior to induction of anaesthesia. Increases the O_2 reserve in the lungs and thus the time to hypoxaemia during subsequent apnoea, e.g. during tracheal intubation. Also increases arterial PO_2, although O_2 content and saturation may not increase by much. Particularly useful when difficulties are anticipated, or in patients at risk from aspiration of gastric contents. Thus a vital part of 'rapid sequence induction'. The optimal technique is uncertain; 3 minutes' administration is thought to be as effective as 5 minutes' administration, or even four vital capacity breaths. A tightly fitting facepiece (to prevent indrawing of room air) and adequate flow of O_2 are vital. Monitoring of end-expiratory O_2 concentration may be a useful guide during preoxygenation; washout of nitrogen from the lungs is indicated by an increase in expired O_2 concentration towards steady-state (near 100% in ideal conditions with no gas leaks or mixing). More effect in obese patients if they are positioned head-up.

See also, Induction, rapid sequence

Pressure. Force per unit area. SI unit is the pascal: 1 Pa = 1 N/m^2.

Pressure generators, *see Ventilators*

Pressure measurement. May be:
- direct:
  - liquid manometers which measure:
    - absolute pressure, e.g. mercury barometer.
    - pressure relative to atmospheric pressure (gauge pressure), e.g. U tube. The sensitivity may be increased by using liquid of low density, inclining the manometer tube or using a different non-miscible liquid in each of the limbs of the U tube (differential liquid manometer).
  - aneroid gauge (one in which there is no liquid). In one form a sealed metal bellows changes size with changes in external or applied pressure, moving a pointer on a scale (e.g. aneroid barometer). In the Bourdon gauge used in anaesthesia, a coiled tube of oval cross-section uncoils as it becomes circular on cross-section, due to the high pressure of the gas inside it, and this moves the pointer.
  - pressure transducers.
- indirect, e.g. in arterial BP measurement.

[Eugene Bourdon (1808–1884), French engineer]

Pressure regulated volume control ventilation. Ventilatory mode combining the benefits of pressure controlled IPPV with a decelerating inspiratory flow pattern and a guaranteed tidal volume. The ventilator automatically monitors the lung's properties and modifies the inspiratory pressure level to deliver a predetermined volume. Maximum inspiratory pressure permitted is just below the preset upper pressure limit and if the tidal volume cannot be delivered with this pressure, the ventilator alarms, indicating that the breath has been pressure limited. Useful mode where lung/chest compliance alters during inspiration, e.g. atelectasis, bronchospasm. Achieves a set tidal/minute volume with the lowest possible inspiratory pressure. The maximum pressure change between two breaths is preset by the ventilator (approximately 3 cmH$_2$O).

Pressure regulators. Formerly called reducing valves, devices for reducing the high pressures delivered by cylinders to anaesthetic machines, and maintaining the reduced pressure at a constant level which is easier to use. Also reduce the requirement for high-pressure tubing.

- May be:
  - direct (Fig. 126a): cylinder pressure tends to open the valve.
  - indirect (Fig. 126b): cylinder pressure P tends to close the valve. The diaphragm moves according to p and the tension in the springs. As p falls, the diaphragm bulges into the regulator, allowing more gas flow into the upper half and thus maintaining p. If p increases, the diaphragm is pushed upwards, decreasing gas flow and

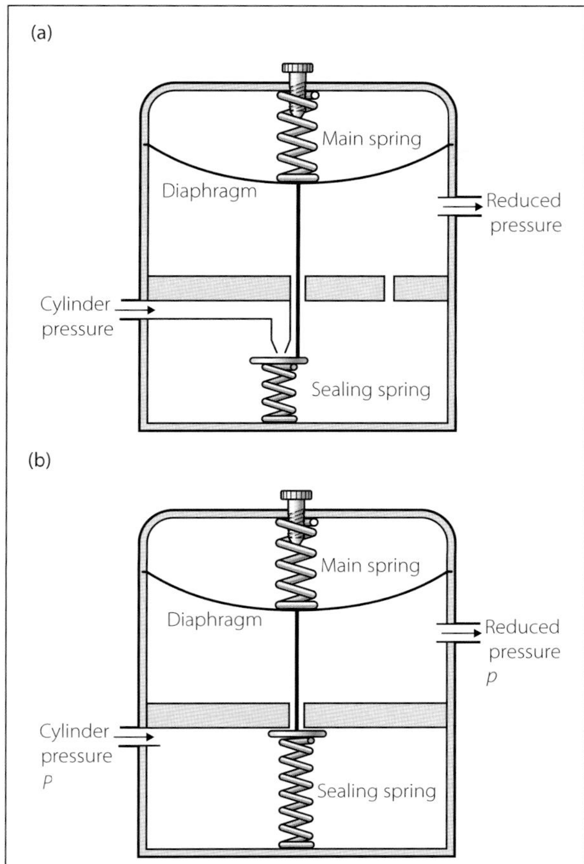

Fig. 126 Diagram of pressure regulators: (a) direct; (b) indirect

again maintaining *p*. Thus pressure is maintained even when there are changes in cylinder pressure or demand.
The regulators are specific for the different gases, and should be labelled accordingly. Pressure relief valves are incorporated in case of excessive pressures. Pressure gauges may also be incorporated.

Two-stage regulators are often used, to reduce wear and tear on the diaphragm and reduce pressure fluctuations, especially if high gas flows are required. The output of one stage is the input of the second. Demand valves may be based on this principle.

Slave regulators are those whose output depends on the output of another regulator. For example, the output of an O_2 regulator may be applied above the diaphragm of a N_2O regulator, keeping the latter's valve open. If the O_2 pressure fails, the N_2O valve closes.

Pressure sores, *see Decubitus ulcers*

Pressure support, *see Inspiratory pressure support*

Priestley, Joseph (1733–1804). English scientist, best known for his work on various gases. A major protagonist of the phlogiston theory, he isolated ammonia (as 'alkaline air'), sulphur dioxide ('vitriolic acid air'), O_2 ('dephlogisticated air'), N_2O ('dephlogisticated nitrous air'), nitrogen dioxide ('nitrous acid air') and methane. Also investigated electrical conduction. Emigrated to the USA in 1794 because of his unpopular religious and political views.

Prilocaine hydrochloride. Amide local anaesthetic agent, introduced in 1959. Slower in onset than lidocaine, but lasts about 1.5 times as long and less toxic. pK_a is 7.9. 55% protein-bound. Undergoes hepatic and renal metabolism. Maximal safe dose: 5 mg/kg alone, 8 mg/kg with adrenaline. Used as 0.5–1.0% solutions for infiltration, 1–2% for nerve blocks and 0.5% for IVRA. Also available as a 4% plain or 3% solution with felypressin for dental infiltration, and in EMLA cream. May cause methaemoglobinaemia in doses above about 600 mg in adults, due to its metabolite *ortho*-toluidine.

Priming principle. Shortening of the time of onset of non-depolarising neuromuscular blockade by administration of a non-depolarising neuromuscular blocking drug in divided aliquots. The priming dose (15–20% of the usual intubating dose) is followed by the remainder of the intubating dose 4–8 min later, depending on the drug used.

- Suggested explanatory theories:
  - the priming dose occupies a proportion of postsynaptic receptors at the neuromuscular junction; the main dose can thus occupy more rapidly the critical mass of receptors for neuromuscular blockade.
  - the priming dose occupies presynaptic receptors, reducing mobilisation and release of acetylcholine; the main dose thus acts faster.

Initially thought to answer the need for rapid tracheal intubation without using suxamethonium. However, the priming dose itself may cause unpleasant symptoms, e.g. diplopia and weakness, and may risk dangerous events, e.g. hypoventilation and aspiration of gastric contents.

Jones RM (1989). Br J Anaesth; 63: 1–3

PRISM, *see Paediatric risk of mortality score*

Proarrhythmias. Arrhythmias caused by or exacerbated by antiarrhythmic drugs. May occur even with standard dosage and normally therapeutic plasma drug levels. Common examples include VT and torsade de pointes.

Probability (*P*). In statistics, the likelihood that the observed result might be expected to occur by chance alone. Analogous to, but distinct from, the chance of a type I error. Statistical significance is usually denoted by a *P* value < 0.05.

Probability limits, *see Confidence intervals*

Procainamide hydrochloride. Class Ia antiarrhythmic drug, chemically related to procaine. Effective against ventricular and supraventricular arrhythmias. Has 85% oral bioavailablity and 15% protein-bound. Undergoes hepatic metabolism (largely via acetylation to *N*-acetylprocainamide) and renal excretion, although 40–50% is excreted unchanged.

- Dosage:
  - up to 50 mg/kg/day orally in 4–8 doses.
  - 25–50 mg/min slowly iv up to 1 g, with ECG monitoring for widened QRS complex or P–R interval prolongation. 2–6 mg/min may follow.
- Side effects: hypotension with iv usage, GIT upset, rash, agranulocytosis, SLE-like syndrome (especially in slow acetylators).

Procaine hydrochloride. Ester local anaesthetic agent, introduced in 1904, now seldom used. The first synthetic local anaesthetic. Less lipid soluble than lidocaine, with slower onset of less intense anaesthesia, and shorter duration of action. pK_a is 8.9. 6% protein-bound. Poorly absorbed from mucous membranes; thus not useful as a surface anaesthetic. Used in 0.25–1.0% solutions for infiltration anaesthesia, and

1–2% for nerve blocks, usually with adrenaline 1:200 000. Maximal safe dose: 12 mg/kg.

Procalcitonin. Propeptide of calcitonin, produced by the C-cells of the thyroid gland but not normally released into the circulation (except in low concentrations) in health. Systemic procalcitonin levels rise significantly during severe infection or inflammation.

Uzzan B, Cohen R, Nicolas P, et al (2006). Crit Care Med; 34: 1996–2003

Prochlorperazine maleate/mesylate. Piperazine phenothiazine with antiemetic, α-adrenergic agonist and weak sedative properties. Used mainly as an antipsychotic and antiemetic drug. Active within 10–20 min of im administration and 30–40 min of oral administration. Action lasts 3–4 h.

- Dosage:
  - 5–20 mg orally/im, 6–12 hourly. Not licensed for iv use in the UK, although it has been safely given by that route. A buccal preparation is also available: dose 3–6 mg.
  - 25 mg rectally 6 hourly.
- Side effects: as for phenothiazines. Extrapyramidal reactions are more likely than following chlorpromazine, especially in children.

Procyclidine hydrochloride. Anticholinergic drug, used in the treatment of Parkinson's disease and drug-induced pyramidal states. Acts centrally to decrease the influence of acetylcholine in the basal ganglia.

- Dosage:
  - 2.5–10 mg orally, 8 hourly.
  - 5–10 mg im, repeated after 20 min up to 20 mg/day.
  - 5 mg iv repeated as necessary; relief is usual after a single dose and within 5 min but may take 30 min.
- Side effects: dry mouth, GIT disturbance, urinary retention, dizziness, blurred vision.

Prodrug. Inactive substance metabolised to active drug within the body, e.g. chloral hydrate (converted to trichloroethanol) and α-methyldopa (converted to α-methylnoradrenaline).

Prokinetic drugs. Group of drugs which increase GIT activity. Include metoclopramide and domperidone, their prokinetic actions mediated via enhancement of GIT cholinergic activity (although dopamine antagonism may contribute). Used clinically in oesophageal reflux, gastric stasis and non-ulcer dyspepsia. Erythromycin has a powerful prokinetic effect via GIT motilin receptors and has been used in ileus. General parasympathomimetic drugs also increase GIT motility but are rarely used for this purpose.

Prolonged Q–T syndromes. Conditions in which the Q–T interval of the ECG exceeds 0.44 s.

- May be:
  - congenital: due to mutation of genes coding for cardiac sodium or potassium ion channels. The autosomal recessive form is often associated with sensineural deafness. Syncope may be provoked by physical exercise and stress.
  - acquired:
    - myocardial disease, e.g. MI, rheumatic fever, 3rd degree heart block, cardiomyopathy.
    - electrolyte disturbance, e.g. hypocalcaemia, hypokalaemia, hypomagnesaemia.
    - drugs, e.g. class Ia, Ic and III antiarrhythmic drugs, phenothiazines, tricyclic antidepressant drugs, selective serotonin reuptake inhibitors and some antibacterial agents, e.g. erythromycin.
    - severe head injury.

Both forms are associated with the development of ventricular arrhythmias including torsade de pointes and VT, causing recurrent syncope or sudden death. This has been associated with anaesthesia. The risk may be greater if there is also increased Q–Tc dispersion. Avoidance of increased sympathetic tone and use of β-adrenergic receptor antagonists is generally recommended; phenytoin and verapamil have been used to treat acute arrhythmias. Long-term treatment is with β-blockers or cardiac pacing.

Kies SJ, Pabelick CM, Hurley HA, et al (2005). Anesthesiology; 102: 204–10

Promethazine hydrochloride/theoclate. Phenothiazine and antihistamine drug, with sedative, anticholinergic and antiemetic properties. Used for antiemesis, allergic reactions, sedation and premedication, especially in children. Also used topically to relieve pruritus, etc. One component of the lytic cocktail. Well absorbed orally but undergoes extensive first-pass metabolism. Excreted renally following hepatic metabolism.

- Dosage:
  - 25–75 mg orally/day; 0.5–1.0 mg/kg for paediatric premedication.
  - 25–50 mg im or by slow iv injection.
- Side effects are those of phenothiazines and anticholinergic drugs.

Prone ventilation. Technique in which patients are turned prone whilst receiving IPPV, used in ARDS. Improves pulmonary function in approximately 50% of patients, especially in early ARDS. Proposed mechanisms for improved oxygenation include increased FRC (via redistribution of secretions, interstitial oedema and atelectasis away from the posterior areas), changes in regional diaphragmatic excursion, and redistribution of perfusion away from more oedematous lung regions. Patients may be turned regularly, e.g. for up to 8 h every 24 h. Disadvantages during turning include accidental displacement of tubes and catheters/cannulae, damage to eyes/face/limbs, etc., stimulation of coughing and cardiovascular instability; once turned the main problems are inaccessibility and care of pressure areas. These practical problems may be reduced by using rotational therapy instead.

Propafenone hydrochloride. Class Ic antiarrhythmic drug, affecting atria, conducting system and ventricles. Has slight β-adrenergic antagonist properties. Used for preventing and treating supraventricular and ventricular arrhythmias. Undergoes hepatic metabolism and renal excretion.

- Dosage: 150–300 mg orally, 8 hourly.
- Side effects are usually mild and include dizziness, GIT disturbances, blurred vision and bradycardia.

Propofol. 2,6-Diisopropylphenol (Fig. 127). IV anaesthetic agent, first used in 1977 and introduced into clinical practice

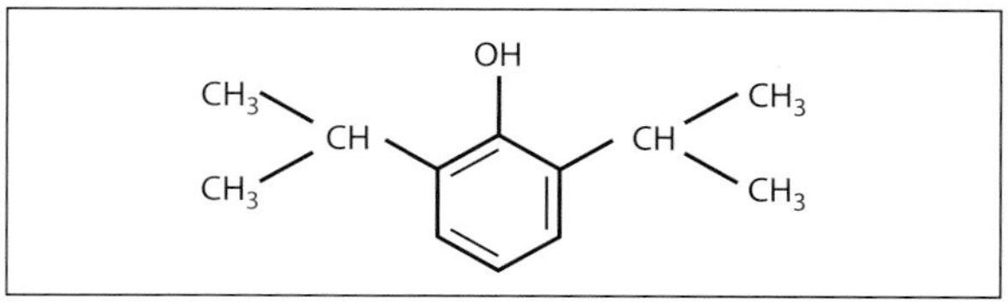

Fig. 127 Structure of propofol

in 1986. Thought to produce anaesthesia by causing potentiation at the $GABA_A$ receptor and possibly by acting on cannabis receptors. Originally prepared with Cremophor EL, but reformulated before commercial release because of fears about allergic reactions. Now presented as an oil–water emulsion: 1% (presented in 20 ml ampoules, 50/100 ml vials and 50 ml prefilled syringes) or 2% (for infusion only and presented in 50 ml vials and 50 ml prefilled syringes), containing 10% soya bean oil, 1.2% egg phosphatide and 2.25% glycerol. A new formulation containing medium-chain triglycerides causes less pain on injection; in addition some formulations contain either 0.005% EDTA or sulphite in an attempt to suppress bacterial growth. Prodrugs and use of alternative drug vehicles have also been studied. pK_a is 11. 98% protein-bound after iv injection. Distribution and elimination half-lives are 1–2 min and 1–5 h respectively; context-sensitive half-life is approximately 20 min after 2 hours' infusion, 30 min after 6 hours' infusion and 50 min after 9 hours' infusion. Metabolised in the liver and excreted renally. Extrahepatic metabolism is suggested by a plasma clearance (25–30 ml/kg/min) which exceeds hepatic blood flow. There are no known active metabolites. Thus recovery is rapid with minimal residual effects, making it a popular agent in short cases, e.g. in day-case surgery. These properties also make it suitable for TIVA and iv sedation.

- Effects:
  - induction:
    - smooth and rapid, with only occasional movements. It has been suggested that loss of response to verbal command is a better indication of adequate dosage than loss of eyelash reflex.
    - pain on injection is common with the standard formulation; it may be reduced by prior injection of, or mixing with, lidocaine.
  - CVS/RS:
    - hypotension is common, although whether caused by direct myocardial depression, reduced SVR or both, is controversial. Normo- or bradycardia is common; resetting of the baroreceptor reflex has been suggested. Reduces the hypertensive response to tracheal intubation.
    - respiratory depression is marked.
    - tends to obtund upper airway reflexes, thus allowing manipulation/instrumentation more readily than thiopental. Thus particularly useful when placing the laryngeal mask airway, etc. Tracheal intubation may be possible after propofol induction without neuromuscular blocking drugs, especially if opioids are also given.
  - CNS:
    - antanalgesia has not been reported.
    - has an antiemetic effect. Increased appetite has been suggested but may reflect the excellent quality of recovery rather than a direct effect.
    - involuntary movements have been reported following propofol, but these are not thought to be epileptiform convulsions. Has been used successfully in intractable epilepsy.
    - reduces cerebral blood flow, ICP and intraocular pressure.
    - dreams may occur. Claims by patients of sexual assault whilst anaesthetised have been made.
  - other: allergic phenomena and delayed recovery have been reported to the Committee on Safety of Medicines.
- Dosage:
  - 1.5–2.5 mg/kg for induction.
  - for maintenance, several regimens have been suggested, based on pharmacokinetic studies, including the Bristol regimen:
    - 10 mg/kg/h for 10 min.
    - 8 mg/kg/h for 10 min.
    - 6 mg/kg/h thereafter, adjusted if required according to clinical response.

    This applies to concurrent use of 66% N_2O, or infusion of alfentanil 30–50 μg/kg/h. More recently a target controlled infusion (TCI) device has been marketed in which prefilled syringes of propofol are loaded and infusion rates automatically adjusted according to the patient's age, weight and required blood concentrations of propofol (in healthy patients, 4–8 μg/ml for induction of anaesthesia and 3–6 μg/ml for maintenance).
  - 1.0–4.0 mg/kg/h for sedation (licensed for up to 3 days).

Contamination during preparation for infusion has led to iatrogenic bacteraemia, and hence the development of the EDTA preparation.

Contains the same energy content as 10% fat emulsion (900 Cal/l). Plasma lipid levels should be monitored in all patients receiving propofol infusions for longer than 3 days.

Not licensed for use in children under 3 years or sedation of children of any age (neurological, cardiac, renal and hepatic impairment have been reported after sedation of children with propofol in ICUs). Myocardial failure and acidosis have been reported after prolonged infusion of high doses in adults, leading to the proposal for a distinct metabolic syndrome, the propofol infusion syndrome.

Propofol infusion syndrome. Progressive myocardial failure, metabolic acidosis, hyperkalaemia and evidence of muscle damage in the absence of other causes, in children and adults receiving infusions of propofol. Typically associated with hyperlipaemia and high infusion rates of propofol (> 4 mg/kg/h) for prolonged periods (> 2 days), it is thought to be related to exacerbation of poor tissue oxygenation and impaired cellular utilisation of glucose, perhaps involving respiratory chain dysfunction. Treatment is supportive and includes withdrawal of propofol; haemodialysis has been used successfully. Mortality is high.

Kam PCA, Cardone D (2007). Anaesthesia; 62: 690–701

Proportional assist ventilation (PAV). Mode of partial ventilatory support in which the ventilator generates an instantaneous inspiratory pressure in proportion to the instantaneous effort of the patient (i.e. does not use preset pressure or volume targets). Intended to facilitate normal neuroventilatory coupling by allowing the patient to control all aspects of breathing (i.e. tidal volume, inspiratory and expiratory durations, and flow patterns), whilst the ventilator functions as an extension of the patient's respiratory muscles. Changes in lung and chest wall impedance may prevent PAV from being fully effective. Has several potential benefits:

- greater patient comfort.
- reduction of peak airway pressure.
- reduced chance of overventilation.
- preservation and enhancement of the patient's own homeostatic control mechanisms.

May be difficult to employ clinically unless facilities for measuring respiratory mechanics are available at the bedside. May have a non-invasive role in COPD.

Propranidid. IV anaesthetic agent, first used in 1956 and withdrawn in 1984. Eugenol (oil of cloves) derivative, prepared in Cremophor EL or polyoxyethylated castor oil. Hydrolysed by plasma and liver esterases. Rapidly acting, with rapid recovery. Hypotension, apnoea following initial hyperventilation, venous thrombosis and adverse drug reactions were common.

Propranolol. β-Adrenergic receptor antagonist (the first to be introduced, in 1964). Non-selective, and without intrinsic sympathomimetic activity. 90–95% protein-bound. Its primary metabolite, 4-hydroxypropanolol, has β-blocking activity. Uses and side effects are as for β-adrenergic receptor antagonists in general.

- Dosage:
  - hypertension, portal hypertension, angina, migraine, phaeochromocytoma: 30–80 mg orally 12 hourly, increased up to 120–320 mg/day.
  - arrhythmias, hypertrophic obstructive cardiomyopathy, anxiety, thyrotoxicosis: 10–40 mg orally 8–12 hourly.
  - acute MI: 40 mg orally 6 hourly for 2–3 days, then 80–160 mg/day.
  - acute iv administration: 1 mg over 1 min, repeated as required up to 5–10 mg.

Propylene glycol. Diol alcohol ($CH_3.CHOH.CH_2OH$), used as a solvent in drugs, e.g. etomidate, GTN, lorazepam. Has been associated with hypotension, lactic acidosis, pulmonary hypertension and haemolysis; these effects are independent of the drug infused.

Prostacyclin. Prostaglandin PGI_2 produced by the intima of blood vessels via the cyclo-oxygenase limb of the arachidonic acid metabolism pathway. The most potent inhibitor of platelet aggregation known, via an increase in cAMP levels. At high doses, may disperse circulating platelet aggregates. Thought to have vital importance in preventing coagulation within normal blood vessels. Also a potent vasodilator drug. Increases renin production and blood glucose levels.

Provided commercially as synthetic epoprostenol sodium, which is reconstituted in saline and glycerine to produce a clear colourless solution of pH 10.5. Used to prevent platelet aggregation during renal dialysis or other forms of extracorporeal circulation; has also been used in pre-eclampsia, pulmonary hypertension, haemolytic uraemic syndrome and septic shock. Half-life is 2–3 min, with cessation of platelet effects within 30 min of stopping an infusion. Its main metabolite is 6-keto-prostaglandin $F_{1\alpha}$.

- Dosage: 2–35 ng/kg/min iv.
- Side effects: flushing, headache, hypotension.

Prostaglandins (PGs). Unsaturated fatty acids containing 20 carbon atoms and a five-membered carbon ring (cyclopentane ring) at one end. Derived from arachidonic acid, and thought to be synthesised in most tissues, although originally isolated from prostatic glands in the 1930s. Named according to the configuration of the cyclopentane ring (e.g. PGA, B, C, etc. to PGI (prostacyclin)), with subscript numbers denoting the number of side-chain double bonds. Involved in many processes throughout the body including immunological and inflammatory responses, temperature regulation, exocrine and endocrine glandular secretion, renal blood flow and renin production, reproductive function, fat metabolism and CNS neurotransmitter activity. They have been implicated in pain perception and local sensitisation of tissues to inflammatory mediators.

Have varying effects on smooth muscle; thus PGE_2, PGI_2 and PGA_2 cause arteriolar dilatation, whilst $PGF_{2\alpha}$ causes vasodilatation in some vascular beds and vasoconstriction in others. $PGF_{2\alpha}$ and PGD_2 cause bronchoconstriction, whereas PGE_2 causes bronchodilatation. PGE_2 and $PGF_{2\alpha}$ cause uterine contraction and are used to induce abortion or labour, e.g. administered vaginally. They may also be given by intra- or extra-amniotic routes for abortion. Oral and iv administration is rarely used, the latter because of side effects including vomiting, diarrhoea, dizziness, pyrexia and rash.

PGE_1 is used iv to maintain patency of the ductus arteriosus in congenital heart disease before corrective surgery. Tachy- or bradycardia, hypotension, pyrexia, DIC and convulsions may occur. It has been studied in the treatment of ARDS. An analogue is available for oral use, to prevent gastric ulcers associated with NSAIDs.

Half-life is at most a few minutes, with local destruction and metabolism of circulating PGs via the pulmonary, hepatic and renal circulations.

Many of the effects of NSAIDs are thought to involve inhibition of PG synthesis.

PGE_2 and $PGF_{2\alpha}$ are given as dinoprostone and carboprost respectively; PGE_1 is given as alprostadil.

Protamine sulphate. Mixture of low molecular weight, cationic, basic proteins prepared from the sperm of salmon and other fish. Used as a heparin antagonist, and in the preparation of protamine zinc insulin. Has an anticoagulant effect when given alone in high doses, via inhibition of formation and action of thromboplastin. Binds and inactivates anionic, acidic heparin, forming a stable salt.

- Dosage: 1 mg iv neutralises 100 U mucous heparin if given within 15 min of the latter's administration; less is required after longer intervals. Dosage is usually adjusted according to the patient's coagulation status. Should be given slowly; individual doses should not exceed 50 mg.
- Side effects: myocardial depression, bradycardia, pulmonary hypertension, histamine release, complement activation, anaphylactic reaction. These effects are more likely following rapid administration. Chronic exposure in diabetics, previous vasectomy or allergy to fish may predispose to allergic reactions.

Protein-binding. Occurs for many blood-borne substances, e.g. bilirubin, mineral ions, hormones, and many drugs. Important in drug pharmacokinetics because only the free unbound fraction is available to cross membranes, produce its effects, or be metabolised or excreted. Free fraction of drug is affected by plasma protein levels, drug concentration, pH and presence of other substances which compete for the same binding sites. Thus one substance may be displaced from protein binding sites by another. The drug–protein complex may act as an antigen in adverse drug reactions.

- The main proteins involved are:
  - albumin: binds acidic drugs, e.g. thiopental, phenytoin, warfarin, salicylates.
  - α_1-acid glycoprotein: binds basic drugs, e.g. local anaesthetic agents, propranolol, quinidine.
  - globulins: bind e.g. tubocurarine.

Protein-binding within the CNS may be involved in the mechanism of action of anaesthetic agents.

See also, Anaesthesia, mechanism of; Drug interactions; Hypoproteinaemia

Protein C. Endogenous plasma protein, capable of promoting fibrinolysis and inhibiting thrombosis and inflammation. The circulating inactive form is activated by the enzyme complex of thrombin coupled with thrombomodulin (an endothelial surface membrane protein). Activated protein C blocks the activated forms of coagulation factors V and VIII, thereby inhibiting prothrombinase and factor X-ase complexes. Activation of protein C may be impaired during sepsis and protein C may also be consumed. Reduced levels of protein C are associated with an increased mortality. Protein C is now available in a recombinant human form (drotrecogin alfa). Early studies suggest a marked reduction in mortality if drotrecogin is given to patients with severe sepsis. Side effects include haemorrhage.

Inherited protein C abnormalities include protein C deficiency and activated protein C resistance (most commonly factor V Leiden), both of which predispose to venous thrombosis.

[Leiden; city in Netherlands where the factor was first identified in 1993]

Bernard GR, Vincent JL, Laterre PF, et al (2001). N Engl J Med; 344: 699–707

Protein:creatinine ratio (PCR). Ratio of protein to creatinine in a random urine sample, used as a more accurate quantitative indicator of proteinuria than simple stick testing whilst not requiring a 24-h urine collection. Has been found to correlate reasonably well with 24-h protein; e.g. PCRs < 1 and > 3 (or $<$ 10 and $>$ 30 mg/mmol, depending on the units of measurement) are consistent with 24-h protein excretions of < 1 g and $>$ 3 g respectively. Albumin:creatinine ratio has also been used.

Proteins. Polypeptide chains of amino acids (usually defined as over 50–500). May incorporate carbohydrates or fats. Present in all cell protoplasm and required for growth and healing. Involved in:

- structure, e.g. collagen, myosin, actin, membranes.
- enzymes.
- hormones and precursors.
- blood components, e.g. immunoglobulins, haemoglobin, albumin.

See also, Nitrogen balance; Nutrition

Prothrombin time, *see Coagulation studies*

Proton pump inhibitors. Group of drugs that selectively inhibit the H^+/K^+-ATPase enzyme located on the luminal surface of the gastric parietal cells, thus virtually abolishing gastric acid production. Used to treat peptic ulcer disease, severe gastro-oesophageal reflux and to decrease the risk from aspiration of gastric contents in high risk patients. Should be used with caution in liver disease. Include omeprazole, lasoprazole, pantoprazole and rabeprazole.

Pruritus. Itch-like sensation in the absence of a normal stimulus; can arise from cutaneous, neurological or psychological triggers. Afferent pathways associated in itching involve a number of inflammatory mediators, in particular histamine peripherally and 5-HT centrally.

- Causes may be:
  - cutaneous:
    - release of histamine, e.g. due to drugs (systemic morphine, cyclizine, antibiotics, anaphylactic/anaphylactoid reactions) or other cutaneous stimuli including trauma, infections/infestations, inflammatory conditions including those associated with systemic disease.
    - deposition of other irritant substances e.g. bile salts, calcium.
    - other skin diseases.
  - neurological:
    - interaction with central neurotransmitters (e.g. epidural/spinal opioids).
    - cerebral lesions.
    - peripheral neuropathy.
  - psychological.

Thus often seen after administration of anaesthetic or related drugs. Although many drugs, especially propofol and ondansetron, have been studied as possible prophylactic or therapeutic agents, there is little evidence to support the use of most. For systemic opioid-induced pruritus, antihistamine drugs may be used, while opioid receptor antagonists are effective following epidural/spinal opioids.

Waxler B, Dadabhoy Z, Stojiljkovic L, Rabito S (2005). Anesthesiology; 103: 168–78

Pseudocholinesterase, *see Cholinesterase, plasma*

Pseudocritical temperature. Temperature at which gas mixtures separate into their component parts. Varies with pressure: for Entonox, highest (−5.5°C) at 117 bar, and decreases above and below this pressure. Thus equals −7°C for Entonox cylinders (135 bar) and −30°C for pipelines (4 bar).

Pseudomembranous colitis. Inflammation of the large bowel characterised by diarrhoea, abdominal pain, fever, and blood and mucus in the stool; presentation ranges from an asymptomatic carrier state to fulminant life-threatening colitis. Caused by toxins produced by *Clostridium difficile*, usually associated with use of antibacterial drugs (especially clindamycin) and immunosuppressive therapy. The use of proton pump inhibitors may be a risk factor. Diagnosis is confirmed by culture of the organism and detection of the toxin in the faeces. Colonoscopy reveals pseudomembranes consisting of fibrin and leucocytes. Infection spreads between patients by environmental contamination and direct cross-infection.

- Management:
  - withdrawal of antibacterial drugs if possible.
  - rehydration.
  - metronidazole 400 mg orally 8 hourly (or 500 mg iv), or vancomycin 125–250 mg orally 6 hourly, for 7–10 days.

Starr J (2005). BMJ; 331: 498–501

Pseudomonas infections. Commonly seen in hospitals since colonisation of the GIT with the Gram-negative organism occurs within days of admission. Systemic effects occur via release of endo- and exotoxins. Spread may result in nosocomial infection including catheter-related sepsis, severe chest infection (especially in those requiring IPPV), meningitis and general features of sepsis. Infection typically results in a characteristic odour. Treatment following culture and sensitivity testing consists of an antipseudomonas penicillin (or third generation cephalosporin) combined with an aminoglycoside.

Psoas compartment block. Used to block the lumbar plexus and part of the sacral plexus, which lie between psoas major anteriorly and quadratus lumborum posteriorly, e.g. for leg surgery.

With the patient in the lateral position with hips flexed, a skin wheal is raised 5 cm lateral to the lower border of the spinous process of L5. A 15 cm needle is inserted perpendicular to the skin until it contacts the transverse process, then withdrawn and redirected slightly cranially to pass the process. A syringe is attached and a loss-of-resistance technique used to identify the psoas compartment (usually at 10–12 cm) as for epidural anaesthesia. 30–40 ml local anaesthetic agent is injected.

Complications include subarachnoid, epidural and iv injection.

Psychological aspects of intensive care, *see Confusion in the intensive care unit; ICU psychosis; Intensive care follow-up; Post-traumatic stress disorder*

Psychoprophylaxis. Technique used in obstetric analgesia and anaesthesia to increase comfort and relaxation during labour. Requires preparation during pregnancy, with education about pregnancy and labour, and training in relaxation and breathing techniques. During labour, deep breathing during contractions, and the concentration this requires, helps the mother to cope with the pain.

PT, Prothrombin time, *see Coagulation studies*

PTS, *see Paediatric trauma score*

PTT, Partial thromboplastin time, *see Coagulation studies*

Pudendal nerve block. Used bilaterally to provide analgesia in obstetric analgesia and anaesthesia, especially for forceps and ventouse delivery. The pudendal nerve (S2–4) arises from the sacral plexus and leaves the pelvis through the greater sciatic foramen, passing behind the ischial spine and sacrospinal ligament to re-enter the pelvis through the lesser sciatic foramen. It supplies the perineum, vulva and lower vagina.

- Techniques:
  - transvaginal approach: with the patient in the lithotomy position, two fingers palpate the ischial spine from within the vagina. A 12.5 cm guarded needle is introduced 1.2 cm beyond the spine, into the sacrospinal ligament, and the needle point extended. After negative aspiration for blood, 10 ml local anaesthetic agent is injected.
  - transperineal approach: a needle is introduced through a point midway between the anus and ischial tuberosity, and directed as above by a finger in the vagina.

Local infiltration of the labia is required to block cutaneous branches of the genitofemoral and ilioinguinal nerves.

Has a high failure rate in obstetrics, exacerbated by inadequate time between performance of the block and attempted delivery.

Pugh, Benjamin (1715–1718). Shropshire-born surgeon and apothecary; practised in Essex. Early advocate of vaccination against smallpox and author of 'A Treatise of Midwifery' in 1754. Advocated the use of an air pipe, inserted into the larynx, to maintain the airway of neonates during delayed breech extraction.

Baskett TF (2000). Resuscitation; 44: 153–5

See also, Cardiopulmonary resuscitation, neonatal

Pulmonary artery catheterisation. Performed using flow-directed balloon-tipped pulmonary artery catheters, introduced into clinical practice in the early 1970s by Swan and Ganz (after whom one commercial device is named) amongst much controversy.

- Catheters may have some of the following features:
  - 70 cm long, marked every 10 cm.
  - channels/lumina:
    - distal (opens at the tip).
    - proximal (opens 30 cm from the tip).
    - for inflating the balloon (1–1.5 ml air used).
    - connections to a thermistor, a few cm from the tip.
    - fibreoptic bundles for continuous oximetry.
    - others include those for cardiac pacing, Doppler imaging, etc.
- Insertion:
  - all lumina are prefilled with heparinised saline, and the balloon checked.
  - aseptic technique is used. The catheter is usually passed through a sterile plastic protective sleeve to allow manipulation without contamination after insertion.
  - insertion is as for central venous cannulation, usually employing the Seldinger technique. The right internal jugular vein is most commonly used. The catheter is threaded down an 8 G introducer sheath, with continuous visible pressure monitoring from the distal lumen. The balloon is inflated in the right atrium and directed by the flow of blood into the pulmonary artery via the right ventricle. Pulmonary capillary wedge pressure is displayed when the balloon occludes a pulmonary vessel; the catheter tip is now separated from the left atrium by a continuous column of blood. Placement is confirmed by the changes in the pressure trace obtained (Fig. 128).
  - coiling and/or knotting of the catheter within the heart may occur if excessive length of catheter is inserted without a change in the pressure trace.
  - once inserted, the balloon is left deflated until wedge pressure measurement is required, to reduce risk of pulmonary artery damage and infarction. The distal lumen pressure should always be displayed, to alert to accidental wedging.
  - use of a catheter is often limited to 2–3 days to reduce risk of complications.
- Information gained:
  - mixed venous, right atrial and ventricular gas tensions and O_2 saturations; e.g. for estimation of cardiac shunt, etc. Continuous monitoring of mixed venous O_2 saturation is possible via fibreoptic bundles.
  - measurement of right atrial and ventricular pressures, pulmonary artery pressure and pulmonary capillary wedge pressure. By convention, measured at end-systole and end-expiration.
  - measurement of right ventricular ejection fraction.
  - cardiac output measurement.
  - derived data:
    - systemic and pulmonary vascular resistance.
    - cardiac index, stroke volume/index.
- Uses, e.g. perioperatively and in ICU:
  - investigating cardiac shunts.
  - monitoring the above pressures and optimising fluid therapy; particularly useful when right atrial pressures do not reflect left heart function; e.g. left ventricular failure or infarction, severe bundle branch block, pulmonary hypertension, cardiac tamponade and constrictive pericarditis, valvular heart disease (*for*

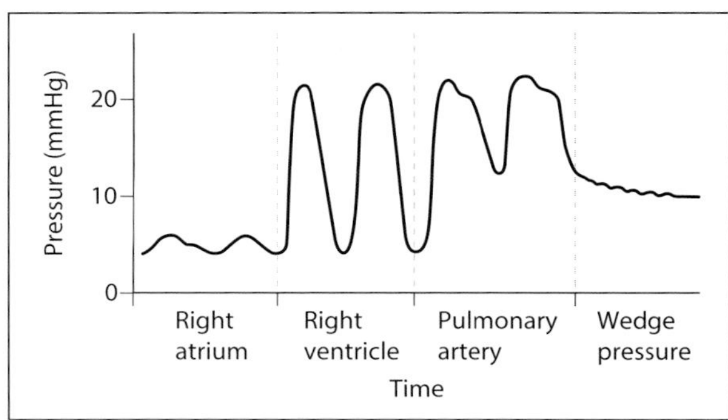

Fig. 128 Pressure trace obtained during placement of a pulmonary artery catheter

interpretation, etc., see Pulmonary capillary wedge pressure).
- measuring cardiac output and derived data.
- monitoring mixed venous O_2 saturation as a continuous indicator of cardiac output and tissue perfusion, e.g. in ICU.
- as a route for cardiac pacing.
- infusion of drugs into the pulmonary circulation, e.g. prostacyclin in pulmonary hypertension.

- Complications:
  - as for central venous cannulation.
  - arrhythmias.
  - infection.
  - catheter knotting.
  - damage to valves, myocardium, etc.
  - pulmonary artery damage or rupture.
  - pulmonary infarction.
  - incorrect positioning, measurement and interpretation.

Although previously widely used in critically ill patients, there is no clear evidence previously that their use reduces overall morbidity and mortality; indeed there is even a suggestion that they are associated with increased mortality. It is generally accepted that the decision to use a pulmonary artery catheter should be based on the risk/benefit ratio for each individual patient, it should be inserted by a well-trained physician, and the data arising from it should be considered in the context of the whole patient and not taken on their own.
[Harold JC Swan (1922–2005), Irish-born US cardiologist; William Ganz, Los Angeles cardiologist]

Pulmonary artery pressure (PAP). Typically one-fifth of systemic circulatory pressure; normal ranges are 15–30 mmHg systolic, 0–8 mmHg diastolic and 10–15 mmHg mean. Usually measured by right-sided cardiac catheterisation. Changes may indicate changes in pulmonary capillary wedge pressure and pulmonary vascular resistance.

Pulmonary capillary wedge pressure (PCWP; Pulmonary wedge pressure, PWP; Pulmonary artery occlusion pressure, PAOP). Pressure measured within the pulmonary arterial system during pulmonary artery catheterisation, with the catheter's tip 'wedged' in a tapering branch of one of the pulmonary arteries. In most patients, represents left atrial filling pressure and thus left ventricular end-diastolic pressure (LVEDP). Thus an indirect indicator of left ventricular end-diastolic volume and myocardial fibre length (*see Starling's law*). Also indicates the likelihood (with measurement of plasma colloid osmotic pressure) of pulmonary oedema formation, assuming normal pulmonary capillary permeability.

- Normal range: 6–12 mmHg; usually 1–4 mmHg less than pulmonary artery diastolic pressure (PADP). Traditionally measured at end-expiration.
- Values should be interpreted with caution in:
  - left ventricular failure: LVEDP may exceed PCWP.
  - mitral valve disease: in stenosis PCWP may exceed LVEDP; in regurgitation large 'v' waves interfere with the PCWP waveform.
  - raised intrathoracic pressure, e.g. PEEP: LVEDP may exceed PCWP.
  - non-compliant left ventricle: LVEDP may exceed PCWP.
  - aortic regurgitation: LVEDP may greatly exceed PCWP.

Gradients between PADP, PCWP and LVEDP may be increased in tachycardia and increased pulmonary vascular resistance. The position of the catheter tip is also important; a continuous column of blood between the catheter and the left ventricle only occurs if the tip lies in zone 3 of the lung (*see Pulmonary circulation*). Although the catheter usually flows to zone 3, especially in the supine position, repositioning of the patient may alter the zonal distribution.

The waveform resembles the venous waveform, with 'a', 'c' and 'v' waves, and swings with respiration. PCWP should not exceed PADP.

As with CVP interpretation, trends are more useful than single values. Response of PCWP to drug or iv fluid administration may be used to indicate intravascular volume status and cardiac function, and guide therapy. Pulmonary oedema is likely at PCWP above 18–20 mmHg, with normal colloid osmotic pressure.
Pinsky MR (2003). Intensive Care Med; 29: 19–22

Pulmonary circulation. Low pressure/low resistance system in series with the systemic circulation; it receives the whole cardiac output. The pulmonary artery divides after about 4 cm into right and left main pulmonary arteries. Pulmonary arteries are thin walled and easily distensible, and lie close to the corresponding airways in connective tissue sheaths, eventually dividing to form capillaries with a total gas exchange interface of about 70 m^2. Venules run close to the septa which separate the lung segments and finally drain into four main pulmonary veins which deliver oxygenated blood into the left atrium.

The separate bronchial circulation supplies the airways down to the respiratory bronchioles, local connective tissue and the visceral pleura; it arises from the aorta and eventually drains via the azygos system into the pulmonary veins, i.e. representing an anatomical shunt.

The diameter of 'extra-alveolar' vessels (those running through lung parenchyma) is affected by lung volume, via the pull of lung parenchyma on their walls. That of 'alveolar' pulmonary vessels (predominantly capillaries) depends on the difference between arterial (P_a), venous (P_v) and alveolar (P_A) pressures, and thus on gravity. Four zones have been described by West, from above downwards:
- zone 1: lung apex; P_A exceeds both P_a and P_v; thus no flow occurs. Does not occur at normal BP in normal lungs.
- zone 2: $P_a > P_A > P_v$; thus flow depends on the difference between P_a and P_A, and not on P_v.
- zone 3: $P_a > P_v > P_A$; i.e. flow depends on the difference between P_a and P_v, as usually occurs in other tissues.
- zone 4: suggested as existing at lung bases; pulmonary interstitial pressure exceeds P_a, thus impairing blood flow.

The vessels are supplied by sympathetic vasoconstrictor (α-receptors) and vasodilator (β_2-receptors) fibres, and by parasympathetic vasodilator fibres. However, resting vascular tone is minimal, with vessels almost maximally dilated in the resting state. Other factors affecting vessel calibre include vascular responses to local changes, e.g. hypoxic pulmonary vasoconstriction and other factors affecting pulmonary vascular resistance.

The pulmonary circulation contains about 10–20% of the total blood volume (i.e. 0.5–1.0 l). It changes during respiration (especially IPPV) and may increase by 25–40% in moving from the erect to the supine position.
[John B West, Californian physiologist]
Fischer LG, van Aken H, Burkle H (2003). Anesth Analg; 96: 1603–16
See also, Starling resistor; Ventilation/perfusion mismatch

Pulmonary embolism (PE). Mechanical obstruction of a pulmonary artery/arteriole; usually refers to blood-borne thrombus. The most common cause of death within the first

10 postoperative days. Thrombus usually arises from a DVT in the legs/pelvis, although the venae cavae and right side of the heart are sometimes sources. The effects depend on the size and distribution of the PE; release of vasoactive mediators, e.g. prostaglandins, may contribute to resultant vasospasm. Massive PEs cause rapid respiratory and cardiovascular collapse, and death. Smaller PEs may cause few haemodynamic effects, but may result in infarction of a section of lung tissue if collateral blood flow is inadequate. Multiple PEs may cause widespread pulmonary vascular obstruction and lead to pulmonary hypertension.

Risk factors are as for DVT.

- Features:
  - pleuritic chest pain, haemoptysis, dyspnoea and mild pyrexia in small PEs.
  - cyanosis, tachypnoea, hypotension, tachycardia, raised JVP and bronchospasm. 3rd and 4th heart sounds may be present. A pleural rub may develop.
  - arterial blood gas analysis reveals hypoxaemia and hypocapnia, with subsequent metabolic acidosis in severe PE. During anaesthesia, end-tidal CO_2 concentration may fall dramatically because of increased dead space and reduced cardiac output.
  - right axis deviation, right bundle branch block and T inversion in leads V_{1-4} may occur in the ECG; both a normal ECG and the 'classic' $S_1Q_3T_3$ pattern are rarely seen.
  - chest X-ray may show enlarged proximal pulmonary arteries with peripheral oligaemia, but is usually non-specific. Wedge-shaped infarcts (Hampton's hump), elevation of the ipsilateral diaphragm and pleural effusion may subsequently develop.

Definitive diagnosis is by pulmonary angiography or ventilation–perfusion scan, with simultaneous inhalation and iv injection of radioisotopes to demonstrate areas of adequate ventilation but absent perfusion. Perfusion-only scans may also be useful. Recent UK guidelines recommend CT angiography as the initial investigation of choice. MRI and echocardiography imaging techniques have also been used.

Features of DVT may be present. A normal D-dimer concentration reliably excludes PE.

- Management:
  - immediate CPR if required. A precordial thump may break up a large PE and improve circulation.
  - O_2 therapy, iv fluids, inotropic drugs, analgesia.
  - anticoagulation: heparin initially (low mw recommended except for the first dose or when rapid anticoagulation and/or the ability to reverse it is required), with substitution by warfarin as for DVT. Fibrinolytic drugs have also been used, especially for large and life-threatening emboli.
  - pulmonary embolectomy may be required for large PEs. Ligation of the inferior vena cava/superficial femoral vein, or insertion of a vena caval umbrella, may be required for recurrent PEs.

[Aubrey Otis Hampton (1900–1955), US radiologist]

Tapson VF (2008). N Engl J Med; 358: 1037–52

See also, Air embolism; Amniotic fluid embolism; Fat embolism

Pulmonary fibrosis. Thickening and infiltration of alveolar walls and perialveolar tissue.

- May result from:
  - localised loss of lung parenchyma, e.g. following infection, infarction or aspiration of irritant substances (e.g. aspiration of gastric contents). Causes decreased movement and breath sounds, dullness to percussion and increased vocal resonance. Neighbouring structures, e.g. trachea, may be pulled towards the affected portion.
  - generalised alveolitis. A degree of fibrosis may remain following ARDS.

Loss of the pulmonary vascular bed may lead to pulmonary hypertension and cor pulmonale. Typically, there is hypoxaemia with hypocapnia due to hyperventilation. $\dot{V}/\dot{Q}$ mismatch is now thought to be responsible for the hypoxaemia, rather than alveolar membrane thickening as previously suspected. Diffusing capacity, compliance and lung volumes are reduced, with normal FEV_1/FVC ratio. Work of breathing is increased; patients usually take small breaths at rapid rates. Chest X-ray may reveal diffuse nodular/reticular shadowing, with local contraction in focal disease.

Treatment is of the underlying cause; corticosteroids are often used.

- Anaesthesia: although the pulmonary defect is restrictive instead of obstructive, principles are as for COPD.

Pulmonary function tests, *see Lung function tests*

Pulmonary hypertension. Definitions vary, but it has been defined as mean pulmonary artery pressure (PAP) > 25 mmHg at rest or > 30 mmHg during exercise. May be primary, but is usually secondary to:

- pulmonary venous/capillary hypertension, e.g. in left ventricular failure, mitral stenosis.
- increased pulmonary blood flow caused by left-to-right cardiac shunts, e.g. ASD, VSD, patent ductus arteriosus.
- increased pulmonary vascular resistance (PVR), e.g. in COPD, recurrent PE, pulmonary fibrosis.

Chronic hypoxaemia, acidosis, polycythaemia and other factors which increase PVR may be involved in development of pulmonary hypertension.

The pulmonary arteries show medial hypertrophy and intimal thickening. The right ventricle becomes hypertrophied and dilates when right ventricular failure supervenes.

- Features:
  - fatigue, dyspnoea, angina, syncope, haemoptysis.
  - low cardiac output, cyanosis, features of right ventricular enlargement/failure, e.g. sternal heave, peripheral oedema. On auscultation: reduced splitting of the second heart sound, with loud pulmonary component.
  - ECG findings: right axis deviation, right bundle branch block, right atrial and ventricular hypertrophy. Chest X-ray: right atrial and ventricular enlargement, large pulmonary arteries with peripheral pruning.

Usually progressive and fatal in primary disease, which is more common in young women. Treatment may include calcium channel blocking drugs, warfarin, and heart–lung transplantation. More recently, prostacyclin analogues (iv or inhaled), endothelin antagonists, e.g. bosentan, nitric oxide and sildenafil have been investigated with some success. Treatment of secondary disease is directed towards the underlying cause.

Anaesthetic management is based on avoidance of factors which further increase PVR. Monitoring of pulmonary capillary wedge pressure is more informative than CVP measurement, but risk of pulmonary artery rupture is increased. Vasodilator drugs have been used, e.g. sodium nitroprusside, GTN and phentolamine, but none is specific to the pulmonary circulation; thus systemic hypotension may occur. Use of prostacyclin and other newer treatments (see above) have been reported.

Blaise G, Langleben D, Hubert B (2003). Anesthesiology 99: 1415–32

See also, Cor pulmonale

Pulmonary irritant receptors. Receptors situated between airway epithelial cells, responsible for initiating bronchospasm and hyperpnoea in response to inhaled noxious gases, smoke, dust and cold air. Afferent impulses pass via the vagi to the medulla. May be involved in initiating asthma attacks.

Pulmonary oedema. Increased pulmonary ECF (normally minimal). Small amounts of fluid normally pass through the capillary wall into the interstitial space of the lung. The junctions between alveolar epithelial cells are relatively resistant to fluid, which is removed by the lymphatic system at about 10 ml/h. Lymphatic removal may increase dramatically if transudation into the interstitial space increases. Net flux into the interstitial space is governed by Starling forces.

- Mechanisms of formation of pulmonary oedema:
  - alteration of Starling forces:
    - increased hydrostatic pressure, e.g. hypervolaemia, left ventricular failure, mitral stenosis.
    - decreased plasma oncotic pressure, e.g. hypoproteinaemia.
    - acute severe subatmospheric airway pressure, e.g. upper airway obstruction.
  - damage to the alveolar–capillary membrane, e.g. ARDS.
  - impairment of lymphatic drainage, e.g. lymphangitis carcinomatosis, silicosis.
  - causes of uncertain aetiology:
    - neurogenic: thought to involve sudden catecholamine release following head injury, with vasoconstriction increasing lung capillary pressures and capillary permeability.
    - following naloxone administration: also thought to involve catecholamine release.
    - in opioid poisoning, possibly related to decreased vascular permeability.
    - following pulmonary surgery or re-expansion of a pneumothorax: probably involves local changes in capillary pressures and permeability.
    - after exposure to high altitude, possibly via pulmonary vasoconstriction.

As fluid clearance mechanisms are overwhelmed, interstitial oedema increases, until alveolar oedema occurs. Eventually, frothy oedema fluid fills the airways, impairing gas exchange. Airways and pulmonary vessels become narrowed by interstitial oedema, and FRC and compliance decrease.

- Features:
  - dyspnoea, tachypnoea, cough with pink frothy sputum, and tachycardia. Respiratory distress is worse lying flat (orthopnoea).
  - wheeze and basal crepitations on auscultation.
  - features of respiratory failure.
  - arterial blood gas analysis usually reveals hypoxaemia, with hypocapnia secondary to hyperventilation. Metabolic acidosis may be present in severe cases.
  - chest X-ray features include those of the underlying condition. Lung oedema itself appears as fluffy shadowing, typically perihilar ('bat's wing') in left ventricular failure and patchy ('cotton-wool') and peripheral in ARDS. Bronchial and vascular markings may appear thickened due to interstitial oedema. Kerley's B lines and fluid in the transverse fissure may be present.

Differentiation between hydrostatic and other causes may be aided by measurement of pulmonary capillary wedge pressure. Alveolar fluid protein content may also be measured. Total lung water content has been measured using radioactive or dye dilution techniques.

- Treatment of severe acute pulmonary oedema:
  - of the underlying condition.
  - O_2 therapy. CPAP may be useful.
  - sitting the patient, with the legs over the edge of the bed.
  - diuretics, e.g. furosemide 20–120 mg iv (causes vasodilatation and diuresis).
  - opioids, e.g. morphine, diamorphine 1–5 mg iv (reduce anxiety and cause vasodilatation).
  - inotropic and vasodilator drugs.
  - IPPV may be required. Gas exchange is usually improved by PEEP.
  - traditionally, venesection has been performed for cardiogenic pulmonary oedema, with removal of 200–500 ml blood. Placing tourniquets on each limb in turn has also been used.

Ware LS, Matthay MA (2005). N Engl J Med; 353: 2788–96

Pulmonary stretch receptors. Mechanoreceptors within the airway smooth muscle; transmit impulses via the vagi to the dorsal medulla. Excitation limits inspiration during pulmonary overinflation (Hering–Breuer reflex). Sensitivity is increased by decreased arterial $P\text{CO}_2$ and increased pulmonary venous pressure. May also be involved in other pulmonary reflexes, e.g. gasp and deflation reflexes.

Pulmonary valve lesions. Include:

- pulmonary stenosis (PS): may occur at the valve (90%), infundibulum or within the artery. Almost always congenital, accounting for 5–10% of congenital heart disease. Other causes include rheumatic fever and carcinoid syndrome. Usually asymptomatic; if severe, PS may cause fatigue, dyspnoea and angina secondary to decreased cardiac output. Right ventricular (and later atrial) hypertrophy may occur. May be associated with right-to-left shunt and cyanosis, e.g. Fallot's tetralogy.

  Features: ejection systolic murmur at the upper left sternal edge, heard best during inspiration. Splitting of the second heart sound is increased, with a quiet pulmonary component in severe PS. Right ventricular and atrial enlargement may be shown on the ECG and chest X-ray; a prominent pulmonary artery and pulmonary oligaemia may appear on the latter.

  During anaesthesia, increased right ventricular O_2 consumption (e.g. caused by tachycardia and increased contractility) should be avoided.
- pulmonary regurgitation (PR): usually a feature of pulmonary hypertension, and results from dilatation of the valve ring. Other causes include congenital absence of the valve, endocarditis (usually in iv drug abusers), and surgical valvotomy. Causes right ventricular hypertrophy, but usually with little clinical effect.

  Features: high-pitched blowing diastolic murmur at the upper left sternal edge.

Pulmonary vascular resistance (PVR). Resistance in the pulmonary circulation, analogous to SVR. May be calculated using the principle of Ohm's law:

$$\text{PVR (dyne s/cm}^5) = \frac{\text{mean pulmonary artery pressure} - \text{left atrial pressure (mmHg)} \times 80}{\text{cardiac output (l/min)}}$$

where 80 is a correction factor.

Normally 20–120 dyne s/cm^5 (n.b. 1 dyne s/cm^5 = 100 N s/m^5).

Resistance is distributed more evenly than in the systemic circulation, with approximately 50% residing in the arteries and arterioles, 30% in the capillaries and 20% in the veins. The pulmonary arteries are thin walled, large in diameter and easily distensible. The pulmonary circulation is therefore more dependent on gravity, posture and the relationship between alveolar and intravascular pressures than on vascular muscular tone.

- PVR is affected by:
  - passive factors:
    - lung expansion: at lung volumes below FRC, the radial forces acting on the extra-alveolar vessels and holding them open are reduced, thus increasing PVR. However, at high lung volumes, the increased airway pressures associated with hyperexpansion may compress the vessels, also increasing PVR. PVR is lowest at lung volumes around FRC.
    - intravascular pressures: PVR falls when either pulmonary artery pressure or pulmonary venous pressure increases, because of recruitment of previously closed vessels or distension of individual capillary segments.
    - cardiac output: as pulmonary blood flow increases, vessel diameter increases, thus reducing PVR.
    - haematocrit and blood viscosity.
  - active factors via changes in muscle tone:
    - hypoxia (*see Hypoxic pulmonary vasoconstriction*), hypercapnia and acidosis increase PVR, especially in combination, whilst their opposites decrease PVR.
    - drugs and biological mediators, e.g. vasoconstrictor drugs, 5-HT and histamine increase PVR whilst vasodilator drugs, nitric oxide, prostacyclin and acetylcholine decrease it. Drugs may also affect PVR via changes in cardiac output and lung volumes.
    - nervous control: sympathetic nervous system supplies vasoconstrictor (α-adrenergic receptor) and vasodilator (β-adrenergic receptor) fibres to the pulmonary vessels, whilst the parasympathetic nervous system supplies cholinergic vasodilator fibres.

  In addition, local vascular resistance may be increased by PE, atelectasis, pleural effusions, surgery, etc.

PVR may be corrected for differences in body size by multiplying by body surface area (PVR index).

See also, Lung; Pulmonary artery catheterisation; Pulmonary hypertension

Pulse. Traditionally palpated at the wrist, but commonly palpated at the head and neck during anaesthesia (*see Carotid arteries*).

- Should be assessed for:
  - heart rate: speed, rhythm, regularity.
  - volume and character, i.e. reflecting pulse pressure and arterial waveform. Pulsus alternans and pulsus paradoxus are two specific abnormalities.
  - simultaneous pulsation at upper and lower limb arteries; femoral delay occurs in coarctation of the aorta.

Pulse deficit. Difference between the auscultated heart rate and palpated pulse rate. Occurs when one heart beat follows another so quickly that ventricular filling is insufficient for a palpable pulsation, e.g. in ventricular ectopic beats and AF.

Pulse detector. Several devices have been used to detect the pulse, e.g. to monitor heart rate or to aid in arterial BP measurement. Each utilises a small transducer positioned over a peripheral artery or attached to a digit:

- microphone or Doppler probe.
- finger probe containing a light source and photocell which detects changes in reflected or transmitted light due to arterial pulsation.

Simple devices emit a noise or flashing light in time with the pulse, or register the pulse rate on a meter. These have been largely replaced by more sophisticated devices displaying a waveform, e.g. pulse oximeter.

Pulse oximeter. Device used to determine arterial O_2 saturation using oximetry. Consists of the following components:

- two light-emitting diodes (LEDs) within the probe emit monochromatic light at red (660 nm) and infra-red (940 nm) wavelengths.
- a photodiode on the opposite side of the probe detects the transmitted light; since it is unable to differentiate between the wavelengths, each LED is alternately switched on and off, the timing of which allows identification of red and infra-red pulses. The periods when both LEDs are off allow compensation for ambient light conditions.
- the signal is converted to a DC component representing tissue background, venous blood and the constant part of arterial blood flow, and an AC component representing pulsatile arterial blood flow. The former is discarded, the latter amplified and averaged over a few seconds.
- the signal is displayed ideally as a continuous trace, showing quality of signal and a numerical value of S_pO_2 (suggested as appropriate notation of S_aO_2 measured by a pulse oximeter). Most modern machines automatically adjust gain to maintain a constant size of trace.

Used in routine monitoring, e.g. during and after anaesthesia and on ICU, but particularly useful during one-lung anaesthesia, poor-risk cases, paediatric anaesthesia, or where observation of cyanosis is difficult, e.g. dark skin, darkened room or poor access to the patient. Oximetry has also been used to monitor sleep apnoea, in cardiac and respiratory function testing, CPR and assessment of peripheral circulation. It has been shown to detect desaturation in patients when clinical assessment reveals no abnormality, e.g. during anaesthesia, recovery and transport of patients.

- Inaccuracy may result from excessive ambient light, movement artifact, low perfusion states, electrical interference, venous congestion, and when S_aO_2 is less than 50%. Coloured nail polish may produce inaccuracies (tend to increase readings). Effects of other pigments, etc.:
  - carboxyhaemoglobin: most is counted as HbO, thus S_pO_2 is falsely high.
  - methaemoglobin and bilirubin: counted as Hb, thus S_pO_2 is falsely low (but may be falsely high if true saturation is very low, i.e. $< 70\%$).
  - methylthioninium chloride (methylene blue), indocyanine green, etc.: may temporarily decrease S_pO_2 for a few minutes after iv injection.
  - fetal haemoglobin, polycythaemia: no effect.

Machines are calibrated during manufacture. Some are preset for low values of carboxyhaemoglobin and methaemoglobin. Others have specific filters.

Burns have been reported following prolonged use, especially with finger probes on children.

Pulse pressure. Difference between systolic and diastolic blood pressures, normally about 35–45 mmHg. Depends on:

- stroke volume.
- compliance of the arterial tree; e.g. increased in the elderly, because of arterial calcification and reduced compliance.
- duration and speed of ventricular ejection.
- aortic valve function.
- site of measurement; increased as the arterial waveform moves peripherally.

See also, Pulse

Pulseless electrical activity (PEA). Cardiac state in which there are myocardial contractions but these are too weak to produce a detectable cardiac output. Should be distinguished from electromechanical dissociation (EMD), in which there are no contractions despite apparently adequate electrical activity. The term pseudo-EMD has been proposed for PEA in which flow is so low it cannot be detected by non-invasive means.
See also, Cardiac arrest

Pulsus alternans. Alternating weak and strong pulses reflecting similar alterations in left ventricular filling and output. Common in left ventricular failure.
See also, Arterial waveform

Pulsus paradoxus. Usually defined as a decrease in arterial BP greater than 10 mmHg on inspiration, caused by reduced left ventricular output secondary to increased negative intrathoracic pressure. May be marked when large negative intrathoracic pressures are generated, e.g. upper or lower airway obstruction, or when diastolic cardiac filling is reduced, e.g. cardiac tamponade, constrictive pericarditis.
See also, Pulse

Pumping effect. Increased vaporiser output when pressure within the breathing system/back bar increases intermittently, e.g. during IPPV or use of the O_2 flush. During the pressure increase, gas within the back bar (i.e. containing the set concentration of volatile agent) is compressed back into the vaporiser chamber, where it becomes saturated with the volatile agent. When the downstream pressure falls, this gas re-expands into the back bar, thus increasing the concentration of volatile agent within the back bar. In addition, saturated vapour in the vaporiser chamber may be forced retrogradely into the vaporiser bypass, increasing the delivered concentration of volatile agent further.

The effect is greatest at low vaporiser settings and low gas flows, and may be minimised by:
- increasing resistance to flow through the vaporiser and bypass.
- lengthening the path through which the retrograde flow must pass before reaching the bypass.
- minimising the volume of the vaporiser chamber.
- placing a non-return valve downstream of the vaporiser.

Pupil. Central orifice of the iris; normally 1–8 mm in size. Contraction (miosis) is caused by parasympathetic stimulation, drugs including opioid analgesic drugs and anaesthesic agents, and pontine lesions. Dilatation (mydriasis) is caused by sympathetic stimulation and anticholinergic drugs. Dilated pupils may occur during awareness or hypercapnia during anaesthesia.
- Abnormal pupils and pupillary reflex may occur in particular lesions, e.g.:
  - ipsilateral fixed dilatation in head injury, followed by bilateral dilatation due to stretching of the 3rd cranial nerve.
  - Horner's syndrome.
  - Argyll Robertson pupil: small and irregular, fixed to light but responsive to accommodation. Classically occurs in tertiary syphilis but may occur in diabetes mellitus and brainstem encephalitis.
  - Holmes–Adie pupil: large and regular, with sluggish light reflex. Often associated with loss of knee reflexes but no other pathology.

[Douglas Argyll Robertson (1837–1909), Scottish surgeon; Gordon M Holmes (1876–1965), Irish-born English neurologist; William J Adie (1886–1935), Australian-born English neurologist]

Pupillary reflex. Easily tested reflex arcs involving the pupils:
- light reflex (Fig. 129): pupillary constriction normally follows direct or contralateral (consensual) illumination. Occasionally, phasic contraction and dilatation occurs (hippus). Pathway: from retina via optic nerve to the optic chiasma, thence to both lateral geniculate bodies via the optic tracts. Fibres then pass to the Edinger–Westphal nuclei of the 3rd cranial nerve. Efferent parasympathetic fibres pass to the ciliary ganglia, then via oculomotor and short ciliary nerves to the iris sphincter muscles of both sides. The cerebral cortex is not involved in the reflex.
- accommodation reflex: constriction normally occurs when the eyes converge. Fibres from the lateral geniculate bodies pass to the visual areas of the cerebral cortex; impulses then pass via superior longitudinal fasciculus and internal capsule to the oculomotor nuclear mass next to the Edinger–Westphal nucleus. When both medial recti are adducted, the pupils constrict.

Impaired reflexes are caused by lesions anywhere along their paths.
[Ludwig Edinger (1855–1918) and Karl FO Westphal (1833–1890), German neurologists]

PVS, *see Persistent vegetative state*

Pyloric stenosis. Stenosis of the gastric outflow. May be:
- congenital:
  - hypertrophy of the circular pyloric muscle; cause is unknown. Occurs in 1:500 births, 80% in males (usually first-born).

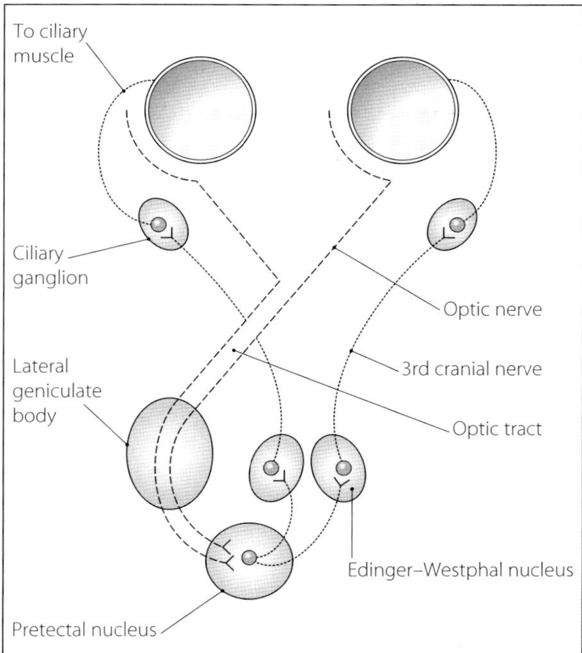

Fig. 129 Pupillary light reflex, showing pathways from one side of the visual field. The right lateral geniculate body and pretectal nucleus have been omitted

- usually presents within 3–12 weeks of age, with persistent projectile vomiting, failure to gain weight and hunger. A 'tumour' may be palpable in the right hypochondrium. The diagnosis is confirmed by ultrasonography.
- marked dehydration and metabolic alkalosis may be present. Resultant aldosterone secretion causes exchange of potassium and hydrogen ions for sodium in the urine, resulting in hypokalaemia and hypochloraemia with paradoxical acid urine.
- treated initially by nasogastric drainage and restoration of electrolyte/fluid balance, e.g. using 0.9% saline followed by dextrose–saline with potassium supplementation according to plasma electrolyte analysis.
- corrective surgery (pyloromyotomy; Ramstedt's procedure) should only be performed following adequate resuscitation, as indicated by absent clinical features of dehydration, good urine output, and normal acid–base and electrolyte (especially chloride) status. Anaesthetic management is as for paediatric anaesthesia, taking measures to avoid aspiration of gastric contents. Rapid sequence induction is usual, but awake intubation and inhalational induction have been used.

- acquired: usually results from gastric carcinoma or ulcer. Metabolic features are similar to those above. Residual gastric contents may be voluminous.

[Wilhelm C Ramstedt (1867–1963), German surgeon]

Pyrazinamide. Bactericidal antituberculous drug used in combination with other drugs. Effectiveness lasts 2–3 months. Useful in tuberculous meningitis because of good penetration into CSF.

- Dosage: 1.5–2.0 g daily for 2 months.
- Side effects: hepatotoxicity, anaemia, vomiting.

Pyrexia. Increased core body temperature, usually taken as ≥ 38°C (100.4°F) although definitions vary. The term implies intact homeostatic mechanisms whereas hyperthermia refers to thermoregulatory failure. Common in ICU patients, it is a feature of the general inflammatory response and brought about by cytokines (especially interleukin-6) and other mediators.

- Caused by:
  - infection including chest infection, urinary tract infection, catheter-related sepsis, sinusitis, etc.
  - others: primary inflammatory diseases e.g. connective tissue disease, drugs e.g. antibacterial drugs, MI, PE, endocrine disorders e.g. hyperthyroidism, acute adrenocortical insufficiency, MH and many others. May occur postoperatively, especially in children (in whom it has been reported in up to 40% of cases).
- Management includes careful examination and investigation (including blood culture and culture of sputum, urine, wound, etc.; X-rays, etc.), removal/replacement of catheters, etc. and review of drug therapy. Symptomatic treatment includes surface or core cooling, simple antipyretics, etc. However, some advocate that antipyretics should not be administered, as they may have deleterious effects (they deny the patient an important host defence mechanism and eliminate an important diagnostic aid). Widespread, empirical use of antibiotics to treat pyrexia is rarely beneficial.

Marik PE (2000). Chest; 117: 855–69

Pyridostigmine bromide. Acetylcholinesterase inhibitor. Pyridine analogue of neostigmine, with slower onset and longer duration of action. Also has weaker nicotinic action on voluntary muscle and less muscarinic action on viscera. Used in myasthenia gravis but less useful than neostigmine for reversing non-depolarising neuromuscular blockade. Half-life is 3–4 h.

- Dosage: 30–120 mg orally 4–12 hourly, up to 1.2 g/day.
- Side effects: as for neostigmine.

Q

Q wave. Initial downward deflection of the QRS complex of the ECG (*see Fig. 57b; Electrocardiography*). Small (q) waves are normal in leads aVL and I when left axis deviation is present, and in leads II, III and aVF with right axis deviation. They may be large in aVR. Pathological (Q) waves are wide (greater than 0.04 s) and deep (greater than 4 mm, or more than a quarter of the height of the R wave in the same lead); in the absence of left bundle branch block they suggest MI.

QRS complex. Represents ventricular depolarisation; normally follows the P wave of the ECG (*see Fig. 57b; Electrocardiography*). Upper case letters are used if a particular wave is considered large, lower case if small. The initial deflection is termed the q (Q) wave if downward, and R wave if upward. The downward S wave follows an R wave. The QRS complex may be used to calculate the electrical axis. Normally has rS pattern in V_1, qR pattern in V_6. The initial small deflection represents left-to-right septal depolarisation; the larger subsequent deflection represents (mainly left) ventricular depolarisation. Normal duration: < 0.12 s. Abnormalities may represent arrhythmias, heart block, bundle branch block, MI, etc.

Q–T interval. Represents the duration of ventricular systole; varies with age, sex and heart rate. Measured from the beginning of the QRS complex to the end of the T wave of the ECG (*see Fig. 57b; Electrocardiography*). Corrected for heart rate by dividing by the square root of the preceding R–R interval (seconds) (Bazett's formula). Normal range is 0.35–0.43.

Shortened in hypercalcaemia, hyperkalaemia and digoxin therapy. Prolonged Q–T syndromes may be caused by hypocalcaemia and hypothermia, and are associated with recurrent syncope or sudden death due to ventricular arrhythmias including VT and torsade de pointes.

[H Cuthbert Bazett (1885–1950), English-born US physiologist]

Q–Tc dispersion. Difference between the longest and shortest measurable corrected Q–T interval on the 12 lead ECG. Originally described using manual calculation, although automatic measuring methods have been described. Has been shown to be a powerful predictor of arrhythmias and sudden cardiac death in several cardiac conditions.

Suggested explanations for Q–Tc dispersion include patchy myocardial fibrosis and left ventricular dilatation, although the exact mechanism is unclear.

Sahu P, Lim PO, Rana BS, Struthers AD (2000). Q J Med; 93: 425–31

Quality assurance. Systematic process by which the quality of care is examined and deficiencies analysed in order to develop strategies for improvement.

- Classically applies to three areas:
  - structure, i.e. the system in place, e.g. assessment of staffng levels, equipment, type of patients, etc.
  - process, i.e. how the care is delivered, e.g. techniques of anaesthesia, monitoring, etc.
  - outcome, i.e. use of quality indicators, e.g. death rates, pain scores, patient satisfaction, etc.

Various methods of investigating each of these areas have been described, often translated from use in industry or commercial business. Audit and risk management are commonly used in medicine. The drive for quality assurance programmes has come from clinical, administrational and political quarters.

See also, Clinical governance; Healthcare Commission; National Institute for Clinical Excellence

Quantal theory. Widely accepted theory proposed in the 1960s to explain miniature end-plate potentials recorded from the neuromuscular junction postsynaptic membrane, at approximately 2 Hz. Postulates that small 'quanta' (packets) of acetylcholine are released randomly from the nerve cell membrane even in the absence of motor nerve activity. Each quantum is thought to be one vesicle's content, about 4–10 000 acetylcholine molecules. During single motor nerve activation about 200 quanta are released into the synaptic cleft.

Quantiflex apparatus. Continuous flow anaesthetic machines that can deliver preset mixtures of O_2 and N_2O, adjusted by a percentage control (minimum of 30% O_2). A single dial adjusts total gas flow delivered. Individual flowmeters indicate flow of O_2 and N_2O; the O_2 flowmeter is usually on the right, and N_2O flowmeter on the left. They are sometimes used in dental surgery.

Quincke, Heinrich Irenaeus (1842–1922). German physician; described and standardised lumbar puncture in 1891, originally as a treatment for hydrocephalus. Used the paramedian approach and suggested 24 hours' bed rest afterwards. His bevelled needle design is still used for lumbar puncture and spinal anaesthesia.

Quinidine. Class Ia antiarrhythmic drug. An isomer of quinine. Used to treat supraventricular and ventricular arrhythmias, but rarely used now because of side effects. Peak plasma levels occur 1–2 h following oral administration; half-life is 5–9 h. Highly protein-bound, it may displace digoxin if the two drugs are given concurrently.

- Dosage: 200–400 mg 6–8 hourly, orally.
- Side effects are common due to a low therapeutic ratio and include ventricular arrhythmias (e.g. torsade de pointes). Anticholinergic effects may result in GIT disturbances; CNS effects (cinchonism) include tinnitus and visual changes. Hypersensitivity reactions include rash, haemolysis and thrombocytopenia. Severe overdose results in confusion and psychosis.

Quinine sulphate/dihydrochloride. Antimalarial drug, reserved for treatment (but not prophylaxis) of falciparum malaria. Also used to treat nocturnal leg cramps.

- Dosage
  - malaria:
    - 600 mg 8 hourly, orally for 7 days.
    - 20 mg/kg over 4 h iv as initial dose (unless a related drug has been given within 24 h), then 10 mg/kg over 4 h every 8–12 h until able to complete the 7-day course with oral therapy.
  - leg cramps: 200–300 mg orally at night.
- Side effects: tinnitus, headache, visual disturbances (cinchonism), GIT disturbances, hypersensitivity (including thrombocytopenia and DIC), arrhythmias, renal failure, hypoglycaemia, convulsions.

4-Quinolones. Class of broad-spectrum antibacterial drugs, which include ciprofloxacin, levofloxacin, moxifloxacin and ofloxacin. More sensitive against Gram-negative than Gram-positive bacteria, they have limited activity against anaerobes. May induce convulsions in susceptible individuals, especially if NSAIDs are taken concurrently. They should be used with caution in hepatic or renal impairment.

Quinupristin/dalfopristin. Antibacterial drugs combined in a 3:7 ratio, presented as a mixture of mesilates. Active against Gram-positive bacteria (including staphylococci but excluding *Enterococcus faecalis*) resistant to other antibacterials. Inactive against Gram-negative organisms.

- Dosage: 7.5 mg/kg iv via central vein 8 hourly for 7–10 days (inflammation, pain and other reactions are common after peripheral administration).
- Side effects: GIT disturbance, myalgia, rash, confusion, hypotension, hepatic impairment; rarely renal impairment and blood dyscrasias.

R

R on T phenomenon. Arises when the R wave of a ventricular ectopic beat falls on the T wave of the preceding beat. At the middle of the T wave, the myocardium is partly depolarised and partly repolarised, and thus vulnerable to establishment of re-entry and circulatory conduction, leading to VF or VT.

R wave. First upward deflection of the QRS complex of the ECG (*see Fig. 57b; Electrocardiography*). Tends to increase in size from V_1 to V_6, with an accompanying reduction in size of S wave across these leads. Loss of this 'R wave progression', with a sudden increase in R wave size in V_5 or V_6, may indicate old anterior MI. In V_{1-6}, at least one normally exceeds 8 mm, but none exceeds 27 mm.

Rabeprazole sodium. Proton-pump inhibitor; actions and effects are similar to those of omeprazole.
- Dosage: 20 mg orally/day.
- Side effects: as for omeprazole.

Rabies. Infection caused by a rhabdovirus, eradicated from Britain in 1902 although occasional cases thought to have originated outside the UK have occurred in animals, e.g. dogs and bats. Spread mainly via domestic dogs and cats, but also by foxes, bats and other wildlife. Transmitted via infected saliva penetrating broken skin or intact mucosa; the virus replicates in local muscle then migrates proximally along peripheral nerves to dorsal root ganglia and the CNS. Incubation period is usually 20–90 days in humans, but may be 4 days to several years.

Malaise, fever, depression and psychosis may be followed by laryngeal spasm, and terror and arousal on drinking fluids. Respiratory failure occurs early and cardiac abnormalities, including myocarditis, are common.

Treatment of established rabies includes injection of human antirabies immunoglobulin, early IPPV, sedation and paralysis, with careful maintenance of acid–base and fluid balance. Almost inevitably fatal once established (death typically occurs 2–10 days after symptoms appear), but may be prevented by wound cleaning and active and passive immunisation.

Rupprecht CE, Hanlon CA, Hemachudha T (2002). Lancet Infect Dis; 2: 327–43

Radford nomogram. Diagram showing the relationship between tidal volume, patient's weight and respiratory frequency. Used to aid appropriate selection of ventilator settings for children and adults. Now rarely used.
[Edward P Radford (1922–2001), US physiologist]

Radial artery. Terminal branch of the brachial artery. Arises in the antecubital fossa, level with the radial neck, and passes downwards on the tendons and muscles attached to the radius (biceps tendon, supinator, pronator teres, flexor digitorum superficialis, flexor pollicis longus, pronator quadratus). Lies deep to brachioradialis muscle in the upper forearm, but subcutaneous in the lower forearm and easily palpable, especially over the distal quarter of the radius. Runs deep to abductor pollicis longus and extensor pollicis brevis tendons at the radial styloid, entering the anatomical snuffbox. Then enters the palm between the 1st and 2nd metacarpals. Branches include a superficial palmar branch (enters the palm superficial to the flexor retinaculum). At the wrist, it is a common site for palpation of the pulse and for arterial cannulation.

Radial nerve (C5–T1). Terminal branch of the posterior cord of the brachial plexus. Descends in the posterior upper arm, passing laterally behind the middle of the humerus in the radial groove. Crosses the antecubital fossa anterior to the elbow joint, between brachialis and brachioradialis. Descends under brachioradialis lateral to the radial artery in the forearm, passing posteriorly proximal to the wrist to end on the dorsum of the hand as digital branches.
- Branches:
  - axillary: to deltoid, teres minor and skin of the posteromedial upper arm.
  - upper arm:
    - to triceps, brachioradialis and extensor carpi radialis longus.
    - skin of the lower posterolateral arm.
  - forearm:
    - to the elbow joint.
    - posterior interosseous nerve arising at the elbow joint: passes posteriorly round the radial neck to supply the elbow, wrist and intercarpal joints, and all extensor muscles of the forearm apart from extensor carpi radialis longus.
    - via digital branches to the lateral side of the dorsum of the hand and posterior aspects of the lateral 2.5 digits up to the distal phalanx.

May be blocked at the elbow, wrist, and at midhumerus with the elbow flexed (the nerve is palpable in the radial groove).

See also, Brachial plexus block; Elbow, nerve blocks; Wrist, nerve blocks

Radiation. Emission of energy in the form of waves or particles. Includes emission of electromagnetic waves, e.g. light, most of which is non-ionising (does not have sufficient energy to overcome electron binding energy). Ionising radiation may result in displacement of electrons in organic material with the potential for tissue damage, and includes:
- α particles: helium nuclei consisting of two protons and two neutrons. Have high energy but penetrate matter poorly.
- β particles: electrons or positrons with variable energy and velocity. Those with high energies are more penetrative than α particles but much less than γ-rays and X-rays.
- γ-rays and X-rays: electromagnetic waves emitted from (γ-rays) or outside (X-rays) the nuclei of excited atoms.

Have extremely high penetration of matter and thus pose a health hazard requiring radiation safety precautions. γ-Rays are used in radiotherapy and imaging, and X-rays in imaging.

Exposure to ionising radiation is kept to a minimum with appropriate storage and handling of radioisotopes, minimal use of X-rays and appropriate use of shielding. Regulations require those performing or directing radiology procedures to have attended a course.

See also, Environmental safety of anaesthetists

Radiography in intensive care. Increasingly used as the range and quality of techniques and equipment available increase. Consultation with radiologists aids the proper selection and interpretation of many imaging techniques. In most cases, the use of mobile equipment results in less than optimal results but may be acceptable given the difficulty of transporting critically ill patients from the ICU; subtle changes between sequential films may be misleading if this is not taken into account. Investigations include chest X-ray, ultrasound and CT and MRI scanning; the latter two require transport to the imaging department. Radioisotope scanning usually requires transfer from the ICU.

Practical considerations include the requirement for sedation and adequate monitoring during transport or the procedure itself, the interference of the procedure with background therapy including the requirement for moving the patient (e.g. to place films underneath, etc.), and the potentially adverse effects of radiological contrast media.

See also, Imaging in intensive care

Radioisotope scanning. Use of radioisotopes to label certain parts of the body in order to investigate organ function, either directly or attached to circulating cells. Includes the following:
- assessment of blood flow: cerebral blood flow, renal blood flow, lung perfusion scans (often in conjunction with ventilation scans in suspected PE).
- nuclear cardiology.
- isolation of lesions: PE, bone metastases/infection/fracture, intra-abdominal sepsis.

The amount of radiation contained within the body after scanning is tiny, posing no risk to medical and nursing staff.

Radioisotopes. Isotopes of elements that undergo disintegration; i.e. the nucleus emits α, β or γ radiation either spontaneously or following a collision. Used clinically as labels to determine fluid compartments, blood flow, pulmonary $\dot{V}/\dot{Q}$ distribution, sites of infection, etc. Technetium-99 m and xenon-133 are often suitable because they are easy to use and their half-lives are short. Also used to label metabolically active substances which are taken up by certain tissues, allowing imaging of the tissue concerned, e.g. fibrinogen labelled with iodine-123 accumulates in a clot and may be used to detect DVT. Therapeutic use includes radiotherapy.

See also, Radioisotope scanning

Radiological contrast media. Contain large molecules which absorb X-rays (e.g. barium (enteral) or iodine (enteral or iv)) or have paramagnetic properties (e.g. gadolinium) for MRI scanning. Adverse reactions may follow iv injection:
- related to high osmolality (up to 7× that of plasma):
  - initial hypervolaemia followed by osmotic diuresis and hypovolaemia.
  - damage to red blood cells and vascular endothelium.
- immunological:
  - direct histamine release is thought to be most likely; complement activation may be involved. True anaphylactic reactions are not thought to occur.
  - reactions range from mild symptoms to cardiovascular collapse and death.
- direct toxicity: myocardial depression and systemic vasodilatation.

Thus initial hypertension may be followed by prolonged hypotension. Renal impairment may result from cardiovascular changes plus direct toxicity.

Incidence of reactions is decreased by using low osmolar, non-ionic media and low doses. Patients at risk of renal impairment should be kept well hydrated and hypovolaemia avoided. Risk of subsequent immune reactions is low, especially with use of antihistamines and corticosteroid therapy. Resuscitation equipment and drugs must always be available.

Dickinson MC, Kam PCA (2008). Anaesthesia; 63: 626–34

See also, Adverse drug reactions

Radiology, anaesthesia for. Most radiological procedures require neither general anaesthesia nor sedation. Anaesthesia may be required for the very young, confused or agitated patients and those with movement disorders. Procedures for which the anaesthetist may be required include CT scanning, MRI, angiography, and invasive procedures, e.g. embolisation of vascular lesions (e.g. in neuroradiology).
- Main anaesthetic considerations:
  - underlying disease process.
  - often cramped conditions, with poor lighting.
  - old or incomplete anaesthetic/monitoring equipment.
  - poor access to the patient.
  - adverse effects of radiological contrast media.
  - specific problems of MRI.

Preoperative assessment and preparation should be as for any anaesthetic procedure.

Radiotherapy. Use of ionising radiation to treat neoplasms. May involve:
- external radiation.
- implantation of internal sources (interstitial radiotherapy), e.g. in gynaecological or CNS tumours.
- administration of radioactive radioisotopes, e.g. iodine-131 in hyperthyroidism, phosphorus-32 in polycythaemia.

- General anaesthesia is rarely required except when patients are uncooperative, e.g. children, patients with movement disorders, etc. Anaesthetic considerations:
  - general condition of the patient: features of malignancy, site and nature of the neoplasm, drug therapy, etc. Haematological abnormalities are common.
  - repeated anaesthetics: multiple treatments are required, e.g. daily for several weeks. Considerations include fear of injections, risk of halothane hepatitis, and repeated periods of starvation (especially important in children). IV cannulation may be difficult, although long-term catheters are often sited.
  - immobilisation of the head may be required, e.g. for CNS tumours; clear plastic masks are often used, with risks of airway obstruction. Head-down positioning may be required. Problems also exist when moulding and making the mask.
  - treatments usually consist of short periods of radiation (e.g. a few minutes), during which time the anaesthetist cannot be present. Monitoring is usually visible via remote-control cameras, but may be restricted.

Techniques available include sedation, neuroleptanaesthesia and formal general anaesthesia. Ketamine is often used, especially in children. Repeated doses may be given as required during positioning and therapy.

Patients formerly treated by radiotherapy may have inflammatory or fibrotic changes in the irradiated area. Pulmonary, cardiac, renal and hepatic involvement may be present. Tissue fibrosis around the airway may make tracheal intubation difficult.

Randomisation. Technique for allocating subjects, e.g. patients to treatment groups in clinical trials, thus overcoming bias when samples are compared. Ensures that factors such as age, sex, weight, etc. are randomly distributed amongst the groups; i.e. any difference in these factors is due to chance alone.

- Randomisation may be:
  - simple: no restriction on allocation. Groups may be unequally sized.
  - block: allocation is performed in blocks, so that groups are equally sized within each block.
  - stratified: factors such as age, sex, etc. are randomised separately, so that they are equally distributed amongst the groups. A more sophisticated method, minimisation, involves the distribution of successive subjects to the groups by taking into account the number of subjects already allocated who have these various factors, using a scoring system. For example, if age, weight and female sex are felt to be important prognostic factors in a particular study, an obese subject may still be allocated to a group which already has several obese subjects in it, if there are fewer older subjects and females than in the other groups.

Computer-generated random numbers are usually employed. Use of coins or dice is tedious and presents the temptation to repeat an allocation if the result is not liked. Other methods, e.g. allocation of alternate patients, or according to patients' birthdays or record numbers, have also been used. However, these methods cannot always be guaranteed free of hidden bias.

Ranitidine hydrochloride. H_2 receptor antagonist; better absorbed and more potent than cimetidine, with fewer side effects. Does not inhibit hepatic enzymes or interfere with metabolism of other drugs. Oral bioavailability is about 80%. Plasma levels peak within 15 min of im injection; effect lasts about 8 h. Half-life is about 2 h. Undergoes hepatic metabolism and is excreted via urine, hence the dose is reduced in renal failure.

- Dosage:
  - 50 mg iv/im 8 hourly. Effective if given 45–60 min preoperatively. If administered iv, 50 mg should be diluted into 20 ml and injected over at least 2 min, since severe bradycardia may occur. May also be given by continuous infusion: 125–250 µg/kg/h.
  - 150–300 mg orally, 12 hourly. For prophylaxis against aspiration pneumonitis, 150 mg orally 6 hourly (e.g. in labour), or 2 h preoperatively (preferably preceded by 150 mg the night before).
- Side effects: blood dyscrasias, impaired liver function and confusion; all are rare.

Ranking, *see Statistical tests*

Raoult's law. The degree of lowering of vapour pressure of a solvent, due to addition of a solute, is proportional to the molar concentration of the solute.
[François M Raoult (1830–1901), French scientist]
See also, Colligative properties of solutions

RAP, Right atrial pressure, *see Cardiac catheterisation; Central venous pressure*

Rapacuronium bromide. Non-depolarising neuromuscular blocking drug, introduced in the US in 1999 and withdrawn in 2001 just before its introduction in the UK, because of reports of severe bronchospasm (in some cases, fatal). Chemically related to vecuronium, it causes rapid onset of neuromuscular blockade (tracheal intubation possible within 60 s) with fast recovery (6–30 min depending on dosage) and was thus suggested as an alternative to suxamethonium.

Rapid opioid detoxification. Technique for treating opioid addiction by precipitating withdrawal using opioid receptor antagonists, e.g. naloxone or naltrexone, supposedly reducing relapse rates compared with conventional management. Ultra-rapid opioid detoxification refers to administration of general anaesthesia or heavy sedation for prolonged periods to reduce awareness or recall of unpleasant withdrawal symptoms whilst the opioid antagonists are given. The technique is controversial (especially the ultra-rapid form) since deaths have occurred and supportive evidence for its efficacy is poor.
Singh J, Basu D (2004). J Postgrad Med; 50: 227–32

Rate–pressure product (RPP). Product of heart rate and systolic BP, used as an indicator of myocardial workload and O_2 consumption. It has been suggested that RPP should be maintained below 15 000 in patients with ischaemic heart disease during anaesthesia. Its usefulness has been questioned, since a proportional increase in rate may increase myocardial O_2 demand more than the same increase in BP. Rate–pressure quotient has been suggested as being a better predictor of myocardial ischaemia: MAP/rate. If under 1, it may indicate ischaemia.

RBBB, Right bundle branch block, *see Bundle branch block*

RDS, *see Respiratory distress syndrome*

Reactance. Portion of impedance to flow of an alternating current not due to resistance; e.g. due to capacitance or inductance. Given the symbol X, and measured in ohms.
[Georg S Ohm (1787–1854), German physicist]

Rebreathing techniques, *see Carbon dioxide measurement*

Receiver operating characteristic (ROC) curves. Curves drawn to indicate the usefulness of a predictive test, originally derived from analysis of radar signals between the World Wars (i.e. did a deflection represent a real signal or just random noise; and if the former, with what degree of certainty?). For the test to be analysed (e.g. the usefulness of ASA physical status to predict mortality after anaesthesia), each cut-off level is examined in turn, and sensitivity and specificity calculated for it. Thus, for example, an ASA grade of 1 has high sensitivity (all deaths have an ASA grade of 1 or above) but low specificity (most patients with a grade of 1 or above do not die). For an ASA grade of 2, sensitivity is a little lower (some patients who die have a grade of 1, and will not be predicted by a grade of 2) whilst specificity is higher although still poor (a grade of 2 is better at predicting death than a grade of 1, although most patients achieving 2 or above still do not die). The process continues until grade 5, which has low sensitivity (few of the deaths have a grade of 5) but high specificity (most patients who are graded 5 do, by definition, die). Sensitivity is plotted against (1 – specificity) and a curve (AUC) obtained (Fig. 130); the area under the curve

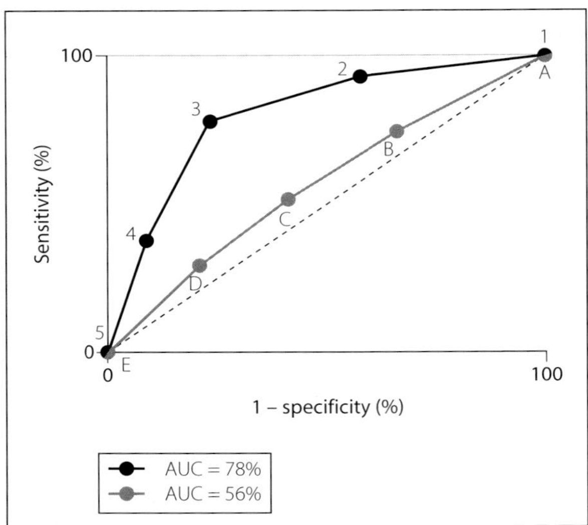

Fig. 130 Examples of two receiver operating characteristic curves for the usefulness of two different 5-point scales (1–5 and A–E) for predicting an outcome. The 1–5 scale performs better than the A–E scale. The dotted line denotes the curve for a test where prediction is no better than chance

represents the usefulness of the test, a perfect test including 100% of the available area and one where prediction is no better than chance, 50%.

ROC curves may be drawn using continuous (e.g. C-reactive protein to predict infection), ordinal (e.g. ASA system) or nominal (e.g. presence of different features on the ECG to diagnose MI) scales. They may also be drawn for different tests in the same plot, allowing comparison between the tests. They also allow selection of the best cut-off to use clinically, usually the uppermost and most left-hand part of the curve, being the best compromise between sensitivity and specificity. They are increasingly used to analyse the usefulness of tests or scoring systems in anaesthesia and intensive care including difficult tracheal intubation and other outcomes.

Galley HF (2004). Br J Anaesth; 93: 623–6

Receptor theory. States that receptors are specific proteins or lipoproteins within cell membranes that interact selectively with extracellular compounds (agonists) to initiate biochemical events within the cell. The structures of the agonist and receptor determine the selectivity and quantitative response. Drugs which interact with the receptor but do not produce the effect of an agonist are antagonists. Degree of binding to receptors is affinity; ability to produce a response is intrinsic activity.

Initial assumptions that the degree of response is proportional to the number of receptors occupied are not universally accepted. Other suggestions include:

- reduced occupancy is required for a potent agonist compared with a less potent agonist, to produce the same response.
- degree of response is proportional to the rate of receptor–agonist interaction and dissociation.

Interaction of drug and receptor may resemble Michaelis–Menten kinetics. Covalent, ionic and hydrogen bonding, and van der Waals forces may be involved.

- Different types of receptor:
  - ligand gated ion channels: direct opening of membrane pores allowing passage of ions (e.g. Na^+, K^+, Ca^{2+}, Cl^-) across the membrane, e.g. nicotinic acetylcholine receptor. Typically fast responses (under a millisecond).
  - G protein-coupled receptors: binding to the receptor causes a change in the guanine binding properties of the neighbouring G protein which then leads to the intracellular response, e.g. adrenergic receptors. Typically of the order of many milliseconds to seconds.
  - ligand operated tyrosine kinases: binding at the cell surface causes activation of tyrosine kinase at the inner surface of the cell, which catalyses phosphation of target proteins via ATP, e.g. insulin receptors. Typically minutes to hours.
  - nuclear receptors: the lipid-soluble effector molecule passes through the cell membrane to interact with the receptor, leading to alteration of DNA transcription, e.g. corticosteroid and thyroid hormones. Typically up to several hours.

Expression of receptor numbers varies. Chronic stimulation (e.g. asthmatics taking β_2-adrenergic receptor agonists) results in a decreased number of receptors (downregulation) whereas understimulation (e.g. following spinal cord injury) leads to an increased number of receptors (upregulation).

See also, Dose–response curves; Pharmacodynamics

Recommended International Nonproprietary Names (RINNs), *see Explanatory Notes at the beginning of this book*

Record-keeping. The first anaesthetic chart was devised by Codman and Cushing in 1894 at the Massachusetts General Hospital, for recording of respiration and pulse rate. BP charting was included in 1901 at Cushing's insistence. Respiration and F_IO_2 were included by McKesson in 1911.

Careful record keeping is now recognised as essential to chart preoperative risk factors, the perioperative course of anaesthesia and postoperative events/instructions. It is particularly useful when taking over another anaesthetist's anaesthetic, and for providing information to those administering anaesthesia subsequently. Similarly, ICU records should chart physiological data, therapy and instructions relating to the stay of any patient in an ICU. Record-keeping is also important for teaching, research and audit, and is extremely important in medicolegal aspects of anaesthesia. Although tending to include similar information, anaesthetic and intensive care charts are not standardised nationally although this has been suggested.

Automated anaesthetic record systems are increasingly used, sometimes incorporated into anaesthetic machines or ICU monitoring systems. They provide accurate, legible and complete documents for data acquisition and subsequent scrutiny. Data from monitoring devices are incorporated with information provided by the anaesthetist/intensive care staff, e.g. drug or other interventions, although lack of familiarity with keyboards or computers may be a hindrance.

Postoperative recovery and progress may be recorded on separate charts, or on the anaesthetic chart.

[Ernest A Codman (1869–1940), US surgeon]

Recovery from anaesthesia. Period from the end of surgery to when the patient is alert and physiologically stable. Definition is difficult because some drowsiness may persist for many hours. Recovery testing is used for more precise investigation. Time to recovery depends on the patient's condition, drugs given, their doses, and the patient's ability to eliminate them. For inhalational anaesthetic agents, similar considerations as for uptake are involved, plus length of operation and degree of redistribution to fat. Thus blood gas solubility is the most important factor initially, but more potent agents, e.g. halothane, are more extensively bound

to fat after prolonged anaesthesia than less potent ones, e.g. enflurane. For iv anaesthetic agents, initial recovery is due to drug redistribution from vessel-rich to vessel-intermediate tissues; subsequent course is related to the rate of clearance from the body. Thus propofol characteristically results in rapid clear-headed wakening, whereas thiopental is more likely to produce drowsiness lasting several hours, especially after repeated dosage. Recommendations for provision of recovery care (Association of Anaesthetists):
- designated recovery rooms or areas should be used.
- during transfer to the recovery area O_2 should be administered, and appropriate monitoring performed.
- the anaesthetist should formally hand over the patient's care to properly trained staff giving details of the operation, anaesthetic technique, perioperative problems including blood loss, and antiemetic and analgesic drugs given.
- all patients should be observed by at least one member of staff until there is a clear airway and cardiovascular stability, and they are able to communicate. The anaesthetist is responsible for removal of tracheal tubes.
- O_2 should be administered at least until awake.
- level of consciousness, arterial O_2 saturation, BP, heart rate, respiratory rate, pain intensity, iv infusions and drugs administered (including O_2) should be recorded, along with other parameters as appropriate (e.g. temperature, urine output, etc.).
- there should be criteria for discharge, including full consciousness, clear airway, respiratory and cardiovascular stability, adequate postoperative analgesia and control of PONV, stable temperature and prescription of postoperative drugs including O_2 and iv fluids as appropriate. There should be adequate handover during discharge from the recovery area.
- children should recover in a designated area.

Patients are often placed on their side, e.g. the recovery position. In the tonsillar position, the pillow is placed under the loin and the trolley tipped head down.

- Problems during recovery:
  - respiratory, e.g. hypoventilation, hypercapnia, hypoxaemia, airway obstruction, bronchospasm, aspiration of gastric contents.
  - cardiovascular, e.g. hypotension, hypertension, arrhythmias.
  - confusion, agitation, etc. Pain and bladder distension are common causes of restlessness and hypertension postoperatively. The above causes must also be excluded.
  - related to anaesthetic drugs, e.g. inadequate reversal of non-depolarising neuromuscular blockade, adverse drugs reactions, MH, dystonic reactions, emergence phenomena, central anticholinergic syndrome, etc.
  - hypothermia, nausea and vomiting, shivering.
  - related to surgery, e.g. bleeding.

The speed and quality of recovery from anaesthesia has been proposed as a possible measure of quality of anaesthesia.

See also, Anaesthetic morbidity and mortality

Recovery position. Position recommended for unconscious but spontaneously breathing subjects, e.g. in CPR or trauma (assuming no contraindication such as fractured neck). Encourages a clear airway and drainage of vomitus, secretions, blood, etc. away from the airway. Often used during recovery from anaesthesia.

Any recovery position is a compromise between the full prone position (better airway and drainage but more diaphragmatic splinting) and the full lateral position (less diaphragmatic splinting but less effective for the airway and less stable; also may be harmful in neck injury). Classically includes flexion of both arms with the upper hand placed under the jaw to support the airway (Fig. 131a). A modified position has been suggested in which the lower arm is kept straight and positioned behind the subject's back, with the hand placed palm upwards and tucked under the lower buttock or thigh; this is to reduce the risk of neurological or vascular damage to the dependent arm caused by the weight of the upper arm crossing it (Fig. 131b). However, this position too may cause problems with the lower arm and thus recent guidelines on CPR have reverted to the traditional position. The actual position adopted should reflect the particular circumstances of the case and the need to protect the airway, stabilise the neck and allow unhindered ventilation. It should be possible to observe the patient at all times and to turn him/her supine easily when required.

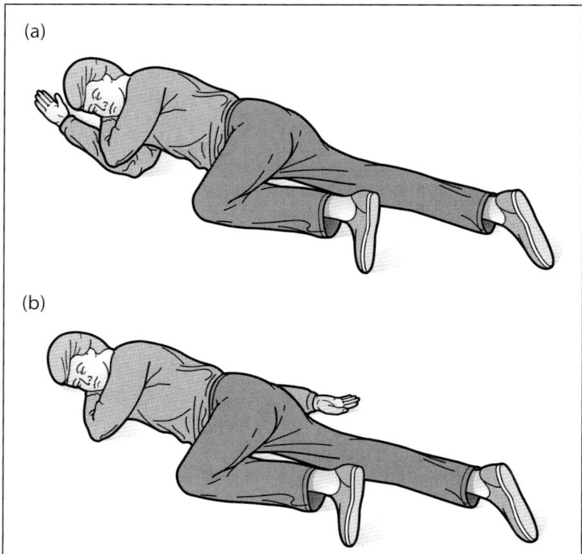

Fig. 131 Recovery position: (a) with lower arm under upper one; (b) with lower arm extended

Recovery room. An area reserved for postoperative care was described by Florence Nightingale in 1863, but the first dedicated recovery room was opened in the USA in 1923. Many more were introduced there after experiences in World War II and the Korean War. First introduced in the UK in 1955.
- Features:
  - placed near the operating suite, if possible near ICU.
  - open ward, allowing good patient observation.
  - at least 2 bays per operating theatre is recommended.
  - each bay is equipped for monitoring (ECG, BP, O_2 saturation, etc.) and patient care (suction, O_2, etc.), also electrical outlets, etc.
  - a full supply of iv equipment and fluids, blankets, airways, etc. should be available.
  - resuscitation equipment, ventilator and drugs should be readily available, with an emergency call system.
  - adequate ventilation is required to remove exhaled anaesthetic gases.
- Drugs available should include:
  - analgesics, antiemetics, sedatives, anticonvulsants, naloxone, flumazenil.
  - doxapram, bronchodilators, corticosteroids, antihistamines.

- anticholinergics, antiarrhythmics, antihypertensives, diuretics, heparin.
- antibiotics, anticholinesterases, neuromuscular blocking drugs, insulin, dextrose, dantrolene.
- local anaesthetics.

[Florence Nightingale (1820–1910), English nurse]
See also, Recovery

Recovery testing. Ranges from simple clinical assessment to more sophisticated methods, e.g. used for comparison between anaesthetic techniques, drugs, etc. Routine testing is usually limited to assessment of general alertness and orientation, and ability to respond, drink, dress and walk where appropriate (e.g. day-case surgery).

- Sophisticated techniques used include tests of:
  - psychomotor function:
    - assessing speed and number of errors made whilst performing set tasks:
      - moving pegs from one set of holes in a board to another set.
      - 'posting' pieces of paper through a slot.
      - deleting every letter 'p' from a page of text.
      - following outlines of shapes with a pen without drawing over their edges, drawing a line from the centre of a maze to the outside, or moving a metal hoop along a tortuous wire without touching it.
      - connecting dots on a page.
    - reaction testing:
      - being faced with four light sources, and pressing the correct switch (out of four choices) when one of them flashes.
      - tracking moving targets with a pen or light.
      - driving simulators.
  - perception:
    - noting the frequency at which a flashing light appears to be continuous (critical flicker–fusion threshold).
    - perception of auditory stimuli in a similar fashion, including discrimination between left and right ears.
  - memory:
    - recall or recognition of objects, pictures, words or word associations shown a short time before.
    - recall of pre- and postoperative events.
    - orientation in time and space.
  - cognitive function, e.g. adding/subtracting numbers, or adding values of different coins.
  - intelligence: standard tests are used.
  - physiological function, e.g. divergence of eyes caused by reductions in extraocular muscle tone.

Many of the above may be performed using computer systems. Problems of detailed recovery testing are related to the time taken, cumbersome equipment required, fatigue, boredom and learning if tests are repeated. Critical flicker–fusion, reaction testing, letter deletion and memory tests are most widely used and thought to be reasonably efficient, the first two especially so. General advice to patients is usually to avoid potentially dangerous activities, e.g. driving, cooking, using machinery, etc., for 24 h following day-case anaesthesia, although subtle changes may persist beyond this period; 48 h has been suggested.

Rectal administration of anaesthetic agents. Results in effective absorption of drugs because of a rich blood supply provided by communicating plexuses formed by the superior, middle and inferior rectal arteries and veins. Drugs undergo less first-pass metabolism than when orally administered, because the plexuses represent anastomoses between portal and systemic circulations. The technique is usually restricted to children. Traditionally used more in Continental Europe, e.g. France. Drugs used have included diazepam 0.4–0.5 mg/kg (widely used for treatment of convulsions in children), methohexital 15–25 mg/kg and thiopental 40–50 mg/kg as 5–10% solutions. Opioids and ketamine have also been given in this way. Diethyl ether was administered rectally by Pirogoff. Bromethol and paraldehyde were used in the 1920s to produce unconsciousness (basal narcosis).

Rectus sheath block. Performed as part of abdominal field block or alone to reduce pain from abdominal incisions. Abdominal contents remain unanaesthetised.

With the patient supine, a blunted needle is introduced 3–6 cm above and lateral to the umbilicus. A gentle 'scratching' motion may aid identification of the tough anterior layer of the sheath, puncture of which is accompanied by a click. The needle is advanced up to the resistance offered by the posterior layer of the sheath, and 15–20 ml local anaesthetic agent injected after negative aspiration. Deposition of solution between rectus muscle and posterior layer allows spread up and down, blocking the lower 5–6 intercostal nerves within the sheath. Spread between the muscle and anterior layer is limited by the tendinous intersections along its length. Multiple injections have been suggested between intersections, to improve spread, but the posterior layer is deficient below a point half-way between the umbilicus and pubis, and peritoneal puncture is more likely below this level.

Recurarisation. Recurrence of non-depolarising neuromuscular blockade after apparent reversal with acetylcholinesterase inhibitors. Originally described with tubocurarine in patients with impaired renal function, where the duration of action of the neuromuscular blocking drug exceeds that of the acetylcholinesterase inhibitor. Has been described with other neuromuscular blocking drugs.

Red cell concentrates, *see Blood products*

Reducing valve, *see Pressure regulators*

Referred pain. Pain felt in a somatic site remote to the source of pain, usually visceral; e.g. diaphragmatic pain is felt in the shoulder tip. The aetiology is obscure, but is thought to be related to the embryological segment from which the organ arose, e.g. diaphragm from the neck region, and heart from the same region as the arm.

- Theories include:
  - convergence: somatic and visceral afferents converge on the same spinothalamic tracts. The brain assumes that neural activity in a particular pathway arises from somatic input, rather than visceral, since the former is far more common than the latter.
  - facilitation: input from visceral afferents increases sensitivity of neurones receiving somatic afferents, thus encouraging somatic sensation.

Effects of local anaesthetic injected at referred areas are inconsistent, supporting both theories (should ease the pain if facilitation is responsible, but not if convergence is responsible).

Reflex arc. Involves predictable, repetitive stereotypic responses to a particular sensory stimulus. Consists of sense organ, afferent neurone, one or more synapses, efferent neurone and effector. The afferent neurones enter the spinal cord via dorsal roots or brain via cranial nerves; the efferent neurones leave via ventral nerve roots or corresponding motor cranial nerves. Also involved in autonomic functions. The simplest reflex arc is monosynaptic, e.g. knee jerk and other stretch reflexes involving muscle spindles. Polysynaptic reflex arcs (two or more synapses) include the withdrawal reflex. Widespread effects may result from activation of a single reflex arc because of ascending, descending, excitatory and inhibitory interneurones.

Reflex sympathetic dystrophy, *see Complex regional pain syndrome type 1*

Reflux, *see Gastro-oesophageal reflux*

Refractometer, *see Interferometer*

Refractory period. Period during and following the action potential during which the neurone is insensitive to further stimulation. Subdivided thus:
- absolute: excited by no stimulus however strong.
- relative: excitation may follow stronger stimuli than normal.

Refrigeration anaesthesia. Use of cold to reduce pain sensation. Used by Larrey in 1807, although the effect of cold on pain has been recognised for centuries. Up to 3 hours' packing in ice was recommended for operations through the thigh. The principle is still used today, e.g. ethyl chloride spray.

Regional anaesthesia. Term originally coined by Cushing to describe techniques of abolishing pain using local anaesthetic agents as opposed to general anaesthesia. Pioneers included Corning and Labat in the USA and Bier, Braun and Lawen in Europe.
- Techniques include:
  - topical anaesthesia.
  - infiltration anaesthesia, Vishnevisky technique and tumescent anaesthesia.
  - peripheral nerve blocks: plexus and single nerve blocks.
  - central neural blockade: epidural and spinal anaesthesia.
  - IVRA and intra-arterial regional anaesthesia.
  - sympathetic nerve blocks.
  - others, e.g. interpleural analgesia.
- Advantages of regional anaesthesia:
  - conscious patient, able to assist in positioning, etc. and warn of adverse effects (e.g. in carotid artery surgery and TURP). There is less interruption of oral intake, especially beneficial in diabetes mellitus.
  - good postoperative analgesia.
  - reduction of certain postoperative complications, e.g. atelectasis and DVT, possibly myocardial ischaemia.
- Contraindications:
  - absolute: patient refusal, anaesthetist's inexperience and localised infection.
  - relative: abnormal anatomy or deformity, coagulation disorders, previous failure of the technique, and neurological disease or other medicolegal considerations.

  Specific contraindications may exist for specific techniques.
- Management:
  - preoperatively:
    - preoperative assessment and preparation as for general anaesthesia.
    - full explanation of the procedure, and consent.
    - preparation of drugs and equipment for general anaesthesia and resuscitation, in addition to those required for the regional technique chosen.
  - perioperatively:
    - monitoring should be applied as for general anaesthesia, i.e. before starting the procedure and continued throughout it.
    - aseptic technique should be observed.
    - for nerve or plexus blocks, short-bevelled needles are traditionally used to minimise nerve contact, although nerve damage may be greater should the nerve be impaled. Nerve stimulators (using 0.3–1.0 mA current lasting 1–2 ms and delivered at 1–3 Hz) increase the success of many blocks and may reduce damage further. A distant ground electrode is required. The needle (preferably sheathed) is placed near the target nerve and stimulated until paraesthesia or twitches are elicited; the output is reduced, the needle repositioned, and the process repeated.

      More recently, ultrasound imaging has been used to indicate the location of nerves and nerve plexi/bundles. The appearance of nerve tissue is variable but usually distinct from that of other tissues. Addition of colour Doppler imaging reveals blood vessels. Claimed advantages include more accurate placement of the needle, especially if anatomy is abnormal, reduced volume of injectate required, greater success rate and reduced complication rate.
    - a single injection of local anaesthetic, repeated boluses (using repeated injections or an indwelling catheter) or continuous infusions may be used.
    - the extent of the block should be assessed (e.g. by response to pinprick or cold) before allowing surgery to start.
    - if sedation is used, care should be taken to ensure that respiratory and cardiovascular depression do not occur. Analgesic drugs (e.g. N_2O or opioid analgesic drugs) may be used to supplement incomplete blockade. General anaesthesia may be used as a planned part of the technique, or if the technique is unsuccessful.
  - postoperatively:
    - close monitoring and supervision should continue as for general anaesthesia.
    - neurological complications may only become apparent once the block has worn off.
- Complications:
  - technical: direct trauma to nerves, blood vessels, pleura, etc., breakage of needles or catheters.
  - associated with positioning of the patient, e.g. compression of an anaesthetised limb.
  - local anaesthetic toxicity: intravascular injection or systemic absorption.
  - excessive spread, e.g. total spinal block during epidural anaesthesia, or phrenic nerve block during brachial plexus block.
  - failure of the technique.
  - those of specific techniques, e.g. hypotension following spinal anaesthesia.
  - others, e.g. injection of the wrong solution through catheters.

See also, specific blocks; Nerve injury during anaesthesia

Regional tissue oxygenation. Important because shock and hypoxaemia cause redistribution of blood flow and alter the metabolic properties of cells; global measurements thus fail to detect areas of local ischaemia. Measurement of regional tissue oxygenation may be required in critically ill patients because deficiencies may be involved in the development and continuation of multiple organ dysfunction. It may be assessed using:

- blood lactate levels (> 2 mmol/l suggests insufficient oxygen delivery): a late marker.
- mixed venous O_2 saturation ($S_{\bar{v}}O_2$), measured using repeated blood sampling or continuous oximetry via a pulmonary artery catheter. Regional S_vO_2 (e.g. hepatic $= S_{hv}O_2$; jugular $= S_{jv}O_2$) can be determined using indwelling catheters.
- intestinal regional capnography (i.e. gastric tonometry). Measures P_{CO_2} in an air- or saline-filled tonometric balloon, placed in the GIT.
- surface or tissue O_2 electrodes: based upon the Clark electrode (*see Oxygen measurement*), they are formed of a noble metal (e.g. gold, silver, platinum). Change in voltage between the anode and cathode is proportional to the amount of O_2 reduced at the cathode.
- optode sensors: use the change in the optical properties (e.g. absorbance or fluorescence) of indicator substances generated by photochemical reactions to measure the concentration of a substance (e.g. O_2) in tissues. Can be mounted in intravascular catheters (e.g. Paratrend monitor).
- near infra-red spectroscopy.
- reflectance spectrophotometry. Measures the absorption of reflected visible light on a tissue surface, e.g. gut wall, fetal scalp.
- nicotinamide adenine dinucleotide (NADH) fluorescence: during tissue hypoxia, NADH accumulates in tissues. The absorption properties of NADH, and its reduced state NAD^+, are different. Tissue catheters have been used in both animal and human models.
- palladium (Pd)-porphyrin phosphorescence: based on the principle that if a Pd-porphyrin molecule is excited by a pulse of light, it can either release the absorbed energy as light or transfer it to molecular O_2. Once excited, the decay in fluorescence is related to the amount of O_2 present (the less O_2, the longer decay). Pd-porphyrin is water soluble and can be injected iv; it has been evaluated in animal models.
- imaging using on-line microscopic observation of the microcirculation.

Regression, *see Statistical tests*

Regurgitation. Term usually describing passive passage of gastric contents into the pharynx. Silent, thus aspiration of gastric contents may occur unnoticed. Normally prevented by the lower oesophageal sphincter; however, swallowed dyes have been found to stain areas of the pharynx and larynx during anaesthesia in normal patients.

Relative analgesia. Technique used in dental surgery involving nasal administration of subanaesthetic concentrations of N_2O, e.g. 10% in O_2 slowly increased to 30–50%. Verbal contact is maintained at all times, and the concentration of N_2O reduced if excessive drowsiness occurs. Performed by the dentist, it depends partly on suggestion.

Relative risk reduction. Indicator of treatment effect in clinical trials. For a reduction in incidence of events from a% to b%, it equals $((a - b) \div a)$%. Gives an overestimated impression of treatment effect if events are rare, and an underestimate if events are common.
See also, Absolute risk reduction; Meta-analysis; Number needed to treat; Odds ratio

Relatives of critically ill patients. Present particular challenges to ICU staff because of the serious nature of the patient's condition, unfamiliarity with the ICU environment and the natural behavioural responses to extreme stress including fear, anger and guilt. The suddenness of many severe conditions may exacerbate relatives' distress. Relatives must be kept informed about the patient's progress, preferably by a consistent single senior doctor accompanied by a member of the nursing staff; they should also feel included in discussions about treatment, etc. Honest and clear explanations, using lay language, may need repeating several times and the potential frustration felt by the medical team must not be transmitted to the relatives. Most ICUs have a separate room for interviews with patients' families and friends, which is preferable to the open ward or corridor. In general, few restrictions are placed on visiting times, and most relatives appreciate and respect the need for staff to perform basic care and procedures during which they may be asked to leave the unit. However, some may choose to stay and participate in some aspects of their relative's care, e.g. washing or shaving. Counselling and religious support may be required and is often best arranged via the ICU staff.

Whether relatives should witness attempts at resuscitation (e.g. in casualty departments) has attracted recent attention, with some welcoming the opportunity for relatives to see that appropriate attempts to save the patient are being made, whilst others argue that their presence may be stressful for medical and nursing staff.

Remifentanil. Ultra-short-acting synthetic opioid analgesic drug, 2000 times more potent than morphine, introduced in the UK in 1997. Available as a whitish powder for reconstitution to a 0.1% solution which is stable for 24 h at room temperature. Further diluted for administration; a 50 µg/ml solution is recommended by the manufacturer. Approximately 70% protein-bound. Metabolised by cholinesterase within erythrocytes to remifentanil acid (very low potency at mu receptors) and excreted renally, its half-life is about 3 min; thus ideally suited to administration by infusion with a rapid recovery when stopped, even after prolonged usage. Because it is cleared so rapidly and completely, patients very soon complain of pain postoperatively unless longer-acting analgesics are given before discontinuation. Has been used via patient controlled analgesia during labour (*see Obstetric analgesia and anaesthesia*). Not recommended for epidural or spinal use since the formulation contains glycine. Postoperative respiratory depression may occur if any drug is left in the dead space of iv lines and subsequently flushed with other drugs or fluids.

- Dosage:
  - to supplement induction of anaesthesia: 0.5–1.0 µg/kg/min, ± initial bolus of 1.0 µg/kg over at least 30 s.
  - during anaesthesia: 0.05–2.0 µg/kg/min during IPPV; 0.025–0.1 µg/kg/min during spontaneous ventilation.

Renal blood flow (RBF). Normally 1200 ml/min (400 ml/100 g/min); i.e. 22% of cardiac output.

- Measurement:
  - direct: circumferential electromagnetic flow measurement, Doppler or thermodilution techniques.
  - indirect:
    - clearance methods: a substance neither metabolised nor taken up by the kidney, and completely cleared, is required, e.g. *para*-amino hippuric acid (PAH). Clearance then equals renal plasma flow. RBF = plasma flow divided by (1 – haematocrit). Continuous iv infusion of PAH is required; inaccuracies may occur since clearance of PAH is only 90% in humans. Radioactive markers have been used; almost 100% cleared, they require only a single injection.

- digital subtraction angiography and radioactive inert gas washout techniques have also been used, the latter indicating regional blood flow.
- Affected by:
  - arterial BP: maintained by autoregulation at MAP between 70 and 170 mmHg in normal subjects.
  - sympathetic nervous system: stimulation causes vasoconstriction and reduction of RBF, and also increases release of renin and prostaglandins. Dopamine is thought to increase RBF by vasodilatation via dopamine receptors.
  - renin/angiotensin system: angiotensin II decreases RBF via vasoconstriction, and increases aldosterone secretion. The latter increases fluid retention which reduces further renin release.
  - vasopressin: causes renal vasoconstriction, especially cortical.
  - intravascular volume: in haemorrhage, autoregulation is overridden, with vasoconstriction and intrarenal redistribution of blood away from the cortex.
  - prostaglandins: increase cortical blood flow, and reduce medullary blood flow.
  - atrial natriuretic peptide: causes vasodilatation, although effects on RBF are unclear. May alter blood flow distribution.

RBF and GFR are reduced by most anaesthetic agents, mainly via reduced cardiac output and BP. Volatile agents are also thought to interfere with autoregulation, although some benefit may arise from the vasodilatation they cause, maintaining blood flow. Urine output therefore often falls perioperatively.

Other factors include pre-existing renal disease or conditions predisposing to renal failure or impairment, e.g. vascular surgery, toxic drugs, trauma, jaundice, hypovolaemia, etc.

Renal failure. Loss of renal function causing increases in plasma urea and creatinine. Divided into acute and chronic renal failure.

- Acute renal failure (ARF):
  - usually occurs over a few days; often reversible although a major cause of death during acute illness, especially in ICU.
  - may develop with or without pre-existing renal impairment. ARF may follow any severe acute illness, trauma or major surgery (especially involving the heart and great vessels), surgery in the presence of hepatic impairment, trauma, obstetric emergencies, and any condition involving hypotension.
  - classically divided thus:
    - prerenal: caused by renal hypoperfusion, e.g. shock, hypovolaemia, cardiac failure, renal artery stenosis.
    - renal: caused by renal disease:
      - glomerular, e.g.:
        - glomerulonephritis.
        - diabetes mellitus.
        - amyloid.
      - tubulointerstitial, e.g.:
        - acute tubular necrosis (ATN): accounts for 75% of hospital ARF. Caused by renal hypoperfusion or ischaemia and/or chemical toxicity, trauma or sepsis. Nephrotoxins include analgesics (e.g. chronic aspirin and paracetamol therapy), NSAIDs, aminoglycosides, immunosuppressive drugs, radiological contrast media and heavy metals. Usually (but not always) associated with oliguria (caused by tubular cell necrosis, tubular obstruction and cortical arteriolar vasoconstriction).
        - acute cortical necrosis: typically associated with placental abruption, pre-eclampsia and septic abortion, but also with factors causing ATN. Confirmed by renal biopsy. Usually irreversible.
        - tubulointerstitial nephritis/pyelonephritis.
        - polycystic renal disease.
        - tubular obstruction, e.g. in myeloma, myoglobinuria.
      - vascular, e.g. hypertension, connective tissue disease.
    - postrenal: caused by obstruction in the urinary collection system, e.g. bladder tumour, prostatic hypertrophy.

    Distinction between renal and pre- or postrenal failure is important since the latter two are potentially treatable before renal failure becomes established.
  - features:
    - oliguria.
    - uraemia and accumulation of other substances (e.g. ammonia): nausea, vomiting, malaise, increased bleeding and susceptibility to infection, decreased healing.
    - reduced sodium and water excretion and oedema, hypertension, hyperkalaemia, acidosis.
  - the following may aid diagnosis:
    - examination of urine: e.g. tubular casts may be seen in ATN, myoglobinuria may be present.
    - plasma and urine indices (Table 31).
    - flushing of the urinary catheter using aseptic technique.
    - assessment of cardiac and fluid volume state to exclude hypovolaemia.
    - effect of a fluid challenge of, e.g. 200–300 ml: increased urine output may occur in incipient prerenal failure.
    - diuretic administration, e.g. furosemide or mannitol: increased urine output may occur in incipient ATN but there is no evidence of a prophylactic or therapeutic effect although reduction in renal O_2 demand (furosemide) and scavenging of free radicals (mannitol) have been suggested as possibly being beneficial.
    - renal ultrasound or biopsy.
  - management:
    - directed at the primary cause, e.g. increasing renal blood flow.
    - monitoring of weight, cardiovascular status including JVP/CVP/pulmonary capillary wedge pressure as appropriate, urea and electrolytes, and acid–base status. Accurate fluid charts are vital.

Table 31 Investigations used to differentiate between prerenal oliguria and acute renal failure

Investigation	*Prerenal oliguria*	*Renal failure*
Specific gravity	>1.020	<1.010
Urine osmolality (mosmol/kg)	>500	<350
Urine sodium (mmol/l)	<20	>40
Urine/plasma osmolality ratio	>2	<1.1
Urine/plasma urea ratio	>20	<10
Urine/plasma creatinine ratio	>40	<20
Fractional sodium excretion (%)	<1	>1
Renal failure index	<1	>1

$$\text{Fractional sodium excretion} = \frac{\text{urine/plasma sodium ratio}}{\text{urea/plasma creatinine ratio}} \times 100\%$$

$$\text{and renal failure index} = \frac{\text{urine sodium}}{\text{urine/plasma creatinine ratio}}$$

- fluid restriction to, e.g. previous hour's urine output + 30 ml/h whilst oliguric.
- H_2 receptor antagonists are commonly administered since GIT haemorrhage is common.
- treatment of hyperkalaemia.
- monitoring of drug levels as clearance may be reduced considerably.
- various dialysis therapies.
- adequate nutrition.

- Chronic renal failure (CRF):
  - irreversible, and often follows ARF.
  - glomerulonephritis is the most common cause, with others including pyelonephritis, diabetes, polycystic disease, vascular disease and hypertension, drugs and familial causes.
  - features (may not be present until GFR falls below 15 ml/min):
    - malaise, anorexia, confusion leading to convulsions and coma. Peripheral and autonomic neuropathy may occur.
    - oedema, pericarditis, hypertension (in 80%; thought to result from increased renin/angiotensin system activity, sodium and water retention, and secondary hyperaldosteronism), peripheral vascular disease, cardiac failure.
    - nausea, vomiting, diarrhoea.
    - osteomalacia, muscle weakness, bone pain, hyperparathyroidism, hyperphosphataemia.
    - amenorrhoea, impotence.
    - pruritus, skin pigmentation, poor healing, increased susceptibility to infection.
    - normocytic normochromic anaemia: caused by reduced erythropoietin production, shortened red cell survival and bone marrow depression. Reduced platelet function may cause bruising and bleeding.
    - hypernatraemia or hyponatraemia may occur. Hyperkalaemia is usual, but hypokalaemia may follow diuretic therapy. Acidosis is common.
  - management:
    - reduction of dietary protein.
    - control of hypertension and cardiac failure.
    - erythropoietin is increasingly used for anaemia.
    - dialysis.
    - renal transplantation.
- Anaesthesia in renal failure:
  - preoperatively:
    - the features of the disease responsible for renal failure must be assessed, e.g. diabetes, hypertension, etc.
    - assessment for the above features of renal failure, in particular cardiovascular complications, fluid and electrolyte and acid–base derangements. Dialysis may be required. Anaemia rarely requires transfusion because of its chronicity with compensatory mechanisms. Patients may be at risk from aspiration of gastric contents if autonomic neuropathy is present.
    - drugs taken commonly include antianginal and antihypertensive drugs, insulin and corticosteroids.
    - pre-existing arteriovenous fistulae or shunts should be noted.
    - premedication as required.
  - perioperatively:
    - iv cannulae should not be sited near arteriovenous fistulae, which should be padded loosely with wool for protection.
    - potassium-containing iv fluids should be avoided.
    - preferred drugs are those that are not primarily excreted renally, and those with short duration of action. Thus a common technique consists of propofol followed by atracurium and isoflurane, sevoflurane or desflurane.
    - drugs which accumulate in renal failure, e.g. morphine, should be used with caution. Patients are thought to be more sensitive to many iv agents including opioids because of smaller volumes of distribution and reduced plasma albumin levels.
    - suxamethonium is not contraindicated unless there is pre-existing peripheral neuropathy or hyperkalaemia.
    - drugs which may impair renal function should be avoided. Enflurane has been avoided because of fluoride ion formation, although the need for this is controversial since plasma levels attained are low.
    - regional techniques are often suitable, e.g. brachial plexus block for fistula formation.
  - postoperatively: close attention to fluid balance is required.

Renal failure index, *see Renal failure*

Renal transplantation. First performed in 1950, and now widespread but limited mainly by the supply of kidneys. Cadaveric graft survival is up to 80–90% at 2 years. Previously considered an emergency and performed on unprepared patients, but the importance of proper preoperative assessment and preparation is now generally accepted. Dialysis is usually performed within 24 h before surgery.

- Anaesthetic problems and techniques are as for chronic renal failure and transplantation. Additional points:
  - general anaesthesia is preferred, although epidural and spinal anaesthesia have been successfully used.
  - direct arterial monitoring is not necessarily required, but CVP monitoring is usual, to guide per- and postoperative fluid therapy. Optimal hydration is vital to encourage graft function.
  - mannitol, furosemide, calcium channel blocking drugs and dopamine are sometimes given before the vessels to the new kidney are unclamped, in order to stimulate urine production and improve renal function.
  - transient hypertension may follow unclamping of the renal vessels.
  - there is an increased incidence of kidney rejection in patients who have received blood transfusion during transplantation.

Both live and cadaveric donors should be well hydrated to maintain urine output before harvesting.
See also, Organ donation

Renal tubular acidosis. Group of conditions characterised by decreased ability of each nephron to excrete hydrogen ions (cf. renal failure, where the overall number of functioning nephrons is reduced, but those that remain excrete more hydrogen ions than normal). Characterised by normal GFR, metabolic acidosis, hyperchloraemia and a normal anion gap. May be associated with distal tubule dysfunction (type 1), proximal tubule dysfunction (type 2; usually associated with other abnormalities of proximal tubule function, e.g. Fanconi's syndrome), or aldosterone deficiency or resistance (type 4). Type 3 is now considered a combination of types 1 and 2 and not a separate entity. Acidosis may be severe, and accompanied by marked hypokalaemia. Treatment includes alkali (e.g. oral sodium bicarbonate) in types 1 and 2, thiazides in type 2, and mineralocorticoid therapy in type 4.
[Guido Fanconi (1892–1979), Swiss paediatrician]

Renin/angiotensin system. Renin, a glycoprotein hormone (mw 37 326), is synthesised and secreted by the

Table 32 Peptides of the renin/angiotensin system

Substance	*Converted to*	*By the action of*	*Site*
Angiotensinogen	Angiotensin I	Renin	Plasma
Angiotensin I	Angiotensin II	Angiotensin converting enzyme	Mainly in lungs
Angiotensin II	Angiotensin III	Aminopeptidase	Many tissues

juxtacapillary apparatus of the renal tubule. Formed from two precursors, prorenin and preprorenin, its half-life is about 80 min. Secretion is increased in hypovolaemia, cardiac failure, cirrhosis and renal artery stenosis. Secretion is decreased by angiotensin II and vasopressin. Renin acts upon the circulating glycoprotein angiotensinogen with subsequent production of the peptides angiotensin I, II and III, involved in arterial BP control and fluid balance (Table 32). Angiotensin I functions as a precursor only. Angiotensin II is a powerful vasoconstrictor with a half-life of a few minutes. It causes aldosterone release from the adrenal cortex, and noradrenaline release from sympathetic nerve endings. It also stimulates thirst and release of vasopressin, and acts directly on renal tubules resulting in sodium and water retention. Some may also be produced in the tissues. Angiotensin III also causes aldosterone release and some vasoconstriction.

Angiotensin converting enzyme inhibitors and angiotensin II receptor antagonists are used to treat hypertension. Aliskiren, a renin inhibitor, has recently been introduced.

Angiotensin II or its analogues have been used as vasopressor drugs when α-agonists are unable to correct severe hypotension, e.g. during surgery for hepatic tumours secreting vasodilator substances.

Reperfusion injury. Paradoxical tissue injury after restoration of blood flow following a period of ischaemia. Thought to involve intracellular calcium excess, cell swelling through osmosis, or free radicals. Although any tissue may be affected, most work has focused on cardiac function following hypoxic insult or hyperfusion. Arrhythmias and myocardial stunning (reversible impairment of cardiac function) may also follow reperfusion.
See also, Isoprostanes, No reflow phenomenon

Reptilase time, *see Coagulation studies*

Reserpine. Antihypertensive drug of the Rauwolfia alkaloid family, first used in the 1950s and rarely used now. Depletes postganglionic adrenergic neurones of noradrenaline by irreversibly preventing its reuptake from axoplasm into storage vesicles. Crosses the blood–brain barrier and depletes central amine stores. Effects may last 1–2 weeks.

Side effects include bradycardia and postural hypotension, depression, sedation, extrapyramidal signs, diarrhoea and weight gain. Directly acting sympathomimetic drugs should be used in preference to indirectly acting ones, if required.
[Leonhard Rauwolf (1535–1596), German botanist]

Reservoir bag. Usually 2 litre capacity in most adult anaesthetic breathing systems and 0.5–1.0 litre for paediatric use; its volume must exceed tidal volume. Movement indicates ventilation, but estimation of tidal volume from the amount of movement is inaccurate. Made of rubber (increasingly, latex-free), distending when under pressure; maximal pressure is thus prevented from rising above about 60 cmH_2O (Laplace's law) unless the bag is particularly stiff or enclosed by string mesh (as required for certain (outdated) ventilating vents/ventilators). Such bags should not be used in routine breathing systems.

Residual volume (RV). Volume of gas remaining in the lungs after maximal expiration. About 1.5 litres in the average 70 kg male; measured as for FRC. Increased RV accounts for most cases of increased FRC.

Resistance. In electrical terms, the ratio between potential difference across a conductor to the current flowing through it (Ohm's law). Measured in ohms (Ω). Resistance to flow of a fluid through a circular tube is analogous to this; it equals the ratio between the pressure gradient along the tube to the flow through it.

Resistance vessels. Term given to those blood vessels involved in regulation of SVR. 50% of resistance to blood flow is due to arterioles, which are thus the main regulators of SVR and therefore distribution of cardiac output.

Resonance. Situation in which an oscillating system responds with maximal amplitude to an alternating external driving force. Occurs when the driving force frequency coincides with the natural oscillatory frequency (resonant frequency) of the system. May occur in pressure transducer systems if long, compliant tubing is used. May give rise to artefacts in the arterial waveform during direct arterial BP measurement.

Resonium, *see Polystyrene sulphonate resins*

Respiration, *see Breathing . . . ; Lung . . . ; Metabolism*

Respirators, *see Ventilators*

Respiratory centres, *see Breathing, control of*

Respiratory depression, *see Hypoventilation*

Respiratory distress syndrome (RDS; Hyaline membrane disease). Occurs in approximately 1% of all live births, almost exclusively in premature babies. Caused by deficiency of surfactant. Surfactant is normally detectable in the fetal lung at 24 weeks' gestation, although reversal of amniotic fluid lecithin/sphingomyelin ratio (related to fetal lung maturity) only occurs at 30 weeks. Decreased lung compliance, increased work of breathing and alveolar collapse may lead to respiratory failure, with characteristic granular appearance of the chest X-ray. Treatment is directed towards preventing hypoxaemia with CPAP initially although IPPV is usually necessary, whilst trying to avoid O_2 toxicity, barotrauma and retinopathy of prematurity. Surfactant given immediately after birth decreases mortality. Extracorporeal membrane oxygenation has been used.

Respiratory exchange ratio. Estimation of respiratory quotient derived from expired CO_2/inspired O_2 measurements, thus dependent on ventilation.

Respiratory failure. Defined as an arterial P_{O_2} at sea level, breathing air and at rest, below 8 kPa (60 mmHg), without intracardiac shunting.

- Divided into:
  - type I failure: hypoxaemia accompanied by normal or low arterial P_{CO_2}. Usually due to $\dot{V}/\dot{Q}$ mismatch, with intrapulmonary right-to-left shunt if severe. Causes

include chest infection, asthma, pulmonary oedema, PE, ARDS, aspiration pneumonitis, etc. O_2 therapy often improves $\dot{V}/\dot{Q}$ mismatch but not shunt; the response to breathing 100% O_2 may indicate the degree of shunt. $P\text{CO}_2$ is often low because of hyperventilation in response to hypoxaemia.
- type II failure (ventilatory failure): hypoxaemia accompanied by arterial $P\text{CO}_2$ exceeding 6.5 kPa (49 mmHg). Causes are as for hypoventilation. Acute exacerbation of COPD is a common cause.

Diagnosis is made by arterial blood gas analysis, but may be suspected clinically by signs of hypoxaemia and hypercapnia, with tachypnoea and use of accessory respiratory muscles.

- Treatment:
  - of underlying cause.
  - sitting the patient up increases FRC and often improves oxygenation.
  - O_2 therapy. Should be used cautiously in type II failure if chronic hypercapnia is suspected.
  - aminophylline may have an inotropic action on the diaphragm and may reduce respiratory muscle fatigue; it is often used in neonates.
  - carbonic anhydrase inhibitors may increase respiratory drive in COPD associated with hypercapnia.
  - respiratory stimulant drugs, e.g. doxapram, have been used to avoid IPPV, e.g. in COPD.
  - CPAP may improve oxygenation and avoid requirement for IPPV.
  - IPPV may be required if $P\text{CO}_2$ is rising or the patient is exhausted. Criteria similar to those used in weaning from ventilators have been suggested for institution of IPPV. Tracheal intubation is usually performed to allow IPPV, although non-invasive positive pressure ventilation and intermittent negative pressure ventilation have been used as alternatives. Tracheostomy may be necessary to aid weaning from mechanical ventilation.
  - intravenous oxygenator, extracorporeal oxygenation and extracorporeal CO_2 removal have been used.

Respiratory function tests, *see Lung function tests*

Respiratory muscle fatigue. Inability of the respiratory muscles to sustain tension with repeated activity. May be caused by:
- decreased central drive, e.g. caused by CNS depressant drugs (e.g. opioid analgesic drugs).
- increased ventilatory load caused by increased airway resistance and reduced compliance (e.g. asthma, COPD, etc.), or increased demand (e.g. exercise, fever, hypoxaemia, etc.).
- respiratory muscle weakness (e.g. following prolonged IPPV, malnutrition, electrolyte imbalance, thyroid disorders, hypoxaemia, sepsis, etc.).

Thought to be involved in hypercapnic respiratory failure and difficulty in weaning from ventilators. Treatment is directed at the underlying cause.

Moxham J (1990). Br J Anaesth; 65: 43–53

Respiratory muscles. Muscle actions during:
- quiet inspiration:
  - diaphragm (the most important muscle of respiration) flattens and moves 1–2 cm caudally.
  - external intercostal muscles (pass downwards and forwards) lift the upper ribs and sternum up and forwards, and the lower ribs mainly up and outwards. The first rib remains fixed.
- forced inspiration: as above, with the diaphragm descending up to 10 cm, plus accessory muscles:
  - scalene muscles.
  - sternomastoid.
  - serratus anterior.
  - pectoralis major.
  - ala nasi.
- quiet expiration: passive recoil of chest and abdomen.
- forced expiration:
  - mainly abdominal muscles (internal and external oblique, rectus abdominis).
  - internal intercostal muscles (pass downwards and backwards); opposite action to the external intercostals, and prevent intercostal bulging.

Respiratory quotient (RQ). Ratio of the volume of CO_2 produced by tissues to the volume of O_2 consumed per unit time. Depends on the type of substrate being utilised: RQ of carbohydrate is 1, RQ of fat 0.7 and that of protein about 0.82. Whole body RQ calculated by measurement of expired CO_2 and inspired O_2 approximates to true RQ, since these volumes are affected by respiration. The term respiratory exchange ratio (R) is therefore becoming more commonly used for this measurement.

Respiratory sounds. Originally detected with the examiner's ear placed against the patient's chest; traditionally assessed with a stethoscope and more recently analysed by digital processing using microphones or accelerometers placed on the chest wall. Sounds arise from vibration of airways and movement of fluid films within them. The nature of the sounds depends on the tissue through which they pass, e.g. quiet or absent in pleural effusion and pneumothorax, increased transmission (e.g. of spoken words) in consolidation. The pitch is related to the size of the airway involved and the density of the gas.
- Classification:
  - basic sounds: arise from:
    - central airways of the lung. Normally audible throughout inspiration and the beginning of expiration, with a gap between the end of the former and the start of the latter.
    - large airways and trachea. Typically audible throughout both inspiration and expiration, with no gap between the phases. Usually audible only over the trachea, this 'bronchial breathing' sound may be heard over the chest if transmitted to the stethoscope via abnormally solid tissue (e.g. consolidation) between it and the large airways.

    Range from under 100 Hz to over 1000–3000 Hz.
  - adventitious sounds:
    - wheezing: musical, arise from the central/lower airways. Sinusoidal, ranging from 100 Hz to over 1000 Hz.
    - rhonchi: snore-like, arise from the larger airways. Typically under 300 Hz and rapidly damped, but lasting over 100 ms. Occur in small airway collapse and secretions.
    - crackles: fine; arise from the central/lower airways. Rapidly damped, typically lasting under 20 ms. Occur in secretions, oedema and fibrosis.

Other sounds may occur, e.g. stridor, although not from the lung itself.

Pasterkamp H, Kraman SS, Wodicka GR (1997). Am J Resp Crit Care Med; 156: 974–87

Respiratory stimulant drugs, *see Analeptic drugs; Opioid receptor antagonists*

Respiratory symbols. By convention, standardised thus:

- general variables:
  - V = gas volume } with a dot above =
  - Q = volume of blood } volume per unit time
  - P = pressure or tension
  - F = fractional concentration in dry gas mixture
  - f = respiratory frequency
  - C = concentration of gas in blood phase
  - D = diffusing capacity
  - R = respiratory exchange ratio
  - S = saturation of haemoglobin with O_2 or CO_2
  - A dash above a symbol indicates mean value.
- localisation (in subscript):
  - I = inspired gas
  - E = expired gas
  - A = alveolar gas
  - T = tidal gas
  - D = dead space gas
  - B = barometric
  - a = arterial blood
  - c = pulmonary capillary blood
  - v = venous blood

e.g. $F_{I}O_2$ = inspired fractional concentration of O_2; $P_{a}O_2$ = arterial O_2 tension.

$S_{p}O_2$ has been suggested as representing haemoglobin saturation as measured by pulse oximetry.

Respirometer. Device for measuring expiratory gas volumes. Examples:

- Wright's anemometer: exhaled air is passed into its chamber through oblique slits, creating circular gas flow, and causing rotation of a double-vaned rotor within the chamber. Rotation is measured and displayed as the volume of gas passing through the device, using an indicator needle attached to the vane, and a dial. Electrical versions are also available; rotations of a disc attached to the vane interrupt passage of light between an emitter and photosensitive cell mounted astride the disc.
- Wright's respirometer: measures gas volume passing in one direction only; thus it may be placed in the 'to and fro' portion of a breathing system. It tends to underestimate at low volumes and overestimate at high volumes, due to inertia/momentum of the vane.
- others: include flowmeters whose signals may be integrated to indicate volume.

[B Martin Wright (1912–2001), London engineer]

See also, Spirometer

Resuscitation, *see Cardiopulmonary resuscitation*

Resuscitation Council (UK). Multiprofessional group formed in 1982 to facilitate education of lay and professional members of the population in the most effective methods of resuscitation. Aims of the Council include encouraging research and study of the techniques of resuscitation, the promotion of training and education in resuscitation, and the establishment and maintenance of standards. The Council has published guidelines for CPR and has set up a series of advanced courses in adult and paediatric resuscitation (i.e. ALS, ILS).

See also, European Resuscitation Council

Resuscitators, *see Self-inflating bags*

Reteplase. Recombinant plasminogen activator, used as a fibrinolytic drug in acute management of MI. Has a longer half-life (13–16 min) than alteplase.

- Dosage: 10 U iv in under 2 min, repeated after 30 min.
- Side effects: as for fibrinolytic drugs. May precipitate with heparin solutions.

Reticular formation/activating system, *see Ascending reticular activating system*

Retinopathy of prematurity (Retrolental fibroplasia). Abnormal proliferation of retinal vessels in response to high arterial P_{O_2} for long periods. Very premature infants of low birth weight are the most susceptible, remaining so until 44 weeks' postconceptual age. O_2 therapy should therefore be monitored closely. Precise mechanisms are unclear, as it may occur in infants who have not received additional O_2. Genetic factors appear to be important. The role of O_2 administered during anaesthesia is controversial, but $F_{I}O_2$ is generally thought to be best restricted to 0.3 unless higher concentrations are required to maintain arterial P_{O_2} of 8.5–11 kPa (60–80 mmHg).

Saugstad OD (2006). J Perinatol 26 Suppl 1: S46–50

Retrobulbar block. Performed to allow surgery to the globe of the eye, e.g. cataract extraction, when combined with facial nerve block and conjunctival anaesthesia. The long and short ciliary nerves are blocked within the cone formed by the extraocular muscles.

With the patient supine and looking straight ahead, a 3.0 cm needle is inserted through the conjunctiva at the lower lateral orbital rim, with the lower lid retracted (injection through the lower eyelid may also be performed). It is passed backward and 10° upward until its tip has passed the midglobe, then angled medially and upward to reach a point behind the globe at the level of the iris (less than 2.0 cm should be inserted). Accidental puncture of the sclera may be signalled by rotation of the globe. After aspiration, 2–4 ml lidocaine with hyaluronidase 5 U/ml, is slowly injected. Produces extraocular muscle paralysis, pupillary dilatation and reduced intraocular pressure.

Complications include retrobulbar haemorrhage causing proptosis, intravascular and subarachnoid injection, the latter causing apnoea and cardiovascular collapse. Peribulbar block and sub-Tenon's block have been suggested as safer alternatives.

See also, Orbital cavity

Retrolental fibroplasia, *see Retinopathy of prematurity*

Retzius cave block. Used to supplement anaesthesia for prostatectomy and bladder surgery. The cave of Retzius is the space between the bladder and pubic symphysis, containing nerves of the sacral plexus and a venous plexus. After subcutaneous infiltration 2–3 cm above the pubis, an 8 cm needle is directed to the back of the symphysis. After careful aspiration, 10 ml local anaesthetic agent with adrenaline is injected in the midline, with a further injection on each side.

[Anders Retzius (1796–1860), Swedish anatomist]

Reuben valve, *see Non-rebreathing valves*

Revised trauma score (RTS). Trauma scale derived from the trauma score but simplified and with greater emphasis on the presence of head injury. Takes the Glasgow coma scale, systolic BP and respiratory rate, each assigned a value of 0–4 according to deviation from normal with 0 representing the most severe score. The values are added to give a total RTS, with a normal of 12. The scoring system has been modified by multiplying each value by a correction factor and the products

added together to give a RTS between 0 and 7.8408, a higher number suggesting a better prognosis. Has been shown to be superior to the trauma score at predicting outcome; a RTS of < 4 has been suggested as indicating the need for transfer to a specialist trauma unit.
Gilpin DA, Nelson PG (1991). Injury; 22: 35–7

Reye's syndrome. Rare condition of unknown aetiology, characterised by vomiting, depression of consciousness and hepatic failure. Jaundice is typically absent or minimal. Usually occurs in children, typically following a viral illness; aspirin has been implicated in epidemiological studies and is thus contraindicated under 16 years of age. Thought to be due to an acquired mitochondrial abnormality. Treatment is mainly supportive, with correction of metabolic disturbances, cerebral oedema and raised ICP. Thought to be improved by administering up to a third of the fluid intake as 10% dextrose.
[R Douglas Reye (1912–1977), Australian pathologist]

Reynolds' number (*Re*). Dimensionless number predicting when flow of a fluid becomes turbulent:

$$Re = \frac{\text{density} \times \text{velocity} \times \text{diameter of tube}}{\textbf{viscosity}}$$

Turbulent flow occurs at $Re > 2000$, laminar flow at < 2000.
[Osborne Reynolds (1842–1912), Irish-born English engineer]

Rhabdomyolysis, *see Myoglobinuria*

Rhesus blood groups. System of blood group antigens first described in 1939 following work on rhesus monkeys. Includes many antigens (agglutinogens) but the terms Rhesus (Rh) positive and negative usually refer to the D agglutinogen, as it is the most antigenic. Rh negative individuals have no D antigen, and form anti-D antibodies when injected with Rh positive blood. 85% of Caucasians are Rh positive, 99% of Orientals.

- Clinical importance:
  - blood transfusion reactions: administration of Rh positive blood to Rh negative individuals who have anti-D antibodies following previous exposure to Rh positive blood.
  - haemolytic disease of the newborn: occurs in Rh positive fetuses of Rh negative mothers. Passage of fetal blood cells into the maternal circulation during pregnancy or labour causes formation of maternal anti-D antibodies. These may pass into subsequent Rh positive fetuses, causing haemolysis which may be fatal. Incidence of primary immunisation in primigravidae is about 15%. Uncommon now with widespread availability of anti-Rh immunoglobulin which is administered to Rh negative mothers at delivery, and after abortion, amniocentesis, etc. Routine administration of anti-Rh to all Rh negative pregnant women has been suggested as a way of reducing the problem further.

Rheumatic fever. Acute disease, thought to be caused by an abnormal immune reaction to certain serotypes of group A streptococci. Most common between 5 and 15 years of age; now rare in the West but still common in developing countries. Typically occurring 2–6 weeks after a sore throat, features include fever, flitting arthritis, carditis, chorea and erythema marginatum (erythema spreading out from a central macule whilst the centre returns to normal). Subcutaneous nodules (Aschoff bodies) may occur over the extensor surfaces of the wrists, elbows and knees. Epistaxis and abdominal pain are common. Diagnosed clinically and by evidence of recent streptococcal infection. Traditionally treated with rest, aspirin and corticosteroids, but the effect of drugs on valve disease is controversial. 50% of patients with carditis progress to valvular heart disease, which may not present until later in life. Mitral and aortic valves are most commonly affected.

Anaesthetic management of patients previously affected is directed towards any existing valve disease, with prophylactic antibiotics as for congenital heart disease.
[Karl Albert Ludwig Aschoff (1866–1942), German pathologist]
Carapetis JR, McDonald M, Wilson NJ (2005). Lancet; 366: 155–68
See also, individual valve lesions

Rheumatoid arthritis (Rheumatoid disease). Systemic inflammatory disease with many features of connective tissue diseases. Characterised by symmetrical polyarthropathy, but affects other organs too. More common in females; peak incidence is at ages 30–50 years. Up to 5% of females over 60 years are affected in the UK. Aetiology is obscure but may involve an immunological process triggered by infectious agents.

- Anaesthetic considerations:
  - systemic effects:
    - skeletal: temporomandibular joint involvement, atlantoaxial subluxation, reduced mobility of the lumbar/cervical spine.
    - neuromuscular: nerve entrapment, sensory/motor neuropathy, myopathy.
    - respiratory: restrictive defect due to pulmonary fibrosis and costochondral disease, pulmonary nodules, pleural effusions, cricoarytenoid arthritis.
    - cardiovascular: pericarditis, conduction defects, coronary arteritis, peripheral vasculitis.
    - haematological: anaemia (usually normochromic normocytic), leucopenia. Felty's syndrome consists of rheumatoid arthritis, splenomegaly and leucopenia; thrombocytopenia, malaise and fever may occur.
    - renal: amyloidosis, pyelonephritis, drug-related impairment.
    - others: ophthalmic complications including Sjögren's syndrome, and atrophic skin and subcutaneous tissues.
  - drug therapy: may include NSAIDs, corticosteroids and immunosuppressive drugs. Gold may cause blood dyscrasias, peripheral neuritis, pulmonary fibrosis, hepatic and renal impairment. Penicillamine may cause blood dyscrasias, renal impairment, neuropathy and a myasthenia gravis-like syndrome.
  - practical considerations:
    - drug administration whilst nil by mouth; rectal or im NSAIDs are useful.
    - venous cannulation may be difficult; skin and veins are fragile, and joints may have reduced mobility.
    - discomfort lying flat; skeletal involvement may make regional techniques unsuitable. Careful positioning and padding are required. Skin is easily damaged.
    - airway maintenance difficulties: caused by involvement of the temporomandibular joint, cervical spine and larynx.

[Augustus R Felty (1895–1963), US physician; Henrik SC Sjögren (1899–1986), Swedish ophthalmologist]
See also, Intubation, difficult

Ribavirin (Tribavirin). Antiviral drug; a nucleoside, it inhibits DNA synthesis and is active against many RNA and DNA viruses although usually reserved for treatment of respiratory syncytial viral infection and Lassa fever. Also used in combination with interferon alfa for the treatment of chronic hepatitis C.

- Dosage: nebulisation or aerosol inhalation of 20 mg/ml solution for 12–18 h for 3–7 days. For hepatitis C, 400–600 mg orally, 12 hourly.
- Side effects are rare but include anaemia and worsening respiration.

Rib fractures. Middle ribs are most commonly affected. Fracture usually occurs at the posterior axillary line, the point of maximal stress. If the first three ribs are affected, injury to the aorta and tracheobronchial tree should be considered. If the lower ribs are involved, damage to liver, spleen and kidneys may occur. Pneumothorax and haemothorax may be present.

Rib fractures cause pain on breathing, with splinting of the chest wall, inability to cough and atelectasis. Multiple fractures may cause flail chest. The mainstay of treatment is good analgesia; this may involve systemic analgesics, epidural anaesthesia or intercostal nerve block.

General management is as for chest trauma and abdominal trauma.

Ribs. Exist in 12 (thoracic) pairs, with occasional additional cervical or lumbar ribs. Attached to thoracic vertebrae posteriorly and costal cartilage anteriorly. Ribs 2–8 are typical (Fig. 132a), consisting of:
  - head: bears two facets for articulation with adjacent vertebrae.
  - neck.
  - tubercle: articulates posteriorly with the transverse process of the corresponding vertebra.
  - shaft: flattened in the vertical plane. Curves forwards and inwards from the angle, lying lateral to the tubercle. The intercostal neurovascular bundle runs in the subcostal groove at the inferior border.
- The first rib is of particular anaesthetic importance because of its relationship to the brachial plexus and other structures (Fig. 132b). Features:
  - short, wide and flattened in the horizontal plane.
  - lower surface is smooth and lies on pleura.
  - upper surface is grooved for the subclavian vessels and brachial plexus.
  - sympathetic chain, superior intercostal artery and upper branch of the first intercostal nerve lie anterior to its neck, between it and the pleura.
  - scalenus anterior and medius attach to the scalene tubercle and body of the rib respectively.

See also, Intercostal nerve block; Intercostal space

Rifabutin. Antituberculous drug used for prophylaxis against *Mycobacterium avium* in immunocompromised patients.

- Dosage: 300 mg orally daily for prophylaxis, 150–450 mg daily for treatment.
- Side effects: blood dyscrasias, nausea, vomiting, hepatic impairment.

Rifampicin. Antibacterial drug, used primarily as an antituberculous drug but also in brucellosis, Legionnaires' disease, severe staphylococcal infection, leprosy and as prophylaxis against meningococcal disease (thus may be given to ICU staff after caring for an infected patient or to household contacts). Causes hepatic enzyme induction and thus decreases the efficacy of oral contraceptives, anticoagulants and phenytoin.

- Dosage: 300 mg orally (iv in severe infections), 6–12 hourly.

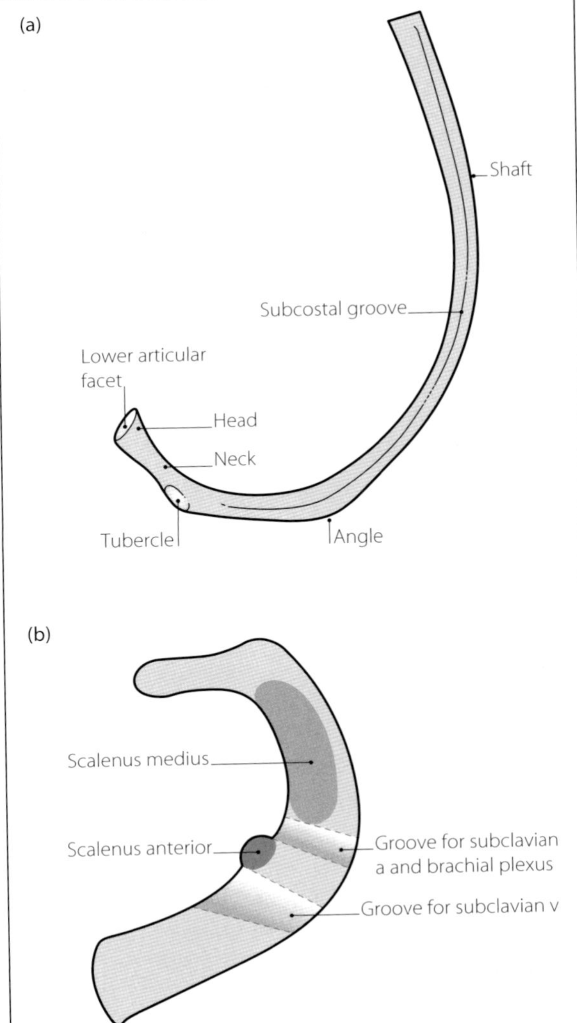

Fig. 132 Anatomy of (a) a typical rib, seen from undersurface; (b) the first rib, seen from above

- Side effects: GIT upset, haemolytic anaemia, dyspnoea, renal and hepatic impairment, rashes, myopathy. Colours body secretions orange.

Right atrial pressure, *see Cardiac catheterisation; Central venous pressure*

Right ventricular function. Increasingly recognised as an important variable in critical illness, although traditionally the left ventricle (LV) has received most attention. The right ventricle (RV) receives blood from systemic and coronary veins, and pumps it into the LV across the pulmonary vascular bed. The pulmonary bed has a low pressure, therefore RV pressures (15–25/8–12 mmHg) are lower than systemic. The low intraventricular pressure permits right coronary blood flow to be continuous throughout the cardiac cycle. The output of the right heart is influenced by its preload, contractility and afterload. The RV is very compliant and when afterload increases (e.g. because of pulmonary vascular resistance secondary to lung injury), the RV dilates. The end-diastolic volume may increase to a greater extent than the preload; consequently, the RV ejection fraction (EF) will decrease markedly with increasing afterload. Changes in the geometry of the RV affect the function of the LV, and vice versa (ventricular interdependence), e.g. impaired RV function (whether acute or chronic) may hinder LV function via RV distension and deviation of the intraventricular septum.

Although the RV is analogous to the LV in terms of control mechanisms it is more difficult to assess; e.g. the relationship between RV preload, RV volume and RV filling pressures is not always constant. In addition, attempts to study RV function are hindered by the greater effect of respiratory excursions on the RV because the pressures involved are less than those on the left side of the heart. RV function may be assessed by RVEF pulmonary artery catheters. A bolus of thermal indicator is distributed to the blood in the right atrium and beat-to-beat blood temperature changes are sensed by a rapid response thermistor on the catheter tip in the pulmonary artery. Temperature changes between each beat can be measured and RVEF calculated using the formula:

$$\text{RVEF} = \frac{1 - (T_2 - T_b)}{(T_1 - T_b)}$$

where T_1 and T_2 = temperatures in the RV during two successive cycles and T_b = basal temperature of blood returning to the heart.

RV function may be altered in acute respiratory failure, sepsis, chest trauma, ischaemic heart disease, and after cardiac surgery. The possibility of RV ischaemia and even infarction in critically ill patients as a cause of RV dysfunction has recently been recognised. During IPPV, decreased venous return subsequent to the increased intrathoracic pressure results in decreased RV end-diastolic volume and thus cardiac output. RV impairment may result in the classic features of right-sided cardiac failure, but may present as a general poor perfusion state.

Ringer's solution. Developed as an *in vitro* medium for tissues and organisms, emphasising the importance of inorganic ions in maintaining cellular integrity. Exact constitution varies between laboratories, but approximates to sodium 137 mmol/l, potassium 4 mmol/l, calcium 3 mmol/l and chloride 142 mmol/l. Modifications include Ringer-lactate (Hartmann's solution) and Ringer's acetate (similar to Hartmann's solution but with acetate instead of lactate).
[Sydney Ringer (1834–1910), English physician]
Lee JA (1981). Anaesthesia; 36: 1115–21

rINNs, Recommended International Non-proprietary Names, *see Explanatory Notes at the beginning of this book*

Risk management. Process for reducing the frequency and cost of adverse events, e.g. complications of anaesthesia. Consists of:
- analysis of risks (e.g. morbidity/mortality meetings, critical incident reporting schemes). Risks are categorised into:
  - individual based (e.g. arising from human error), e.g. wrong drug given.
  - operating room based (arising from the interaction between anaesthetists and their working environment, e.g. operating theatre), e.g. disconnection of breathing system.
  - system based (human actions superimposed on inherent flaws in a system or process), e.g. because of alterations to the operating list caused by cancellations due to lack of beds, a patient arrives in the anaesthetic room without the diseased limb marked and has the wrong leg amputated.
- prevention of risks associated with routine activities (e.g. proper training and supervision, provision of trained anaesthetic assistants).
- avoidance of particularly high risk activities (e.g. wider use of regional anaesthesia for Caesarean section).
- minimising the severity of adverse events should they occur (e.g. training in defibrillation, maintenance of emergency drugs and equipment).
- risk financing (e.g. indemnity).
- having a system for dealing with disasters and complaints, to reduce both psychological and legal sequelae.

Audit of preventative measures is usually an integral part of a risk management programme, the costs of which may be considerable although the avoidance of legal action is an attractive benefit. Protocols may contribute to risk management by standardising care although they are not universally viewed with approval.
See also, Clinical governance; Quality assurance

Ritrodine hydrochloride. β-Adrenergic receptor agonist, used as a tocolytic drug in premature labour.
- Dosage:
  - 50–350 μg/min iv (or 10 mg 3–8 hourly, im), continued for 12–48 h after contractions have ceased.
  - 10 mg orally, 30 min before stopping iv infusion, repeated 2 hourly for 24 h then 10–20 mg 4–6 hourly.
- Side effects: nausea, vomiting, sweating, tremor, hypokalaemia, tachycardia, hypotension, pulmonary oedema, arrhythmias, increased uterine bleeding after Caesarean section, blood dyscrasias and hepatic impairment on prolonged therapy. Administration of excessive volumes of iv fluids may increase the risk of pulmonary oedema.

Rivastigmine, *see Acetylcholinesterase inhibitors*

ROC curves, *see Receiver operating characteristic curves*

Rocuronium bromide. Non-depolarising neuromuscular blocking drug, introduced in 1994. Chemically related to vecuronium, with similar lack of cardiovascular effects, although tachycardia may accompany very large doses. Has been suggested as the drug of choice when suxamethonium is contraindicated. Good intubating conditions occur 60 s after an initial dose of 0.6 mg/kg; relaxation lasts for about 30–40 min (about 20 min after 0.45 mg/kg). Supplementary dose: 0.15 mg/kg; effects last for about 15 min. May be infused iv at 0.3–0.6 mg/kg/h after a loading dose. Primarily excreted by the liver. Cumulation is unlikely at recommended doses. Reversed by sugammadex.

Ropivacaine hydrochloride. Amide local anaesthetic agent, introduced in 1997. Chemically related to bupivacaine (a propyl group replacing a butyl group) but less lipid soluble and less toxic, being associated with fewer and less severe CNS and CVS adverse effects. pK_a is 8.1. Prepared as the (S)-enantiomer (*see Isomerism*). Used in 0.2–1.0% concentrations; initially reported to be approximately equipotent to bupivacaine in terms of analgesia whilst producing less motor block, e.g. for epidural anaesthesia. However, this has been disputed, the lesser motor block seen with ropivacaine being related to its lower potency and thus selection of non-comparable solutions in comparative studies. In addition, comparable concentrations contain slightly less ropivacaine than bupivacaine. Has vasoconstrictor properties; thus relatively unaffected by addition of vasoconstrictor drugs. About 94% protein-bound; undergoes hepatic metabolism with 1% excreted unchanged in the urine. Has about 40%

greater clearance than bupivacaine. Maximal safe dose has been estimated at 3.5 mg/kg.

Rotameter. Refers to the trade name of a type of flowmeter commonly used on anaesthetic machines; first fitted in the 1930s.

- Features include:
  - constant pressure, variable orifice.
  - consists of a needle valve, below a bobbin within a tapered tube. Gas flow rates are marked along the tube's length. Readings are taken from the top of the bobbin. Tubes are arranged in banks at the back of the anaesthetic machine, traditionally for O_2, CO_2 and cyclopropane (the last two on older machines only), N_2O, and air, from left to right in the UK (see below).
  - accurate to within 2%.
  - bobbins are made of light metal alloy; each is individually matched to its particular tube, and specific for a certain gas.
  - the tube's taper is narrower at the bottom to allow accurate measurement of low flow rates, and wider above to measure higher flows.
  - the space between the bobbin and walls of tube is narrow at the bottom of the tube; gas flow behaves as through a tube, i.e. is largely laminar. Thus gas viscosity is important at low flow rates. Higher up the tube, the space between the bobbin and tube is wide compared with the length of the bobbin, because of the tube's taper. Gas flow behaves as through an orifice, i.e. is turbulent. Thus gas density is important at high flow rates.
  - inaccuracies may result from sticking of the bobbin against the sides of the tube. This is reduced by:
    - keeping the tube vertical to reduce friction between bobbin and tube.
    - angular notches in the bobbin, causing it to rotate when gas flows.
    - regular cleaning to prevent dirt accumulating within the tube.
    - reduction of static charge building up within the tube. Many are internally coated with a thin layer of gold. Alternatively, regular spraying with antistatic solution may be performed.
  - the O_2 control knob is larger than the others and differently shaped to aid recognition. All are colour-coded as for cylinders.
  - on some older machines, the CO_2 bobbin could be hidden at the top of the tube if the CO_2 valve was accidentally left fully open.
  - with the traditional arrangement of rotameters, i.e. O_2 upstream, O_2 may be lost if there is a leak from a tube downstream. This may be prevented by placing the O_2 inlet downstream from the others, e.g. by fitting a baffle across the top of the rotameter tubes so that N_2O enters first, and O_2 last.
  - in modern machines, N_2O and O_2 rotameters are mechanically linked such that less than 25% O_2 cannot be delivered.

Rotational therapy (Kinetic therapy). Technique in which critically ill patients are turned laterally from the horizontal to an angle of about 40°, often several times per hour on a programmable bed. Thought to reduce the incidence of nosocomial pneumonia, decubitus ulcers, DVT and PE. Also reported to shorten duration of both IPPV and ICU stay. May share mechanisms of action with prone ventilation techniques. Compared with the prone position, it has less chance of accidental displacement of tubes and catheters/cannulae, damage to eyes/face/limbs, etc., stimulation of coughing and cardiovascular instability. Accessibility to the patient remains good.

Goldhill DR, Imhoff M, McLean B, Waldmann C (2007). Am J Crit Care; 16: 50–61

Rowbotham, Edgar Stanley (1890–1979). English pioneer of anaesthesia. With Magill, developed tracheal intubation including blind nasal intubation, and endotracheal anaesthesia. Also pioneered basal narcosis with rectal paraldehyde, and local and intravenous techniques. The first anaesthetist in the UK to use cyclopropane. Designed several pieces of apparatus, including a vaporiser, airway, local anaesthetic needles and other equipment. Latterly worked at Charing Cross, London. Particularly interested in anaesthesia for thyroid surgery.

Condon HA, Gilchrist E (1986). Anaesthesia; 41: 46–52

Royal College of Anaesthetists. Arose from the granting of a Charter to the College of Anaesthetists by Queen Elizabeth II in March 1992. Regulates and promotes research, training, education and maintenance of standards in anaesthesia. Administers the FRCA examination. Has around 6500 Fellows (including overseas); together with Members (non-trainees without the Final FRCA, a membership category introduced in 2001) and registered trainees, this amounts to ~12 000 members in total. Created a Faculty of Pain Medicine in 2007. The *British Journal of Anaesthesia* has been its official journal since 1990; it also publishes guidelines, a regular *Bulletin* and *CEPD Reviews*.

Spence AA (1992). Br J Anaesth; 68: 457–8

R–R interval. Time between successive R waves on the ECG. Thus heart rate =

$$\frac{60}{\text{R} - \text{R interval(s)}}$$

Normally varies by less than 0.16 s at rest (sinus arrhythmia). Useful in the diagnosis of autonomic neuropathy.

RT, Reptilase time, *see Coagulation studies*

RTS, *see Revised trauma score*

Rule of nines. Guide to the percentage of body surface area represented by various parts of the body; used in assessment and treatment of burns:

- head: 9%.
- arms: 9% each.
- trunk: 18% front; 18% back.
- legs: 18% each.
- perineum: 1%.

For small areas, the patient's palmar surface represents about 1% of surface area.

- For children, proportions of body parts are different:
  - head: 15%.
  - arms: 10% each.
  - trunk: 20% front; 20% back.
  - legs: 12% each.

S

S-100β protein. Calcium-binding protein present in glial cells, studied as an early marker of neurological damage after CVA, head injury, cardiac surgery and neurosurgery. Metabolised in the kidney with a half-life of ~25 min, the serum concentration is usually negligible but increases after brain injury, although it is thought that S-100β may also be produced from other tissues and its relationship with functional impairment is uncertain.
Hall RI (2004). Can J Anaesth; 51: 645–8

S wave. Downward deflection following the R wave of the ECG (*see Fig. 57b; Electrocardiography*). Its size usually decreases from V_2 to V_6; the deepest wave is normally less than 30 mm. Prominence in standard leads I, II and III ($S_1S_2S_3$ pattern) may be normal in young people but may be associated with right ventricular hypertrophy. May also be seen in MI along with other changes.
See also, QRS complex

SA node, Sinoatrial node, *see Heart, conducting system*

Sacral canal. Cavity, 10–15 cm long and triangular in section, running the length of the sacrum, itself formed from five fused sacral vertebrae (Fig. 133). Continuous cranially with the lumbar vertebral canal. The anterior wall is formed by the fused bodies of the sacral vertebrae, and the posterior walls by the fused sacral laminae. Due to failure of fusion of the fifth laminar arch, the posterior wall is deficient between the cornua, forming the sacral hiatus, which is covered by the sacrococcygeal membrane (punctured during caudal analgesia). Congenital variants of fusion are common, e.g. deficient fusion of several laminae; this is thought to be a contributing cause of unreliability of caudal analgesia. The canal contains the termination of the dural sac at S2, the sacral nerves and coccygeal nerve, the internal vertebral venous plexus and fat. Its average volume in adults is 32 ml in females and 34 ml in males.
Crighton IM, Barry BP, Hobbs GJ (1997). Br J Anaesth; 78: 391–5

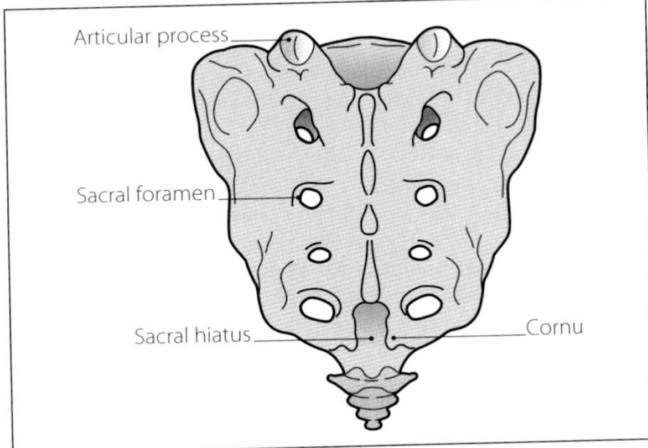

Fig. 133 Anatomy of the sacrum (posterior view)

Sacral nerve block, *see Caudal analgesia*

Sacral plexus. Supplies the pelvic and hip muscles, and the skin of the buttock and posterior thigh. Lies in front of the sacrum deep to the pelvic fascia, and formed from the anterior primary rami of L4–S4 (Fig. 134). Its major branch is the sciatic nerve.
See also, Sciatic nerve block

Saddle block, *see Spinal anaesthesia*

Safe transport and retrieval (STaR). Course conceived by the Advanced Life Support Group and first run in 1998. Teaches a systematic approach to the safe transfer and retrieval of critically ill and injured patients. Aimed at doctors, nurses and paramedics.
See also, Transportation of critically ill patients

Salbutamol. β-Adrenergic receptor agonist, used mainly as a bronchodilator drug. Relatively selective for β_2-receptors, although it does cause slight β_1-receptor stimulation. Undergoes extensive first-pass metabolism if given orally, thus usually administered by inhalation or iv. Produces bronchodilatation within 15 min; effects last 3–4 h. May also reduce the release of histamine and inflammatory mediators from mast cells sensitised with IgE, hence its particular use in asthma.

Also used as a tocolytic drug in premature labour and to improve cardiac output in low perfusion states, via β_2-receptor mediated smooth muscle relaxation in the uterus and blood vessels respectively.

- Dosage:
  - 2–4 mg orally, 6–8 hourly.
  - 500 µg im/sc, 4 hourly as required.
  - 250 µg iv slowly, repeated as required. 3–20 µg/min

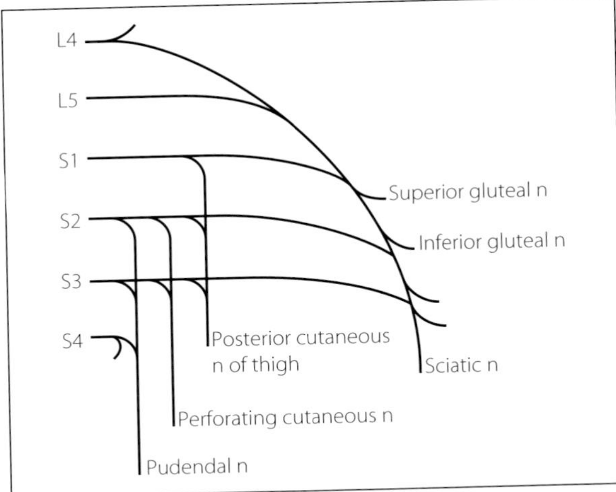

Fig. 134 Plan of the sacral plexus

infusion may be used. IV injection has been claimed to be more effective than inhalation in severe asthma, but this is controversial. Up to 45 μg/min may be required in premature labour.
- 1–2 puffs by aerosol (100–200 μg) 6–8 hourly. 200–400 μg is recommended for dry powder inhalation, since bioavailability for the latter is lower.
- 2.5–5 mg by nebulised solution, 4–6 hourly.
- Side effects: tachycardia, tremor, headache. Hypokalaemia may occur with prolonged use. Pulmonary oedema may occur after use for tocolysis.

Salicylate poisoning. Usually acute but may be chronic, especially in children.
- Features:
  - nausea, vomiting, haematemesis, sweating, tinnitus, deafness, confusion, hallucinations. Loss of consciousness is uncommon unless poisoning is severe.
  - hyperventilation results from direct respiratory centre stimulation, possibly via central uncoupling of oxidative phosphorylation. Respiratory alkalosis results. Compensatory renal excretion of bicarbonate results in urinary water and potassium loss with dehydration and hypokalaemia.
  - metabolic acidosis is caused by the salicylic acid, and its metabolic effects (increased production of ketone bodies, lactic acid and pyruvic acid, hyperglycaemia or hypoglycaemia). Thus the urine, initially alkaline, becomes acid.
  - arrhythmias, hypotension.
  - convulsions, pulmonary oedema, hyperthermia and renal failure may occur.
  - impaired coagulation is rarely significant.
- Treatment:
  - general measures as for poisoning and overdose, e.g. O_2 therapy, iv fluid administration. Activated charcoal (1 mg/kg) should be given to all patients who have ingested > 150 mg/kg or those who are symptomatic. Additional doses may be given if serum salicylate levels continue to rise.
  - increased elimination may be indicated if plasma levels exceed 500 mg/l (3.6 mmol/l) in adults or 300 g/l (2.2 mmol/l) in children. Techniques include forced alkaline diuresis, dialysis and haemoperfusion.

Mortality of acute overdose is approximately 2%; mortality of chronic overdose about 25%.
See also, Forced diuresis

Salicylates. Group of NSAIDs derived from salicylic acid. Aspirin (acetylsalicylic acid) is the most commonly prescribed; others, e.g. sodium salicylate, are also available but less potent. Have anti-inflammatory and antipyretic effects; they act via inhibition of synthesis and release of prostaglandins. Thought to act (at least partly) centrally, since they are effective when injected into the brains of experimental animals. Uncouple oxidative phosphorylation in the mitochondria of cartilage and induce formation of nitric oxide sensitising leucocytes to fight infection more effectively. Inhibit platelet and vascular endothelial cyclo-oxygenase; at low dosage, they selectively inhibit platelet cyclo-oxygenase. They are thus used as antiplatelet drugs. Effects on platelets are irreversible, lasting until new platelets are synthesised (7–10 days).

Used for mild to moderate pain, pyrexia, rheumatic fever, rheumatoid arthritis, and peripheral and coronary artery disease including after coronary artery bypass graft. They are contraindicated in gout because urinary excretion of uric acid may be decreased.

Absorbed rapidly from the upper GIT after therapeutic dosage, with peak plasma levels within 2 h of ingestion. Absorption is determined by the composition of tablets, intestinal pH and gastric emptying. About 90% protein-bound, they compete with other substances for protein binding sites, e.g. thyroxine, penicillin, phenytoin. Biotransformation occurs in hepatic endoplasmic reticulum and mitochondria. Excreted mainly in the urine, especially if the latter is alkaline. Half-life is about 15 min, but is very dependent on the dose taken.
- Side effects: as for NSAIDs and salicylate poisoning. They have been implicated in causing Reye's syndrome in children.

Salicylates should not be given to children under 16 years, patients with peptic ulcer disease or coagulation disorders, or those taking anticoagulant drugs.

Saline solutions. IV fluids containing sodium chloride, used extensively to replace sodium and ECF losses, e.g. in dehydration, and perioperatively. A 0.9% solution is most commonly used ('physiological saline', often erroneously called 'normal saline'); other saline-containing solutions include Hartmann's solution and dextrose/saline mixtures. Twice 'normal' saline (1.8%) is used in hyponatraemia, and up to 7.5% solutions have been used (largely experimentally) in hypovolaemic shock.

Administration of large volumes of saline may result in hyperchloraemic acidosis, the clinical significance of which is unclear.
See also, Hypertonic intravenous solutions; Normal solution

Samples, statistical. Parts of populations, selected for statistical tests or analysis. In order to represent the true population, samples should be as large as possible, and free of bias; i.e. should be random. Matched samples refer to groups matched for possible confounding variables, allowing better comparison of the desired measurements. Optimum matching occurs when subjects act as their own controls (i.e. measurements are paired).
See also, Clinical trials; Randomisation; Statistics

Sanders oxygen injector, *see Injector techniques*

Saphenous nerve block, *see Ankle, nerve blocks; Knee, nerve blocks*

SAPS, *see Simplified acute physiology score*

Sarcoidosis. Systemic disease, possibly caused by an infective agent or immunological derangement, characterised by non-necrotising granuloma formation. The lungs or hilar lymph nodes are affected in over 80% of patients, but the disease may involve the eyes, skin, musculoskeletal system, abdominal organs, heart or nervous system. Often acute in onset and self-limiting.

Diagnosed on clinical grounds, supported by tissue biopsy, chest X-ray, hypercalcaemia (due to derangement of vitamin D metabolism), raised angiotensin converting enzyme levels and positive Kveim test (granuloma formation following intradermal injection of sarcoid tissue suspension).

Anaesthetic and ICU considerations include the possibility of pulmonary fibrosis, cardiac failure, heart block, laryngeal fibrosis, renal failure and hypercalcaemia. Corticosteroids are often prescribed.
[Morten A Kveim (1892–1967), Norwegian pathologist]
Iannuzzi MC, Rybicki BA, Teirstein AS (2007). N Engl J Med; 357: 2153–65

SARS, *see Severe acute respiratory syndrome*

Saturated vapour pressure (SVP). Pressure exerted by the vapour phase of a substance, when in equilibrium with the liquid phase. Indicates the degree of volatility; e.g. for inhalational anaesthetic agents, diethyl ether (SVP 59 kPa (425 mmHg)) is more volatile and easier to vaporise than halothane (SVP 32 kPa (243 mmHg)). SVP increases with temperature, therefore SVPs of volatile agents are quoted at standard temperature (usually 20°C). At boiling point, SVP equals atmospheric pressure.
See also, Vapour pressure

Scalp, nerve blocks. Local anaesthetic infiltration is usually performed with added vasoconstrictor, e.g. adrenaline, because of the rich vascular supply of the scalp. Injection is performed first in the subcutaneous tissue above the aponeurosis (where nerves and vessels lie), then below. Infiltration in a band around the head, above the ears and eyebrows, provides anaesthesia of the scalp. Individual branches of the maxillary nerve may also be blocked. The occipital nerves supplying the posterior scalp may be blocked by infiltrating between the mastoid process and occipital protuberance on each side.

Scavenging. Removal of waste gases from the expiratory port of anaesthetic breathing systems; desirable because of the possible adverse effects of chronic and short-term exposure to inhalational anaesthetic agents. Adsorption of volatile agents using activated charcoal (Aldasorber device) has been used but is ineffective at removing N_2O.

- Scavenging systems consist of:
  - collecting system: usually a shroud enclosing the adjustable pressure limiting valve. For paediatric breathing systems, several attachments have been described, including various connectors and funnels.
  - tubing: standard plastic tubing is usual; all connections should be 30 mm to avoid accidental connection to the breathing system.
  - receiving system: incorporates a reservoir to enable adequate removal of gases even if the volume cleared per minute is less than peak expiratory flow rate. May use rubber bags or rigid bottles, etc. If the system is closed, a dumping valve and pressure-relief valve are required to prevent excess negative or positive pressure, respectively, being applied to the patient's airway. Vents are often present in rigid reservoirs. Requirements:
    - negative pressure: maximum 0.5 cmH_2O at 30 l/min gas flow.
    - positive pressure: maximum 5 cmH_2O at 30 l/min gas flow, and 10 cmH_2O at 90 l/min. Ideally, the relief valve should be as near to the expiratory valve as possible.
  - disposal system: may be:
    - passive: no external energy supply; the gases pass through wide bore tubing to the roof of the building, terminating in a ventile. Maximal resistance should be 0.5 cmH_2O at 30 l/min. The least efficient system, since it depends on wind direction. Requires a water trap to remove condensed water vapour.
    - assisted passive: employs the air-conditioning system's extractor ducts.
    - active: uses a dedicated fan system or ejector flowmeter. Requires a low pressure high volume system (able to remove 75 l/min with a peak flow of 130 l/min); thus hospital suction equipment is unsuitable.

The Health and Safety Commission in 1996 set occupational exposure standards at a maximum of 100 ppm N_2O, 50 ppm enflurane/isoflurane and 10 ppm halothane (each over an 8-h period). Different levels have been set in different Western countries.
See also, COSHH regulations; Environmental safety of anaesthetists; Pollution

SCCM, *see Society of Critical Care Medicine*

Schimmelbusch mask, *see Open-drop techniques*

Sciatic nerve block. Used for surgery to the lower leg, usually combined with femoral nerve block, obturator nerve block and lateral cutaneous nerve of the thigh block (*see Fig. 65; Femoral nerve block*). May also be performed to provide analgesia after fractures, or sympathetic nerve block of the foot.

The sciatic nerve (L4–S3) arises from the sacral plexus, leaving the pelvis through the greater sciatic foramen beneath the piriformis muscle, and between the ischial tuberosity and the greater trochanter of the femur. It becomes superficial at the lower border of gluteus maximus, and runs down the posterior aspect of the thigh to the popliteal fossa, where it divides into tibial and common peroneal nerves. It supplies the hip and knee joints, posterior muscles of the leg, and skin of the leg and foot below the knee except for the medial calf. The posterior cutaneous nerve of the thigh runs close to it and is usually blocked with it.

- Four different approaches are commonly used:
  - posterior: with the patient lying with the side to be blocked uppermost, and the uppermost knee flexed, a line is drawn between the greater trochanter and posterior superior iliac spine. At the line's midpoint, a perpendicular is dropped 3 cm, and a 12 cm needle introduced at this point, at right angles to the skin. The nerve lies on the ischial spine; traditionally it is identified by its feel and by elicitation of paraesthesia although a nerve stimulator (seeking contraction of the hamstrings and muscles of the back of the lower leg and foot) is usually recommended nowadays. 15–30 ml local anaesthetic agent is injected. Onset of blockade may take 30 min.
  - anterior: with the patient lying supine, a line is drawn between the pubic tubercle and anterior superior iliac spine, and divided into thirds. A perpendicular is dropped from the junction of the medial and middle thirds. Another line, parallel with the original line, is drawn from the greater trochanter; its intersection with the perpendicular marks the site of needle insertion. A 12 cm needle is directed slightly laterally to encounter the femur, then withdrawn and directed medial to the femur to a depth of 5 cm from the femur's anterior edge. 15–30 ml solution is injected. This approach is particularly useful if movement is painful, e.g. fractured femur.
  - lithotomy: with the hip and knee on the side to be blocked flexed to 90°, a needle is inserted perpendicular to the skin at the midpoint of a line between the greater trochanter and the ischial tuberosity. 15–20 ml solution is injected at a depth of 5–6 cm. The posterior cutaneous branch (supplying the posterior thigh) may be missed.
  - lateral: with the patient lying supine, a needle is inserted horizontally at a point 2–3 cm below and 4–5 cm distal to the greater trochanter. When the femur is encountered it is withdrawn and redirected posteriorly ~30° and cranially ~30–45°, to reach the nerve at 8–10 cm. 20–30 ml solution is injected.

See also, Regional anaesthesia

Scleroderma, *see Systemic sclerosis*

Scoliosis, *see Kyphoscoliosis*

Scopolamine, *see Hyoscine*

Scribner shunt, *see Shunt procedures*

SCUF, Slow continuous ultrafiltration, *see Ultrafiltration*

SDD, *see Selective decontamination of the digestive tract*

Second. SI unit of time; defined according to the frequency of radiation emitted by caesium-133 in its lowest energy (ground) state.

Second gas effect. Increased alveolar concentration of one inhalational anaesthetic agent caused by uptake of a second inhalational agent. Most marked when the second gas occupies a large volume, e.g. N_2O. Analogous but opposite to the Fink effect at the end of anaesthesia.

Second messenger. Intracellular substance, e.g. cAMP, calcium ions, linking extracellular chemical messengers (first messengers) with the physiological response. G protein-coupled receptors are often involved in second messenger systems.

Sedation. State of reduced consciousness in which verbal contact with the patient may be maintained. Used to reduce discomfort during unpleasant procedures, e.g. regional anaesthesia, dental surgery, endoscopy, cardiac catheterisation, etc., and on ICU. For short procedures, drugs of short duration of action and causing minimal cardiorespiratory depression are preferable. Best control is usually achieved with iv administration, although other routes may be used, e.g. oral premedication. Full monitoring should be employed during procedures as for general anaesthesia. Drugs may be given by small bolus repeated as necessary, or by continuous infusion; the latter is easier to titrate. The level of sedation required depends on the individual patient and the procedure performed. Patient-controlled sedation has been used during procedures performed under local or regional anaesthesia; the patient uses a patient-controlled analgesia device containing e.g. propofol as required.

On ICU, sedative and analgesic drugs are given to reduce pain, distress and anxiety, and to aid tolerance of tracheal tubes, IPPV, tracheal suction, physiotherapy, etc. Cardiovascular depression is particularly undesirable, although respiratory depression may be an advantage if IPPV is required. Long-term administration is often required; thus side effects not seen after brief administration may occur, and drugs with long half-lives may cumulate. The desired end-point is usually a peaceful, cooperative patient who can respond to commands, with deeper levels of sedation provided for stimulating procedures, e.g. physiotherapy. Sedation scoring systems have been devised to assist titration of drugs.

- The following drugs have been used for sedation in ICU or for short procedures:
  - opioid analgesic drugs: commonly used on ICU. Provide analgesia and euphoria, and aid toleration of IPPV. All produce respiratory depression; thus they should be used cautiously in patients breathing spontaneously. Hypotension is particularly likely if hypovolaemia is present and following rapid iv injection. GIT motility is reduced. Drugs used include:
    - morphine 2.5–5 mg boluses (20–60 μg/kg/h infusion). Cumulation of metabolites may occur after prolonged infusion, especially in renal failure. Increased susceptibility to infection has been shown in experimental animals receiving very large doses.
    - pethidine 0.5–2 mg/kg/h. Myocardial depression may occur at high levels. Cumulation is particularly likely in hepatic failure, and cumulation of norpethidine (has convulsant properties) in renal failure.
    - fentanyl 1–5 μg/kg/h; cumulation readily occurs after prolonged infusion, since its short duration of action initially is due to redistribution, and clearance is slower than that of morphine.
    - alfentanil 30–60 μg/kg/h; cumulation is less likely than with fentanyl.
    - remifentanil 0.025–0.1 mg/kg/min (with or without an initial dose of e.g. 0.5 mg/kg/min) has also been used, either alone or in combination with propofol/midazolam.
  - benzodiazepines: often used in conjunction with opioids. Widely used for short procedures. May produce cardiorespiratory depression, and may cumulate in impaired hepatic/renal function and after prolonged administration. Verbal contact with the patient may be impaired. Flumazenil has been used to reverse sedation. Commonly used drugs:
    - diazepam 2.5–10 mg boluses. It and its metabolites have long duration of action.
    - midazolam 2–5 mg boluses (50–200 μg/kg/h infusion). Particularly likely to cause hypotension.
  - iv anaesthetic agents, e.g.:
    - ketamine 5–10 mg boluses (1–2 mg/kg/h infusion). Has been used during regional anaesthesia, but rarely used in ICU except in asthma.
    - thiopental 1–3 mg/kg/h; mainly used in neurological disease. Recovery may be prolonged.
    - propofol 0.3–4.0 mg/kg/h; allows rapid recovery. For patient-controlled sedation: boluses of 10–20 mg with no background infusion and a lockout of 2–5 min. Target-controlled infusion (TCI) has also been used: 0.5–3.0 μg/ml target with or without patient-controlled increases as required. Propofol is licensed for 3 days' sedation of adults (but should be avoided in children). It is licensed for longer use in neurosurgical patients. Propofol has been associated with metabolic disturbance, the propofol infusion syndrome.
    - etomidate: no longer used in ICU because of adrenal suppression.
  - inhalational anaesthetic agents:
    - N_2O up to 70% is commonly used during regional anaesthesia, but haematological side effects preclude prolonged or frequent use.
    - isoflurane has been used on ICU with good results, although high plasma levels of fluoride ions have been reported after prolonged use. Has recently been administered using a conserving device combining direct addition of liquid agent with a carbon filter/evaporator system that conserves and recycles ~90% of the administered agent; it fits into the patient's breathing system without the need for anaesthetic machines.
  - others:
    - dexmedetomidine has been used successfully for the sedation of ICU patients, in whom it has been found to be as effective as propofol.
    - clomethiazole, droperidol, chlorpromazine; rarely used. Chloral hydrate, 30–50 mg orally/rectally repeated as required, may be useful in children.

Neuromuscular blocking drugs are sometimes used in ICU to facilitate IPPV, especially if chest compliance is reduced or ICP is raised. Their use has declined in recent years because of the risk of paralysis with concurrent inadequate sedation, increased risk from accidental disconnection, possible increased incidence of DVT, PE, critical illness polyneuropathy and impaired communication. Atracurium and vecuronium are most commonly used.

NSAIDs, etc. and regional techniques may also be used to provide analgesia in ICU.

Kress JP, Hall JB (2006). Crit Care Med; 34: 2541–6

Sedation scoring systems. Used in intensive care to assess the level of sedation of patients in order to balance its beneficial (reduced stress, cardiovascular stability, ventilator synchrony, etc.) and adverse (increased risk of ventilator associated pneumonia, deep vein thrombosis, etc.) effects. Provide an opportunity to titrate the level of sedation against predefined end-points (e.g. assessments of consciousness, agitation and/or ventilator synchrony). Other parameters assessed include pain, anxiety, muscle tone and reaction to tracheal suction. Most systems use single numerical scores:

- Ramsay scale: described in 1974. Score ranges from 1 (awake) to 6 (no response).
- comfort scale: described in 1992. Comprises eight items with responses ranging from 1 to 5. Measures level of consciousness, facial grimacing, muscle tone, level of agitation and physiological parameters (e.g. heart rate, BP).
- sedation–agitation scale: described in 1999. Score ranges from 1 (minimal or no response to noxious stimuli) to 7 (pulling at tracheal tube, trying to remove catheters, etc.).
- Motor Activity Assessment Scale (MAAS): developed in surgical patients in 1999. Score ranges from 0 (unresponsive) to 6 (dangerously agitated and uncooperative).

[Michael AE Ramsay, US anaesthetist]

De Jonghe B, Cook D, Appere-De-Vecchi C, et al (2000). Intensive Care Med; 26: 275–85

Seebeck effect, *see Temperature measurement*

Seldinger technique. Method of percutaneous cannulation of a blood vessel, described in 1953. A needle is inserted into the vessel, and a guidewire passed through it. After removal of the needle, the cannula is introduced into the vessel over the wire, which is then removed. Refinements include the use of a dilator, passed over the wire to enlarge the hole made by the needle, before the cannula is inserted. Widely used for central venous cannulation; favoured by many as being safer and more reliable than using cannula-over-needle techniques, although more costly.

Has also been used to cannulate other body cavities, e.g. the trachea in percutaneous tracheostomy formation, the chest for insertion of a chest drain or the abdominal cavity in paracentesis.

[Sven-Ivar Seldinger (1921–1998), Swedish radiologist]

Selective decontamination of the digestive tract (SDD; Selective parenteral and enteral antisepsis regimen, SPEAR). Technique for preventing endogenous infections in patients requiring ventilatory support on ICU. SDD aims to prevent colonisation of the GIT by potentially pathogenic organisms, based on the premise that most infections on ICU are endogenous.

Non-absorbable antibacterial drugs (e.g. tobramycin, colistin, amphotericin, neomycin) are administered to the pharynx/mouth/upper GIT, whilst another (e.g. cefotaxime) is administered iv. Sparing of the normal anaerobic GIT organisms prevents overgrowth by pathogens. SDD significantly reduces nosocomial pneumonia, although it has not consistently decreased mortality. Its place in ICU is therefore yet to be determined.

D'Amico R, Pifferi S, Leonetti C, et al (1998). BMJ; 316: 1275–85

Selective serotonin reuptake inhibitors (SSRIs). Antidepressant drugs, introduced in 1987 and increasingly replacing tricyclic antidepressant drugs as the main group of drugs used in depression and other disorders. Inhibit the presynaptic reuptake of 5-HT from the synaptic cleft in the CNS, leading via desensitisation of the presynaptic membrane to an increase in 5-HT activity. Include citalopram, escitalopram, fluoxetine, fluvoxamine, paroxetine and sertraline; they have similar actions and are metabolised in the liver with half-lives of about a day (1–4 days for fluoxetine).

Side effects are fewer than for the tricyclic antidepressants since muscarinic, dopamine, histamine and noradrenergic receptors are unaffected. However, GIT upset, insomnia and agitation may occur; the syndrome of inappropriate antidiuretic hormone and impaired platelet function have been reported. In overdose, severe adverse effects are uncommon although the serotonin syndrome may occur if tricyclics or monoamine oxidase inhibitors are also taken.

May cause hepatic enzyme inhibition, thus increasing the action of certain tricyclics, type Ic anti-arrhythmic drugs (especially lipid-soluble β-adrenergic receptor antagonists), phenytoin and benzodiazepines. Increased bleeding may occur in warfarin therapy. Concurrent administration of drugs which have 5-HT reuptake blocking effects, e.g. pethidine, may provoke the serotonin syndrome.

Selenium. Trace element found in meat, chicken and fish; normal intake ~60–75 μg/day. Selenoproteins are antioxidants and are involved in certain biological reactions, e.g. conversion of thyroxine to triiodothyronine. Low blood selenium levels have been recorded in ICU patients, especially those with septic shock. Low selenium levels are associated with a high ICU mortality; the replenishment of plasma selenium is associated with a decrease in nosocomial infections and a decreased mortality in patients with sepsis.

Berger MM, Shenkin A (2007). Crit Care Med; 35: 306–7

Self-inflating bags. Rubber or silicone bags used for IPPV, which reinflate when released after compression. Thus may be used for IPPV without requiring an external gas supply, e.g. during draw-over anaesthesia, transfer of ventilated patients, or CPR. May be thick-walled or lined with foam-rubber. Usually assembled with a non-rebreathing valve at the outlet and a one-way valve at the inlet; thus fresh air is drawn in during refilling. O_2 may be added through a port at the inlet; a reservoir bag may also be added to the inlet to increase F_IO_2. Available in adult and paediatric sizes. Bellows may be used in a similar way, but are less convenient to use.

Sellick's manoeuvre, *see Cricoid pressure*

Semon's law, *see Laryngeal nerves*

Sengstaken–Blakemore tube. Double-cuffed gastric tube designed to compress gastro-oesophageal varices, thereby controlling bleeding. Passed via the mouth into the stomach; the distal balloon is then inflated with 150–250 ml air,

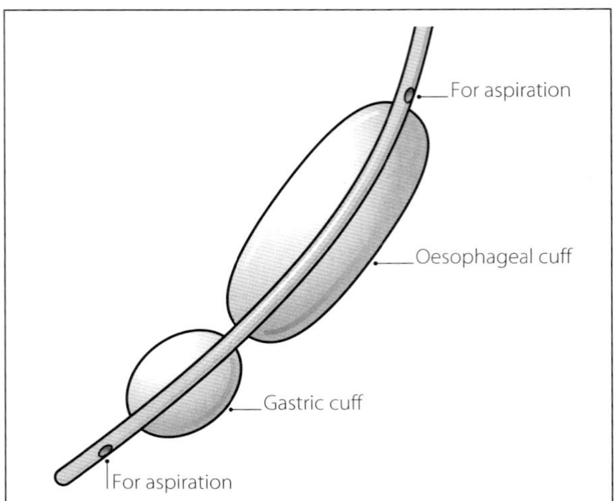

Fig. 135 Distal end of Sengstaken–Blakemore tube

preventing accidental removal. The proximal balloon is then inflated to 30–40 mmHg (4–5 kPa), compressing the varices. Traction has been advocated but is rarely used. Newer versions include channels for aspiration of gastric and oesophageal contents (Fig. 135); the latter may be aspirated continuously to reduce pulmonary soiling. Thus four lumina may be present:
- for aspiration above the oesophageal balloon.
- for aspiration from the stomach.
- for inflation of each balloon.

Usually kept inflated for 12–24 h; the oesophageal balloon is deflated first. Careful placement is essential to avoid airway obstruction, pulmonary aspiration, ischaemic necrosis of gastric mucosa, oesophageal rupture, etc. The tubes are very uncomfortable.

[Robert W Sengstaken and Arthur H Blakemore (1879–1970), US surgeons]

Sensitivity. In statistics, the ability of a test to exclude false negatives. Equals:

$$\frac{\text{the number correctly identified as positive}}{\text{total with the condition}}$$

See also, Errors; Predictive value; Specificity

Sensory evoked potentials, *see Evoked potentials*

Sensory pathways. The sensory system includes the special senses, visceral sensation and general somatic sensation. The latter is divided into:
- exteroreceptive sensation: provides information about the external environment and includes modalities such as touch, pressure, temperature and pain.
- proprioceptive sensation: provides information about body position and movement.

Free nerve endings may be associated with nociception. Some nerve endings are 'specialised', e.g. Meissner's corpuscles (touch), Pacinian corpuscles (vibration and joint position) and Ruffini corpuscles (joint position). The last two may be involved with muscle spindles.

- The sensory fibres enter the spinal cord through the dorsal root, their cell bodies lying in the dorsal root ganglia. Subsequent pathways (Fig. 136):
  - proprioception, vibration and ½ touch sensation:
    - first order neurones turn medially and ascend in the ipsilateral posterior columns to the lower medulla, where they synapse with cells in the cuneate or gracile nuclei.
    - second order neurones cross the contralateral side of the medulla and ascend in the medial lemniscus to the ventral posterolateral nucleus of the thalamus.
    - third order neurones project to the sensory cortex.
  - pain, temperature and the remainder of touch sensation:
    - first order neurones synapse in the dorsal horn of the spinal cord (mainly in laminae VI and VII).
    - most of the second order neurones cross (either at the same level or 1–2 segments higher) to reach the spinothalamic tracts. In the medulla, the latter form the spinal lemniscus, which ascends to the thalamus.
    - third order neurones project to the sensory cortex.

The primary somatosensory area of the cerebral cortex is in the postcentral gyrus, although there is a large distribution of sensory fibres in other areas. Regions of greatest importance (e.g. face, mouth, hands) have a disproportionately greater representation than other areas.

- Signs of sensory pathway loss:
  - peripheral nerve lesion: complete loss of sensation in the nerve's distribution (although the zone of loss may be limited because of overlap between nerves).
  - posterior root lesion: pain and paraesthesia are experienced in the dermatomal distribution. If the root involves a reflex arc, the reflex will be diminished or lost.
  - posterior column lesion: ipsilateral loss of position and vibration sense with preservation of pain, touch and temperature sensation.
  - spinothalamic tract lesion: contralateral loss of pain and temperature sensation.
  - brainstem and thalamus lesions: upper brainstem or thalamic lesions may cause complete hemisensory disturbance with loss of postural sense, light touch and pain sensation. 'Pure' thalamic lesions may result in central pain.
  - sensory cortex lesions: paraesthesia may be felt, with or without disturbed appreciation of sensation, e.g. inability to distinguish between heat and pain, or inability to identify objects by touch, etc.

[Georg Meissner (1829–1905), German anatomist; Filippo Pacini (1812–1883), Italian anatomist; Angelo Ruffini (1864–1929), Italian histologist]

See also, Dermatomes; Spinal cord injury

Sepsis. SIRS as a result of proven or suspected infection (i.e. invasion of normally sterile host tissue by micro-organisms or the inflammatory response to their presence). Severe sepsis has been defined as sepsis plus organ dysfunction, hypoperfusion or hypotension, and has been suggested as a replacement for the now obsolete term septicaemia (bacteraemia is the presence of viable circulating bacteria). A major cause of organ failure in ICU, severe sepsis is directly or indirectly responsible for 75% of all ICU deaths.

Most ICU infections are endogenous, caused by colonisation of the patient's GIT by pathogenic organisms. Gram-negative bacteria (e.g. *Escherichia coli*, klebsiella, pseudomonas and proteus species) have traditionally been most commonly responsible, because of their widespread presence, their tendency to acquire resistance to antibacterial drugs and their resistance to drying and disinfecting agents. Gram-positive bacteria (e.g. streptococci, staphylococci) are increasingly common, especially associated with invasive cannulation; other organisms (e.g. fungi) may also be responsible. The inflammatory response involves cytokines, nitric oxide, thromboxanes, leukotrienes, platelet activating factor, prostaglandins and complement. Endothelial and neutrophil adhesion molecule expression increases, resulting in cellular infiltration into the tissues.

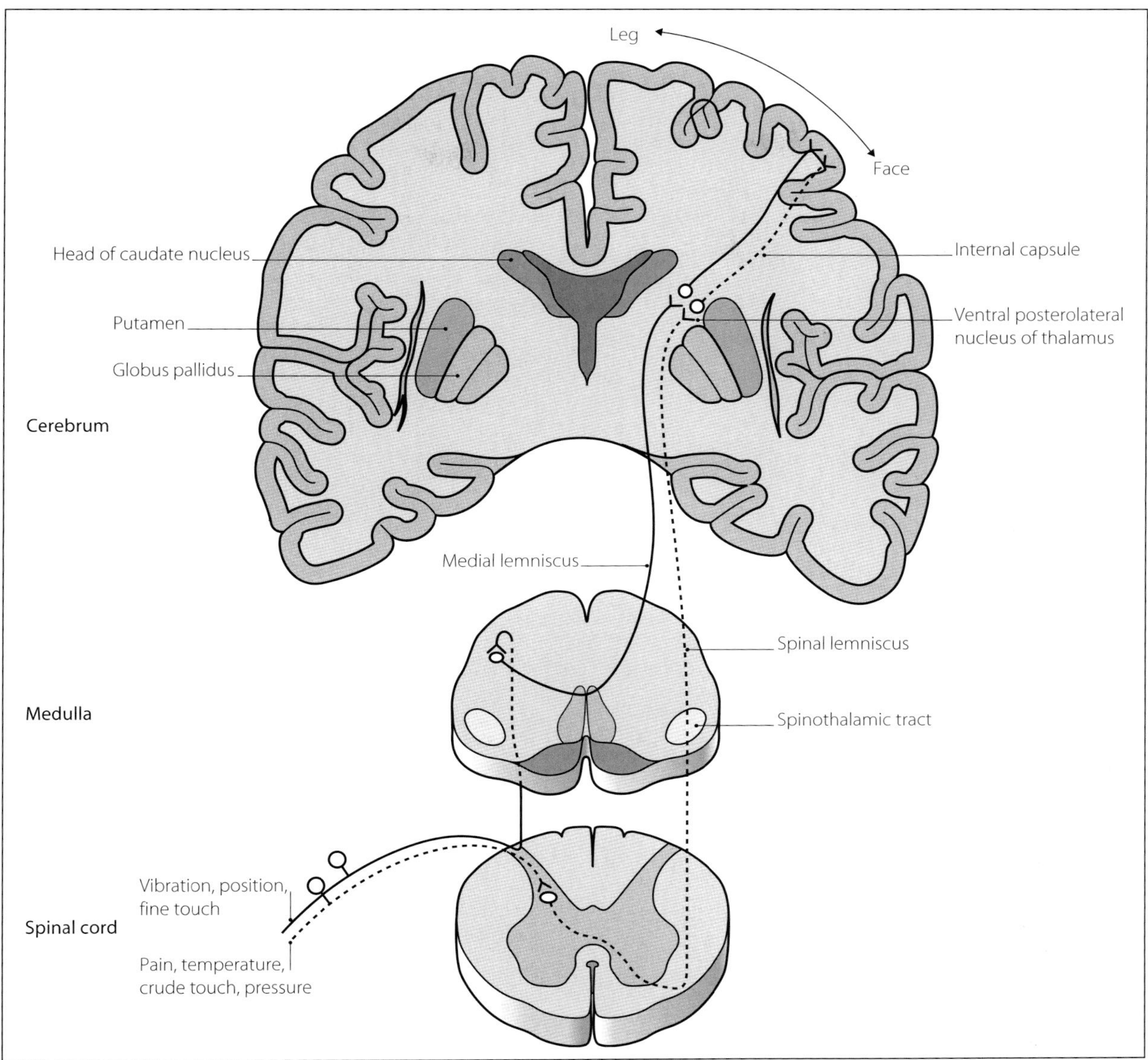

Fig. 136 Anatomy of sensory pathways

- Critically ill patients are susceptible to sepsis because of:
  - impaired local defences, e.g. anatomical barriers, ciliary activity, coughing, gastric pH. Presence of tracheal tubes and indwelling catheters and cannulae provide routes for infection.
  - impaired neutrophil function, humoral immunity (especially following splenectomy) and cell-mediated immunity. Contributory factors include drugs, malnutrition, old age, malignancy, organ failure and infection itself. Infection control is important in reducing sepsis in the ICU.
- Management:
  - supportive, e.g. iv fluids, O_2 therapy, inotropic drugs, etc. Nutrition is important as hypercatabolism is common.
  - early use of antibacterial and antifungal drugs, etc. Initial choice is based on the most likely infective organisms in each particular situation. Samples of urine, sputum, blood, CSF, etc. should be taken before starting therapy.
  - various new immunomodulatory treatments have been investigated, e.g. anti-endotoxin antibodies, anti-cytokine products, but most have produced disappointing results clinically despite encouraging results experimentally. This may represent the heterogeneous patient population and/or the complex nature of the inflammatory network responsible for the features of sepsis. Drotrecogin alfa has been recommended in severe sepsis.
  - surgical drainage, debridement, removal of cause e.g. infected lines, etc.

Complications include septic shock and multiple organ failure including ARDS, renal failure, hepatic failure, pancreatitis and diabetes mellitus, DIC, cardiac failure and coma. GIT haemorrhage is common; preventative measures include H_2 receptor antagonists, antacids and sucralfate.

Lever A, Mackenzie I (2007). Br Med J; 335: 879–83 and 929–32

See also, Catheter-related sepsis; Fungal infection in the ICU; Nosocomial infection; Sepsis-related organ failure assessment; Sepsis score; Sepsis severity score

Sepsis-related organ failure assessment (SOFA). Scoring system devised in 1994 to describe quantitatively and objectively the degree of organ dysfunction in sepsis over time. Intended to improve the understanding of organ dysfunction/failure and to assess the effect of particular therapies on its course. The function of six different organ systems (respiratory, cardiovascular, central nervous, coagulation, hepatic and renal systems) is weighted (each scored 1–4) according to the degree of physiological derangement observed. Minimum SOFA score is 6; maximum 24.
Vincent JL, Moreno R, Takala J, et al (1996). Intensive Care Med; 22: 707–10

Sepsis score. Index of severity of sepsis, devised in 1983 by assigning scores to each of four arbitrarily selected categories: local infection, pyrexia, systemic response and laboratory results. The maximum score awarded in each category varies from 6 to 22.
Elebute EA, Stoner HB (1983). Br J Surg; 70: 29–31

Sepsis severity score. Index of severity of sepsis, devised in 1983 by assigning scores of 1–5 according to the degree of impairment of each of the following organ systems: lung, kidney, coagulation, CVS, liver, GIT and neurological. The three highest (worst) scores are then squared to produce the final score.
Stevens LE (1983). Arch Surg; 118: 1190–2

Sepsis syndrome. Obsolete term for the systemic response to infection.
See also, Sepsis; Septic shock; Septicaemia; Systemic inflammatory response syndrome

Septic shock. Hypotension (or the requirement for inotropic or vasopressor drugs) despite adequate fluid resuscitation, together with evidence of perfusion abnormalities (e.g. lactic acidosis, oliguria, mental impairment), associated with sepsis. Initially, features include hyperthermia, tachycardia, tachypnoea, hypotension and vasodilatation with a hyperdynamic circulation and increased cardiac output. In later stages, or if hypovolaemia or poor myocardial function is present, hypotension with vasoconstriction supervenes. Mortality is about 50% although it varies with age and the nature of the sepsis. Most cases are caused by bacteria (nowadays approximately equally split between Gram-positive and -negative, although traditionally associated with Gram-negative organisms); other organisms may also be responsible. Risk factors for developing septic shock include age (< 10 years and > 70 years), diabetes mellitus, alcoholic liver disease, ischaemic heart disease, malignancy, immunosuppression, prolonged hospital stay, invasive monitoring, tracheal intubation and prior use of antibacterial agents. The underlying pathophysiology is as for sepsis; microvascular abnormalities supervene including impaired autoregulation, altered blood cell morphology, endothelial swelling, increased endothelial permeability and opening of arteriovenous shunts.

- Cardiovascular features include:
  - reduced SVR with relative hypovolaemia.
  - increased pulmonary vascular resistance.
  - increased capillary permeability.
  - reduced myocardial contractility caused by circulating depressant factors, acidaemia and hypoxaemia.
  - O_2 consumption may be normal but O_2 extraction and utilisation are reduced.
- Management:
  - as for sepsis.
  - corticosteroids have been associated with increased mortality although recent evidence suggests that they may improve outcome in selected patients with impaired pituitary–adrenal axis function, e.g. those not responding to a corticotropin stimulation test.
  - prostaglandins, naloxone and thyrotrophin releasing hormone have been used but their benefit has not been proven.
- Complications: as for sepsis.

Annane D, Bellissant E, Cavaillon JM (2005). Lancet; 365: 63–78

Septicaemia, *see Sepsis*

Sequential analysis, *see Statistical tests*

Serotonin, *see 5-Hydroxytryptamine*

Serotonin syndrome. Impaired mental state, increased muscle activity and autonomic instability arising from excessive 5-HT activity in the brainstem and spinal cord. Seen in selective serotonin reuptake inhibitor (SSRI) overdose, especially in combination with other antidepressant drugs. Also associated with the use of tramadol, pethidine and cocaine. Features include confusion, agitation, convulsions, myoclonus, rigidity, hyperreflexia, fever, diarrhoea, hyper- or hypotension and tachycardia. DIC, renal and cardiac failure may also occur. Treatment is supportive; 5-HT antagonists, e.g. methysergide, cyproheptadine, have been used. Usually lasts for under 24 h but deaths have been reported.

A washout period of several weeks has been suggested between monoamine oxidase inhibitor and SSRI therapy.
Boyer EW, Shannon M (2005). N Engl J Med; 352: 1112–20

Servomechanisms. Control systems involving continuous assessment of output and its automated modification, to maintain constancy. Used in ventilators and other computerised equipment. Have also been used to control iv infusions, e.g. of sodium nitroprusside to reduce BP; continuous measurement of BP is used as input for a computer-controlled infusion device. Fuzzy logic is increasingly used in these systems.

Severe acute respiratory syndrome (SARS). Infectious respiratory condition caused by a new coronavirus, first reported in East Asia in early 2003 and thought to have spread via air travellers to Europe and North America. Has mostly affected previously healthy adults, with an incubation period 2–11 days. Spread is thought to be mainly via droplets, usually via air, with most cases of transmission thought to involve close exposure to an affected individual. Features include high fever initially with malaise, myalgia and headache; after 3–7 days dry cough and dyspnoea may occur leading to acute respiratory failure in 10–20% of cases and a mortality ranging from 1% in patients < 24 years to > 50% in those > 65 years. Chest X-ray, initially normal, may show focal interstitial infiltrates which may become generalised. Thrombocytopenia and leucopenia are common; raised liver function tests may occur but renal function usually remains normal. Treatment is largely supportive, although the following have been used empirically:

- ribavirin 8 mg/kg iv, 8 hourly (n.b. not licensed for this use in UK) or 1.2 g orally, 12 hourly after a loading dose of 4 g orally, for 7–14 days (caution in impaired renal function).
- hydrocortisone 2–4 mg/kg iv, 6–8 hourly, for ~7 days. Methylprednisolone 10 mg/kg/day iv has been used for 2 days before hydrocortisone.
- antibacterial prophylaxis.

Staff require protection from infection since several cases of transmission to healthcare workers have occurred.

Peng PWH, Wong DT, Bevan D, Gardam M (2003). Can J Anaesth; 50: 989–97

Sevoflurane. 1,1,1,3,3,3-hexafluoroisopropyl fluoromethyl ether (Fig. 137). Inhalational anaesthetic agent, first synthesised in 1968 but not introduced in the UK until 1995 because of the development of isoflurane in preference.

- Properties:
  - colourless liquid with pleasant smelling vapour, 7.5 times heavier than air.
  - mw 200.
  - boiling point 58°C.
  - SVP at 20°C 21 kPa (160 mmHg).
  - partition coefficients:
    - blood/gas 0.69.
    - oil/gas 53.
  - MAC 1.4% (80 years) – 2.5% (children/young adults); up to 3.3% in neonates.
  - non-flammable, non-corrosive.
  - supplied in liquid form with no additive.
  - interacts with soda lime at temperature of 65°C to produce Compounds A, B, C, D and E, the first two the only ones produced in clinical practice. Production is more likely at high temperatures, high concentrations of sevoflurane, use of baralyme and low gas flows. The significance of Compound A (pentafluoroisopropenyl fluoromethyl ether) continues to excite controversy since it has been shown to be toxic in rats, causing renal, hepatic and cerebral damage. However, clinical experience has never implicated Compound A in causing harm in humans, even with sevoflurane at low fresh gas flows (maximal concentrations of Compound A around 30 parts per million; minimal levels for human toxicity thought to be around 150–200 parts per million).
- Effects:
  - CNS:
    - smooth, extremely rapid induction and recovery. Concentrations of 4–8% produce anaesthesia within a few vital capacity breaths. Pain and restlessness may occur postoperatively if adequate analgesia is not provided, since excretion is so rapid.
    - anticonvulsant properties as for isoflurane.
    - at concentration of $<$ 1 MAC has minimal effect on ICP in patients with normal ICP. Studies suggest that autoregulation is preserved in patients with cerebrovascular disease, in contrast to other inhalational agents.
    - reduces $CMRO_2$ as for isoflurane, with about a 50% reduction at 2 MAC.
    - decreases intraocular pressure.
    - has poor analgesic properties.
  - RS:
    - well tolerated vapour with minimal airway irritation.
    - respiratory depressant, with increased rate and decreased tidal volume.
    - causes bronchodilatation.
  - CVS:
    - vasodilatation and hypotension may occur, but less than with isoflurane and with little myocardial depression. Little compensatory tachycardia, unlike isoflurane.
    - myocardial O_2 demand decreases. Coronary steal is not thought to occur.
    - arrhythmias uncommon as for isoflurane. Little myocardial sensitisation to catecholamines.
    - renal and hepatic blood flow generally preserved.
  - other:
    - dose-dependent uterine relaxation.
    - nausea/vomiting occurs in up to 25% of cases.
    - skeletal muscle relaxation; non-depolarising neuromuscular blockade may be potentiated.
    - may precipitate MH.

```
        F            CF3
        |           /
   H -- C -- O -- C -- H
        |           \
        H            CF3
```

Fig. 137 Structure of sevoflurane

Under 5% metabolised in the liver to hexafluoroisopropanol and inorganic fluoride ions, the rest being excreted by the lungs. High levels of fluoride have never been reported, even after prolonged surgery, but avoidance in renal impairment has been suggested. Inducers of the particular cytochrome P_{450} enzyme involved (e.g. isoniazid, alcohol) increase metabolism of sevoflurane, but barbiturates do not.

0.5–3.0% is usually adequate for maintenance of anaesthesia, with higher concentrations for induction. Tracheal intubation may be performed easily with spontaneous respiration. Considered the agent of choice for inhalational induction in paediatrics because of its rapid and smooth induction characteristics. Has also been used for the difficult airway including airway obstruction.

See also, Vaporisers

Shivering, postoperative. Tremors were first described after barbiturate administration, but they may occur following all types of general anaesthesia. Traditionally said to be more common following halothane ('halothane shakes'). Rarer in elderly patients due to decreased thermoregulatory control. May increase metabolic rate by up to six times and triple O_2 consumption. Can also aggravate postoperative pain, damage surgical wounds and increase intraocular and intracranial pressures. Damage to teeth may occur, especially in the presence of an oral airway.

EMG studies suggest that postoperative shivering differs from shivering due to cold. It has been suggested that anaesthetic agents suppress descending pathways which normally inhibit spinal reflexes; this may be more likely than a response to intraoperative hypothermia, although the latter may be of importance if severe.

- Suggested treatment:
  - O_2 administration.
  - pethidine 10–25 mg iv has been successfully used, possibly by stimulating central α_2 receptors. Pentazocine 30 mg or doxapram 1 mg/kg or pre-induction ondansetron have also been used.

Shivering after epidural anaesthesia is common, and is thought to be caused by differential nerve blockade, either suppressing descending inhibition of spinal reflexes, or allowing selective transmission of cold sensation. Shivering is rare in spinal anaesthesia, where blockade is more dense. Warming of epidural injectate has produced conflicting results. Epidural administration of opioid analgesic drugs, e.g. sufentanil 50 μg, fentanyl 25 μg, pethidine 25 mg, may be an effective remedy.

De Witte J, Sessler DI (2002). Anesthesiology; 96: 467–84

Shock. Syndrome in which tissue perfusion is inadequate for the tissues' metabolic requirements. Sympathetic compensatory mechanisms may preserve organ perfusion initially, but subsequent organ dysfunction may lead to irreversible organ damage and death.

- Classically divided into:
  - hypovolaemic shock, e.g. following haemorrhage, burns, dehydration, etc.
  - cardiogenic shock, e.g. following MI.
  - septic shock.
  - others, e.g. anaphylactic reaction, adrenocortical insufficiency, neurogenic shock (e.g. in high spinal cord injury).

Division into hypovolaemia, myocardial failure and peripheral vascular failure has been suggested as being more indicative of underlying mechanisms. Thus shock may arise from inadequate cardiac output or maldistribution of blood flow; the latter has been increasingly implicated by studies of O_2 delivery ($\dot{D}O_2$) and total body O_2 consumption ($\dot{V}O_2$). A decrease in $\dot{V}O_2$ is thought to represent maldistribution rather than an absolute decrease in blood flow. In cardiogenic shock both $\dot{V}O_2$ and cardiac output are reduced; in septic shock they may both increase initially. Features depend on the aetiology but include hypotension, tachycardia, oliguria and metabolic acidosis. MODS may follow, with renal failure and ARDS common. Hepatic, gastrointestinal and pancreatic impairment, and DIC may occur.

- Management:
  - directed at the primary cause.
  - support of the cardiovascular system. Haemodynamic monitoring has traditionally relied on measurement of BP, pulse rate, CVP, urine output, pulmonary capillary wedge pressure and cardiac output. Lactate has also been measured. Recently, $\dot{D}O_2$, $\dot{V}O_2$ and gastric tonometry have been used to guide therapy. Cardiovascular support is achieved with iv fluids, inotropic drugs and vasodilator drugs.
  - support of other organs: as for renal failure, ARDS, etc. O_2 therapy is mandatory.
  - corticosteroids were advocated for sepsis in the past but have been associated with increased mortality, and should now be reserved for proven adrenocortical insufficiency.

Mortality exceeds 50% for cardiogenic and septic shock.

Shock index (SI). Ratio of heart rate to systolic blood pressure; has been used to identify and monitor haemorrhage in trauma patients. An elevated shock index (> 0.9) has been suggested as an indication for admission to ICU.

Shock lung, *see Acute respiratory distress syndrome*

Shunt. One extreme form of $\dot{V}/\dot{Q}$ mismatch, causing hypoxaemia. Refers to the actual amount of venous blood bypassing ventilated alveoli and mixing with pulmonary end-capillary blood (cf. venous admixture, the calculated amount of shunt required to produce the observed arterial PO_2).

- May be:
  - intrapulmonary, e.g. atelectasis, chest infection, etc.
  - extrapulmonary, e.g. congenital heart disease.

Physiological shunt (venous admixture) = shunt-like effect of $\dot{V}/\dot{Q}$ mismatch + anatomical shunt (actual shunt). The latter includes pathological shunt and normal mixing of bronchial and Thebesian venous blood with oxygenated pulmonary venous blood.

Hypoxaemia due to shunt responds poorly to increased F_IO_2, since the O_2 content of pulmonary end-capillary blood is already near maximum, because of the shape of the oxyhaemoglobin dissociation curve. Some benefit is derived from increased dissolved O_2. Thus the amount of shunt may be estimated from the response to breathing high concentrations of O_2, assuming a haemoglobin concentration of 10–14 g/100 ml, arterial PCO_2 of 3.3–5.3 kPa (25–40 mmHg), and arteriovenous O_2 difference of 5 ml/100 ml (Fig. 138). Amount of shunt may also be estimated from the shunt equation.

[Adam Thebesius (1686–1732), German physician]

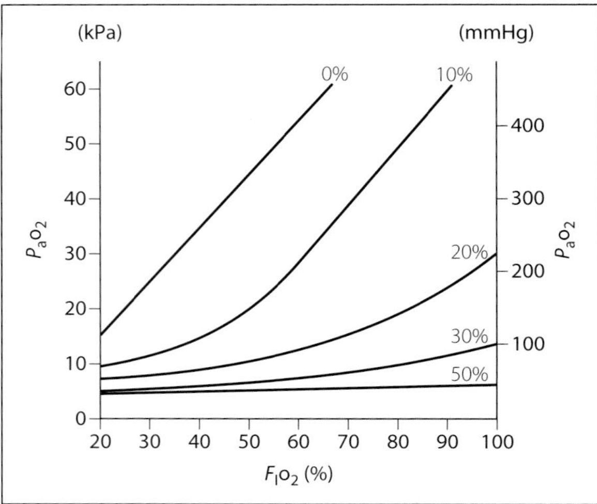

Fig. 138 P_aO_2 at varying F_IO_2 for different percentages of shunt

Shunt equation.

$$\frac{\dot{Q}_S}{\dot{Q}_T} = \frac{(C_cO_2 - C_aO_2)}{(C_cO_2 - C_{\bar{v}}O_2)}$$

Allows calculation of shunt. Derived as follows. Total pulmonary blood flow equals $\dot{Q}_T$, made up of blood flow to unventilated alveoli ($\dot{Q}_S$) and blood flow to ventilated alveoli ($\dot{Q}_T - \dot{Q}_S$; Fig. 139).

In unit time, the volume of O_2 leaving the lungs equals the volume of O_2 in blood draining ventilated alveoli plus the volume of O_2 in shunted blood. Or,

$$\dot{Q}_T \times C_aO_2 = [(\dot{Q}_T - \dot{Q}_S) \times C_cO_2] + [\dot{Q}_S \times C_{\bar{v}}O_2],$$

where C_aO_2 = arterial O_2 content,
C_cO_2 = end-capillary O_2 content,
$C_{\bar{v}}O_2$ = mixed venous O_2 content.

Thus $\dot{Q}_T \times C_aO_2 = (\dot{Q}_T \times C_cO_2) - (\dot{Q}_S \times C_cO_2) + (\dot{Q}_S \times C_{\bar{v}}O_2)$,
or $(\dot{Q}_S \times C_cO_2) - (\dot{Q}_S \times C_{\bar{v}}O_2) = (\dot{Q}_T \times C_cO_2) - (\dot{Q}_T \times C_aO_2)$,
or $\dot{Q}_S\,(C_cO_2 - C_{\bar{v}}O_2) = \dot{Q}_T\,(C_cO_2 - C_aO_2)$.

Therefore

$$\frac{\dot{Q}_S}{\dot{Q}_T} = \frac{(C_cO_2 - C_aO_2)}{(C_cO_2 - C_{\bar{v}}O_2)} = \text{shunt fraction.}$$

Arterial and venous O_2 contents may be estimated thus:

$$C_aO_2 = (P_aO_2 \times S) + (Hb \times 1.34 \times S_aO_2),$$
$$C_vO_2 = (P_{\bar{v}}O_2 \times S) + (Hb \times 1.34 \times S_{\bar{v}}O_2),$$

where P_aO_2 and S_aO_2 = arterial PO_2 and haemoglobin saturation respectively,
$P_{\bar{v}}O_2$ and $S_{\bar{v}}O_2$ = mixed venous PO_2 and haemoglobin saturation respectively,
S = volume of O_2 dissolved in 100 ml blood per kPa applied O_2 tension (0.0225) or mmHg (0.003),
Hb = haemoglobin content in g/100 ml, 1.34 = Hüfner's constant.

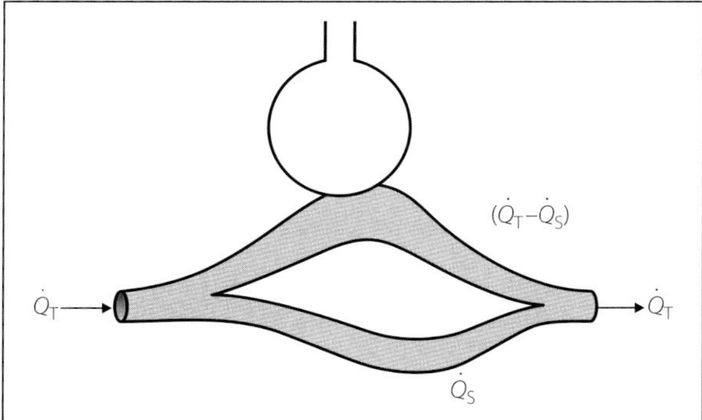

Fig. 139 Calculation of shunt equation

End-capillary O_2 content cannot be measured directly, but is estimated from calculation of the alveolar air equation:

$$C_cO_2 = (P_AO_2 \times S) + (Hb \times 1.34),$$

where P_AO_2 = 'ideal' alveolar PO_2, and saturation is assumed to be 100%.

Shunt procedures. Performed to provide access to the circulation for haemodialysis and related procedures, thus requiring the capacity for high flow rates of blood both out of and back into the circulation. May involve:

- temporary cannulation of vessel(s), e.g. central venous cannulation with a double-lumen catheter (or two single ones). Choice of vessel, technique, etc. is as for placement of any central line, although the catheter is usually required for a longer time. Venous stenosis or thrombosis may be more common if the subclavian vein is used. Most double-lumen dialysis catheters are designed with one channel for withdrawal and one for return of blood; the latter opens proximal to the former to reduce the withdrawal of freshly dialysed blood from the return channel via the withdrawal channel, and thus inefficiency.
- surgical creation of a permanent arteriovenous shunt between adjacent vessels, e.g. radial artery/cephalic vein, using either direct anastomosis of the vessels (fistula) or insertion of a silastic catheter (Scribner shunt). Venous wall thickening allows repeated cannulation although thrombosis and venous stenosis may occur. Other complications include infection, pseudoaneurysm and arm ischaemia. Surgical shunts may be performed under local infiltration anaesthesia, regional anaesthesia (e.g. brachial plexus block) or general anaesthesia. Anaesthetic considerations are as for renal failure.

[Belding H Scribner (1921–2003), Seattle nephrologist]

Shy–Drager syndrome, *see Autonomic neuropathy*

SI units, Units of the Système International d'Unités, *see Units, SI*

SIADH, *see Syndrome of inappropriate antidiuretic hormone secretion*

Siamese twins, *see Conjoined twins*

Sick Doctor Scheme. Scheme set up in 1981 in the UK by the Association of Anaesthetists and Royal College of Psychiatrists, to encourage voluntary reporting of sick doctors practising anaesthesia and thus potentially putting patients at risk. The anonymous reporter, having contacted the Association, is given the name and telephone number of a referee. The latter contacts an appointed psychiatrist from another Region, who in turn contacts the sick doctor. A similar scheme (The National Counselling Service for Sick Doctors) is now available to doctors from all specialties. Intended as an alternative to the more formal scheme available via the Department of Health (previously involving appropriate action taken via a subcommittee ('three wise men' procedure); more recently replaced by a framework involving the National Clinical Assessment Service) and General Medical Council (assesses doctors on health and performance as well as conduct).

A scheme of the same name exists in Ireland, to help doctors afflicted by substance abuse.

Sick euthyroid syndrome. Abnormal thyroid function tests occurring in critically ill patients. Low triiodothyronine (T_3) with normal or raised thyroxine (T_4) is the most common pattern. Low T_3 and T_4 are generally associated with more severe disease and worse prognosis. Most patients are clinically euthyroid. Thought to result from reduced thyroid stimulating hormone secretion, reduced peripheral conversion of T_4 to T_3 and reduced plasma protein binding.

Sick sinus syndrome. Syndrome caused by impaired sinoatrial node activity or conduction; may lead to periods of severe bradycardia with intermittent loss of P waves or sinus arrest, and may alternate with periods of SVT or AF (bradycardia–tachycardia syndrome; bradytachy syndrome). Usually occurs in elderly patients with ischaemic heart disease. May be precipitated by anaesthesia. Requires cardiac pacing if diagnosed preoperatively or if it occurs perioperatively.

See also, Heart, conducting system

Sickle cell anaemia. Haemoglobinopathy, first described in 1910 in Chicago. Caused by substitution of glutamic acid by valine in the sixth amino acid from the N-terminal of haemoglobin β chains. Inherited as an autosomal gene; heterozygotes (genotype HbAS; sickle cell trait) possess both normal (HbA) and abnormal (HbS) haemoglobins (though they may also possess other abnormal haemoglobin combinations (e.g. HbSC)); homozygotes (HbSS) contain only abnormal haemoglobin. Thought to have originated from spontaneous genetic mutation, with subsequent selection owing to the relative resistance conferred by sickle cell trait against malaria. Most common in West Central Africa, North-East Saudi Arabia and East Central India, but has been described in Southern Mediterranean populations. Incidence of HbSS in US Blacks is under 1%; incidence of HbAS is 8–10%.

Deoxygenated HbS polymerises and precipitates within red blood cells, with distortion and increased rigidity. Sickle-shaped red cells are characteristic. The distorted cells increase blood viscosity, impair blood flow and cause capillary and venous thrombosis and organ infarction. They have shortened survival time. O_2 affinity of dissolved HbS is normal, but overall affinity is reduced if some of the HbS is polymerised. HbS polymerises at PO_2 of 5–6 kPa (40–50 mmHg); thus HbSS patients are continuously sickling. HbAS patients' red cells contain both HbS and HbA and sickle at 2.5–4.0 kPa (20–30 mmHg).

- Features:
  - HbSS:
    - haemolysis causing anaemia and hyperbilirubinaemia. Gallstones may occur. Enlargement of the skull and long bones is common, due to compensatory bone marrow hyperplasia. Acute aplastic crises may occur, and sequestration crises in children.
    - impaired tissue blood flow may result in CVA, papillary necrosis of the kidney, ulcers, pulmonary infarcts,

priapism, and avascular necrosis of bone. Crises are caused by acute vascular occlusion, and may feature neurological lesions and severe pain, e.g. abdominal, back, chest (the sickle chest syndrome is a common cause of death and includes cough, fever and severe hypoxaemia). They may be precipitated by hypothermia, dehydration, infection, exertion and hypoxaemia. Treatment is with analgesia (often requiring opioids, e.g. by PCA), O_2 and rehydration. Exchange blood transfusion may be required.
   - increased susceptibility to infection. Osteomyelitis is typically caused by unusual organisms, e.g. salmonella.
- HbAS: usually asymptomatic, since arterial $P\text{O}_2$ is unlikely to reach the level required to induce sickling.
- combinations of HbS with other haemoglobins usually produce mild disease. In heterozygotes for HbS and haemoglobin C (HbC), red cells may sickle at around 4 kPa (30 mmHg) because HbC itself is less soluble than HbA, and makes red cells more rigid.

Diagnosis is by detection of HbS in the blood. The Sickledex test involves addition of reagent to blood, with observation for turbidity. It detects HbS but provides no information about other haemoglobins. A sodium metabisulphite test induces sickling in susceptible cells, which are then counted. Haemoglobin electrophoresis is the only method of determining the nature of the haemoglobinopathy.

Sickle cells are usually present in peripheral blood in HbSS.

- Anaesthetic considerations:
  - preoperatively:
    - all races at risk should be screened for HbS, ideally by electrophoresis. In the UK, Sickledex testing is usual initially, with progression to electrophoresis if positive. In emergencies, if the Sickledex test is positive, diagnosis may be aided by blood counts and peripheral film. If the history does not suggest HbSS, and haemoglobin/reticulocyte count and peripheral film are normal with no red cell fragments, HbAS is likely, although HbSC and other heterozygous variants may still be present. Management ultimately depends on the nature of the surgery, availability of blood, etc.
    - preoperative assessment is directed towards the above complications, especially impairment of pulmonary and renal function. Preoperative folic acid has been suggested. Exchange transfusion is often used in HbSS patients before major surgery, to reduce HbS concentrations to 20–40%.
    - hypoxaemia, dehydration, hypothermia and acidosis should be prevented at all times perioperatively. Prophylactic antibiotics are often administered.
  - perioperatively:
    - standard techniques may be used, apart from tourniquets which cause tissue ischaemia (IVRA is contraindicated). Heat loss should be prevented and cardiovascular stability maintained. Preoxygenation and $F_{I}O_2$ of 50% reduces the risk of hypoxaemia by increasing arterial $P\text{O}_2$ and pulmonary O_2 reserve. IV hydration should be maintained. Frequent analysis of acid–base status is required in HbSS patients. Prophylactic bicarbonate administration has been suggested, but administration according to acid–base analysis is usually preferred.
    - intraoperative crises may present with changes in breathing pattern or BP, acidosis and hypoxaemia. Detection may be difficult.
  - postoperatively: the precautions already instituted should continue, since complications may occur postoperatively. Patients are generally considered unsuitable for most day-case surgery. O_2 administration for at least 24 h is usually advocated.

Firth PG, Head CA (2004). Anesthesiology; 101: 766–85

SID, *see Strong ion difference*

Siggaard-Andersen nomogram. Diagram derived from analysis of many blood samples, showing the plot of log arterial $P\text{CO}_2$ against plasma pH, with base excess, standard bicarbonate and buffer base illustrated as additional lines (Fig. 140). Allows determination of arterial $P\text{CO}_2$ by equilibrating a blood sample with two known concentrations of CO_2, and measuring the sample pH at each concentration. The points are plotted on the diagram and joined by a line, and the $P\text{CO}_2$ read from the vertical scale according to the pH of the original sample. Alternatively, if arterial $P\text{CO}_2$ can be measured directly, a single measurement of pH and $P\text{CO}_2$, together with haemoglobin concentration (since haemoglobin is a major blood buffer), allows determination of the derived data. Modern blood-gas machines automatically perform the required calculations, making such plotting unnecessary.
[Ole Siggaard-Andersen, Danish biochemist]

Sigh, *see Intermittent positive pressure ventilation*

Significance, *see Statistical significance*

Sildenafil (Viagra). Orally active selective phosphodiesterase inhibitor, used in male erectile dysfunction. Catastrophic interactions with nitrates (e.g. GTN) have been reported, resulting in severe hypotension and death; thus a history must be obtained in suspected ischaemic heart disease before administering nitrates.

Has also been investigated as a treatment for pulmonary hypertension. Tadalfil and vardenafil are related drugs.

Simplified acute physiology score (SAPS). Scoring system used to assess severity of illness by determining the degree of deviation of physiological variables from normal values. Originally incorporating 14 variables and excluding pre-existing disease, a modified version (SAPS II) has been developed in which 12 variables are weighted according to age and underlying disease. SAPS III uses a new, improved model for risk adjustment. Used in a similar way to APACHE.

Le Gall JR, Lemeshow S, Leleu G, et al (1995). JAMA; 273: 644–50

See also, Mortality/survival prediction on intensive care unit

Simpson, James Young (1811–1870). Scottish obstetrician; Professor of Midwifery at Edinburgh. The first to administer an anaesthetic for obstetrics in 1847, using diethyl ether. Following a suggestion by Waldie later that year, he used chloroform for the same purpose. Encountered stiff opposition from the clergy and others, who maintained that painful childbirth was either God's will, beneficial to the patient, or both; this continued until Snow's administration of chloroform to Queen Victoria in 1853 ('chloroform à la reine'). Helped popularise chloroform as the replacement for ether. Created baronet in 1866.
[David Waldie (1813–1889), Scottish-born Liverpool doctor and chemist]

Rae SM, Wildsmith JAW (1997). Br J Anaesth; 79: 271–3

Simulators in anaesthesia, *see Anaesthetic simulators*

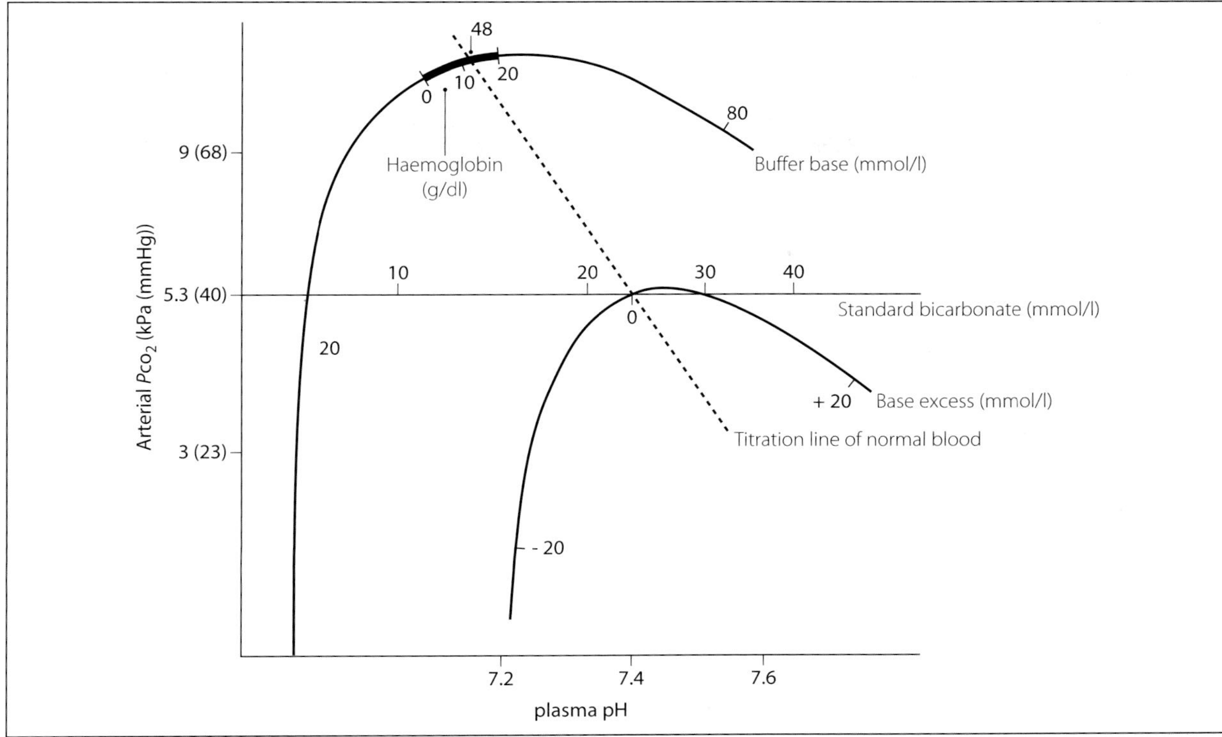

Fig. 140 Siggaard-Andersen nomogram

SIMV, Synchronised intermittent mandatory ventilation, *see Intermittent mandatory ventilation*

Single pass albumin dialysis, *see Liver dialysis*

Sinoatrial node, *see Heart, conducting system*

Sinus arrhythmia. Normal phenomenon (especially in young people) characterised by alternating periods of slow and rapid heart rates. The ECG shows sinus rhythm with irregular spacing of normal complexes. Most commonly related to respiration, with a rapid rate at end-inspiration and a slower rate at end-expiration. Thought to be caused by activation of pulmonary stretch receptors during inspiration, causing inhibition of the cardioinhibitory centre via vagal afferents, with resultant speeding of heart rate; the opposite occurs during expiration. May also involve direct impulse conduction between medullary respiratory and cardiac neurones. Also seen in patients treated with digoxin. Abolished by atropine.

Sinus bradycardia. Usually defined as sinus rhythm at less than 60 beats/min. The ECG shows normal P waves and QRS complexes occurring at a slow rate.

- Caused by:
  - physiological slowing, e.g. in athletes, or during sleep.
  - disease states, e.g. hypothyroidism, raised ICP, acute MI, sick sinus syndrome, jaundice.
  - activation of vagal reflexes, e.g. carotid sinus massage, Valsalva manoeuvre. During anaesthesia, it may follow skin incision, stretching or dilatation of the anus, cervix, mesentery and bladder (Brewer–Luckhardt reflex), pulling on the ocular muscles (oculocardiac reflex), etc. May occur in critically ill patients during tracheobronchial suctioning, etc.
  - hypoxaemia, especially in children. Thought to be caused by central depression of the vasomotor centre.
  - blockade of the cardiac sympathetic innervation during high spinal or epidural anaesthesia.
  - drugs, e.g. halothane, neostigmine, digoxin, opioid analgesic drugs, β-adrenergic receptor antagonists.

If it occurs, the stimulus should be stopped. It may be treated with anticholinergic drugs (e.g. atropine), β-adrenergic receptor agonists or cardiac pacing, but treatment is only required if accompanied by symptoms, hypotension or escape beats.

Sinus rhythm. Normal heart rhythm in which each P wave is followed by a QRS complex on the ECG; i.e. each impulse originates in the sinoatrial node, which has the fastest inherent rhythmicity of all cardiac pacemaker cells. Normal heart rate is usually defined as 60–100 beats/min.
See also, Cardiac cycle; Heart, conducting system; Sinus arrhythmia; Sinus bradycardia; Sinus tachycardia

Sinus tachycardia. Usually defined as sinus rhythm at over 100 beats/min. The ECG shows regular normal P waves and QRS complexes at a rapid rate.

- Caused by:
  - increased sympathetic activity, e.g. fear, anxiety; during anaesthesia, it may represent hypoxaemia, hypercapnia, and inadequate anaesthesia or neuromuscular blockade. It may also occur as a compensatory mechanism, e.g. in anaemia, hypovolaemia, air embolism/PE, etc.
  - increased metabolic rate, e.g. hyperthyroidism, fever, pregnancy, MH.
  - drugs, e.g. sevoflurane, isoflurane, pancuronium, sympathomimetic drugs, cocaine, anticholinergic drugs.

Reduces the time available for ventricular filling and coronary blood flow; it may precipitate myocardial ischaemia if severe. Treatment is usually directed at the cause; β-adrenergic receptor antagonists may be required if the patient is at risk of myocardial ischaemia.

Sinusitis. Infection of the nasal sinuses of the skull. May occur as a consequence of upper respiratory tract infection, trauma or, especially relevant to ICU, prolonged tracheal intubation; has been reported in 2–40% of patients requiring IPPV. Up to 10 times more common if nasotracheal or nasogastric tubes are in place; thought to be related to obstruction of drainage through the sinus ostia (although in a third of cases the contralateral side is affected). Also more common in immunosuppressed and diabetic patients. Usually affects the maxillary or sphenoid sinuses, although ethmoid and frontal sinusitis may also occur (and may result in cerebral venous thrombosis).

May present with non-specific features of sepsis; diagnosed by CT scanning (although plain X-rays may be helpful), ± antral puncture and aspiration. Ultrasound examination may be useful, but requires specialised equipment. Organisms involved are usually Gram-negative bacteria, staphylococci or anaerobes. Management includes extubation, antibacterial drugs ± surgical drainage. Antihistamines and decongestants have also been used. Usually resolves within a week of extubation.

See also, Intubation, complications of

SIRS, *see Systemic inflammatory response syndrome*

Skin diseases. Anaesthetic considerations may be related to:

- diseases with cutaneous and systemic manifestations, e.g. connective tissue diseases, porphyria, polymyositis, neurofibromatosis, severe skin disease with anaemia and malnutrition, etc.
- scarring or fibrosis of tissues around the face, mouth or neck causing difficulty with tracheal intubation, e.g. systemic sclerosis, epidermolysis bullosa dystrophica. In the latter, bullous lesion formation may follow instrumentation (e.g. laryngoscopy), and may be followed by scarring.
- involvement of the immune system causing airway obstruction (e.g. hereditary angioedema) or severe manifestations of histamine release (e.g. urticaria pigmentosa). Histamine-releasing drugs should be avoided.
- increased heat loss during anaesthesia if large areas of erythema are present.
- susceptibility to skin trauma following handling, laryngoscopy, and use of sticking plaster, ECG electrodes, etc.
- effect of drug therapy, e.g. corticosteroids, immunosuppressive drugs.

In addition, anaesthetic agents may precipitate cutaneous lesions (e.g. in adverse drugs reactions, bullous eruption following barbiturate poisoning, porphyria).

Skull. The upper part contains the brain, whilst the lower anterior portion forms the facial skeleton:

- superior aspect: divided from left to right by the coronal suture, separating the frontal bone anteriorly and the parietal bones posteriorly. The sagittal suture separates the two parietal bones in the midline, and the lambdoid suture separates the parietal bones and occipital bone posteriorly. The anterior fontanelle closes at about 18 months of age.
- lateral aspect: consists of parietal and occipital bones posteriorly, temporal and sphenoid bones inferiorly, and frontal bone, with the zygomatic and maxillary bones below, anteriorly. The mandible articulates with the temporal bone at the temporomandibular joint.
- anterior aspect: consists of frontal bone superiorly, zygomatic bones at the inferolateral edges of the orbits, and maxilla centrally, with the mandible inferiorly. Nerves and vessels pass through the anterior foramina and the inferior and superior orbital fissures (Fig. 141a). In addition, the foramen rotundum (below and medial to the superior orbital fissure's medial end) transmits the maxillary division of the 5th cranial nerve.
- inferior aspect: especially important because of the structures transmitted by its foramina (Fig. 141b).

In addition, branches of the 1st cranial nerve pass through the cribriform plate's perforations.

See also, Mandibular nerve blocks; Maxillary nerve blocks; Ophthalmic nerve blocks; Orbital cavity

Skull X-ray. Useful investigation for the detection of linear and depressed skull fractures following head injury, for classifying facial trauma and planning of maxillofacial surgery. Although the presence of a fracture increases the likelihood of intracranial damage, significant injury may be present with a normal X-ray. Investigation of choice for demonstrating basal skull fractures which are poorly visualised by CT scanning. Pneumocephalus is easily evident on a plain skull X-ray.

Sleep. Naturally occurring state of unconsciousness; the response to external stimuli is decreased, but the subject may usually be readily roused. Two patterns are described:

- non-rapid eye movement (NREM) sleep, divided into four stages according to EEG activity:
  - stage 1: occurs as the subject falls asleep; characterised by low amplitude, high frequency theta waves (3–12 Hz).
  - stage 2: sleep spindles occur (12–14 Hz) and high amplitude K complexes).
  - stages 3 and 4: known as slow wave sleep with high amplitude, low frequency delta waves (0.5–2 Hz, 75 μV).
  - stage 4: represents deep sleep, with rhythmic slow waves.
- rapid eye movement (REM) sleep (paradoxical sleep): rapid, irregular, low amplitude waves occur, similar to those seen in awake subjects. Dreaming occurs. The eyes make rapid movement, accompanied by tachycardia, tachypnoea, skeletal muscle relaxation and penile erection.

In a typical night's sleep, a young adult rapidly passes through stages 1 and 2, spending about 60–90 min in stages 3 and 4. A period of REM sleep follows, lasting 60–90 min. This cycle repeats, thus providing about five episodes of REM sleep per night (25% of total sleep time). Sleep disruption is common in the ICU and may be related to:

- pre-existing disease: e.g. patients with COPD show decreased total sleep time and REM sleep with frequent arousals caused by hypoxaemia, hypercapnia and coughing.
- drugs: e.g. benzodiazepines abolish stages 3 and 4 NREM sleep; opioid analgesic drugs increase arousal frequency; tricyclic antidepressant drugs, barbiturates and amfetamines inhibit REM sleep. Catecholamines increase wakefulness.
- anaesthesia and surgery: the stress response to surgery, fever, pain, opioids, starvation and age decrease stages 3 and 4 NREM sleep and abolish REM sleep on subsequent nights.
- environmental factors: noise (e.g. telephones, conversations, alarms, etc.), bright lighting, high temperatures etc.

Sleep deprivation may result in ICU psychosis, increased catabolism, upper airway muscle dysfunction and failure in weaning from ventilators.

Parthasarathy S, Tobin MJ (2004). Intensive Care Med; 30: 197–206

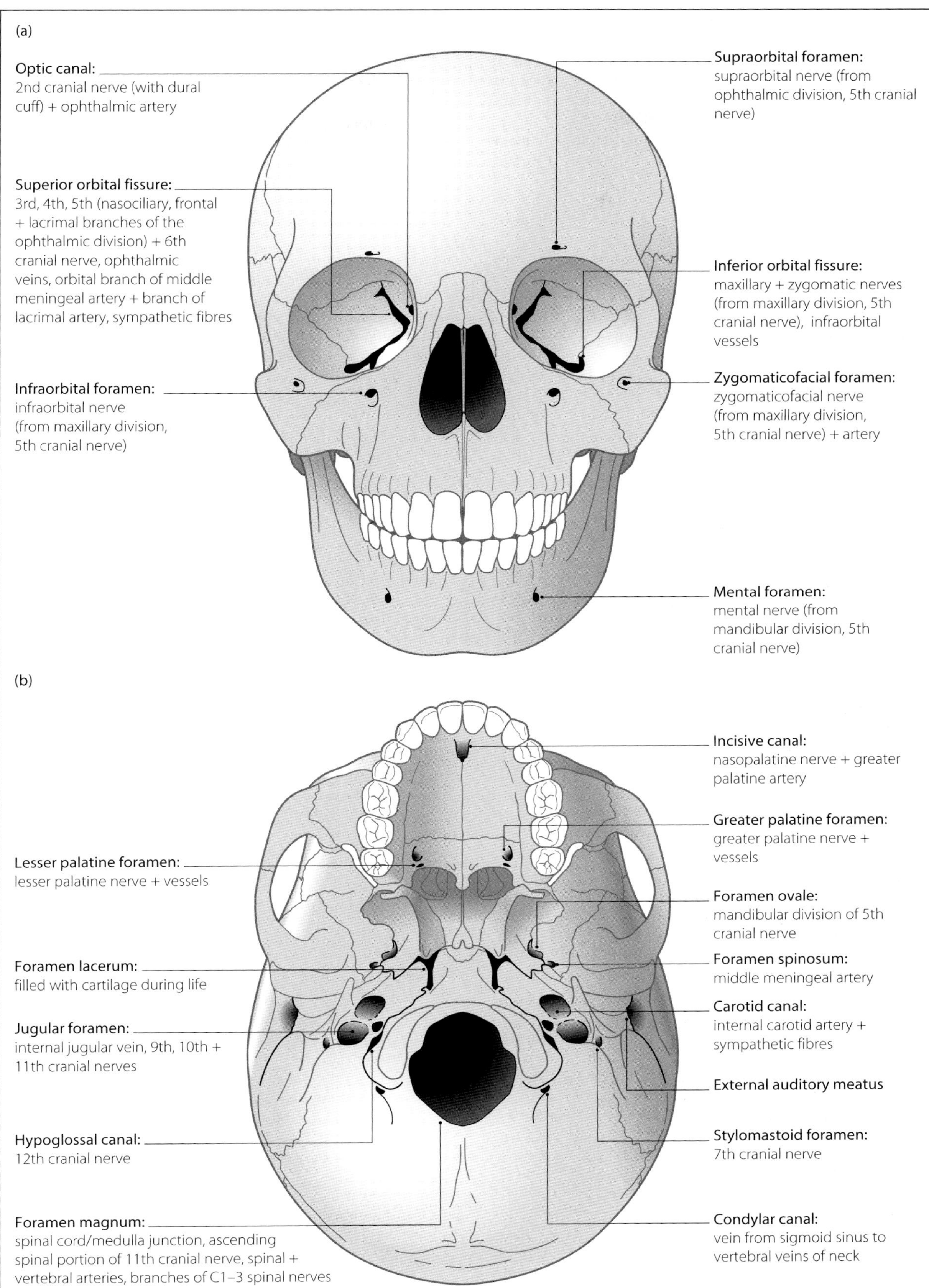

Fig. 141 Skull: (a) anterior aspect; (b) base, showing foramina

Sleep apnoea/hypnoea. Cessation (apnoea) or reduction of > 50% (hypopnoea) for > 10 s occurring during sleep. May have a central mechanism (caused by lack of respiratory drive, e.g. Ondine's curse) or may be obstructive (obstructive sleep apnoea; OSA). OSA is caused by passive collapse of the pharyngeal airway during the deeper planes of sleep, resulting in intermittent upper airway obstruction. Resultant hypoxaemia and hypercapnia results in arousal to lighter planes, thus disrupting normal sleep architecture. Prevalence in adult males is about 3%. Associated with obesity, pharyngeal abnormalities (e.g. retrognathia, tonsillar hypertrophy, acromegaly) and other conditions (e.g. hypothyroidism). A neck circumference of > 42 cm (17 in) is a good predictor of OSA. Sedative drugs (including alcohol) can precipitate or exacerbate the condition. Features include loud (heroic) snoring, restlessness, morning headaches and daytime somnolence. Severe OSA may result in cor pulmonale (obesity hypoventilation syndrome). Diagnosis requires monitoring of nasal and oral airflow, chest and abdominal movements, EEG and oximetry. Treatment includes weight loss, nasal CPAP and removal of tonsils if enlarged. Uvulopharyngopalatoplasty (UVPP) is of dubious benefit. Tracheostomy may be indicated in severe cases.

- Anaesthetic implications:
  - of any predisposing cause.
  - premedication may precipitate complete airway obstruction and should be avoided.
  - maintenance of the airway during induction of anaesthesia and tracheal intubation may be difficult.
  - airway obstruction may readily occur postoperatively; patients should be nursed in an ICU or HDU.

Loadsman JA, Hillman DR (2001). Br J Anaesth; 86: 254–66

Slow reacting substance-A, *see Leukotrienes*

Smallpox, *see Biological weapons*

Smoke inhalation. Resultant pulmonary insufficiency is the commonest cause of death in patients admitted to hospital with burns.

- Problems are related to:
  - low F_IO_2 of inspired gas, and inhalation of carbon monoxide, cyanide, nitrogen oxides and other substances. All may result in hypoxaemia.
  - inhaled carbon particles coated with irritant substances, e.g. aldehydes, which may cause laryngospasm, bronchospasm and inhibition of ciliary activity.
  - $\dot{V}/\dot{Q}$ mismatch, shunt and pulmonary oedema may occur.
  - thermal injury to the airway may be followed by upper airway obstruction, bronchospasm, tracheal and bronchial oedema and sloughing.

Further respiratory impairment may occur if infection and ARDS supervene.

- Management: as for burns, carbon monoxide poisoning, cyanide poisoning, respiratory failure.

See also, Nitrogen, higher oxides of

Smoking. Common cause of cardiovascular and respiratory pathology in surgical and non-surgical patients.

- Effects:
  - cardiovascular:
    - nicotine is an adrenergic agonist; it increases heart rate, SVR and thus BP. It also increases myocardial O_2 demand, and possibly decreases coronary blood flow.
    - carbon monoxide combines with up to 15% of haemoglobin to form carboxyhaemoglobin, reducing the O_2-carrying ability of blood. Causes shift of the oxyhaemoglobin dissociation curve to the right, further impeding release of O_2. Thus haemoglobin concentration and packed cell volume are often increased, increasing blood viscosity and hindering oxygen delivery further.
    - increased risk of ischaemic heart disease and frequency of ventricular arrhythmias.
    - increased risk of DVT has been suggested but this is disputed.
  - pulmonary:
    - impaired ciliary activity.
    - reduced immunological defence mechanisms, e.g. neutrophil, macrophage and lymphocyte activity.
    - increased risk of bronchial carcinoma.
    - increased bronchial reactivity and COPD.

Smokers are more likely to suffer increased sputum production and retention, bronchospasm, coughing, atelectasis and chest infection perioperatively. Poor wound and bone healing is also more common.

Stopping smoking is thought to be beneficial preoperatively, in order to minimise its acute adverse effects. Effects of carbon monoxide and nicotine are significantly reduced after 12–24 h abstinence; up to 6–8 weeks is thought to be necessary for restoration of ciliary and immunological activity.

See also, Carbon monoxide poisoning

Snake bites, *see Bites and stings*

Snow, John (1813–1858). Pioneer of English anaesthesia, born in York. Moved to London in 1836. Developed the science and art of anaesthesia, describing five stages of anaesthesia in 1847. Designed inhalers for diethyl ether and chloroform, and wrote two famous textbooks on the use of these agents (his book on chloroform was published posthumously). Widely regarded as the expert in his field, he administered chloroform to Queen Victoria during childbirth in 1853 and 1857. Also famous for demonstrating that cholera was spread by contaminated drinking water, not by foul air as previously believed. Removal of the Broad Street water pump handle on his suggestion is said to have stopped the London epidemic of 1854. One of the heraldic supporters of the Royal College of Anaesthetists (with Clover).

Society of Critical Care Medicine (SCCM). Founded in 1970 to support the specialty of critical care as a separate but interdisciplinary entity, with *Critical Care Medicine* as its official journal. Supports research, education and provision of resources.

Soda lime. Mixture used for CO_2 absorption in anaesthetic breathing systems, composed of calcium hydroxide (~90%), sodium hydroxide (4–5%), potassium hydroxide (traditionally 1%; in the UK modern preparations do not contain potassium hydroxide), silicates (for binding; less than 1%) and indicators. Used with 14–19% water content. CO_2 in solution reacts with sodium (± potassium) hydroxides to form the respective carbonates, which then react with calcium hydroxide to produce calcium carbonate, replenishing sodium and potassium hydroxides. Heat is produced during the reaction. Exhaustion of its activity is indicated by dyes; several have been used but the most common one changes from pink to white.

Provided in granules of size 4–8 mesh (will pass through a mesh of 4–8 strands per inch in each axis; i.e. pore size of 1⁄16–1⁄64 in^2). Cannisters should be tightly packed to reduce channelling of gases through large gaps. The total volume of space between granules should equal the volume of the granules themselves. Dust may be inhaled using older systems, especially the 'to-and-fro' system. Large cannisters containing up to 2 kg soda lime are commonly employed.

Known to react with trichloroethylene, with the risk of neurological damage. The modern inhalational anaesthetic agents, especially sevoflurane, may react with soda lime if the latter is warm and very dry. Compound A, carbon monoxide, formic acid and formaldehyde may be produced. Compound A is a particular product of sevoflurane, leading to fears over its use in circle systems, although evidence of toxic levels of compound A within such systems has not been found. Significant levels of carbon monoxide have been reported. Furthermore, the temperature in the absorber may increase to dangerous levels and there may be some absorption of the volatile agent itself. The minimal level of moisture that will prevent such reactions is 2% for sodium hydroxide and 4.7% for potassium hydroxide, leading to the latter's removal from modern preparations in the UK. Normal use of circle systems is not thought to result in such low levels of moisture, but they have been found after prolonged passage of dry gas through the absorber, e.g. at the start of a Monday morning operating session if gases are left running over the weekend.

Attempts to prevent the soda lime drying out include shutting off anaesthetic machines after use, changing the soda lime regularly and not relying on colour changes to indicate dehydration, checking for unusually hot absorption cannisters or unexpectedly low concentrations of volatile agent, and addition of zeolites that can physically trap water, or inorganic chlorides that crystallise water within the soda lime. A new mixture (calcium hydroxide lime) consisting of calcium hydroxide with calcium chloride (plus calcium sulphate and polyvinylpyrrolidone to improve hardness and porosity) has been developed which does not contain sodium or potassium hydroxide and does not react with any of the currently used volatile agents.

Sodium (Na^+). Principal cation in the ECF, accounting for 90% of the osmotically active solute in plasma and interstitial fluid. Thus the prime determinant of ECF volume. Total body content is about 4000 mmol, of which 50% is in bone, 40% in ECF, and 10% intracellular. About 70% is available for exchange. Normal plasma levels: 135–145 mmol/l. Of central importance in the function of excitable cells, e.g. concerning membrane potentials and action potentials.

Actively absorbed from the small intestine and colon, facilitated by aldosterone and the presence of glucose in the gut lumen. The kidney filters approximately 26 000 mmol Na^+/day, of which 99.5% is reabsorbed by passage through the nephron (mostly at the proximal convoluted tubule). Reabsorption is influenced by renal tubular hydrostatic and oncotic gradients, aldosterone, adrenocortical hormones, atrial natriuretic hormone, and the rate of secretion of hydrogen and potassium ions.

- Daily losses: about 150 mmol in the urine, with 10 mmol via each of faeces, sweat and skin. Saliva contains 10 mmol/l, sweat 50 mmol/l, gastric secretions 60 mmol/l, and the rest of the GIT about 130 mmol/l.
- Daily requirement: about 1 mmol/kg/day.
- Regulated via changes in:
  - ECF sodium concentration and osmolality via osmoreceptors, affecting the renin/angiotensin system and aldosterone secretion.
  - ECF volume changes: via baroreceptors, affecting atrial natriuretic peptide secretion in addition to the above hormones.

See also, Hypernatraemia; Hyponatraemia

Sodium bicarbonate, *see Bicarbonate*

Sodium calcium edetate. Chelating agent, used in the treatment of acute and chronic lead poisoning. Has also been used successfully in poisoning with copper and radioactive materials.

- Dosage: 40 mg/kg iv 12 hourly for 5 days; repeated if necessary after a 2-day break.
- Side effects: nephrotoxicity, nausea and vomiting, myalgia, hypotension, T wave abnormalities on the ECG.

Sodium citrate. Non-particulate antacid, widely used preoperatively to increase gastric pH in patients at risk of aspiration of gastric contents, e.g. in obstetrics. Thought to be less harmful than magnesium trisilicate if inhaled. Effective for 30–50 min following oral intake of 30 ml 0.3 molar solution.

Also used to relieve discomfort from urinary tract infection by raising urinary pH.

Sodium clodronate, *see Bisphosphonates*

Sodium cromoglicate (Cromoglycate). Drug used in the prophylaxis of asthma. Thought to stabilise mast cells by preventing calcium ion entry, thus preventing IgE mediated release of inflammatory substances from granules. Particularly useful in allergic and exercise-induced asthma, especially in children. Should be taken regularly; will not terminate an acute attack. Administered as a powder, aerosol or nebulised solutions, usually 10–20 mg 4–8 times daily.

See also, Bronchodilator drugs

Sodium dichloroacetate. Activator of pyruvate dehydrogenase, resulting in increased oxidation of lactate to acetyl-coenzyme A and CO_2. Has been used to treat lactic acidosis although randomised trials have not found an increase in survival.

Sodium nitrite, *see Cyanide poisoning*

Sodium nitroprusside (SNP). Vasodilator drug, used as an antihypertensive drug, e.g. in hypotensive anaesthesia. Also used in cardiac failure. Presented as a powder for reconstitution in 5% dextrose. Unstable in solution, with decomposition to highly coloured products. Solutions require protection from light and should be used within 24 h of preparation.

Reacts with thiol groups in vascular smooth muscle and converted to nitrite, which reacts with hydrogen ions to produce nitric oxide. Acts mainly on arteries, although veins are also affected. Thus reduces SVR, maintaining cardiac output and tissue perfusion. Also reduces myocardial O_2 consumption whilst increasing coronary blood flow, although coronary steal has been reported. Compensatory tachycardia is common. Hepatic blood flow remains constant, whilst renal blood flow and cerebral blood flow increase. Active within 30 s of administration. Broken down non-enzymatically within red blood cells (catalysed by haemoglobin) to produce five cyanide ions from each molecule, some of which combine with haemoglobin to form methaemoglobin; the remainder are converted to thiocyanate in the liver by rhodonase and then excreted in the urine. Plasma half-life of SNP is about 2 min.

- Dosage: usually 0.1–5 µg/kg/min iv, to a maximum of 8 µg/kg/min (maximal total dose of 1 mg/kg over 2–3 h). Tachyphylaxis may occur.
- Side effects:
  - rebound hypertension following its abrupt withdrawal. Caused by activation of the renin/angiotensin system and increased plasma catecholamine levels.
  - raised ICP may occur.
  - platelet aggregation may be inhibited.
  - pulmonary shunt may be increased in normal lungs via impairment of pulmonary hypoxic vasoconstriction.
  - cyanide toxicity (hence limitation of dose). More likely in vitamin B_{12} deficiency. May present with metabolic acidosis, and reduced arteriovenous O_2 difference. Treated as for cyanide poisoning. Combination of SNP with trimetaphan, and prophylactic administration of thiosulphate have been suggested as methods for reducing risk of cyanide toxicity.
  - thiocyanate may cumulate after more than 3 days' infusion, with possible interference with thyroid function.

Sodium/potassium pump. Protein pump system present in every cell membrane, responsible for active transport of sodium out of cells and potassium into cells. The protein is an enzyme which catalyses hydrolysis of ATP to ADP, providing the energy required for the transport. Consists of two α subunits (mw 95 000) which extend through the membrane and provide the binding site for ATP, and two β subunits (mw 40 000). Three sodium ions are transported for every two potassium ions, creating a net negative charge within the cell. Required for maintenance of body fluid and cell volumes and composition. Inhibited by cardiac glycosides.

Sodium thiosulphate, *see Cyanide poisoning*

Sodium valproate. Anticonvulsant drug used for all forms of epilepsy. Acts mainly by blocking neuronal sodium channels but also by inhibiting calcium channels in thalamic neurons and enhanching GABA activity. Rapidly absorbed by mouth and largely protein-bound (90%), its half-life is approximately 12 h.

- Dosage:
  - 20–30 mg/kg/day orally.
  - 400–800 mg (up to 10 mg/kg) iv over 3–5 min followed by iv infusion up to 2.5 g/day. Plasma levels are poor indicators of efficacy but are useful in monitoring toxicity at high doses.
- Side effects: GIT disturbances, transient hair loss, rarely thrombocytopenia and impaired platelet function, pancreatitis and severe hepatitis. An increase in plasma ammonia level occurs in 20% of patients but is usually transient.

SOFA, *see Sepsis-related organ failure assessment*

Solubility. Extent to which a substance dissolves in another substance.

- Examples of clinical relevance:
  - inhalational anaesthetic agents: uptake depends on their solubility in blood, and potency depends on their solubility in lipids (Meyer–Overton rule). The ability of N_2O to expand gas-containing cavities depends on its greater blood solubility than nitrogen. For a gas dissolving in a liquid, solubility depends on the temperature (solubility decreases as temperature increases), and the properties of the gas and liquid (expressed by the solubility coefficient). Some volatile agents, e.g. halothane, may also dissolve in rubber anaesthetic tubing, producing significant concentrations even when the vaporiser is turned off.
  - non-gaseous drugs: solubility in water determines requirements for other solvents, e.g. Cremophor EL or propylene glycol for parenteral injection. Solubility in lipid membranes affects the extent to which a drug crosses membranes, e.g. GIT wall, blood–brain barrier.

See also, Partition coefficient

Solubility coefficients. Expression of solubility. Two coefficients are commonly used:

- Bunsen solubility coefficient: volume of gas measured at STP which dissolves in unit volume of liquid at the stated temperature and pressure.
- Ostwald solubility coefficient: volume of gas dissolved in unit volume of liquid at the stated temperature and pressure, i.e. equals the partition coefficient between liquid and gas phases. If measured at 0°C, it equals the Bunsen solubility coefficient.

For solubility of inhalational anaesthetic agents, the Ostwald solubility coefficient (at 37°C) is usually used as it is independent of pressure.

[Robert WE Bunsen (1811–1899) and Wilhelm Ostwald (1853–1932), German chemists]

Solvent abuse. Form of substance abuse involving the intake (usually by inhalation) of a variety of solvents used in glues, paints and similar products; include toluene, petroleum products and carbon tetrachloride. Acute problems may include depressed consciousness and arrhythmias, the latter probably related to myocardial sensitisation to endogenous catecholamines. Sudden death has occurred. Specific organ damage (renal, hepatic) may occur with specific substances, e.g. toluene after prolonged usage. Management is largely supportive.

Harris D (2006). Arch Dis Child Educ Pract Ed; 91: ep93–100

Somatostatin (Growth hormone inhibiting hormone). Hormone secreted by the median eminence of the hypothalamus. Exists in two forms, with either 14 or 28 amino acid residues. Thought to be a neurotransmitter in the brain and spinal cord (especially substantia gelatinosa, where it may be involved in pain transmission – somatostatin has been shown to produce analgesia when injected epidurally). Other actions include:

- inhibition of release of growth hormone and thyroid stimulating hormone.
- suppression of release of GIT hormones e.g. gastrin, cholecystokinin, vasoactive intestinal peptide.
- inhibition of release of insulin and glucagon.

Analogues (lanreotide and octreotide) have been used to control diarrhoea and flushing in the carcinoid syndrome, possibly via inhibition of 5-HT release; they have been used in the management of bleeding oesophageal varices.

Sonoclot, *see Coagulation studies*

Sore throat, postoperative. Reported in up to 90% of cases in some studies, and in up to 25% of patients following spontaneous breathing via a facepiece.

- May be related to:
  - tracheal intubation:
    - use of suxamethonium.

- shape and type of tracheal tube and cuff; larger tubes are associated with a greater incidence of sore throat and hoarse voice than smaller ones.
- trauma on laryngoscopy, intubation and extubation.
- use of stylets or bougies.
- pharyngeal suction.
- use of throat packs.
- use of lubricating/local anaesthetic gel or spray.

- use of nasogastric tubes.
- anticholinergic premedication.
- use of oro-/nasopharyngeal airways.
- use of unhumidified gases.

Also common after tracheal intubation in the ICU, especially after prolonged IPPV.
McHardy FE, Chung F (1999). Anaesthesia; 54: 444–53

Sotalol hydrochloride. Water soluble non-selective β-adrenergic receptor antagonist and class III antiarrhythmic drug, available for oral and iv administration. Used for prophylaxis and treatment of supraventricular and ventricular arrhythmias.

- Dosage:
  - 80 mg orally/day in 1–2 doses (with ECG monitoring), increased up to 160–320 mg/day.
  - 20–120 mg iv over 10 min, repeated 6 hourly as required.
- Side effects: as for β-adrenergic receptor antagonists.

Prolonged Q–T interval and torsades de pointes may occur, especially in the presence of hypokalaemia.

SPAD, Single pass albumin dialysis, *see Liver dialysis*

SPEAR, Selective parenteral and enteral antisepsis regimen, *see Selective decontamination of the digestive tract*

Specific dynamic action. Energy required to assimilate food into the body, manifested as an increase in metabolic rate following intake. Thus the net total amount of energy obtained from foodstuffs is reduced (by 30% for protein, 6% for carbohydrates and 4% for fats).
See also, Nutrition

Specific gravity (Relative density). The density of a substance divided by that of water. Still used to indicate urinary concentration because measurement is easy (using a hydrometer), although not as useful clinically as osmolality. Depends on the nature and number of solute particles, whereas osmolality depends only on number of particles. Thus heavy molecules, e.g. radiographic contrast media, greatly increase specific gravity with only small increases in osmolality. Normal values: for urine, 1.002–1.035; for plasma, 1.010.

Glucose 2.7 g/l and protein 4 g/l each increase specific gravity by 0.001.

For a gas, the ratio of substance to that of air is often used. Most anaesthetic-related gases and vapours are heavier than air, e.g. isoflurane, enflurane, sevoflurane and desflurane (× 7.5), halothane (× 6.8), N_2O (× 1.53), CO_2 (× 1.5), O_2 (× 1.1).

Specific heat capacity, *see Heat capacity*

Specific latent heat, *see Latent heat*

Specificity. In statistics, the ability of a test to exclude false positives. Equals:

$$\frac{\text{the number correctly identified as negative}}{\text{total without the condition}}$$

See also, Errors; Predictive value; Sensitivity

SPECT, Single photon emission computed tomography, *see Positron emission tomography*

Spectroscopy. In anaesthesia, used for gas analysis, especially for estimation of CO_2, N_2O and volatile agent concentrations. Different types:

- infra-red spectroscopy: depends on the ability of gases containing different atoms to absorb infra-red light (thus O_2 and nitrogen cannot be analysed):
  - side stream: sample gas is drawn into a chamber through which half of a split infra-red beam is passed, the other half passing through a reference chamber containing air. The amount of infra-red light absorbed by the sample gas depends on the amount of gas present, and is determined by comparing the emergent beams from the sample and reference chambers. This is done with photoelectric cells behind each chamber, or by passing the beams through two further chambers containing e.g. CO_2, separated by a diaphragm. The heating effect of the infra-red light causes pressure to rise within these chambers; the difference in pressure between them depends on the amount of infra-red light absorbed by the original gas sample. Some devices employ a single chamber instead of two, and some use a rotating perforated wheel to divide the beam(s) of light into pulses. The wheel may incorporate different filters to measure different substances. The technique may be used for multiple simultaneous gas analysis. Interference by other gases, e.g. methane (produced in significant amounts in up to 30% of patients), may be reduced by using either a different wavelength or more than one wavelength for each volatile agent.
  - main stream: analysis takes place at the breathing system itself, by incorporating a special connector near the patient end of the tubing. An emitter/detector is attached to the connector and light is passed through small sapphire windows in the connector. Although more rapid and not requiring sample tubing, the device may be bulky and heavy.
- photoacoustic spectroscopy: relies on absorption of infra-red light of different wavelengths by different molecules, with subsequent emission of sound at the wavelengths concerned for each molecule. Detection is with a microphone. Multiple simultaneous gas analysis may be performed.
- Raman spectroscopy: relies on Raman scattering, the absorption and immediate emission of light by gases in a pattern specific to the individual molecules. All gaseous molecules may be analysed in this way (but not single atoms). Since most light passed through a gas does not produce this effect, powerful light sources, e.g. lasers, are required to give an adequate signal. Multiple simultaneous gas analysis may be performed.
- ultraviolet spectroscopy: has been used to measure halothane concentrations. Requires lengthy warming-up and frequent calibration; now rarely used routinely.
- gas discharge meter: used to measure nitrogen concentration. 1500 V potential is passed across the gas sample in a tube. Intensity of purple light at a specific wavelength is measured.
- mass spectroscopy: now usually referred to as mass spectrometry (*see Mass spectrometer*).

[Chandrasekhara V Raman (1888–1970), Indian physicist]
See also, Carbon dioxide, end-tidal; Carbon dioxide measurement; Near infra-red spectroscopy

Spider bites, *see Bites and stings*

Spinal anaesthesia (Subarachnoid/intrathecal anaesthesia). Probably first performed by Corning in 1885, but first performed for surgery by Bier in 1899. Initial use of cocaine was associated with tremor, headache and muscle spasms. The less toxic procaine was first used by Braun in 1905 and was soon used widely. Hyperbaric solutions were introduced by Barker in 1907. Further refinements were related to new local anaesthetic agents. Continuous spinal techniques were described in the 1940s, initially via rubber tubing connected to the needle left in situ.

Popularity waned in the late 1940s following reports of neurological damage and the introduction of neuromuscular blocking drugs for general anaesthesia (GA). In the classic Woolley and Roe case in the UK in 1947, two cases of paraplegia during the same operating list followed spinal anaesthesia. Phenol contamination via cracks in the cinchocaine ampoules was blamed at the time, although contamination of the syringes and needles with acidic descaler solution from the steriliser has been suggested as being more likely.

Increasing popularity over the last 40–50 years has followed better understanding of the technique, and acceptance that the incidence of side effects is low when spinal anaesthesia is correctly performed.

- Indications: surgical procedures to the lower body, especially perineum and legs. Considered the method of choice (with epidural anaesthesia) by many anaesthetists for TURP, Caesarean section and orthopaedic surgery, e.g. of the hip. Has been used for upper abdominal surgery. Deliberate high or total spinal anaesthesia was formerly used for hypotensive anaesthesia, and to provide abdominal muscle relaxation.
- Anatomy:
  - the spinal cord ends at L1–2 in adults, lower levels in children. The dura ends at S2; therefore lumbar puncture is usually performed at the L3–4, L4–5 or L5–S1 interspaces (n.b. the actual interspace used may be higher than that intended).
  - the L4 or L4–5 interspace is usually crossed by a line drawn between the iliac crests, although this is not very reliable. The spinous process of T12 has a notched lower edge.
  - the course taken by the needle is as for reaching the epidural space, plus the dura (*see also, Meninges; Vertebrae; Vertebral canal; Vertebral ligaments*).
- Technique:
  - preoperative assessment, preparation and premedication are as for GA. Facilities for resuscitation and progression to GA must be available.
  - monitoring is as for GA. An iv cannula must be placed. Preloading with fluid is controversial (see below).
  - the patient is placed in the lateral position, with chin on the chest and knees drawn up, or sitting on the edge of the trolley. Back flexion opens the intervertebral spaces. An assistant is required to steady the patient.
  - sterile gloves are considered mandatory. The back is cleaned, avoiding contamination of gloves and needles with cleaning solution (implicated in causing arachnoiditis and meningitis). Masks reduce both forward and downward dispersal of the anaesthetist's oral bacteria during talking and are usually recommended. Use of gown and drapes is controversial; they are usually employed in the UK, but less so in the USA.
  - median approach:
    - the chosen interspace is infiltrated with local anaesthetic.
    - the spinal needle is inserted in the midline, aiming slightly cranially. Non-cutting needles, e.g. Sprotte (smooth-sided pointed tip, with wide lateral hole proximal to the tip), Whitacre (pencil-tip-shaped, with the hole just proximal to the tip) or Greene (oblique bevel, with bevel edges rounded) are associated with a lower incidence of post-dural puncture headache and are often used (Fig. 142). The Quincke needle point, with its short-bevelled cutting tip, is less often used nowadays except in patients at low risk of headache, e.g. the elderly. 22–29 G needles are commonly used; the larger are easier to use but increase the risk of headache. Thinner needles are often inserted through a 19 G iv needle or introducer, e.g. Sise introducer. The bevel (if present) is faced laterally to reduce the risk of headache.

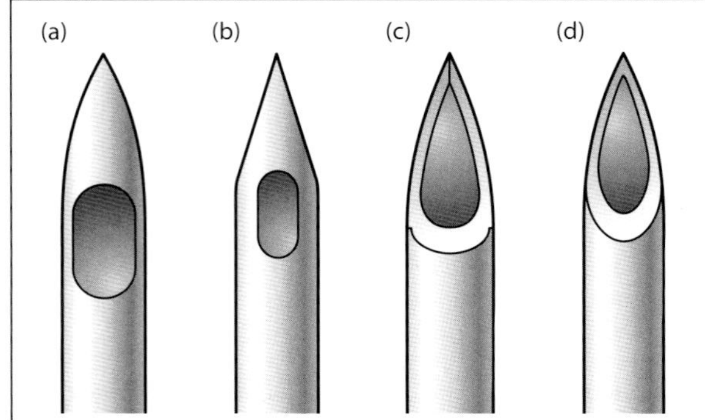

Fig. 142 Different types of spinal needles: (a) Sprotte; (b) Whitacre; (c) Greene: (d) Quincke

    - resistance increases as the ligamentum flavum is entered and when dura is encountered, with a sudden give as the dura is pierced. Correct location is confirmed by CSF at the needle hub; aspiration may be required with very fine needles. Rotation of the needle in 90° steps may produce CSF if none is obtained initially.

    Hanging drop and other techniques have been used to identify the epidural space prior to dural puncture.
    - with the other hand securing the needle against the patient's back to avoid dislodgement, the solution is injected, with aspiration before, during and after injection to confirm correct placement. Injection should cease if pain is experienced.
  - paramedian approach: requires less back flexion, and is easier if the vertebral ligaments are calcified:
    - infiltration is performed 1.5 cm lateral to the cranial border of the spinous process at the selected interspace.
    - the needle is inserted, aiming medially and cranially until the resistance of the ligamentum flavum is felt. If the lamina is encountered, the needle is walked off its cranial edge.
    - dural puncture and injection as before.
  - a continuous catheter technique may be used as for epidural anaesthesia; it has been unpopular because of fears over infection and CSF leak, difficulty of handling the very fine catheters (28–32 G), and the occurrence of cauda equina syndrome following use of lidocaine, but allows incremental injection of solution and therefore greater cardiovascular stability during onset of block. Both catheter-through-needle and catheter-over-needle systems are available.
- Solutions used (Table 33):
  - only hyperbaric bupivacaine 0.5% + 8% glucose is available specifically for spinal anaesthesia in the UK. In the USA, hyperbaric 0.75% bupivacaine + 8.25%

Table 33 Doses (mg) of local anaesthetics required for spinal blockade of different heights

Agent	*L4*	*T10*	*T4–6*	*Duration (h)*
Bupivacaine 0.5% (heavy)	5–10	10–15	15–20	1.5–2.5
Cinchocaine 0.5% (heavy)	4–6	6–8	10–12	2–3
Lidocaine 5% (heavy)	25–50	50–75	75–100	1–1.5
Tetracaine 1.0% (heavy; mixed with equal volumes of CSF)	4–6	8–12	14–16	1.5–2.5

glucose, tetracaine (amethocaine) 1% + 10% glucose, and lidocaine 5% are available (the latter for dilution to 2.5% before administration because of fears over transient radicular irritation syndrome or damage).

- larger volumes are required for plain solutions than for heavy ones. Duration of block may be extended by addition of vasopressors; adrenaline 0.2–0.5 ml 1:1000 and phenylephrine 0.5–5 mg have been used although rarely in the UK. Fears have been expressed concerning possible cord ischaemia provoked by their use. L5–S2 segments remain blocked for the longest.
- low dose techniques are increasingly used, e.g. in obstetrics; a common combination for labour consists of 1 ml bupivacaine 0.25% with fentanyl 10–25 μg.
- spread of solution and extent of blockade are affected by many factors, including:
  - dose: thought to be the most important; increased variability may occur with altered concentration and volume.
  - site of injection.
  - baricity of solution and position: thus hyperbaric solutions affect dependent parts, hypobaric solutions, e.g. tetracaine 0.1%, affect upper parts. Plain bupivacaine 0.5% is slightly hypobaric; tetracaine 1% is isobaric.

    Use of hyper- or hypobaric solutions relies on lateral/supine positioning and head-up/down tilt, combined with the normal curvature of the spine:
    - thoracic curve is concave anteriorly; T4 is traditionally held to be the most posterior part (most dependent in the supine position) but recent imaging studies suggest T8 instead.
    - lumbar curve is convex anteriorly; L3–4 is the most anterior part (uppermost in the supine position). This curve may be abolished by flexing the hips in the supine position.

      In addition, the greater width of females' hips compared with their shoulders tends to tip their spinal canal head down, in the lateral position; in males, the opposite occurs.

      Thus slow injection of 1 ml hyperbaric solution at L5–S1 with the patient sitting produces saddle block suitable for perineal surgery, with minimal hypotension. Blocks may be restricted to one side by injection in the lateral position, although 'fixing' of local anaesthetic may require up to 40 min. Injection of hyperbaric solution in the lateral position with immediate turning into the supine position usually produces blockade to T4–6.
  - patient factors, e.g. weight, height, sex, age, are not thought to be as critical as previously suspected, but they have a small influence. Large variability of blockade between patients is normally found. Recently, volume of CSF has been implicated at least partly in this variability. Reduced volumes of agent are required in obstetric analgesia and anaesthesia.
  - technical factors, e.g. speed of injection, barbotage (repeated aspiration of CSF into syringe, mixing it with local anaesthetic before re-injection), direction of the needle, etc., tend to affect variability of blocks; thus slow injection without barbotage produces the most reliable results.
- spinal opioids improve the quality and duration of analgesia but at the risk of specific side effects.
- other drugs have been studied, e.g. ketamine, midazolam and clonidine, but these are not licensed.

- Effects:
  - results in rapid onset of block (usually within 3–5 min), although maximal effect may take up to 30 min. Vasodilatation in the feet is usually seen first, with flushing and increased warmth.
  - thought to act mainly at spinal nerve roots, although some effect is possible at the spinal cord itself. Differential blockade of different motor and sensory modalities is traditionally thought to be related to the size and therefore sensitivity of different neurones to local anaesthetics. Thus the smaller sympathetic preganglionic fibres are more easily blocked than larger sensory and motor fibres, with the sympathetic 'level' higher than the sensory level. Assessment of the sympathetic level is difficult; the galvanic skin response has been used. The level of blockade for touch sensation is usually 1–2 segments below that for pinprick, whilst that for motor innervation is 1–2 segments lower than that for sensory innervation.
  - CVS:
    - sympathetic blockade causes vasodilatation below the level of block. Reductions in cardiac output and BP are thought to be caused mainly by reduced venous return consequent to venous dilatation, although the fall in SVR contributes. Increased or unaltered cardiac output has also been reported. Reflex vasoconstriction occurs above the level of block. Hypotension is particularly likely in hypovolaemia, since cardiac output in this case is dependent on resting vasoconstriction.

      Hypotension is also more likely in obstetrics, when aortocaval compression may occur. Hypotension may be exacerbated by bradycardia and sedative drugs (depressant effects of local anaesthetic are minimal). The drop in BP may be greater with higher levels of blockade, but this is not always so.
    - bradycardia may be due to block of sympathetic cardiac innervation (T1–4), vagal stimulation during surgery, or a reflex response to decreased venous return. Cardiac arrest has been reported, possibly involving the Bezold–Jarisch reflex.
    - cardiac work and O_2 demand are reduced.
    - renal, hepatic, cerebral and coronary blood flows are maintained if marked hypotension does not occur.
    - reduction in perioperative bleeding is thought to be due to reduced BP, lack of venous hypertension secondary to venoconstriction, and pooling of blood in dependent vessels.
    - reduction of postoperative DVT is thought to be due to vasodilatation, haemodilution and reduced viscosity secondary to iv fluid administration, increased fibrinolysis, and possible effects of local anaesthetics themselves.
    - absorbed adrenaline may have systemic effects, if used.
  - RS: intercostal and abdominal weakness may impair active exhalation and coughing, although tidal volume and inspiratory pressure are maintained by intact diaphragmatic innervation (C3–5). FRC is reduced when

supine, and hypoventilation may follow sedation; thus O_2 is usually administered via a facepiece as a precaution, and to allow concurrent N_2O administration if required.
- GIT: bowel contraction results from dominant parasympathetic tone following sympathetic blockade. Sphincters relax and peristalsis increases.
- urinary retention may occur.
- stress response to surgery is attenuated.

Injected drug is eliminated via absorption by subarachnoid and epidural vessels.

- Management:
  - assessment: level of sensory blockade is usually determined by testing for temperature (e.g. using ice or ethyl chloride spray) or pinprick sensation, though touch may be more reliable. Knowledge of appropriate dermatomes is required. Motor block is assessed by testing muscle groups of appropriate myotomes. The Bromage scale is commonly used for assessment of motor block:
    - 0: full flexion possible at knees and feet.
    - 1: cannot raise extended leg, but can move knees and feet.
    - 2: cannot flex knee, but can move feet.
    - 3: cannot move any part of leg or foot.
  - positioning of the patient may be used to extend or reduce spread of the block as required, until fixed.
  - a high level of block may produce feelings of impaired breathing and nasal stuffiness, plus impaired sensation or power in the arms. Total spinal blockade results in apnoea and loss of consciousness, with fixed dilated pupils. Treatment is as for hypotension, plus tracheal intubation and IPPV. Recovery is complete if BP and oxygenation are maintained.
  - preloading with iv fluid prior to performing spinal anaesthesia is controversial, with some authorities favouring the use of vasoconstrictors as being equally efficacious and more logical. In addition, fears have been expressed concerning fluid overload, especially in the elderly.

    A drop in systolic BP by one-third normal value is usually considered acceptable in healthy patients. Management of larger decreases:
    - positioning the patient head-down: increases venous return but risks higher level of block unless the head is raised.
    - iv fluid administration. Crystalloids are usually acceptable initially.
    - use of vasopressor drugs. May increase myocardial work and O_2 demand secondary to increases in SVR. Ephedrine (3–6 mg iv repeated as required) is commonly used; effects on venous tone may be greater than with other drugs, e.g. phenylephrine (10–50 μg increments iv), metaraminol (0.5–1 mg increments iv).
    - atropine 0.3–0.6 mg or glycopyrronium 0.2–0.3 mg if bradycardia occurs.
  - nausea: may be related to vagal stimulation, e.g. during handling of the bowel. Hypotension is an important cause.
  - sedation is commonly administered, by infusion or bolus. Benzodiazepines are commonly used; ketamine provides some analgesia, e.g. whilst positioning for injection in trauma cases. Propofol infusions may also be used. Advantages include reduced awareness and a smoother procedure if unpleasant sensations are not completely abolished. Disadvantages include respiratory and cardiovascular depression and confusion, especially if sedation is excessive. General and spinal anaesthesia may be combined, not necessarily with increased risk of hypotension.
- Complications:
  - hypotension and high blockade as above.
  - post-dural puncture headache.
  - neurological damage:
    - transient radicular irritation: more common with lidocaine.
    - direct trauma is extremely rare. Injection should stop immediately if pain is felt.
    - haematoma formation with spinal cord compression is extremely rare with normal coagulation. It may be masked by regional blockade. Permanent neurological damage may occur if surgical decompression is delayed > 8–12 h.
    - cord ischaemia, e.g. anterior spinal artery syndrome, thought usually to occur with severe hypotension. Vasopressor drugs have been implicated but their role is unclear.
    - infection/aseptic meningitis.
    - cauda equina syndrome.
    - arachnoiditis.
  - backache (the contribution of spinal anaesthesia itself is doubtful but muscular relaxation with possible stretching of ligaments etc. has been suggested rather than direct trauma).
- Contraindications:
  - non-acceptance by the patient.
  - infection, both generalised and local.
  - hypovolaemia/shock.
  - neurological disease: raised ICP is an absolute contraindication because of the risk of coning. Other disease is controversial; medicolegal implications are usually quoted (e.g. fear of being blamed if a naturally progressive lesion becomes worse).
  - abnormal coagulation: full anticoagulation or coagulation disorders are considered absolute contraindications. Low dose heparin therapy is controversial; the decision usually depends on consideration of individual risks and benefits, and immediately preoperative coagulation studies. Widely accepted guidelines state that a spinal or epidural needle or catheter should not be inserted (or a catheter manipulated or removed) within 6 h after unfractionated prophylactic heparin or 12 h after low molecular weight heparin. Heparin should not be given until 2–4 h after an epidural or spinal. It is generally accepted that these guidelines are not based on strong evidence although they are widely followed (but frequently overridden if the clinical circumstances suggest the benefit outweighs the risk).

    A platelet count of 80–100 × 10^9/l is usually taken as the lower safe limit, but the true safe value is unknown. Platelet function is also important, but effects of antiplatelet drugs, e.g. salicylates, are unclear. A bleeding time of 10 min has been suggested as the lower safe limit although performance of the test may vary between investigators, making it unreliable. Aspirin's effects on bleeding time are diminished after 48 h in healthy volunteers.

    Spinal anaesthesia has been claimed to be safer than epidural anaesthesia, since the needles are finer.
  - emergency abdominal surgery, especially intestinal obstruction: hypovolaemia may be present, and increased GIT activity following spinal anaesthesia may increase the risk of perforation. The patient may also be actively vomiting.

[Albert Woolley (1891–?) and Cecil Roe(1902–?), English labourers; Nicholas Greene and Lincoln F Sise (1874–1942),

US anaesthetists; G Sprotte, German anaesthetist; Rolland J Whitacre (1909–1956), US anaesthetist; Philip R Bromage, Canadian anaesthetist]
Liu SS, McDonald SB (2001). Anesthesiology; 94: 888–906

Spinal cord. Cylindrical structure beginning superiorly at the foramen magnum and terminating inferiorly level with L1–2 (L3 at birth, rising to the adult level by 20 years). May rarely end at T12 or L3. Continuous superiorly with the medulla oblongata, it tapers inferiorly to form the conus medullaris. The filum terminale, an extension of the pia mater, attaches the lower end to the back of the coccyx. Has cervical and lumbar enlargements corresponding to innervation of the upper and lower limbs respectively. Lies within the vertebral canal, surrounded by the meninges and bathed in CSF. The anterior median fissure is a deep longitudinal fissure and the posterior median sulcus is a shallow furrow. Gives off 31 pairs of spinal nerves throughout its length. On cross-section, consists of central H-shaped grey matter surrounded by white matter. The grey matter is composed of anterior and posterior horns, with lateral horns (sympathetic columns) in the thoracic region. The two halves are joined across the midline by the grey commissure which contains the central canal (Fig. 143).

- Main ascending tracts:
  - posterior (dorsal) columns: convey ipsilateral touch and vibration/proprioception sensation, from the lower body via the fasciculus gracilis and upper body via the fasciculus cuneatus.
  - posterior and anterior spinocerebellar tracts: convey proprioception sensation to the cerebellum via inferior and superior cerebellar peduncles respectively.
  - lateral and anterior spinothalamic tracts: the former conveys contralateral pain and temperature sensation; the latter conveys contralateral touch and pressure sensation.
  - spinotectal tract: conveys information to the brainstem involved in spinovisual reflexes.
- Main descending tracts:
  - lateral and anterior corticospinal tracts: convey motor innervation from the cerebral cortex; the former via crossed (pyramidal) fibres and the latter via uncrossed (extrapyramidal) fibres.
  - rubrospinal, tectospinal and vestibulospinal tracts: contain extrapyramidal fibres passing from brainstem nuclei to lower motor neurones.
- Blood supply:
  - anterior spinal artery: formed from two branches of the vertebral arteries, and descends in the anterior median fissure from the brainstem to the conus medullaris. Supplies the anterior ⅔ of the cord.
  - posterior spinal arteries: arise from the vertebral arteries, each dividing into two branches which descend along the side of the cord, one anterior and one posterior to the dorsal nerve roots. Supply the posterior ⅓ of the cord.
  - radicular branches: arise from local arteries, e.g. intercostal, lumbar, and feed the spinal arteries. The most important are at T1 and the lower thoracic/upper lumbar level (artery of Adamkiewicz). The cord at T3–5 and T12–L1 is thought to be most at risk from ischaemia.

[Albert Adamkiewicz (1850–1921), Polish pathologist]
See also, Anterior spinal artery syndrome; Motor pathways; Sensory pathways; Spinal cord injury

Spinal cord injury. Most commonly occurs in males aged 15–35, mostly caused by motor vehicle accidents. C5–6 and T12–L1 levels of the spinal cord are affected most often. Associated injuries (especially head injury) occur in 25–65% of cases.

- Features of acute injury:
  - initial hypertension and peripheral vasoconstriction. Arrhythmias are common. Hypotension and bradycardia may occur in lesions above T6 and T1 respectively, caused by sympathetic disruption (spinal shock). Autonomic hyperreflexia may occur after 4–6 weeks if the lesion is above T5–6.

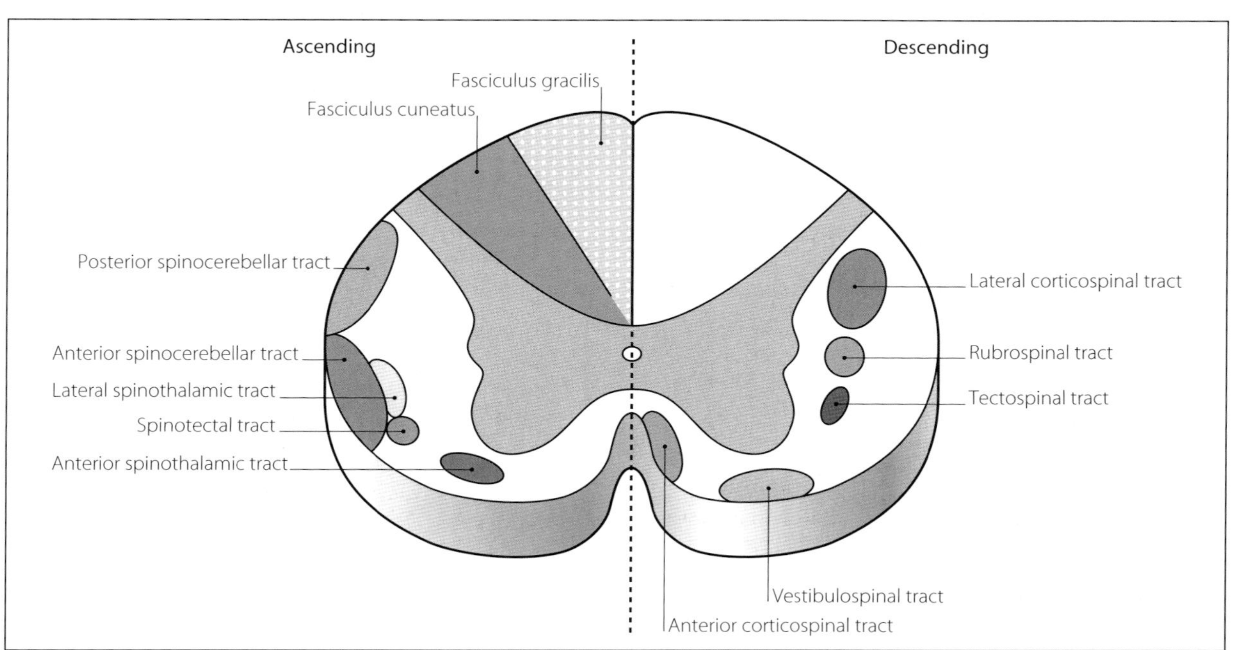

Fig. 143 Anatomy of spinal cord showing ascending and descending tracts

- neurogenic pulmonary oedema is common with cervical lesions.
- initial flaccid paralysis is followed after 2–3 weeks by spastic paralysis. Paralytic ileus is common for 2–3 weeks.

- Certain clinical syndromes may occur:
  - complete injury, with loss of motor or sensory function below a certain level.
  - incomplete injury syndromes:
    - central cord: arms paralysed more than legs, with bladder dysfunction and variable sensory loss.
    - anterior cord: paralysis below the level of lesion, with proprioception, touch and vibration sense preserved.
    - posterior cord: only touch and temperature sensation impaired.
    - hemisection of cord (Brown-Séquard): ipsilateral paralysis and loss of proprioception, touch and vibration sensation, with loss of contralateral pain and temperature sensation.

Primary damage is from the initial injury; the following have been suggested as causing secondary damage: ischaemia, compression, oedema, release of free radicals, arachidonic acid metabolites and excitatory amino acids, and leakage of calcium into cells and potassium out of cells. Thus initial treatment is aimed at reducing ischaemia, inflammation and oedema formation.

- Management:
  - as for any trauma, with particular emphasis on the airway, maintenance of cardiac output and oxygenation, and stabilisation of the spine.
  - high dose methylprednisolone (30 mg/kg iv, followed by 5.4 mg/kg/h for 24–48 h) within 8 h of injury has been shown to reduce the incidence and severity of long-term sequelae.
  - IPPV is required in lesions above C3–5.
  - prevention of DVT, stress ulcers, bedsores, etc.

Mortality is highest in patients under 1 year and over 70 years. Pulmonary complications (e.g. hypoventilation, aspiration pneumonitis, chest infection, PE) are the commonest causes of death within the first 3 months of injury. Other complications are related to nutrition, urinary function and sepsis, osteoporosis, psychological problems and pain syndromes.

- Anaesthetic management is related to:
  - other injuries and cardiorespiratory impairment.
  - potential difficult intubation and risk of aspiration.
  - hyperkalaemic response to suxamethonium within 10 days–6 months of injury.
  - positioning of the patient.
  - impaired temperature regulation.
  - requirement for postoperative IPPV.
  - impaired cardiovascular responses and autonomic hyperreflexia.

[Charles E Brown-Séquard (1818–1894), Mauritius-born US, English and French physician]

See also, Anterior spinal artery syndrome

Spinal headache, *see Post-dural puncture headache*

Spinal nerves. Consist of pairs of nerves (8 cervical, 12 thoracic, 5 lumbar, 5 sacral and 1 coccygeal). Formed within the vertebral canal from anterior (ventral) and posterior (dorsal) roots, themselves formed from rootlets which emerge from the antero- and posterolateral aspects of the spinal cord. The anterior roots convey efferent motor fibres from the cord, and the posterior roots convey afferent sensory fibres to the cord; thus they are mixed nerves. Each spinal nerve leaves the vertebral canal through an intervertebral foramen. The posterior (dorsal) root ganglia lie within the foramina except for C1 and C2 (lie on the posterior vertebral arches) and the sacral and coccygeal ganglia (lie within the canal). The first cervical nerve emerges between the occiput and the arch of the atlas; C2–7 emerge above their respective vertebrae and C8 emerges between C7 and T1. Below this, each spinal nerve emerges below its corresponding vertebra. After giving off a small meningeal branch, each divides into a large anterior and smaller posterior primary ramus (Fig. 144).

- Anterior primary rami:
  - supply cutaneous and motor innervation of the limbs, and front and sides of the neck, thorax and abdomen.
  - cervical: C1–4 form the cervical plexus, C5–8 the brachial plexus.
  - thoracic: termed the intercostal nerves.
  - lumbar: L1–4 form the lumbar plexus.
  - sacral and coccygeal: contribute to the sacral plexus.
- Posterior primary rami:
  - supply motor and sensory innervation to the muscles and skin of the back.
  - do not contribute to limb innervation or plexus formation.
  - divide into medial and lateral branches (except for C1, S4, S5 and coccygeal rami). Cutaneous innervation of T6 and above is contained in the medial branch, below this in the lateral branch.
  - cervical:
    - C1: entirely motor, supplying the muscles of the upper neck.
    - C2: supplies the skin of the back of the head via the greater occipital nerve; motor supply to the neck muscles.
    - C3–8: sensory supply to the lower occiput and neck; motor fibres to the neck muscles.
  - thoracic, lumbar, sacral and coccygeal: unremarkable.

Embryonic segmental distribution of nerves to the skin and muscles is represented by the segmental distribution of cutaneous and motor innervation (dermatomes and myotomes respectively).

Spinal opioids. Spinal or epidural administration of opioid analgesic drugs has become widespread since the first report of epidural morphine administration in man in 1979. Opioids given in this way are thought to bind to opioid receptors in the substantia gelatinosa of the spinal cord, interfering with pain pathways. Although systemic absorption of opioid may contribute to the analgesia, selective spinal block is suggested

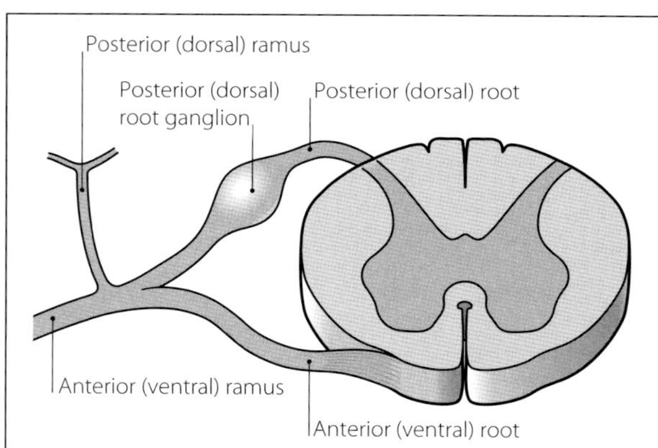

Fig. 144 Typical spinal nerve

by a high CSF:plasma drug ratio and the low doses required compared with those used for parenteral administration. A segmental effect has been reported, i.e. maximal analgesia is related to the site of injection, although lumbar administration has been used for analgesia after thoracic surgery. This may be related to the lipid solubility of the opioid used; thus morphine diffuses further in the CSF than less soluble drugs.

The main advantage of spinal opioids over systemic opioids is profound analgesia which lasts longer. Advantages over spinal or epidural local anaesthetic agents are the lack of sympathetic, motor or sensory blockade, and the ability to provide analgesia distant to the level of injection (e.g. lumbar injection is effective for pain following thoracotomy).

Onset and duration of action are closely related to the lipid solubility of the drug. Highly lipid-soluble drugs, e.g. fentanyl and methadone, cross the CSF and bind to the spinal cord rapidly (molecular shape is also important). Only a small amount is thus available to diffuse throughout the CSF. However, their duration of action is short since they are more rapidly absorbed into the bloodstream. They are more likely to act (at least partially) via systemic absorption. Poorly lipid-soluble drugs, e.g. morphine, have slower onset time (up to 1 h) and their actions last for up to 24 h (Table 34).

Opioids are often mixed with local anaesthetics since combination has been shown to be synergistic. Such mixtures may be given by bolus or by infusion, especially epidural infusion; commonly used mixtures for the latter include 0.1–0.2% bupivacaine plus fentanyl 2–4 µg/ml or diamorphine 50–100 µg/ml, infused at 5–15 ml/h for e.g. postoperative analgesia and chronic pain management. In obstetric analgesia and anaesthesia, fentanyl (and to a lesser extent, diamorphine and morphine) is widely used in the UK for bolus and infusion in labour; in the USA sufentanil is commonly used. Epidural infusion of opioids alone is less commonly used:

- diamorphine 0.25–2.0 mg/h.
- fentanyl 40–100 µg/h.
- methadone 0.5 mg/h.
- morphine 0.5 mg/h.
- sufentanil 20–50 µg/h.
- pethidine 10–15 mg/h.

Pethidine is unique in that it has local anaesthetic properties and has thus been used as the sole agent e.g. for spinal anaesthesia and epidural infusion.

Recently, a preparation of morphine in a naturally occurring lipid lysosomal carrier (extended-release epidural morphine) has been introduced, which increases the duration of analgesia to up to 48 h.

- Side effects of spinal opioids:
  - respiratory depression:
    - early (within an hour of administration): thought to be related to high plasma levels of the drug; thus more common if highly soluble drugs are used. Also more common if sedative drugs have also been given.
    - late (4–15 h after administration, depending on the drug used): thought to be caused by rostral spread of the drug within the CSF to the medullary respiratory centre. More likely with poorly lipid-soluble drugs (e.g. morphine), after intrathecal administration, in the elderly, and if parenteral opioids are administered at the same time. Highly lipid-soluble drugs, e.g. fentanyl, bind more avidly to the spinal cord, with less drug available to spread within the CSF. Although uncommon (0.5–3.0%), late respiratory depression may occur when the patient is unattended, e.g. at night, hence the requirement for close monitoring for up to 24 h after administration, especially if morphine is used. Respiratory rate alone is a poor indicator of the degree of depression; arterial oxygen saturation and level of sedation may be more useful. Naloxone may reverse respiratory depression without affecting analgesia; prophylactic low dose infusion has been used.
  - urinary retention: occurs in 30–40% of cases, although its occurrence in up to 90% of males has been reported. Presence of vesical opioid receptors has been suggested.
  - pruritus: affects up to 70% of patients after morphine, 10% after fentanyl. More common after intrathecal administration. May be helped by antihistamine drugs and naloxone. The cause is unknown.
  - nausea and vomiting: similar incidence to that after parenteral administration, although more common after intrathecal opioids.
  - herpes simplex virus reactivation has been described in obstetric patients.

Table 34 Extradural and spinal doses of commonly used opioids

Drug	*Extradural dose*	*Spinal dose*	*Duration (h)*
Buprenorphine	60–300 µg	25–50 µg	8–10
Diamorphine	1–5 mg	100–300 µg	6–8
Fentanyl	50–150 µg	10–25 µg	2–4
Methadone	4–8 mg	0.5–2.0 mg	4–6
Morphine	1–8 mg	100–400 µg	12–18
Pethidine	25–100 mg	10–100 mg	6–8
Sufentanil	10–75 µg	5–20 µg	2–6

Spinal shock. Syndrome following sudden spinal cord injury, characterised by hypotension (if the level of injury is above T6) and bradycardia (if the level is above T1). Hypotension arises from interrupted sympathetic vasoconstrictor tone, and is greatest in the upright position. Usually replaced by autonomic hyperreflexia after 4–6 weeks. Hypotension may be dramatic on induction of anaesthesia and institution of IPPV.

See also, Valsalva manoeuvre

Spinal surgery. May be required for kyphoscoliosis, trauma, laminectomy, tumours, abscess, etc.

- Anaesthetic management is as for kyphoscoliosis and neurosurgery; main points:
  - preoperative assessment for associated disease, ventilatory impairment, neurological damage, etc.
  - traction and impaired movement may hinder access and tracheal intubation, especially for cervical spine surgery.
  - severe hyperkalaemia may follow suxamethonium if neurological damage is present. Period of risk: 10 days–6 months.
  - surgery may be prolonged with risk of excessive blood loss, hypothermia, etc. Damage to inferior vena cava, aorta and iliac arteries may lead to rapid exsanguination without obvious bleeding from the operation site.
  - hypotensive anaesthesia reduces blood loss but may risk spinal cord ischaemia. Infiltration with vasopressors has been used.
  - epidural anaesthesia has been used, e.g. for laminectomy, with good results.
  - cord function may be assessed by the wake-up test or by monitoring evoked potentials.

- airway obstruction may follow anterior cervical spine surgery if extensive. Ondine's curse may also occur.

Admission to ICU/HDU may be required if there is a risk of airway obstruction, respiratory impairment or excessive bleeding.

Spirometer. Device for measuring lung volumes. The wet spirometer consists of a lightweight cylinder suspended over a breathing chamber with a water seal (Fig. 145). Vertical movement of the cylinder corresponding to respiratory movements is recorded on a rotating drum via a pen attached to the cylinder.

May be used to measure volumes directly, or using dilution techniques. Also used to calculate flow rates and basal metabolic rate. Inaccuracies may arise from inertia of the system at high respiratory rates, and the dissolution of small amounts of gas into the water of the seal.

Dry spirometers, e.g. the Vitalograph, are more convenient for bedside use. It contains bellows attached to a pen, with a sheet of recording paper automatically moved by a motor during expiration. The best results from three attempts are usually recorded.

Spironolactone. Diuretic, acting via competitive antagonism of aldosterone. Inhibits sodium/potassium exchange in the distal renal tubule, with retention of potassium and hydrogen ions. Used to treat oedema due to secondary hyperaldosteronism, e.g. associated with hepatic failure and cardiac failure, and in primary hyperaldosteronism. Diuresis occurs 2–3 h after oral administration.

- Dosage: 100–400 mg daily, orally.
- Side effects: GIT disturbances, gynaecomastia, hyperkalaemia.

Splitting ratio. Ratio of gas flow bypassing an anaesthetic vaporiser to the gas flow entering it. At a splitting ratio of zero, the total gas flow passes through the vaporiser; at a ratio of infinity, none passes through (i.e. the vaporiser is switched off).

Sprays. In anaesthesia, usually employed to deliver local anaesthetic agent (usually 4% lidocaine) to the larynx and trachea, e.g. for awake tracheal intubation, and to reduce stimulation during positioning and tracheal extubation. Spraying the cords at laryngoscopy does not attenuate the hypertensive response to laryngoscopy itself. Common laryngeal sprays include the Forrester, Macintosh and Swerdlow sprays (Fig. 146). A metered-dose aerosol is also available, delivering 10 mg of 10% lidocaine per spray; its nozzle may be too short to reach the larynx. Syringes with long perforated nozzles are also available.

Sprays may also be used to spray cocaine into the nose, to produce anaesthesia and vasoconstriction.

Other sprays used in anaesthesia include the ethyl chloride spray for refrigeration anaesthesia and testing regional anaesthesia, and disinfectant sprays, dressings, etc.

Problems include blockage, bacterial contamination of the local anaesthetic agent, parts of the spray becoming detached and entering the airway (e.g. the tip of the Macintosh spray), and excessive administration of local anaesthetic agent.
[Alexander C Forrester (1907–1996), Glasgow anaesthetist; Mark Swerdlow (1918–2003), Manchester anaesthetist]

SRS-A, Slow reacting substance-A, *see Leukotrienes*

SSRIs, *see Selective serotonin reuptake inhibitors*

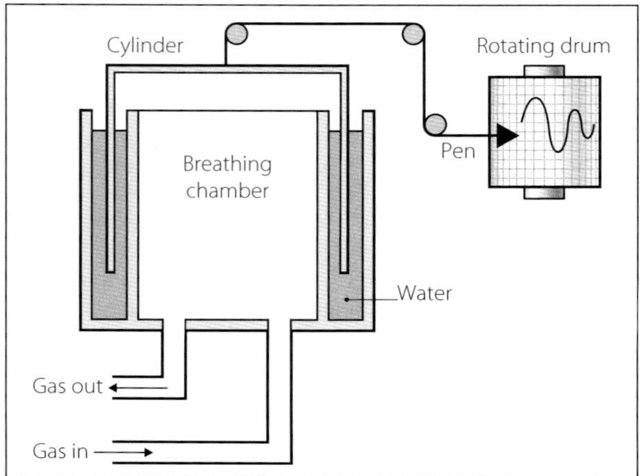

Fig. 145 Wet spirometer

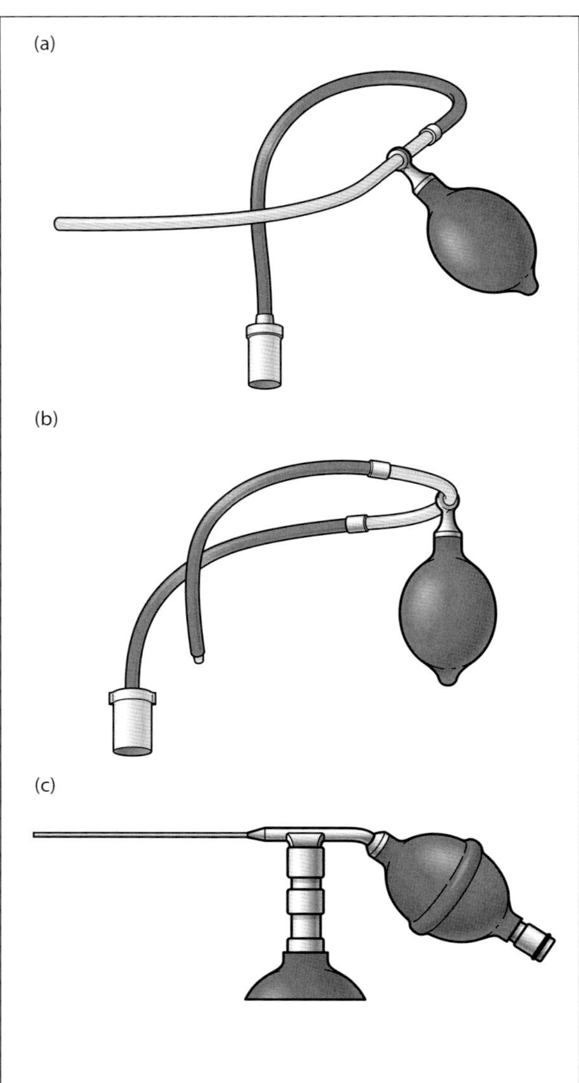

Fig. 146 Commonly used anaesthetic sprays: (a) Forrester; (b) Macintosh: (c) Swerdlow

S–T segment. Portion of the ECG between the end of the QRS complex and the beginning of the T wave (*see Fig. 57b; Electrocardiography*). Represents ventricular repolarisation. Average duration is 0.32 s. Normally within 1 mm of the height of the isoelectric line (between the T wave and following P wave). Elevated following acute myocardial damage, e.g. MI and pericarditis. Depressed by myocardial ischaemia, hypokalaemia and digoxin therapy, the latter typically producing a 'reverse tick' pattern. May also be depressed in reciprocal leads following MI.

Stages of anaesthesia, *see Anaesthesia, stages of*

Standard bicarbonate. Plasma concentration of bicarbonate when arterial $P\text{CO}_2$ has been corrected to 5.3 kPa (40 mmHg), with haemoglobin fully saturated and at a temperature of 37°C. Thus eliminates the respiratory component of acidosis or alkalosis. Normally 24–33 mmol/l.
See also, Acid–base balance

Standard deviation (SD). Expression of the variability of a population or sample. Equals the square root of variance, i.e.

$$\text{SD} = \sqrt{\frac{\Sigma(x-\bar{x})^2}{n-1}}$$

Squaring $(x-\bar{x})$ eliminates any minus signs, i.e. for those values of x less than $\bar{x}$.

In a sample of normal distribution, a range of 1 SD on either side of the mean includes about 68% of all observations, 2 SDs on either side include about 95%, and 3 SDs on either side include about 99.7%.
See also, Statistical frequency distributions; Statistics

Standard error of the mean (SE). Indication of how well the mean of a sample represents the true population mean.

$$\text{SE} = \frac{\text{standard deviation (SD)}}{\sqrt{n}}$$

where n = number of values.

SE is large when n is small, i.e. the sample mean is less likely to represent the population mean.

Often presented with the mean in statistical data, because the data appear tidier, and mean ± SE has a smaller spread than mean ± SD. Apart from this, SE has no advantage over SD.
See also, Statistical tests; Statistics

Staphylococcal infections. Caused by members of the Staphylococcus genus of Gram-positive bacteria. *S. aureus* is the major pathogen, causing a spectrum of infections including boils, abscesses, cellulitis, wound infection, osteomyelitis, chest infection and septic shock. Infection is especially problematic in immunodeficiency, e.g. in critically ill patients. Other conditions arise from exotoxin production, e.g. toxic shock syndrome, scalded skin syndrome and food poisoning.

S. aureus produces an enzyme (coagulase) which converts fibrinogen to fibrin and thus clots blood. Strains may be typed by viral bacteriophages; up to 65% of strains produce exotoxins. Nasal carriage of *S. aureus* occurs in about a third of normal subjects; the organism may also be present on the skin, especially perineum. Over 30 coagulase negative staphylococcus species exist, mostly as skin commensals although they may cause clinical infection, especially *S. epidermidis* (typically associated with prosthesis- and catheter-related sepsis) and *S. saprophyticus* (typically causing urinary tract infection).

Bacterial resistance is an increasing problem, with 90% of hospital staphylococci resistant to benzylpenicillin and related drugs via production of β-lactamase. Meticillin-resistant *S. aureus* (MRSA) is a particular problem in hospitals and increasingly in the community too. Glycopeptides are usually reserved for its treatment although resistance has been reported. Strict infection control is required to reduce cross-contamination and spread of infection.

STaR, *see Safe transport and retrieval*

Starling forces. Factors determining the movement of fluid across the capillary wall endothelium. Movement into the interstitial space is encouraged by the hydrostatic pressure gradient (capillary hydrostatic pressure (P_c) – interstitial fluid hydrostatic pressure (P_i)). This flow is counteracted by the colloid osmotic gradient (capillary colloid osmotic pressure (π_c) – interstitial fluid colloid osmotic pressure (π_i)):

$$\dot{Q} = K\,[(P_c - P_i) - \sigma(\pi_c - \pi_i)]$$

where $\dot{Q}$ = net flow of fluid for a given surface area
K = permeability or filtration coefficient (flow rate per unit pressure gradient across the endothelium)
σ = reflection coefficient (represents permeability of the endothelium to plasma proteins).

The equation does not account for active transport of solutes and effects of surface tension in the lung.

Capillary hydrostatic pressure falls from about 30 mmHg at the arteriolar end (favouring net flow of fluid out of the capillary) to 15 mmHg at the venous end (favouring net flow in). In health, the volume of fluid leaving the capillary exceeds that being reabsorbed by about 10%, the excess being absorbed by the lymphatic system. Greater imbalance may result in oedema.
[Ernest H Starling (1866–1927), London physiologist]

Starling resistor. Model consisting of a length of collapsible tubing passing through a rigid box (Fig. 147). The effects of different upstream pressures (P_1), pressures in the chamber (P_2) and downstream pressures (P_3) on flow through the tubing can be studied. Used to illustrate the effect of gravity on regional pulmonary circulation, P_1, P_2 and P_3 representing arterial, alveolar and venous pressures respectively.
See also, Ventilation/perfusion mismatch

Starling's law (Frank–Starling law). Intrinsic regulatory mechanism of the heart stating that force of myocardial contraction is proportional to initial fibre length, up to a point (Fig. 148). Neither variable is easily measured; hence myocardial contraction is often represented by cardiac output, stroke volume, stroke index or stroke work (y-axis) and initial fibre length is represented by left ventricular end-diastolic volume, left ventricular end-diastolic pressure or pulmonary capillary wedge pressure (x-axis).

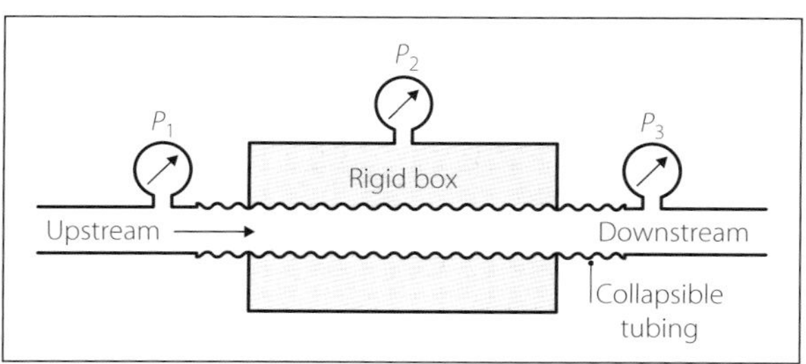

Fig. 147 Starling resistor (see text)

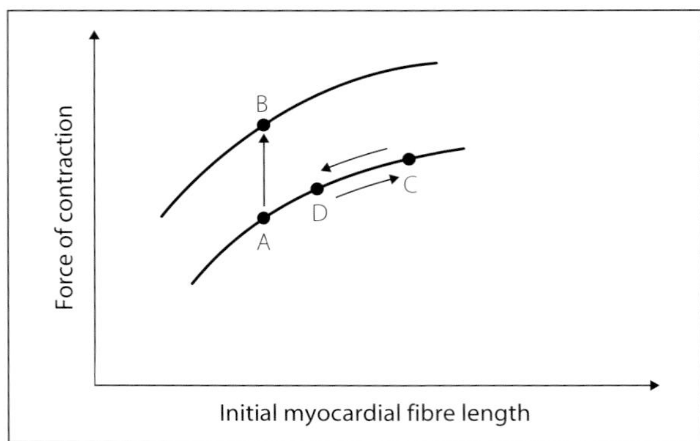

Fig. 148 Starling's law

The law explains how right and left ventricular outputs remain matched, i.e. if right ventricular output increases, the increase in pulmonary venous pressure in turn increases left ventricular filling; the resultant increased stretch increases left ventricular output in line with that of the right ventricle.

Changes in myocardial contractility shift the curve's position; e.g. in cardiac failure and MI it is moved downwards and to the right (e.g. in Fig. 148, from the upper curve to the lower curve). Cardiac dilatation compensates initially, by moving along the curve to the right.

The (Starling) curves may be plotted for individual patients, and have been used to guide management of reduced output states. Therapeutic measures alter the heart's position on the curve, e.g. use of inotropic drugs moves heart function from A to B, venodilators move it from C to D, and a fluid bolus challenge moves it from D to C (see Fig. 148).
[Otto Frank (1865–1944), German physiologist]
O'Rourke MF (1984). Aust N Z J Med; 14: 879–87

Starvation, *see Malnutrition*

Static electricity, *see Antistatic precautions; Explosions and fires*

Statistical frequency distributions. In statistics, relationships between measured variables and the frequency with which each value occurs. For continuous data, the resultant curve may often be described by a mathematical equation, allowing statistical tests and other analyses to be performed. Many types of biological data have a 'normal' (Gaussian) distribution (Fig. 149). Such data are described by the mean and standard deviation (SD). The standard normal deviate (z) describes any individual value by relating it to the mean and SD, and can be used to calculate the probability that such a value lies within the 'normal' range. Parametric statistical tests may be used to test the hypothesis that different samples of normally distributed data are in fact taken from the same population (null hypothesis). They compare within-group variability with between-group differences; e.g. two samples are likely to represent different populations if the scatter (SD) of each is small and their means are very different.

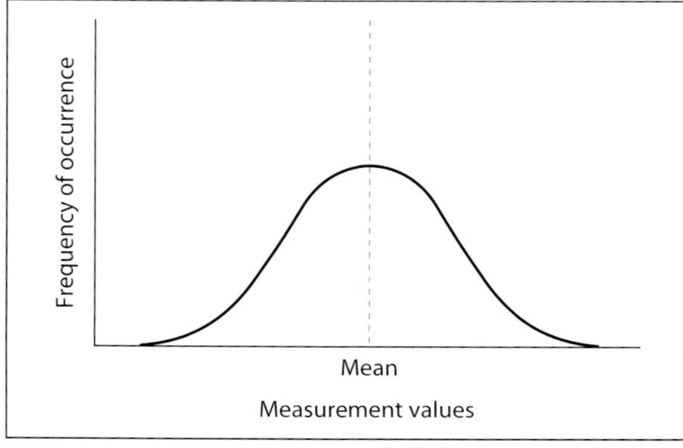

Fig. 149 Normal frequency distribution curve

Data which are not normally distributed (e.g. skewed) may often be 'normalised', e.g. by logarithmic transformation, allowing application of parametric tests which are more sensitive than non-parametric tests.

Other types of distribution include the binomial (in which there are two possibilities for each measurement, e.g. yes or no, dead or alive, etc.), multinomial, and Poisson distribution (which describes random events where non-events cannot be counted, e.g. radioactive decay).
[Karl F Gauss (1777–1855), German mathematician; Simeon D Poisson (1781–1840), French mathematician]
See also, Samples, statistical

Statistical significance. Term denoting a probability of less than 0.05 ($P < 0.05$) for a statistical test or a result of inferential statistics. Represents an arbitrary cut-off without reference to practical or clinical significance, but widely used by convention. More stringent 'levels' of probability are sometimes used (e.g. $P < 0.01$), e.g. to account for the increased likelihood of a significant result due to chance alone when large numbers of comparisons are made. The terms 'very' or 'highly' significant to describe very small P values should not be used when presenting data, but the P value itself should be provided.
See also, Errors

Statistical tests. Methods of comparing or extrapolating data in inferential statistics, e.g. in clinical trials. Involve mathematical calculations depending on the descriptive statistics of each sample group. Results are traditionally expressed as the probability that any observed differences between groups are due to chance alone, i.e. the likelihood that the samples are taken from the same population (null hypothesis). Increasingly, confidence intervals are being used to indicate the range within which a real difference is likely to lie.

- Many different tests have been described, applicable to specific types of data and situations, e.g.:
  - comparing groups consisting of:
    - different subjects with different treatments:
      - two groups:
        - parametric (for normally distributed continuous data): unpaired (Student's) t test. Compares the mean and standard deviation for each group. Two-tailed tests allow for either an increase or a decrease in the variable measured.
        - non-parametric:
          - nominal data: chi-squared test (contingency table) with Yates's correction for continuity. Compares the observed frequency of events with the expected frequency. Fisher's exact test is used if any expected frequency is less than 5.
          - ordinal data: Mann–Whitney rank sum test. Ranks all the results in ascending order and compares the group's distributions within the ranking.
          - all types of data: sequential analysis. Relies on the relationship between the size of difference between groups, and the number of subjects

required to achieve statistical significance for that difference (as the size of difference increases, fewer subjects are required). A graph is drawn with precalculated 'significance' boundaries, with an indicator of sample size on the *x*-axis and an indicator of size of difference on the *y*-axis. Results are analysed at intervals as the study progresses, and points plotted on the graph; the study is stopped when a boundary is crossed, thus minimising the number of subjects required to achieve a significant result.

- more than two groups:
  - parametric: analysis of variance (ANOVA). Similar basis to the *t* test. Only indicates that a significant difference exists, not between which groups it exists. Student–Neuman–Keuls, Tukey's and other tests are used to indicate which of the comparisons achieve statistical significance.
  - non-parametric:
    - nominal data: chi-squared test as above (Yates's correction is not required).
    - ordinal data: Kruskal–Wallis test. Similar basis to the Mann–Whitney test.
- same subjects before and after a treatment:
  - two groups:
    - parametric: paired *t* test. More powerful than the unpaired test because intersubject variability is reduced, since each subject acts as his or her own control.
    - non-parametric:
      - nominal data: McNemar's test.
      - ordinal data: Wilcoxon signed-rank sum test. Ranks the differences between the paired results.
- serial measurements following a treatment:
  - parametric: repeated-measure ANOVA.
  - non-parametric:
    - nominal data: Cochrane's test.
    - ordinal data: Friedman statistic.

- comparing two variables for association:
  - parametric: linear regression analysis and correlation. Regression analysis determines the magnitude of change of one variable produced by the other variable. Expressed as the slope of the line of best fit, the equation relating the two variables, indicators of scatter, or statistical differences from the line of no association. Correlation indicates the degree of association only and is expressed as the Pearson correlation coefficient (r). An r of +1 or –1 indicates complete positive or negative association respectively, whilst an r of 0 indicates no association. For comparison of two methods of measurement (e.g. invasive and non-invasive arterial BP measurement), the difference between the two values obtained at each measurement is calculated. Bias and precision (mean and standard deviation respectively of the differences) indicate the degree of agreement between the two methods (Bland and Altman plot).
  - non-parametric:
    - nominal data: contingency coefficient.
    - ordinal data: Spearman rank correlation.

Non-normally distributed interval data may be transformed and normalised before application of parametric tests, otherwise weaker non-parametric tests must be applied.

- Inappropriate study design or tests may result in errors and incorrect conclusions. Common examples include:
  - multiple testing without correction. With a probability (P) of 0.05 taken as representing statistical significance, one test in 20 would be expected to produce a 'significant' result by chance. The Bonferroni correction is commonly used to account for multiple comparisons between groups.
  - insufficient power.
  - application of the incorrect test, e.g. use of the *t* test to compare ordinal data.

The tests and modifications are usually named after the mathematicians that described or developed them (apart from Student's *t* test).

[Student: pseudonym used by William S Gosset (1876–1937), English chemist, in order to publish his work (publication of papers on any subject was banned by his employers, Guinness, after trade secrets had been included in a paper published by another employee); Arthur Guinness (1725–1803), Irish brewer]

See also, Statistical frequency distributions

Statistics. Collection, analysis and interpretation of numerical data, used to describe and compare samples and populations. May be:

- descriptive; i.e. describes sample data without extrapolation to the whole population. Descriptive terms vary according to the type and distribution of data but include measures of:
  - central tendency, e.g. mean, mode, median.
  - scatter, e.g. standard deviation, percentiles.

  Thus normally distributed data are described by their mean and standard deviation, ordinal data by the median and percentiles (usually 25th–75th (i.e. interquartile range)) and range, and nominal by the mode and a list of possible categories.
- inferential (analytical); i.e. used to relate sample data to the whole population. Applications include the use of clinical or laboratory measurements to define disease, and determining whether different samples are from the same population (null hypothesis). The latter is commonly performed in clinical trials, using statistical tests.

See also, Confidence intervals; Predictive value; Sensitivity; Specificity; Standard error of the mean; Statistical frequency distributions; Statistical significance

Status asthmaticus. Has been variously defined as acute severe asthma which is refractory to medical treatment, or which persists for 12 or 24 h. Acute severe asthma is now the preferred term.

Status epilepticus. Continuous or rapidly repeating convulsions persisting for > 30 min without regaining consciousness. Generalised convulsive status epilepticus (GCSE) is the most common form; in one-third of cases it is the first presentation of epilepsy. After 30 minutes' seizures, increased ICP, hypotension and failure of cerebral autoregulation result in decreased cerebral perfusion pressure. Failure of central control of breathing causes hypoxaemia, pulmonary hypertension and cardiac failure. At this stage, visible seizures may be absent despite continuing cerebral seizure activity.

- Aetiology:
  - acute processes, e.g. electrolyte imbalance, renal failure, sepsis, head injury, CVA, drug abuse (e.g. alcohol, cocaine), CNS infection (e.g. encephalitis, meningitis), hypoxic brain injury.
  - chronic disease, e.g. pre-existing epilepsy ± low anticonvulsant drug levels, chronic alcoholism, cerebral lesions.

- Management:
  - general:
    - initial rapid assessment and CPR. O_2 and iv cannulation are mandatory and tracheal intubation often necessary. Monitoring of BP, ECG, temperature, etc. should be instituted.
    - 50 ml of 50% glucose should be given iv with thiamine 100 mg if alcoholism/malnutrition is present.
    - acidosis may require bicarbonate therapy although it usually corrects itself with resuscitation.
    - hyperthermia may require active cooling.
  - common UK and US regimen for anticonvulsant therapy:
    - premonitory stage (status may be heralded by increasing seizure frequency and intensity): diazepam 10–20 mg iv (or midazolam 5–10 mg im if the route is not available; rectal diazepam has also been used), repeated once after 15 min if seizures continue. In the past, clonazepam and paraldehyde have also been used.
    - early status (< 30 min): lorazepam 100 μg/kg iv.
    - established status: phenytoin 15–20 mg/kg iv ± phenobarbital 10 mg/kg iv. Fosphenytoin may also be used; 1.5 mg is equivalent to 1 mg phenytoin.
    - refractory status (seizures continue despite therapeutic levels of above anticonvulsants): requires transfer to a specialised unit with EEG monitoring and anaesthesia with thiopental or propofol.

Finney SJ, Hirsch NP (2005). Curr Anaesth Crit Care; 16: 123–31

Status lymphaticus. 'Syndrome' supposedly occurring in children who died unexpectedly under anaesthesia; said to have characteristic associated pathological findings. Now thought not to exist, and merely an excuse for poor management.

Macintosh RR, Pratt FB (1995). Paediatr Anaesth; 5: 354 and 388

Stellate ganglion block. Performed for painful arm conditions, e.g. complex regional pain syndrome type 1, herpes zoster, phantom limb, shoulder/hand syndrome, and to improve circulation, e.g. in Raynaud's syndrome, postembolectomy. Has formerly been performed in quinine poisoning, angina and asthma.

The ganglion represents the fused inferior cervical and first thoracic sympathetic ganglions, and is present in 80% of subjects. It usually lies on or above the neck of the first rib. Some sympathetic fibres may leave the sympathetic chain below the ganglion of T1, and run directly to the brachial plexus, bypassing the ganglion. The precise site of action of the block is controversial, since studies using dye have shown that the ganglion itself may not be affected by injected solution.

With the patient supine and the neck extended, Chassaignac's tubercle (transverse process of C6) is palpated level with the cricoid cartilage. The carotid sheath is retracted laterally with the fingers, and a skin wheal raised over the tubercle. A 5 cm needle is inserted directly posteriorly to contact the tubercle, passing medial to the retracted carotid sheath. It is withdrawn 1–2 mm and 5–10 ml local anaesthetic agent is injected after careful aspiration. A 2 ml test dose has been suggested before injection of the main dose. Successful block is signalled by Horner's syndrome.

Complications include intravascular injection (including into the vertebral artery), recurrent laryngeal nerve and brachial plexus blocks, pneumothorax, subarachnoid and epidural injection, and haematoma formation.

[Maurice Raynaud (1834–1881), French physician]

See also, Sympathetic nerve blocks; Sympathetic nervous system

Sterilisation of breathing equipment, *see Contamination of breathing equipment*

Steroid therapy, *see Corticosteroids*

Stethoscope. Invented in its monaural form (as a wooden trumpet-shaped tube) by Laennec in 1819; Cammann's binaural model appeared in 1852. During anaesthesia, allows continuous auscultation of breath sounds and heart sounds. May indicate air embolism. Two forms are commonly used in anaesthesia:

- precordial stethoscope: often connected to a monoaural earpiece to allow the anaesthetist greater freedom.
- oesophageal stethoscope: a modified nasogastric tube. Widely used in the USA; less so in the UK, apart from paediatric anaesthesia. Addition of temperature probe, ECG electrodes and pacing wires has been described.

[Rene TH Laennec (1781–1826), French physician; George Cammann (1804–1863), US physician]

Stevens–Johnson syndrome. Immune-complex mediated hypersensitivity skin disorder resulting in the separation of the epidermis from the dermis. Erythema multiforme and toxic epidermal necrolysis are respectively considered lesser and more severe forms of the same condition. Caused by drugs (especially anticonvulsant and antibacterial agents), viral infections and malignancy, although in 50% of cases the cause is unknown. Treatment is mainly supportive but includes careful fluid and electrolyte replacement; skin lesions are treated as burns. Specific treatment with cyclophosphamide, plasmapheresis and intravenous immunoglobulins has been used. Mortality is 15%.

[Albert M Stevens (1884–1945), Frank C Johnson (1894–1934), New York paediatricians]

Stewart–Hamilton equation. Formula used in cardiac output measurement when using thermodilution techniques:

$$\dot{Q} = \frac{V(T_B - T_I)K_1K_2}{T_B(t)dt}$$

where $\dot{Q}$ = cardiac output
V = volume of injectate
T_B = blood temperature
T_I = injectate temperature
K_1 and K_2 = computer constants
$T_B(t)dt$ = change in blood temperature over time.

[GN Stewart (1860–1930), Canadian-born US scientist; WF Hamilton (1893–1964), US physiologist]

Stings, *see Bites and stings*

Stoichiometric mixture. Mixture of reactants in such proportions that none remains at the end of the reaction. Stoichiometric mixtures often react violently, and are thus more likely to be involved in explosions and fires.

Stokes–Adams attack. Syncope occurring in complete heart block; may be due to transient asystole or VF. Occurs suddenly, and may progress to convulsions. Recovery is typically rapid. Differential diagnosis includes vasovagal syncope, transient ischaemic attack, micturition and cough syncope, and postural hypotension. Requires cardiac pacing.

[William Stokes (1804–1878), Irish physician; Robert Adams (1791–1875), Irish surgeon]

Stovaine. Local anaesthetic drug, introduced in 1904, as a less toxic alternative to cocaine. Slightly irritant, and replaced in turn by procaine.
[Ernest Forneau (1872–1949), French chemist; *forneau* is French for stove]

STP/STPD. Standard temperature and pressure (0°C; 101.3 kPa (760 mmHg)) and STP dry. Used for standardising gas volume measurements.

Streptococcal infections. Caused by members of the Streptococcus genus of Gram-positive bacteria. Several species exist, usually as normal commensals in the upper respiratory tract, but they may cause a wide range of clinical infections. Classified according to the type of haemolysis they cause on blood agar (none, α and β), the latter also subclassified according to cell wall antigens into groups A–H and K–V.

- Important pathogenic streptococci:
  - *S. pyogenes* (Group A β-haemolytic): the major pathogen, causing pharyngitis, cellulitis, necrotising fasciitis, erysipelas, scarlet fever and septic shock. The organism is further subdivided into strains and types according to surface antigens. The M antigen confers particular virulence. Several exotoxins may contribute to the clinical features of infection, e.g. scarlet fever, toxic shock syndrome. In addition, cross-reactivity between anti-streptococcal antibodies and host tissue may result in disease, e.g. rheumatic fever and glomerulonephritis.
  - Group B β-haemolytic: especially important in neonates/infants (arthritis, meningitis, peritonitis) and obstetrics/gynaecology (septic abortion, chorioamnionitis, etc.). May also cause adult meningitis, endocarditis, osteomyelitis, etc.
  - Group C and G β-haemolytic: similar to Group A organisms; Group D are different and have been renamed enterococci (e.g. *E. faecalis*; may cause nosocomial infection).
  - *S. viridans*: a group of partial α- or non-haemolytic streptococci; may cause endocarditis and abscesses, especially in immunodeficiency, e.g. on the ICU and in the elderly. Includes *S. mitis*, *S. sanguis*, *S. mutans* and *S. milleri*.
  - *S. pneumoniae* (pneumococcus): α-haemolytic organism present in up to 70% of the population's oropharynx. May cause pneumonia (the most common cause in the community; in hospital it is especially common in impaired protective reflexes, e.g. the elderly and infirm, CNS depression), otitis media, meningitis and septic shock. Prophylactic pneumococcal vaccine is recommended for those at risk, e.g. those with immunodeficiency or diabetes, following splenectomy and in the elderly.

Usually sensitive to penicillins amongst other antibacterial drugs.

Streptokinase. Enzyme obtained from group C β-haemolytic streptococci; used as a fibrinolytic drug in life-threatening arterial or venous thromboembolism, especially acute PE and MI. Binds to plasminogen to form an activator complex, resulting in breakdown of plasminogen to form plasmin, which causes fibrinolysis. Since most individuals have antibodies to streptokinase, a loading dose is required to overcome this natural resistance. Resultant immune complexes are rapidly cleared from the bloodstream; subsequent streptokinase is split into fragments during its action and cleared.

- Dosage: MI: 1 500 000 units iv over 60 min; otherwise 250 000 iv over 30 min, then 100 000/h for up to 24–72 h.
- Side effects: nausea, vomiting, bleeding (including CVA), embolic complications from break-up of thrombi, allergic reactions (including anaphylactic reactions). Guillain–Barré syndrome has been reported. Contraindicated in conditions where bleeding is likely.

Streptomycin. Aminoglycoside and antibacterial drug; now used as an antituberculous drug in drug-resistant TB or in brucellosis. Half-life is about 2.5 h with normal renal function.

- Dosage: 15 mg/kg daily (up to 1 g) by deep im injection, 1–3 daily.
- Side effects: as for aminoglycosides. Hypersensitivity may occur. Plasma concentrations should be monitored, especially in renal impairment; peak and trough levels should not exceed 40 μg/ml and 3 μg/ml respectively.

Stress response to surgery. Term used to encompass the metabolic and hormonal changes following surgery, although the same may occur after trauma, burns, haemorrhage, etc. The response has been suggested as being necessary for survival and recovery after trauma.

Tissue trauma (involving release of polypeptides from the wound site), hypovolaemia and pain initiate a neuroendocrine reflex involving secretion of ACTH, endorphins, growth hormone, vasopressin and prolactin. Stimulation of the sympathetic nervous system increases plasma catecholamines. Plasma cortisol and aldosterone increase, with increased renin/angiotensin system activity. Increase in these hormones produces a period of intense catabolism, the magnitude and duration of which are proportional to the extent of injury. Fatty acids are mobilised and utilised, amino acids are converted to carbohydrate, and negative nitrogen balance occurs. Plasma glucose is raised, with impaired insulin production. Metabolic rate, body temperature, O_2 consumption and CO_2 production increase. Water and sodium retention occurs, with increased urinary potassium loss. Immunological and haematological changes include increased cytokine production, acute phase reactions, leucocytosis and lymphocytosis.

- Effects of anaesthesia:
  - inhalational anaesthetic agents have little effect.
  - opioid analgesic drugs in high dosage (e.g. 50–100 μg/kg fentanyl, 2–4 mg/kg morphine) attenuate the response to abdominal and pelvic surgery, but do not abolish the response to initiation of cardiopulmonary bypass.
  - etomidate infusion prevents the cortisol response, but with little other effect.
  - spinal and epidural anaesthesia with local anaesthetic agents abolish the response to surgery on the lower part of the body. The effect on upper abdominal and thoracic surgery is less clear, with suppression of the glucose response but not of the cortisol response. Block of autonomic and somatic afferent pathways is thought to be required for complete prevention. Spinal opioids do not prevent the response despite good analgesia, although slight modification may occur.

    To be effective, the above require administration before the surgical stimulus; their effects last for several hours after single dosage.

The benefit of attenuating the stress response is controversial, although improved outcome has been claimed in critically ill patients.

Desborough JP (2000). Br J Anaesth; 85: 109–17

Stress ulcers. Acute gastric ulceration secondary to any severe medical or surgical illness, e.g. classically burns (Curling's ulcers) and head injury (Cushing's ulcers). Usually involve the fundus and may be multiple. Associated with hypovolaemia, reduced cardiac output and splanchnic hypoperfusion. Gastric mucosal ischaemia and acid production are thought to be involved, although the aetiology is unclear. Prophylaxis is usual in ICU.
Daley RJ, Rebuck JA, Welage LS, Rogers FB (2004). Crit Care Med; 32: 2008–13
See also, Peptic ulcer disease

Stridor. Harsh high-pitched sound occurring in upper airway obstruction. Inspiratory stridor suggests obstruction at or above the upper trachea (e.g. epiglottitis), since extrathoracic obstruction is exacerbated by the negative intrathoracic pressures generated during inspiration. Expiratory stridor suggests obstruction of the lower trachea or bronchi with exacerbation as the airways are compressed during forced expiration. Typically present on exertion initially, progressing to stridor at rest as obstruction worsens.

More common in children because of the smaller diameter of their airways. Slight narrowing thus has a proportionately greater effect.

Treatment is as for airway obstruction. Helium/O_2 mixtures may decrease work of breathing and improve oxygenation.

Stroke, *see Cerebrovascular accident*

Stroke index. Stroke volume divided by body surface area, thus accounting for the effect of body size. Normally 30–50 ml/m^2.

Stroke volume (SV). Volume of blood ejected by the ventricle per heart beat; i.e.

$$SV = \frac{\text{cardiac output}}{\text{heart rate}}$$

Also equals end-diastolic volume – end-systolic volume. Normally 70–80 ml for a 70 kg man at rest.

Affected by ventricular filling and preload, myocardial contractility, and outflow resistance and SVR.

Stroke work. Measurement of (usually left) ventricular performance, indicating the work done by the ventricle. Increased in hypertension and hypervolaemia, and decreased in shock, cardiac failure and aortic stenosis.

Stroke work (g) = stroke volume (ml) × (MAP – PCWP (mmHg)) × 0.0136

where PCWP = pulmonary capillary wedge pressure
0.0136 = correction factor for units

Normally 60–80 g. Stroke work index = stroke work divided by body surface area; normally 40–80 g/m^2.

Strong ion difference (SID). Difference between the concentrations of the strong cations (those that dissociate almost totally at the pH of interest – e.g. in blood, Na^+, K^+, Ca^{2+}, Mg^{2+}) and strong anions (e.g. Cl^-, lactate, SO_4^{2-}) in a solution. Based on the concept of electroneutrality, proposed in the 1980s by Stewart as part of his 'alternative approach' to acid–base balance, in which the number of positive ions in a solution equals the number of negative ones. A SID > 0 represents the presence of unmeasured anions; the normal value is 40–44 mmol/l in plasma, this value representing the contribution made by weak acids (mostly albumin) and carbon dioxide. As SID falls it results in increased dissociation of water to maintain electroneutrality, leading to increased H^+ and therefore reduced pH, i.e. metabolic acidosis. As SID increases, plasma pH rises.

The strong ion gap (SIG) accounts for the effect of other anions not included in the SID equation; i.e. SIG = SID – [HCO_3^-] – [albumin$^-$].

[Peter A Stewart (1921–1993), Canadian-born US physiologist]

Sirker AA, Rhodes A, Grounds RM, Bennett ED (2002). Anaesthesia; 57: 348–56

Stuffing box, *see Cylinders*

Stump pressure, *see Carotid artery surgery*

Subarachnoid block, *see Spinal anaesthesia*

Subarachnoid haemorrhage (SAH). Bleeding into the subarachnoid space. Commonest cause is trauma although non-traumatic SAH usually results from rupture of an intracranial (Berry) aneurysm (75–80%) or arteriovenous malformation (5%). Incidence of aneurysmal SAH is 10–30 per 100 000 population/year. Most frequent at 40–60 years of age. Risk factors include hypertension, smoking, oral contraceptive pill and cocaine abuse.

- Features:
  - 50% of patients have warning symptoms for 2–3 weeks beforehand (sentinel headache).
  - initial rupture: sudden, severe headache (ipsilateral in 30%), vomiting, syncope, loss of consciousness.
  - focal neurological deficit, especially cranial nerve III. Ocular haemorrhage may accompany diplopia.
  - meningism within 6–24 h.
  - cerebral vasospasm within 3–12 days (peaks at 6–8 days); may cause reversible or irreversible neurological damage. Degree depends on the volume of blood in the subarachnoid space. A major cause of morbidity and mortality in those surviving the initial bleed, causing symptoms in 20–30% of cases, especially those with grades 3–5 haemorrhage (see below).
  - hydrocephalus (20%): caused by obstruction of CSF circulation by blood.
- Patients are graded thus (Hunt and Hess scale):
  - grade 0: unruptured aneurysm.
  - grade 1: asymptomatic or mild headache and neck stiffness. Mortality 0–5%.
  - grade 2: severe headache, neck stiffness, cranial nerve palsy. Mortality 2–10%.
  - grade 3: mild focal deficit, lethargy, confusion. Mortality 8–15%.
  - grade 4: stupor, hemiparesis, early decerebrate rigidity. Mortality 60–70%.
  - grade 5: deep coma, decerebrate posture. Mortality 70–100%.

CT scanning detects SAH in 95% of cases; it may indicate the volume of blood present, allow rough localisation of the aneurysm and demonstrate hydrocephalus. Lumbar puncture (revealing xanthochromic CSF) is only necessary in questionable circumstances. Cerebral angiography demonstrates an aneurysm in 80% of cases; the anterior (30%) and posterior (25%) communicating arteries, middle cerebral (20%) and basilar (10%) arteries are most commonly affected (*see Cerebral circulation*). It may also demonstrate vasospasm.

- Management:
  - admission with careful monitoring. ECG changes occur in 50% of cases (typically T wave inversion, ST

segment changes or arrhythmias; caused by increased catecholamine secretion).
- unconscious patients are managed as for coma.
- maintenance of good hydration and control of severe hypertension.
- drainage of hydrocephalus with an intraventricular catheter, which also allows measurement of ICP and cerebral perfusion pressure.
- nimodipine to relieve vasospasm: 60 mg orally, 4 hourly, for 21 days as prophylaxis; 15 μg/kg/h iv, doubled after 2 h if BP is stable and continued for 5–14 days in established vasospasm, along with expansion of plasma volume and maintenance of BP (using inotropes if necessary).
- analgesia and anticonvulsant drugs as necessary.
- surgery is often delayed for 7–10 days to allow stabilisation, despite the risk of rebleeding. More recently, earlier surgery has been advocated, especially in low grade SAH. Percutaneous embolisation of the aneurysm may be possible.

- Complications:
  - death (10–15% of patients before reaching hospital). Brainstem death may follow hours to days after ICU admission.
  - rebleeding: most common on the first day (4% of cases), with 15–20% occurring within 2 weeks and 50% within 6 months.
  - neurological deficit resulting from vasospasm.
  - hyponatraemia may result from the syndrome of inappropriate antidiuretic hormone secretion or cerebral salt wasting syndrome.
- Anaesthetic considerations:
  - as for neurosurgery.
  - hypotensive anaesthesia has been traditionally employed but now normotension is favoured to maintain cerebral perfusion pressure. Cerebral perfusion may be further impaired if hypotension is profound.

[Sir James Berry (1860–1946), Canadian surgeon; Robert H Hess and William Hunt (1921–1999), US neurosurgeons]

Wilson SR, Hirsch NP, Appleby I (2005). Anaesthesia; 60: 470–85

See also, Transcranial Doppler ultrasound

Subclavian venous cannulation. The subclavian vein is the continuation of the axillary vein and arises at the lateral border of the first rib (*see Fig. 84; Internal jugular venous cannulation*). It passes over the first rib anterior to the subclavian artery, separated from it by scalenus anterior, to join with the internal jugular vein at the medial end of the clavicle. It receives the external jugular vein at the clavicle's midpoint. The right phrenic nerve lies between the vein and scalenus anterior, the left phrenic nerve between the vein and artery.

- Technique:
  - head-down position distends the vein and reduces risk of air embolism. The head is turned to the contralateral side. Aseptic techniques are used.
  - a finger is run medially in the subclavian groove until an 'obstruction' is felt (subclavius muscle), also marked by a notch on the under surface of the clavicle. This point lies between the midpoint of the clavicle and a point dividing its middle and medial thirds.
  - after local anaesthetic infiltration, a needle is introduced under the clavicle and directed towards the sternal notch, aspirating during advancement. When the vein has been entered, the cannula is advanced or a wire inserted (Seldinger technique).

The approach is contraindicated in patients with coagulopathy, since direct pressure cannot be applied to the bleeding vessel.

See also, Central venous cannulation, for complications and comparison with other techniques

Subdural haemorrhage. Haemorrhage between the pia and arachnoid layers of the meninges. May be:

- cranial:
  - acute: usually caused by acceleration–deceleration head injury resulting in tearing of surface or bridging vessels. Patients usually present with confusion or loss of consciousness following a lucid interval. CT scanning shows a hyperdense mass, often with surrounding oedema. Mortality ranges from 60 to 90% depending on the underlying brain injury, Glasgow coma scale on admission, patient's age and concurrent anticoagulant therapy.
  - chronic: usually occurs in elderly patients, with head injury identified in < 50%. Present with a variety of symptoms including headaches, confusion, dementia, language difficulties, convulsions and transient ischaemic attacks. CT scanning shows an isodense lesion; bilateral haematomata occur in 25% of cases.
- spinal (very rare), e.g. following lumbar puncture.

Treated by surgical evacuation.

See also, Neurosurgery

Substance abuse. Difficult to define, since society tolerates intake of certain substances (e.g. alcohol, tobacco) but not others (illicit drugs); in addition, excessive intake of otherwise acceptable substances (e.g. alcohol) is generally considered as abuse. Addiction is a state of compulsive use associated with physical, psychological or social harm and despite evidence of that harm; dependence is a physiological adaptation associated with withdrawal symptoms when ingestion ceases.

- Potential problems for anaesthesia or intensive care:
  - alcohol poisoning and alcoholism commonly accompany abuse of other substances. Solvent abuse is more common in young patients.
  - malnutrition may accompany chronic substance abuse.
  - effects of iv administration, often with non-sterile needles (e.g. opioid analgesic drugs, barbiturates):
    - high risk of sepsis, thrombophlebitis, cellulitis, bacterial endocarditis and septic systemic and pulmonary embolism.
    - veins are often difficult to find and cannulate.
    - high risk group for hepatitis and HIV infection.
  - chronic effects of the substance, e.g. hepatic impairment/enzyme induction (e.g. opioids, barbiturates); cardiomyopathy (cocaine). Thrombocytopenia may occur in cocaine and opioid abuse.
  - acute effects:
    - depressant, e.g. opioids, barbiturates: respiratory depression, hypotension.
    - excitatory, e.g. amfetamines, cocaine, lysergic acid diethylamide (LSD): tachycardia, hypertension, arrhythmias, pyrexia. Hallucinations may occur postoperatively. Anticholinergic drugs, drugs which sensitise the myocardium to catecholamines, and indirectly acting sympathomimetic drugs should be avoided. LSD may impair plasma cholinesterase.
  - effects of withdrawal:
    - opioids: tachycardia, tremor, acute anxiety, GIT symptoms, piloerection and sweating ('cold turkey'). Unpleasant but rarely life-threatening.
    - barbiturates: anxiety, tremor, hallucinations and convulsions. May be life-threatening.

- Conduct of anaesthesia:
  - patients may be resistant to iv anaesthetic agents, with rapid recovery.
  - surgical cut-down, central venous cannulation or inhalational induction may be required if peripheral venous cannulation is impossible.
  - estimation of appropriate doses of opioids may be difficult, especially in opioid addicts. Inhalational and regional techniques are often preferred. **Opioid antagonists** may provoke acute withdrawal and should be avoided.
  - withdrawal states may occur postoperatively.

See also, Abuse of anaesthetic agents; Barbiturate poisoning; Misuse of Drugs Act; Opioid poisoning; Rapid opioid detoxification; Solvent abuse

Substance P. 11-amino-acid **tachykinin** neuropeptide, involved in pain pathways (*see Gate control theory of pain*). High levels are found in axons and cell bodies of primary afferent fibres in the dorsal root ganglia, also in the superficial levels of the dorsal horn of the **spinal cord**.

- Evidence for its involvement in pain transmission includes:
  - distribution in the regions of pain pathways.
  - depletion by **capsaicin**, a red pepper extract, renders animals insensitive to noxious thermal and chemical stimuli, without affecting other sensory modalities.

Also involved in the regulation of the respiratory rhythm, nausea and vomiting, and mood.

Substantia gelatinosa, *see Sensory pathways; Spinal cord*

Sub-Tenon's block. Used in **ophthalmic surgery** as an alternative to **retrobulbar block** and **peribulbar block**. Tenon's capsule is a connective tissue layer surrounding the eye and extraocular muscles. The posterior part separates the globe from the retrobulbar space; injection of local anaesthetic between the capsule and sclera posteriorly results in spread along the extraocular muscles and diffusion into the retrobulbar space.

Topical anaesthesia is applied first. With the patient looking up, the conjunctiva and anterior Tenon's capsule are picked up with toothed forceps, 5–6 mm inferomedial to the limbus (the junction of the cornea and sclera). A small incision is made with scissors which are then passed backwards around the globe underneath Tenon's capsule to reach the posterior part. A special cannula is then passed into this space and 3–4 ml solution slowly injected. Gentle external pressure is applied to the eye and further injections made if required. Suitable solutions include a mixture of **lidocaine** 2% and **bupivacaine** 0.5–0.75% in equal volumes with or without **adrenaline** 1:400 000 and **hyaluronidase** 5 units/ml.

Provides rapid anaesthesia with less risk of perforating the globe or retrobulbar haemorrhage than retrobulbar block. Subconjunctival oedema may occur but the block is usually less uncomfortable than others.

[Jacques R Tenon (1724–1816), French ophthalmologist]

Kumar CM, Williamson S, Manickam B (2005). Eur J Anaesthesiol; 22: 567–77

Succinylcholine, *see Suxamethonium*

Sucralfate. Ulcer-healing drug, a complex of aluminium hydroxide and sulphated sucrose. Provides mucosal protection from gastric acid. Has no antacid effect. Used in **peptic ulcer disease**, and has been used on **ICU** as prophylaxis against peptic ulceration; thought to be associated with fewer nosocomial infections than the **H_2 receptor antagonists**.

- Dosage: 1 g 6 hourly, orally/nasogastrically.
- Side effects are rare; include constipation, nausea, vomiting, rash.

Suction equipment. Consists of:
  - pump to generate a vacuum. Efficiency of the system is related to the degree of subatmospheric pressure generated, and the volume of air that can be moved in unit time (displacement). Pumps may employ pistons (usually low displacement), rotating fans (high displacement), foot-operated bellows and compressed gases using the **Venturi principle**. Piped suction systems use a high displacement pump connected to a large central reservoir, with traps to prevent contamination.
  - reservoir: must be large enough to enable aspiration of large volumes, but not so large that the desired vacuum takes too long to achieve. A filter and float valve prevent contamination of the pump with aspirated liquid.
  - delivery tubing; usually disposable, attached to rigid (Yankauer) or flexible catheters. Smooth-tipped catheters may reduce the mucosal damage following endotracheal suctioning. Prolonged **tracheobronchial suctioning** may cause lung collapse and hypoxaemia; bradycardia is common in critically ill patients. Preoxygenation should thus precede tracheal suction. Enclosed suction catheters which do not require detachment of the patient from the breathing system are available; the catheter is handled through a plastic sleeve, maintaining sterility. Hypoxaemia and dispersal of infectious droplets have thus been reduced.

Minimal flow rate of 35 l/min air, and generation of at least 80 kPa (600 mmHg) negative pressure, have been suggested for apparatus for anaesthetic use.

[Sidney Yankauer (1872–1932), US surgeon]

Sudeck's atrophy, *see Complex regional pain syndrome type 1*

Sufentanil citrate. Synthetic **opioid analgesic drug**, introduced in 1984. Available in the USA but not the UK, for marketing reasons. An analogue of **fentanyl**, with 5–7 times the latter's potency. Of shorter elimination **half-life** (about 2–3 h) than fentanyl, with similar clearance and slightly smaller volume of distribution. Has similar clinical effects to fentanyl, including cardiovascular stability and lack of **histamine** release. Usual dose is 0.1–0.5 μg/kg for minor surgery, up to 8 μg/kg for longer procedures and up to 30 μg/kg as the sole agent for, e.g. **cardiac surgery**. Has been given epidurally (10–75 μg) and spinally (5–20 μg), effects lasting 2–6 h.

Sugammadex. Reversal agent currently under investigation for reversal of **non-depolarising neuromuscular blockade** caused by **rocuronium**. A modified **γ-cyclodextrin** molecule, each sugammadex molecule has a ring-shaped structure that binds a molecule of rocuronium tightly within it to form a water-soluble complex, thus favouring removal of rocuronium molecules from the neuromuscular junction into the plasma. Has a lesser binding effect on **vecuronium** and a much lesser effect on **pancuronium**. Studies suggest that sugammadex has a good safety profile and can reverse rocuronium-induced neuromuscular blockade within a few minutes, even when given a few minutes after the neuromuscular blocking drug. Suggested clinical usage includes treatment of overdose, allowing maintenance of optimal relaxation until the very end of surgery without residual postoperative weakness, and allowing rapid reversal of paralysis when higher dose rocuronium is used for rapid sequence induction.

Naguib M (2007). Anesth Analg; 104: 575–81

Sulfadiazine (Sulphadiazine). Sulphonamide and antibacterial drug, used as prophylaxis against rheumatic fever and in toxoplasmosis.

- Dosage: 500 mg–1.0 g orally/iv daily.
- Side effects: as for sulphonamides.

Sulphaemoglobinaemia. Presence of an abnormal haemoglobin of uncertain chemical structure, but which may be produced by adding hydrogen sulphide *in vitro*. Often coexists with methaemoglobinaemia. Reduces O_2-carrying capacity of blood and shifts the oxyhaemoglobin dissociation curve to the left, decreasing O_2 delivery to the tissues. Usually due to ingestion of phenacetin, sulphonamides, primaquine or metoclopramide. Treatment includes O_2 therapy; normal haemoglobin cannot be regenerated from sulphaemoglobin.

Sulphonamides. Group of broad spectrum antibacterial drugs, less commonly used now because of bacterial resistance and side effects. Also active against certain protozoa, e.g. toxoplasma and pneumocystis. Act by inhibiting bacterial dihydrofolate synthesis; their action is enhanced by trimethoprim which inhibits tetrahydrofolate production from dihydrofolate. Toxic effects include renal impairment, blood dyscrasias and allergic reactions.

Sulphonylureas. Group of oral hypoglycaemic drugs, used in non-insulin-dependent diabetes mellitus. Act by encouraging surviving β cells of the pancreas to secrete insulin, and possibly by increasing peripheral uptake of glucose. Several are available, e.g.:

- chlorpropamide: half-life 35–45 h.
- glibenclamide, gliclazide and glibornuride: half-life 8–12 h.
- tolbutamide, tolazamide, , glimepiride: half-life 5–8 h.
- glipizide: half-life 2–4 h.
- gliquidone: half-life 1–2 h.

All of the above are excreted by the liver except chlorpropamide, which is excreted renally.

The shorter-acting drugs may be stopped on the day of surgery; perioperative hypoglycaemia is most likely with long-acting drugs, e.g. chlorpropamide, and in the elderly.

Sumatriptan. 5-HT_{1D} receptor agonist, used to treat acute migraine and cluster headache. Should not be used for prophylaxis. Has also been used in post-dural puncture headache although evidence is anecdotal only. Almotriptan, eletriptan, frovatriptan, naratriptan, rizatriptan and zolmitriptan are newer, related drugs.

- Dosage: 50–100 mg orally, 6 mg sc or 20 mg intranasally as soon as possible after onset; the dose may be repeated (not during the same attack) if migraine recurs up to 300 mg orally, 12 mg sc or 40 mg intranasally in 24 h.
- Side effects: tingling, heaviness, tightness including chest discomfort, flushing, dizziness, nausea, drowsiness, hypotension, brady- or tachycardia, convulsions, hepatic dysfunction. Contraindicated in ischaemic heart disease and concurrent therapy with related drugs or ergotamine. Coronary vasospasm may follow iv injection.

Superior vena caval obstruction (Superior vena caval syndrome). 80–90% of cases are caused by malignancy, especially bronchial carcinoma and lymphoma. Other causes include mediastinal fibrosis and thrombosis. Results in distended veins, oedema and cyanosis in the arm, head and neck, with prominent collateral vessels in the chest wall. Visual disturbances and headache may occur. Most patients have dyspnoea and orthopnoea. Emergency radiotherapy may be required if malignancy is the cause. Steroids have also been used to reduce oedema.

- Anaesthetic considerations:
  - patients should be nursed sitting up preoperatively, to minimise facial and neck swelling.
  - induction of anaesthesia with iv agents may be prolonged if an arm vein is used.
  - tracheal intubation may be difficult. Laryngeal oedema may be present.
  - bleeding may be torrential, especially during median sternotomy.

Supine hypotension syndrome, *see Aortocaval compression*

Supraorbital nerve block, *see Ophthalmic nerve blocks*

Suprascapular nerve block. Performed for analgesia in painful shoulders. A needle is inserted 1–2 cm cranial to the scapular spine, on a line bisecting the inferior scapular angle. 5 ml local anaesthetic agent is injected when the scapular notch is identified.

Supraventricular tachycardia (SVT). Paroxysmal tachycardia with a rate of 140–250 beats/min, caused by a rapidly firing ectopic focus in the atria or atrioventricular node. Circular conduction of impulses via abnormal anatomical pathways or within the node itself results in re-entry and perpetuation of the arrhythmia. Occurs in otherwise healthy individuals although it may be associated with heart disease, Wolff–Parkinson–White and Lown–Ganong–Levine syndromes, hyperthyroidism, and excessive consumption of caffeine, nicotine or alcohol. Typically sudden in onset. May cause palpitations, dyspnoea, lightheadedness, and polyuria if prolonged.

- Features: regular narrow QRS complexes on the ECG (Fig. 150), unless bundle branch block is also present. A degree of atrioventricular block may be present, especially when associated with digoxin toxicity. It may be difficult to distinguish SVT from VT.
- Treatment: European Resuscitation Council guidelines:
  - supportive treatment: O_2 therapy, iv cannulation.
  - carotid sinus massage, Valsalva manoeuvre, and other methods of vagal stimulation (e.g. holding ice to the face); may abolish SVT or slow the rate if atrioventricular block is present.
  - antiarrhythmic drugs:
    - adenosine 3 mg iv, repeated after 1–2 min using 6 mg then 12 mg if required.

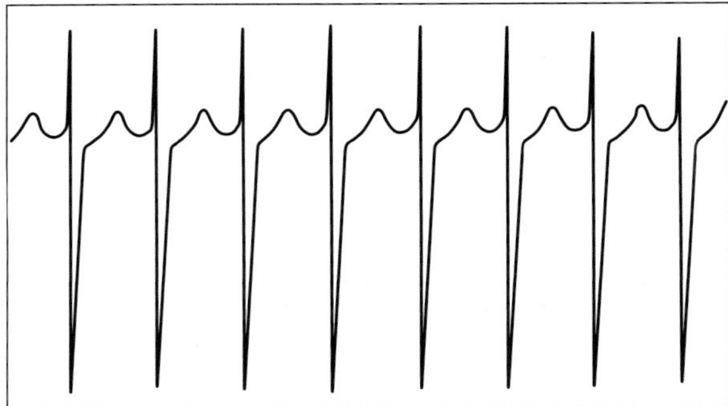

Fig. 150 SVT

- if heart rate is still above 200, or there is hypotension, chest pain, cardiac failure or impaired consciousness, one or more of the following may be used:
  - esmolol 40 mg iv over a minute followed by 4 mg/min, repeated and increased up to 12 mg/min respectively.
  - digoxin up to two iv doses of 0.5 mg over 30 min (not in Wolff–Parkinson–White syndrome).
  - verapamil 5–10 mg iv.
  - amiodarone 900 mg iv over an hour.
- overdrive cardiac pacing (not in atrial fibrillation).
- if there are severe features: cardioversion followed by amiodarone 300 mg over 15 min and 600 mg over the next hour.

Other drugs, e.g. β-adrenergic receptor antagonists, disopyramide, diltiazem, have also been used. Ablation therapy or surgery may be required.

Delacrétaz E (2006). N Engl J Med; 354: 1039–51

See also, Atrial flutter

Sural nerve block, *see Ankle, nerve blocks*

Surface area, body. Used to estimate drug doses, and in physiological calculations, e.g. cardiac index, basal metabolic rate, etc., since it reflects body requirements and activity more accurately than weight, height, etc.; however, use of basal metabolic rate has been suggested as being more logical.

The rule of nines is used to estimate surface area of parts of the body. Nomograms for total surface area (Fig. 151) are based on the formula:

$$\text{surface area (m}^2) = \text{weight}^{0.425}(\text{kg}) \times \text{height}^{0.725}(\text{cm}) \times 0.007184$$

Surface tension. Tangential force in the surface of a liquid, defined in terms of the force acting perpendicularly across a line of unit length. Caused by attraction between the liquid molecules; whereas molecules in the bulk of the liquid are attracted in all directions, those at the surface are only attracted inwards. Thus the surface tends to contract to the smallest possible area, e.g. a free drop tends to be spherical. Has important implications in lung mechanics; normally reduced by pulmonary surfactant. Measured in N/m.

See also, Laplace's law

Surfactant. Complex material composed of dipalmitoyl phosphatidyl choline (DPPC), protein and carbohydrate, which prevents alveolar collapse at lower lung volumes by reducing alveolar surface tension. Thought to do this by alignment of the hydrophilic parts of the DPPC molecules on the surface of the alveolar fluid lining, with repulsion between adjacent molecules. Repulsion increases as the molecules are pressed together at low volumes. Compliance is increased, alveoli are held open, and alveolar fluid is reduced.

Produced by type II pneumocytes, partly under control of the hypothalamic–pituitary–adrenal axis. Appears at about 24 weeks' gestation. Deficiency due to immaturity causes the respiratory distress syndrome (RDS). It may also be deficient in areas of lung affected by PE, bronchial obstruction, and in heavy smokers.

Administration of synthetic surfactant has been used in neonatal RDS, and has been investigated in ARDS.

Suxamethonium chloride (Succinylcholine). Depolarising neuromuscular blocking drug, introduced in 1951. Formerly available as the bromide/iodide. Structurally composed of two acetylcholine molecules joined together (Fig. 152). Stored at 4°C to prevent hydrolysis. Incompatible with thiopental.

- Dosage:
  - 0.5–1.5 mg/kg iv depending on the relaxation required. Usual initial dose is 1 mg/kg iv, producing paralysis within 30–90 s which lasts 2–5 min. Subsequent doses: 0.2–0.5 mg/kg. Low doses (5–10 mg) have been used for treatment of laryngospasm.
  - has been used by infusion of 0.1% solution with 5% dextrose or 0.9% saline at 2–5 mg/min.
  - may also be given im (2 mg/kg) or sc.

Rapidly hydrolysed by plasma cholinesterase to succinyl monocholine and choline, then to succinic acid and choline. Succinyl monocholine has weak blocking properties.

Hexafluorenium and tetrahydroaminocrine have been used to prolong suxamethonium's action.

- Side effects:
  - prolonged paralysis. May be caused by:
    - reduced cholinesterase activity (*see Cholinesterase, plasma*) due to:
      - inherited atypical cholinesterase.
      - reduced amount of cholinesterase.
      - inhibition of cholinesterase by drugs.
    - excessive dosage, cumulation of succinylcholine and production of dual block. The latter may occur after 200–500 mg in adults.

    Dual block may also develop with reduced enzyme activity. Management of prolonged paralysis:
    - maintenance of anaesthesia and oxygenation.
    - diagnosis of the nature of block using neuromuscular blockade monitoring. Edrophonium has been suggested to distinguish non-depolarising from depolarising blockade, but is less commonly used.
    - neostigmine has been used to reverse dual block.
    - in prolonged depolarising blockade ('suxamethonium or Scoline apnoea'), recovery usually occurs within 4 h. It may be speeded by administering fresh frozen plasma, but spontaneous recovery is usually preferable.
    - blood may be analysed for cholinesterase activity, and screening of relatives performed.
  - muscle fasciculations, coinciding with initial depolarisation of muscle fibres. They are painful if the patient is awake. Thought to contribute to:
    - postoperative muscle pains, typically around the neck, back and upper arms, and occurring on the 2nd–3rd day. Most common in young fit women and after early ambulation.
    - increased intraocular pressure. Suxamethonium causes contraction of the extraocular muscles, but may also cause choroidal vasodilatation; the response may still occur if the extrinsic muscles are cut. The increase usually lasts for under 10 min. Suxamethonium is usually avoided in penetrating eye injuries but this is controversial (*see Eye, penetrating injury*).
    - increased intragastric pressure. Formerly thought to increase risk of aspiration of gastric contents, but an accompanying increase in lower oesophageal sphincter tone maintains barrier pressure.
    - increased plasma potassium. Although this arises mainly from depolarisation (see below), leakage of potassium from damaged muscle fibres may contribute. Plasma myoglobin and creatine phosphokinase (normally intracellular) are increased after injection of suxamethonium.

  Fasciculations and the resulting complications may be reduced by pretreatment with other drugs, although not

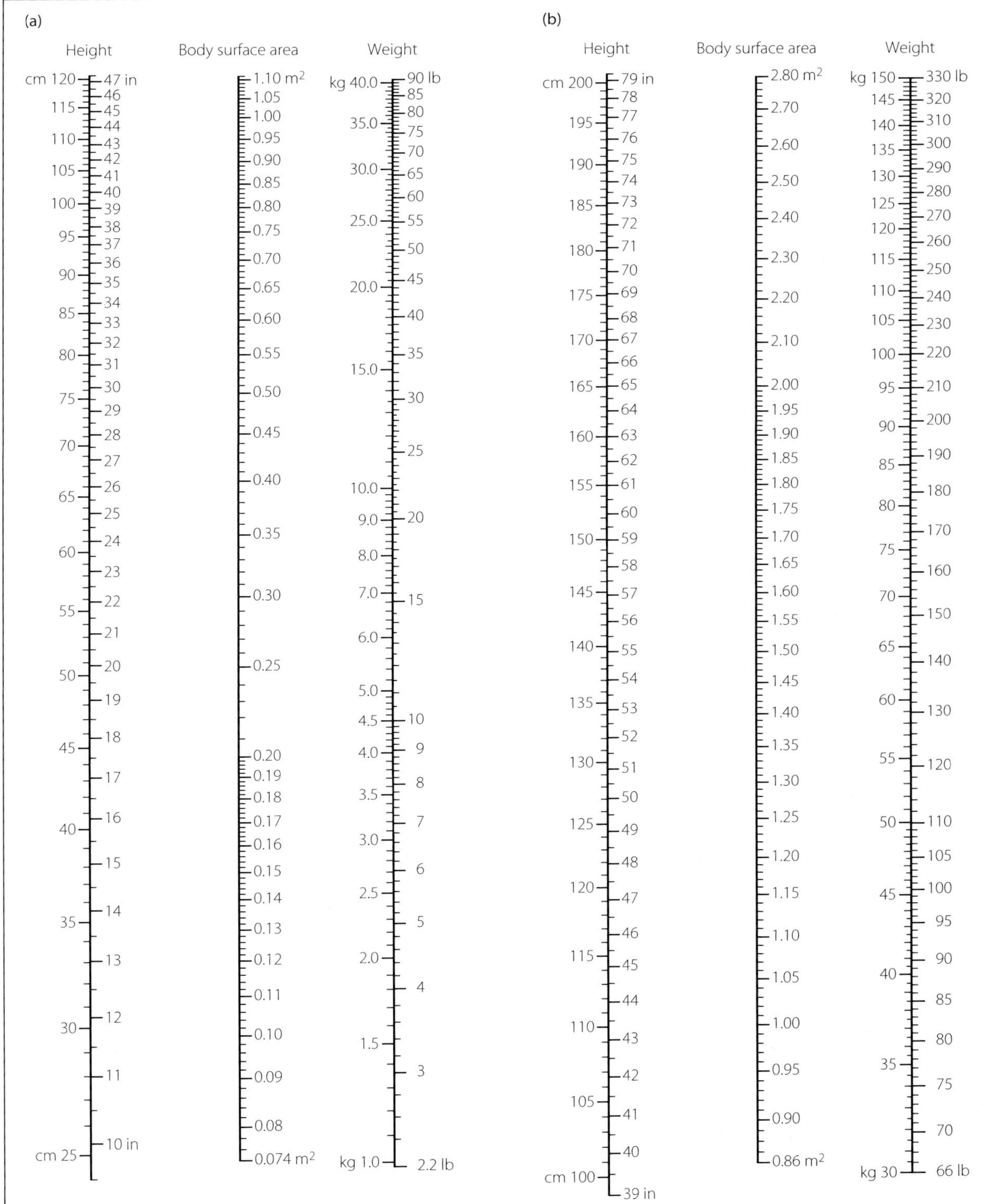

Fig. 151 Body surface area nomograms: (a) children; (b) adults

$$(CH_3)_3\overset{+}{N}-CH_2-CH_2-O-\overset{O}{\overset{\|}{C}}-CH_2-CH_2-\overset{O}{\overset{\|}{C}}-O-CH_2-CH_2-\overset{+}{N}(CH_3)_3$$

Fig. 152 Structure of suxamethonium

consistently. Adverse effects may also still occur despite lack of fasciculations. Drugs that have been described include:
- non-depolarising neuromuscular blocking drugs (usually 1/10 usual intubating dose), given 2–3 min before suxamethonium, which may be required in increased dosage. Tubocurarine is the best studied, although others have been used. The possibility of aspiration pneumonitis precludes this technique in rapid sequence induction.
- lidocaine 1–2 mg/kg iv, given 2–3 min before suxamethonium.
- diazepam 10 mg iv.
- dantrolene 100–200 mg orally, 2 h preoperatively.
- suxamethonium 0.1 mg/kg iv 1–2 min before the main dose.
- calcium 10 mmol iv. Arrhythmias may occur.
- magnesium sulphate 1–2 g iv.
- chlorpromazine 0.1 mg/kg.
- hexafluorenium.

- hyperkalaemia. Plasma potassium increases usually by 0.5 mmol/l in normal patients, and lasts for 3–5 min. This follows normal movement of potassium out of muscle cells during depolarisation at the neuromuscular junction, with some leakage due to trauma following fasciculations as above. The increase may be dangerous in patients whose plasma potassium levels are already high (typically renal failure, although the response is of normal magnitude unless neuropathy is present). Increases of several mmol/l may occur if the acetylcholine receptors are not confined to the neuromuscular junction, but have spread along the whole length of the muscle fibres, as occurs in denervation hypersensitivity. This process is also thought to occur in other conditions in which massive hyperkalaemia may follow administration of suxamethonium for certain periods after the lesion:
  - burns: 9 days–2 months.
  - spinal cord injury, intracranial lesions (e.g. CVA, subarachnoid haemorrhage, head injury) and muscle trauma: 10 days–6–7 months.
  - peripheral nerve injury: 4 days–6–7 months.
  - peripheral neuropathy, tetanus and severe infection: uncertain period of risk.

  Maximal risk occurs at 14–28 days. Severe arrhythmias and cardiac arrest may occur, usually responding well to CPR. The same drugs used to attenuate the fasciculations have been used to reduce the hyperkalaemic response, with varying success. Salbutamol has also been used.

  The risk of hyperkalaemia in disseminated sclerosis and Parkinson's disease is unclear. It has been described in muscular dystrophies (related to massive rhabdomyolysis and possibly MH), but not in motor neurone disease.
- bradycardia: common after the second dose, but may occur after the first dose, especially in children. Other muscarinic effects may occur, e.g. increased GIT motility and secretion.
- adverse drug reactions. Although rare, they may be severe. Anaphylactic and anaphylactoid reactions are well described.
- MH.
- masseter spasm.
- abnormal sustained contraction in myotonic syndromes.

Resistance may occur in myasthenia gravis, and increased sensitivity in the myasthenic syndrome.

Its use has declined because of its many disadvantages and the introduction of alternative drugs, e.g. atracurium, vecuronium, rocuronium and mivacurium. However, the conditions suxamethonium provides for tracheal intubation are generally considered superior and occur faster than those attained by other drugs. Its short duration of action allows tracheal intubation with subsequent spontaneous ventilation, and is especially advantageous if intubation is difficult.

See also, Depolarising neuromuscular blockade

Suxethonium bromide/iodide. Depolarising neuromuscular blocking drug, introduced with suxamethonium in 1951. Similar to suxamethonium, but the quaternary ammonium group at each end of the molecule contains two methyl and one ethyl group instead of three methyl groups.

SVP, *see Saturated vapour pressure*

SVR, *see Systemic vascular resistance*

SVT, *see Supraventricular tachycardia*

Swallowing (Deglutition). Active passage of liquid or food bolus from mouth to stomach. Initiated voluntarily by the tongue pressing against the palate from the tip back, pushing food into the oropharynx. Continues by reflex activity, with afferent fibres in the 9th and 10th cranial nerves; impulses pass to the tractus solitarius and nucleus ambiguus of the medulla, with efferent fibres to pharyngeal and tongue muscles via 9th, 10th and 12th nerves. The nasopharynx is sealed by soft palate elevation and superior constrictor contraction, and the larynx by elevation and glottic closure. The epiglottis moves posteriorly but does not seal the glottic opening as formerly suspected. Respiration ceases. Food is propelled by the inferior constrictor into the upper oesophagus where it initiates peristalsis (*see Oesophageal contractility*).

Suppressed in plane 1 of surgical anaesthesia; its reappearance may herald the onset of vomiting.

Difficulty with swallowing (dysphagia) may be caused by anatomical (e.g. local tumours, inflammation, achalasia) or neurological (e.g. myasthenia gravis, bulbar palsies) factors; pulmonary aspiration of food and saliva may lead to repeated chest infection.

Swan–Ganz catheter, *see Pulmonary artery catheterisation*

Sympathetic nerve blocks. Although blockade of sympathetic nerves commonly accompanies various regional techniques (e.g. epidural or spinal anaesthesia, brachial plexus block), selective blockade of sympathetic fibres is used for:
- pain management: certain pain syndromes are thought to involve abnormal sympathetic activity, e.g. complex regional pain syndromes type 1 and 2 (formerly reflex sympathetic dystrophy and causalgia respectively), phantom limb pain. The underlying mechanism is unknown but may involve abnormal linkage between mechanoreceptors and sympathetic neurones. Recent evidence suggests that sympathetic blocks may not actually improve outcome as traditionally believed.
- improvement of blood flow, e.g. in peripheral ischaemia, Raynaud's disease, accidental intra-arterial injection of thiopental.

Sympathetic ganglia may be blocked at three levels: the cervicothoracic ganglia (stellate ganglion block), coeliac plexus (coeliac plexus block) and lumbar ganglia (lumbar sympathetic block). Blockade may be short-term (using

local anaesthetic agents) or permanent (chemical sympathectomy), when neurolytic agents such as phenol or alcohol are used. IVRA using guanethidine is also used.
[Maurice Raynaud (1834–1881), French physician]

Sympathetic nervous system. Part of the autonomic nervous system. Myelinated preganglionic efferent fibres emerge from spinal segments T1–L2 into the corresponding primary ramus at each level, and pass via a white ramus communicans into the sympathetic trunk (*see Fig. 20; Autonomic nervous system*). They may then:
- synapse in the corresponding ganglion and pass via a grey ramus communicans to the corresponding spinal nerve for distribution.
- ascend or descend in the sympathetic chain, and synapse at a distant ganglion.
- pass without synapsing to a peripheral ganglion, to synapse there.

The sympathetic trunk is a ganglionated nerve chain extending from the base of the skull to the coccyx, and lying about 2–3 cm lateral to the vertebral column. The portion above T1 does not receive any rami communicantes; i.e. the cervical sympathetic outflow must descend to T1, then into the sympathetic trunk and ascend to the cervical ganglia. The trunk descends in the neck behind the carotid sheath and enters the thorax anterior to the neck of the first rib. It passes over the heads of the upper ribs and overlies the sides of the lower four thoracic vertebrae. It enters the abdomen behind the medial arcuate ligament (*see Diaphragm*) and lies between the lumbar vertebral bodies and psoas major, passing into the pelvis anterior to the sacral ala. The two chains meet and terminate on the anterior surface of the coccyx.

- Ganglia:
  - cervical:
    - superior:
      - lies opposite C2–3.
      - branches: superior cardiac nerve, and branches to the upper four cervical nerves, internal carotid plexus and cranial nerves VII, IX, X and XII.
    - middle:
      - lies opposite C6.
      - branches: middle cardiac nerve, and branches to C5 and C6.
    - inferior:
      - lies opposite C7; often fused with the first thoracic ganglion to form the stellate ganglion on the neck of the first rib.
      - branches: inferior cardiac nerve, and branches to C7 and C8.
  - thoracic:
    - usually 12 although variable.
    - branches: to splanchnic and intercostal nerves.
  - lumbar: usually four ganglia.
  - sacral: usually four ganglia.
- Sympathetic innervation of viscera is via the cardiac, coeliac and hypogastric plexuses. The sympathetic nervous system is concerned with the 'flight or fight' response to stress. Stimulation causes:
  - pupillary dilatation and ciliary muscle relaxation.
  - tachycardia and increased myocardial contractility and velocity of conduction of impulses.
  - α-adrenergic receptor-mediated vasoconstriction (β_2-receptor-mediated vasodilatation in skeletal muscle, abdominal viscera, and coronary, pulmonary and renal circulations).
  - bronchodilatation and reduced bronchial secretion.
  - decreased GIT motility, contraction of sphincters and reduction of secretions (thick viscous secretion from salivary glands). Mixed effects on insulin and glucagon secretion (decreased by α-receptor stimulation, increased by β_2-receptor stimulation).
  - bladder relaxation and sphincteric contraction. Increased renin secretion.
  - variable effect on the uterus.
  - ejaculation of semen.
  - piloerection and sweating of palms.
  - hepatic glycogenolysis and adipose lipolysis.

Acetylcholine is the neurotransmitter at ganglia and the adrenal medulla; noradrenaline is the neurotransmitter at postganglionic nerve endings (except for sweat glands, where acetylcholine is the transmitter). The adrenal medulla represents a sympathetic ganglion which secretes directly into the bloodstream.

Central control for sympathetic activity is from the medulla, pons and hypothalamus.

See also, Acetylcholine receptors; Sympathetic nerve blocks

Sympathomimetic drugs. Refer to drugs that stimulate adrenergic receptors. Actions of individual drugs vary depending on whether they affect predominantly α- or β- receptors, or both. Some stimulate receptors directly; others act indirectly via release of endogenous catecholamines (Table 35).

Used clinically as vasopressor, inotropic and bronchodilator drugs. Amfetamine is used in narcolepsy for its CNS stimulant action.

See also, individual drugs

Synapse. Junction between a neurone (presynaptic cell) and another (postsynaptic) cell, usually another neurone but also muscle or glandular cells. Allows unidirectional transmission of action potentials between cells (synaptic transmission), usually by neurotransmitter release although electrical transmission across gap junctions may also occur. One presynaptic neurone may contribute to over 1000 synapses. Most presynaptic nerve endings bear terminal buttons (synaptic knobs), with up to several thousand from different cells contacting each postsynaptic neurone. The terminal buttons contain many mitochondria and vesicles containing neurotransmitter, and are separated from the postsynaptic membrane by the synaptic cleft (30–50 nm wide). Neurotransmitter receptors are present in high concentrations in the postsynaptic membrane opposite the terminal buttons.

See also, Neuromuscular junction

Table 35 Actions of sympathomimetic drugs

	Direct stimulation		
Drug	α	β	*Indirect activity*
Adrenaline	+	++	–
Noradrenaline	++	+	–
Isoprenaline	–	++	–
Phenylephrine	++	–	–
Methoxamine	++	–	–
Salbutamol	–	++	–
Ephedrine	+	+	+
Metaraminol	++	+	++
Amfetamine	+	+	++

Synaptic transmission. Usually involves release from presynaptic cells of a neurotransmitter which passes across the synaptic cleft and binds to specific receptors in the postsynaptic membrane. This initiates a change in membrane potential in the postsynaptic cell; the neurotransmitter is then broken down by a specific enzyme (e.g. acetylcholinesterase), diffuses into surrounding tissues, or is taken up by the presynaptic nerve ending (e.g. noradrenaline). Initiation of an action potential in the postsynaptic cell depends on the number and frequency of impulses arriving from different presynaptic cells; impulses may be excitatory or inhibitory. In addition, presynaptic inhibition and facilitation may occur, via neurones forming synapses at the presynaptic nerve ending.

Some synapses are electrical, with transmission across gap junctions; some are both electrical and chemical. A synaptic delay of at least 0.5 ms occurs at chemical synapses, but not at electrical ones.

See also, Neuromuscular transmission

Synchronised intermittent mandatory ventilation, *see Intermittent mandatory ventilation*

Syndrome of inappropriate antidiuretic hormone secretion (SIADH). Increased plasma vasopressin levels and water retention despite plasma hypo-osmolality and expanded or normal ECF.

- Caused by:
  - ectopic production of vasopressin, e.g. by carcinoma of bronchus, pancreas, prostate, colon and other tissue, or lymphoma.
  - pulmonary disease, e.g. chest infection, TB, abscess.
  - CNS disorders, e.g. brain tumour, CVA, head injury, encephalitis, meningitis, surgery.
  - stress, e.g. pain, severe illness, trauma.
  - acute intermittent porphyria.
  - drugs, e.g. vasopressin overtreatment, oxytocin, indometacin, antidepressants, chlorpropamide, carbamazepine.
- Features: those of hyponatraemia. Urinary sodium exceeds 20 mmol/l (often 50–150 mmol/l), plasma osmolality is low (< 280 mosm/kg), and urinary/plasma osmolality ratio exceeds 1.
- Treatment:
  - of primary cause.
  - water restriction; demeclocycline 600–1200 mg daily in divided doses if persistent (thought to block the renal effects of vasopressin). Furosemide and phenytoin have been used.
  - as for hyponatraemia if severe.

See also, Cerebral salt wasting syndrome

Syphilis. Sexually transmitted infection caused by the spirochaete *Treponema pallidum*.

- Divided clinically into:
  - primary stage: appearance of chancre at site of infection, 10 days–10 weeks after inoculation.
  - secondary stage: faint macular rash, condylomata and lymphadenopathy.
  - tertiary stage: lesions in skin, subcutaneous tissue, bone, tongue, testes, liver and CNS (meningovascular syphilis, tabes dorsalis, general paralysis of the insane).

Carditis and aortitis may occur, leading to ascending or arch aortic aneurysm and aortic regurgitation. Angina may occur in 50% of patients with aortitis.

Serological tests are strongly positive after 3 months in untreated cases. Treatment is usually with penicillin. Anaesthetic considerations are mainly related to the CVS effects. Blood donors are screened for syphilis before donation.

Syringe labels. Until recently, the system of colour-coded labels widely used in the UK differed from that in use in the USA, Canada, Australia and New Zealand. In 2003 the Royal College of Anaesthetists, Association of Anaesthetists, Faculty of Accident & Emergency Medicine, and Intensive Care Society agreed to recommend the international system, updated in 2004:

- sedatives/tranquillisers: orange.
- induction agents: yellow.
- neuromuscular blocking drugs: red.
- opioids: blue.
- vasopressors: violet.
- local anaesthetics: grey.
- anticholinergics: green.
- antiemetics: salmon.
- others: white. Antagonists are marked by appropriately coloured oblique stripes on the label's upper and side edges.

Because of the importance of recognising suxamethonium and adrenaline rapidly, these two drugs are highlighted by their labels bearing a black upper half with the drug's name in reverse colour. Combinations of drugs bear both relevant colours.

Syringes. First use is attributed to both Wood and Pravaz in 1855, although parenteral administration of drugs had been described earlier. Disposable polystyrene or polypropylene syringes are now widely used. Glass syringes are used for injecting drugs which are incompatible with plastic, e.g. paraldehyde, and for location of the epidural space. Plastic 'loss of resistance devices' resemble syringes but do not meet the required standards to be termed as such.

[Alexander Wood (1817–1884), Scottish physician; Charles Gabriel Pravaz (1791–1853), French surgeon]

Ball C, Westhorpe R (2000). Anaesth Intensive Care; 28: 125

Systemic inflammatory response syndrome (SIRS). Term used to describe the clinical state resulting from many different disease processes (e.g. trauma, pancreatitis, burns, infection) but which are all thought to involve activation of the cytokine cascade. Defined as two or more of:

- hypothermia (< 36°C) or hyperthermia (> 38°C).
- heart rate > 90 beats/min.
- tachypnoea (> 20 breaths/min.)
- leucopenia (< 4000/mm^3), leucocytosis (> 12 000/mm^3), or the presence of greater than 10% immature neutrophils.

See also, Sepsis

Systemic lupus erythematosus (SLE). Connective tissue disease most commonly affecting women aged 15–55, with a prevalence of up to 250 per 100 000. More common in the Afro-Caribbean population. Its aetiology is unknown; both genetic and environmental factors have been implicated. May also be drug induced; classic causes include methyldopa, procainamide and hydralazine. Involves many abnormalities of the immune system, with autoantibodies a central feature; they may affect tissues directly or via immune complex deposition. General features and anaesthetic considerations are as for connective tissue diseases; the most common features of SLE are fatigue, fever, arthralgia and myalgia, skin rashes, psychological involvement and haematological abnormalities (thrombocytopenia and anaemia in about 50% and lupus anticoagulant in about 10%; the latter may prolong coagulation, especially the intrinsic pathway. Risk of bleeding is not increased if other factors and platelets are normal, but risk of thrombosis is increased, possibly via inhibition of prostacyclin production and platelet aggregation.)

Renal, cardiac and pulmonary involvement each occur in about 50% of cases. Patients may present with acute complications requiring admission to the ICU.

Diagnosed according to clinical features and results of investigations, especially autoantibody titres (e.g. antinuclear and anti-double stranded DNA antibodies), although autoantibodies may also be present in other connective tissue diseases and other conditions.

Treatment includes corticosteroids, NSAIDs, immunosuppressive drugs and antimalarial drugs. Prognosis is generally good although long-term treatment is usually required; prognosis is worse in CNS involvement, hypertension and early onset.

D'Cruz DP (2006). Brit Med J; 332: 890–4

Systemic sclerosis (SS; Scleroderma). Rare connective tissue disease most commonly affecting women in their 40s. Its aetiology is unknown. Involves increased deposition of connective tissue components and fibrosis affecting small vessels, skin and other tissues. General features and anaesthetic considerations are as for connective tissue diseases; the disease may be limited to the skin or be truly systemic, involving:

- peripheral vasculature and skin: calluses, ulceration or ischaemia of the extremities may occur. The tight skin may make iv cannulation or mouth opening difficult.
- oesophagus: impaired motility occurs in about 90% of cases, with potential risk of aspiration of gastric contents.
- lungs: pleurisy, effusions, fibrosis and pulmonary hypertension are common.
- kidneys: affected to some degree in most patients with diffuse SS. Hypertension may signal accelerated renal impairment and the need for angiotensin converting enzyme inhibitor therapy. Function may recover after many years' dysfunction.
- heart: involved in over 90% of cases, usually pericardial effusion.
- others: joints, muscle peripheral nerves.

The CREST syndrome comprises calcinosis, Raynaud's phenomenon, (o)esophagitis, sclerodactyly and telangiectasia.

Treatment includes penicillamine, colchicine and immunosuppressive drugs including corticosteroids.

[Maurice Raynaud (1834–1881), French physician]

Systemic vascular resistance (SVR; Peripheral vascular resistance, PVR; Total peripheral resistance, TPR). Resistance against which the heart pumps. May be calculated using the principle of Ohm's law:

$$\text{SVR (dyne s/cm}^5) = \frac{\text{MAP} - \text{CVP (mmHg)}}{\text{cardiac output (1/min)}} \times 80 \text{ (correction factor)}$$

Normally 1000–1500 dyne s/cm^5 (n.b. 1 dyne s/cm^5 = 100 N s/m^5).

The above equation ignores the effects of blood viscosity, pulsatile flow and the different results of pressure changes on different vascular beds.

- SVR is mainly determined by the diameter of the arterioles, small changes in their calibre producing large changes in resistance. Arteriolar calibre may be affected by:
  - intrinsic contractile response of vascular smooth muscle to increased intravascular pressure (myogenic theory of autoregulation).
  - locally produced substances causing vasodilatation (e.g. CO_2, potassium and hydrogen ions, lactic acid, histamine, nitric oxide, adenosine, prostaglandins and kinins; metabolic theory of autoregulation), or vasoconstriction, e.g. 5-HT. Hypoxia causes vasodilatation peripherally and vasoconstriction in the lungs. Increased temperature causes vasodilatation, whilst cold causes vasoconstriction.
  - neural innervation:
    - α-adrenergic receptors: the most important type, affecting most vessels. Stimulation causes vasoconstriction.
    - β_2-adrenergic receptors: stimulation causes vasodilatation of arterioles to muscle and viscera.
    - dopamine receptors: stimulation causes vasodilatation of renal and splanchnic vessels.
    - sympathetic cholinergic receptors: stimulation causes vasodilatation in skeletal muscle.
    - other neurotransmitters may be involved, e.g. substance P, vasoactive intestinal peptide, etc.
  - circulating substances, e.g. noradrenaline, angiotensin II, vasopressin, vasopressor drugs (causing vasoconstriction); vasodilator drugs, atrial natriuretic peptide (causing vasodilatation). Adrenaline causes vasodilatation in skeletal muscle and the liver. Toxins released in septic shock may cause vasodilatation. The locally produced substances above may also cause systemic effects.

SVR increases progressively with age. Chronically increased SVR is the hallmark of essential hypertension.

SVR ÷ body surface area (SVR index; SVRI) adjusts for differences in body size between individuals.

See also, Arterial blood pressure; Renin/angiotensin system

Systole, *see Cardiac cycle*

Systolic time intervals. Measurements derived from the systolic phase of the cardiac cycle, obtained from simultaneous phonocardiography and recording of ECG and carotid artery tracing. Allow evaluation of left ventricular function.

- Include:
  - QS_2 (qA_2): interval between the ECG QRS complex and the aortic component of the second heart sound.
  - left ventricular ejection time (LVET): period from the beginning of the carotid upstroke to the dicrotic notch.
  - pre-ejection period (PEP): QS_2 – LVET. Represents the rate of ventricular isometric pressure change, i.e. dp/dt.
  - others, e.g. duration of mechanical systole, are less commonly measured. Ratios of the intervals have been calculated, e.g. PEP ÷ LVET.

T

t½, *see Half-life*

T-piece breathing systems, *see Anaesthetic breathing systems*

t tests, *see Statistical tests*

T wave. Wave on the ECG representing ventricular repolarisation (*see Fig. 57b; Electrocardiography*). Normally upright in leads I, II and V_{3-6}; the upper height limit is 5 mm in the standard leads and 10 mm in the chest leads.

- Abnormalities:
  - may be inverted in myocardial ischaemia, ventricular hypertrophy, mitral valve prolapse, bundle branch block and digoxin toxicity.
  - may be notched in pericarditis.
  - tall peaked waves may occur in hyperkalaemia.

Tachycardias, *see Sinus tachycardia; Supraventricular tachycardia; Ventricular tachycardia*

Tachykinins. Group of neuropeptides involved in cardiovascular, respiratory, endocrine and behavioural responses. Include substance P, neurokinin A and neurokinin B, which are natural agonists at NK1, NK2 and NK3 receptors, respectively. Particular interest has focused on NK1 and NK2 receptor activation, which results in bronchoconstriction, and on development of neurokinin-1 receptor antagonists as antiemetic drugs.

Tachyphylaxis. Term usually referring to tolerance that develops rapidly.

Tacrine, *see Tetrahydroaminocrine*

Tacrolimus. Immunosuppressive drug; acts by inhibiting cytotoxic lymphocyte proliferation and cytokine expression. Used to prevent graft rejection after liver and renal transplantation. A topical preparation is available for treatment of dermatitis. Extensively bound to red blood cells and plasma proteins. Achieves steady-state concentrations after about 3 days' administration; half-life varies from 3 to 40 h with mainly hepatic metabolism and biliary excretion.

- Dosage: 100–300 μg/kg orally in two doses or iv over 24 h.
- Side effects: renal impairment, various central and peripheral neurological disturbances, cardiomyopathy, diabetes.

Tamponade, *see Cardiac tamponade*

Target-controlled infusion, *see Propofol*

TB, *see Tuberculosis*

TCD, *see Transcranial Doppler ultrasound*

TCI, Target-controlled infusion, *see Propofol*

TEE, Transesophageal echocardiography, *see Transoesophageal echocardiography*

Teeth. Comprised of the crown (consisting of enamel, dentine and pulp from outside inwards) and root. All parts may be damaged during anaesthesia; the deeper the damage, the more extensive is the treatment required. Traumatic damage is involved in about 30% of malpractice claims against anaesthetists. Damage most commonly occurs during intubation or postoperatively when the patient bites on an oral airway. Preoperative assessment of the teeth is essential, noting any loose, chipped or false teeth. Patients with caries, prostheses and periodontal disease, and those in whom tracheal intubation is difficult, are at particular risk. Appropriate warnings should be given and noted on the anaesthetic chart preoperatively.

Dentures and removable bridges, etc. are traditionally removed before anaesthesia, in case they should become dislodged and obstruct or pass into the airway. However, the need for routine preoperative removal of dentures has been questioned since this may cause distress to many patients, especially women. If damage to teeth does occur, the extent of damage should be carefully documented and the patient referred as soon as possible to a dentist (ideally in the same hospital) who can carry out necessary emergency treatment and decide whether further treatment is necessary.

Owen H, Waddell-Smith I (2000). Anaesth Intensive Care; 28: 133–45

See also, Dental surgery; Mandibular nerve blocks; Maxillary nerve blocks

Teicoplanin. Glycopeptide and antibacterial drug, related to vancomycin but longer acting. Wide spectrum of activity as for vancomycin. 90% protein-bound, with a half-life of 7 days. Excreted unmetabolised in urine.

- Dosage: 400 mg iv then 200 mg once daily; 400 mg 12 hourly × 3 then once daily for severe infections. 400 mg may also be given for prophylaxis before surgery.
- Side effects: GIT disturbance, allergic reactions, blood dyscrasias, hepatic and renal impairment, erythema.

Temazepam. Benzodiazepine used in insomnia, and commonly used for premedication, especially in day-case surgery. Shorter acting than diazepam, with faster onset of action. Half-life is 8 h.

10–40 mg given orally, 45–60 min preoperatively, is usually an effective anxiolytic. For children, 0.5 mg/kg may be given. Gel-filled capsules were withdrawn from NHS use in 1995 because of abuse by iv drug users, the liquefied gel causing marked vascular damage on injection. Temazepam became a Schedule 3 Controlled Drug in 1996, although without special prescription requirements.

See also, Misuse of Drugs Act

Temperature. Property of a system which determines whether heat is transferred to or from other systems. Three

Table 36 Corresponding points on different temperature scales

	Kelvin (K)	*Celsius (°C)*	*Fahrenheit (°F)*
Absolute zero	0	−273	−459
Melting point of ice	273	0	32
Boiling point of water	373	100	212

temperature scales are recognised: Kelvin (formerly Absolute) scale, Celsius (formerly Centigrade) scale and Fahrenheit scale (Table 36). The SI unit of temperature is the kelvin. [Anders Celsius (1701–1744), Swedish scientist; Gabriel D Fahrenheit (1686–1736), German scientist]

Temperature measurement. Methods used may be:
- electrical:
  - thermocouple: relies on the Seebeck effect; i.e. the production of voltage at the junction of two different conductors, the magnitude of which is proportional to temperature. A circuit may consist of a measuring thermocouple junction (e.g. as a needle) and a reference junction, with measurement of the voltage produced at the measuring probe. Because voltage is also produced at the reference junction, electrical manipulation is required to compensate for changes in temperature at the latter.
  - thermistor: resistance falls exponentially with temperature. Consists of a metal oxide semiconductor bead which may be small enough to be placed within body cavities. Calibration may be difficult.
  - platinum resistance wire: resistance increases proportionally with temperature. Very accurate but fragile.
- non-electrical:
  - liquid thermometers: the liquid (usually mercury) expands as temperature increases, and moves out of its glass bulb and up the barrel of the instrument. Temperature is read from a scale along its length. A constriction just above the bulb prevents the mercury from withdrawing back into the bulb. Alcohol is used for very low temperatures.
  - gas expansion thermometers, e.g. an anaeroid gauge used for pressure measurement is calibrated in units of temperature. Accuracy is poor and calibration may be difficult.
  - bimetallic strip, arranged in a coil. A pointer is moved by coiling or uncoiling of the strip as temperature changes.
  - infra-red thermometry: relies on the principle that the maximal amount of radiation (black box radiation) emitted by a body depends only on that body's temperature. The radiation emitted by a surface is less than that emitted by a black body at the same temperature; the ratio is defined as emissivity of the surface. Measurement of radiation emitted by a surface plus knowledge of its emissivity allows calculation of the surface's temperature. Infra-red thermometers detect infra-red radiation emitted by the tympanic membrane and calculate its temperature in under a second, allowing for heat loss in the ear canal. They may also be used to measure surface temperature at other sites, e.g. skin, or to estimate temperature at these sites from tympanic membrane temperature.
  - chemical thermometers: consist of a plastic strip containing a number of cells, each holding liquid crystals which melt and change colour according to temperature. Accurate to 0.5°C.
- Sites of measurement:
  - tympanic membrane: correlates most closely with hypothalamic temperature, and has rapid response time. Carries risk of tympanic perforation if direct contact techniques are used.
  - oesophageal: accurate if the lower third is used, otherwise measured temperature is influenced by the temperature of inspired gases.
  - nasopharyngeal and bladder: similar to oesophageal.
  - rectal: usually 0.5–1.0°C higher than core temperature, because of bacterial fermentation. Response time is slow because of insulation by faeces.
  - blood: thermistors incorporated into pulmonary artery catheters allow continuous measurement.
  - skin: does not reflect core temperature. The difference between core and skin temperatures gives some indication of peripheral perfusion, and is commonly used in the ICU.

Performed routinely as part of basic monitoring in ICUs. Used perioperatively to monitor heat loss during anaesthesia or to warn of hyperthermia.
[Thomas J Seebeck (1770–1831), Russian-born German physicist]

Temperature regulation. Humans are homeothermic, maintaining body core temperature at 37°C ± 1°C. The core usually includes cranial, thoracic, abdominal and pelvic contents, and variable amounts of the deep portions of the limbs. Temperature is lowest at night and highest in mid-afternoon, also varying with the menstrual cycle.

Constant temperature is required for optimal enzyme activity. Denaturation of proteins occurs at 42°C. Loss of consciousness occurs at hypothermia below 30°C.
- Mechanisms of heat loss/gain:
  - heat gain:
    - from the environment.
    - from metabolism (mainly in the brain, liver and kidneys): approximately 80 W is produced in an average man under resting conditions. This would raise body temperature by about 1°C per hour if totally insulated. Vigorous muscular activity may increase heat production by up to 20 times. In babies, brown fat produces much heat.
  - heat loss:
    - radiation from the skin. May account for 40% of total loss.
    - convection: related to airflow (e.g. 'wind-chill'). Accounts for up to 40% of total loss.
    - evaporation from the respiratory tract and skin: the latter is increased by sweating, which normally accounts for 20% of total loss but this figure may increase markedly.
    - conduction: of little importance in air, but significant in water.

Temperature-sensitive cells are present in the anterior hypothalamus (thought to be the most important site), brainstem, spinal cord, skin, skeletal muscle and abdominal viscera. Peripheral temperature receptors are primary afferent nerve endings and respond to cold and hot stimuli via Aδ and C fibres respectively. Central control of thermoregulation is by the hypothalamus. Efferents pass via the sympathetic nervous system to blood vessels, sweat glands and piloerector muscles. Local reflexes are also involved. Efferents also pass to somatic motor centres in the lower brainstem to cause shivering, and to higher centres.

- Regulatory mechanisms:
  - behavioural, e.g. curling up in the cold, etc.
  - skin blood flow: may be altered by vasodilatation or vasoconstriction of skin vessels, and by opening or closing of arteriovenous anastomoses in the skin. Affects all routes of heat loss. Alteration alone is sufficient to maintain constant body temperature in environments of 20–28°C in adults and 35–37°C in neonates (thermoneutral range).
  - shivering and piloerection (reduced or absent in babies, brown fat metabolism occurring instead).
  - sweating.

Buggy DJ, Crossley AWA (2000). Br J Anaesth; 84: 615–28
See also, Heat loss during anaesthesia

Temporomandibular joint (TMJ). Synovial joint between the mandibular condyle and the articular surface of the squamous temporal bone. Protrusion, retraction and grinding movements of the lower jaw occur by a gliding mechanism whereas mouth opening and closing involves gliding and hinging movements. Joint stability is least when the mouth is fully open (e.g. during laryngoscopy) and forward dislocation may occur. Affected by rheumatoid arthritis, degenerative disease, ankylosing spondylitis and systemic sclerosis. Mouth opening may be severely limited, hindering laryngoscopy.
See also, Intubation, difficult; Trismus

Tenecteplase. Fibrinolytic drug, used in acute management of MI. Binds to fibrin, the resultant complex converting plasminogen to plasmin, which dissolves the fibrin.

- Dosage: 0.5–0.6 mg/kg (to a maximum of 50 mg) iv over 10 s.
- Side effects: as for fibrinolytic drugs.

TENS, *see Transcutaneous electrical nerve stimulation*

Tensilon test, *see Edrophonium*

Tension. In physics, another word for force, implying stretching (cf. compression). Also refers to the partial pressure of a gas in solution.

Tension time index. Area between tracings of left ventricular pressure and aortic root pressure during systole, multiplied by heart rate (*see Fig. 60; Endocardial viability ratio*). Represents myocardial workload and hence O_2 demand; when taken in conjunction with diastolic pressure time index, it may indicate the myocardial O_2 supply/demand ratio and the likelihood of myocardial ischaemia.

Terbutaline sulphate. β-Adrenergic receptor agonist, used as a bronchodilator drug and tocolytic drug. Has similar effects to salbutamol, but possibly has less cardiac effect.

- Dosage:
  - 2.5 mg orally, 8–12 hourly.
  - 250–500 μg im/sc, 6 hourly as required.
  - 250–500 μg iv slowly, repeated as required. 1–5 μg/min infusion may be used (containing 3–5 μg/ml). Up to 25 μg/min may be required in premature labour (*see Ritodrine*).
  - 1–2 puffs by aerosol (250–500 μg), 6–8 hourly.
  - 5–10 mg by nebulised solution, 6–12 hourly.
- Side effects: as for salbutamol.

Terlipressin, *see Vasopressin*

Terminal care, *see Palliative care; Withdrawal of treatment in ICU*

Test dose, epidural. In epidural anaesthesia, injection of a small amount of local anaesthetic agent through the catheter before injection of the main dose, in order to identify accidental subarachnoid or iv placement of the catheter. Less commonly performed before 'through the needle' epidural block, since leakage of CSF or blood should be more easily noticeable.

Controversial, since it is not always reliable. The volume and strength of the test solution is also controversial. 3 ml 2% lidocaine with adrenaline 1:200 000 has been suggested as the ideal solution; subarachnoid injection produces spinal anaesthesia within 2–3 min, and iv injection produces tachycardia within 90 s. Injection of fentanyl 50–100 μg or 1 ml air (with Doppler monitoring) has also been used. In modern 'low-dose' techniques, e.g. epidural analgesia for labour, each dose 'acts as its own test' since a standard dose of e.g. 10 ml bupivacaine 0.1% with 20 μg fentanyl would be expected to produce noticeable effects were it to be injected subarachnoid or iv without causing a dangerously high block or severe systemic toxicity.
Guay J (2006). Anesth Analg; 102: 921–9

Tetanic contraction. Sustained muscle contraction caused by repetitive electrical stimulation of a motor nerve. About 25 Hz stimulation is required for frequent enough action potentials to produce it, although the necessary rate varies according to the muscle studied. The force produced exceeds that of single muscle twitches. During tetanic contraction, acetylcholine is mobilised from reserve stores to the readily available pool.

Produced during neuromuscular blockade monitoring.
See also, Neuromuscular junction; Neuromuscular transmission; Post-tetanic potentiation

Tetanus. Rare in developed countries following immunisation programmes, but accounts for up to 1 million deaths annually worldwide. Caused by infection with *Clostridium tetani*, a widely occurring spore-forming Gram-positive bacillus found in soil, dust and faeces. Inoculation may be via minor injury. Recently reported in drug abusers 'skin-popping' contaminated heroin. Clinical features are caused by a potent exotoxin, tetanospasmin, which moves along peripheral nerves to the spinal cord, where it blocks release of neurotransmitters especially at inhibitory neurones causing muscle spasm. Incubation period is 3–21 days (average 7 days). Local infection may cause muscle spasm around the site of injury; generalised tetanus is characterised by trismus, irritability, rigidity and opisthotonos. Cardiac arrhythmias/arrest and hypertension may follow sympathetic hyperactivity. As binding of tetanospasmin is irreversible, recovery depends on formation of new nerve terminals.

- Treatment:
  - human anti-tetanus immunoglobulin (5000–10 000 units): neutralises circulating toxin.
  - surgical excision and debridement of the wound.
  - metronidazole to eradicate existing organisms.
  - sedation, neuromuscular blocking drugs and IPPV may be required. Dantrolene and magnesium sulphate have been used. The latter reduces sympathetic overactivity and reduces spasm by decreasing presynaptic activity.
  - of cardiovascular complications.

Overall mortality is up to 55% (greater in previously unvaccinated individuals, if age exceeds 50, and if generalised spasms rapidly follow initial symptoms).

Active immunisation with tetanus vaccine should always be performed in trauma and burns unless within 5–10 years of previous administration. Anti-tetanus immunoglobulin is given to non-immune patients with heavily contaminated or old wounds.

Cook TM, Protheroe RT, Handel JM (2001). Br J Anaesth; 87: 477–87

See also, Clostridial infections

Tetany. Increased sensitivity of excitable cells, manifested as peripheral muscle spasm. Usually facial and carpopedal, the shape of the hand in the latter termed *main d'accoucheur* (French: obstetrician's hand). Usually caused by hypocalcaemia; it also occurs in hypomagnesaemia and may be hereditary.

Tetracaine hydrochloride (Amethocaine). Ester local anaesthetic agent, introduced in 1931. Widely used in the USA for spinal anaesthesia; in the UK, used only for surface anaesthesia, e.g. in ophthalmology. More potent and longer lasting than lidocaine, but more toxic. Toxicity resembles that of cocaine. Rapidly absorbed from mucous membranes. Hydrolysed completely by plasma cholinesterase to form butylaminobenzoic acid and dimethylaminoethanol. Administration: 0.5–1% solution for spinal anaesthesia; 0.4–0.5% for epidural anaesthesia; 0.1–0.2% solution for infiltration, usually with adrenaline; 0.5–1% solutions for surface analgesia.

Available in a 4% gel (available over the counter without prescription) for topical anaesthesia of the skin, e.g. before venepuncture. The melting point of the drug is lowered by the formation of specific hydrates within the gel. The resultant oil globules penetrate the skin readily with onset of action about 30–45 min; effects last 4–6 h. Skin blistering may occur. Has been combined with lidocaine together with a heating compound in a plaster, designed to be used for surface anaesthesia before venepuncture.

Maximal safe dose: 1.5 mg/kg.

Tetracycline. Broad spectrum antibacterial drug, used mainly for chlamydia, rickettsia, spirochaete and brucella infections, certain mycoplasma infections, acne, acute exacerbations of COPD and leptospirosis. Several tetracyclines exist, with tetracycline itself the only one administered iv. Has also been instilled into the pleural cavity to treat recurrent pleural effusions.

- Dosage:
  - 250–500 mg orally 6–8 hourly.
  - 500 mg iv 12 hourly.
- Side effects: stained teeth (if given to children), renal impairment, GIT upset, benign intracranial hypertension, hepatic impairment.

Tetrahydroaminocrine hydrochloride (Tacrine). Acetylcholinesterase inhibitor formerly used to prolong the action of suxamethonium. Also used prophylactically to reduce muscle pains following suxamethonium, and as a central stimulant. Has recently been investigated as a treatment for Alzheimer's disease.

[Alois Alzheimer (1864–1915), German neurologist and pathologist]

Tetrodotoxin. Toxin obtained from puffer fish which selectively blocks voltage-gated fast sodium channels in nerves. Useful experimentally, e.g. for investigating neuromuscular transmission.

Thalassaemia. Group of autosomally inherited disorders involving decreased production of the α or β chains of haemoglobin (Hb). More common in Mediterranean, African and Asian areas. Severity is related to the pattern of inheritance of the Hb genes (normally, one β gene and two α genes are inherited from each parent).

- Divided into:
  - β thalassaemia:
    - not apparent immediately as fetal haemoglobin does not contain β chains.
    - heterozygous β thalassaemia (thalassaemia minor) produces mild (often asymptomatic) anaemia, but may be associated with other types of Hb (e.g. HbC, HbE, HbS); resultant anaemia may vary from mild to severe.
    - homozygous β thalassaemia (Cooley's anaemia; thalassaemia major) results in severe anaemia in infancy, with no production of HbA. Features include craniofacial bone hyperplasia, hepatosplenomegaly and cardiac failure. Haemosiderosis may occur due to repeated blood transfusion. Usually fatal before adulthood although bone marrow transplantation may offer a cure. Some genetic subtypes are associated with a milder clinical course (thalassaemia intermedia).
  - α thalassaemia: severity varies, depending on the number of gene deletions. Usually causes mild anaemia; deletion of all four α genes is incompatible with life.

[Thomas B Cooley (1871–1945), US paediatrician]

THAM, tris-(hydroxymethyl)-aminomethane, *see 2-Amino-2-hydroxymethyl-1,3-propanediol*

Theophylline. Bronchodilator drug, used alone or in combination with ethylenediamine as aminophylline.

Actions and effects: as for aminophylline.

- Dosage: 125–250 mg orally, 6–8 hourly; 175–500 mg slow-release preparation 12 hourly.

Therapeutic intervention scoring system (TISS). Scoring system for assessing the severity of critical illness according to the number of interventions a patient receives. Originally comprising over 70 interventions which were scored 1–4 according to complexity and invasiveness; more recent modifications have reduced this number to under 30. Although of value in an individual clinician's practice, the score for a particular patient may vary between clinicians and units according to differences in treatment strategies. Has been used as a means of assessing the need for ICU resources.

Miranda DR (1997). Intensive Care Med; 23: 615–17

Therapeutic ratio/index. Relationship between the doses of a drug required to produce undesirable and desirable effects. A drug with a high therapeutic ratio has a greater margin of safety than one with low therapeutic ratio. Defined experimentally as the ratio of median lethal dose to median effective dose:

$$\frac{LD_{50}}{ED_{50}}$$

Thermal conductivity detector, *see Katharometer*

Thermistor, *see Temperature measurement*

Thermocouple, *see Temperature measurement*

Thermodilution cardiac output measurement, *see Cardiac output measurement*

Thermoneutral range. Temperature range in which temperature regulation may be maintained by changes in skin blood flow alone. Corresponds to the temperature that feels 'comfortable'. About 20–28°C in adults and 35–37°C in neonates. Neonatal metabolic rate and mortality are reduced if body temperature is kept within the thermoneutral range.

Thiamylal sodium. IV anaesthetic agent, with similar properties to thiopental. Unavailable in the UK.

Thiazide diuretics. Group of diuretics used to treat mild hypertension and oedema caused by cardiac failure. Chlorothiazide was the first to be studied but many now exist, e.g. bendroflumethiazide (bendrofluazide), chlortalidone. Act mainly at the proximal part of the distal convoluted tubule of the nephron, where they inhibit sodium resorption. They also act at the proximal tubule, causing weak inhibition of carbonic anhydrase and increasing bicarbonate and potassium excretion, and have a direct vasodilator action. Their antihypertensive action increases only slightly as dosage is increased. Rapidly absorbed from the GIT with onset of action within 1–2 h, lasting 12–24 h.

Side effects include hypokalaemia, hyponatraemia, hyperuricaemia, hypomagnesaemia, hypochloraemic alkalosis, hyperglycaemia, hypercholesterolaemia, exacerbation of renal and hepatic impairment, impotence, and rarely rashes and thrombocytopenia.

Thiazolidinediones. Oral hypoglycaemic drugs used in management of type II diabetes mellitus. Bind to a nuclear receptor, PPARγ, in adipose cells, liver and skeletal muscle, increasing sensitivity to insulin. Not indicated for monotherapy; usually used in combination with a biguanide or sulphonylurea. Two available agents are pioglitazone and rosiglitazone (the latter may be associated with increased mortality due to cardiovascular events). They are expensive compared with other oral hypoglycaemic agents.

Thigh, lateral cutaneous nerve block. Provides analgesia of the anterolateral thigh/knee, e.g. for leg surgery (especially skin graft harvesting) and diagnosis of meralgia paraesthetica (numbness and paraesthesia caused by lateral cutaneous nerve compression by the inguinal ligament, under which it passes).

With the patient supine, a needle is introduced perpendicular to the skin, 2 cm medial and caudal to the anterior superior iliac spine. A click is felt as the fascia lata is pierced. 10–15 ml local anaesthetic agent is injected in a fan shape laterally.

Thiopental sodium (Thiopentone; 5-ethyl-5-(1-methylbutyl)-2-thiobarbiturate). Widely used iv anaesthetic agent, synthesised in 1932 and first used in 1934 by Lundy and Waters. Also used in severe convulsions and status epilepticus. The sulphur analogue of pentobarbitone (Fig. 153).

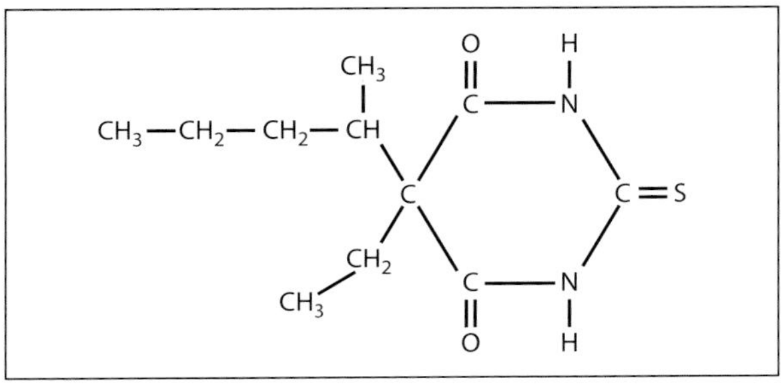

Fig. 153 Structure of thiopental

Stored as the sodium salt, a yellow powder with a faint garlic smell, with 6% anhydrous sodium carbonate added to prevent formation of (insoluble) free acid when exposed to atmospheric CO_2. Presented in an atmosphere of nitrogen. Readily soluble in water; the solution is stable for 24–36 h after mixing although the manufacturers recommend discarding after 7 h. Most commonly used as a 2.5% solution, with pH of 10.5. pK_a is 7.6; about 60% is non-ionised at a pH of 7.4. About 85% bound to plasma proteins after injection. Follows a multicompartmental pharmacokinetic model after a single iv injection, with redistribution from vessel-rich tissues (e.g. brain) to lean body tissues (e.g. muscle), with return of consciousness. Slower redistribution then occurs to vessel-poor tissues (e.g. fat (*see Fig. 86; Intravenous anaesthetic agents*)).

- Effects:
  - induction:
    - smooth, occurring within one arm–brain circulation time. Involuntary movements and painful injection are rare.
    - recovery within 5–10 min after a single dose.
  - CVS:
    - causes dose-related direct myocardial depression, decreasing cardiac output and causing compensatory tachycardia with increased myocardial O_2 demand. Cardiovascular depression is related to speed of injection and is exacerbated by hypovolaemia.
    - has little effect on SVR but may decrease venous vascular tone, reducing venous return.
  - RS:
    - causes dose-related depression of the respiratory centre, decreasing the responsiveness to CO_2 and hypoxia. Apnoea is common after induction.
    - laryngospasm readily occurs following laryngeal stimulation.
    - has been implicated in causing bronchospasm, but this is disputed.
  - CNS:
    - anticonvulsant.
    - decreases pain threshold (antanalgesia).
    - reduces cerebral perfusion pressure, ICP and cerebral metabolism.
  - other:
    - causes brief skeletal muscle relaxation at peak CNS effect.
    - reduces renal and hepatic blood flow secondary to reduced cardiac output. Causes hepatic enzyme induction.
    - reduces intraocular pressure.
    - has no effect on uterine tone.

Metabolised by oxidisation in the liver (10–15% per hour), with under 1% appearing unchanged in the urine. Desulphuration to pentobarbitone may also occur following prolonged administration. Elimination half-life is 5–10 h. Up to 30% may remain in the body after 24 h. Cumulation may occur on repeated dosage.

- Complications:
  - extravenous injection causes pain and erythema.
  - intra-arterial injection causes intense pain, and may cause distal blistering, oedema and gangrene, traditionally attributed to crystallisation of thiopental within arterioles and capillaries, with local noradrenaline release and vasospasm. Endothelial damage and subsequent inflammatory reaction have been suggested as being more likely. Particularly hazardous with the 5% solution, now rarely used. Treatment: leaving the needle/cannula in the artery, the following may be injected:

- saline, to dilute the drug.
- vasodilators, traditionally papaverine 40 mg, tolazoline 40 mg, phentolamine 2–5 mg, to reduce arterial spasm.
- local anaesthetic, traditionally procaine 50–100 mg (also a vasodilator), to reduce pain.
- heparin, to reduce subsequent thrombosis.

Brachial plexus block and stellate ganglion block have been used to encourage vasodilatation (before heparinisation). Postponement of surgery has been suggested. Injection of thiopental should always stop after 1–2 ml, to ask whether there is any pain.

- respiratory/cardiovascular depression as above.
- adverse drug reactions. Severe anaphylactic reactions are rare (1:14 000 to 35 000), typically occurring after several previous exposures.

Contraindicated in porphyria.

- Dosage:
  - 3–6 mg/kg iv. Requirements are reduced in hypoproteinaemia, hypovolaemia, the elderly and critically ill patients. Injection should always proceed slowly, with a pause after the expected adequate dose before further administration.
  - Has also been given rectally: 40–50 mg/kg as 5–10% solution.
  - By infusion for convulsions: 2–3 mg/kg/h.

Thiosulphate, *see Cyanide poisoning*

Third gas effect, *see Fink effect*

Third space. 'Non-functional' interstitial fluid compartment, to which fluid is transferred following trauma, burns, surgery and other conditions including infection, pancreatitis, etc. Most of the fluid originates from the ECF, but some movement from intracellular fluid also occurs. Includes fluid lost to the transcellular fluid compartment, e.g. ascites, bowel contents, etc. Although not lost from the body, fluid shifts to the third space are equivalent to functional ECF losses and must be accounted for when estimating fluid balance. Losses may exceed 10 ml/kg/h during abdominal surgery, and should be replaced initially with 0.9% saline or Hartmann's solution, although colloids may also be used.
See also, Stress response to surgery

Thoracic inlet. Kidney-shaped superior (cranial) opening of the thorax, bounded by the superior border of the manubrium sternum anteriorly, 1st thoracic vertebra posteriorly, and the first ribs laterally. Anteroposterior diameter is about 5 cm; transverse diameter about 10 cm. Its plane slopes downward (60° to the horizontal) and forward.

- Contents (*see Fig. 24; Brachial plexus and Fig. 102; Mediastinum*):
  - median plane (from anterior to posterior): sternohyoid and sternothyroid muscles; remains of thymus; inferior thyroid ± braciocephalic veins; trachea; oesophagus; recurrent laryngeal nerve; thoracic duct.
  - laterally:
    - both sides: upper pleura/apex of lung; sympathetic trunk, superior intercostal artery and ventral ramus of T1 (from medial to lateral) between the pleura and neck of the first rib; internal thoracic artery anteriorly.
    - right side: brachiocephalic vessels; vagus; phrenic nerve.
    - left side: common carotid/subclavian arteries; vagus; brachiocephalic vein; phrenic nerve.

Thoracic inlet X-ray views may be useful if tracheal compression or displacement is suspected.

Thoracic surgery. The first pneumonectomy was performed in in 1895 by Macewan. Surgical and anaesthetic techniques improved with experience of treating chest injuries during World War II. The commonest indication for thoracic surgery was formerly TB and empyema but is now malignancy, especially bronchial carcinoma.

- Main anaesthetic principles:
  - preoperatively:
    - preoperative assessment of exercise tolerance, cough, haemoptysis, etc. Ischaemic heart disease secondary to smoking is common. Cyanosis, tracheal deviation, stridor, abnormal chest wall movement, pleural effusion and systemic features of malignancy may be present.
    - investigations include chest X-ray, CT scanning and MRI. Rarely, bronchography is performed, e.g. in bronchiectasis. Arterial blood gas analysis and lung function tests are routinely performed, e.g. spirometry, flow–volume loops, etc. A poor postoperative course following pneumonectomy is suggested by FVC, FEV_1, maximal voluntary ventilation or residual volume:total lung capacity ratio under 50% of predicted value. Poor outcome is also likely if resting pulmonary artery pressure is raised, or diffusing capacity is low.
    - preparation includes antibiotic therapy, physiotherapy and use of bronchodilator drugs as appropriate. Digoxin is sometimes given prophylactically, especially in older patients.
    - premedication commonly includes anticholinergic drugs to reduce secretions.
  - perioperatively:
    - specific diagnostic procedures include bronchoscopy, mediastinoscopy, bronchography and oesophagoscopy.
    - preoxygenation is usually employed. IV induction of anaesthesia is usually suitable; difficulties may include cardiovascular instability, airway obstruction, difficult tracheal intubation, risk of aspiration of gastric contents in oesophageal disease, and problems of lesions affecting the mediastinum.
    - endobronchial tubes are often used, although standard tracheal tubes are usually acceptable unless isolation of lung segments is required. Endobronchial blockers may also be used.
    - large bore iv cannulae are vital, since blood loss may be severe.
    - standard monitoring is used; arterial and central venous cannulation are often employed.
    - maintenance of anaesthesia is usually with standard agents and techniques. Spontaneous ventilation is rarely allowed, since ventilation of the affected lung is poor once the chest is opened. Pendelluft, $\dot{V}/\dot{Q}$ mismatch and decreased venous return secondary to mediastinal shift may also occur. Hypoxaemia is common during one-lung anaesthesia. Injector techniques and high frequency ventilation have been used for tracheal resection.
    - positioning of the patient: the lateral position is usually employed, with the affected lung uppermost. The arm is placed over the head, displacing the scapula upwards. Drainage of secretions from the affected lung without soiling the unaffected lung may be achieved using the Parry Brown position (prone, with

a pillow under the pelvis and a 10 cm rest under the chest; the arm on the operated side overhangs the table's edge with the head turned to the opposite side, and the table is tipped head down so that the trachea slopes downwards).
- at closure of the chest, the lung is re-expanded after endobronchial suction. Up to 40 cmH_2O airway pressure may be requested by the surgeon to test bronchial sutures. Tubes are placed for chest drainage. After pneumonectomy, chest drains are often not used; air is introduced or removed to equalise the intrapleural pressures on both sides and centralise the mediastinum. The pleural space slowly fills with fluid postoperatively, with eventual fibrosis.

- postoperatively:
  - IPPV is usually avoided if possible, as it risks leakage from the bronchial stump with possible fistula formation.
  - postoperative analgesia is vital to ensure adequate ventilation. Standard techniques are used, especially continuous iv opioid infusions (including patient-controlled analgesia), thoracic epidural anaesthesia and use of spinal opioids. Cryoanalgesia and intercostal nerve block may be performed by the surgeon whilst the chest is open.
  - physiotherapy is important postoperatively.

Specific procedures and conditions include removal of inhaled foreign body, bronchopleural fistula, chest trauma, bronchopulmonary lavage.

Similar considerations apply to oesophageal surgery. Ivor Lewis oesophagectomy (performed for carcinoma of the middle third of the oesophagus) involves laparotomy to mobilise the stomach and duodenum, followed by turning of the patient and right thoracotomy. Patients are often malnourished.

[Arthur I Parry Brown (1908–2007), London anaesthetist; Ivor Lewis (1895–1982), London surgeon]

See also, Pneumothorax

Thoracocardiography, *see Inductance cardiography*

Three-in-one block, *see Femoral nerve block; Lumbar plexus*

Thrombelastography, *see Coagulation studies*

Thrombin inhibitors. Group of compounds that bind to various sites on the thrombin molecule, investigated as alternatives to heparin. Includes hirudin and related substances. Ximelagatran, a prodrug for melagatran, was extensively investigated as an oral anticoagulant but withdrawn in 2006 following reports of hepatic impairment. Dabigatran was introduced in the UK in 2008 for the prevention of deep vein thrombosis in adults undergoing elective hip or knee replacement. Rivaroxaban is currently under development.

Kam PCA, Kaur N, Thong CL (2005). Anaesthesia; 60: 565–74

Thrombin time, *see Coagulation studies*

Thrombocytopenia. Defined as a platelet count below 100 × 10^9/l. Common in critically ill patients.

- Caused by:
  - decreased production: e.g. bone marrow depression (by drugs, infection, etc.), vitamin B_{12}/folate deficiency, hereditary defects, paroxysmal nocturnal haemoglobinuria, thiazide diuretics, alcoholism.
  - shortened survival:
    - immune, e.g. autoantibodies (e.g. idiopathic thrombocytopaenic purpura, SLE, rheumatoid arthritis, malignancy, drugs (e.g. quinine, heparin, α-methyldopa), infection (e.g. HIV), alloantibodies (e.g. post-transfusion).
    - non-immune, e.g. DIC, thrombotic thrombocytopenic purpura, cardiopulmonary bypass, haemolytic uraemic syndrome.
  - abnormal distribution, e.g. hypersplenism, hypothermia.

Patients with platelet counts above 50 × 10^9/l are usually asymptomatic. Bleeding time increases progressively as the count falls below 100 × 10^9/l. Counts below 20–30 × 10^9/l are associated with spontaneous bleeding, e.g. mucocutaneous, gastrointestinal, cerebral. Diagnosis of the underlying condition requires examination of the blood film and bone marrow, coagulation studies, etc.

- Treatment: according to the underlying cause. Platelet transfusion is required for counts below 20–30 × 10^9/l or if bleeding occurs; transfusion may be ineffective if increased platelet destruction is responsible.

Regional anaesthesia in the presence of thrombocytopenia (e.g. in obstetric analgesia and anaesthesia) is controversial, with any benefits weighed against the potential risk of spinal haematoma. Many anaesthetists would consider a platelet count above 70–80 × 10^9/l acceptable if there was no clinical evidence of impaired function (e.g. bruising or noticeably prolonged bleeding), coagulation studies were normal, the count had been stable for at least several days and there was a particular clinical advantage of regional anaesthesia.

Thromboelastography, *see Coagulation studies*

Thromboembolism, *see Coagulation; Deep vein thrombosis*

Thrombolytic drugs, *see Fibrinolytic drugs*

Thrombophlebitis, *see Intravenous fluid administration*

Thromboplastin time, *see Coagulation studies*

Thrombotic thrombocytopenic purpura (TTP). Rare disorder characterised by intravascular thrombosis, consumptive thrombocytopenia, and haemolytic anaemia (due to mechanical damage to red cells). May be difficult to distinguish from haemolytic-uraemic syndrome (with which it is thought to overlap) and DIC. Often associated with increased levels of large von Willebrand factor multimers in the plasma and a deficiency of a specific metalloprotease that cleaves it, ADAMTS13. Has been associated with pregnancy.

Typically presents with abdominal pain, nausea/vomiting and weakness. Neurological symptoms (e.g. CVA, convulsions) may also occur. Diagnosed largely clinically.

Treated by plasmapheresis, for which there is good evidence of efficacy. Immunosuppressive drugs have also been used, e.g. corticosteroids. Untreated, may rapidly progress to death in ~80% of cases; mortality with treatment is ~20%.

George JN (2006). New Engl J Med; 18: 1927–35

Thromboxanes. Substances related to prostaglandins, synthesised by the action of cyclo-oxygenase on arachidonic acid. Thromboxane A_2 is released by platelets at sites of injury, causing vasoconstriction and platelet aggregation, and is opposed by prostacyclin. It is metabolised to thromboxane B_2, which has little activity.

Thymol. Aromatic hydrocarbon used as an antioxidant in halothane and trichloroethylene. May build up inside vaporisers unless cleaned regularly. Also used as a disinfectant and deodorant, e.g. in mouthwashes.

Thyroid crisis (Thyroid storm). Rare manifestation of severe hyperthyroidism. May be triggered by stress including surgery and infection. Features include tachycardia, arrhythmias (including VT, VF and AF), cardiac failure, fever, diarrhoea, sweating, hyperventilation, confusion and coma.

- Treatment:
  - supportive, e.g. cooling, sedation, rehydration, treatment of arrhythmias (β-adrenergic receptor antagonists are usually employed). IPPV may be required in respiratory failure.
  - hydrocortisone 100 mg iv 6 hourly.
  - antithyroid drugs:
    - 200 mg potassium iodide orally/iv 6 hourly.
    - 60–120 mg carbimazole or 600–1200 mg propylthiouracil orally/day.
  - plasmapheresis and exchange transfusion have been used in severe cases.

Thyroid gland. Largest endocrine gland, extending from the attachment of sternothyroid muscle to the thyroid cartilage superiorly, to the 6th tracheal ring inferiorly. The two lateral lobes lie lateral to the oesophagus and pharynx, with the isthmus overlying the 2nd–4th tracheal rings anteriorly. Arterial supply is via the superior and inferior thyroid arteries (branches of the external carotid arteries and thyrocervical trunk of the subclavian artery respectively). The external and recurrent laryngeal nerves are closely related to the superior and inferior thyroid arteries respectively.

Produces thyroxine (T_4) and triiodothyronine (T_3), which increase tissue metabolism and growth. They also increase the effects of catecholamines by increasing the number and sensitivity of β-adrenergic receptors. Iodine is absorbed from the GIT as iodide and actively transported into the thyroid gland, where it is oxidised by a peroxidase and bound to thyroglobulin. Iodination of tyrosine residues of thyroglobulin produces T_3 and T_4, which are cleaved from the parent molecule. Both hormones are more than 99% bound to plasma proteins including thyroxine-binding globulin (TBG) and albumin. T_3 is secreted in smaller amounts than T_4, is 3–5 times as potent, is faster acting, and has a shorter half-life. T_4 is converted to T_3 peripherally.

Control of T_3 and T_4 production is by thyroid stimulating hormone (TSH), secreted by the pituitary gland. Secretion is inhibited by T_3, T_4 and stress, and stimulated by thyrotrophin releasing hormone (TRH), secreted by the hypothalamus. TRH secretion is also inhibited by T_3 and T_4.

- Tests of thyroid function:
  - radioactive iodine uptake.
  - total plasma T_3 and T_4 (normally 1–3 nmol/l and 60–150 nmol/l respectively). Increased in hyperthyroidism, and when TBG levels are raised, e.g. in pregnancy, hepatitis. Decreased in hypothyroidism and when TBG levels are reduced, e.g. corticosteroid therapy, or when binding of T_3 and T_4 is inhibited, e.g. by phenytoin and salicylates.
  - free T_3 or T_4 index: obtained by adding radioactive T_3/T_4 to plasma, then adding a hormone-binding resin. Any radioactive T_3/T_4 not bound to TBG is taken up by the resin. Free T_3/T_4 index is the product of the resin uptake and plasma T_3/T_4 levels.
  - plasma TSH: indicates the level of hypersecretion in hyperthyroidism (usually depressed, due to negative feedback by T_3 and T_4). High in primary hypothyroidism. May be measured after injection of TRH.

The gland also secretes calcitonin, important in calcium homeostasis, from parafollicular (C) cells.

Anaesthetic considerations of thyroid surgery: as for hyper-/hypothyroidism.

See also, Neck, cross-sectional anatomy; Sick euthyroid syndrome

Thyroidectomy, *see Hyperthyroidism; Thyroid gland*

Thyrotoxicosis, *see Hyperthyroidism; Thyroid crisis*

Tibial nerve block, *see Ankle, nerve blocks; Knee, nerve blocks*

Ticarcillin. Carboxypenicillin antibacterial drug, used primarily for pseudomonas infections although also active against other Gram-negative organisms. Available in the UK only in combination with clavulanic acid.

- Dosage: 3.2 g 4–8 hourly (depending on severity), iv 3.2 g contains 3 g ticarcillin and 200 mg clavulanic acid.
- Side effects: as for benzylpenicillin.

Tick-borne diseases. Common worldwide although uncommon in the UK; soft ticks cause a variety of skin lesions and transmit spirochaetal relapsing fevers whilst hard ticks are the vectors for arboviral haemorrhagic fevers, encephalitis, typhus and Lyme disease. Rarely, tick bites may result in ascending flaccid paralysis leading to respiratory and bulbar involvement within a few days unless the tick is removed. The causative agent is unknown.

Spach DH, Liles WC, Campbell GL, et al (1993). N Engl J Med; 329: 936–47

Tidal volume. Volume of gas inspired and expired with each breath. Normally 7 ml/kg. Measured using spirometers or respirometers. 'Effective' tidal volume equals tidal volume minus dead space volume.

See also, Lung volumes

Tigecycline. Antibacterial drug related to tetracycline; active against Gram-positive and -negative organisms and some anaerobic bacteria. Reserved for complicated soft tissue and abdominal infections.

- Dosage: 100 mg iv initially, then 50 mg 12 hourly.
- Side effects: as for tetracyclines.

Time constant (τ). Expression used to describe an exponential process. Equals the time in which the process would be completed if the rate of change were maintained at its initial value. At 1 τ the process is 63% complete (i.e. 37% of the initial quantity remains), at 2 τ it is 86.5% complete, and at 3 τ it is 95% complete. After 6 τ the process is 99.75% complete.

When used to refer to expiration of air from the lungs, τ equals compliance × resistance; thus stiff alveoli served by narrow airways empty at similar rates to compliant alveoli served by wide airways.

See also, Half-life

Time to sustained respiration. Time for adequate regular respiration to occur in the neonate after delivery, without stimulation. Related to fetal wellbeing and respiratory depression caused by drugs administered to the mother before delivery.

See also, Fetus, effects of anaesthetic drugs on; Obstetric analgesia and anaesthesia

Tinzaparin sodium, *see Heparin*

Tirofiban. Antiplatelet drug, used in unstable angina or non-Q wave MI, within 12 h of the last episode of chest pain. Acts by reversibly inhibiting activation of the glycoprotein IIb/IIIa complex on the surface of platelets.

- Dosage: 400 ng/kg/min iv for 30 min, followed by 100 ng/kg/min for at least 48 h (and during and 12–24 h after percutaneous coronary intervention if performed), up to 108 h maximum.
- Side effects are related to increased bleeding. Platelet function takes up to 2–4 h to return to normal after discontinuation of therapy.

TISS, *see Therapeutic intervention scoring system*

Tissue oxygen tension, *see Oxygen, tissue tension*

TIVA, *see Total intravenous anaesthesia*

TMJ, *see Temporomandibular joint*

TNS, Transcutaneous nerve stimulation, *see Transcutaneous electrical nerve stimulation*

Tobramycin. Aminoglycoside and antibacterial drug with similar activity to gentamicin but more active against pseudomonas although less active against other Gram-negative organisms.

- Dosage: 1 mg/kg im/slowly iv, 8 hourly; increased to up to 5 mg/kg/day in severe infections (decreased again as soon as possible). Blood concentrations: 1 h post-dose < 10 mg/l; pre-dose < 2 mg/l.
- Side effects: as for aminoglycosides.

Tocainide hydrochloride. Class Ib antiarrhythmic drug reserved for life-threatening ventricular arrhythmias because of its toxicity. An analogue of lidocaine, but undergoes less first-pass metabolism when given orally, and with longer elimination half-life (10–12 h).

- Dosage:
  - 400–800 mg 8 hourly, orally.
  - 500–750 mg iv over 30 min. Hypotension and bradycardia may occur.
- Side effects: as for lidocaine; also GIT disturbances, agranulocytosis, aplastic anaemia, thrombocytopenia, hepatitis, pulmonary fibrosis, pneumonitis and an SLE-like syndrome.

Tocolytic drugs. Used to inhibit uterine contractions when premature delivery of the fetus is threatened, to prevent uterine activity during/after incidental maternal surgery or fetal surgery, and to relax the uterus acutely, e.g. in fetal distress, obstructed delivery or uterine inversion. Drugs traditionally used are β_2-adrenergic receptor agonists and include ritodrine, salbutamol and terbutaline. Side effects may persist after discontinuation of the infusion; these include tachycardia, arrhythmias, hypotension and occasionally pulmonary oedema (thought to be caused by increased pulmonary hydrostatic pressure; fluid administration and concomitant corticosteroids may also contribute). Arrhythmias may occur if halothane is subsequently used.

Other tocolytic drugs include oxytocin antagonists (e.g. atosiban, introduced in the UK in 2000). Atosiban has fewer side effects than β_2-agonists in preterm labour, although it is expensive; thus often reserved for cases at particular risk from the side effects of β_2-agonists (although it may cause nausea, vomiting, tachycardia and hypotension). Nifedipine, magnesium sulphate and inhibitors of prostaglandin synthesis, e.g. indometacin, also cause tocolysis but are not widely used in the UK. GTN patches have also been used. Acutely, GTN 100–400 μg iv or sublingually has been successfully used.
See also, Obstetric analgesia and anaesthesia

TOE, *see Transoesophageal echocardiography*

Tolazoline hydrochloride. α-Adrenergic receptor antagonist, structurally related to phentolamine. Traditionally used by iv infusion to relieve arterial spasm following accidental intra-arterial injection of thiopental. Also used to reduce pulmonary vascular resistance, e.g. in congenital diaphragmatic hernia.

- Dosage: 1 mg/kg.

Tolerance. Progressively decreasing response to repeated dosage of a drug. May result from altered number of receptors, altered response to receptor activation, altered pharmacokinetics (e.g. enzyme induction) or development of physiological compensatory mechanisms. Classically occurs with morphine.
See also, Tachyphylaxis

Tongue. Muscular organ attached to the hyoid bone and mandible. Covered by mucous membrane and divided into anterior ⅔ and posterior ⅓ by a V-shaped groove, the sulcus terminalis. At the latter's apex is a small depression, the foramen caecum. The lower surface is attached to the floor of the mouth by the frenulum.

- Muscles of the tongue:
  - genioglossus: fibres fan back from the superior genial spine of the mandible to the tip and whole length of the dorsum of the tongue. The lowest fibres attach to the hyoid bone.
  - hyoglossus: attached to the body and greater horns of the hyoid bone, passing upwards and forwards into the sides of the tongue.
  - palatoglossus and styloglossus: pass from the palate and styloid process respectively.
  - intrinsic muscles: include vertical, longitudinal and transverse fibres.
- Nerve supply:
  - sensory: glossopharyngeal nerve to the posterior ⅔ and facial nerve to the anterior ⅓.
  - motor: hypoglossal nerve.

The tone of genioglossus is important in preventing approximation of the tongue and posterior pharyngeal wall which results in airway obstruction. Genioglossus tone varies with respiration and is maximal in inspiration. It also decreases during sleep; this may contribute to the development of sleep apnoea. Anaesthetic and sedative agents decrease this tone and thus predispose to obstruction, which may be relieved by elevating the jaw, placing the patient in the lateral position, and use of pharyngeal airways.

Macroglossia predisposes to respiratory obstruction and may hinder tracheal intubation, e.g. in acromegaly and Down's syndrome. It may also occur after posterior fossa neurosurgery. Tongue piercing studs should be removed preoperatively.

Tongue forceps, *see Forceps*

Tonicity. Refers to the effective osmotic pressure of solutions in relation to that of plasma. Thus a urea solution may be isosmotic with plasma but its effective osmotic pressure (and thus tonicity) falls after infusion because urea distributes

evenly across cell membranes. Similarly, 5% dextrose solution is isosmotic with plasma but hypotonic when infused since the dextrose is metabolised by red blood cells leaving water.
See also, Intravenous fluids

Tonometry, gastric, *see Gastric tonometry*

Tonsil, bleeding. Haemorrhage usually occurs within a few hours postoperatively, but may be delayed.

- Problems include:
  - hidden blood loss if the patient (usually a child) swallows it; hypovolaemia may thus be severe before diagnosis is made.
  - risk of aspiration of gastric contents (mostly altered blood).
  - airway management and tracheal intubation may be difficult if bleeding is torrential.
  - significant amounts of the anaesthetic agents used previously may still be present.
  - possibility of an undiagnosed coagulation disorder.
- Management:
  - preoperative assessment of coagulation and cardiovascular status, with iv resuscitation. Nasogastric aspiration is controversial, since it may exacerbate bleeding.
  - experienced assistance is required. Each of the following techniques has its advocates:
    - inhalational induction in the left lateral position (with suction available), traditionally using halothane (but nowadays, often sevoflurane) in O_2, and tracheal intubation during spontaneous ventilation. The main advantage is the maintenance of spontaneous ventilation if intubation is difficult. However, induction may be prolonged and hindered by bleeding, gagging, etc., and the high concentrations of volatile agent required plus hypovolaemia may cause significant hypotension.
    - rapid sequence induction using a small dose of iv agent, e.g. thiopental followed by suxamethonium and intubation. Advantages of this technique include rapidity of intubation and the greater familiarity of most anaesthetists with it. However, it should only be attempted if intubation was easy at the initial operation. Hypotension may follow induction, and laryngoscopy may be difficult in torrential haemorrhage.
  - nasogastric aspiration is performed before extubation. This should be performed when the patient is awake and laryngeal reflexes have returned.

See also, Ear, nose and throat surgery; Induction, rapid sequence

Topical anaesthesia. Application of local anaesthetic agent to skin or mucous membranes to produce anaesthesia. Used on the skin, conjunctiva, nasal passages, larynx and pharynx, tracheobronchial tree, rectum and urethra. Local anaesthetic has also been instilled into the bladder, pleural cavity, peritoneal cavity and synovial fluid of joints.

Application may be via direct instillation, soaked swabs, pastes/ointments or sprays. Agents used include cocaine, lidocaine, tetracaine (amethocaine) and benzocaine. Systemic absorption may be rapid and the maximal safe doses should not be exceeded.
See also, EMLA cream; Iontophoresis

Torr. Unit of pressure; 1 torr = 1/760 atmosphere = 1 mmHg. [Evangelista Torricelli (1608–1647), Italian physicist]

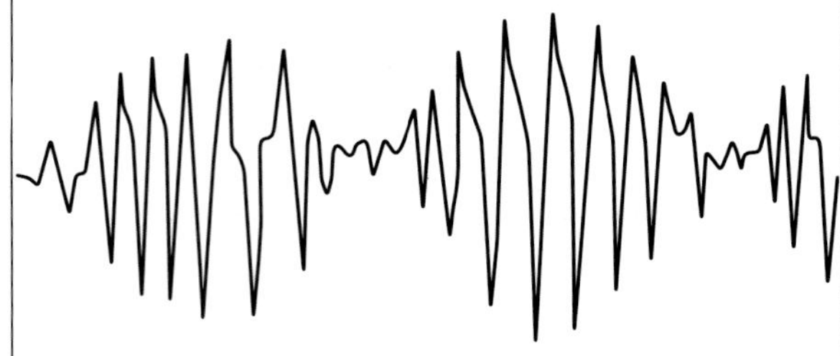

Fig. 154 Torsade de pointes

Torsade de pointes. Atypical VT characterised by polymorphic QRS complexes with repeated fluctuations of QRS axis, the complexes appearing to twist about the baseline (Fig. 154). Often associated with a prolonged Q–T interval. Initiated by a ventricular ectopic beat occurring during a prolonged pause after a previous ectopic.

- Causes include:
  - electrolyte abnormalities, e.g. hypokalaemia, hypomagnesaemia, hypocalcaemia.
  - drugs, e.g. class I antiarrhythmic drugs, tricyclic antidepressant drugs, phenothiazines.
  - heart disease.
- Treatment:
  - of predisposing condition.
  - cardioversion.
  - magnesium sulphate.
  - increasing the heart rate, e.g. isoprenaline, cardiac pacing.

Class I antiarrhythmic drugs should be avoided.

Total intravenous anaesthesia (TIVA). Anaesthetic technique employing iv agents alone, and avoiding the use of inhalational agents. Drugs are given usually by infusion to achieve hypnosis, analgesia and neuromuscular blockade (where required). The patient breathes O_2, air or a mixture of the two. The drugs chosen are usually of short action and half-life to reduce risk of accumulation and prolonged recovery. Examples include propofol, together with alfentanil, fentanyl or remifentanil. Ketamine has been used for its analgesic properties, e.g. together with midazolam. Neuroleptanaesthesia has also been used.

- Advantages:
  - avoids unwanted effects of inhalational anaesthetic agents.
  - avoids pollution by gases and vapours.
  - may be used without complex apparatus such as anaesthetic machines, cylinders, vaporisers, etc., e.g. in wars, etc.
- Disadvantages:
  - requires repeated injections or infusion devices, e.g. syringe pumps, etc.
  - prediction of plasma levels of anaesthetic agents is more difficult than with inhalational agents, because of the more complicated pharmacokinetics. Thus awareness or excessive dosage may occur unless one is familiar with the technique. Computer-assisted infusion has been employed to provide steady plasma levels according to pharmacokinetic data collected from hundreds of patients. The target-controlled infusion (TCI) device employs similar data to run a special syringe driver according to the patient's age, weight and desired blood propofol concentration, which are entered by the anaesthetist.

- once a drug has been infused, it cannot be removed from the body other than by metabolism and excretion. Thus there is less control than with inhalational agents, which may be removed by ventilation.

Total lung capacity. Volume of gas in the lungs after maximal inspiration. Normally approximately 6 litres. Determined by helium dilution (does not measure gas in poorly ventilated regions) or with the body plethysmograph.
See also, Lung volumes

Total parenteral nutrition, *see Nutrition, total parenteral*

Tourniquets. Used to reduce bleeding during limb surgery, and to allow IVRA. Inflated following exsanguination of the limb, e.g. by raising it for 2–3 min with the artery compressed, or by using a rubber Esmarch bandage. The latter increases CVP and may provoke cardiac failure in susceptible patients. It may also dislodge emboli from DVTs.

- Measures suggested to reduce compression and ischaemic damage:
  - inflation pressures:
    - arm: systolic BP + 50 mmHg (+ 100 mmHg for IVRA).
    - leg: systolic BP × 2.

    Suggested values vary, and depend partly on age, weight, etc.
  - inflation time: 2 h maximum is the most common recommendation, although 60 min for the arm and 90 min for the leg are often quoted. Periodic deflation and reinflation may allow longer use.

Equipment should be checked before use. Tourniquets should not be used in sickle cell anaemia (avoidance in sickle trait has also been suggested). Careful padding is required under the tourniquet. Skin preparation solutions may cause chemical burns if allowed to soak into the padding.
[Johann FA von Esmarch (1823–1908), German surgeon]
Kam PCA, Kavanaugh R, Yoong FFY (2001). Anaesthesia; 56: 534–45
See also, Compartment syndromes

Toxic epidermal necrolysis. Severe adverse drug reaction characterised by widespread epidermal erythema, blistering and necrosis. Fever and membrane involvement (e.g. pharyngitis, conjunctivitis) may precede the generalised skin reaction by 2–3 days. May rarely involve the oesophagus, rest of the GIT, tracheobronchial tree and kidney. Similar to, but more severe than, bullous ethythema multiforme and Stevens–Johnson syndrome but clinical features may overlap with the latter. Most common in the elderly and patients with HIV infection, SLE and following bone marrow transplantation.

Results in significant fluid loss, altered temperature regulation and increased susceptibility to infection. Management is supportive and along the lines of burns management. Corticosteroids have been used but without supporting evidence.
Chave TA, Mortimer NJ, Sladden MJ, et al (2005). Br J Dermatol; 153: 241–53

Toxic shock syndrome. Systemic illness associated with certain *Staphylococcus aureus* strains, thought to be caused by exotoxins (possibly with concurrent Gram-negative endotoxin production). Streptococci have also been implicated.

First described in 1978; the reported incidence increased around 1980, especially associated with menstruation and use of tampons. Features typically occur rapidly and include fever, hypotension, GIT upset, headache and myalgia. Generalised rash and/or oedema leads to desquamation 10–20 days later. Multiorgan failure may occur. Treatment is supportive, with antibacterial drug therapy.

TPN, Total parenteral nutrition, *see Nutrition, total parenteral*

TPR, Total peripheral resistance, *see Systemic vascular resistance*

Trachea, *see Tracheobronchial tree*

Tracheal administration of drugs. Has been used when iv administration is not possible, e.g. cardiac arrest. 2–3 times the iv dose, diluted in 10 ml saline, is injected via a catheter placed through the tracheal tube. Five manual hyperinflations aid dispersal of the drug. Atropine, adrenaline and lidocaine are the drugs most commonly administered in this way; isoprenaline and naloxone have also been given. Solutions which may cause local tissue damage should be avoided, e.g. calcium, bicarbonate. Many respiratory drugs are administered using inhalers and nebulisers.

Tracheal extubation, *see Extubation, tracheal*

Tracheal intubation, *see Intubation, tracheal*

Tracheal tubes. Developed along with techniques for tracheal intubation. O'Dwyer described his intubating tube in 1885, although various tubes had been used previously, e.g. for CPR. The modern wide bore tracheal tube was developed by Magill and Rowbotham after World War I, following the use of thin gum-elastic tubes for insufflation techniques. Separate tubes were placed into the trachea for delivery and removal of gases; these were eventually replaced by a single rubber ('Magill') tube. Red rubber tracheal tubes have largely been replaced by sterile disposable polyvinyl chloride tubes, since the former deteriorate on repeated sterilisation, are more costly to use, and are irritant to the respiratory mucosa. Plastic tubes soften as they warm, e.g. in the trachea; they may be softened in warm water, e.g. before nasal intubation.

- Features of 'typical' modern tracheal tubes (Fig. 155a):
  - marked with the following information:
    - size (internal diameter in mm; the external diameter may be marked in smaller lettering).
    - the letters IT or Z79-IT (for plastic tubes) denote that the material has been implantation tested in rabbit muscle for tissue compatibility, according to the American National Standards Committee which met in committee room no. Z79 in 1956.
    - the distance from the tip of the tube is marked at intervals along the tube's length. Most plastic tubes are longer than is usually required, and may be cut to size.
    - other markings may refer to the manufacturer, the trade name of the type of tube, and whether it is intended for oral or nasal use.

    A radio-opaque line is incorporated in most modern tubes, to aid detection on chest X-rays.
  - curved with a left-facing bevel at the distal end. There may be a hole in the wall opposite the bevel (Murphy eye) to allow ventilation should the end become obstructed by the tracheal wall or mucus.
  - attached to a tracheal tube connector at the proximal end.
  - may bear a cuff near the distal end, with a pilot balloon running towards the proximal end.

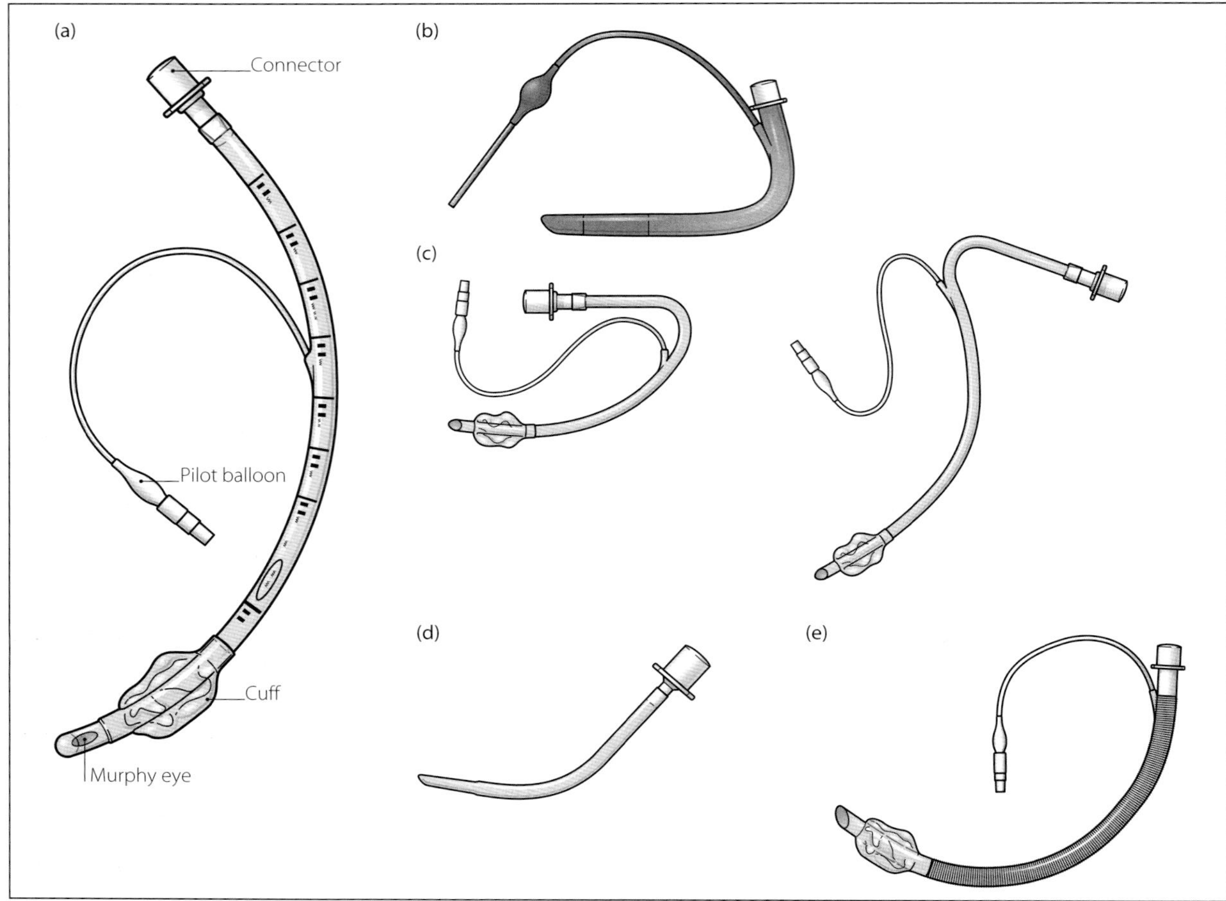

Fig. 155 Tracheal tubes: (a) 'typical'; (b) Oxford; (c) oral and nasal RAE; (d) Cole; (e) reinforced (not to scale)

- Other shapes and types of tubes (Fig. 155b–e):
  - Oxford tube: conforms more closely with the shape of the mouth and pharynx, thus less liable to kink. The bevel faces posteriorly; insertion of the tube is aided by a gum-elastic bougie protruding a short distance from the distal end. Traditionally made of red rubber, they are thicker walled than traditional red rubber tubes. Available with or without cuffs.
  - RAE tube: plastic; designed to be even more 'anatomically' shaped than the Oxford tube. Nasal RAE tubes are also available, as are other manufacturers' versions. Available with or without cuffs.
  - Cole tube: used in neonates. Shouldered, with thickened walls to prevent kinking. Designed to minimise resistance to flow of gas by virtue of their wide proximal portion; however, they increase resistance by causing turbulence at the junction with the narrow portion. They also may cause damage to the larynx and trachea if the shoulder is forced too far distally. Their avoidance has therefore been repeatedly suggested.
  - reinforced tubes: resemble standard tubes but contain a spiral of metal or nylon in the tube wall. Used where kinking of the tube may otherwise occur, e.g. neurosurgery, faciomaxillary surgery. Originally made of latex rubber, they are now commonly made of plastic. They cannot be cut to size. Available with or without cuffs. The silicone tube supplied with the intubating laryngeal mask airway is reinforced and has a tapered tip, making it easier to pass through the device without catching on the vocal cords or arytenoids. This tube is also easier to railroad over a fibreoptic scope than standard tracheal tubes.

Tubes may bear an extra channel for sampling of distal gases or for jet ventilation. A directional tube has also been described, in which traction on a ring at the proximal end flexes the distal end, aiding placement during tracheal intubation. Laser-protected tubes include tubes made totally out of metal and those coated with 'laser-proof' substances.

Size 9 mm and 8 mm tubes are often employed for men and women respectively, although smaller tubes have been suggested since larger tubes are associated with greater incidence of sore throat and hoarse voice. Average suitable length is 22–25 cm for oral tubes, and 25–28 cm for nasal tubes (*for sizes of tubes for children, see Paediatric anaesthesia*).

[Francis J Murphy (1900–1972), Detroit anaesthetist; Frank Cole (1918–1977), US anaesthetist; RAE: Wallace H Ring, John C Adair, Richard A Elwyn, Salt Lake City anaesthetists]

See also, Endobronchial tubes; Intubation, tracheal; Tracheostomy

Tracheobronchial suctioning. Required in patients who have a tracheal tube in place because of inability to mobilise secretions effectively. Also useful for investigative purposes, e.g. for obtaining sputum samples. The catheter should be inserted gently until resistance is felt, withdrawn slightly and suction applied whilst withdrawing. 'Closed' suction systems are used in the ICU setting to reduce the risk of bacterial contamination of the airway.

- Complications:
  - hypoxaemia: may be related to rapid removal of airway gases causing atelectasis, bronchospasm/coughing or disconnection from the ventilator. Particularly likely if the patient is PEEP dependent. Reduced by preoxygenation before and after suctioning, limitation of catheter size and use of self-contained suction catheters within the breathing system which avoid the need for disconnection.
  - atelectasis: reduced by avoiding excessive negative pressures and prolonged suction, and limiting the catheter size, e.g. appropriate size (FG) = 3 × (tracheal tube internal diameter ÷ 2).
  - trauma to airway mucosa, haemorrhage and oedema: reduced by careful technique, avoidance of excessive negative pressure, use of rounded-tipped catheters and intermittent rather than continuous suction. Special care should be taken in the presence of coagulopathy.
  - cross-infection/dispersal of infected material: reduced by sterile technique and self-contained suction equipment incorporating a catheter within the breathing tubing.
  - arrhythmias: may be related to hypoxaemia. Sinus bradycardia is especially common, via vagal stimulation.
  - increased ICP: inevitably follows suction; especially detrimental in patients with pre-existing raised ICP. May be reduced by increased sedation.

See also, Ciliary activity

Tracheobronchial tree. Branching system consisting of 23 generations of passages from trachea to alveoli, comprising:

- conducting airways: make up anatomical dead space:
  - trachea (generation 0): 10 cm long and 2 cm wide in the adult. Descends from the larynx level with C6, passing through the neck and thorax to its bifurcation level with T4–5 (at the level of the angle of Louis). Its walls are formed of fibrous tissue reinforced by 15–20 U-shaped cartilaginous rings (deficient posteriorly), united behind by fibrous tissue and smooth muscle. Lined with ciliated epithelium.

    Relations: lies anterior to the oesophagus, with the recurrent laryngeal nerve in the groove between them. In the neck (*see Fig. 110; Neck, cross-sectional anatomy*) it is crossed anteriorly by the isthmus of the thyroid gland. Laterally lie the lateral lobes of the thyroid, the inferior thyroid artery and carotid sheath (containing the internal jugular vein, common carotid artery and vagus nerve). In the thorax (*see Fig. 102b; Mediastinum*) it is crossed anteriorly by the brachiocephalic artery and vein. On the left lie the common carotid and subclavian arteries above, and the aorta below. On the right lie the mediastinal pleura, right vagus nerve and azygous vein.
  - right and left main bronchi (generation 1): arise at T4–5:
    - right: 3 cm long, and wider and more vertical than the left, and therefore likelier to receive inhaled foreign bodies. The right upper main bronchus arises about 2.5 cm from its origin.

      Relations: separated from the pericardium and superior vena cava by the right pulmonary artery. The azygous vein lies above.
    - left: about 5 cm long.

      Relations: separated from the left atrium by the left pulmonary artery. The aortic arch lies above, and the bronchial vessels posteriorly (separating it from the oesophagus and descending thoracic aorta).
  - lobar and segmental bronchi (generations 2–4) (Fig. 156).
  - small bronchi to terminal bronchioles (generations 5–16).
- respiratory airways:
  - respiratory bronchioles (generations 17–19): bear occasional alveoli.
  - alveolar ducts (generations 20–22): lined with alveoli.
  - alveoli (generation 23).

[Pierre CA Louis (1787–1872), French physician]

See also, Alveolus; Ciliary activity; Lung

Tracheo-oesophageal fistula (TOF). Oesophageal atresia occurs in 1:3000 births, with TOF in 25% of cases. Different forms exist (Fig. 157). Babies may be premature and have other congenital abnormalities. TOF may present with

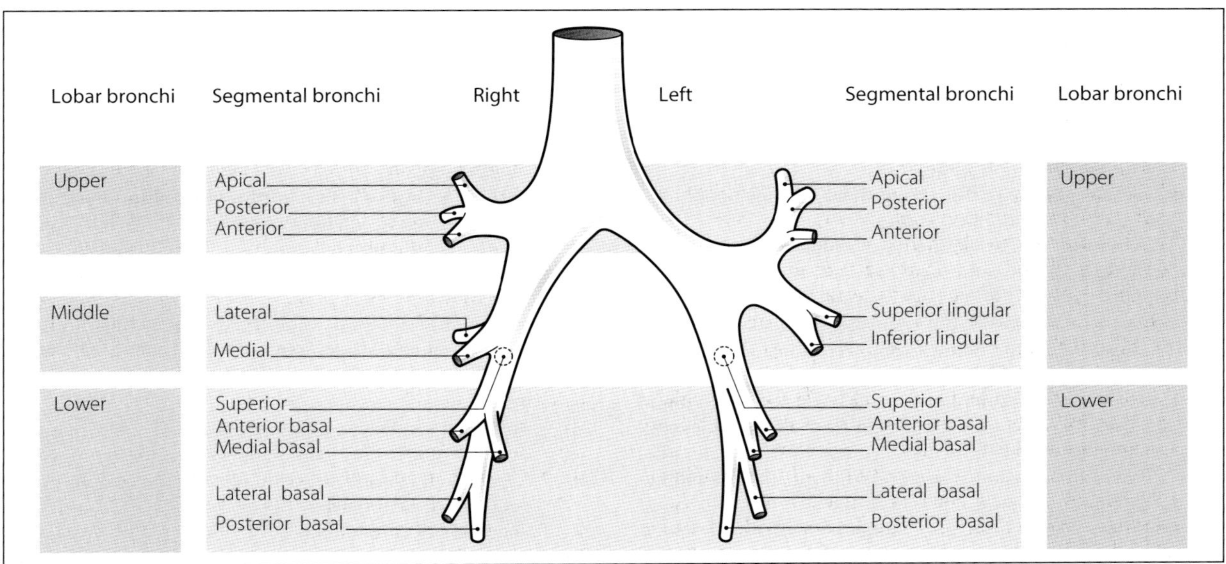

Fig. 156 Lobar and segmental bronchi

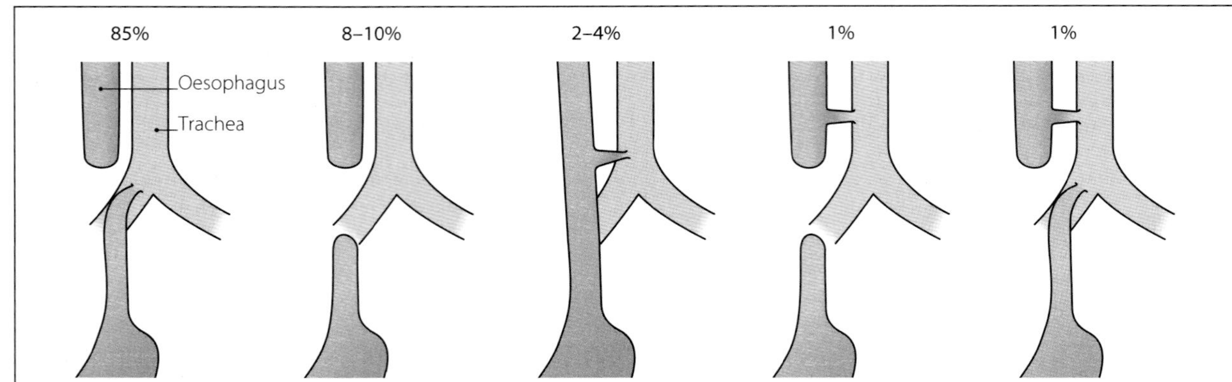

Fig. 157 Different forms of tracheo-oesophageal fistulae and their incidence

choking during feeds, production of copious frothy mucus from the mouth, or repeated chest infections following pulmonary aspiration. It is diagnosed by passing a radio-opaque nasogastric tube into the blind pouch; contrast medium is avoided because of risk of aspiration. Treated by surgery, performed via right thoracotomy. Primary anastomosis of the oesophagus is performed if possible.

- Anaesthesia is as for paediatric anaesthesia. In particular:
  - preoperatively:
    - the baby is nursed head-up, with continuous suction to the blind pouch to prevent pulmonary aspiration.
    - correction of electrolyte imbalance may be required.
  - perioperatively:
    - traditionally, tracheal intubation is performed awake, avoiding IPPV by facepiece to prevent gastric inflation. Intubation of the fistula may occur; if this happens the tracheal tube may be withdrawn and reinserted with the bevel direction altered. Positioning of the tip of the tube distal to the fistula prevents gastric inflation; this may be achieved by deliberate endobronchial intubation, followed by careful withdrawal of the tracheal tube until breath sounds are heard on both sides of the chest.
    - classically, neuromuscular blockade and IPPV are avoided until the chest is open, to prevent gastric distension. Many paediatric anaesthetists use gentle manual IPPV, since gastric distension is rare.
    - surgical manipulation may cause sudden increases in airway pressures or reductions in cardiac output.
  - postoperatively: IPPV may be required.

After repair, a blind passage may remain at the site of the fistula, making subsequent tracheal intubation difficult. Tracheomalacia may also occur.

Tracheostomy. First performed in the 1700s for upper airway obstruction. Modern indications:
  - prophylactic or therapeutic relief of airway obstruction.
  - to protect the tracheobronchial tree against aspiration of food, saliva, etc. when pharyngeal and laryngeal reflexes are obtunded, e.g. neurological disease.
  - to allow suction and removal of secretions.
  - prolonged IPPV in ICU. Cited advantages over conventional tracheal intubation include easier nursing management, improved patient comfort, ability for oral nutrition and speech, decreased incidence of sinusitis, and possibly assistance of weaning by a 30–50% reduction in dead space.

The traditional open procedure may be performed under general or local anaesthesia. The patient lies supine with the neck hyperextended, and a horizontal incision is made 1.5 cm below the level of the cricoid cartilage. After location of the trachea, a vertical incision is made through the 2nd, 3rd and 4th tracheal rings. A slit or circular opening is made in the trachea (creation of a tracheal flap has been implicated in causing tracheal stenosis). During general anaesthesia, ventilation with 100% O_2 should precede withdrawal of the tracheal tube (which is withdrawn into the larynx only, in case readvancement is required). The tracheostomy tube is then inserted. Stay sutures may be brought out on to the skin from the trachea, to aid subsequent tube reinsertion.

Increasingly, surgical tracheostomy is being replaced by the percutaneous procedure, especially in critically ill patients receiving IPPV (*see Tracheostomy, percutaneous*).

- Tracheostomy tubes:
  - uncuffed: plastic or metal (usually silver). They may allow speech if a one-way valve is used; air is drawn into the lungs through the tracheostomy and exhaled through the larynx and mouth. A fenestration in the tube improves the strength of the voice.
  - cuffed: plastic, with low pressure, high volume cuffs to minimise tracheal mucosal damage. The cuff may be deflated and the tube occluded with a finger during expiration, to allow speech. Cuffed tubes may also be fenestrated. Some incorporate a separate catheter opening just above the cuff, through which O_2 may be diverted using a manual control to allow speech. The catheter may also be used for suction.
- Complications may be early or late:
  - early:
    - haemorrhage, especially from branches of the anterior jugular veins or thyroid isthmus.
    - displacement of the tube: extrusion or endobronchial intubation.
    - blockage, e.g. by secretions, compression by the cuff or occlusion against the carina.
    - subcutaneous emphysema.
    - pneumothorax.
  - late:
    - infection, including superficial wound infection, tracheitis and chest infection.
    - tracheal erosion and ulceration, e.g. into blood vessels, oesophagus, etc.
    - tracheal stenosis; usually occurs level with the stoma or the tube's cuff, although subglottic stenosis may also occur. Surgical resection may be required.
    - tracheal dilatation may occur.
- Tracheostomy care includes:
  - humidification: vital to reduce risk of obstruction by viscous secretions.

- tracheobronchial suctioning: sterile technique is mandatory. The suction catheter's diameter should not exceed half that of the tracheostomy tube. Suction is applied on withdrawal, not insertion, of the catheter.
- daily cleaning and dressing to reduce risk of infection.
- secure fixation, e.g. with double tapes.
- presence of tracheal dilators, spare tracheostomy tubes, and equipment for manual ventilation and tracheal intubation, in case of displacement.
- provision of a means of communication, e.g. pen and paper.

The initial tube is usually left in situ for at least a week, to allow formation of a tract. Changing may be assisted by removing and inserting tubes over a thin catheter. Once decannulated, the stoma usually closes spontaneously within a few days, but surgical closure may be required.
See also, Minitracheotomy

Tracheostomy, percutaneous. Increasingly used in critically ill patients requiring tracheostomy instead of the traditional open procedure because of the following advantages:
- may be performed in the ICU or other clinical area, thus avoiding transfer of critically ill patients to the operating suite.
- does not require a surgeon.
- may be quicker in skilled hands.
- may be associated with fewer complications.
- provides an opportunity for teaching emergency access to the airway (i.e. percutaneous location of the trachea).

Generally avoided in children and in the presence of coagulopathy, localised infection and difficult anatomy.
- Methods:
  - initial preparation and positioning as for the open procedure.
  - following infiltration with local anaesthetic, a small vertical incision is made over the space between the first/second tracheal rings and the trachea located with a syringe and cannula (the tracheal tube is withdrawn into the larynx under direct vision to avoid damage). Fibreoptic endoscopy has been used to confirm correct needle placement but may result in damage to the 'scope.
  - the cannula is left in the trachea, a wire advanced through it and the cannula withdrawn.
  - blunt dissection of the superficial tissues is performed using artery forceps. Some operators would regard blunt dissection down to the trachea, prior to location of the tracheal lumen with the needle and subsequent cannulation, as being a safer technique. Once the wire is in place in the trachea, different methods of passing the tracheostomy tube have been described:
    - serial dilatation method: special dilators are slid over the wire, starting with 12 FG and proceeding up to 36 FG depending on the size of tracheostomy tube, which is finally passed into the trachea mounted on the appropriate dilator.
    - single dilatation (Ciaglia) method: a specially formed smooth dilator, with a progressively larger diameter along its length, is slid over the wire. After a single-pass dilatation, the tracheostomy tube is passed into the trachea mounted on the same dilator. A related method involves a conical threaded dilator that is 'screwed' into place over a guidewire akin to a self-tapping screw.
    - dilating forceps (Griggs) method: a special pair of curved forceps, incorporating a groove in the opposing surfaces of its jaws, is slid over the wire with the jaws closed. The forceps are then opened outside the trachea to dilate the soft tissues before being closed and passed into the trachea. They are then opened forcibly within the trachea and removed whilst still open; the tracheostomy tube is then passed over the wire into the trachea.
    - translaryngeal tracheostomy method: a guidewire is passed retrogradely into the mouth via a percutaneous needle in the trachea, under bronchoscopic control. A reinforced flexible tube with a cuff at its proximal end and a cone-shaped dilator fixed to its distal end is then passed over the guidewire from the mouth and pulled out through the front of the neck; the cone portion is then removed and the tube manipulated so that the intratracheal portion (bearing the cuff) passes caudally to lie in the standard tracheostomy tube position.

Complications are as for open surgery; initial studies suggest their incidence is low. Tracheal tears may occur with all the above methods.
[Pasquale Ciaglia (1912–2000), US thoracic surgeon; Bill Griggs, Australian intensivist]

Train-of-four nerve stimulation, *see Neuromuscular blockade monitoring*

TRALI, Transfusion related acute lung injury, *see Blood transfusion*

Tramadol hydrochloride. Opioid analgesic drug, introduced in the UK in 1994 but used in continental Europe for several years. A pure agonist at mu opioid receptors, it is also a delta and kappa receptor agonist; it also inhibits noradrenaline uptake and enhances 5-HT release. Undergoes renal and metabolic elimination. Half-life is about 6 h (increased in the elderly).
- Dosage:
  - 50–100 mg orally 4–6 hourly up to 400 mg/day for short courses. A slow-release formulation is available: 100–200 mg once/twice daily. A combined preparation with paracetamol is also available (37.5 mg tramadol with 325 mg paracetamol): 1–2 tablets 6 hourly.
  - 50–100 mg im/slowly iv 4–6 hourly (up to 250 mg in divided doses as initial dose for postoperative pain, up to 600 mg/day).
- Side effects: nausea, vomiting, dizziness, dry mouth, sweating, confusion and hallucinations, respiratory depression, sedation (the latter two less commonly than with morphine). Drug dependence and withdrawal have been reported, especially following prolonged treatment. Convulsions have been reported, especially in combination with other drugs known to reduce seizure threshold, e.g. tricyclic antidepressants and selective serotonin reuptake inhibitors. Has been implicated in increasing awareness if given during anaesthesia.

Tranexamic acid. Antifibrinolytic drug, used to reduce bleeding, e.g. in prostatectomy, menorrhagia or dental extraction in haemophiliacs; it has also been used in streptokinase overdose and hereditary angioneurotic oedema.
- Dosage: 1.0–1.5 g orally, 6–8 hourly for 3–4 days; 0.5–1.0 g slowly iv, 8 hourly.
- Side effects: GIT disturbances, dizziness. Contraindicated in thromboembolic disease.

Transcranial Doppler ultrasound (TCD). Application of ultrasound to visualise cerebral vessels. A low frequency (2 MHz) pulse range-gated ultrasound beam is directed

through the thin-boned transtemporal window; this allows assessment of the middle and anterior cerebral arteries of the cerebral circulation. Using the Doppler effect, flow velocities within these vessels can be determined. Uses include the detection of cerebral vasospasm following subarachnoid haemorrhage, assessment of cerebral blood flow (e.g. in head injury, carotid artery surgery) and the detection of air embolism. Has also been used to assess cerebral autoregulation.
Moppett IK, Mahajan RP (2004). Br J Anaesth; 93: 710–24

Transcutaneous electrical nerve stimulation (TENS). Stimulation of peripheral nerves via cutaneous electrodes, to relieve pain. Based on the gate control theory of pain transmission; i.e. stimulation of Aβ fibres (by high frequency TENS) and Aδ fibres (by low frequency TENS) inhibits pain transmission by C fibres. Current is provided by a battery-powered pulse generator which typically delivers a range of currents (0–50 mA), frequencies (0–200 Hz) and pulse widths (0.1–0.5 ms). Rectangular pulses are usually employed. Surface electrodes are usually carbon-impregnated silicone rubber.

The electrodes are placed either side of the painful area or its supplying nerves, and the current increased until tingling is felt. Experimentation with timing and duration is usually required to achieve maximal effects.

Has been used successfully in acute pain (e.g. for fractured ribs, labour, postoperatively, etc.), but is usually employed for chronic pain management (peripheral nerve disorders, spinal cord and root disorders, muscle pain and joint pain). Efficacy is difficult to assess as there is significant placebo effect, but TENS may significantly reduce analgesic requirements.

Allergic dermatitis at electrode sites may occur. Contraindicated in patients with pacemakers.

Transducers. Devices which convert one form of energy to another, usually to electricity in monitoring systems.
- May be:
  - passive: involving changes in:
    - resistance, e.g. strain gauge, thermistor, photoresistor.
    - inductance, e.g. pressure transducers.
    - capacitance, e.g. condenser microphone.
  - active, i.e. involving generation of potentials:
    - piezoelectric effect: generation of voltage across the faces of a quartz crystal when deformed.
    - photoelectric cell.
    - thermocouple.
    - radiation counters.
    - electrode potentials, e.g. pH electrode.
    - electromagnetic induction.

See also, Arterial blood pressure measurement; Damping; pH measurement; Pressure measurement; Temperature measurement

Transfer factor, *see Diffusing capacity*

Transfusion, *see Blood transfusion*

Transfusion-related acute lung injury, *see Blood transfusion*

Transient radicular irritation syndrome (Transient neurologic syndrome). Pain and dysaesthesia in the buttock, thighs or calves following spinal anaesthesia; usually occurs within 24 h of the block and typically resolves within 72 h. Related especially to the use of lidocaine, particularly associated with hyperbaric solutions in higher concentrations (2.5–5%) and use of very narrow-gauge needles or microcatheters, which result in pooling of the drug around sensitive nerve roots. The lithotomy position has also been implicated, via stretching of the lumbosacral nerve roots and increasing their vulnerability. The syndrome may reflect a transient form of cauda equina syndrome following continuous spinal anaesthesia.
Pollock JE (2002). Reg Anesth Pain Med; 27: 581–6

Transoesophageal echocardiography (TOE). Form of echocardiography allowing imaging of the heart in a variety of different planes without requiring access to the chest. Increasingly used to assess cardiac function in awake, anaesthetised and critically ill patients. Basic principles are as for echocardiography and ultrasound, combined with the ability to manipulate the probe's tip and place it under the heart within the stomach, behind the heart in the oesophagus or anywhere in between. Views may be obtained of the left and right atria and ventricles (both transversely and longitudinally), all valves and outflow tracts, and proximal aorta and pulmonary vessels.

Can be used to detect structural abnormalities, myocardial ischaemia or MI (manifest by changes in segmental wall motion), presence of valve vegetations, pericarditis, aortic abnormalities, etc. Doppler analysis allows estimation of blood flows and cardiac output. Commonly used perioperatively during cardiac surgery, especially for:
- assessment of the mitral valve pre- and post-repair.
- detecting perivalvular leaks after valve replacement.
- determining the position/extent of aortic atheromatous plaques or dissection.
- removal of intracardiac air before coming off cardiopulmonary bypass.
- guiding fluid therapy and assessing myocardial contractility.
- guiding the position of an intra-arterial balloon pump distal to the left subclavian artery.

Also used in high-risk patients undergoing non-cardiac surgery, and in ICU and emergency departments.

Complications include dental, pharyngeal and oesophageal trauma and cardiovascular disturbances. Contraindicated in oesophageal disease and upper GIT bleeding.
Kneeshaw JD (2006). Br J Anaes; 97: 77–84

Transplantation. Use of cadaveric or live donor tissues has increased with improved techniques and introduction of immunosuppressive drugs such as ciclosporin.
- Main points:
  - identification of donors and matching with recipients. There may be underutilisation of potential donor organs following brainstem death in some ICUs.
  - organ donation.
  - preoperative state of the recipient, surgical procedure and postoperative course.
  - chronic physical and psychological effects of transplantation, drug therapy and possible organ rejection.

See also, Heart–lung transplantation; Heart transplantation; Liver transplantation; Lung transplantation; Renal transplantation

Transportation of critically ill patients. May be primary (from site of injury or illness to hospital, e.g. by ambulance) or secondary (from one ICU to another). Up to 10 000 interhospital transfers of critically ill patients occur per year in the UK.
- Reasons include:
  - upgrade in the level of care required (e.g. for specialist surgery, dialysis, etc.).

- to obtain a specialised investigation unavailable in the base hospital.
- local lack of ICU resources (no bed available).
- repatriation of ICU patients to units closer to the patient's normal residence.

Ideally, transfer and retrieval systems should be planned and coordinated at local, regional and national levels, with adequate funding, clear guidelines and communication channels, and a transport coordinator (Consultant) identified in each hospital. Considerable stabilisation may be required prior to transfer, avoiding transfer of unstable patients. All relevant notes and radiographs should accompany the patient.

- Requirements:
  - vehicle: standard ambulance or a specifically designed mobile ICU. Dedicated aircraft have been used.
  - team: should be experienced in transporting critically ill patients. Includes a suitably senior doctor, assistant (ICU nurse, ODP, nurse, etc.) and driver/pilot, ± other staff for ongoing training. All team members should be clearly identified using special clothing.
  - equipment: should be robust, lightweight and portable, including a ventilator (allowing SIMV and PEEP), monitors (as for any anaesthetic/ICU), O_2 (possibly liquid), defibrillator, infusion pumps/syringe drivers, anaesthetic/resuscitation drugs and all necessary disposables. All equipment should be battery operated with battery lengths appropriate to the journey duration. Adequate communication includes a mobile telephone. A mobile ICU stretcher makes transfer easier.

Other aspects include audit of transfers (there should be documentation of transfer events and any critical incidents) and team insurance. Although in general, patients' relatives should not travel with the patient, arrangements should be made for them to travel and be warmly received at the receiving hospital. Patients may also require transfer between departments in a single hospital, e.g. from ICU to the radiology department for imaging. Similar considerations apply to those above.

See also, Safe transport and retrieval

Transposition of the great arteries. Accounts for 5% of congenital heart disease. Caused by failure of the truncus arteriosus to rotate during embryological development. The aorta arises from the right ventricle and the pulmonary artery from the left ventricle. Thus the pulmonary and systemic circulations work independently, resulting in severe hypoxaemia. Survival is only possible if a connection exists between the two circulations, e.g. ASD, VSD or patent ductus arteriosus. Other malpositions of the great arteries may occur.

Features include cyanosis, early cardiac failure and right ventricular hypertrophy, with normal pulmonary and systemic pressures. 85–90% of infants die within a year without treatment.

- Treatment:
  - palliation: shunt procedures, e.g. creation of an ASD by balloon septostomy or surgery.
  - correction: use of baffles, e.g. Mustard procedure: redirection of vena caval flow into the left atrium, and pulmonary venous blood into the right atrium, using a pericardial patch. The right ventricle thus supplies the systemic circulation. Systemic venous obstruction and poor long-term right ventricular function have led to increased use of procedures which switch the pulmonary and systemic circulations, at ventricular or arterial levels.

[William T Mustard (1914–1987), Toronto surgeon]

Transpulmonary thermodilution cardiac output measurement, *see Cardiac output measurement*

Transurethral resection of the prostate (TURP). Cystoscopic procedure for the removal of hypertrophied prostatic tissue; concerns about increased long-term morbidity have led to a recent increase in open prostatectomy although this is controversial.

- Anaesthetic considerations:
  - preoperative assessment: most patients are elderly, with coexisting disease. Some may have prostatic malignancy with systemic manifestations; oestrogen therapy may cause fluid retention. Renal impairment may be present.
  - use of irrigating solution (usually glycine) may result in the TURP syndrome. Absorption rates of irrigating solution of up to 240 ml/min have been reported. Suggested monitoring includes measurement of the volume of irrigation in and out of the patient, the patient's weight, or plasma sodium, osmolality, isotopes (for research only) or ethanol added to the irrigation bag (10%), the latter usually measured via a breath analyser which gives an estimation of plasma ethanol concentration. A drop in plasma sodium concentration of > 10 mmol/l or a plasma ethanol concentration of > 0.6 mg/ml suggests absorption of more than 2 l fluid, and surgery should be stopped.

    Use of saline is possible with bipolar diathermy and reduces the risk of dilutional hyponatraemia, though fluid (saline) overload may still occur.
  - positioning of the patient in lithotomy position, with restricted ventilation and increased venous return. Venous pooling in the legs may occur when the legs are brought down at the end of the procedure, with possible hypotension.
  - blood loss may be major but is difficult to assess. Portable photometric devices may be used to estimate haemoglobin concentration in the irrigating fluid. Transfusion has been suggested if resection time exceeds 1 h.
  - hypothermia may contribute to the features of the TURP syndrome. Irrigating fluid should be warmed since this may be a major route of heat loss.
  - postoperative complications are common and include urinary and chest infections, sepsis and haemorrhage.
  - mortality is up to 6%, usually due to peri- and postoperative MI.

General or regional techniques may be used. Postoperative course is generally considered to be better with the latter (spinal or epidural anaesthesia), which also allow monitoring of CNS function during the procedure.

Transversus abdominis plane block. Block of the nerves supplying the anterior abdominal wall by deposition of local anaesthetic agent in the fascial plane between the internal oblique and transversus abdominis muscles.

With the patient supine, a blunt needle is inserted perpendicular to the skin just cranial to the iliac crest and just anterior to the edge of the latissimus dorsi muscle. A resistance is felt as the external oblique aponeurosis is encountered, followed by a 'give' as it is pierced and a second 'give' as the needle passes through the internal oblique aponeurosis. After aspiration, 20 ml solution (e.g. 0.25–0.5% bupivacaine) is injected.

McDonnell JG, O'Donnell BD, Farrell T, et al (2007). Reg Anesth Pain Med; 32: 399–404

See also, Abdominal field block, Rectus sheath block

Trauma. Most common cause of death in young adults in the UK and USA, and the third commonest cause overall.

Management has been consistently shown to be inadequate in many cases, exacerbated by poor coordination of resources. Care in some countries, e.g. USA, West Germany and Australia, is better organised than in the UK (e.g. 20% of deaths were considered preventable in recent Royal College of Surgeons of England reports). Hypoxia and missed diagnoses were common.

- Improved results are thought to require:
  - improved prehospital care and transport, e.g. involving helicopters (used in many countries); possibly doctors should accompany emergency vehicles. The debate concerning stabilisation at the scene of the accident versus 'scoop and run' continues.
  - centralised trauma centres, with full facilities for CPR, imaging and surgery within one unit, to handle severe injuries. Patients would present directly from accidents or via referring hospitals, which would deal with less severe trauma cases. Emergency, anaesthetic, ICU, orthopaedic, neurosurgical, cardiothoracic and general surgical staff should be available at all times.
  - use of trauma scales and triage to facilitate appropriate management, especially in major incidents.
- Management of individual cases:
  - initial rapid assessment and CPR. O_2 administration and large iv cannulae are mandatory. Cervical spine injury should be assumed until proven otherwise, and the neck immobilised with a collar. Full stomach and alcohol intake are likely. Antigravity suits may be useful in severe blood loss, especially prior to hospital. Life-threatening conditions requiring immediate detection and treatment include:
    - airway obstruction.
    - tension or open pneumothorax, haemothorax.
    - flail chest.
    - hypovolaemia.
    - cardiac tamponade.
  - further assessment:
    - examination of the patient's face and head, spine, chest, abdomen and limbs, including the back (the patient should be unclothed).
    - type of injury is important, e.g.:
      - penetrating injury: internal damage is likely, especially with high velocity missiles.
      - blunt injury: crushing, shearing damage and fractures may result. Speed of collision, height of fall, etc. are important.
      - burns/blast injury, etc.
    - trauma scales/triage.
  - specific management as for haemorrhage, head injury, chest trauma, spinal cord injury, abdominal trauma, pelvic trauma; coexistent conditions, e.g. smoke inhalation, aspiration of gastric contents, hypothermia, eye injury may be present. Intra-abdominal bleeding may be revealed by peritoneal lavage.
  - continuous monitoring of pulse, BP, urine output, neurological signs, CVP, etc. Pulse oximetry is particularly useful.
  - imaging, e.g. X-ray, CT scanning, etc., as appropriate.
  - analgesia, e.g. Entonox, local blocks, iv opioids.
  - late problems:
    - fat embolism: classically occurs on the second day; its incidence may be reduced if fractures are fixed early.
    - DVT: classically during the second week.
    - wound infection: tetanus prophylaxis and antibiotics are given as appropriate; staphylococcal, streptococcal and anaerobic infections are most common.
    - chest infection/ARDS.
    - those associated with massive blood transfusion.
    - renal impairment, e.g. associated with hypotension, crush syndrome, etc.
    - catabolism may be marked after multiple trauma.
- Anaesthesia may be required for fixation of fractures, removal of foreign bodies, cleaning/debridement/suturing of wounds, evacuation of clot, control of internal haemorrhage, skin grafting, etc. Problems:
  - nature of injury.
  - alcohol or other drugs.
  - gastric emptying is reduced by trauma; the time between last oral intake and injury is more important than the time between intake and surgery.
  - hypovolaemia.
  - risk of massive hyperkalaemia following suxamethonium administration; time of onset is related to the nature of injury.

Adequate resuscitation is required first unless surgery is lifesaving; risks of delayed surgery are weighed against anaesthetic risks. Regional techniques may be useful if no contraindications exist. Sedation should be avoided in head injury. Postoperative care should be on ICU/HDU unless injury is minor.

Recommendations now exist for the uniform reporting of data following major trauma using an Utstein style system.

See also, Emergency surgery; Transportation of critically ill patients

Trauma scales. Scoring systems developed to aid assessment and triage of trauma cases, prediction of outcome, comparison between centres/countries. Several have been described:

- primarily used for triage: need to be simple and quick to perform; examples include:
  - Glasgow coma scale.
  - trauma score and revised trauma score.
  - circulation, respiration, abdomen, motor and speech scale.
  - prehospital index.
  - AVPU.
  - paediatric trauma score.
- primarily used for outcome prediction: need to be more detailed; examples include:
  - injury severity score.
  - trauma revised injury severity score.
  - abbreviated injury scale.
  - a severity characterisation of trauma.
  - international classification injury severity score.

Steele A, Bocconi GA, Oggioni R, Tulli G (1998). Curr Anaesth Crit Care; 9: 8–15

See also, Audit; Mortality/survival prediction on intensive care unit

Trauma score. Scoring system based on the Glasgow coma score, systolic BP, respiratory rate and effort, and capillary refill. Each is awarded points between 0–1 and 1–5, giving a total of 1–16 with 16 the best possible. Originally presented as a means of triage, with transfer of patients scoring under 12 to a trauma centre. Since capillary refill and respiratory effort may be difficult to assess in the field, they have been removed in the revised trauma score.

Trauma revised injury severity score (TRISS). Trauma scale combining the revised trauma score (RTS), injury severity score (ISS), age and type of injury in an attempt to improve the individual scoring systems' usefulness. Used primarily in audit since it provides a probability of survival and thus comparison against actual survival rates. Revised trauma and injury severity scores are each weighted by a coefficient depending on whether injury was blunt or penetrating, and the result adjusted again by a factor accounting for the patient's age.

Traumatic neurotic syndrome. Psychological diagnosis applied to patients whose claims of awareness during anaesthesia were met with professional denial, before the possibility of awareness was fully appreciated by anaesthetists. Sharing features with a general post-traumatic stress syndrome, it was characterised by recurrent nightmares, anxiety, irritability, preoccupation with death, and fear of insanity. An excellent prognosis was possible once the patient's experience was accepted by health workers.

Treacher Collins syndrome, *see Facial deformities, congenital*

TREM-1 (Triggering receptor expressed on myeloid cells-1). Immunoglobulin molecule thought to be involved in, and to amplify, the inflammatory pathway that is activated in sepsis. Cohen J (2001). Lancet; 358: 776–7

Triage. Sorting of patients according to severity of injury in order to maximise total number of survivors. Usually refers to trauma cases in battles or major incidents, although similar approaches have been used in other fields of acute medicine, e.g. chest pain. First used during Napoleon's Russian campaign by Larrey, who scored soldiers according to their need for medical treatment, treating the most severely injured first. Modern triage systems give first priority to those patients who might survive only if treated, leaving until later those expected to die even if treated, and those expected to survive even without treatment.

- Many systems exist, but most divide survivors into:
  - 1st priority: immediate treatment/transfer required.
  - 2nd priority: treatment urgent, but with stabilisation first.
  - 3rd priority: minor injury, e.g. 'walking wounded'.
  - 4th priority: expected to die, therefore low priority.

Triage is helped by using trauma scales, with sorting according to score. Attention is also paid to the mechanism of injury. Some systems include colour-coded labels with details of injuries, treatments, etc., to be attached to patients. Triage may be repeated at different stages of retrieval and treatment, e.g. at the scene of accident, at the receiving hospital, on wards, etc.; thus patients may change in priority as circumstances change.

Trials, clinical, *see Clinical trials*

Tribavirin, *see Ribavirin*

Tricarboxylic acid cycle (Citric acid cycle; Krebs cycle). Final common pathway for oxidation of carbohydrate, fat and some amino acids to CO_2 and water. Consists of a sequence of reactions which occur within mitochondria and require O_2. Acetylcoenzyme A (containing two carbon atoms) enters the cycle, having been formed from fat metabolism or glycolysis via pyruvate (Fig. 158). At each step where a carbon atom is lost, CO_2 is produced. For each turn of the cycle, 15 ATP molecules are formed via transfer of hydrogen atoms to the cytochrome oxidase system or formation of guanosine triphosphate (including the two ATP molecules generated by conversion of pyruvate to acetylcoenzyme A).

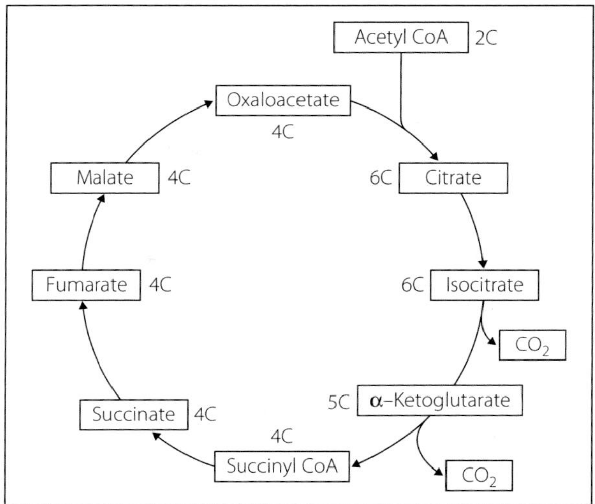

Fig. 158 Tricarboxylic acid cycle

[Hans A Krebs (1900–1981), German-born English biochemist]

Trichloroethylene. CCl_2CHCl. Inhalational anaesthetic agent, synthesised in 1864 and used clinically in 1935; withdrawn from commercial manufacture in the UK in 1988. Similar smell and properties to chloroform (hence coloured with waxoline blue to distinguish them). Decomposed by light, and stabilised by thymol 0.01%. Interacts with soda lime to form dichloroacetylene (C_2Cl_2) at 60°C. The latter compound is a potent neurotoxin, and may cause temporary or permanent damage to the cranial nerves, especially V and VII. Very soluble in blood (blood/gas partition coefficient of 9); induction and recovery are thus slow. Extremely potent (MAC 0.17) and a powerful analgesic. Previously popular in obstetrics as an analgesic agent, and for providing analgesia during IPPV; traditionally used instead of N_2O by the Armed Forces (e.g. in the triservice apparatus). Cardiovascularly stable, it sensitises the myocardium to catecholamines and PONV are common.

Triclofos. Related drug to chloral hydrate. Metabolised to trichloroethanol as is chloral hydrate.

- Dosage: 1–2 g orally in adults; 25–30 mg/kg in children < 1 year; 250 mg–1.0 g in children aged 1–12 years.
- Side effects: as for chloral hydrate but causes fewer GIT side effects.

Tricuspid valve lesions. Tricuspid stenosis is usually associated with mitral stenosis and aortic valve disease resulting from rheumatic fever; may also coexist with pulmonary stenosis in the carcinoid syndrome. Isolated tricuspid stenosis is very rare.

- Features:
  - increased right atrial pressure with peripheral oedema and hepatomegaly.
  - prominent 'a' wave in the jugular venous waveform.
  - mid- and late diastolic heart murmur, heard best in inspiration at the left lower sternal edge.
  - right atrial enlargement may be shown on chest X-ray and ECG.

Tricuspid regurgitation usually results from right ventricular enlargement, e.g. in right-sided cardiac failure. Usually causes little clinical impairment.

- Features:
  - large systolic wave in the jugular venous waveform.
  - pansystolic murmur at the left lower sternal edge.

Anaesthetic considerations are related more to the accompanying mitral and aortic lesions than to the tricuspid lesion itself.

See also, Ebstein's anomaly

Tricyclic antidepressant drug poisoning. Accounts for about 10% of cases of poisoning. Newer drugs (e.g. selective serotonin reuptake inhibitors) have better safety profiles.

- Features:
  - tachycardia, hypotension; impaired myocardial contractility and conduction may cause AF, widening of the QRS complex, heart block, VT and VF.
  - severe metabolic acidosis may occur.
  - agitation, hyperreflexia, hallucinations, convulsions, coma, blurred vision, urinary retention, pyrexia.
- Management:
  - ICU admission has been suggested at plasma levels > 1 mg/ml or when QRS complex duration exceeds 100 ms.
  - as for general poisoning and overdoses, including measures to prevent gastric absorption.
  - ECG monitoring is usually recommended for at least 12–24 h.
  - induction of alkalaemia (pH > 7.5) has been used to reduce the amount of free drug, e.g. with bicarbonate or hyperventilation. β-Adrenergic receptor antagonists have been used in ventricular tachyarrhythmias; cardiac pacing may be required for bradyarrhythmias. Physostigmine has been used to restore consciousness and slow the heart rate although this is controversial and convulsions have occurred following its use.

See also, Tricyclic antidepressant drugs

Tricyclic antidepressant drugs. Group of antidepressant drugs; the term includes several newer 1-, 2- and 4-ring structured drugs with similar actions. Competitively block reuptake of noradrenaline by postganglionic sympathetic nerve endings. Also have CNS anticholinergic properties. Used in depression and pain management; analgesic properties are thought to be associated with impairment of 5-HT reuptake (e.g. especially by amitriptyline and clomipramine). Many cause sedation, e.g. amitriptyline, dosulepin (dothiepin), mianserin, trazodone and trimipramine. Sedation is less likely with clomipramine, nortriptyline, imipramine and desipramine.

2–4 weeks' therapy is required before their effect is apparent. Half-lives may be up to 48 h. Metabolised in the liver and excreted renally.

- Anaesthetic considerations: increased sensitivity to catecholamines may result in hypertension and arrhythmias following administration of sympathomimetic drugs. Ventricular arrhythmias may occur with high concentrations of volatile anaesthetic agents, especially halothane.

See also, Tricyclic antidepressant drug poisoning

Trigeminal nerve blocks, *see Gasserian ganglion block; Mandibular nerve blocks; Maxillary nerve blocks; Nose; Ophthalmic nerve blocks*

Trigeminal neuralgia (Tic douloureux). Chronic pain state characterised by brief, severe lancinating pain involving the trigeminal nerve distribution. Usually involves the mandibular division; may also involve the glossopharyngeal nerve. Pain tends to be unilateral during the acute attack, which may be triggered by non-noxious stimulation of the ipsilateral nasal or perioral region (sometimes restricted to one specific zone). There is minimal or no sensory loss in the trigeminal distribution. Pain-free intervals typically separate attacks, which may be so severe as to cause suicide. Aetiology is uncertain although it may involve a structural abnormality in the trigeminal root adjacent to the pons.

- Treatment includes:
  - drugs, including carbamazepine (beneficial in 70% of cases), phenytoin, clonazepam, tricyclic antidepressant drugs, gabapentin and simple analgesics.
  - trigeminal nerve blocks.
  - surgical decompression of the trigeminal nerve.
  - destructive lesions, e.g. with alcohol injection, radiofrequency coagulation, or surgical destruction. Anaesthesia dolorosa may ensue.
  - acupuncture.

Nurmikko TJ, Eldridge PR (2001). Br J Anaesth; 87: 117–32

See also, Gasserian ganglion block

Trigger points. Areas in muscle or fascia; may be latent (tender when palpated) or active (painful at rest or on exertion or stretching). Mechanical stimulation may cause muscle weakness and/or local twitching. Pain is often referred, giving rise to myofascial pain syndromes. Examination may reveal tender nodules within taut bands of muscle, felt especially if the fingertips are moved perpendicular to the direction of muscle fibres. May be numerous, and may correspond to traditional acupuncture points. Local anaesthetic injection and acupuncture may relieve symptoms.

Trimeprazine, *see Alimemazine*

Trimetaphan camsylate. Ganglion blocking drug, no longer generally available in the UK, used to lower BP during hypotensive anaesthesia. Its hypotensive effect is enhanced by a direct relaxant action on vascular smooth muscle and by histamine release from mast cells. Rapid onset and offset, thus usually given by iv infusion. Compensatory tachycardia is common. Tachyphylaxis may occur. Partially broken down by plasma cholinesterase and may have prolonged action in patients with decreased activity of this enzyme.

Trimethoprim. Antibacterial drug used especially in urinary tract infections, exacerbations of COPD and in combination with the sulphonamide sulfamethoxazole (co-trimoxazole). Reversibly inhibits bacterial dihydrofolate dehydrogenase.

- Dosage:
  - 200 mg orally, 12 hourly.
  - 150–250 mg slowly iv, 12 hourly.
- Side effects: GIT upset, pruritus.

Triple point. Temperature and pressure at which the solid, liquid and gas phases of a substance exist in equilibrium. The kelvin is defined according to the triple point of water (273.16 K at 611.2 Pa).

Triservice apparatus. Anaesthetic apparatus adopted by the Armed Forces for battle use. Consists of (in order, starting at the patient):

- facepiece with non-rebreathing valve fitted.
- short length of ordinary tubing connected to a self-inflating bag.
- another length of tubing.
- two Oxford miniature vaporisers in series.

- an O_2 cylinder may be attached, between the vaporisers and a further length of tubing which acts as a reservoir.

For spontaneous ventilation, a draw-over technique is employed. Controlled ventilation may be performed by squeezing the bag, or replacing it with a suitable ventilator. A variety of volatile agents may be used in the vaporisers, the calibration scales of which may be changed accordingly. They are specially adapted to contain more liquid (50 ml), and are fitted with extendable feet. Halothane, enflurane or isoflurane are traditionally used in the upstream vaporiser, and trichloroethylene (to compensate for the absence of N_2O) in the downstream one.

Trismus. Spasm of the masseter muscles, resulting in impaired mouth opening (lockjaw).

- Causes may be:
  - local:
    - abscess/infection around jaw, teeth, etc.
    - mandibular fractures.
    - parotitis.
    - temporomandibular joint disease.
  - systemic:
    - tetanus.
    - strychnine poisoning.
    - phenothiazines.
    - CVA.
    - hysteria.

May occur after administration of suxamethonium (e.g. masseter spasm or in dystrophia myotonica).

Anaesthesia in the presence of trismus is as for airway obstruction and difficult intubation. Injection of local anaesthetic into the masseter muscle may relieve the spasm.

See also, Intubation, difficult

Trisodium edetate. Chelating agent used in severe hypercalcaemia. Rarely used because of the risk of renal damage.

- Dosage: up to 70 mg/kg iv (diluted to 10 mg/ml) over 2–3 h, daily.
- Side effects: hypocalcaemia, nausea, diarrhoea, pain on injection, renal impairment.

TRISS, *see Trauma revised injury severity score*

Tropical diseases. Many diseases are restricted to tropical and subtropical regions. Several are considered 'tropical' because they have been largely eradicated in the West. Diseases may be imported by travellers. Anaesthetic involvement may be related to management of severe cases on ICU, or surgery related to, or incidental to, the disease concerned.

- Common diseases or those of particular anaesthetic interest may share anaemia and malnutrition as common features, and include:
  - malaria.
  - diarrhoeal illness (e.g. typhoid, giardiasis, amoebic dysentery, cholera): cause electrolyte imbalance and dehydration.
  - amoebiasis: may cause systemic illness, diarrhoea, bowel perforation and hepatic abscesses. Treatment may include surgery.
  - hydatid disease: parasites may form cysts, usually in the liver but occasionally in the lungs, heart, kidneys or brain. Spillage of hydatic fluid intraoperatively may cause allergic reactions.
  - leprosy: chronic infective granulomatous disease affecting peripheral nerves, skin and upper respiratory tract mucosa. Patients may be taking corticosteroids. Areas of skin may be anaesthetic.
  - trypanosomiasis:
    - African (sleeping sickness): parasitic CNS invasion with confusion, coma and death. Myocarditis and hepatitis may occur.
    - American (Chagas' disease): meningoencephalitis, hepatic failure, cardiomyopathy and achalasia of the cardia may occur.
- Other diseases much more common in underdeveloped countries include:
  - syphilis.
  - tetanus.
  - hepatitis.
  - HIV infection.
  - TB.
  - poliomyelitis.
  - rabies.

[Carlos Chagas (1879–1934), Brazilian physician]

Tropisetron hydrochloride. 5-HT_3 receptor antagonist, licensed as an antiemetic drug in chemotherapy-induced nausea and vomiting. Similar to ondansetron but with longer duration of action.

- Dosage: 2–5 mg orally or slowly iv.

Trypanosomiasis, *see Tropical diseases*

TS, *see Trauma score*

TSR, *see Time to sustained respiration*

TT, Thrombin time, *see Coagulation studies*

TTP, *see Thrombotic thrombocytopenic purpura*

Tuberculosis (TB). Infection with the acid- and alcohol-fast bacillus *Mycobacterium tuberculosis* which mainly affects the lungs and lymph nodes, although any tissues may be affected. Once a common cause of death in the West, it has been declining for much of the 20th century until a recent upsurge in incidence in the 1980s/90s, thought to be related to an increase in the world's population, increased population movement, increasing resistance to antituberculous drugs (itself related to poor compliance with treatment), and an increase in HIV infection, with which it is often associated. It has been estimated that one-third of the world's population is infected with TB. In the UK, it is still largely restricted to migrants from underdeveloped countries, immunosuppressed patients and the homeless and destitute.

- Classified into:
  - primary TB: occurs in patients not previously infected (i.e. tuberculin-negative). Following a mild inflammatory reaction at the site of infection (e.g. lung or GIT), infection spreads to the regional lymph nodes. The lesions usually heal and calcify without further sequelae, but occasionally active organisms enter the bloodstream. This may cause 'haematogenous lesions' especially involving the lungs, bones, joints and kidneys. Rarely, a tuberculous focus ruptures into a vein causing acute dissemination (acute miliary TB).

    Patients may be asymptomatic, with evidence of infection provided by routine chest X-ray or conversion of the tuberculin test from negative to positive. Primary infection may be accompanied by a febrile illness. Occasionally primary TB is progressive and may cause pleurisy, pleural effusions and meningitis.
  - postprimary pulmonary TB: occurs in patients previously infected (i.e. tuberculin-positive). Usually affects

the upper lobes. Reactivation (or reinfection) causes a brisk inflammatory response; resultant fibrosis tends to limit the spread of infection. Regional lymph node involvement is therefore unusual. Again the lesion usually heals, but it may rupture into a bronchus causing cavitation. It may then spread throughout the lung, or rarely via the bloodstream causing miliary TB.

Usually insidious in onset, features include productive cough, haemoptysis (early) and dyspnoea (late). Pleuritic pain may be caused by pleurisy or pneumothorax.

Diagnosis includes history and examination (based on a high index of suspicion), chest X-ray, examination and culture of sputum for acid-fast bacilli (both may be negative), and tuberculin test (in primary TB).

- Management includes isolation, testing of contacts, and antituberculous drug therapy (isoniazid, rifampicin, pyrazinamide, ethambutol, streptomycin, capreomycin, cycloserine, azithromycin, clarithromycin and 4-quinolones). Programmes of supervised drug administration have been instituted in many countries to improve compliance. Multidrug resistance occurs in about 2% of cases in the UK but this is thought to be increasing.

Anaesthetic and respiratory equipment used for patients with active TB should be cleaned and sterilised before reuse. Cases of spread to other patients have been reported in the ICUs of UK hospitals.

See also, Contamination of anaesthetic equipment

Tubocurarine chloride (D-tubocurarine chloride). Non-depolarising neuromuscular blocking drug, isolated from curare in 1935. Its name is derived from the early classification of curare according to the means of storage ('tubes' refers to tubular bamboo canes). Initial dose is 0.3–0.5 mg/kg; this causes relaxation within 3–5 min, lasting for 30–50 min. Supplementary dose: 0.5–1 mg/kg. Commonly causes histamine release and ganglion blockade, causing vasodilatation and hypotension. Severe anaphylactoid reactions are rare. Excreted mainly in the urine, but 30% via the liver. No longer supplied in the UK from 1996.

Tumescent anaesthesia. Method of infiltrating large volumes of dilute local anaesthetic agent into tissues until they become swollen, used mainly for plastic surgery, e.g. liposuction. Typical solutions contain 0.05–0.1% lidocaine ± 1:1 000 000–1:2 000 000 adrenaline; bicarbonate, steroids and antibiotics have also been added. The volumes may exceed several litres, leading to the risk of local anaesthetic toxicity and fluid overload. PE and surgical complications have also been reported. May be used alone or in combination with sedation or general anaesthesia. Monitoring of patients for at least 24 h postoperatively has been suggested.

Tumour lysis syndrome. Condition in which medical treatment of an aggressive malignancy (typically haematological) results in sudden liberation of intracellular contents with resultant severe and potentially life-threatening hyperkalaemia, hypocalcaemia, hyperphosphataemia, lactic acidosis and hyperuricaemia. May occasionally occur spontaneously. Individual electrolyte abnormalities are managed along standard lines. Good hydration and prevention of renal uric acid precipitation by alkalisation of the urine (e.g. with bicarbonate or acetazolamide) and allopurinol administration may prevent renal failure from developing.

Davidson MB, Thakkar S, Hix JK (2004). Am J Med; 116: 546–54

Tumour necrosis factor, *see Cytokines*

Turbulence, *see Flow*

Turner's syndrome (Gonadal dysgenesis). Congenital absence of the second X chromosome. Sufferers are female in appearance, but with primary amenorrhoea and immature genitalia. Other features include short stature, short webbed neck and high palate; thus tracheal intubation may be difficult. Renal abnormalities, hypertension and coarctation of the aorta may occur.

[Henry H Turner (1892–1970), US physician]

TURP, *see Transurethral resection of the prostate*

TURP syndrome. Syndrome following TURP, thought to occur in a mild form in up to 8% of cases but severe in only 1–2%. Caused by absorption of irrigating fluid (usually hypotonic glycine 1.5%) through open prostatic vessels or from the extra-prostatic tissues. Has also been reported following other procedures involving irrigation with electrolyte-free solutions, e.g. percutaneous lithotripsy and hysteroscopic endometrial resection.

Symptoms are caused by intravascular volume overload, dilutional hyponatraemia and intracellular oedema. Additional effects are caused by glycine and its metabolites, e.g. ammonia.

Features include bradycardia, hypotension (often preceded by hypertension), angina, dyspnoea, visual and mental changes, convulsions and coma. Severity depends on the volume of irrigant absorbed (e.g. lethargy and nausea after 1–2 litres glycine; severe symptoms after > 2 litres) and the rate of absorption (faster onset if absorbed via prostatic veins; slower if absorbed from the extravascular tissues). Features may occur shortly after starting surgery, or postoperatively.

- Preventative measures:
  - limiting the height of the reservoir bag of irrigant to 60 cm.
  - limiting the volume of irrigant infused.
  - restriction of resection time to 60 min.
  - resection by experienced surgeons.
  - avoidance of hypotonic iv fluids.
- Measures to aid its detection:
  - use of spinal or epidural anaesthesia, allowing respiratory monitoring and detection of mental changes.
  - CVP measurement for patients at risk.
  - monitoring of plasma sodium concentration (more than a 10 mmol/l drop indicating > 2 litres irrigating fluid absorbed) or osmolality gap.
  - monitoring of tracer substances, e.g. ethanol 10% added to the irrigating fluid and measured in the blood or breath (over 0.6 mg/ml indicating > 2 litres fluid absorbed).
- Management: as for hyponatraemia, convulsions, raised ICP, acidosis, etc. Diuretics, e.g. furosemide, are usually advocated. Hypertonic saline solutions have been used. Vasopressor drugs may be required. Mannitol has been suggested to treat oliguria.

Hahn RG (2006). Br J Anaesth; 96: 8–20

Twilight sleep. Technique formerly popular in obstetrics as a means of easing labour pain and reducing subsequent recall. Injection of morphine and hyoscine was followed by hyoscine alone. Apart from causing maternal restlessness, it often caused neonatal respiratory depression. Now rarely used.

See also, Obstetric analgesia and anaesthesia

U

U wave. Low amplitude positive deflection following the T wave of the ECG, possibly representing slow repolarisation of papillary muscle. Seen best in the right chest leads and at slow heart rates but not always present. Made more prominent by hypokalaemia. Reversed polarity may indicate myocardial ischaemia.

U–D interval. During Caesarean section, the time between incision of the uterus and delivery of the baby. As the interval increases, so fetal wellbeing is compromised, probably due to disruption of placental blood flow. Fetal acidosis is thought to be unlikely at U–D intervals of 1.5–3 min.
See also, I–D interval

UEMS, European Union of Medical Specialties (Union Européenne des Médecins Spécialistes; UEMS), *see European Board of Anaesthesiology*

Ulcerative colitis, *see Inflammatory bowel disease*

Ulnar artery. A terminal branch of the brachial artery, arising at the apex of the antecubital fossa. Lies superficial to flexor digitorum profundus and deep to the superficial flexors in the forearm. Then passes deep to flexor carpi ulnaris, lateral to the ulnar nerve. At the wrist, it lies between flexor carpi ulnaris and flexor digitorum profundus tendons. Passes anterior to the flexor retinaculum to end lateral to the pisiform bone. Branches supply the deep extensor and ulnar muscles of the forearm, the wrist and elbow joints, and the deep and superficial palmar arches. May be cannulated for arterial BP measurement but the radial artery is preferred because the latter is thought to be associated with a lower risk of digital ischaemia.

Ulnar nerve (C7–T1). A terminal branch of the medial cord of the brachial plexus. Descends on the medial side of the upper arm, first in the anterior, and later in the posterior compartment. Passes behind the medial epicondyle to enter the forearm; descends on the medial side deep to flexor carpi ulnaris, medial to the ulnar artery. Divides into cutaneous branches 5 cm above the wrist. Dorsal and palmar cutaneous sensory branches supply the skin of the ulnar half of the hand and palm, and the medial 2½ fingers. Also supplies the elbow joint, flexor carpi ulnaris and the ulnar side of flexor digitorum profundus. In the hand, it supplies the hypothenar muscles, interossei, third and fourth lumbricals and adductor pollicis.

The nerve may be damaged by stretcher poles hitting the elbow, or if the elbows rest on unpadded surfaces during prolonged anaesthesia in the supine position. Injury results in loss of cutaneous sensation on the ulnar 1½ fingers and the ulnar side of the hand. Paralysis of the small muscles of the hand results in clawing.

May be blocked at various sites (*see Brachial plexus block; Elbow, nerve blocks; Wrist, nerve blocks*).

Ultrafiltration. Process by which water is removed from the blood during various forms of dialysis. Water passes across the semipermeable membrane as a result of positive pressure on the blood side of the membrane (e.g. the patient's BP or use of a pump), negative pressure on the other side, or an osmotic gradient from use of dialysate fluid. Rates of up to 1.5 l/h may be removed by intermittent isolated ultrafiltration (IIUF) in which a haemodialysis circuit is used but without dialysate, but more controlled removal of fluid (100–150 ml/h) may be achieved in slow continuous ultrafiltration (SCUF), with greater haemodynamic stability and without the need for fluid replacement. Combination with dialysis may also be employed (SCUF-D) but removal of larger molecules is less efficient than with continuous haemofiltration.

Ultra-rapid opioid detoxification, *see Rapid opioid detoxification*

Ultrasound. Technique originally developed for use in industry, now established as a valuable tool for imaging soft tissues. Relies on the transmission of high frequency vibrations and the detection of echoes resulting from their reflection at tissue interfaces. The simplest system provides information concerning tissue depth (amplitude or A scan). If the vibrations are repeated rapidly, the echoes are capable of detecting movement at tissue interfaces (movement or M mode). If the direction of the ultrasound source is then varied, a two-dimensional tomogram may be produced (B mode).

Uses include diagnostic and fetal imaging, assessment of cardiac function (echocardiography) and transcranial Doppler ultrasound. It has also been used to assess the depth of the epidural space and locate nerves for regional anaesthesia, and has been recommended by NICE as a means of localising the internal jugular vein prior to central venous cannulation.

Hatfield A, Bodenham A (1999). Br J Anaesth; 83: 789–800

See also, Doppler effect; Imaging in intensive care; Transoesophageal echocardiography

Unconsciousness, *see Coma*

Units, SI. System of units (Système Internationale d'Unités) introduced in 1960 by the General Conference of Weights and Measures (Conférence Générale des Poids et Mesures) and based on the metric system. There are seven base units: metre, second, kilogram, ampere, kelvin, candela and mole. Derived units include the newton, pascal, joule, watt and hertz. Standard terms denote multiples and divisions of units, e.g. kilo- ($\times 10^3$), mega- ($\times 10^6$), giga- ($\times 10^9$) tera- ($\times 10^{12}$) and peta- ($\times 10^{15}$); and milli- ($\times 10^{-3}$), micro- ($\times 10^{-6}$), nano- ($\times 10^{-9}$), pico- ($\times 10^{-12}$) and femto- ($\times 10^{-15}$) respectively

Manohin A, Manohin M (2003). Eur J Anaesth; 20: 259–81

Universal gas constant. Constant (symbol R) in the ideal gas law equation $PV = RT$, where P = pressure, V = volume and T = temperature of a perfect gas. Equals 8.3144 J/K/mol (1.987 cal/K/mol).

Uraemia. Strictly, a plasma urea exceeding 7.0 mmol/l; the term was formerly used to describe the clinical picture in renal failure.

Urapidil. α_1-Adrenergic receptor antagonist with central 5-HT_{1A} receptor agonist activity. Causes reduction in preload and afterload by causing arterial and vasodilatation with little reflex tachycardia. Has little effect on the coronary vessels. Although studied experimentally with promising results, it is not available commercially.

Urea. NH_2CONH_2; a product of hepatic amino acid breakdown to ammonia. Produced in the urea cycle from hydrolysis of arginine; ornithine is also produced and reacts with carbamoyl phosphate and then aspartate to reform arginine. Ammonia and CO_2 are introduced into the cycle by 'carrier' molecules. Freely filtered at the glomerulus of the nephron; about 50% is reabsorbed in the proximal tubule. Excretion in the urine accounts for 85% of daily nitrogen excretion. Normal plasma levels: 2.5–7.0 mmol/l. Increased production (e.g. from increased protein intake or catabolism) may increase plasma urea slightly, but levels above 13 mmol/l usually represent impaired renal function. Creatinine measurement or clearance studies may aid diagnosis.
See also, Nitrogen balance

Urinalysis, *see Urine*

Urinary retention. Inability to pass urine. May be either acute or chronic (the latter often leading to retention with overflow). May occur with prostatic enlargement, urethral stricture, spinal or epidural anaesthesia (including use of spinal opioids), after abdominal or pelvic surgery, and following administration of drugs with anticholinergic effects. Neurological causes are rarer but include spinal cord injury, cauda equina syndrome, Guillain–Barré syndrome and autonomic neuropathies (e.g. diabetic). Signs include a full bladder, tender to palpation and dull to percussion. May cause agitation and confusion postoperatively; can cause hypertension, tachycardia and raised ICP in unconscious patients. May cause acute pyelonephritis.

Urinary catheterisation (either urethral or, occasionally, suprapubic) may be required if encouragement (running taps, etc.) is unsuccessful.
See also, Oliguria

Urinary tract infection (UTI). Most common nosocomial infection seen in critically ill patients and a common cause of generalised sepsis. Almost always associated with urinary catheterisation, with the risk increasing the longer the catheter is in place. Gram-negative organisms (e.g. *Escherichia coli*, pseudomonas) are commonly involved, gaining entry to the bladder either through the catheter's lumen or along its surface. Diagnosis is confirmed by the presence of white blood cells and > 100 000 organisms/mm^3 on urine microscopy. Urinary catheterisation should only be performed when necessary, aseptic technique used and the catheter removed as soon as possible. Treatment of established UTI is with antibacterial drugs according to the results of urine culture.

Urine. Liquid containing urea and other waste products, excreted by the kidneys. Normal output in temperate climates is 800–2500 ml/day. Coloured yellowish by the pigments urochrome and uroerythrin, it darkens on standing by oxidation of urobilinogen to urobilin (colour does not necessarily reflect urine's concentration). Coloured red by haemoglobin or myoglobin. Specific gravity is normally 1.002–1.035. Osmolality may range between 30 and 1400 mosmol/kg, depending on fluid and hormonal status. pH is usually below 5.3. Normally contains under 150 mg protein/24 h. Abnormal constituents include glucose, ketones, bilirubin, erythrocytes, large numbers of leucocytes and casts.

Urinalysis is usually performed using reagent sticks; the reagents change colour according to the presence and amount of various normal and abnormal constituents in the sample. Specific gravity, electrolytic and solute content and pH can also be quantified.

Despite the kidneys' ability to concentrate the urine, a minimum of 500 ml/day is required to eliminate urea and other electrolytes. Oliguria is usually defined as less than 0.5 ml/kg/h and may indicate hypovolaemia or renal failure; anuria is complete cessation of urine flow and may indicate obstruction or urinary retention in addition. Polyuria occurs in diabetes insipidus, renal failure, diuretic therapy, diabetes mellitus (because of the osmotically active glucose load) and excessive water intake (water diuresis).

Urine output is often measured during critical illness and major surgery, since it reflects tissue perfusion and volume status of the circulation (assuming normal renal and cardiac function). Although renal blood flow is often reduced and circulating levels of vasopressin are high during surgery, urine output is usually maintained. An hourly urine output of > 0.5 ml/kg/h is regarded as the minimum acceptable during critical illness or surgery by most anaesthetists.
See also, Nephron

Urokinase. Enzyme extracted from male human urine, used as a fibrinolytic drug mainly for thrombolysis in the eye and arteriovenous shunts, although also indicated in PE or DVT. Acts via activation of plasminogen.
- Dosage:
  - 5000–25 500 iu instilled into the shunt.
  - PE/DVT: 4400 iu/kg iv over 10 min, then 4400 iu/kg/h for 12–24 h.
- Side effects: nausea, vomiting, back pain. Allergic reactions are rare.

Urotensin II. Peptide hormone found in fish and discovered in human tissues in 1999, with specific receptors in the heart and arterial vessels and possibly CNS. Has extremely potent vasoconstrictive properties that vary according to vessel type. Its role as a major mediator in cardiovascular regulation and a potential role for urotensin II antagonists have been suggested.
Affolter J, Webb DJ (2001). Lancet; 358: 774–5

Uterus. Pear-shaped pelvic organ, 7.5 cm long, 5 cm wide and 2.5 cm thick when non-gravid. Divided into the upper body and lower cervix, separated by the isthmus. Separated from the bladder anteriorly by the uterovesical pouch, and from the rectum posteriorly by the uterorectal pouch. The broad ligaments lie laterally.

Blood supply is from the uterine artery, a branch of the internal iliac artery. The uterine vein drains into the internal iliac vein.
- Nerve supply:
  - sympathetic motor preganglionic fibres from T1–L2 and parasympathetic motor preganglionic fibres from S2–4 via the paracervical plexus. Actions are variable, depending on the stage of the menstrual cycle and pregnancy.
  - sensory fibres via sympathetic pathways, emerging in the paracervical tissues and passing through the hypogastric plexus to T11–12, sometimes also to T10 and L1.

- Actions of drugs on the pregnant uterus:
  - α-adrenergic receptor agonists, e.g. noradrenaline: increase uterine tone and strength of contraction.
  - β-adrenergic receptor agonists, e.g. adrenaline, salbutamol: decrease uterine tone and strength of contraction. Agonists specific for β_2-receptors are used as tocolytic drugs to delay premature labour.
  - oxytocin and ergometrine: produce powerful contraction. Atosiban (oxytocin antagonist) causes uterine relaxation.
  - prostaglandins PGE_2 and $PGF_{2\alpha}$: stimulate uterine contraction.
  - volatile inhalational anaesthetic agents: cause dose-related reduction of uterine tone.
  - iv anaesthetic agents, sedative and analgesic drugs, neuromuscular blocking drugs, acetylcholinesterase inhibitors: no effect on uterine tone.
  - others: acetylcholine, bradykinin, histamine and 5-HT increase contraction. Smooth muscle relaxants, e.g. amyl nitrite, GTN and papaverine, cause relaxation. Alcohol has a direct relaxant action and suppresses oxytocin secretion from the pituitary gland.

See also, Obstetric analgesia and anaesthesia

UTI, *see Urinary tract infection*

Utstein style. Uniform system of reporting data for out-of-hospital cardiac arrests, arising from a meeting of representatives of international Resuscitation Councils in Utstein Abbey on the Island of Mosteroy off Norway in June 1990. A second meeting (The Utstein II conference) in London the same year resulted in the publication of recommended guidelines for uniform reporting of such data, the 'Utstein style'. This 'style' has been recommended for in-hospital CPR attempts, paediatric CPR, laboratory CPR research and trauma.

Dick WF, Baskett PJF (1999). Resuscitation 42: 81–100

V

Vacuum insulated evaporator (VIE). Container for storage of liquid O_2 and maintenance of piped gas supply. An outer carbon steel shell is separated by a vacuum from an inner stainless steel shell which contains O_2. The inner temperature varies between −160 and −180°C. Gaseous O_2 is withdrawn and heated to ambient temperature (and thus expanded) as required (Fig. 159). If pressure within the container falls, liquid O_2 may be withdrawn, vaporised in an evaporator and returned to the system, restoring working pressure. If passage of heat across the insulation causes vaporisation of liquid O_2 and a rise in pressure, gas is allowed to escape through a safety valve. The contents are indicated by a weighing device incorporated into the chamber's supports.
Howells RS (1980). Anaesthesia; 35: 676–98

Vagus nerve. Tenth cranial nerve. Arises in the medulla from the:
- dorsal nucleus of the vagus (parasympathetic).
- nucleus ambiguus (motor fibres to laryngeal, pharyngeal and palatal muscles).
- nucleus of the tractus solitarius (sensory fibres from the larynx, pharynx, GIT, heart and lungs, including taste).

Leaves the medulla between the olive and inferior cerebellar peduncle, and passes through the jugular foramen of the skull. Descends in the neck within the carotid sheath between the internal jugular vein and internal/common carotid arteries (*see Fig. 110; Neck, cross-sectional anatomy, and Fig. 102a; Mediastinum*). Passes behind the root of the lung to form the pulmonary plexus, then on to the oesophagus to form the oesophageal plexus with the vagus from the other side. Both pass through the oesophageal opening of the diaphragm to supply the abdominal contents and GIT as far as the splenic flexure (*see Fig. 20; Autonomic nervous system*).
- Branches:
  - to the external auditory meatus and tympanic membrane.
  - to muscles of the pharynx and soft palate.
  - laryngeal nerves.
  - to cardiac, pulmonary and oesophageal plexuses.
  - to intra-abdominal organs.

The vagi form a major part of the parasympathetic nervous system. Vagal reflexes causing bradycardia, laryngospasm and bronchospasm may be troublesome during anaesthesia. Intense stimulation may result in partial or complete heart block or even asystole. Anal and cervical stretching (e.g. Brewer–Luckhardt reflex) and traction on the extraocular muscles (oculocardiac reflex) are particularly intense stimuli, but it may also follow skin incision and stimulation (e.g. surgical) of the mesentery, biliary tract, uterus, bladder, urethra, testes, larynx, glottis, bronchial tree and carotid sinus. Also involved in the diving reflex.

Anticholinergic drugs help prevent vagal reflexes during surgery. Should they occur, surgical activity should cease, and atropine or glycopyrronium administered if necessary.

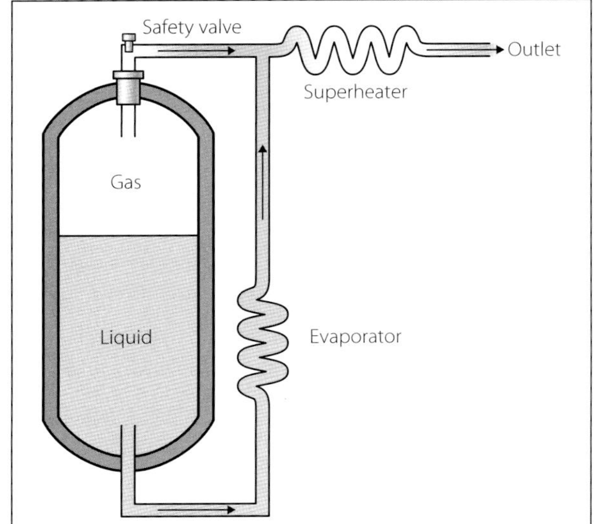

Fig. 159 Vacuum insulated evaporator

Valence. Capacity of an atom or group of atoms to combine with others in definite proportions; compared with that of hydrogen (value of 1). Dependent on the number of electrons in the outer shell of the atom; covalent bonds are formed when electrons are shared between different atoms, e.g. water: H–O–H.

VALI, *see Ventilator-associated lung injury*

Valproate/valproic acid, *see Sodium valproate*

Valsalva manoeuvre. Forced expiration against a closed glottis after a full inspiration, originally described as a technique for expelling pus from the middle ear. In its standardised form, 40 mmHg pressure is held for 10 s.
- Direct arterial BP tracings in normal subjects show four phases (Fig. 160):
  - phase I: increase in intrathoracic pressure expels blood from thoracic vessels.
  - phase II: decrease in BP due to reduction of venous return; activation of the baroreceptor reflex causes tachycardia and vasoconstriction, raising BP towards normal.
  - phase III: further drop in BP as intrathoracic pressure suddenly drops, with pooling of blood in the pulmonary vessels.
  - phase IV: overshoot, as compensatory mechanisms continue to operate with venous return restored. Increased BP causes bradycardia.
- Abnormal responses:
  - 'square wave' response, seen in cardiac failure, constrictive pericarditis, cardiac tamponade and valvular

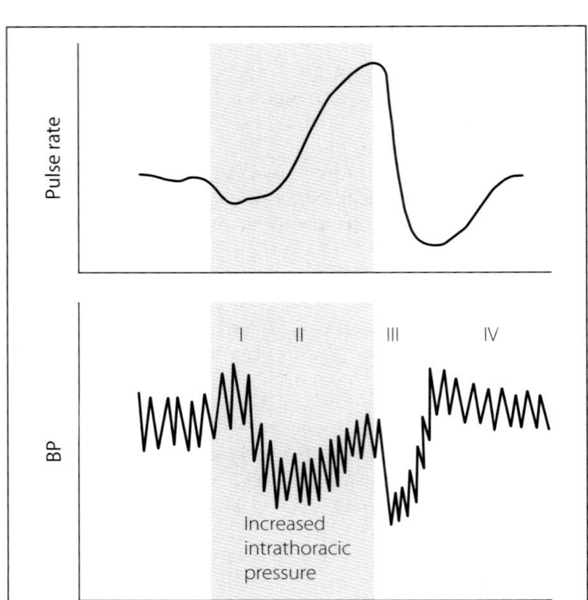

Fig. 160 Normal Valsalva response (see text)

heart disease, when CVP is markedly raised. BP rises, remains high throughout the manoeuvre, and returns to its previous level at the end.
- autonomic dysfunction, e.g. autonomic neuropathy, drugs. BP falls and stays low until intrathoracic pressure is released. Pulse rate changes and overshoot are absent.
- an exaggerated reduction in BP may be seen in hypovolaemia, e.g. during IPPV.

Useful as a bedside test of autonomic function. Concurrent ECG tracing allows accurate measurement of changes in heart rate. The manoeuvre may be useful in evaluating heart murmurs, and may be successful in terminating SVT (because of increased vagal tone in phase IV).
[Antonio Valsalva (1666–1723), Italian anatomist]

Valtis–Kennedy effect. Shift to the left of the oxyhaemoglobin dissociation curve during blood storage, originally described in 1954 for acid–citrate–dextrose storage. The shift reflects progressive depletion of 2,3-DPG.
[DJ Valtis, Greek physician; Arthur C Kennedy, Glasgow physician]

Valveless anaesthetic breathing systems. Anaesthetic breathing systems designed to eliminate resistance which inevitably results from adjustable pressure-limiting valves. In the Samson system, the valve is replaced by an adjustable orifice; in the Hafnia systems, expired gases pass through a port, assisted by an ejector flowmeter.
[Heyman H Samson, South African anaesthetist; *Hafnia*: Latin name for Copenhagen]

Valves, *see Adjustable pressure-limiting valves; Demand valves; Non-rebreathing valves*

Valvular heart disease. Causes, features and anaesthetic management: as for congenital heart disease and individual lesions. Valve replacement: as for cardiac surgery. Many prosthetic valves are available in different sizes, e.g. silastic ball-and-cage, metal flaps and porcine valves. Thrombosis may form on prostheses, hence the requirement for long-term anticoagulation. Patients with prosthetic valves also require prophylactic antibiotics as for congenital heart disease.

Van der Waals equation of state. Modification of the ideal gas law, accounting for the forces of attraction between gas molecules, and also the volume of the molecules:

$$RT = (P + a/V^2)(V - b)$$

where R = universal gas constant
T = temperature
P = pressure exerted by the gas
V = molar volume of gas
a and b = correction terms.

[Johannes van der Waals (1837–1923), Dutch physicist]

Van der Waals forces. Weak attractive forces between neutral molecules and atoms, caused by electric polarisation of the particles induced by the presence of other particles.
See also, Van der Waals equation of state

Van Slyke apparatus. Device used to measure blood gas partial pressures. O_2 and CO_2 are released into a burette from the blood by addition of a liberating solution. Each gas in turn is converted to a non-gaseous substance by chemical reaction, and the pressure drop in the burette measured for each. The same reagents may be used as in the Haldane apparatus.
[Donald D van Slyke (1883–1971), US chemist]
See also, Carbon dioxide measurement; Gas analysis; Oxygen measurement

Vancomycin. Glycopeptide and antibacterial drug with bactericidal activity against aerobic and anaerobic Gram-positive bacteria (including multiresistant staphylococci), although resistant enterococci are increasingly reported. Usually reserved for severe infections, resistant organisms or penicillin allergy. Not absorbed orally.

- Dosage:
  - 500 mg iv over an hour, 6 hourly, or 1 g over 100 min 12 hourly.
  - 125–250 mg 6 hourly, orally, in pseudomembranous colitis (for 7–10 days).
- Side effects: renal impairment, ototoxicity, blood dyscrasias, nausea, fever, allergic reactions, phlebitis. Rapid infusion may cause hypotension, urticaria, pruritus, flushing ('red man syndrome'), dyspnoea and cardiac arrest. Plasma levels should be monitored; the pre-dose level should be < 10 mg/l and the peak should be < 30 mg/l 2 hours post-dose.

See also, Infection control

Vancomycin resistant enterococci, *see Infection control; Vancomycin*

VAP, *see Ventilator-associated pneumonia*

Vaporisers. Devices for delivering accurate and safe concentrations of volatile inhalational anaesthetic agents to the patient.

- Classified into:
  - plenum vaporisers (*plenum = chamber*): widely used in modern anaesthesia despite their cost and complexity, because of their reliability, safety features and accuracy:
    - gas passes through the vaporiser under pressure at the back bar of the anaesthetic machine.
    - in modern types, e.g. 'Tec' (temperature compensated) vaporisers, fresh gas is divided by the control dial into two streams, one of which enters the vaporisation

chamber, becomes fully saturated with agent, and rejoins the other stream at the outlet (Fig. 161a). The ratio of the two streams (splitting ratio) determines the final delivered concentration (n.b. a different mechanism exists for the Tec 6 desflurane vaporiser (see below). In older vaporisers the delivered concentration was also affected by various other factors (see below). In the obsolete 'copper kettle' type, a separate supply of O_2 was passed through the vaporiser, becoming fully saturated. It was then added to the main fresh gas flow, at a rate calculated according to desired final concentration and vaporiser temperature. The original design included a large mass of copper as a heat sink, hence its name.

- have high resistance so unsuitable for positioning in a circle system.
- performance is not affected by whether ventilation is spontaneous or controlled.
- include the Tec series of vaporisers. Features of the Mark 4 over the Mark 3 (Fig. 161b):
  - flow of liquid agent into the delivery line is prevented if the vaporiser is inverted.
  - interlock system prevents use of more than one vaporiser at a time, if mounted side by side.
  - fitted with the key filling system (not fitted to all Mark 3 models).

  Features of the Mark 5 over the Mark 4:
  - increased capacity.
  - improved filling system.

  Features of the Mark 6 (desflurane vaporiser):
  - cannot use the above mechanism since desflurane's BP is very close to room temperature, such that small variations in the latter result in large changes in SVP.
  - requires an electrical power supply for the heating elements and control mechanisms.
  - the fresh gas does not enter the vaporising chamber, but passes along a separate path to mix with pure desflurane vapour leaving the chamber at the outlet (produced by heating the vaporising chamber to 39°C, thus ensuring complete vaporisation).
  - fresh gas encounters a flow restriction within the vaporiser, causing back pressure which varies according to fresh gas flow.
  - a system of pressure transducers and internal circuitry is used to monitor and adjust the performance to produce a consistent output even if fresh gas flow alters (detected by a change in back pressure). Internal switches cut out the system if temperature increases above 57°C or if the vaporiser is tilted or becomes empty.

  Features of the Mark 7 over the Mark 5 (all modern agents but desflurane):
  - more accurate and easily controllable output throughout different flow ranges.
  - improved filling options and protection against spillage and contamination.

- draw-over vaporisers: despite their variable output, often preferred in the battlefield (e.g. triservice apparatus) and developing countries because they are cheap, simple and portable:
  - gas is drawn into the vaporising chamber by the patient's inspiratory effort.
  - resistance must be low.
  - performance is affected by minute ventilation, the output falling as ventilation increases.
  - may be suitable for use within circle systems, e.g. Goldman vaporiser (Fig. 161b), a small, light, uncompensated device with a glass container (originally adapted from a motor vehicle fuel pump). Similar vaporisers were designed by McKesson and Rowbotham, the latter's containing a wire gauze wick.
  - also used for draw-over techniques, e.g. (Fig. 161b):
    - EMO (Epstein and Macintosh of Oxford) diethyl ether inhaler: large vaporiser, incorporating a large vaporisation chamber, a water jacket for a heat sink, and a temperature-compensating fluid-filled bellows at the outlet.
    - OMV (Oxford miniature vaporiser): small uncompensated device, containing a water-filled heat sink (with antifreeze). Contains wire wicks; may thus be emptied of one agent, flushed and refilled with another. Different calibration scales may be fixed to the control valve for the various agents. A modified form is used in the triservice apparatus.
  - obsolete types, used formerly for obstetric analgesia:
    - Emotril (Epstein and Macintosh of Oxford/Trilene) trichloroethylene apparatus: incorporated within a metal box.
    - Cardiff methoxyflurane inhaler: free-standing on a base.
- systems involving addition of liquid volatile agent directly to the fresh gas stream:
  - require delivery of liquid agent at a rate calculated automatically to produce the desired concentration.
  - incorporated into computerised anaesthetic machines.
  - combined with a carbon filter/evaporator system that fits into the patient's breathing system, conserving and recycling ~90% of the administered agent. Have been used for sedation on ICU without the need for anaesthetic machines.

- Factors affecting the delivered concentration:
  - splitting ratio (plenum vaporisers).
  - SVP of the volatile agent: equals the partial pressure of the agent within the vaporiser. Agents with high SVP, e.g. diethyl ether, are easier to vaporise than those with low SVPs, e.g. methoxyflurane.

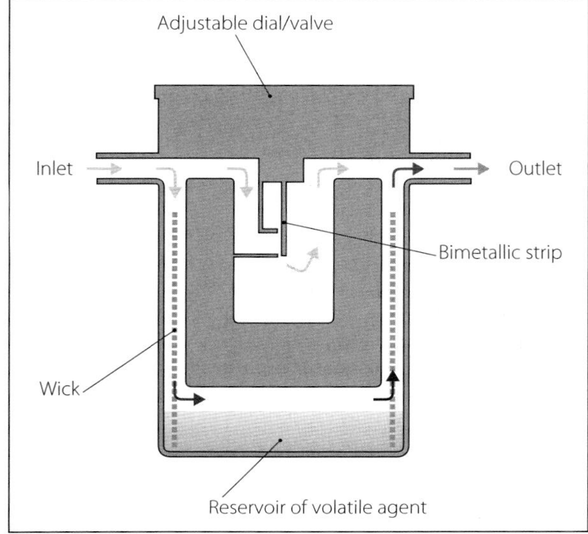

Fig. 161 (a) Principles of modern Tec vaporiser (considerably simplified). When the dial/valve is adjusted, it alters the 'splitting ratio' of the gas that passes through the two paths shown. When it is in the 'off' position, all the gas passes via an additional route through the top (not shown) that bypasses these two paths completely. Pale arrows: no volatile agent vapour; dark arrows: containing vapour.

(Continued)

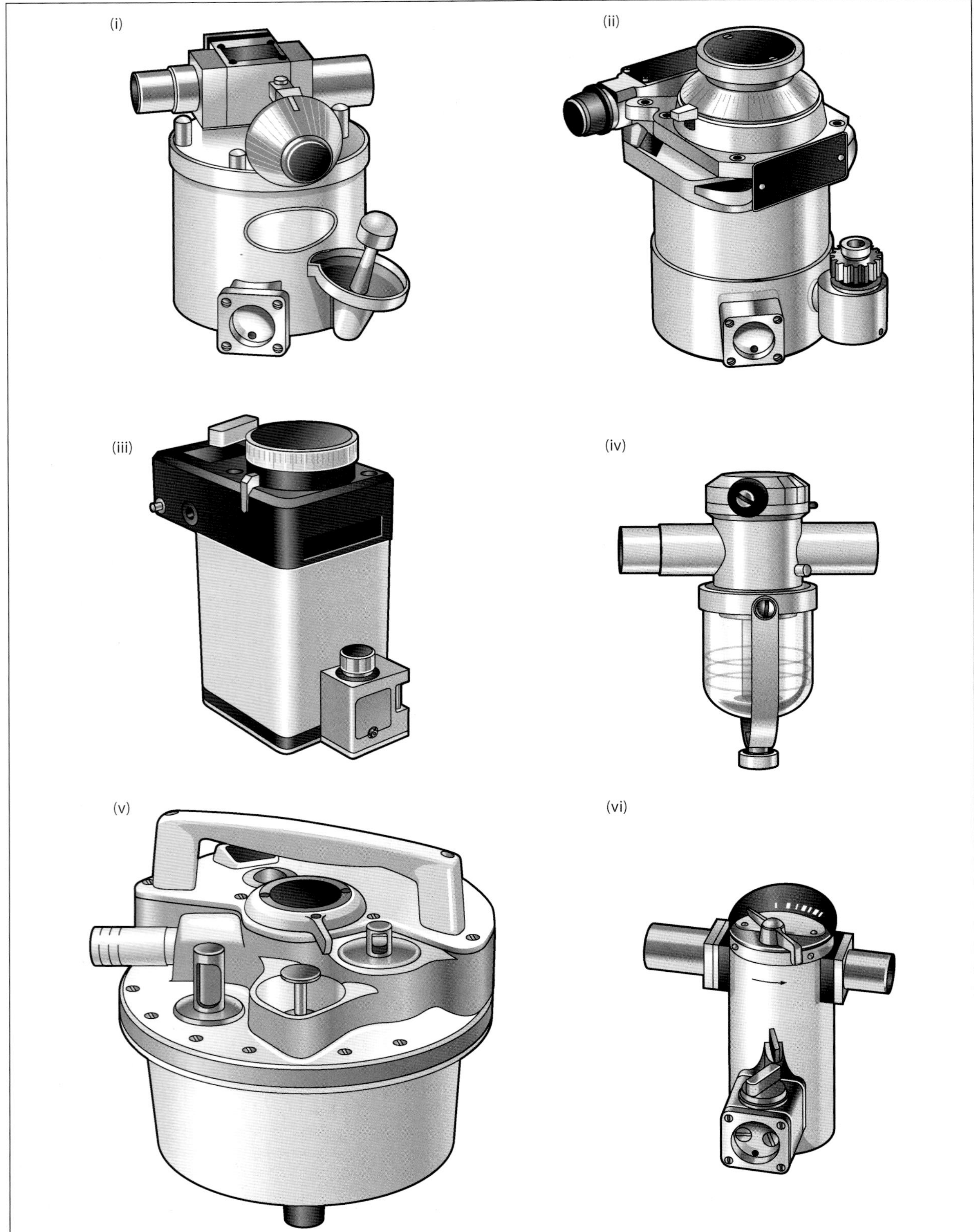

Fig. 161 Cont'd. (b) 'Classic' types of vaporiser: (i) Tec Mark 2; (ii) Tec Mark 3; (iii) Tec Mark 4; (iv) Goldman; (v) EMO; (vi) OMV (see text). (n.b. the external appearance of the Tec Mark 5 and onwards did not change significantly from that of the Mark 4)

- temperature of the liquid: affects the SVP. As liquid vaporises, latent heat of vaporisation is lost, and temperature and thus SVP falls. Delivered concentration of agent would therefore fall if not for temperature compensation devices, e.g.:
  - bimetallic strip at the outlet (Tec Mark 2) or inlet (subsequent Tec models) of the vaporisation chamber.
  - fluid-filled bellows at the gas outlet, e.g. EMO inhaler (see below); expands as temperature rises.
  - longitudinally expanding metal rod at the gas outlet, e.g. Dräger models.

  Temperature loss is reduced by providing heat sinks of metal (e.g. Tec) or water (EMO). Older vaporisers incorporated heating devices or thermometers to allow adjustment as temperature changed.
- surface area of the gas/liquid interface: increased with:
  - wicks and baffles, e.g. most plenum vaporisers (see below). Wicks maintain surface area despite gradual emptying of the vaporiser (level compensation).
  - a cowl to direct gas flow on to or into the liquid (e.g. the original Boyle's bottle).
  - production of many tiny bubbles with a sintered brass or glass diffuser, e.g. copper kettle type vaporisers.
- fresh gas flow: the output of older devices varied considerably with gas flow (e.g. the Tec Mark 2 was supplied with charts showing the delivered versus the set concentrations at various flow rates); modern plenum vaporisers perform more consistently. Draw-over vaporisers are more efficient at lower gas flows.
- pumping effect.

For vaporisers in series: contamination of the second with vapour from the first may occur if both are turned on simultaneously. Although this cannot occur with modern vaporisers, for other types the one containing the less volatile agent (i.e. with lower SVP) should be placed upstream, because:

- it requires proportionally more of the fresh gas flow than the vaporiser containing the more volatile agent, and would thus receive more contaminant if placed downstream.
- the more volatile agent, being easier to vaporise, would attain higher (and thus potentially dangerous) concentrations than those set if it contaminated the vaporiser designed for a less volatile agent.

Vaporisers have been associated with many hazards, and require regular servicing.

[Heinrich Dräger (1847–1917), German engineer; Victor Goldman (1903–1993), London anaesthetist; Hans G Epstein (1909–2002), Berlin-born Oxford physicist]

See also, Altitude, high

Vapour. Matter in the gaseous form below its critical temperature; i.e. its constituent particles may enter the liquid form. As liquid vaporises, heat is required (latent heat of vaporisation); as vapour condenses, an equal amount of heat is produced. These processes occur continuously above the surface of a liquid at equilibrium.

See also, Vapour pressure

Vapour pressure. Pressure exerted by molecules escaping from the surface of a liquid to enter the gaseous phase. When equilibrium is reached at any temperature, the number of molecules leaving the liquid phase equals the number entering it; the vapour pressure now equals SVP. Raising the temperature of the liquid increases the molecules' kinetic energy, allowing more of them to escape and raising the vapour pressure. When SVP equals atmospheric pressure, the liquid boils.

Variance. Standard deviation squared. Thus an indicator of spread of values within a sample. Although standard deviation is commonly used when describing data, many statistical calculations employ its square, hence the use of variance as a meaningful term (e.g. analysis of variance, ANOVA).

See also, Statistics

VAS, Visual analogue scale, *see Linear analogue scale*

Vascular access, *see Central venous cannulation; Intravenous fluid administration*

Vascular resistance, *see Pulmonary vascular resistance; Systemic vascular resistance*

Vasculitides. Group of conditions characterised by inflammation of blood vessels. All except giant cell arteritis are uncommon and associated with connective tissue diseases or drug hypersensitivity. Diagnosis requires biopsy which often shows granuloma formation associated with vessel inflammation.

- Classification:
  - group 1: systemic necrotising arteritis of small/medium arteries:
    - polyarteritis nodosa.
    - Kawasaki's disease.
    - Wegener's granulomatosis.
    - connective tissue disease associated arteritis.
  - group 2: small vessel vasculitis:
    - Henoch–Schönlein purpura: usually occurs in childhood following an upper respiratory tract infection. Features include fever, headache, macular/urticarial rash becoming purpuric, over the buttocks and posterior of the limbs. Inflammatory synovitis is common. Focal glomerulonephritis may lead to nephrotic syndrome and rarely renal failure.
    - mixed cryoglobulinaemic vasculitis.
    - connective tissue disease associated vasculitis.
  - group 3: giant cell arteritis/large artery vasculitis:
    - temporal arteritis: usually affects the elderly and often associated with polymyalgia rheumatica. Headache, often localised, is the predominant symptom. Blindness may result if corticosteroids are not given as soon as possible.
    - Takayasu's arteritis: rare large vessel arteritis affecting young women. Affects the aorta and its branches causing inflammation and then stenosis of affected vessels. Features include cerebrovascular insufficiency (fainting, dizziness, etc.) and reduced peripheral pulses. Treatment depends on the underlying condition but usually includes immunosuppressive drugs.

[Eduard H Henoch (1820–1910), German physician; Johann L Schönlein (1793–1864), German paediatrician; Michishige Takayasu (1860–1938), Japanese ophthalmologist]

Vasoactive intestinal peptide (VIP). GIT hormone, also found in the hypothalamus, cortex, primary afferent neurones, spinal cord, retina and bloodstream. Causes oesophageal relaxation preceding a peristaltic wave, relaxation of sphincters, stimulation of intestinal electrolyte and water secretion and inhibition of gastric secretion. Dilates peripheral blood vessels and causes bronchodilatation. Has positive inotropic and chronotropic action on the heart and causes coronary vasodilatation. Has an important role in the regulation of circadian rhythms. Tumours secreting VIP (VIPomas) may cause severe diarrhoea and hypotension.

Vasoconstrictor drugs, *see Vasopressor drugs*

Vasodilator drugs. Drugs causing vasodilatation as their main effect (cf. isoflurane, morphine). The term is sometimes reserved for drugs acting directly at vascular smooth muscle itself. Nitric oxide is thought to be a common end pathway for most drugs.

- May be divided according to their main site of action, although considerable overlap occurs:
  - venous system: GTN, isosorbide.
  - arterial system: hydralazine, calcium channel blocking drugs, salbutamol, diazoxide, minoxidil, adenosine.
  - venous and arterial systems: sodium nitroprusside, α-adrenergic receptor antagonists, angiotensin converting enzyme inhibitors, ganglion blocking drugs, potassium channel activators.
- Used to reduce SVR and thus:
  - systemic BP, e.g. in hypotensive anaesthesia, hypertensive crisis, pre-eclampsia. Their effect is sometimes offset by reflex tachycardia.
  - afterload and ventricular work, e.g. in cardiac failure, shock. Increase stroke volume and reduce myocardial O_2 demand. Also reduce preload via venous dilatation.

Also used to reduce pulmonary vascular resistance in pulmonary hypertension, although the systemic circulation is usually affected too.

See also, Antihypertensive drugs; Inotropic drugs

Vasomotor centre. Group of neurones in the ventrolateral medulla, involved in the control of arterial BP. Projects to sympathetic preganglionic neurones in the spinal cord. Normal continuous discharge causes partial contraction of vascular smooth muscle (vasomotor tone) and resting sympathetic stimulation of the heart.

- Discharge is increased by:
  - chemoreceptor discharge.
  - pain, emotion.
  - hypoxia (causes direct stimulation initially, but depression follows).
- Discharge is decreased by:
  - baroreceptor discharge.
  - lung inflation.
  - prolonged pain, emotion.

Thus responds to hypotension (reduced baroreceptor discharge) by increasing sympathetic activity.

Dorsal and medial neurones functionally constitute the cardioinhibitory centre, stimulation of which inhibits the vasomotor centre and increases vagal activity.

Vasopressin (Arginine vasopressin, AVP; Antidiuretic hormone, ADH). Neuropeptide synthesised in the cell bodies of the supraoptic and paraventricular nuclei of the hypothalamus. Transported down their axons to the posterior lobe of the pituitary gland, from which it is secreted. Metabolised in the kidney and liver, it has a circulatory half-life of 10–30 min.

- Main effects:
  - water retention by the kidney, via increased adenylate cyclase activity and cAMP levels. Increases the permeability of renal collecting ducts, allowing water to pass back into the renal interstitium. Urine volume decreases; its concentration increases. Conversely, plasma volume increases; its concentration decreases.
  - vasoconstriction due to a direct effect on vascular smooth muscle; increases BP if given in high doses. Thought to have a minor role in normal BP regulation.
  - has a role in temperature regulation, control of circadian rhythm and memory function.
  - increased plasma levels of coagulation factor VIII.

There are at least three types of vasopressin receptor, which are G protein-coupled: V_1 (sometimes called V_{1a}) receptors are primarily vascular but also present on platelets; V_2 receptors are responsible for vasopressin's antidiuretic actions on the kidney; and V_3 (V_{1b}) receptors are located centrally and involved in vasopressin's neurotransmitter actions.

- Release is increased by:
  - increased plasma osmolality; detected by osmoreceptors in the anterior hypothalamus.
  - decreased ECF volume (e.g. in haemorrhage); detected by baroreceptors.
  - pain, nausea, hypoxaemia, emotional and physical stress.
  - drugs, e.g. morphine, barbiturates.
  - angiotensin II.
- Release is inhibited by:
  - decreased plasma osmolality.
  - increased ECF volume.
  - drugs, e.g. alcohol, butorphanol.
- Used therapeutically in various forms:
  - argipressin: synthetic vasopressin; used in pituitary diabetes insipidus (DI; 5–20 U sc/im, 4 hourly) and for control of bleeding oesophageal varices (20 U iv over 15 min). Side effects include pallor, nausea, abdominal cramps and myocardial ischaemia. GTN (patch or iv) has been used to reduce the incidence and severity of side effects.
  - terlipressin: a prodrug, it is enzymatically cleaved to release vasopressin. Dosage: 2 mg iv followed by 1–2 mg 4–6 hourly for up to 72 h. Side effects are milder than after argipressin.
  - lypressin: used as a nasal spray in pituitary DI: 5–10 U 6–8 hourly. Side effects are milder than after argipressin.
  - desmopressin: minimal vasoconstrictor activity; used in pituitary DI and to boost factor VIII levels in haemophilia and von Willebrand's disease.
  - felypressin: used as a vasoconstrictor in local anaesthesia.

Vasopressin has been suggested as an alternative to adrenaline in the treatment of cardiac arrest and sepsis-induced hypotension, and as a means of preserving organ function in brainstem-dead donors. Vasopressin antagonists (e.g. tolvaptan, conivaptan and lixivaptan) have been studied for use in cardiac failure and hyponatraemia.

Treschan TA, Peters J (2006). Anesthesiology; 105: 599–612

See also, Syndrome of inappropriate antidiuretic hormone secretion

Vasopressor drugs. Drugs causing vasoconstriction; used to increase arterial BP, e.g. during anaesthesia, intensive care or CPR, or to prolong the action of local anaesthetic agents by preventing their systemic absorption. Formerly used rather indiscriminately to increase BP, they are now reserved for situations where vasodilatation is a specific problem, e.g. anaphylactic reaction, spinal anaesthesia, etc.

- Mostly sympathomimetic drugs:
  - catecholamines, e.g. adrenaline, noradrenaline, dopamine.
  - non-catecholamines, e.g. ephedrine, metaraminol, phenylephrine.
- Directly acting vasopressor hormones and their analogues have also been used, e.g. in hypotension refractory to other potent vasopressors:

- vasopressin and its synthetic analogues.
- angiotensin (*see Renin/angiotensin system*).

See also, Inotropic drugs

Vasovagal syncope. Fainting, often caused by emotion. May occur in patients undergoing venous cannulation or regional anaesthesia. Vasodilatation in muscle (sympathetic discharge) and bradycardia (vagal discharge) cause hypotension and loss of consciousness, usually short lived.

Kapoor WN (2002). Circulation; 106: 1606–9

vCJD, *see Creutzfeldt–Jakob disease*

Vecuronium bromide. Non-depolarising neuromuscular blocking drug, introduced in the UK in 1983. A monoquaternary aminosteroid, similar in structure to pancuronium. Initial dose is 80–100 μg/kg; good intubating conditions occur within 90 s. Relaxation lasts for 20–30 min; duration is increased to 50 min if 150 μg/kg is used, and 80 min if 250 μg/kg is used. Supplementary dose: 30–50 μg/kg. May also be given by infusion, at 50–80 μg/kg/h. Causes minimal histamine release, ganglion or vagal blockade even at several times the usual doses. Thus has minimal effects on BP and pulse, but may allow unopposed vagal stimulation to cause bradycardia. Metabolised in the liver to the active 3-desacetylvecuronium. Excreted mainly in bile, but also in urine. Reversal of action is fast, and acetylcholinesterase inhibitors may not always be required. Cumulation is unlikely.

Venous admixture. Refers to lowering of arterial $P\text{O}_2$ from the 'ideal' level which would occur if there were no shunt or $\dot{V}/\dot{Q}$ mismatch, either of which may lower $P\text{O}_2$. Defined as the amount of true shunt which alone would give the observed $P\text{O}_2$. May be calculated from the shunt equation.

Venous cannulation, *see Central venous cannulation; Intravenous fluid administration*

Venous drainage of arm. Deep veins accompany the arteries. Superficial veins on the back of the hand form the dorsal venous arch, from which the basilic and cephalic veins arise. Smaller veins arise from the anterior aspect of the arm (Fig. 162). The anatomy of the veins may vary considerably, especially that of the cephalic vein.

- Main veins of the forearm:
  - basilic vein: ascends on the posteromedial side of the forearm, passing to the anterior side below the elbow. Passes along the medial side of the biceps muscle and pierces the deep fascia. Becomes the axillary vein at the axilla.
  - cephalic vein: ascends on the lateral side of the forearm, passing anterior to the elbow. Runs on the lateral aspect of biceps, along the groove between deltoid and biceps, and pierces the clavipectoral fascia at the lower border of pectoralis major, to join the axillary vein. The angle at which the vessels meet, and the presence of valves at the junction, may cause difficulty in 'feeding' an iv catheter past this point.

See also, Antecubital fossa

Venous drainage of head and neck, *see Cerebral circulation; Jugular veins*

Venous drainage of leg. The main veins are superficial and deep (Fig. 163):

- the important superficial veins arise at the ankle:

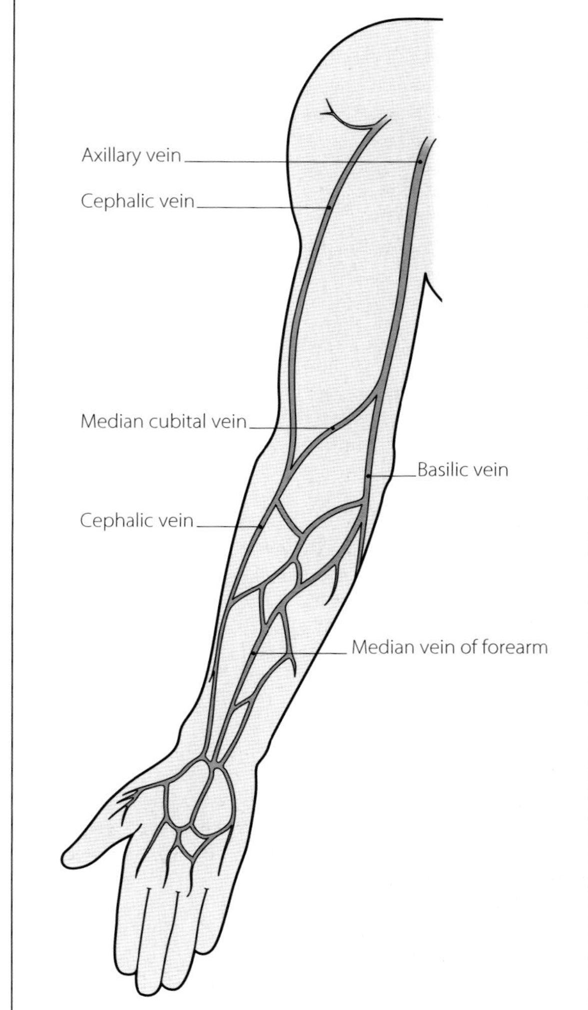

Fig. 162 Venous drainage of the arm

  - long (great) saphenous vein: passes anterior to the medial malleolus behind the saphenous nerve. Ascends behind the medial condyles of the tibia and femur, passing into the thigh and through the saphenous opening in the deep fascia to end in the femoral vein.
  - short (small) saphenous vein: passes behind the lateral malleolus, piercing the deep fascia to join the popliteal vein.
- deep veins start as digital and metatarsal veins in the sole, forming the lateral and medial plantar veins. These form the posterior tibial veins. The anterior tibial veins pass through the interosseus membrane, joining the posterior tibial veins to form the popliteal vein. This ascends through the popliteal fossa to form the femoral vein, which becomes the external iliac vein deep to the inguinal ligament.

Venous pressure, *see Central venous pressure; Jugular venous pressure; Venous waveform*

Venous return. Refers to the volume of blood entering the right atrium per minute. A major determinant of cardiac output as described by Starling's law.

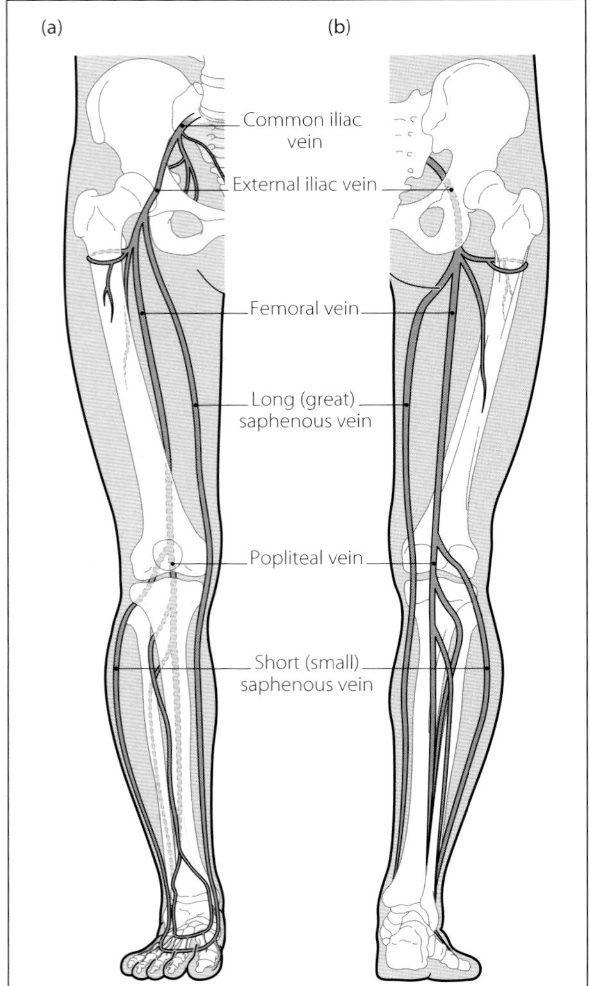

Fig. 163 Venous drainage of the leg: (a) anterior; (b) posterior

- Depends on:
  - venous tone.
  - intrathoracic pressure.
  - intra-abdominal pressure.
  - blood volume.
  - right and left ventricular function.
  - muscular activity (muscle pump).
  - posture.
  - vasodilator/vasopressor drug therapy.

See also, Preload

Venous waveform. Obtained from the tracing of CVP. Can be seen but not felt in the neck as the JVP. Consists of named waves and descents (Fig. 164):

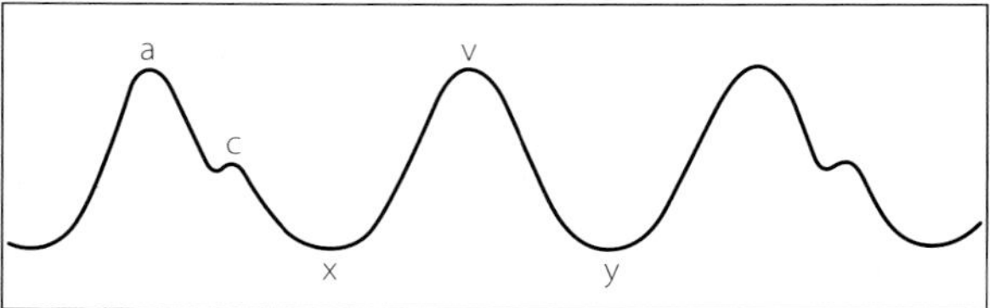

Fig. 164 Venous waveform

  - 'a' wave is due to atrial contraction.
  - 'c' wave is thought to be due to transmitted pulsation from the carotid arteries, or to bulging of the tricuspid valve into the right atrium.
  - 'v' wave is due to the rise in atrial pressure before tricuspid opening.
  - 'x' descent is due to atrial relaxation.
  - 'y' descent is due to atrial emptying as blood enters the ventricle.
- Abnormalities seen in the JVP wave may assist diagnosis of certain valve and rhythm disorders:
  - no 'a' wave: AF.
  - enlarged 'a' wave:
    - tricuspid stenosis.
    - stiff right ventricle, e.g. pulmonary stenosis, pulmonary hypertension.
  - enlarged 'v' wave: tricuspid regurgitation, e.g. due to cardiac failure.
  - cannon waves (large waves, not corresponding to 'a', 'v' or 'c' waves):
    - complete heart block (irregular).
    - junctional arrhythmias (regular).

A similar waveform is seen in the left atrial pressure tracing.
See also, Cardiac cycle

Ventilation, controlled, *see Airway pressure release ventilation; Assisted ventilation; High frequency ventilation; Inspiratory pressure support; Inspiratory volume support; Intermittent mandatory ventilation; Intermittent negative pressure ventilation; Intermittent positive pressure ventilation; Inverse ratio ventilation; Mandatory minute ventilation; Pressure regulated volume control ventilation; Proportional assist ventilation; Synchronised intermittent mandatory ventilation*

Ventilation, liquid, *see Liquid ventilation*

Ventilation, spontaneous, *see Breathing, control of; Breathing, work of; Respiratory muscles*

Ventilation/perfusion mismatch ($\dot{V}/\dot{Q}$ mismatch). Imbalance between alveolar ventilation ($\dot{V}$) and pulmonary capillary blood flow ($\dot{Q}$). In the ideal lung model, ventilation would be distributed uniformly to all parts of the lung and would be matched by uniform distribution of blood flow (i.e. $\dot{V}/\dot{Q} = 1$). However, even in a healthy 70 kg male, alveolar ventilation and blood flow are unequal (4 l/min and 5 l/min respectively), giving a $\dot{V}/\dot{Q}$ ratio of 0.8.

In addition, gravitational forces result in a gradient of $\dot{V}/\dot{Q}$ ratios in the lung as one travels from the apex to the base in the upright position. Both ventilation and perfusion increase from apex to base, but ventilation to a lesser extent than perfusion. Thus the $\dot{V}/\dot{Q}$ ratio is higher at the apex ($\dot{V}/\dot{Q} = 3.3$) than at the base ($\dot{V}/\dot{Q} = 0.63$). Similar but smaller changes occur across the lung in the supine position.

$\dot{V}/\dot{Q}$ mismatch may result in $\dot{V}/\dot{Q}$ ratios ranging from zero (perfusion but no ventilation; shunt) to infinity (ventilation but no perfusion; dead space). Its effects on gas exchange are those of shunt and dead space, and can be assessed by determining venous admixture and physiological dead space. $\dot{V}/\dot{Q}$ mismatch is a common cause of hypoxaemia in pulmonary disease, e.g. COPD, asthma, chest infection, pulmonary oedema, etc. and circulatory disorders, e.g. PE.

Mismatch may be measured using radioisotope scanning of ventilation and perfusion separately, e.g. with xenon and technetium.
See also, Pulmonary circulation

Ventilator-associated lung injury (VALI). Condition sharing symptomatic and pathological features of ALI and ARDS. Thought to be due to use of inappropriate ventilator settings (large tidal volumes and high peak inspiratory pressures) that induce high shear forces in small airways and alveoli. Epithelial overstretching and the repeated collapse and overdistension of airways and alveoli result in local and systemic inflammation with activation of neutrophils and release of cytokines. Its existence has led to the development of lung protection strategies.

Pinhu L, Whitehead T, Evans T, Griffiths M (2003). Lancet; 361: 332–40

See also, Barotrauma; Intermittent positive pressure ventilation

Ventilator-associated pneumonia (VAP). Nosocomial pneumonia developing more than 48 h after tracheal intubation and IPPV. Causes ~50% of ICU infections. Early infections are most often due to common respiratory flora, late infections often due to pseudomonas species, resistant staphylococci and acinetobacter species. Viruses and fungi may also be causal agents.

- Risk factors:
  - patient-related: age, cardiorespiratory disease, ARDS, coma, multiple organ dysfunction syndrome.
  - ventilator-related: duration of IPPV > 7 days, tracheal cuff pressure < 20 cmH_2O, reintubation, tracheostomy.
  - general ICU care: supine position, invasive devices, aspiration, H_2-receptor antagonists, indiscriminate use of broad-spectrum antibiotics.

Diagnosis is difficult due to non-specific signs, e.g. chest X-ray infiltrates, fever, leucocytosis, purulent sputum. Diagnosis may be facilitated by quantitative cultures of specimens obtained by tracheobronchial aspiration, lavage or brush specimens. Differential diagnosis includes pulmonary oedema, atelectasis, PE, ARDS and pulmonary haemorrhage.

Treatment employs 'best guess' or, preferably, specific antibimicrobial therapy.

Preventative measures include good oral care, head-up tilt and possibly selective decontamination of the digestive tract though this is controversial.

Porzecanski I, Bowton DL (2006). Chest; 130: 597–604

See also Chest infection; Intubation, tracheal; Nosocomial infections; Sepsis

Ventilators. Mechanical devices for delivering ventilation to the lungs. First described in the early 1900s as an alternative to resuscitation equipment incorporating bellows. Many developments took place alongside those in thoracic surgery in the first half of the century; the polio epidemics in Denmark in the 1950s were a major impetus to the development of reliable positive pressure ventilators.

- Divided into:
  - negative pressure devices used for intermittent negative pressure ventilation: the negative pressure around the thorax causes chest expansion and draws in air:
    - tank ventilators ('iron lungs'):
      - enclose the whole body (apart from the head and neck) within an airtight casing.
      - efficient, but access to the patient is very restricted.
    - cuirass ventilators:
      - enclose the thorax and upper abdomen. Inflatable jacket versions have been described.
      - less restrictive but less efficient.

    Do not protect against aspiration of gastric contents. Their efficiency may be reduced by indrawing of the soft tissues of the upper airway during inspiration. Tracheostomy may be required if this occurs.
  - positive pressure devices used for IPPV: deliver positive pressure to the lungs via a tracheal tube, tracheostomy, injector device or, more recently, facemask or nasal mask (non-invasive positive pressure ventilation).

    Positive pressure ventilators are widely used during anaesthesia and in ICU. They may be powered:
    - electrically, e.g. employing a crankshaft (e.g. Cape ventilator) or solenoid (e.g. Siemens or Engström ventilators).
    - by a separate supply of compressed air or O_2 employing fluidics or pneumatics (e.g. Penlon Nuffield ventilator).
    - by anaesthetic gases (e.g. Manley ventilator). These types are 'minute volume dividers' (see below).
- Classification of positive pressure ventilators: many different classifications have been suggested, e.g. according to the mechanism of action:
  - 'mechanical thumbs': intermittent occlusion of the open limb of a T-piece, e.g. by a solenoid, e.g. the Sheffield infant ventilator. 'Intermittent blowers' may be used to achieve a similar effect by moving a column of driving gas forwards and backwards along a length of tubing connecting the ventilator with the T-piece, e.g. the Penlon Nuffield ventilator attached to the Bain coaxial anaesthetic breathing system. Anaesthetic gases are delivered separately through the other limb of the T-piece. A similar technique may be used with a circle system.
  - 'minute volume dividers': supply only the minute volume of anaesthetic gas delivered to them, by dividing the preset minute volume into equally sized breaths, e.g. Manley ventilators. Delivered minute volume may be read directly from the anaesthetic machine flowmeters.

    The East–Freeman automatic vent is a small device containing a magnetised bobbin, and is placed at the patient end of an anaesthetic breathing system (e.g. Magill system) whose adjustable pressure-limiting valve is closed. The reservoir bag distends until the upstream pressure exceeds a certain limit, and gas is delivered to the patient. As upstream pressure falls, the bobbin closes the vent, and the cycle repeats. Such vents, typically reserved for emergency or temporary use, are rarely used now. Similar obsolete devices include the Flowmasta and Minivent ventilators.
  - 'bag-squeezers': employ mechanical or pneumatic force to compress the bag or bellows intermittently, e.g. Airshields ventilator, Oxford ventilator (pneumatic), Cape ventilator (mechanical). Widely used with modern circle systems. Bellows which ascend during filling are preferable to those that descend during filling, since the former will not fill if there is a disconnection or leak whereas the latter will still descend.
  - 'intermittent blowers': produce intermittent flow from a high pressure source, e.g. cylinders. Include the Bird ventilators used on ICU, and small devices used for transportation of ventilated patients, e.g. Pneupac ventilator. The Penlon Nuffield ventilator is suitable for use with the Bain and circle systems; it may also be used for children (with a paediatric pressure release valve) using the T-piece.
  - jet ventilators: include those used for injector techniques and high frequency ventilation.
- Another widely used classification is that suggested by Mapleson in 1969, according to the characteristics during the inspiratory phase and inspiratory to expiratory (I to E) cycling:
  - inspiratory characteristics:
    - flow generators: produce a high generating pressure (e.g. 400 kPa) and are thus able to deliver flow which is

unaffected by patient characteristics. The flow produced may be constant or non-constant (usually the former). Non-constant flow generators include the Cape ventilator, in which flow is sinusoidal because of the crank mechanism employed. These ventilators are able to produce the high inflation pressures required to achieve the preset flow in non-compliant lungs, e.g. in bronchospasm, and most ICU ventilators are therefore flow generators (Fig. 165a). Barotrauma may occur if high airway pressures are reached.
- pressure generators: produce low generating pressure (e.g. 1.5 kPa); thus the flow delivered is affected by patient characteristics (Fig. 165b). The pressure produced may be constant or non-constant (usually the former; non-constant pressure generators include the East–Freeman automatic vent, in which the tension in the stretched reservoir bag falls as the reservoir bag empties). Since the airway pressure attainable is preset, the risk of barotrauma is reduced. However, the tidal volume delivered depends on the resistance of the tubing and the patient's respiratory mechanics, e.g. compliance, airway resistance, etc. Pressure generators are usually employed in paediatric anaesthesia, to reduce the risk of barotrauma. Examples of constant pressure generators are the Manley and East Radcliffe ventilators.

- I to E cycling:
  - time cycled: the duration of inspiration is preset, e.g. Manley MP2, Penlon Nuffield, Siemens Servo 900 series.
  - pressure cycled: expiration begins when a preset airway pressure is reached, e.g. Bird ventilator.
  - volume cycled: expiration begins when a preset tidal volume has been delivered, e.g. Manley Pulmovent ventilator.
  - flow cycled (pressure generators only): expiration begins when a preset inspiratory flow is reached, e.g. Bennett PR-2 ventilator. Rarely used as a method of cycling.

Many of the above have been replaced by more sophisticated ventilators which may be employed as either flow generators or pressure generators, with a choice of cycling methods.

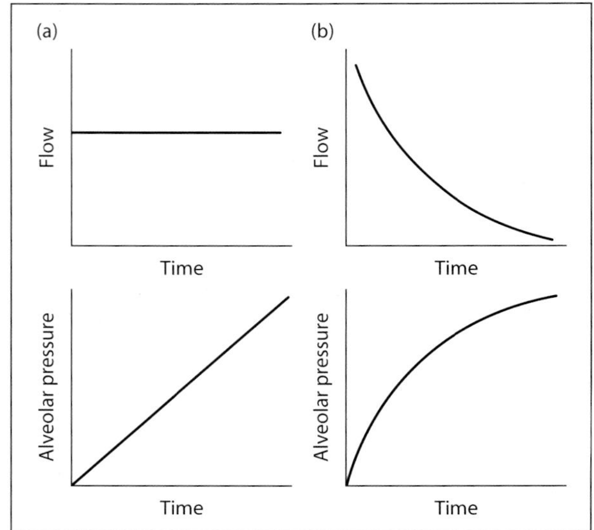

Fig. 165 Inspiratory characteristics of (a) constant flow and (b) constant pressure generators

Thus they may be used both for anaesthesia and (with more complex features) for different clinical situations, e.g. on ICU.

The expiratory phase usually involves passive recoil of the lungs to atmospheric pressure. Many ventilators allow application of PEEP if required. Negative end-expiratory pressure is no longer used. The changeover from expiratory to inspiratory phases is usually time cycled, although it may be triggered by the patient in some modes.

The ideal ventilator for use on ICU should include flexibility in flow or pressure generation and cycling as above, allow PEEP and special modes to be used, e.g. for weaning, allow humidification and administration of nebulised drugs, be easy to sterilise and incorporate monitors and alarms. Specific advanced ventilator modes used in ICU include airway pressure release ventilation, inspiratory pressure support, inspiratory volume support, intermittent mandatory ventilation, inverse ratio ventilation, mandatory minute ventilation, pressure regulated volume control ventilation, proportional assist ventilation, synchronised intermittent mandatory ventilation. Many permit alteration of the I:E ratio, inspiratory waveform, PEEP, etc.

[Ernst W von Siemens (1816–1892), German engineer; Carl-Gunnar Engström (1912–1987), Swedish physician; Roger EW Manley (1930–1991), UK anaesthetist and engineer; William W Mapleson, Cardiff physicist]

Smallwood RW (1988). Anaesth Intensive Care; 14: 251–7

See also, Monitoring

Ventile, *see Scavenging*

Ventricular ectopic beats (VEs, VEBs; Premature ventricular contractions/beats, PVCs/PCBs). Contraction of ventricular muscle caused by an ectopic focus instead of normal impulse conduction. The ventricles discharge early; the next sinus impulse finds the ventricular muscle refractory, causing a pause before the next beat. VEs typically appear as wide bizarre complexes on the ECG (Fig. 166); VEs arising from different sites (i.e. multifocal) may have different configurations.

They may occur in normal hearts, but may also indicate organic heart disease. Other causes include drugs, e.g. halothane, digoxin, antiarrhythmic drugs, electrolyte and acid–base disturbances, hypoxaemia, hypercapnia and pain. Common during anaesthesia, especially with spontaneous ventilation with halothane. May occur at regular intervals, e.g. every 2nd or 3rd beat. Usually do not require treatment, apart from correction of the cause. Antiarrhythmic drugs (usually lidocaine) are usually recommended for VEs more common than 5 per minute, or if multifocal or close to the preceding T wave with risk of the R on T phenomenon.

See also, Arrhythmias

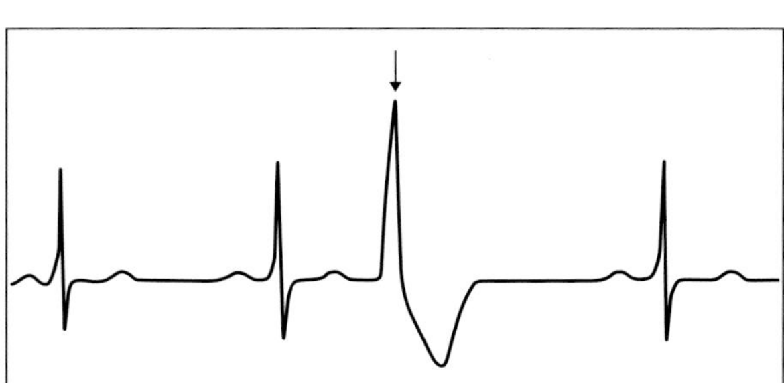

Fig. 166 Ventricular ectopic beat (arrowed)

Ventricular fibrillation (VF). Incoordinated and ineffective ventricular contraction caused by completely irregular ventricular depolarisation. Usually follows the R on T phenomenon. Causes include myocardial ischaemia, MI, hypoxaemia, electrocution, electrolyte imbalance, hypothermia and drug toxicity (e.g. adrenaline, digoxin). There is no cardiac output; asystole therefore follows unless treated. VF is the most common cause of cardiac arrest. The ECG shows continuous random electrical activity without QRS complexes (Fig. 167).

Treated by defibrillation although a single precordial thump is advocated for witnessed or monitored arrests.

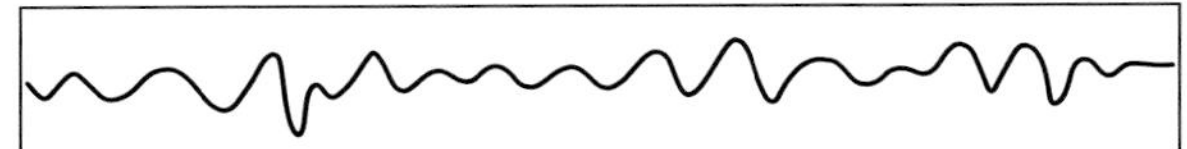

Fig. 167 Ventricular fibrillation

Ventricular septal defect (VSD). Accounts for 20–30% of congenital heart disease; may also follow MI or trauma. The commonest congenital form involves the membranous septum immediately below the tricuspid valve; bulbar or muscular septal involvement is rarer. Blood flows across the defect from left to right during systole. As right ventricular pressures decrease after birth, shunt increases. May cause cardiac failure in infancy. Small defects with normal pulmonary artery pressures are often asymptomatic (Maladie de Roger) and may close spontaneously. Large defects may lead to pulmonary hypertension and Eisenmenger's syndrome.

- Features:
  - harsh pansystolic murmur, heard best in the left 4th intercostal space (louder with small defects). Splitting of the second heart sound.
  - of Eisenmenger's syndrome if present.
  - of left and right ventricular hypertrophy on ECG and chest X-ray.

  Up to 25% of patients may be affected by bacterial endocarditis at some time.
- Treated by surgery. Anaesthesia is as for congenital heart disease and cardiac surgery.

[Henri L Roger (1809–1891), French physician]

Ventricular stretch receptors, *see Baroreceptors*

Ventricular tachycardia (VT). Rapid series of ventricular ectopic beats (usually defined as more than three in succession). The pulse rate usually lies between 130 and 250 beats/min. Normal atrial activity may continue independently, or the ventricular impulses may pass retrogradely to the atria.

- Distinguished from SVT by the following features (Fig. 168):
  - QRS complexes are usually wide and bizzare.
  - retrograde conduction to the atria may result in inverted P waves (which may be hidden by the QRS complexes).
  - independent atrial activity may be suggested by:
    - occasional P waves.
    - capture beats (normal QRS complexes following occasional normal atrioventricular conduction).
    - fusion beats (with combined features of normal and ectopic QRS complexes, representing simultaneous atrially conducted and ectopic ventricular activity).
  - marked left axis deviation, with all of the chest leads either negative or positive.

  Both VT and SVT may be regular, and associated with normotension or hypotension. Differentiation between broad-complex VT and SVT may be particularly difficult. The response to adenosine may aid diagnosis.

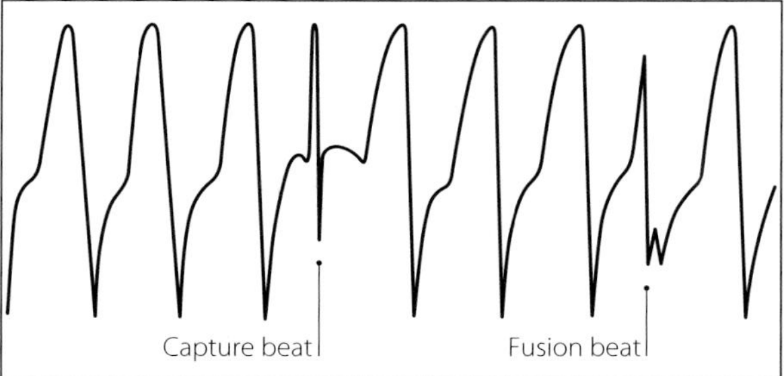

Fig. 168 Ventricular tachycardia, showing capture and fusion beats

Causes are as for ventricular ectopic beats.

- Treatment (following CPR if necessary):
  - antiarrhythmic drugs, e.g. lidocaine and related drugs, amiodarone.
  - cardioversion, especially if VT causes hypotension or drugs are contraindicated or ineffective.
  - cardiac pacing has also been used.
  - prophylaxis of recurrent VT includes antiarrhythmic drugs, surgical excision of the ectopic focus, and implantable defibrillators.

See also, Torsade de pointes

Venturi principle. Entrainment of a fluid through a side-arm into an area of low pressure caused by a constriction in a tube (Bernoulli effect). Entrainment depends on careful positioning of the side-arm, a suitably shaped constriction, and the gradual increase in diameter of the limb distal to the constriction.

The principle is employed in gas mixing devices (including fixed performance oxygen therapy devices), suction equipment, ejector flowmeters, scavenging equipment, and devices used to circulate gases round breathing systems.

[Giovanni Venturi (1746–1822), Italian physicist]

Verapamil hydrochloride. Calcium channel blocking drug, mainly used as an antiarrhythmic drug to treat SVT. Acts by prolonging conduction through the atrioventricular node. Also used in angina and hypertension, including following tracheal intubation. Undergoes extensive first-pass metabolism when given orally. Excreted renally.

- Dosage:
  - 5 mg by slow iv injection, repeated up to 15–20 mg at 5-min intervals.
  - 40–120 mg 8 hourly, orally.
- Side effects: hypotension, bradycardia, complete heart block and asystole, especially if the patient has received β-adrenergic receptor antagonists. Contraindicated in Wolff–Parkinson–White syndrome, since atrioventricular block may encourage conduction through accessory pathways with resultant arrhythmia. Its action may be potentiated by inhalational anaesthetic agents, especially halothane.

Veratridine. Steroidal alkaloid, which binds specifically to activated (open) sodium channels and prevents them from closing. Has been used experimentally to block unmyelinated C fibres preferentially.

Vertebrae. Bony components of the vertebral column. The latter is about 70 cm long in the adult male and is flexed

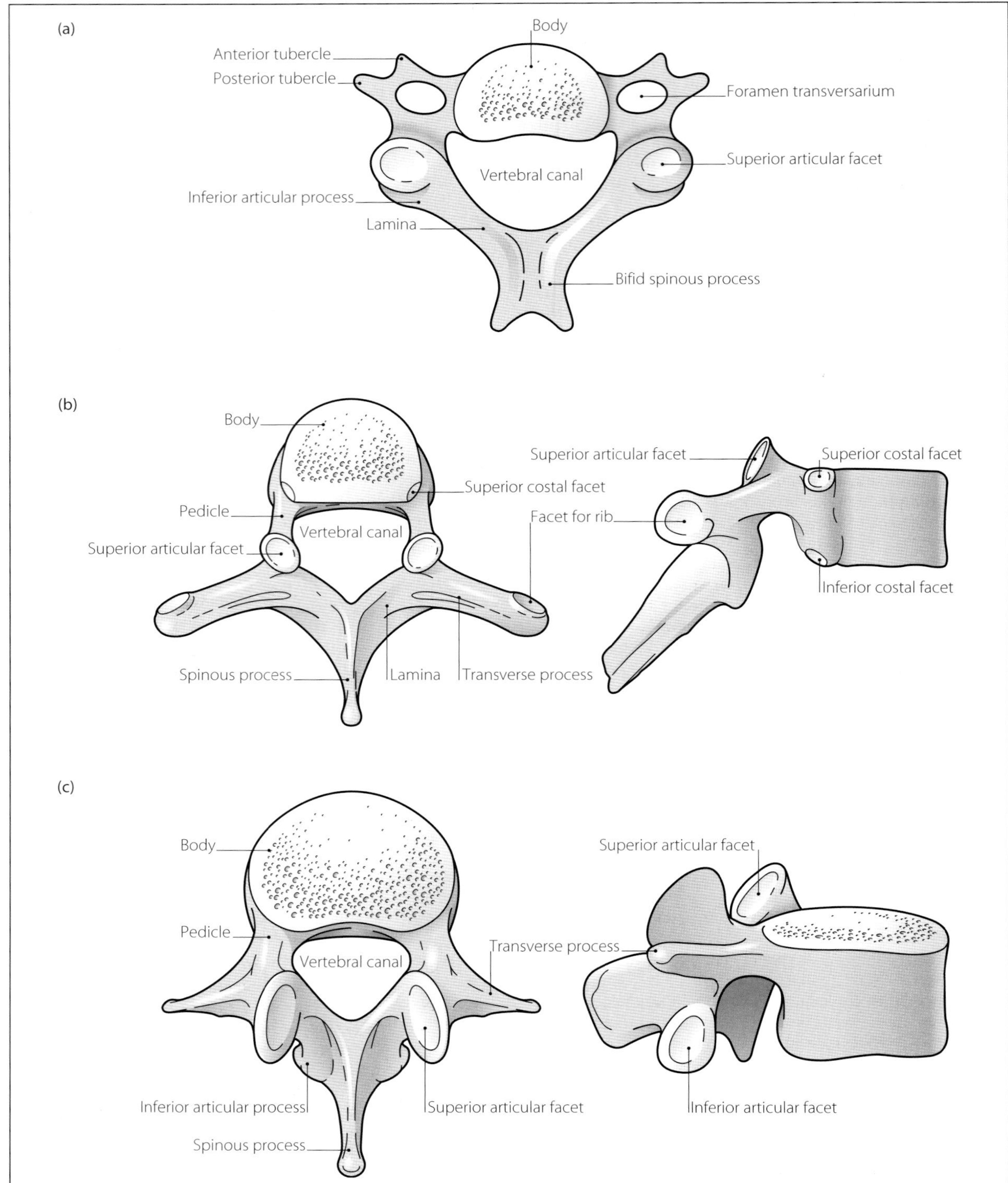

Fig. 169 Typical vertebrae: (a) cervical, superior view; (b) thoracic, superior and lateral views; (c) lumbar, superior and lateral views

throughout its length in the fetus; after birth two secondary curves appear so that the cervical and lumbar regions are convex forwards and the thoracic and sacral regions are concave. There are 7 cervical vertebrae, 12 thoracic, 5 lumbar, 5 fused sacral and 3–5 fused coccygeal. Vertebral bodies of C2 to L5 are separated by fibrocartilaginous vertebral discs, accounting for about 25% of the spine's total length. Each has an outer fibrous annulus fibrosus, and the more fluid inner nucleus pulposus. The latter may prolapse through the former, impinging upon the **spinal cord** or spinal nerves. Discs thin with age, resulting in reduced height. Vertebrae and discs are united by the **vertebral ligaments**.

- Structure of a typical vertebra:
  - body: short and cylindrical and lies anteriorly.
  - arch: encloses the **vertebral canal** and lies posteriorly. Composed of the rounded pedicles anteriorly and the

flattened laminae posteriorly. The laminae are united in the midline by the spinous process. They also bear transverse processes and superior and inferior articular processes which bear facets for articulation with adjacent vertebrae.

- Regional differences:
  - cervical (Fig. 169a):
    - each has the foramen transversarium passing through its transverse processes, through which pass the vertebral arteries.
    - C1 (atlas):
      - has neither body nor spine.
      - articular facets articulate superiorly with the base of the skull.
      - facet on the anterior edge of the vertebral canal articulates with the odontoid peg.
    - C2 (axis): odontoid peg projects from the superior surface of the body, held against the body of the atlas by the transverse ligament. The gap between the peg and atlas is normally less than 3 mm on neck flexion (5 mm in children).
    - C2–6: bifid spinous processes.
    - C7 (vertebra prominens): non-bifid spine (the first easily palpable spine encountered, feeling from the skull downwards; T1 below it has a more prominent spine).
  - thoracic (Fig. 169b):
    - body: heart-shaped, articulating with the ribs via superior and inferior costal facets at the rear of the body.
    - transverse processes: large, passing backwards and laterally, and bearing facets which articulate with the ribs' tubercles (except the last two thoracic vertebrae).
    - spinous processes: long, inclined at about 60° to the horizontal.
    - anatomical variations:
      - T1: has a longer upper facet for the 1st rib and a smaller lower facet for the 2nd rib.
      - T10–12: usually bear single costal facets on their bodies.
      - T12: spinous process has notched lower edge.
  - lumbar (Fig. 169c):
    - body: kidney-shaped.
    - transverse processes: thick, passing laterally. Bear the accessory processes posteriorly at their bases.
    - spines: project horizontally backwards.
    - L5: short but massive transverse processes, arising from the sides of the body and pedicles. The body is deeper anteriorly than posteriorly.
  - sacral: fused to form the sacrum, enclosing the sacral canal.
  - coccygeal: fused to form the triangular coccyx, the base of which articulates with the sacrum.

Vertebral arteries. Arise from the subclavian arteries, passing upwards through the foramina transversaria of the upper six cervical vertebrae and passing medially behind the lateral mass of the atlas. They enter the skull through the foramen magnum, uniting to form the basilar artery after piercing the dura. Vertebrobasilar insufficiency typically results in dizziness, vertigo, diplopia and hemiparesis.

May be damaged or entered during central venous cannulation and brachial plexus block.

See also, Cerebral circulation

Vertebral canal. Triangular canal within the vertebrae, with its base posteriorly. Contains:

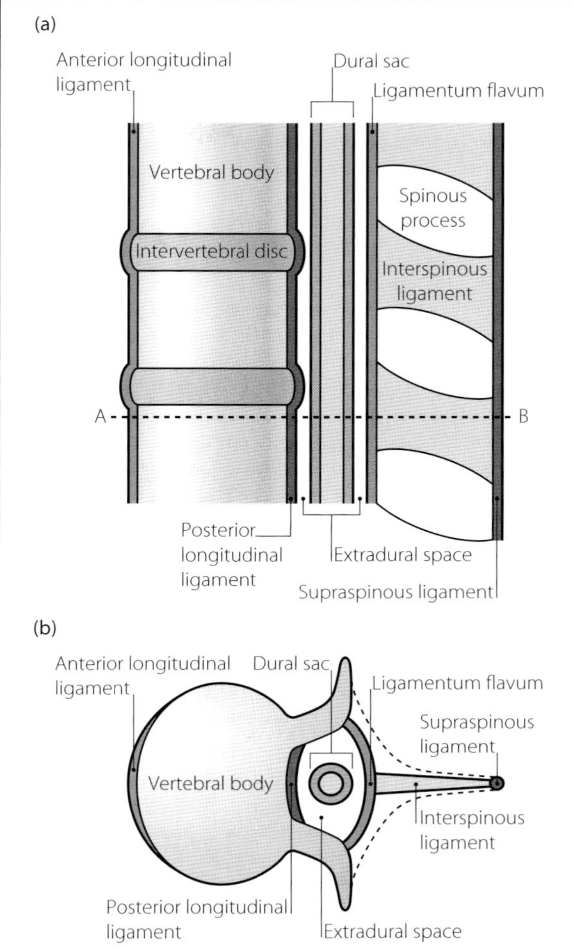

Fig. 170 Vertebral ligaments: (a) longitudinal section of vertebral column; (b) transverse section through A–B

- epidural space and contents.
- spinal cord and spinal nerves/roots.

Vertebral ligaments. Individual vertebrae are linked by a number of ligaments (Fig. 170):

- anterior longitudinal ligament: runs from C2 to the sacrum, attached to the anterior aspects of the vertebral bodies. Continues superiorly to form the anterior atlanto-occipital membrane.
- posterior longitudinal ligament: as for the anterior, but attached to the posterior vertebral aspects. Continues superiorly to form the membrana tectoria between the axis and occiput.
- ligamenta flava (yellow ligaments): run between the laminae of adjacent vertebrae. More developed in the lumbar than thoracic regions. Continue superiorly as the posterior atlanto-occipital membrane.
- interspinous ligaments: run between the spines of adjacent vertebrae.
- supraspinous ligament: runs from C7 to the sacrum, attached to the tips of the spines.

- Additional ligaments at the atlanto-occipito-axial complex:
  - transverse ligament of the atlas: runs between medial aspects of the atlas' lateral masses, securing the odontoid peg.

- alar ligaments: pass from the sides of the odontoid peg to the occipital condyles.
- apical ligament: thin band, connecting the odontoid's tip to the anterior aspect of the foramen magnum.

● Sacrococcygeal ligaments:
- posterior: overlies the sacral hiatus.
- anterior: passes over the anterior aspect of the sacrum and coccyx.
- lateral: joins the lateral angle of the sacrum to the transverse processes of the coccyx.

VF, *see Ventricular fibrillation*

Viagra, *see Sildenafil*

Victoria, Queen (1819–1901). British monarch, given chloroform by Snow during the births of her eighth and ninth children: Prince Leopold in 1853, and Princess Beatrice in 1857 (on the latter occasion, Prince Albert administered chloroform himself prior to Snow's arrival). This gave respectability to pain relief during labour, which had been criticised as being against God's will.
[Leopold (1853–1884), Beatrice (1857–1944), Albert (1819–1861)]
See also, Obstetric analgesia and anaesthesia

VIE, *see Vacuum insulated evaporator*

Vigabatrin. Anticonvulsant drug used as second line treatment for partial and generalised secondary seizures. Its efficacy in tonic–clonic seizures is less well documented. Irreversibly inhibits γ-aminobutyric acid transaminase (GABA-T), the enzyme responsible for breakdown of GABA. Duration of action approximately 24 h with elimination half-life of 7 h. Excreted unchanged in the urine.

● Dosage: 1 g initially, increased up to 2–3 g/day, orally.
● Side effects: sedation, dizziness, headache, agitation, psychosis, visual disturbances.

VIP, *see Vasoactive intestinal peptide*

Viscosity (η). Tendency of fluids to resist flow. Measured in poise. Equal to shear force (force per unit surface area) divided by velocity gradient between adjacent fluid layers. Dependent on intermolecular attractive forces, e.g. van der Waals forces, and entanglement of bulky molecules. Decreased at high temperatures; particles have more kinetic energy and may escape from their neighbours more easily. Laminar flow is inversely proportional to viscosity.

Blood viscosity depends largely on haematocrit (increasing exponentially as haematocrit increases), red cell characteristics and blood protein concentration. It rises with age and smoking. It is increased slightly by volatile anaesthetic agents. Blood viscosity alters with different flow rates; i.e. blood is a non-Newtonian fluid. At vessel diameters of less than 0.3 mm, it drops markedly, resulting in greater flow than with a Newtonian fluid. The reason is unclear, but may involve 'plasma skimming' (the tendency of cellular components of blood to remain in the middle of vessels whilst plasma passes into branches arising from the vessel wall). Blood cell deformability may also be important. At very low blood flow, viscosity increases as the cells clump together.

Relative viscosity (compared with water) of normal plasma is 1.5; that of normal whole blood is 3.5.

Viscosity may be derived by measuring the time taken for a liquid to drain through a narrow tube. Alternatively, the torque on an inner drum may be measured when an outer drum is rotated, the specimen liquid filling the space between the drums.
[Sir Isaac Newton (1642–1727), English scientist]

Vishnevskiy technique (Transverse injection anaesthesia). Injection of local anaesthetic agent into a transverse 'slice' of a limb; originally described using procaine. Infiltration is performed from skin to bone, using large volumes of agent. Has been called the 'squirt and cut' technique.
[Aleksandr V Vishnevskiy (1874–1948), Russian surgeon]

Vital capacity. The largest volume of air that can be expired slowly after maximal inspiration; measured by a spirometer. Reduced in the supine position. Also reduced in the elderly, and in patients with restrictive lung disease, muscle weakness, abdominal swelling and pain.
See also, Forced vital capacity; Lung function tests; Lung volumes

Vitamin B_{12} (Cobalamin). Water-soluble vitamin present in many animal tissues, especially eggs and liver. Exists as various related compounds, e.g. hydroxo- or cyanocobalamin. Combines with gastric intrinsic factor, enabling its absorption from the terminal ileum. Required for red blood cell maturation and as a cofactor by methionine synthase. Deficiency may be caused by failure of intrinsic factor production due to atrophic gastritis (pernicious anaemia) or gastric resection, or by disease/resection of the ileum. Dietary deficiency is rare. Inhibited by N_2O. Deficiency results in macrocytic megaloblastic anaemia and subacute combined degeneration of the cord.

Administered im 3 monthly as hydroxocobalamin; cyanocobalamin requires more frequent administration. It has been used in the treatment of cyanide poisoning.

Vitamin deficiency. May occur in:
- inadequate intake relative to requirements, e.g. malnutrition (including inadequate provision during TPN).
- malabsorption, e.g. due to gastric disease (vitamin B_{12}), pancreatic disease (fat-soluble vitamins: A, D, E and K).
- impaired metabolism of precursors, e.g. osteomalacia in renal failure.
- antagonism by drugs, e.g. warfarin (vitamin K), N_2O (folate and vitamin B_{12}).

● Specific deficiency states of possible anaesthetic importance:
- vitamin A: night blindness, dry skin.
- vitamin B_1 (thiamine): peripheral neuropathy, encephalopathy, cardiomyopathy (beriberi). May accompany chronic alcoholism. Vitamin B_1 is used in ethylene glycol poisoning.
- vitamin B_2 (riboflavin): anaemia, mouth lesions.
- vitamin B_6 (pyridoxine): convulsions, anaemia. May accompany chronic alcoholism. Vitamin B_6 is used in ethylene glycol poisoning and isoniazid therapy.
- niacin: dermatitis, diarrhoea, dementia (pellagra).
- vitamin B_{12}: anaemia, subacute combined degeneration of the cord.
- vitamin C: generalised bleeding (especially gums), anaemia, weakness, poor wound healing (scurvy).
- vitamin D: hypocalcaemia, hyperphosphataemia, muscle weakness, rickets (in children), osteomalacia (in adults).
- vitamin E: haemolysis, oedema.
- vitamin K: bleeding tendency.

Vitamin K. Fat-soluble group of vitamins which catalyse the carboxylation of glutamic acid residues to activate coagulation factors II, VII, IX and X. Deficiency results in increased tendency to bleed and may result from:

- inadequate intake: rare in adults, common in the newborn.
- inadequate absorption, e.g. malabsorption syndromes, biliary obstruction.
- inadequate utilisation, e.g. liver disease.
- drug therapy: especially warfarin and similar drugs which act as vitamin K antagonists.

May be given orally, iv or im to help correct deficiency; takes up to 12 h to work. May cause several weeks' upset to coagulation control in patients on long-term warfarin therapy. Available as a synthetic analogue (menadiol sodium phosphate) or as phytomenadione (vitamin K_1).

- Dosage: 2.5–10 mg, repeated as necessary. Prothrombin time should be monitored.

Anaphylactoid reactions may follow rapid iv injection.
See also, Coagulation studies

Vitamins. Term derived from 'vital amins'. Group of dietary compounds necessary for health and growth but which do not supply energy (Table 37). Lack of one or more produces vitamin deficiency states. Vitamins A, D, E and K are fat soluble; the rest are water soluble.

Vocal cords, *see Larynx*

Volatile anaesthetic agents, *see Inhalational anaesthetic agents*

Volt. Unit of electrical potential. One volt is the potential difference between two points when 1 joule of work is done per coulomb of electricity passing from one point to the other. [Alessandro Volta (1745–1827), Italian physicist]

Volume of distribution (V_d). Mathematical concept indicating the amount of a drug in the tissues; equal to the volume of water in which an injected dose would have to be diluted in order to give the measured plasma concentration. For a drug confined to plasma, V_d equals blood volume. For a drug distributed equally throughout the body, it equals total body water volume. For a drug concentrated in the tissues, V_d exceeds total body water volume. May be calculated from the graph of plasma drug concentration against time after iv injection:

$$V_d = \frac{\text{dose}}{\text{concentration at time 0}}$$

Examples (approximate values for a 70 kg man):

- digoxin: $V_d = 500$ litres
- propranolol: $V_d = 250$ litres
- lidocaine: $V_d = 120$ litres
- insulin: $V_d = 50$ litres
- aspirin: $V_d = 12$ litres
- warfarin: $V_d = 9$ litres

Drugs or poisons with a small V_d are easily cleared from the plasma by haemodialysis or haemoperfusion; those with large V_d may be cleared from the plasma but levels tend to rise again (with possible recurrence of toxic effects) following cessation of dialytic therapy.
See also, Pharmacokinetics

Volume support, *see Inspiratory volume support*

Vomiting. Reflex involving retrograde passage of gastric contents through the mouth. The vomiting centre in the lateral medullary reticular formation receives afferent impulses from the:

- GIT, abdominal organs and peritoneum via the vagus and sympathetic nerves.
- heart mainly via the vagus nerve.
- vestibular apparatus.
- chemoreceptor trigger zone (CTZ).
- higher centres.

Chemical irritants, e.g. strong saline, stimulate the vomiting centre via receptors in the GIT. Drugs (e.g. apomorphine) and neurotransmitters (e.g. dopamine, noradrenaline, acetylcholine, 5-HT) stimulate the CTZ. Raised ICP is thought to cause vomiting via increased pressure on the floor of the fourth ventricle.

Motor impulses travel through cranial nerves V, VII, IX, X and XII to the upper GIT and through spinal nerves to the diaphragm and abdominal muscles.

- Sequence of events:
  - salivation increases.
  - breathing deepens.
  - glottis closes.
  - breath is held in mid-inspiration.
  - abdominal muscles contract.
  - oesophageal sphincters relax.
  - gastric contents are expelled.

Nausea is a sensation that may or may not be associated with the act of vomiting itself, although the two are usually considered together since the neurological pathways are similar. The incidence of PONV has been found to vary from

Table 37 Functions, sources and adult daily requirements of vitamins

Vitamin	*Function*	*Sources*	*Daily requirements*
A	Visual pigmentation, fetal development	Yellow vegetables and fruit	15–20 μg/kg
B_1 (Thiamine)	Cofactor in decarboxylation	Liver, cereals	20 μg/kg
B_2 (Riboflavin)	Flavoproteins	Liver, milk	20 μg/kg
Niacin	Constituent of NAD and NADP	Yeast and lean meat	0.4 mg/kg
B_6 (Pyridoxine)	Decarboxylases and transaminases	Yeast, wheat and liver	20 μg/kg
Pantothenic acid	Constituent of coenzyme A	Eggs, liver	0.3–0.8 mg/kg
Biotin	Fatty acid synthesis	Egg yolk, liver	2–3 μg/kg
Folic acid	Methylating reactions	Green vegetables	2–3 μg/kg
Vitamin B_{12}	Amino acid metabolism, erythropoiesis	Liver, meat, eggs	0.04–0.1 μg/kg
Vitamin C (ascorbic acid)	Collagen synthesis	Citrus fruits	1.0 mg/kg
Vitamin D	Intestinal absorption of calcium and phosphate	Fish, liver	0.1–0.2 μg/kg
Vitamin E	Antioxidants	Milk, eggs, meat	0.1–0.2 μg/kg
Vitamin K	Blood coagulation	Green vegetables	1.0 μg/kg

15 to 90%. Usually distressing, it is particularly undesirable in ear and ophthalmic surgery, and neurosurgery.

- Effects of prolonged vomiting:
  - loss of hydrogen, chloride, potassium and sodium ions, and water.
  - renal bicarbonate loss to restore pH, causing alkaline urine.
  - fall in sodium and ECF causing aldosterone release, which causes renal sodium and fluid retention, in exchange for potassium and hydrogen ions. If hypokalaemia is severe, hydrogen ion loss predominates, with paradoxical acid urine.
  - thus dehydration, metabolic alkalosis and total body potassium depletion may occur.

Von Recklinghausen's disease, *see Neurofibromatosis*

Von Willebrand's disease. Commonest inherited coagulation disorder (affects ~1:100–1000 people but may be very mild); first described in 1926, with autosomal dominant transmission. Abnormality of von Willebrand factor, a protein involved in platelet adhesion and carriage of coagulation factor VIII, leads to factor VIII deficiency, abnormal platelet adhesiveness and abnormal vascular endothelium. Epistaxis and bruising are more common than haemarthrosis and haematoma, although there is marked variation in clinical severity.

Classified into three main types; type I (quantitative reduction in von Willebrand factor) accounts for about 90% of cases whilst types II (qualitative abnormality of von Willebrand factor) and III (similar to type I but a severe autosomal recessive form) account for about 10% and $< 1\%$ respectively.

- Investigations:
  - platelet count: low or normal.
  - prothrombin time: normal.
  - partial thromboplastin time: prolonged.
  - bleeding time: prolonged.

Fresh frozen plasma or cryoprecipitate may be given prior to surgery. Desmopressin administration may boost levels of factor VIII and von Willebrand factor, and may be used preoperatively (0.4 µg/kg iv). Tranexamic acid 1 g orally has also been advocated. Antiplatelet drugs must be avoided.

During pregnancy, levels of factor VIII and von Willebrand factor increase, but they may fall rapidly after delivery.

[Erik von Willebrand (1870–1949), Swedish physician]

Mannucci PM (2004). N Engl J Med; 351: 683–94

See also, Blood products; Coagulation studies

Voriconazole. Broad-spectrum triazole antifungal drug, related to fluconazole and used for severe fungal infections.

- Dosage: 400–800 mg orally or 4–6 mg/kg iv, daily.
- Side effects: as for fluconazole, though most organ systems can be affected.

$\dot{V}/\dot{Q}$ mismatch, *see Ventilation/perfusion mismatch*

VRE, Vancomycin resistant enterococci, *see Infection control; Vancomycin*

VSD, *see Ventricular septal defect*

VT, *see Ventricular tachycardia*

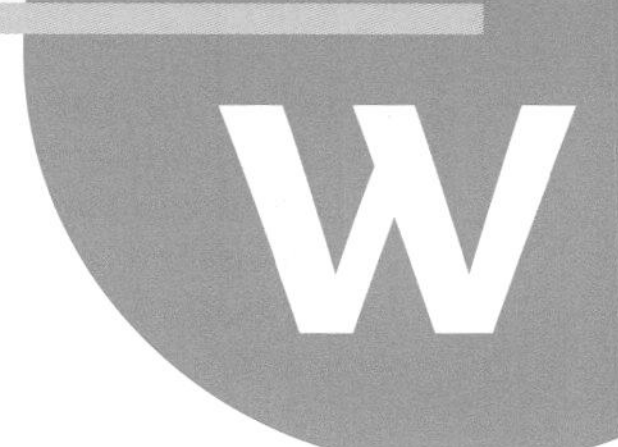

Wakefulness, *see Awareness*

Wake-up test. Intraoperative awakening to allow assessment of spinal cord function during spinal surgery. Has also been used to assess cerebral function during basilar artery clipping.

Warfarin sodium. Oral anticoagulant drug, first synthesised in 1944. Rapidly absorbed by mouth and almost totally protein-bound. Competes with vitamin K in the synthesis of coagulation factors II, VII, IX and X in the liver; therefore requires 1–2 days for its effect to develop. Also inhibits protein C and S. Metabolised in the liver and excreted in urine and faeces. Half-life is about 30 h. Dosage is adjusted according to results of coagulation studies: the International Normalised Ratio (INR) is maintained at about 2–3 for prophylaxis and treatment of DVT, PE, transient ischaemic attacks and in patients with atrial fibrillation and a high risk of embolisation; 3–4.5 for recurrent DVT/PE, cardiac and arterial prostheses. The usual maintenance dose is 3–9 mg/day. The INR is usually checked daily or on alternate days initially, but thereafter up to every 2 months, depending on the response.

Drugs causing hepatic enzyme induction, e.g. phenobarbital and phenytoin, reduce its effect. If the second drug is withdrawn without reducing the dose of warfarin, haemorrhage may occur. Effects may be enhanced by drugs that displace it from protein binding sites, e.g. sulphonamides, NSAIDs. Emergency treatment of haemorrhage due to excessive warfarin effect involves use of vitamin K injection (up to 5 mg iv) and the administration of factors II, VII, IX and X (prothrombin complex concentrate, or fresh frozen plasma).

Teratogenic; thus traditionally avoided in the first trimester of pregnancy, although there is evidence it may be more effective than heparin at preventing valve thrombosis and thus safer for pregnant women with prosthetic heart valves. Warfarin crosses the placenta, risking placental or fetal haemorrhage if given in the third trimester.

Patients taking warfarin who present for surgery may pose problems with perioperative coagulation. Suggested guidelines:

- heart valves: maintain warfarin therapy for short (under 30 min) surgery, with fresh frozen plasma available. Otherwise, stop warfarin 3 days preoperatively, and start heparin infusion 24 h later (about 15 000 units/12 h), maintaining activated partial thromboplastin time (APPT) at 2–3 times normal. Stop heparin 6 h preoperatively, and check INR and APTT 1 hour preoperatively. Surgery may be delayed, or plasma administered, if INR exceeds 1.5. Restart warfarin as soon as possible postoperatively, or heparin if nil by mouth for over 48 h. Extra precautions have been suggested for prosthetic mitral valves, since the risk of emboli is greater than for other valves: aspirin 75 mg or dipyridamole 300 mg/day is started when warfarin is stopped. Heparin is restarted 6–12 h postoperatively until able to take warfarin.
- other conditions: stop warfarin for 48 h before surgery. The INR should be less than 1.5. Heparin may be given perioperatively sc to reduce thromboembolism until warfarin is restarted, or iv infusion used postoperatively in high risk cases, e.g. recurrent PE.
- emergency surgery: give vitamin K, and wait for synthesis of new clotting factors (about 6–12 h); this may interfere with subsequent anticoagulation for weeks afterwards. Alternatively, fresh frozen plasma may be given (though specific factors are better). The INR is monitored throughout.

[Wisconsin Alumni Research Foundation, where warfarin was developed]

Warren, John C (1778–1856). Professor of Surgery and Anatomy at Harvard Medical School. It was at Warren's invitation that Wells gave his demonstration of N_2O anaesthesia, which ended in failure. Later, at Morton's first public demonstration of diethyl ether, Warren performed the surgery.

Washout curves. Graphs displaying the exponential decline in concentration of a substance which is continuously being removed from a system. The substance may be 'washed out' by blood flow, in the case of dye dilution cardiac output measurement, or by ventilation of the lungs, in the case of nitrogen washout. The term is sometimes used to describe any exponential process.

Water, *see Fluid balance; Fluids, body*

Water balance, *see Fluid balance*

Water diuresis. Diuresis occurring about 15 min after the intake of a large volume of hypotonic fluid. Absorption of the fluid is followed by inhibition of vasopressin secretion and by increased urinary water loss.

Water intoxication, *see Hyponatraemia*

Waterhouse–Friderichsen syndrome, *see Adrenocortical insufficiency*

Waters bag, *see Anaesthetic breathing systems*

Waters cannister, *see Carbon dioxide absorption in anaesthetic breathing systems*

Waters, Ralph Milton (1883–1979). US anaesthetist; became Assistant Professor of Surgery in charge of anaesthetics at University of Wisconsin, leading to his appointment as the first university Professor of Anaesthesia in the USA (1933). Was the first to establish a resident training programme in anaesthesia and the first to use cyclopropane clinically (1930). Re-examined chloroform toxicity, advocated the use of inflatable cuffs on tracheal tubes, and was involved in many aspects of anaesthesia, including the use of thiopental and endobronchial intubation. Designed his 'to-and-fro' cannister for CO_2 absorption in anaesthetic breathing systems, and the Waters airway, a metal oropharyngeal airway with a side-arm for attachment to a gas supply.

Waterton, Charles (1783–1865). Squire of Walton Hall, Yorkshire; made his first voyage to South America in 1812. Described the preparation of curare and the blow pipes, darts, bows and arrows used by the Indians of the Amazon and Orinoco basins. Experimented with the drug on his return to England, and maintained life in a paralysed donkey by employing artificial ventilation. Published details of his work and travels in *Wanderings in South America* (1825).

Watt. Unit of power. One watt (W) = 1 joule per second (J/s).
[James Watt (1736–1819), Scottish engineer]

Waveforms. Repetitive patterns plotted against time produce waveforms which may be complex, e.g. ECG, or simple, as in the sine wave. All waveforms may ultimately be broken down into component sine waves (Fourier analysis). For any sine wave, there is oscillation about a mean value, the maximal displacement from which is the amplitude. The number of complete oscillations per second is the frequency, and the distance between successive points at the same stage of the cycle, e.g. successive peaks, is the wavelength. Waveform monitoring is very common in anaesthesia and intensive care, e.g. cardiovascular (ECG, intravascular pressures, plethysmography, etc.), respiratory (rate, depth, pattern, etc.), ventilatory (gas flow, pressure, etc.), neurological (intracranial pressure, EEG, nerve conduction studies, etc.).

Weaning from ventilators. Process of gradual withdrawal of ventilatory support. Usually presents no problems after less than a few days' support; following longer periods, rapid weaning is less likely.

- Criteria for beginning weaning vary considerably; the following have been suggested:
  - absence of major organ or system failure, particularly CVS.
  - precipitating illness is successfully treated.
  - absence of severe infection or fever.
  - adequate nutrition.
  - low intra-abdominal pressure.
  - absence of severe fluid, acid–base or electrolyte imbalance, e.g. of potassium, magnesium, calcium or phosphate, or endocrine disturbance, e.g. hypothyroidism.
  - minimal sedation with absence of severe pain.
  - respiratory function:
    - arterial blood gases are near premorbid values.
    - respiratory rate < 35/min.
    - maximal negative inspiratory airway pressure attainable exceeds −25 cmH_2O.
    - airway occlusion pressure greater than 6 cmH_2O below atmospheric.
    - tidal volume > 5 ml/kg.
    - minute ventilation < 10 litres.
    - vital capacity > 10–15 ml/kg.
    - FRC > 50% of predicted value.
    - ratio of breaths/min to tidal volume < 100.

After long-term ventilation, scoring systems have been proposed, reflecting F_IO_2 and level of PEEP required, lung compliance, work of breathing, temperature, pulse rate and arterial BP, etc.

- Techniques of weaning:
  - humidification of inspired air is important.
  - sitting the patient up increases FRC and diaphragmatic efficiency.
  - the lowest F_IO_2 necessary to maintain adequate oxygenation should be used, to decrease the risk of absorption atelectasis, and possibly promote hypoxic pulmonary vasoconstriction. High F_IO_2 must be avoided in patients with COPD.
  - a simple T-piece is often used when IPPV has been for a short duration. A 30 cm expiratory limb and fresh gas flow of twice minute volume will prevent indrawing of room air with lowering of F_IO_2, and rebreathing. Use should be limited in duration as the loss of physiological positive end-expiratory pressure may increase the risk of atelectasis.
  - CPAP is often preferred, especially following PEEP, in ARDS and in left ventricular dysfunction.
  - specific ventilatory modes:
    - IMV and variants: the set mandatory ventilator rate is decreased as patient spontaneous rate increases. Spontaneous breaths are usually augmented with inspiratory pressure support (see below). Allows closer monitoring of recovery and reduces complications of IPPV.
    - airway pressure release ventilation, inspiratory pressure support, pressure regulated volume control ventilation, mandatory minute ventilation, inspiratory volume support, high frequency ventilation and variants and negative pressure ventilation have also been used.
  - overall time for completion of weaning may not be reduced by the above methods, but sedation and complications of IPPV may be reduced, and patient morale may benefit from 'coming off' the ventilator sooner. Assessment is also made easier.
  - short periods of spontaneous or assisted ventilation may be introduced and gradually increased, with clinical monitoring, assessment of S_pO_2 and frequent arterial blood gas measurements. Inspiratory muscle resistance training may be incorporated. Recommencement of IPPV should be considered if tachypnoea (> 30/min), tachycardia (> 110/min), fatigue, restlessness, distress or falling S_pO_2 occur.
  - extubation may be performed when the patient is stable and able to guard the airway. Excessive secretions may be removed via minitracheotomy. Elective formation of a tracheostomy may assist in weaning by reducing dead space, allowing easy access for tracheobronchial toilet and permitting a reduction in sedation.
  - non-invasive positive pressure ventilation may allow tracheal extubation while providing ventilatory support.

Work of breathing is increased by demand and expiratory valves, tubing, etc., especially using CPAP and IMV circuits through certain ventilators. Sophisticated modern ventilators generally provide circuits of low resistance, with minimal exertion required to open demand valves. Weaning may be impaired by respiratory muscle fatigue, especially of the diaphragm, e.g. due to electrolyte abnormalities, prolonged illness (particularly involving infection), failing cardiac function, acidosis, hypoxia and critical illness polyneuropathy and myopathy.

Wedge pressure, *see Pulmonary capillary wedge pressure*

Wegener's granulomatosis. Necrotising small vessel granulomatous vasculitis, particularly involving pulmonary and renal vessels. Features include non-specific symptoms (malaise, weight loss, fever, night sweats), nasal discharge and ulceration, pleurisy, haemoptysis, myalgia, arthralgia and renal failure. Progression is variable but some cases develop rapid multiorgan failure requiring ICU admission for IPPV and haemofiltration/dialysis. The diagnosis may be suspected clinically if both lungs and kidneys are involved, supported by detecting antineutrophil cytoplasmic antibodies (ANCA). Tissue biopsies are frequently unhelpful as granulomatous deposits are difficult to locate in life, even in the kidney.

Treatment of organ failure is supportive; Wegener's itself is treated with cyclophosphamide and corticosteroids. Eventual remission is complete in approximately 75% of cases.

[Friedrich Wegener (1907–1990); German pathologist]

See also, Vasculitides

Weight. The force a body exerts on anything which supports it. The weight of a body of mass 1 kilogram is 1 kilogram weight (kilogram force).

Weil's disease, *see Leptospirosis*

Wells, Horace (1815–1848). US dentist, present at Colton's demonstration of N_2O in Hartford, Connecticut on 10th December 1844. Noticing that a member of the audience (Samuel Cooley) had knocked his shin under the gas' influence and felt no pain, he suggested its use for dental extraction. Wells had one of his own teeth pulled out by John Riggs the following day, whilst breathing N_2O prepared by Colton. Performed successful painless extractions in several patients over subsequent days, before his ill-fated demonstration of N_2O before Warren at Harvard Medical School, Boston, at which the patient complained of pain and Wells was denounced as a fraud. Continued to practise dentistry, but became increasingly disillusioned as acceptance of N_2O was overshadowed by Morton's discovery of diethyl ether. Later a chloroform addict, he committed suicide by cutting his femoral artery whilst in prison.

[Samuel Cooley (1809–?), druggist's assistant; John Riggs (1810–1885), US dentist]

Wenckebach phenomenon, *see Heart block*

WFSA, *see World Federation of Societies of Anaesthesiologists*

Wheezing. Sustained, musical whistling respiratory sound produced usually during expiration, indicating narrowing of the natural or artificial airway. Distinguished from stridor by being lower pitched and composed of a wider range of frequencies, and usually represents smaller airways' obstruction. May be generalised or localised.

- Caused by:
  - narrowed bronchi: bronchospasm, bronchiolitis, pulmonary oedema, aspiration of gastric contents, inhaled foreign body, airway tumour, pneumothorax, coughing or straining (causing airway collapse via increased intrathoracic pressure).
  - narrowed artificial airway: kinked tracheal tube, overinflated tracheal/tracheostomy tube cuff, placement of the tracheal tube's bevel against the posterior wall of the trachea, inadvertent endobronchial intubation, kinked/obstructed respiratory tubing, malfunction of breathing system or ventilator valves.

Bronchospasm should be diagnosed only when other causes have been excluded.

Whistle discriminator. Device used to confirm correct attachment of N_2O and O_2 supplies to an anaesthetic machine. Placed at the fresh gas outlet; when O_2 passes through it, the whistle sounds at a higher pitch than with N_2O at the same flow rate, because O_2 has lower density.

Whole bowel irrigation. Technique of GIT decontamination used in the treatment of poisoning and overdoses, especially with metals and delayed-release drug preparations, although convincing evidence for its efficacy is lacking. Employs large volumes (up to 2 l/h in adults) of polyethylene glycol administered via mouth or nasogastric tube until the rectal effluent is clear. Should not be used in debilitated patients or in the presence of gastrointestinal ileus, intestinal obstruction, perforation or haemorrhage. Electrolyte disturbances have not been reported with polyethylene glycol, unlike preoperative bowel preparations which were studied initially.

Wilcoxon signed rank test, *see Statistical tests*

Willis, circle of, *see Cerebral circulation*

'Wind-up'. Phenomenon in which the electrophysiological response of central pain-carrying neurones (e.g. those in the dorsal horn of the spinal cord) to stimuli from nociceptive neurones increases as the stimuli are repeated; in addition the receptive fields of the individual neurones expand. Used to describe the hyperexcitability that may occur in acute and chronic pain states, and the concept of plasticity within the CNS by which painful input may alter the connections and activities of central neurones. Excitatory amino acids such as glutamic and aspartic acids are thought to be involved in the phenomenon, acting especially via NMDA receptors although other receptor types are also thought to be involved, as are other modulating substances such as dynorphin, substance P and calcitonin gene-related peptide. Intracellular accumulation of these and other substances via gene induction is also thought to be important. Prevention of wind-up is a central tenet of pre-emptive analgesia.

Withdrawal of treatment in ICU. Cessation of all or individual components of treatment is a frequent mode of death in the ICU. In general, treatment is withdrawn when it has ceased or failed to achieve the benefits for which it was employed. It usually takes place when there is confirmed brainstem death or the patient's prognosis is poor with no prospect of returning to a reasonable quality of life. Occasionally, even a treatment which might produce benefit may be withheld or withdrawn if the patient is suffering from a terminal illness. The withdrawal of each individual medical treatment should be considered from the patient's perspective in the context of benefit. Withdrawal of treatment should not be regarded as 'causing' death, rather permitting the dying process to continue.

Factors taken into account in the decision to withdraw treatment include the patient's age, diagnosis, severity of disease, coexisting illnesses, prognosis, response to current treatment, physiological reserve, anticipated quality of life and wishes, if known.

- Ethical issues include:
  - the wishes (often unknown) of an unconscious (and therefore incapacitous) patient.
  - the validity and legality of decisions made by a surrogate.
  - the diversion of limited resources from patients with a good chance of survival to those who are unlikely to benefit.
  - the definition of futility.
  - the definition of a good quality of life.

- the nature of medical treatment, i.e. feeding, hydration, etc.
- consideration of religious beliefs.

- Prior to withdrawal of treatment, the following should be undertaken/sought:
  - full discussion between all medical, nursing and paramedical staff treating the patient during which consensus should be obtained that the patient is dying.
  - the views of the family and the legal status of any elected or appointed representative and advance decision of the patient.
  - consensus on the mode, extent and timing of treatment withdrawal by clinical staff and patient's family.

If brainstem death is diagnosed and organ donation is intended, withdrawal of support takes place after organ removal (beating heart donation). Otherwise, observations, monitoring, drugs, procedures and routine care (apart from comfort relief) can be withdrawn once clinical staff and the patient's family have reached a consensus. IPPV may continue unchanged during this period or the technique of 'terminal weaning' of ventilation may be employed, in which inspired oxygen concentration is reduced to an $F_{I}O_2$ of 0.21. Feeding/antibiotics are stopped and inotropic support, etc. terminated. Sedation and analgesia are maintained, or increased if the patient becomes distressed, to ensure a peaceful, humane, comfortable and dignified death for the patient and to diminish distress for the family. Privacy is important for the patient and family during the dying process. Organ donation after death is known as non-beating heart donation.

Where the condition which precipitated the patient's admission to ICU involves suspicious circumstances (poisoning, assault, etc.), contact with the coroner is advised prior to treatment withdrawal. Whatever the circumstances, good clinical records should be kept.

See also, Ethics; Euthanasia; Mental Capacity Act; Palliative care

Wolff–Parkinson–White syndrome. Condition in which a congenital accessory connection between the atria and ventricles conducts more rapidly than the atrioventricular (AV) node, but has a longer refractory period. An atrial extrasystole finds the accessory bundle still refractory, but when the impulse passes via the AV node to the ventricles, the accessory bundle has recovered, and can conduct the impulse back to the atria. Circular conduction can continue with resultant SVT. AF and atrial flutter may also occur, but less commonly.

The ECG classically shows a short P–R interval and wide QRS complexes with δ waves (Fig. 171). A positive QRS complex in lead V_1 denotes type A (accessory bundle on the left side of the heart); if negative, type B (right side of heart).

Anaesthetic management of known cases should be directed at avoiding increased sympathetic activity, including that due to anxiety. Antiarrhythmic drugs should be continued perioperatively. Drugs causing tachycardia (e.g. atropine, ketamine, pancuronium) should be avoided. Isoflurane is probably the volatile anaesthetic agent of choice as it suppresses accessory pathway conduction.

Treatment of arrhythmias (including perioperatively) follows standard measures. Digoxin and verapamil may increase impulse conduction through accessory pathways by blocking conduction through the AV node, and should be avoided. Management of established cases includes electrophysiological assessment (accessory pathway mapping), long-term prophylactic therapy (e.g. with flecainide, sotalol) and radiofrequency ablation of the accessory pathway.

[Sir John Parkinson (1885–1976), London cardiologist; Louis Wolff (1898–1972) and Paul White (1886–1973), US cardiologists]

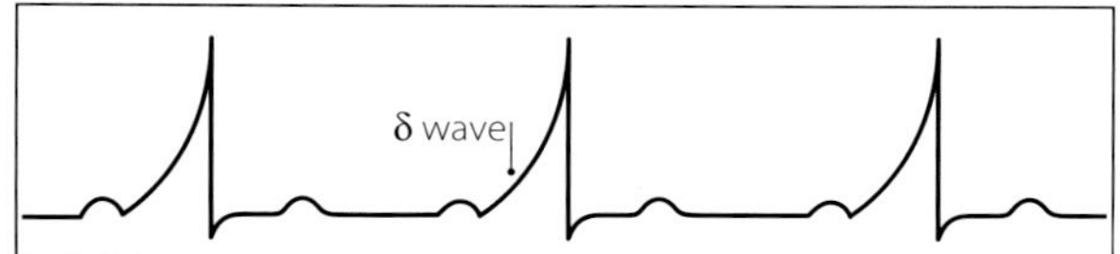

Fig. 171 ECG showing δ waves

Work. Product of force and distance. SI unit is the joule. Work is done whenever the point of application of a force moves in the direction of that force.

Work of breathing, *see Breathing, work of*

World Federation of Societies of Anaesthesiologists (WFSA). Founded in 1955 at the first World Congress of Anaesthesiologists in The Hague, Holland, in order to promote anaesthetic education, research, training and safety standards throughout the world. World Congresses are held every 4 years (since 1960). Membership is via 40 anaesthetic societies in different countries. Has three regional sections: Latin American, Asia/Australian and European. The last of these was founded in 1966 and renamed the Confederation of European National Societies of Anaesthesiology in 1998.

Baird WLM (1995). Acta Anaesthesiol Scand; 39: 436–7

Wrist, nerve blocks. Used for minor surgery to the hand.

- The following nerves are blocked (Fig. 172):
  - median nerve (C6–T1): at the level of the proximal skin crease, it lies between flexor carpi radialis tendon laterally and palmaris longus tendon medially. With the wrist dorsiflexed, 2–5 ml local anaesthetic agent is injected just lateral to the palmaris longus tendon, at a depth of 0.5–1 cm.
  - ulnar nerve (C7–T1): lies under flexor carpi ulnaris tendon proximal to the pisiform bone, medial and deep to the ulnar artery. At the level of the ulnar styloid process, a needle is inserted between flexor carpi ulnaris tendon and the ulnar artery, and 2–5 ml solution injected. The two cutaneous branches of the nerve may be blocked by subcutaneous infiltration around the ulnar side of the wrist from the flexor carpi ulnaris tendon.
  - radial nerve (C5–T1): its branches pass along the radial and dorsal aspects of the wrist. At the level of the proximal skin crease, a needle is inserted lateral to the radial artery, and 3 ml solution injected. Infiltration around the radial border of the wrist blocks superficial branches.

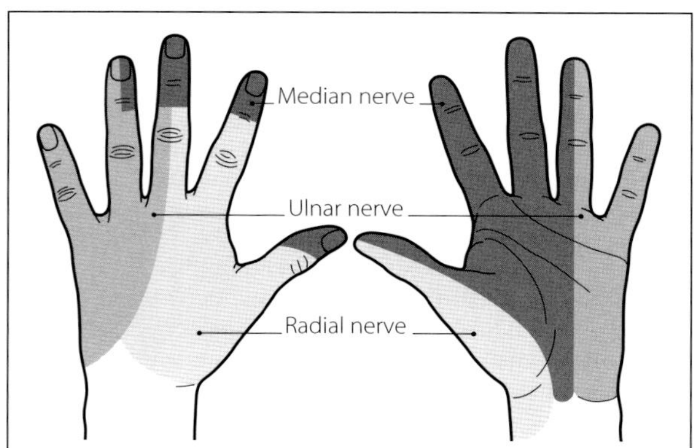

Fig. 172 Cutaneous innervation of the hand

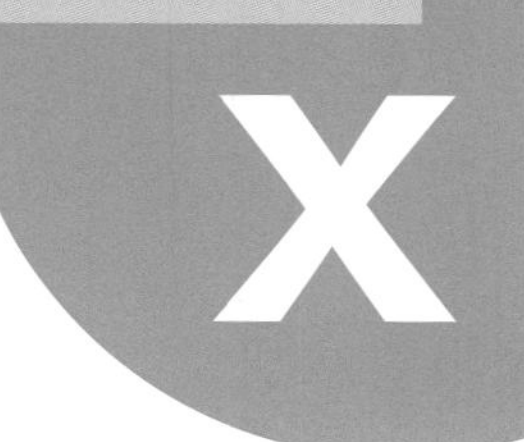

Xamoterol fumarate. Orally active partial β_1-adrenergic receptor agonist, introduced to treat mild cardiac failure. Has inotropic effects at low resting sympathetic tone, increasing myocardial contractility and cardiac output. At high resting sympathetic tone (e.g. moderate/severe cardiac failure), associated with detrimental β-receptor antagonist effects and increased mortality. Discontinued in the UK in 2000.

Xanthines (Methylxanthines). Derivatives of dioxypurine; they include caffeine and theophylline. Phosphodiesterase inhibitors, with wide spectra of activity including CNS stimulation, diuresis, increased myocardial contractility and smooth muscle relaxation. May also inhibit adenosine and reduce noradrenaline release.

Xenon. Inert gas, making up less than 0.00001% of air. Shown to have anaesthetic properties (MAC 71) with a blood/gas solubility of 0.14, resulting in extremely rapid uptake and excretion regardless of duration of use. Oil/gas solubility is 20, with a MAC of 71%. Has respiratory depressant effects but little effect on cardiovascular stability. Increases cerebral blood flow and intracranial pressure but may have neuroprotective properties through its inhibition of NMDA receptors. These features, plus its lack of adverse environmental properties (unlike N_2O), have led to investigations into its use as an anaesthetic agent, despite its high cost.

Its radioactive isotope ^{133}Xe is used in estimations of organ blood flow (e.g. Xe computed tomography for assessment of cerebral blood flow) and in analysis of distribution of ventilation in lung perfusion/ventilation scans.

Harris PD, Barnes R (2008). Anaesthesia; 63: 284–93

Xylometazoline. Vasoconstrictor sympathomimetic drug, acting via α-adrenergic receptor agonism. Used as a nasal decongestant and to reduce bleeding in nasal intubation, including awake intubation. Instilled into each nostril as either drops or a spray of a 0.1% solution. Hypertension may rarely occur in susceptible patients, e.g. those taking monoamine oxidase inhibitors. Should be avoided in angle-closure glaucoma.

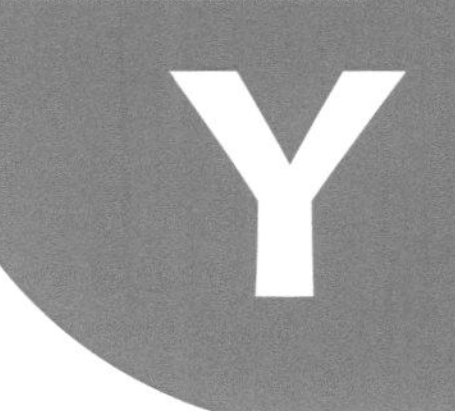

Yates's correction, *see Statistical tests*

Yohimbine, *see α-Adrenergic receptor antagonists*

Z

Zeolite. Hydrous silicate, used for ion- or molecule trapping. An artificial zeolite is used in O_2 concentrators, to retain nitrogen from compressed air. Has also been added to soda lime to retain water and prevent drying out.

Zero, absolute. The lowest possible temperature that can be attained: 0 kelvin (corresponds to −273°C).

Zero order kinetics, *see Pharmacokinetics*

Ziconotide acetate. Synthetic form of a peptide derived from the venomous sea snail *Conus magus*, introduced in 2006 for the treatment of chronic pain. Acts as a neurone-specific N-type calcium channel blocking drug and thought to interrupt ascending pain pathways in the spinal cord.

- Dosage: 2.4 μg/day by continuous intrathecal infusion, increased up to 21.6 μg/day.
- Side effects: confusion, dizziness, headache, visual disturbances, nausea/vomiting, agitation and psychiatric symptoms.

Zidovudine (Azidothymidine; AZT). Nucleoside reverse transcriptase inhibitor; a thymidine derivative, it inhibits DNA synthesis via incorporation into DNA. The first anti-HIV drug used; other similar drugs are now available but zidovudine is still used for prevention and treatment of HIV infection and AIDS. Traditionally used in cases of needle-stick injury to medical/nursing staff.

- Dosage:
  - various oral regimens have been used, usually 0.5–1.0 g/day.
  - 1–2 mg/kg iv over an hour, 4 hourly.
- Side effects include bone marrow depression, nausea and vomiting, anorexia, GIT disturbance, neuropathy, convulsions, myopathy, hepatic impairment.

Zinc deficiency. May occur in patients with inadequate diets, malabsorption, catabolism and during TPN. Causes angular stomatitis, eczematous eruptions and impaired wound healing. Normal plasma zinc level (assuming normal serum albumin) is 12–20 μmol/l; daily requirement is 2.5–6.4 mg/day.

Replacement therapy dosage: 60–125 mg zinc sulphate monohydrate 1–3 times daily. Side effects of therapy include abdominal pain and dyspepsia.

Zoledronic acid, *see Bisphosphonates*

Zone of risk. Area of the operating room in which mixtures of anaesthetic agents may be explosive. Originally defined in the UK in 1956 as extending to a height of 4 ft 6 in above the floor, and 4 ft laterally from the anaesthetic equipment. Redefined subsequently as extending 25 cm from any part of the apparatus or patient's airways that contain the anaesthetic mixture. Any flame or potential source of sparks should be placed outside this zone.
See also, Explosions and fires